17th Edition

HARRISON'S
MANUAL
of MEDICINE

EDITORS

Anthony S. Fauci, MD, ScD(HON)

Chief, Laboratory of Immunoregulation; Director,
National Institute of Allergy and Infectious Diseases,
National Institutes of Health, Bethesda

Eugene Braunwald, MD, ScD(HON)

Distinguished Hersey Professor of Medicine,
Harvard Medical School; Chairman, TIMI Study Group,
Brigham and Women's Hospital, Boston

Dennis L. Kasper, MD, MA(HON)

William Ellery Channing Professor of Medicine,
Professor of Microbiology and Molecular Genetics,
Harvard Medical School; Director, Channing Laboratory,
Department of Medicine, Brigham and Women's Hospital, Boston

Stephen L. Hauser, MD

Robert A. Fishman Distinguished Professor and Chairman,
Department of Neurology, University of California, San Francisco,
San Francisco

Dan L. Longo, MD

Scientific Director, National Institute on Aging,
National Institutes of Health, Bethesda and Baltimore

J. Larry Jameson, MD, PhD

Professor of Medicine;
Vice President for Medical Affairs and Lewis Landsberg Dean,
Northwestern University Feinberg School of Medicine, Chicago

Joseph Loscalzo, MD, PhD

Hersey Professor of the Theory and Practice of Medicine,
Harvard Medical School; Chairman, Department of Medicine;
Physician-in-Chief, Brigham and Women's Hospital, Boston

17th Edition

HARRISON'S MANUAL of MEDICINE

EDITORS

Anthony S. Fauci, MD

Eugene Braunwald, MD

Dennis L. Kasper, MD

Stephen L. Hauser, MD

Dan L. Longo, MD

J. Larry Jameson, MD, PhD

Joseph Loscalzo, MD, PhD

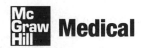

New York   Chicago   San Francisco   Lisbon   London   Madrid
Mexico City   New Delhi   San Juan   Seoul   Singapore   Sydney   Toronto

Harrison's
PRINCIPLES OF INTERNAL MEDICINE
Seventeenth Edition
MANUAL OF MEDICINE
Copyright © 2009, 2005, 2002, 1998, 1995, 1991, 1988 by *The McGraw-Hill Companies*. All rights reserved. Printed in the United States of America. Except as permitted under the United States Copyright Act of 1976, no part of this publication may be reproduced or distributed in any form or by any means, or stored in a data base or retrieval system, without the prior written consent of the author.

1 2 3 4 5 6 7 8 9 0   DOC/DOC   12 11 10 9
ISBN 978-0-07-147743-7
MHID 0-07-147743-8

The editors were James Shanahan and Mariapaz Ramos Englis; the production supervisor was Catherine H. Saggese; the designer was Alan Barnett. The index was prepared by Barbara Littlewood. RR Donnelley was printer and binder.

Library of Congress Cataloging-in-Publication Data
Harrison's manual of medicine / editors, Anthony S. Fauci ... [et al.]. --
17th ed. p. ; cm.
  Abridgement of : Harrison's principles of internal medicine / editors, Anthony S. Fauci ... [et al.]. 17th ed. c2008.
  Includes bibliographical references and index.
  ISBN-13: 978-0-07-147743-7 (pbk. : alk. paper)
  ISBN-10: 0-07-147743-8 (pbk. : alk. paper) 1. Internal medicine— Handbooks, manuals, etc. I. Fauci, Anthony S. II. Harrison, Tinsley Rudolph, 1900-1978. III. Harrison's principles of internal medicine. IV. Title: Manual of medicine.
  [DNLM: 1. Clinical Medicine—Handbooks. 2. Internal Medicine— Handbooks. WB 39 H323 2008J
  RC46.H333 2008 Suppl.
  616—dc22

2008053640

ISBN 978-0-07-163511-0; MHID 0-07-163511-4
Exclusive rights by The McGraw-Hill Companies, Inc., for manufacture and export. This book cannot be re-exported from the country to which it is consigned by McGraw-Hill. The International Edition is not available in North America.

CONTENTS

Contributors xiii
Preface. xv
Acknowledgments. xvii

SECTION 1   CARE OF THE HOSPITALIZED PATIENT

1   Initial Evaluation and Admission Orders
for the General Medicine Patient 1
2   Electrolytes/Acid-Base Balance. 3
3   Diagnostic Imaging in Internal Medicine. 22
4   Procedures Commonly Performed by Internists 25
5   Principles of Critical Care Medicine 30
6   Pain and Its Management. 34
7   Assessment of Nutritional Status 39
8   Enteral and Parenteral Nutrition 41
9   Transfusion and Pheresis Therapy. 44
10   Palliative and End-of-Life Care 46

SECTION 2   MEDICAL EMERGENCIES

11   Cardiovascular Collapse and Sudden Death 55
12   Shock. 58
13   Sepsis and Septic Shock 63
14   Acute Pulmonary Edema. 66
15   Acute Respiratory Distress Syndrome 69
16   Respiratory Failure 71
17   Confusion, Stupor, and Coma 74
18   Stroke 79
19   Subarachnoid Hemorrhage 88
20   Increased Intracranial Pressure and Head Trauma 90
21   Spinal Cord Compression. 94
22   Hypoxic-Ischemic Encephalopathy 96
23   Status Epilepticus 98
24   Diabetic Ketoacidosis and Hyperosmolar Coma 100
25   Hypoglycemia 103
26   Infectious Disease Emergencies 105
27   Oncologic Emergencies 112
28   Anaphylaxis 116
29   Bites, Venoms, Stings, and Marine Poisonings 117
30   Hypothermia and Frostbite 127

31 Poisoning and Drug Overdose 130
32 Bioterrorism 160

SECTION 3 COMMON PATIENT PRESENTATIONS

33 Chest Pain 175
34 Abdominal Pain 179
35 Headache 183
36 Back and Neck Pain 189
37 Fever, Hyperthermia, Chills, and Rash 199
38 Pain and Swelling of Joints 203
39 Syncope 207
40 Dizziness and Vertigo 211
41 Acute Visual Loss and Double Vision 215
42 Weakness and Paralysis 218
43 Tremor and Movement Disorders 222
44 Aphasias and Related Disorders 224
45 Sleep Disorders 226
46 Dyspnea 231
47 Cough and Hemoptysis 233
48 Cyanosis 239
49 Edema 240
50 Nausea, Vomiting, and Indigestion 244
51 Weight Loss 247
52 Dysphagia 249
53 Diarrhea, Constipation, and Malabsorption 253
54 Gastrointestinal Bleeding 259
55 Jaundice and Evaluation of Liver Function 263
56 Ascites 271
57 Azotemia and Urinary Abnormalities 274
58 Anemia and Polycythemia 280
59 Lymphadenopathy and Splenomegaly 283
60 Generalized Fatigue 288

SECTION 4 OPHTHALMOLOGY AND OTOLARYNGOLOGY

61 Common Disorders of Vision and Hearing 293
62 Sinusitis, Pharyngitis, Otitis, and Other Upper
Respiratory Infections 301

SECTION 5   DERMATOLOGY

63 General Examination of the Skin 309
64 Common Skin Conditions 314

SECTION 6   HEMATOLOGY AND ONCOLOGY

65 Examination of Blood Smears and Bone Marrow 321
66 Red Blood Cell Disorders 323
67 Leukocytosis and Leukopenia 329
68 Bleeding and Thrombotic Disorders 332
69 Cancer Chemotherapy 339
70 Myeloid Leukemias, Myelodysplasia,
and Myeloproliferative Syndromes 344
71 Lymphoid Malignancies 352
72 Skin Cancer 364
73 Head and Neck Cancer 367
74 Lung Cancer 368
75 Breast Cancer 374
76 Tumors of the Gastrointestinal Tract 379
77 Genitourinary Tract Cancer 391
78 Gynecologic Cancer 395
79 Prostate Hyperplasia and Carcinoma 399
80 Cancer of Unknown Primary Site 401
81 Paraneoplastic Endocrine Syndromes 405
82 Neurologic Paraneoplastic Syndromes 407

SECTION 7   INFECTIOUS DISEASES

83 Diagnosis of Infectious Diseases 411
84 Antibacterial Therapy 422
85 Health Care–Associated Infections 428
86 Infections in the Immunocompromised Host 432
87 Infective Endocarditis 440
88 Intraabdominal Infections 448
89 Infectious Diarrheas 451
90 Sexually Transmitted Diseases and
Reproductive Tract Infections 462
91 Infections of the Skin, Soft Tissues, Joints, and Bones 477
92 Pneumococcal Infections 486

93 Staphylococcal Infections 489
94 Streptococcal/Enterococcal Infections, Diphtheria, and Other Infections Caused by Corynebacteria and Related Species 496
95 Meningococcal and Listerial Infections 504
96 Infections Caused by *Haemophilus*, *Bordetella*, *Moraxella*, and HACEK Group Organisms................ 508
97 Diseases Caused by Gram-Negative Enteric Bacteria, *Pseudomonas*, and *Legionella* 513
98 Infections Caused by Miscellaneous Gram-Negative Bacilli .. 522
99 Anaerobic Infections 528
100 Nocardiosis and Actinomycosis 535
101 Tuberculosis and Other Mycobacterial Infections 538
102 Lyme Disease and Other Nonsyphilitic Spirochetal Infections 549
103 Rickettsial Diseases 554
104 *Mycoplasma* Infections 560
105 Chlamydial Infections 561
106 Herpesvirus Infections.............................. 564
107 Cytomegalovirus and Epstein-Barr Virus Infections........ 572
108 Influenza and Other Viral Respiratory Diseases........... 577
109 Rubeola, Rubella, Mumps, and Parvovirus Infections 584
110 Enteroviral Infections............................... 588
111 Insect- and Animal-Borne Viral Infections............... 592
112 HIV Infection and AIDS 600
113 Fungal Infections.................................. 618
114 *Pneumocystis* Infections 633
115 Protozoal Infections................................ 636
116 Helminthic Infections and Ectoparasite Infestations 648

SECTION 8 CARDIOLOGY

117 Physical Examination of the Heart 661
118 Electrocardiography................................ 665
119 Noninvasive Examination of the Heart 669
120 Congenital Heart Disease in the Adult 674
121 Valvular Heart Disease 678
122 Cardiomyopathies and Myocarditis..................... 684
123 Pericardial Disease 688
124 Hypertension...................................... 693
125 Metabolic Syndrome 699

126 ST-Segment Elevation Myocardial Infarction (STEMI) 700
127 Unstable Angina and Non-ST-Elevation
Myocardial Infarction................................ 709
128 Chronic Stable Angina............................... 712
129 Bradyarrhythmias 717
130 Tachyarrhythmias 720
131 Congestive Heart Failure and Cor Pulmonale 730
132 Diseases of the Aorta 736
133 Peripheral Vascular Disease 739
134 Pulmonary Hypertension............................. 742

SECTION 9 **PULMONOLOGY**

135 Respiratory Function and Pulmonary
Diagnostic Procedures............................... 747
136 Asthma 753
137 Environmental Lung Diseases 756
138 Chronic Obstructive Pulmonary Disease 759
139 Pneumonia and Lung Abscess......................... 764
140 Pulmonary Thromboembolism and
Deep-Vein Thrombosis 769
141 Interstitial Lung Disease 772
142 Diseases of the Pleura and Mediastinum 777
143 Disorders of Ventilation............................. 781
144 Sleep Apnea 783

SECTION 10 **NEPHROLOGY**

145 Approach to the Patient with Renal Disease 785
146 Acute Renal Failure................................. 789
147 Chronic Kidney Disease and Uremia 794
148 Dialysis 796
149 Renal Transplantation 798
150 Glomerular Diseases 801
151 Renal Tubular Disease............................... 808
152 Urinary Tract Infections 815
153 Renovascular Disease 820
154 Nephrolithiasis 826
155 Urinary Tract Obstruction............................ 829

SECTION 11 GASTROENTEROLOGY

156 Peptic Ulcer and Related Disorders 831
157 Inflammatory Bowel Diseases 836
158 Colonic and Anorectal Diseases 840
159 Cholelithiasis, Cholecystitis, and Cholangitis 844
160 Pancreatitis 849
161 Acute Hepatitis 854
162 Chronic Hepatitis 859
163 Cirrhosis and Alcoholic Liver Disease 868
164 Portal Hypertension 872

SECTION 12 ALLERGY, CLINICAL IMMUNOLOGY, AND RHEUMATOLOGY

165 Diseases of Immediate Type Hypersensitivity 877
166 Primary Immune Deficiency Diseases 881
167 SLE, RA, and Other Connective Tissue Diseases 885
168 Vasculitis 891
169 Ankylosing Spondylitis 895
170 Psoriatic Arthritis 897
171 Reactive Arthritis 899
172 Osteoarthritis 900
173 Gout, Pseudogout, and Related Diseases 903
174 Other Musculoskeletal Disorders 907
175 Sarcoidosis 910
176 Amyloidosis 913

SECTION 13 ENDOCRINOLOGY AND METABOLISM

177 Disorders of the Anterior Pituitary and Hypothalamus 917
178 Diabetes Insipidus and SIADH 923
179 Thyroid Gland Disorders 925
180 Adrenal Gland Disorders 933
181 Obesity 939
182 Diabetes Mellitus 942
183 Disorders of the Male Reproductive System 947
184 Disorders of the Female Reproductive System 952
185 Hypercalcemia and Hypocalcemia 959
186 Osteoporosis and Osteomalacia 965

187 Hypercholesterolemia and Hypertriglyceridemia 968
188 Hemochromatosis, Porphyrias, and Wilson's Disease 975

SECTION 14 NEUROLOGY

189 The Neurologic Examination 979
190 Neuroimaging 986
191 Seizures and Epilepsy 988
192 Alzheimer's Disease and Other Dementias 995
193 Parkinson's Disease 1002
194 Ataxic Disorders 1007
195 ALS and Other Motor Neuron Diseases 1010
196 Autonomic Nervous System Disorders 1013
197 Trigeminal Neuralgia, Bell's Palsy,
     and Other Cranial Nerve Disorders 1020
198 Spinal Cord Diseases 1026
199 Tumors of the Nervous System 1031
200 Multiple Sclerosis (MS) 1035
201 Acute Meningitis and Encephalitis 1042
202 Chronic Meningitis 1052
203 Peripheral Neuropathies, Including
     Guillain-Barré Syndrome (GBS) 1055
204 Myasthenia Gravis (MG) 1065
205 Muscle Diseases 1068

SECTION 15 PSYCHIATRY AND SUBSTANCE ABUSE

206 Psychiatric Disorders 1077
207 Psychiatric Medications 1085
208 Eating Disorders 1093
209 Alcoholism 1095
210 Narcotic Abuse 1099

SECTION 16 DISEASE PREVENTION AND HEALTH MAINTENANCE

211 Routine Disease Screening 1103
212 Immunization and Advice to Travelers 1107
213 Cardiovascular Disease Prevention 1118
214 Prevention and Early Detection of Cancer 1121
215 Smoking Cessation 1126
216 Women's Health 1128

SECTION 17   ADVERSE DRUG REACTIONS

217 Adverse Drug Reactions 1131

SECTION 18   LABORATORY VALUES

218 Laboratory Values of Clinical Importance 1141

Index 1173

ASSOCIATE EDITORS

TAMAR F. BARLAM, MD
Associate Professor of Medicine
Boston University School of Medicine, Boston

ANNE R. CAPPOLA, MD, SCM
Assistant Professor of Medicine
Division of Endocrinology, Diabetes, and Metabolism
University of Pennsylvania School of Medicine
Philadelphia

S. ANDREW JOSEPHSON, MD
Assistant Professor of Neurology, Director, Neurohospitalist Program
University of California, San Francisco
San Francisco

CAROL A. LANGFORD, MD, MHS
Director, Center for Vasculitis Care and Research
Department of Rheumatic and Immunologic Diseases
Cleveland Clinic Foundation, Cleveland

LEONARD S. LILLY, MD
Associate Professor of Medicine
Harvard Medical School
Chief, Brigham/Faulkner Cardiology
Brigham & Women's Hospital, Boston

DAVID B. MOUNT, MD
Assistant Professor of Medicine
Harvard Medical School
Associate Physician, Brigham & Women's Hospital
Renal Division Staff Physician, VA Boston Healthcare System, Boston

EDWIN K. SILVERMAN, MD, PHD
Associate Professor of Medicine
Channing Laboratory and Pulmonary and Critical Care Division
Department of Medicine, Brigham & Women's Hospital
Harvard Medical School, Boston

Numbers indicate the chapters written or co-written by the contributor.

TAMAR F. BARLAM, MD
13, 26, 29, 37, 62, 83–111, 113–116, 139, 152, 212

EUGENE BRAUNWALD, MD
11, 12, 14, 33, 46–49, 117–124, 126–131, 134, 143, 144, 217

ANNE R. CAPPOLA, MD, SCM
7, 8, 24, 25, 30, 51, 177–188, 216

ANTHONY S. FAUCI, MD
28, 32, 38, 55, 56, 63, 64, 112, 159–176

STEPHEN L. HAUSER, MD
6, 17–23, 35, 36, 39–45, 61, 82, 189–207, 209, 210, 215

J. LARRY JAMESON, MD, PHD
1, 3, 4, 7, 8, 24, 25, 30, 31, 51, 60, 125, 177–188, 208, 211, 216, 218

S. ANDREW JOSEPHSON, MD
6, 17–23, 35, 36, 39–45, 61, 82, 189–207, 209, 210, 215

DENNIS L. KASPER, MD
13, 26, 29, 37, 62, 83–111, 113–116, 139, 152, 212

CAROL A. LANGFORD, MD
28, 32, 38, 55, 56, 63, 64, 112, 159–176

LEONARD S. LILLY, MD
11, 33, 117–124, 127–133, 213

DAN L. LONGO, MD
9, 10, 27, 34, 50, 52–54, 58, 59, 65–81, 156–158, 214

JOSEPH LOSCALZO, MD, PHD
2, 5, 15, 16, 57, 132, 133, 135–138, 140–142, 145–151, 153–155

DAVID B. MOUNT, MD
2, 57, 145–151, 153–155

EDWIN K. SILVERMAN, MD, PHD
5, 15, 16, 135–138, 140–142

PREFACE

Harrison's Principles of Internal Medicine (HPIM) provides a comprehensive body of information important to an understanding of the biological and clinical aspects of quality patient care. It remains the premier medical textbook for students and clinicians. With the rapidly expanding base of medical knowledge and the time constraints associated with heavy patient-care responsibilities in modern health care settings, it is not always possible to read a comprehensive account of diseases and their presentations, clinical manifestations, and treatments before or even immediately after encountering the patient. It was for these reasons, among others, that in 1988 the Editors first condensed the clinical portions of *HPIM* into a pocket-sized volume, *Harrison's Manual of Medicine.* Similar to the prior 6 editions, this new edition of the *Manual,* drawn from the 17th edition of *HPIM,* presents the key features of the diagnosis, clinical manifestations, and treatment of the major diseases that are likely to be encountered on a medical service.

The Editors stress that the *Manual* should not substitute for in-depth analysis of the clinical problem, but should serve as a ready source of well-crafted and informative summaries that will be useful "on-the-spot" and that will prepare the reader for a more in-depth analysis drawn from more extensive reading at a later time. The *Manual* has met with increasing popularity over the years; its popularity and value relate in part to its abbreviated format, which has proven to be extremely useful for initial diagnosis, brief description of pathogenesis, and outline of management in time-restricted clinical settings. The most obvious change in this new edition of the *Manual* is its appearance: full-color format will increase the speed with which readers can locate and use information within its chapters. The *Manual* has been written for easy and seamless reference to the full text of the 17th edition of *HPIM,* and the Editors recommend that the full textbook—or *Harrison's On Line*—be consulted as soon as time allows.

As with previous editions, this latest edition of the *Manual* attempts to keep up with the continual and sometimes rapid evolution of internal medicine practices. In this regard, every chapter has received a close review and has been updated from the prior edition, with substantial revisions and new chapters provided where appropriate. In Section 1 on *Care of the Hospitalized Patient,* a new chapter entitled "End-of-Life Care" has been added. Section 2 on *Medical Emergencies* now includes a chapter entitled "Spinal Cord Compression." Chapters on "Tremor and Movement Disorders" and "Generalized Fatigue" appear in Section 3 on *Common Patient Presentations.* In Section 7 on *Infectious Diseases,* the chapter on "HIV Infection and AIDS" has been extensively revised to reflect important advances in therapy since the last edition. In Section 8 on *Cardiology,* there are new chapters on "Noninvasive Examination of the Heart," "Congenital Heart Disease in the Adult," and "Metabolic Syndrome." In Section 9 on *Pulmonology,* there is a new chapter on "Sleep Apnea," and in Section 16 on *Disease Prevention and Health Maintenance,* there are important new chapters on "Cardiovascular Disease Prevention" and "Smoking Cessation."

In full recognition of the important role of digital information delivery in alleviating the increasing time demands put on clinicians, the last 3 editions of the *Manual,* including the current edition, have been made available in PDA format. In addition, a version of the *Manual* for use with the iPhone platform is available for the 17th edition.

In 2006, in recognition of the increasing use of electronic health records systems in hospitals, *Harrison's Practice* made its debut. This innovative, digital point-of-care resource delivers substantial clinical reference data to the bedside. Its outline format and telescopic nature make it an ideal tool for finding and employing complex medical reference information quickly. Taken as a complete portfolio, *Harrison's* is now available in a variety of formats designed to be suitable for all levels of medical training and for all varieties of health care settings.

ACKNOWLEDGMENTS

The Editors and McGraw-Hill wish to thank their editorial staff whose assistance and patience made this edition come out in a timely manner:

From the Editors' offices: Pat Duffey; Gregory K. Folkers; Julie McCoy; Elizabeth Robbins, MD; Kathryn Saxon; Kristine Shontz; and Stephanie Tribuna.

From McGraw-Hill: James F. Shanahan, Mariapaz Ramos Englis, Catherine Saggese, M. Lorraine Andrews, and Eileen Scott who has been a part of HMOM since the 11th edition.

The Editors also wish to acknowledge contributors to past editions of this Manual, whose work formed the basis for many of the chapters herein: Joseph B. Martin, MD, PhD; Kurt Isselbacher, MD; Jean Wilson, MD; Daryl R. Gress, MD; Michael Sneller, MD; John W. Engstrom, MD; Kenneth Tyler, MD; Sophia Vinogradov, MD; Dan B. Evans, MD; Punit Chadha, MD; Glenn Chertow, MD; James Woodrow Weiss, MD.

NOTICE

Medicine is an ever-changing science. As new research and clinical experience broaden our knowledge, changes in treatment and drug therapy are required. The authors and the publisher of this work have checked with sources believed to be reliable in their efforts to provide information that is complete and generally in accord with the standards accepted at the time of publication. However, in view of the possibility of human error or changes in medical sciences, neither the authors nor the publisher nor any other party who has been involved in the preparation or publication of this work warrants that the information contained herein is in every respect accurate or complete, and they disclaim all responsibility for any errors or omissions or for the results obtained from use of the information contained in this work. Readers are encouraged to confirm the information contained herein with other sources. For example and in particular, readers are advised to check the product information sheet included in the package of each drug they plan to administer to be certain that the information contained in this work is accurate and that changes have not been made in the recommended dose or in the contraindications for administration. This recommendation is of particular importance in connection with new or infrequently used drugs.

1 Initial Evaluation and Admission Orders for the General Medicine Patient

Patients are admitted to the hospital when (1) they present the physician with a complex diagnostic challenge that cannot be safely or efficiently performed in the outpatient setting; or (2) they are acutely ill and require inpatient diagnostic tests, interventions, and treatments. The decision to admit a patient includes identifying the optimal clinical service (e.g., medicine, urology, neurology), the level of care (observation, general floor, telemetry, ICU), and necessary consultants. Admission should always be accompanied by clear communication with the patient and family, both to obtain information and to outline the anticipated events in the hospital. Patients often have multiple physicians, and based on the nature of the clinical problems, they should be contacted to procure relevant medical history and to assist with clinical care during or after admission.

The scope of illnesses cared for by internists is enormous. During a single day on a typical general medical service, it is not unusual for physicians, especially residents in training, to admit ten patients with ten different diagnoses affecting ten different organ systems. Given this diversity of disease, it is important to be systematic and consistent in the approach to any new admission.

Physicians are often concerned about making errors of commission. Examples would include prescribing an improper antibiotic for a patient with pneumonia or miscalculating the dose of heparin for a patient with new deep venous thrombosis (DVT). However, errors of omission are also common and can result in patients being denied life-saving interventions. Simple examples include: not checking a lipid panel for a patient with coronary heart disease, not prescribing an angiotensin-converting enzyme (ACE) inhibitor to a diabetic with documented albuminuria, or forgetting to give a patient with an osteoporotic hip fracture calcium, vitamin D, and an oral bisphosphonate.

Inpatient medicine typically focuses on the diagnosis and treatment of acute medical problems. However, most patients have multiple medical problems affecting different organ systems, and it is equally important to prevent nosocomial complications. Prevention of common hospital complications, such as DVT, peptic ulcers, line infections, falls, delirium, and pressure ulcers, is an important aspect of the care of all general medicine patients.

A consistent approach to the admission process helps to ensure comprehensive and clear orders that can be written and implemented in a timely manner. Several mnemonics serve as useful reminders when writing admission orders. A suggested checklist for admission orders is shown below and it includes several interventions targeted to prevent common nosocomial complications. Computerized order entry systems are also useful when designed to prompt structured sets of admission orders. However, these should not be used to the exclusion of orders tailored for the needs of an individual patient.

Checklist mnemonic: ADMIT VITALS AND PHYSICAL EXAM

- *A*dmit to: service (Medicine, Oncology, ICU); provide status (acute or observation).
- *D*iagnosis: state the working diagnosis prompting this particular hospitalization.
- *M*D: name the attending, resident, intern, student, primary care MD, and consultants.
- *I*solation requirements: state respiratory or contact isolation and reason for order.
- *T*elemetry: state indications for telemetry and specify monitor parameters.
- *V*ital signs (VS): frequency of VS; also specify need for pulse oximetry and orthostatic VS.
- *I*V access and IV fluid or TPN orders (see Chap. 2).
- *T*herapists: respiratory, speech, physical, and/or occupational therapy needs.
- *A*llergies: also specify type of adverse reaction.
- *L*abs: blood count, chemistries, coagulation tests, type & screen, UA, special tests.
- *S*tudies: CT scans (also order contrast), ultrasounds, angiograms, endoscopies, etc.
- *A*ctivity: weight bear/ambulating instructions, fall/seizure precautions and restraints.
- *N*ursing Orders: call intern if (x/y/z), also order I/Os, daily weights, and blood glucose.
- *D*iet: include NPO orders and tube feeding. State whether to resume diet after tests.
- *P*eptic ulcer prevention: proton-pump inhibitor or misoprostil for high-risk patients.
- *H*eparin or other modality (warfarin, compression boots, support hose) for DVT prophylaxis.
- *Y*ank all Foley catheters and nonessential central lines to prevent iatrogenic infections.
- *S*kin care: prevent pressure sores with heel guards, air mattresses, and RN wound care.
- *I*ncentive spirometry: prevent atelectasis and hospital-acquired pneumonia.
- *C*alcium, vitamin D, and bisphosphonates if steroid use, bone fracture, or osteoporosis.
- *A*CE inhibitor and aspirin: use for nearly all patients with coronary disease or diabetes.
- *L*ipid panel: assess and treat all cardiac and vascular patients for hyperlipidemia.
- *E*CG: for nearly every patient >50 years at the time of admission.
- *X*-rays: chest x-ray, abdominal series; evaluate central lines and endotracheal tubes.
- *A*dvanced directives: Full code or DNR; specify whether to rescind for any procedures.
- *M*edications: be specific with your medication orders.

It may be helpful to remember the medication mnemonic "Stat DRIP" for different routes of administration (*s*tat, *d*aily, *r*ound-the-clock, *I*V, and *p*rn medications). For the sake of cross-covering colleagues, provide relevant prn orders for acetaminophen, diphenhydramine, stool softeners or laxatives, and sleeping pills. Specify any stat medications since routine medication orders entered as "once daily" may not be dispensed until the following day unless ordered as stat or "first dose now."

2 Electrolytes/Acid-Base Balance

SODIUM

Disturbances of sodium concentration [Na^+] result in most cases from abnormalities of H_2O homeostasis, which change the relative ratio of Na^+ to H_2O. Disorders of Na^+ balance per se are, in contrast, associated with changes in extracellular fluid volume, either hypo- or hypervolemia. Maintenance of the "effective circulating volume" is achieved in large part by changes in urinary sodium excretion, whereas H_2O balance is achieved by changes in both H_2O intake and urinary H_2O excretion (Table 2-1). Confusion can result from the coexistence of defects in both H_2O and Na^+ balance. For example, a hypovolemic pt may have an appropriately low urinary Na^+ due to increased renal tubular reabsorption of filtered NaCl; a concomitant increase in circulating arginine vasopressin (AVP)—part of the defense of effective circulating volume (Table 2-1)—will cause the renal retention of ingested H_2O and the development of hyponatremia.

Hyponatremia   This is defined as a serum [Na^+] <135 mmol/L and is among the most common electrolyte abnormalities encountered in hospitalized pts. Symptoms include nausea, vomiting, confusion, lethargy, and disorientation; if severe (<120 mmol/L) and/or abrupt, seizures, central herniation, coma, or death may result (see Acute Symptomatic Hyponatremia, below). Hyponatremia is almost always the result of an increase in circulating AVP and/or increased renal sensitivity to AVP; a notable exception is in the setting of low solute intake ("beer potomania"), wherein a markedly reduced urinary solute excretion is inadequate to support the excretion of sufficient free H_2O. The serum [Na^+] by itself does not yield diagnostic information regarding total-body Na^+ content; hyponatremia is primarily a disorder of H_2O homeostasis. Pts with hyponatremia are thus categorized diagnostically into three groups, depending on their clinical volume status: hypovolemic, euvolemic, and hypervolemic hyponatremia (Fig. 2-1). All three forms of hyponatremia share an

TABLE 2-1	**OSMOREGULATION VERSUS VOLUME REGULATION**	
	Osmoregulation	Volume Regulation
What is sensed	Plasma osmolality	"Effective" circulating volume
Sensors	Hypothalamic osmoreceptors	Carotid sinus
		Afferent arteriole
		Atria
Effectors	AVP	Sympathetic nervous system
	Thirst	Renin-angiotensin-aldosterone system
		ANP/BNP
		AVP
What is affected	Urine osmolality	Urinary sodium excretion
	H_2O intake	Vascular tone

Note: See text for details. AVP, arginine vasopressin; ANP, atrial natriuretic peptide; BNP, brain natriuretic peptide.
Source: Adapted from Rose BD, Black RM (eds): *Manual of Clinical Problems in Nephrology.* Boston, Little Brown, 1988; with permission.

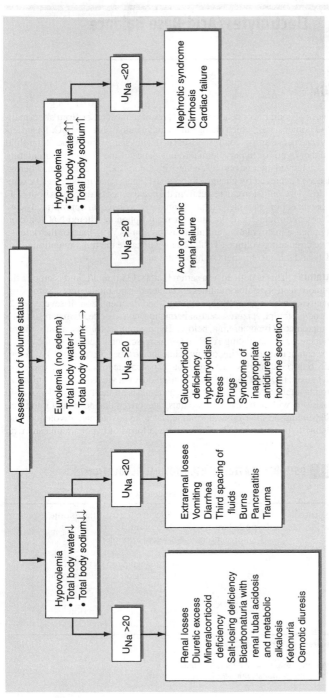

FIGURE 2-1 The diagnostic approach to hyponatremia. See text for details. *(From Schrier RW: Atlas of Diseases of the Kidney. Philadelphia, Blackwell Science, 1999; with permission.)*

exaggerated, "nonosmotic" increase in circulating AVP, in the setting of reduced serum osmolality. Notably, hyponatremia is often multifactorial; clinically important nonosmotic stimuli that can cause a release of AVP and increase the risk of hyponatremia include drugs, pain, nausea, and strenuous exercise.

Laboratory investigation of a pt with hyponatremia should include a measurement of serum osmolality to exclude "pseudohyponatremia" due to hyperlipidemia or hyperproteinemia. Serum glucose also should be measured; serum Na^+ falls by 1.4 mM for every 100-mg/dL increase in glucose, due to glucose-induced H_2O efflux from cells. Hyperkalemia may suggest adrenal insufficiency or hypoaldosteronism; increased blood urea nitrogen (BUN) and creatinine may suggest a renal cause. Urine electrolytes and osmolality are also critical tests in the initial evaluation of hyponatremia. In particular, a urine Na^+ <20 meq/L is consistent with hypovolemic hyponatremia in the clinical absence of a "hypervolemic," Na^+-avid syndrome such as congestive heart failure (CHF) (Fig. 2-1). Urine osmolality <100 mosmol/kg is suggestive of polydipsia or, in rare cases, of decreased solute intake; urine osmolality >400 mosmol/kg suggests that AVP excess is playing a more dominant role, whereas intermediate values are more consistent with multifactorial pathophysiology (e.g., AVP excess with a component of polydipsia). Finally, in the right clinical setting, thyroid, adrenal, and pituitary function should also be tested.

Hypovolemic Hyponatremia Hypovolemia from both renal and extrarenal causes is associated with hyponatremia. Renal causes of hypovolemia include primary adrenal insufficiency and hypoaldosteronism, salt-losing nephropathies (e.g., reflux nephropathy, nonoliguric acute tubular necrosis), diuretics, and osmotic diuresis. Random "spot" urine Na^+ is typically >20 meq/L in these cases but may be <20 meq/L in diuretic-associated hyponatremia if tested long after administration of the drug. Nonrenal causes of hypovolemic hyponatremia include GI loss (e.g., vomiting, diarrhea, tube drainage) and integumentary loss (sweating, burns); urine Na^+ is typically <20 meq/L in these cases.

Hypovolemia causes profound neurohumoral activation, inducing systems that preserve effective circulating volume, such as the renin-angiotensin-aldosterone axis (RAA), the sympathetic nervous system, and AVP (Table 2-1). The increase in circulating AVP serves to increase the retention of ingested free H_2O, leading to hyponatremia. The optimal treatment of hypovolemic hyponatremia is volume administration, generally as isotonic crystalloid, i.e., 0.9% NaCl ("normal saline"). If the history suggests that hyponatremia has been "chronic," i.e., present for 48 hours, care should be taken to avoid overcorrection (see below), which can easily occur as AVP levels plummet in response to volume-resuscitation; if necessary, the administration of desmopressin (DDAVP) and free water can reinduce or arrest the correction of hyponatremia (see below).

Hypervolemic Hyponatremia The edematous disorders (CHF, hepatic cirrhosis, and nephrotic syndrome) are often associated with mild to moderate degrees of hyponatremia ([Na^+] = 125–135 mmol/L); occasionally, pts with severe CHF or cirrhosis may present with serum [Na^+] <120 mmol/L. The pathophysiology is similar to that in hypovolemic hyponatremia, except that "effective circulating volume" is decreased due to the specific etiologic factors, i.e., cardiac dysfunction, peripheral vasodilation in cirrhosis, and hypoalbuminemia in nephrotic syndrome. The degree of hyponatremia is an indirect index of the associated neurohumoral activation (Table 2-1) and an important prognostic indicator in hypervolemic hyponatremia.

Management consists of treatment of the underlying disorder (e.g., afterload reduction in heart failure, large-volume paracentesis in cirrhosis, immunomodulatory therapy in some forms of nephrotic syndrome), Na^+ restriction, diuretic therapy, and, in some pts, H_2O restriction. Vasopressin antagonists (e.g., tolvaptan and conivaptan) are also effective in normalizing hyponatremia associated with both cirrhosis and CHF.

Euvolemic Hyponatremia The syndrome of inappropriate ADH secretion (SIADH) characterizes most cases of euvolemic hyponatremia. Other causes of euvolemic hyponatremia include hypothyroidism and secondary adrenal insufficiency due to pituitary disease; notably, repletion of glucocorticoid levels in the latter may cause a rapid drop in circulating AVP levels and overcorrection of serum $[Na^+]$ (see below).

Common causes of SIADH include pulmonary disease (e.g., pneumonia, tuberculosis, pleural effusion) and central nervous system (CNS) diseases (e.g., tumor, subarachnoid hemorrhage, meningitis); SIADH also occurs with malignancies (e.g., small cell carcinoma of the lung) and drugs (e.g., selective serotonin reuptake inhibitors, tricyclic antidepressants, nicotine, vincristine, chlorpropamide, carbamazepine, narcotic analgesics, antipsychotic drugs, cyclophosphamide, ifosfamide). Optimal treatment of euvolemic hyponatremia includes treatment of the underlying disorder. H_2O restriction to <1 L/d is a cornerstone of therapy but may be ineffective or poorly tolerated. However, vasopressin antagonists are predictably effective in normalizing serum $[Na^+]$ in SIADH. Alternatives include the coadministration of loop diuretics to inhibit the countercurrent mechanism and reduce urinary concentration, combined with oral salt tablets to abrogate diuretic-induced salt loss and attendant hypovolemia.

Acute Symptomatic Hyponatremia Acute symptomatic hyponatremia is a medical emergency; a sudden drop in serum $[Na^+]$ can overwhelm the capacity of the brain to regulate cell volume, leading to cerebral edema, seizures, and death. Women, particularly premenopausal women, are particularly prone to such sequelae; neurologic consequences are comparatively rare in male pts. Many of these pts develop hyponatremia from iatrogenic causes, including hypotonic fluids in the postoperative period, prescription of a thiazide diuretic, colonoscopy preparation, or intraoperative use of glycine irrigants. Polydipsia with an associated cause of increased AVP may also cause acute hyponatremia, as can increased H_2O intake in the setting of strenuous exercise, e.g., a marathon. The recreational drug ecstasy [methylenedioxymethamphetamine (MDMA)] can cause acute hyponatremia, rapidly inducing both AVP release and increased thirst.

Severe symptoms may occur at relatively modest levels of serum $[Na^+]$, e.g., in the mid-120s. Nausea and vomiting are common premonitory symptoms of more severe sequelae. An important concomitant is respiratory failure, which may be hypercapnic due to CNS depression or normocapnic due to neurogenic, noncardiogenic pulmonary edema; the attendant hypoxia amplifies the impact of hyponatremic encephalopathy.

R_X Hyponatremia

Three considerations are critical in the therapy of hyponatremia. First, the presence, absence, and/or severity of symptoms determine the urgency of therapy (see above for acute symptomatic hyponatremia). Second, pts with hyponatremia that has been present for >48 h ("chronic hyponatremia") are at risk for osmotic demyelination syndrome, typically central pontine myelinolysis, if serum Na^+ is corrected by >10–12 mM within the first 24 h and/or by >18 mM within the first 48 h. Third, the response to interventions, such as hypertonic saline or vasopressin antagonists, can be highly unpredictable, such that frequent monitoring of serum Na^+ (every 2–4 h) is imperative.

Treatment of acute symptomatic hyponatremia should include hypertonic saline to acutely increase serum Na^+ by 1–2 mM/h to a total increase of 4–6 mM; this increase is typically sufficient to alleviate acute symptoms, after which corrective guidelines for "chronic" hyponatremia are appropriate (see below). A number of equations and algorithms have been developed to estimate the required rate of hypertonic solution; one popular approach is to calculate a "Na^+ deficit," where the Na^+ deficit $= 0.6 \times$ body weight $\times$ (target $[Na^+]$ – starting $[Na^+]$). Regardless of the method used to determine the rate of administered hypertonic saline, the increase in serum $[Na^+]$ can be highly unpredictable, as the underlying physiology rapidly changes; serum $[Na^+]$ should be monitored every 2–4 h during and after treatment with hypertonic saline. The administration of supplemental O_2 and ventilatory support can also be critical in acute hyponatremia, if pts develop acute pulmonary edema or hypercapnic respiratory failure. IV loop diuretics will help treat acute pulmonary edema and will also increase free H_2O excretion by interfering with the renal countercurrent multiplier system. It is noteworthy that vasopressin antagonists do not have a role in the management of acute hyponatremia.

The rate of correction should be comparatively slow in *chronic* hyponatremia (<10–12 mM in the first 24 h and <18 mM in the first 48 h), so as to avoid osmotic demyelination syndrome. Vasopressin antagonists are highly effective in SIADH and in hypervolemic hyponatremia due to heart failure or cirrhosis. Should pts overcorrect serum $[Na^+]$ in response to vasopressin antagonists, hypertonic saline, or isotonic saline (in chronic hypovolemic hyponatremia), hyponatremia can be safely reinduced or stabilized by the administration of the vasopressin *agonist* DDAVP and the administration of free H_2O, typically IV D_5W; again, close monitoring of the response of serum $[Na^+]$ is essential to adjust therapy.

Hypernatremia This is rarely associated with hypervolemia, where the association is typically iatrogenic, e.g., administration of hypertonic sodium bicarbonate. More commonly, hypernatremia is the result of a combined H_2O and volume deficit, with losses of H_2O in excess of Na^+. Elderly individuals with reduced thirst and/or diminished access to fluids are at the highest risk of hypernatremia due to decreased free H_2O intake. Common causes of renal H_2O loss are osmotic diuresis secondary to hyperglycemia, postobstructive diuresis, or drugs (radiocontrast, mannitol, etc.); H_2O diuresis occurs in central or nephrogenic diabetes insipidus (DI) (Chap. 58). In pts with hypernatremia due to renal loss of H_2O, it is critical to quantify *ongoing* daily losses in addition to calculation of the baseline H_2O deficit (Table 2-2).

℞ Hypernatremia

The approach to correction of hypernatremia is outlined in Table 2-2. As with hyponatremia, it is advisable to correct the H_2O deficit slowly to avoid neurologic compromise, decreasing the serum $[Na^+]$ over 48–72 h. Depending on the blood pressure or clinical volume status, it may be appropriate to initially treat with hypotonic saline solutions (1/4 or 1/2 normal saline); blood glucose should be monitored in pts treated with large volumes of D_5W, should hyperglycemia ensue. Calculation of urinary electrolyte-free H_2O clearance is helpful to estimate daily, ongoing loss of free H_2O in pts with nephrogenic or central DI (Table 2-2). Other forms of therapy may be helpful in selected cases of hypernatremia. Pts with central DI may respond to the administration of intranasal DDAVP. Stable pts with nephrogenic DI due to lithium may reduce

TABLE 2-2　CORRECTION OF HYPERNATREMIA

H₂O Deficit

1. Estimate total-body water (TBW): 50–60% body weight (kg) depending on body composition
2. Calculate free-water deficit: $[(Na^+ 140)/140] \times TBW$
3. Administer deficit over 48–72 h

Ongoing H₂O Losses

4. Calculate free-water clearance, C_eH_2O:

$$C_eH_2O = V\left(1 - \frac{U_{Na} + U_K}{S_{Na}}\right)$$

where V is urinary volume, U_{Na} is urinary $[Na^+]$, U_K is urinary $[K^+]$, and SNa is serum $[Na^+]$.

Insensible Losses

5. ~10 mL/kg per day: less if ventilated, more if febrile

Total

6. Add components to determine H_2O deficit and ongoing H_2O loss; correct the H_2O deficit over 48–72 h and replace daily H_2O loss.

their polyuria with amiloride (2.5–10 mg/d) or hydrochlorothiazide (12.5–50 mg/d) or both in combination. These diuretics are thought to increase proximal H_2O reabsorption and decrease distal solute delivery, thus reducing polyuria; amiloride may also decrease entry of lithium into principal cells in the distal nephron by inhibiting the amiloride-sensitive epithelial sodium channel (ENaC). Notably, however, most patients with lithium-induced nephrogenic DI can adequately accommodate by increasing their H_2O intake. Occasionally, nonsteroidal anti-inflammatory drugs (NSAIDs) have also been used to treat polyuria associated with nephrogenic DI, reducing the negative effect of local prostaglandins on urinary concentration; however, the nephrotoxic potential of NSAIDs typically makes them a less attractive therapeutic option.

POTASSIUM

Since potassium (K^+) is the major intracellular cation, discussion of disorders of K^+ balance must take into consideration changes in the exchange of intra- and extracellular K^+ stores. (Extracellular K^+ constitutes <2% of total-body K^+ content.) Insulin, β_2-adrenergic agonists, and alkalosis tend to promote K^+ uptake by cells; acidosis, insulinopenia, or acute hyperosmolality (e.g., after treatment with mannitol or D50W) promote the efflux or reduced uptake of K^+. A corollary is that tissue necrosis and the attendant release of K^+ can cause severe hyperkalemia, particularly in the setting of acute kidney injury. Hyperkalemia due to rhabdomyolysis is thus particularly common, due to the enormous store of K^+ in muscle; hyperkalemia may also be prominent in tumor lysis syndrome.

The kidney plays a dominant role in K^+ excretion. Although K^+ is transported along the entire nephron, it is the principal cells of the connecting segment and cortical collecting duct that play a dominant role in K^+ excretion. Apical Na^+ entry into principal cells via the amiloride-sensitive epithelial Na^+ channel (ENaC) generates a lumen-negative potential difference, which drives passive

K^+ exit through apical K^+ channels. *This relationship is key to the bedside understanding of potassium disorders.* For example, decreased distal delivery of Na^+ tends to blunt the ability to excrete K^+, leading to hyperkalemia. Abnormalities in the RAA can cause both hypo- and hyperkalemia; aldosterone has a major influence on potassium excretion, increasing the activity of ENaC channels and thus amplifying the driving force for K^+ secretion across the luminal membrane of principal cells.

Hypokalemia Major causes of hypokalemia are outlined in Table 2-3. Atrial and ventricular arrhythmias are the most serious health consequences of hypokalemia. Pts with concurrent Mg deficit and/or digoxin therapy are at a particularly increased risk of arrhythmias. Other clinical manifestations include muscle weakness, which may be profound at serum $[K^+]$ <2.5 mmol/L, and, if hypokalemia is sustained, hypertension, ileus, polyuria, renal cysts, and even renal failure.

TABLE 2-3	CAUSES OF HYPOKALEMIA

I. Decreased intake
  A. Starvation
  B. Clay ingestion
II. Redistribution into cells
  A. Acid-base
    1. Metabolic alkalosis
  B. Hormonal
    1. Insulin
    2. β_2-Adrenergic agonists (endogenous or exogenous)
    3. α-Adrenergic antagonists
  C. Anabolic state
    1. Vitamin B_{12} or folic acid administration (red blood cell production)
    2. Granulocyte-macrophage colony-stimulating factor (white blood cell production)
    3. Total parenteral nutrition
  D. Other
    1. Pseudohypokalemia
    2. Hypothermia
    3. Hypokalemic periodic paralysis
    4. Thyrotoxic periodic paralysis
    5. Barium toxicity
II. Increased loss
  A. Nonrenal
    1. Gastrointestinal loss (diarrhea)
    2. Integumentary loss (sweat)
  B. Renal
    1. Increased distal flow: diuretics, osmotic diuresis, salt-wasting nephropathies
    2. Increased secretion of potassium
      a. Mineralocorticoid excess: primary hyperaldosteronism, secondary hyperaldosteronism (malignant hypertension, renin-secreting tumors, renal artery stenosis, hypovolemia), apparent mineralocorticoid excess (hereditary, licorice, chewing tobacco, carbenoxolone), congenital adrenal hyperplasia, Cushing's syndrome, Bartter's syndrome, Gitelman's syndrome
      b. Distal delivery of non-reabsorbed anions: vomiting, nasogastric suction, proximal (type 2) renal tubular acidosis, diabetic ketoacidosis, glue-sniffing (toluene abuse), penicillin derivatives
      c. Other: amphotericin B, Liddle's syndrome, hypomagnesemia

The cause of hypokalemia is usually obvious from history, physical examination, and/or basic laboratory tests. However, persistent hypokalemia may require a more thorough, systematic evaluation (Fig. 2-2). Initial laboratory evaluation should include electrolytes, BUN, creatinine, serum osmolality, Mg^{2+}, and Ca^{2+}, a complete blood count, and urinary pH, osmolality, creatinine, and electrolytes. Serum and urine osmolality are required for calculation of the transtubular K^+ gradient (TTKG), which should be <3 in the presence of hypokalemia (see also Hyperkalemia). Further tests such as urinary Mg^{2+} and Ca^{2+} and/or plasma renin and aldosterone levels may be necessary in specific cases.

R_X Hypokalemia

Hypokalemia can generally be managed by correction of the underlying disease process (e.g., diarrhea) or withdrawal of an offending medication (e.g., loop or thiazide diuretic), combined with oral KCl supplementation. However, hypokalemia is refractory to correction in the presence of Mg deficiency, which should also be corrected when present; renal wasting of both cations may be particularly prominent after renal tubular injury, e.g., from cisplatin nephrotoxicity. If loop or thiazide diuretic therapy cannot be discontinued, a distal tubular K-sparing agent, such as amiloride or spironolactone, can be added to the regimen. Angiotensin-converting enzyme (ACE) inhibition in pts with CHF attenuates diuretic-induced hypokalemia and protects against cardiac arrhythmia. If hypokalemia is severe (<2.5 mmol/L) and/or if oral supplementation is not feasible or tolerated, IV KCl can be administered through a central vein with cardiac monitoring in an intensive care setting, at rates that should not exceed 20 mmol/h. KCl should always be administered in saline solutions, rather than dextrose; the dextrose-induced increase in insulin can acutely exacerbate hypokalemia.

Hyperkalemia Causes are outlined in Table 2-4; in most cases, hyperkalemia is due to decreased renal K^+ excretion. However, increases in dietary K^+ intake can have a major effect in susceptible pts, e.g., diabetics with hyporeninemic hypoaldosteronism and chronic kidney disease. Drugs that impact on the renin-angiotensin-aldosterone axis are also a major cause of hyperkalemia, particularly given recent trends to coadminister these agents, e.g., spironolactone or angiotensin receptor blockers with an ACE inhibitor in cardiac and/or renal disease.

The first priority in the management of hyperkalemia is to assess the need for emergency treatment (ECG changes and/or K^+ ≥6.0 mM). This should be followed by a comprehensive workup to determine the cause (Fig. 2-3). History and physical examination should focus on medications (e.g., ACE inhibitors, NSAIDs, trimethoprim/sulfamethoxazole), diet and dietary supplements (e.g., salt substitute), risk factors for acute kidney failure, reduction in urine output, blood pressure, and volume status. Initial laboratory tests should include electrolytes, BUN, creatinine, serum osmolality, Mg^{2+}, and Ca^{2+}, a complete blood count, and urinary pH, osmolality, creatinine, and electrolytes. A urine [Na^+] <20 meq/L suggests that distal Na^+ delivery is a limiting factor in K^+ excretion; volume repletion with 0.9% saline or treatment with furosemide may then be effective in reducing serum [K^+] by increasing distal Na^+ delivery. Serum and urine osmolality are required for calculation of the TTKG. The expected values of the TTKG are largely based on historic data: <3 in the presence of hypokalemia and >7–8 in the presence of hyperkalemia.

$$\text{TTKG} = \frac{[K^+]_{urine} \times Osm_{serum}}{[K^+]_{serum} \times Osm_{urine}}$$

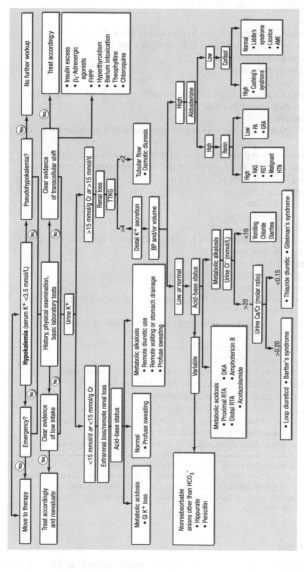

FIGURE 2-2 The diagnostic approach to hypokalemia. See text for details. FHPP, familial hypokalemic periodic paralysis; GI, gastrointestinal; TTKG, transtubular potassium gradient; CCD, cortical collecting duct; BP, blood pressure; RTA, renal tubular acidosis; DKA, diabetic ketoacidosis; RAS, renal artery stenosis; RST, renin-secreting tumor; HTN, hypertension; PA, primary aldosteronism; GRA, glucocorticoid-remediable aldosteronism; AME, apparent mineralocorticoid excess. [*From Mount DB, Zandi-Nejad K: Disorders of potassium balance, in The Kidney, 8th ed, BM Brenner (ed). Philadelphia, Saunders, 2008; with permission.*]

TABLE 2-4   **MAJOR CAUSES OF HYPERKALEMIA**

I. "Pseudo"-hyperkalemia
 A. Cellular efflux; thrombocytosis, leukocytosis, in vitro hemolysis
 B. Hereditary defects in red cell membrane transport
II. Intra- to extracellular shift
 A. Acidosis
 B. Hyperosmolality; radiocontrast, hypertonic dextrose, mannitol
 C. β_2-adrenergic antagonists (noncardioselective agents)
 D. Digoxin or ouabain poisoning
 E. Hyperkalemic periodic paralysis
III. Inadequate excretion
 A. Inhibition of the renin-angiotensin-aldosterone axis; ↑ risk of hyperkalemia when used in combination
   1. ACE inhibitors
   2. Renin inhibitors; aliskiren (in combination with ACE inhibitors or ARBs)
   3. ARBs
   4. Blockade of the mineralocorticoid receptor; spironolactone, eplerenone
   5. Blockade of the ENaC; amiloride, triamterene, trimethoprim, pentamidine
 B. Decreased distal delivery
   1. Congestive heart failure
   2. Volume depletion
   3. NSAIDs, cyclosporine
 C. Hyporeninemic hypoaldosteronism
   1. Tubulointerstitial diseases; SLE, sickle cell anemia, obstructive uropathy
   2. Diabetes, diabetic nephropathy
   3. Drugs; NSAIDs, beta blockers, cyclosporine
   4. Chronic kidney disease, advanced age
 D. Renal resistance to mineralocorticoid
   1. Tubulointerstitial diseases; SLE, amyloidosis, sickle cell anemia, obstructive uropathy, post-ATN
   2. Hereditary; pseudohypoaldosteronism type I—defects in the mineralocorticoid receptor *or* ENaC
 E. Advanced renal insufficiency with low GFR
 F. Primary adrenal insufficiency
   1. Autoimmune; Addison's disease, polyglandular endocrinopathy
   2. Infectious; HIV, CMV, TB, disseminated fungal infection
   3. Infiltrative; amyloidosis, malignancy, metastatic cancer
   4. Drug-associated; heparin, low-molecular-weight heparin
   5. Hereditary; adrenal hypoplasia congenita, congenital lipoid adrenal hyperplasia, aldosterone synthase deficiency
   6. Adrenal hemorrhage or infarction; may occur in antiphospholipid syndrome

Note: ACE, angiotensin-converting enzyme; ARBs, angiotensin receptor blockers; ATN, acute tubular necrosis; CMV, cytomegalovirus; ENaC, epithelial sodium channel; GFR, glomerular filtration rate; HIV, human immunodeficiency virus; NSAIDs, nonsteroidal anti-inflammatory drugs; SLE, systemic lupus erythematosus; TB, tuberculosis.

℞ Hyperkalemia

The most important consequence of hyperkalemia is altered cardiac conduction, with the risk of bradycardic cardiac arrest. Figure 2-4 shows serial ECG patterns of hyperkalemia; ECG manifestations of hyperkalemia should be considered a true medical emergency and treated urgently. However, ECG changes of hyperkalemia are notoriously insensitive, particularly in pts with

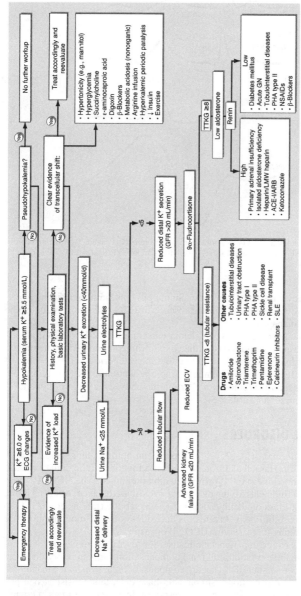

FIGURE 2-3 The diagnostic approach to hyperkalemia. See text for details. ECG, electrocardiogram; TTKG, transtubular potassium gradient; GFR, glomerular filtration rate; ECV, effective circulatory volume; GN, glomerulonephritis; NSAIDs, nonsteroidal anti-inflammatory drugs; LMW heparin, low-molecular-weight heparin; ACE-I, angiotensin-converting enzyme inhibitor; ARB, angiotensin II receptor blocker; PHA, pseudohypoaldosteronism; SLE, systemic lupus erythematosus. [*From Mount DB, Zandi-Nejad K: Disorders of potassium balance, in The Kidney, 8th ed, BM Brenner (ed). Philadelphia, Saunders, 2008; with permission.*]

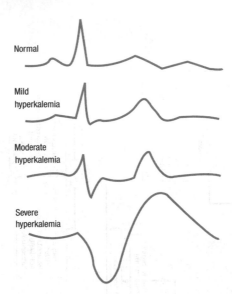

FIGURE 2-4 Diagrammatic ECGs at normal and high serum K. Peaked T waves (precordial leads) are followed by diminished R wave, wide QRS, prolonged P-R, loss of P wave, and ultimately a sine wave.

chronic kidney disease; given these limitations, pts with significant hyperkalemia ($K^+ \geq 6$–6.5 mmol/L) in the absence of ECG changes should also be aggressively managed.

Urgent management of hyperkalemia constitutes a 12-lead ECG, admission to the hospital, continuous cardiac monitoring, and immediate treatment. Treatment of hyperkalemia is divided into three categories: (1) antagonism of the cardiac effects of hyperkalemia, (2) rapid reduction in $[K^+]$ by redistribution into cells, and (3) removal of K^+ from the body. Treatment of hyperkalemia is summarized in Table 2-5.

ACID-BASE DISORDERS   (Fig. 2-5)

Regulation of normal pH (7.35–7.45) depends on both the lungs and kidneys. By the Henderson-Hasselbalch equation, pH is a function of the ratio of HCO_3^- (regulated by the kidney) to P_{CO_2} (regulated by the lungs). The HCO_3/P_{CO_2} relationship is useful in classifying disorders of acid-base balance. Acidosis is due to gain of acid or loss of alkali; causes may be metabolic (fall in serum HCO_3^-) or respiratory (rise in P_{CO_2}). Alkalosis is due to loss of acid or addition of base and is either metabolic ($\uparrow$ serum $[HCO_3^-]$) or respiratory ($\downarrow P_{CO_2}$).

To limit the change in pH, metabolic disorders evoke an immediate compensatory response in ventilation; full renal compensation for respiratory disorders is a slower process, such that "acute" compensations are of lesser magnitude than "chronic" compensations. Simple acid-base disorders consist of one primary disturbance and its compensatory response. In mixed disorders, a combination of primary disturbances is present.

The cause of simple acid-base disorders is usually obvious from history, physical examination, and/or basic laboratory tests. Initial laboratory evaluation

TABLE 2-5 TREATMENT OF HYPERKALEMIA

Mechanism	Therapy	Dose	Onset	Duration	Comments
Stabilize membrane potential	Calcium	10% Ca gluconate, 10 mL over 10 min	1–3 min	30–60 min	Repeat in 5 min if persistent electrocardiographic changes; avoid in digoxin toxicity.
Cellular K$^+$ uptake	Insulin	10 U R with 50 mL of D50, if blood sugar <250	30 min	4–6 h	Can repeat in 15 min; initiate D10W IV at 50–75 mL/h to avoid rebound hypoglycemia.
	β$_2$-agonist	Nebulized albuterol, 10–20 mg in 4 mL saline	30 min	2–4 h	Can be synergistic/additive to insulin; should not be used as sole therapy; use with caution in cardiac disease; may cause tachycardia/hyperglycemia.
K$^+$ removal	Kayexalate	30–60 g PO in 20% sorbitol	1–2 h	4–6 h	May cause ischemic colitis and colonic necrosis, particularly in enema form and postoperative state.
	Furosemide Hemodialysis	20–250 mg IV	15 min Immediate	4–6 h	Depends on adequate renal response/function. Efficacy depends on pretreatment of hyperkalemia (with attendant decrease in serum K$^+$), the dialyzer used, blood flow and dialysate flow rates, duration, and serum to dialysate K$^+$ gradient.

15

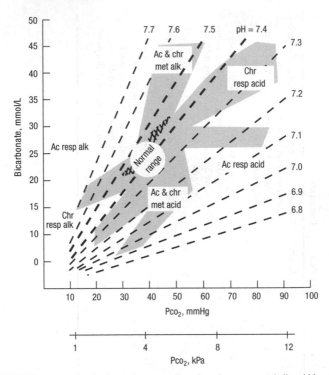

FIGURE 2-5 Nomogram showing bands for uncomplicated respiratory or metabolic acid-base disturbances in intact subjects. Each confidence band represents the mean ±2 SD for the compensatory response of normal subjects or pts to a given primary disorder. Ac, acute; chr, chronic; resp, respiratory; met, metabolic; acid, acidosis; alk, alkalosis. (*From Levinsky NG: HPIM-12, p. 290; modified from Arbus GS: Can Med Assoc J 109:291, 1973.*)

depends on the dominant acid-base disorder, but for metabolic acidosis and alkalosis this should include electrolytes, BUN, creatinine, albumin, urinary pH, and urinary electrolytes. An arterial blood gas (ABG) is not always required for pts with a simple acid-base disorder, e.g., mild metabolic acidosis in the context of chronic renal failure. However, concomitant ABG and serum electrolytes are necessary to fully evaluate more complex acid-base disorders. The compensatory response should be estimated from the ABG; Winter's formula [$P_{aCO_2} = (1.5 \times [HCO_3^-]) + 8 \pm 2$] is particularly useful for assessing the respiratory response to metabolic acidosis. The anion gap should also be calculated; the anion gap = $[Na^+] - ([HCO_3^-]+[Cl^-])$ = unmeasured anions – unmeasured cations. The anion gap should be adjusted for changes in the concentration of albumin, a dominant unmeasured anion; the "adjusted anion gap" = anion gap + ~2.5 × (4 – albumin mg/dL). Other supportive tests will elucidate the specific form of anion-gap acidosis (see below).

Metabolic Acidosis The low HCO_3^- in metabolic acidosis results from the addition of acids (organic or inorganic) or from a loss of HCO_3^-; causes of metabolic acidosis are classically categorized by presence or absence of an increase in the anion gap (Table 2-6). Increased anion-gap acidosis (>12 mmol/L) is due to addition of acid (other than HCl) and unmeasured anions to the body. Com-

TABLE 2-6 METABOLIC ACIDOSIS

Non-Anion-Gap Acidosis		Anion-Gap Acidosis	
Cause	Clue	Cause	Clue
Diarrhea	Hx; ↑ K⁺	DKA	Hyperglycemia, ketones
Enterostomy	Drainage	RF	Late chronic kidney disease
RF	Early chronic kidney disease	Lactic acidosis (L-lactate)	Clinical setting + ↑ serum lactate
RTA		Alcoholic ketoacidosis	Hx; weak + ketones; + osm gap
Proximal	↓ K⁺, presence of other proximal tubular defects (Fanconi Syndrome)	Starvation	Hx; mild acidosis; + ketones
Distal—hypokalemic	↓ K⁺; hypercalciuria; UpH >5.5	Salicylates	Hx; tinnitus; high serum level; + ketones; + lactate
Distal—hyperkalemic	↑ K⁺; nl PRA/aldo; UpH >5.5	Methanol	Large AG; concomitant respiratory alkalosis; retinitis; + toxic screen; + osm gap
Distal—hyporeninemic hypoaldosteronism	↑ K⁺; ↓ PRA/aldo; UpH <5.5	Ethylene glycol	RF; CNS symptoms; + toxic screen; crystalluria; + osm gap
Dilutional	Massive volume expansion with saline	D-lactic acidosis	Small-bowel disease; prominent neuro symptoms
Ureterosigmoidostomy	Obstructed ileal loop	Propylene glycol	IV infusions, e.g., lorazepam; + osm gap; RF
Hyperalimentation	Amino acid infusion	Pyroglutamic aciduria, 5-oxoprolinuria	Large AG; chronic acetaminophen
Acetazolamide, NH₄Cl, lysine HCl, arginine HCl, sevelamer-HCl	Hx of administration of these agents		

Note: RTA, renal tubular acidosis; PRA, plasma renin activity; UpH, urinary pH; DKA, diabetic ketoacidosis; RF, renal failure; CNS, central nervous system; AG, anion gap; osm gap, osmolar gap.

mon causes include ketoacidosis [diabetes mellitus (DKA), starvation, alcohol], lactic acidosis, poisoning (salicylates, ethylene glycol, and methanol), and renal failure.

Rare and newly appreciated causes of anion-gap acidosis include D-lactic acidosis, propylene glycol toxicity, and 5-oxoprolinuria (also known as pyroglutamic aciduria). D-Lactic acidosis (an increase in the D-enantiomer of lactate) can occur in pts with removal, disease, or bypass of the short bowel, leading to increased delivery of carbohydrates to colon. Intestinal overgrowth of organisms that metabolize carbohydrate to D-lactate results in D-lactic acidosis; a wide variety of neurologic symptoms can ensue, with resolution following treatment with appropriate antibiotics to change the intestinal flora. Propylene glycol is a common solvent for IV preparations of a number of drugs, most prominently lorazepam. Pts receiving high rates of these drugs may develop a hyperosmolar anion-gap metabolic acidosis, due mostly to increased lactate, often accompanied by acute kidney failure. Pyroglutamic aciduria (5-oxoprolinuria) is a high anion-gap acidosis caused by dysfunction of the γ-glutamyl cycle that replenishes intracellular glutathione; 5-oxoproline is an intermediate product of the cycle. Hereditary defects in the γ-glutamyl cycle are associated with 5-oxoprolinuria; acquired defects occur in the context of acetaminophen therapy, due to derepression of the cycle by reduced glutathione and overproduction of 5-oxoproline. Resolution occurs after withdrawal of acetaminophen; treatment with N-acetyl cysteine to replenish glutathione stores may hasten recovery.

The differentiation of the various anion-gap acidoses depends on the clinical scenario and routine laboratory tests (Table 2-6) in conjunction with measurement of serum lactate, ketones, toxicology screens (if ethylene glycol or methanol ingestion are suspected), and serum osmolality. D-Lactic acidosis can be diagnosed by a specific assay for the D-enantiomer; 5-oxoprolinuria can be diagnosed by the clinical scenario and confirmed by gas chromatographic/mass spectroscopic (GC/MS) analysis of urine, a widely available pediatric screening test for inborn errors of metabolism (typically "urine for organic acids").

Pts with ethylene glycol, methanol, or propylene glycol toxicity may have an "osmolar gap," defined as a >10-mosm/kg difference between calculated and measured serum osmolality. Calculated osmolality = $2 \times Na^+$ + glucose/18 + BUN/2.8. Of note, pts with alcoholic ketoacidosis and lactic acidosis may also exhibit a modest elevation in the osmolar gap; pts may alternatively metabolize ethylene glycol or methanol to completion by presentation, with an increased anion gap and no increase in the osmolar gap. However, the rapid availability of a measured serum osmolality may aid in the urgent assessment and management of pts with these medical emergencies.

Normal anion-gap acidosis can result from HCO_3^- loss from the GI tract. Diarrhea is by far the most common cause, but other GI conditions associated with external losses of bicarbonate-rich fluids may lead to large alkali losses—e.g., in ileus secondary to intestinal obstruction, in which liters of alkaline fluid may accumulate within the intestinal lumen. Various forms of kidney disease are associated with non-anion-gap acidosis due to reduced tubular reabsorption of filtered bicarbonate and/or reduced excretion of ammonium (NH_4^+). The early stages of progressive renal disease are frequently associated with a non-anion-gap acidosis, with development of an anion-gap component in more advanced renal failure. Non-anion-gap acidosis is also seen in renal tubular acidosis or in the context of tubulointerstitial injury, e.g., after acute tubular necrosis, allergic interstitial nephritis, or urinary tract obstruction. Finally, non-anion-gap acidosis due to exogenous acid loads may occur after rapid volume expansion with saline-containing solutions, the administration of NH_4Cl (a component of cough syrup), lysine HCl, or treatment with the phosphate binder sevelamer hydrochloride.

Calculation of the urinary anion gap may be helpful in the evaluation of hyperchloremic metabolic acidosis, along with a measurement of urine pH. The urinary anion gap is defined as urinary ($[Na^+] + [K^+]$) − $[Cl^-]$ = [unmeasured anions] − [unmeasured cations]); the NH_4^+ ion is the major unmeasured urinary cation in metabolic acidosis, wherein the urinary anion gap should be strongly negative. A negative anion gap thus suggests GI losses of bicarbonate, with appropriate renal response and increased NH_4^+ excretion; a positive anion gap suggests altered urinary acidification, as seen in renal failure or distal renal tubular acidoses. An important caveat is that the rapid renal excretion of unmeasured anions in anion-gap acidosis, classically seen in DKA, may reduce the serum anion gap and generate a positive value for the urinary anion gap, despite the adequate excretion of urinary NH_4^+; this may lead to misdiagnosis as a renal tubular acidosis.

Rx Metabolic Acidosis

Treatment of metabolic acidosis depends on the cause and severity. DKA responds to insulin therapy and aggressive hydration; close attention to serum $[K^+]$ and administration of KCl is essential, given that the correction of insulinopenia can cause profound hypokalemia. The administration of alkali in anion-gap acidoses is controversial and is rarely appropriate in DKA. It is reasonable to treat severe lactic acidosis with IV HCO_3^- at a rate sufficient to maintain a pH >7.20; treatment of moderate lactic acidosis with HCO_3^- is controversial. IV HCO_3 is however appropriate to reduce acidosis in D-lactic acidosis, ethylene glycol and methanol toxicity, and 5-oxoprolinuria.

Chronic metabolic acidosis should be treated when HCO_3^- is <18–20 mmol/L. In pts with chronic kidney disease, there is some evidence that acidosis promotes protein catabolism and may worsen bone disease. Sodium citrate may be more palatable than oral $NaHCO_3$, although the former should be avoided in pts with advanced renal insufficiency, as it augments aluminum absorption. Oral therapy with $NaHCO_3$ usually begins with 650 mg tid and is titrated upward to maintain serum $[HCO_3^-]$.

Metabolic Alkalosis   Metabolic alkalosis is due to a primary increase in serum $[HCO_3^-]$, distinguished from chronic respiratory acidosis—with a compensatory increase in renal HCO_3^- reabsorption—by the associated increase in arterial pH (normal or decreased in chronic respiratory acidosis). Administered, exogenous alkali (HCO_3^-, acetate, citrate, or lactate) may cause alkalosis if the normal capacity to excrete HCO_3^- is reduced or if renal HCO_3^- reabsorption is enhanced. A recently resurgent problem is "milk alkali syndrome," a triad of hypercalcemia, metabolic alkalosis, and acute renal failure due to ingested calcium carbonate, typically taken for the treatment or prevention of osteoporosis.

Metabolic alkalosis is primarily caused by renal retention of HCO_3^- and is due to a variety of underlying mechanisms. Pts are typically separated into two major subtypes: Cl^--responsive and Cl^--resistant. Measurement of urine Cl^- affords this separation in the clinical setting (Fig. 2-6). The quintessential causes of Cl^--responsive alkalosis are GI-induced from vomiting or gastric aspiration through a nasogastric tube, and renal-induced from diuretic therapy. Hypovolemia, chloride deficiency, activation of the renin-angiotensin-aldosterone axis, and hypokalemia play interrelated roles in the maintenance of this hypochloremic or "contraction" alkalosis. The various syndromes of true or apparent

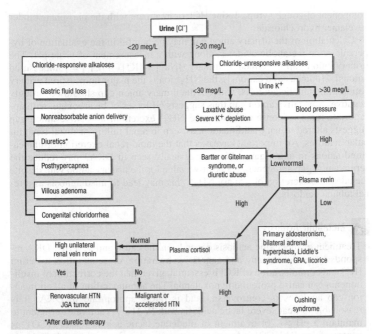

FIGURE 2-6 The diagnostic approach to metabolic alkalosis. See text for details. JGA, juxtaglomerular apparatus; GRA, glucocorticoid-remediable aldosteronism; HTN, hypertension. [*Modified from Dubose TD: Disorders of acid-base balance, in The Kidney, 8th ed, BM Brenner (ed). Philadelphia, Saunders, 2008; with permission.*]

mineralocorticoid excess cause Cl^--resistant metabolic alkalosis (Fig. 2-6); most of these pts are hypokalemic, volume-expanded, and/or hypertensive.

Common forms of metabolic alkalosis are generally diagnosed from the history, physical examination, and/or basic laboratory tests. ABGs will help determine whether an elevated $[HCO_3^-]$ is reflective of metabolic alkalosis or chronic respiratory acidosis; ABGs are required for the diagnosis of mixed acid-base disorders. Measurement of urinary electrolytes will aid in separating Cl^--responsive and Cl^--resistant forms. Urinary $[Na^+]$ may thus be >20 meq/L in Cl^--responsive alkalosis despite the presence of hypovolemia; however, urinary $[Cl^-]$ will be very low. Notably, urinary $[Cl^-]$ may be variable in pts with diuretic-associated alkalosis, depending on the temporal relationship to diuretic administration. Other diagnostic tests—e.g., plasma renin, aldosterone, cortisol—may be appropriate in Cl^--resistant forms with high urinary $[Cl^-]$ (Fig. 2-6).

℞ Metabolic Alkalosis

The acid-base disorder in Cl^--responsive alkalosis will typically respond to saline infusion; however, the associated hypokalemia should also be corrected. Pts with true or apparent mineralocorticoid excess require specific treatment of the underlying disorder. For example, hyperactive amiloride-sensitive ENaC channels cause Liddle's syndrome, which can respond to therapy with amiloride and related drugs; pts with hyperaldosteronism may in turn respond to blockade of the mineralocorticoid receptor with spironolactone or eplerenone. Finally, severe alkalosis in the critical care setting may require treatment with acidifying agents such as acetazolamide or HCl.

Respiratory Acidosis Respiratory acidosis is characterized by CO_2 retention due to ventilatory failure. Causes include sedatives, stroke, chronic pulmonary disease, airway obstruction, severe pulmonary edema, neuromuscular disorders, and cardiopulmonary arrest. Symptoms include confusion, asterixis, and obtundation.

℞ Respiratory Acidosis

The goal is to improve ventilation through pulmonary toilet and reversal of bronchospasm. Intubation or noninvasive positive pressure ventilation (NP-PV) may be required in severe acute cases. Acidosis due to hypercapnia is usually mild; however, combined respiratory and metabolic acidosis may cause a profound reduction in pH. Respiratory acidosis may accompany low tidal volume ventilation in ICU pts and may require metabolic "overcorrection" to maintain a neutral pH.

Respiratory Alkalosis Excessive ventilation causes a primary reduction in CO_2 and ↑ pH in pneumonia, pulmonary edema, interstitial lung disease, and asthma. Pain and psychogenic causes are common; other etiologies include fever, hypoxemia, sepsis, delirium tremens, salicylates, hepatic failure, mechanical overventilation, and CNS lesions. Pregnancy is associated with a mild respiratory alkalosis. Severe respiratory alkalosis may acutely cause seizures, tetany, cardiac arrhythmias, or loss of consciousness.

℞ Respiratory Alkalosis

Treatment should be directed at the underlying disorders. In psychogenic cases, sedation or a rebreathing bag may be required.

"Mixed" Disorders In many circumstances, more than a single acid-base disturbance exists. Examples include combined metabolic and respiratory acidosis with cardiogenic shock; metabolic alkalosis and anion-gap acidosis in pts with vomiting and diabetic ketoacidosis; and anion-gap metabolic acidosis with respiratory alkalosis in pts with salicylate toxicity. The diagnosis may be clinically evident and/or suggested by relationships between the P_{CO_2} and $[HCO_3^-]$ that diverge from those found in simple disorders. For example, the P_{CO_2} in a pt with metabolic acidosis and respiratory alkalosis will be considerably less than that predicted from the $[HCO_3^-]$ and Winter's formula $[P_{aCO_2} = (1.5 \times [HCO_3^-]) + 8 \pm 2]$.

In "simple" anion-gap acidosis, the anion gap increases in proportion to the fall in $[HCO_3^-]$. A lesser drop in serum $[HCO_3^-]$ than in the anion gap suggests a coexisting metabolic alkalosis. Conversely, a proportionately *larger* drop in $[HCO_3^-]$ than in the anion gap suggests the presence of a mixed anion-gap and non-anion-gap metabolic acidosis. Notably, however, these interpretations assume 1:1 relationships between unmeasured anions and the fall in $[HCO_3^-]$, which are not uniformly present in individual pts or as acidoses evolve. For example, volume resuscitation of pts with DKA will typically increase glomerular filtration and the urinary excretion of ketones, resulting in a decrease in the anion gap in the absence of a supervening non-anion-gap acidosis.

For a more detailed discussion, see Singer GG, Brenner BM: Fluid and Electrolyte Disturbances, Chap. 46, p. 274; and DuBose TD Jr: Acidosis and Alkalosis, Chap. 48, p. 287, in HPIM-17. See also Mount DB, Zandi-Nejad K: Disorders of potassium balance, in *The Kidney*, 8th ed, BM Brenner (ed). Philadelphia, Saunders, 2008; and Ellison DH, Berl T: Clinical practice. The syndrome of inappropriate antidiuresis. N Engl J Med 356:2064, 2007.

3   Diagnostic Imaging in Internal Medicine

Clinicians have a wide array of radiologic modalities at their disposal to aid them in noninvasive diagnosis. Despite the introduction of highly specialized imaging modalities, radiologic tests such as chest radiographs and ultrasound continue to serve a vital role in the diagnostic approach to patient care. At most institutions, CT is available on an emergent basis and is invaluable for initial evaluation of patients with trauma, stroke, suspected CNS hemorrhage, or ischemic stroke. MRI and related techniques (MR angiography, functional MRI, MR spectroscopy) provide remarkable resolution of many tissues including the brain, vascular system, joints, and most large organs.

This chapter will review the indications and utility of the most commonly utilized radiologic studies used by internists.

CHEST RADIOGRAPHY   See Fig. 3-1.

- Can be obtained quickly and should be part of the standard evaluation for patients with cardiopulmonary complaints.
- Is able to identify life-threatening conditions such as pneumothorax, intraperitoneal air, pulmonary edema, and aortic dissection.
- Is most often normal in a patient with an acute pulmonary embolus.
- Should be repeated in 4–6 weeks in a patient with an acute pneumonic process to document resolution of the radiographic infiltrate.
- Is used in conjunction with the physical exam to support the diagnosis of congestive heart failure. Radiographic findings supporting the diagnosis of heart failure include cardiomegaly, cephalization, Kerley B lines, and pleural effusions.
- Should be obtained daily in intubated patients to examine endotracheal tube position and the possibility of barotrauma.
- Helps to identify alveolar or airspace disease. Radiographic features of such diseases include inhomogeneous, patchy opacities and air-bronchograms.
- Helps to document the free-flowing nature of pleural effusions. Decubitus views should be obtained to exclude loculated pleural fluid prior to attempts to extract such fluid.

ABDOMINAL RADIOGRAPHY

- Should be the initial imaging modality in a patient with suspected bowel obstruction. Signs of small-bowel obstruction on plain radiographs include

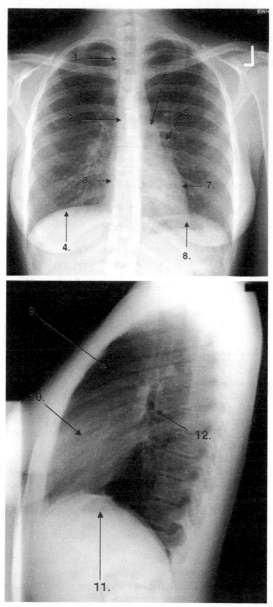

FIGURE 3-1 Normal chest radiograph-review of anatomy. **1.** Trachea. **2.** Carina. **3.** Right atrium. **4.** Right hemi-diaphragm. **5.** Aortic knob. **6.** Left hilum. **7.** Left ventricle. **8.** Left hemi-diaphragm (with stomach bubble). **9.** Retrosternal clear space. **10.** Right ventricle. **11.** Left hemi-diaphragm (with stomach bubble). **12.** Left upper lobe bronchus.

multiple air-fluid levels, absence of colonic distention, and a "stepladder" appearance of small-bowel loops.
- Should not be performed with barium enhancement when perforated bowel, portal venous gas, or toxic megacolon is suspected.
- Is used to evaluate the size of bowel:
  1. Normal small bowel is <3 cm in diameter.
  2. Normal caliber of the cecum is up to 9 cm, with the rest of the large bowel up to 6 cm in diameter.

ULTRASOUND

- Is more sensitive and specific than CT scanning in evaluating for the presence of gallstone disease.
- Can readily identify the size of the kidneys in a patient with renal insufficiency and can exclude the presence of hydronephrosis.
- Can expeditiously evaluate for the presence of peritoneal fluid in a patient with blunt abdominal trauma.
- Is used in conjunction with doppler studies to evaluate for the presence of arterial atherosclerotic disease.
- Is used to evaluate cardiac valves and wall motion.
- Should be used to localize loculated pleural and peritoneal fluid prior to draining such fluid.
- Can determine the size of thyroid nodules and guide fine-needle aspiration biopsy.
- Is the modality of choice for assessing known or suspected scrotal pathology.
- Should be the first imaging modality utilized when evaluating the ovaries.

COMPUTED TOMOGRAPHY

- CT of the brain should be initial radiographic modality in evaluating a patient with a potential stroke.
- Is highly sensitive for diagnosing an acute subarachnoid hemorrhage and in the acute setting is more sensitive than MRI.
- CT of the brain is an essential test in evaluating a patient with mental status changes to exclude entities such as intracranial bleeding, mass effect, subdural or epidural hematomas, and hydrocephalus.
- Is better than MRI for evaluating osseous lesions of the skull and spine.
- CT of the chest should be considered in the evaluation of a patient with chest pain to rule out entities such as pulmonary embolus or aortic dissection.
- CT of the chest is essential for evaluating lung nodules to assess for the presence of thoracic lymphadenopathy.
- CT with high-resolution cuts through the lungs is the imaging modality of choice for evaluating the lung interstitium in a patient with interstitial lung disease.
- Can be used to evaluate for presence of pleural and pericardial fluid and to localize loculated effusions.
- Is useful in a patient with unexplained abdominal pain to evaluate for conditions such as appendicitis, mesenteric ischemia or infarction, diverticulitis, or pancreatitis.
- CT of the abdomen is also the test of choice for evaluating for nephrolithiasis in a patient with renal colic.
- Is the test of choice for evaluating for the presence of an abscess in the chest or abdomen.
- In conjunction with abdominal radiography, CT can help identify the cause of bowel obstruction.

- Can identify abdominal conditions such as intussusception and volvulus in a patient with abdominal pain.
- Is the imaging modality of choice for evaluating the retroperitoneum.
- Should be obtained expeditiously in a patient with abdominal trauma to evaluate for the presence of intraabdominal hemorrhage and to assess injury to abdominal organs.

MAGNETIC RESONANCE IMAGING

- Is more useful than CT in the evaluation of ischemic infarction, dementia, mass lesions, demyelinating diseases, and most nonosseous spinal disorders.
- Provides excellent imaging of large joints including the knee, hip, and shoulder.
- Can be used, often with CT or angiography, to assess possible dissecting aortic aneurysms and congenital anomalies of the cardiovascular system.
- Cardiac MRI is proving useful to evaluate cardiac wall motion and for assessing cardiac muscle viability in ischemic heart disease.
- Is preferable to CT for evaluating adrenal masses such as pheochromocytoma and for helping to distinguish benign and malignant adrenal masses.

4 Procedures Commonly Performed by Internists

Internists perform a wide range of medical procedures, although practices vary widely among institutions and by specialty. Internists, nurses, or other ancillary health care professionals perform venipuncture for blood testing, arterial puncture for blood gases, endotracheal intubation, and flexible sigmoidoscopy, and insert IV lines, nasogastric (NG) tubes, and urinary catheters. These procedures are not covered here but require skill and practice to minimize patient discomfort and potential complications. Here, we review more invasive diagnostic and therapeutic procedures performed by internists—thoracentesis, lumbar puncture, and paracentesis. Many additional procedures are performed by specialists and require additional training and credentialing, including the following:

- Allergy—skin testing, rhinoscopy
- Cardiology—stress testing, echocardiograms, coronary catheterization, angioplasty, stent insertion, pacemakers, electrophysiology testing and ablation, implantable defibrillators, cardioversion
- Endocrinology—thyroid biopsy, dynamic hormone testing, bone densitometry
- Gastroenterology—upper and lower endoscopy, esophageal manometry, endoscopic retrograde cholangiopancreatography, stent insertion, endoscopic ultrasound, liver biopsy
- Hematology/Oncology—bone marrow biopsy, stem cell transplant, lymph node biopsy, plasmapheresis
- Pulmonary—intubation and ventilator management, bronchoscopy
- Renal—kidney biopsy, dialysis
- Rheumatology—joint aspiration

Increasingly, ultrasound, CT, and MRI are being used to guide invasive procedures, and flexible fiberoptic instruments are extending the reach into the body. For most invasive medical procedures, including those reviewed below, informed consent should be obtained in writing before beginning the procedure.

THORACENTESIS

Drainage of the pleural space can be performed at the bedside. Indications for this procedure include diagnostic evaluation of pleural fluid, removal of pleural fluid for symptomatic relief, and instillation of sclerosing agents in pts with recurrent, usually malignant pleural effusions.

Preparatory Work   Familiarity with the components of a thoracentesis tray is a prerequisite to performing a thoracentesis successfully. Recent PA and lateral chest radiographs with bilateral decubitus views should be obtained to document the free-flowing nature of the pleural effusion. Loculated pleural effusions should be localized by ultrasound or CT prior to drainage.

Technique   A posterior approach is the preferred means of accessing pleural fluid. Comfortable positioning is a key to success for both pt and physician. The pt should sit on the edge of the bed, leaning forward with the arms abducted onto a pillow on a bedside stand. Pts undergoing thoracentesis frequently have severe dyspnea, and it is important to assess if they can maintain this positioning for at least 10 min. The entry site for the thoracentesis is based on the physical exam and radiographic findings. Percussion of dullness is utilized to ascertain the extent of the pleural effusion with the site of entry being the first or second highest interspace in this area. The entry site for the thoracentesis is at the superior aspect of the rib, thus avoiding the intercostal nerve, artery, and vein, which run along the inferior aspect of the rib (Fig. 4-1).

The site of entry should be marked with a pen to guide the thoracentesis. The skin is then prepped and draped in a sterile fashion with the operator observing sterile technique at all times. A small-gauge needle is used to anesthetize the skin, and a larger-gauge needle is used to anesthetize down to the superior aspect

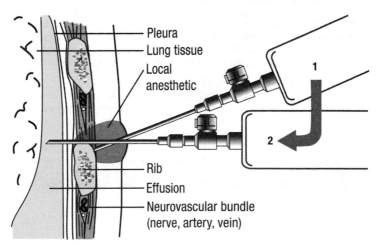

Pleura
Lung tissue
Local anesthetic
1
2
Rib
Effusion
Neurovascular bundle (nerve, artery, vein)

FIGURE 4-1 In thoracentesis, the needle is passed over the top of the rib to avoid the neurovascular bundle. (*From LG Gomella, SA Haist: Clinician's Pocket Reference, 11th ed. New York, McGraw-Hill, 2007.*)

of the rib. The needle should then be directed over the upper margin of the rib to anesthetize down to the parietal pleura. The pleural space should be entered with the anesthetizing needle, all the while using liberal amounts of lidocaine.

A dedicated thoracentesis needle with an attached syringe should next be utilized to penetrate the skin. This needle should be advanced to the superior aspect of the rib. While maintaining gentle negative pressure, the needle should be slowly advanced into the pleural space. If a diagnostic tap is being performed, aspiration of only 30–50 mL of fluid is necessary before termination of the procedure. If a therapeutic thoracentesis is being performed, a three-way stopcock is utilized to direct the aspirated pleural fluid into collection bottles or bags. No more than 1 L of pleural fluid should be withdrawn at any given time as quantities >1–1.5 L can result in reexpansion pulmonary edema.

After all specimens have been collected, the thoracentesis needle should be withdrawn and the needle site occluded for at least 1 min.

Specimen Collection   The diagnostic evaluation of pleural fluid depends on the clinical situation. All pleural fluid samples should be sent for cell count and differential, Gram stain, and bacterial cultures. LDH and protein determinations should also be made to differentiate between exudative and transudative pleural effusions. The pH should be determined if empyema is a diagnostic consideration. Other studies on pleural fluid include mycobacterial and fungal cultures, glucose, triglyceride level, amylase, and cytologic determination.

Post-Procedure   A post-procedural chest radiograph should be obtained to evaluate for a pneumothorax, and the pt should be instructed to notify the physician if new shortness of breath develops.

LUMBAR PUNCTURE

Evaluation of CSF is essential for the diagnosis of suspected meningeal infection, subarachnoid hemorrhage, leptomeningeal neoplastic disease, and noninfectious meningitis. Relative contraindications to LP include local skin infection in the lumbar area, suspected spinal cord mass lesion, and a suspected intracranial mass lesion. Any bleeding diathesis should also be corrected prior to performing LP to prevent the possible occurrence of an epidural hematoma. A functional platelet count > 50,000/μL and an INR < 1.5 are advisable to perform LP safely.

Preparatory Work   Familiarity with the components of a lumbar puncture tray is a prerequisite to performing LP successfully. In pts with focal neurologic deficits or with evidence of papilledema on physical exam, a CT scan of the head should be obtained prior to performing LP.

Technique   Proper positioning of the pt is important to ensure a successful LP. Two different pt positions can be used: the lateral decubitus position and the sitting position. Most routine LPs should be performed using the lateral decubitus position (Fig. 4-2). The sitting position may be preferable in obese pts. With either position, the pt should be instructed to flex the spine as much as possible. In the lateral decubitus position, the pt is instructed to assume the fetal position with the knees flexed toward the abdomen. In the sitting position, the pt should bend over a bedside table with the head resting on folded arms.

The entry site for a LP is below the level of the conus medullaris, which extends to L1-L2 in most adults. Thus, either the L3-L4 or L4-L5 interspace can be utilized as the entry site. The posterior superior iliac crest should be identified and the spine palpated at this level. This represents the L3-L4 interspace, with the other interspaces referenced from this landmark. The midpoint of the interspace be-

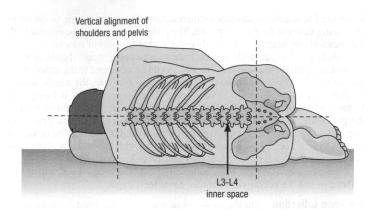

FIGURE 4-2 Proper positioning of a patient in the lateral decubitus position. Note that the shoulders and hips are in a vertical plane; the torso is perpendicular to the bed. (*From SE Strauss et al: JAMA 296:2012, 2006; with permission.*)

tween the spinous processes represents the entry point for the thoracentesis needle. This entry site should be marked with a pen to guide the LP. The skin is then prepped and draped in a sterile fashion with the operator observing sterile technique at all times. A small-gauge needle is then used to anesthetize the skin and subcutaneous tissue. The spinal needle should be introduced perpendicular to the skin in the midline and should be advanced slowly. The needle stylette should be withdrawn frequently as the spinal needle is advanced. As the needle enters the subarachnoid space, a "popping" sensation can sometimes be felt. If bone is encountered, the needle should be withdrawn to just below the skin and then redirected more caudally. Once CSF begins to flow, the opening pressure can be measured. This should be measured in the lateral decubitus position with the pt shifted to this position if the procedure was begun with the pt in the sitting position. After the opening pressure is measured, the CSF should be collected in a series of specimen tubes for various tests. At a minimum, a total of 10–15 mL of CSF should be collected in the different specimen tubes.

Once the required spinal fluid is collected, the stylette should be replaced and the spinal needle removed.

Specimen Collection   Diagnostic evaluation of CSF is based on the clinical scenario. In general, spinal fluid should always be sent for cell count with differential, protein, glucose, and bacterial cultures. Other specialized studies that can be obtained on CSF include viral cultures, fungal and mycobacterial cultures, VDRL, cryptococcal antigen, oligoclonal bands, and cytology.

Post-Procedure   To reduce the chance of a post-LP headache, the pt should be instructed to lie prone for at least 3 h. If a headache does develop, bedrest, hydration, and oral analgesics are often helpful. If an intractable post-LP headache ensues, the pt may have a persistent CSF leak. In this case, consultation with an anesthesiologist should be considered for the placement of a blood patch.

PARACENTESIS

Removal and analysis of peritoneal fluid is invaluable in evaluating pts with new-onset ascites or ascites of unknown etiology. It is also requisite in pts with known ascites who have a decompensation in their clinical status. Relative contraindications include bleeding diathesis, prior abdominal surgery, distended bowel, or known loculated ascites.

Preparatory Work　Prior to performing a paracentesis, any severe bleeding diathesis should be corrected. Bowel distention should also be relieved by placement of a nasogastric tube, and the bladder should also be emptied before beginning the procedure. If a large-volume paracentesis is being performed, large vacuum bottles with the appropriate connecting tubing should be obtained.

Technique　Proper pt positioning greatly improves the ease with which a paracentesis can be performed. The pt should be instructed to lie supine with the head of the bed elevated to 45°. This position should be maintained for ~15 min to allow ascitic fluid to accumulate in the dependent portion of the abdomen.

The preferred entry site for paracentesis is a midline puncture halfway between the pubic symphysis and the umbilicus; this correlates with the location of the relatively avascular linea alba. The midline puncture should be avoided if there is a previous midline surgical scar, as neovascularization may have occurred. Alternative sites of entry include the lower quadrants, lateral to the rectus abdominis, but caution should be used to avoid collateral blood vessels that may have formed in patients with portal hypertension.

The skin is prepped and draped in a sterile fashion. The skin, subcutaneous tissue, and the abdominal wall down to the peritoneum should be infiltrated with an anesthetic agent. The paracentesis needle with an attached syringe is then introduced in the midline perpendicular to the skin. To prevent leaking of ascitic fluid, "Z-tracking" can sometimes be helpful: after penetrating the skin, the needle is inserted 1–2 cm before advancing further. The needle is then advanced slowly while continuous aspiration is performed. As the peritoneum is pierced, the needle will give noticeably. Fluid should flow freely into the syringe soon thereafter. For a diagnostic paracentesis, removal of 50 mL of ascitic fluid is adequate. For a large-volume paracentesis, direct drainage into large vacuum containers using connecting tubing is a commonly utilized option.

After all samples have been collected, the paracentesis needle should be removed and firm pressure applied to the puncture site.

Specimen Collection　Peritoneal fluid should be sent for cell count with differential, Gram stain, and bacterial cultures. Albumin measurement of ascitic fluid is also necessary for calculating the serum–ascitic albumin gradient. Depending on the clinical scenario, other studies that can be obtained include mycobacterial cultures, amylase, adenosine deaminase, triglycerides, and cytology.

Post-Procedure　The pt should be monitored carefully post-procedure and should be instructed to lie supine in bed for several hours. If persistent fluid leakage occurs, continued bedrest with pressure dressings at the puncture site can be helpful. For pts with hepatic dysfunction undergoing large-volume paracentesis, the sudden reduction in intravascular volume can precipitate hepatorenal syndrome. Administration of 25 g IV albumin following large-volume paracentesis has been shown to decrease the incidence of renal failure post-procedure. Finally, if the ascites fluid analysis shows evidence of spontaneous bacterial peritonitis, then antibiotics (directed toward gram-negative gut bacteria) and IV albumin should be administered as soon as possible.

5 Principles of Critical Care Medicine

INITIAL EVALUATION OF THE CRITICALLY ILL PATIENT

Initial care of critically ill pts must often be performed rapidly and before a thorough medical history has been obtained. Physiologic stabilization begins with the principles of advanced cardiovascular life support and frequently involves invasive techniques such as mechanical ventilation and renal replacement therapy to support organ systems that are failing. A variety of severity-of-illness scoring systems, such as APACHE II, have been developed. Although these tools are useful for ensuring similarity among groups of pts involved in clinical trials or in quality assurance monitoring, their relevance to individual pts is less clear. These scoring systems are not typically used to guide clinical management.

SHOCK

Shock, which is characterized by multisystem end-organ hypoperfusion and tissue hypoxia, is a frequent problem requiring ICU admission. A variety of clinical indicators of shock exist, including reduced mean arterial pressure, tachycardia, tachypnea, cool extremities, altered mental status, oliguria, and lactic acidosis. Although hypotension is usually observed in shock, there is not a specific blood pressure threshold that is used to define it. Shock can result from decreased cardiac output, decreased systemic vascular resistance, or both. The three main categories of shock are hypovolemic, cardiogenic, and high cardiac output/low systemic vascular resistance. Clinical evaluation can be useful to assess the adequacy of cardiac output, with narrow pulse pressure, cool extremities, and delayed capillary refill suggestive of reduced cardiac output. Indicators of high cardiac output (e.g., widened pulse pressure, warm extremities) associated with shock suggest reduced systemic vascular resistance. Reduced cardiac output can be due to intravascular volume depletion (e.g., hemorrhage) or cardiac dysfunction. Reduced systemic vascular resistance is often caused by sepsis, but high cardiac output hypotension is also seen in pancreatitis, burns, anaphylaxis, peripheral arteriovenous shunts, and thyrotoxicosis. Early resuscitation of septic and cardiogenic shock may improve survival; objective assessments such as echocardiography and/or invasive vascular monitoring should be used to complement clinical evaluation. The approach to the pt in shock is outlined in Fig. 5-1.

MECHANICAL VENTILATORY SUPPORT

Critically ill pts often require mechanical ventilation. During initial resuscitation, standard principles of advanced cardiovascular life support should be followed. Mechanical ventilation should be considered for acute hypoxemic respiratory failure, which may occur with cardiogenic shock, pulmonary edema (cardiogenic or noncardiogenic), or pneumonia. Mechanical ventilation should also be considered with ventilatory failure, which can result from an increased load on the respiratory system—often manifested by lactic acidosis or decreased lung compliance. Mechanical ventilation may decrease respiratory work, improve arterial oxygenation with improved tissue O_2 delivery, and reduce acidosis. Reduction in mean arterial pressure after institution of mechanical ventilation commonly occurs due to reduced venous return from positive pressure ventilation, reduced en-

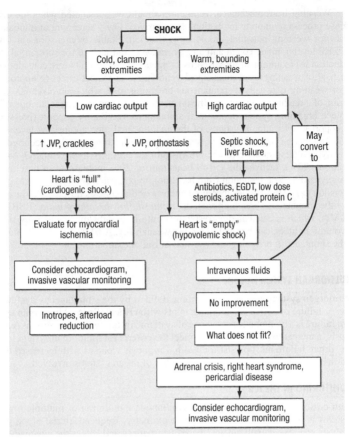

FIGURE 5-1 Approach to patient in shock. JVP, jugular venous pulse; EGDT, early goal-directed therapy.

dogenous catecholamine secretion, and administration of drugs used to facilitate intubation. Since hypovolemia often contributes to postintubation hypotension, IV volume administration should be considered. The major types of respiratory failure are discussed in Chap. 16.

℞ The Mechanically Ventilated Patient

Many pts receiving mechanical ventilation require treatment for pain (typically with narcotics) and for anxiety (typically with benzodiazepines, which also have the benefit of providing amnesia). Less commonly, neuromuscular blocking agents are required to facilitate ventilation when there is extreme dyssynchrony between the pt's respiratory efforts and the ventilator that cannot be corrected with manipulation of the ventilator settings; aggressive sedation is required during treatment with neuromuscular blockers. Neuromuscular blocking agents should be used with caution because a myopathy associated with prolonged weakness can result.

Weaning from mechanical ventilation should be considered when the disease process prompting intubation has improved. Daily screening of intubated pts for weaning potential should be performed. Stable oxygenation (at low PEEP levels), intact cough and airway reflexes, and lack of (or substantial reduction in) requirement for vasopressor agents are required before considering a trial of weaning from mechanical ventilation. The most effective approach for weaning is usually a spontaneous breathing trial, which involves 30–120 min of breathing without significant ventilatory support. Either an open T-piece breathing system or minimal amounts of ventilatory support (pressure support to overcome resistance of the endotracheal tube and/or low levels of CPAP) can be used. Failure of a spontaneous breathing trial has occurred if tachypnea (respiratory rate >35 breaths/min for >5 min), hypoxemia (O_2 saturation <90%), tachycardia (>140 beats/min or 20% increase from baseline), bradycardia (20% reduction from baseline), hypotension (<90 mmHg), hypertension (>180 mmHg), or increased anxiety or diaphoresis develop. At the end of the spontaneous breathing trial, the *rapid shallow breathing index* (RSBI or f/VT), which is calculated as respiratory rate in breaths/min divided by tidal volume in liters, can be used to predict weanability. A f/VT <105 at the end of the spontaneous breathing test warrants a trial of extubation.

MULTIORGAN SYSTEM FAILURE

Multiorgan system failure is a syndrome defined by the simultaneous dysfunction or failure of two or more organs in pts with critical illness. Multiorgan system failure is a common consequence of systemic inflammatory conditions (e.g., sepsis, pancreatitis, and trauma). To meet the criteria for multiorgan system failure, organ failure must persist for >24 h. Prognosis worsens with increased duration of organ failure and increased number of organ systems involved.

MONITORING IN THE ICU

With critical illness, close and often continuous monitoring of multiple organ systems is required. In addition to pulse oximetry, frequent arterial blood gas analysis can reveal evolving acid-base disturbances and assess the adequacy of ventilation. Intra-arterial pressure monitoring is frequently performed to follow blood pressure and to provide arterial blood gases and other blood samples. Pulmonary artery (Swan-Ganz) catheters can provide pulmonary artery pressure, cardiac output, and systemic vascular resistance measurements. However, no morbidity or mortality benefit from pulmonary artery catheter use has been demonstrated, and rare but significant complications from placement of central venous access (e.g., pneumothorax, infection) or the pulmonary artery catheter (e.g., cardiac arrhythmias, pulmonary artery rupture) can result. Thus, routine pulmonary artery catheterization in critically ill pts is not recommended.

For intubated pts receiving volume-controlled modes of mechanical ventilation, respiratory mechanics can be followed easily. The peak airway pressure is regularly measured by mechanical ventilators, and the plateau pressure can be assessed by including an end-inspiratory pause. The inspiratory airway resistance is calculated as the difference between the peak and plateau airway pressures (with adjustment for flow rate). Increased airway resistance can result from bronchospasm, respiratory secretions, or a kinked endotracheal tube. Static compliance of the respiratory system is calculated as the tidal volume divided by the gradient in airway pressure (plateau pressure minus PEEP). Reduced respiratory system compliance can result from pleural effusions, pneumothorax, pneumonia, pulmonary edema, or auto-PEEP.

PREVENTION OF CRITICAL ILLNESS COMPLICATIONS

Critically ill pts are prone to a number of complications, including the following:

- Sepsis—Often is related to the invasive monitoring performed of critically ill pts.
- Anemia—Usually is due to chronic inflammation as well as iatrogenic blood loss.
- Deep-venous thrombosis—May occur despite standard prophylaxis with SC heparin or sequential compression devices and may occur at the site of central venous catheters.
- GI bleeding—Stress ulcers of the gastric mucosa frequently develop in pts with bleeding diatheses, shock, or respiratory failure, necessitating prophylactic acid neutralization in such pts.
- Acute renal failure—A tendency exacerbated by nephrotoxic medications and dye studies. The most common etiology is acute tubular necrosis. Low-dose dopamine treatment does not protect against the development of acute renal failure.
- Hyperglycemia—Frequently occurs with parenteral nutrition; intensive insulin therapy to provide normoglycemia improves survival in surgical ICU pts.
- ICU-acquired weakness—Neuropathies and myopathies have been described; they are especially common in sepsis.

NEUROLOGIC DYSFUNCTION IN CRITICALLY ILL PATIENTS

A variety of neurologic problems can develop in critically ill pts. Most ICU pts develop delirium, which is characterized by acute changes in mental status, inattention, disorganized thinking, and an altered level of consciousness. Less common but important neurologic complications include anoxic brain injury, stroke, and status epilepticus.

LIMITATION OR WITHDRAWAL OF CARE

Withholding or withdrawing care commonly occurs in the ICU. Technological advances have allowed many pts to be maintained in the ICU with little or no chance of recovery. Increasingly, pts, families, and caregivers have acknowledged the ethical validity of withdrawal of care when the pt or surrogate decision-maker determines that the pt's goals for care are no longer achievable with the clinical situation.

For a more detailed discussion, see Kress JP, Hall JB: Principles of Critical Care Medicine, Chap. 261, p. 1673, in HPIM-17.

6   Pain and Its Management

APPROACH TO THE PATIENT: PAIN

Pain is the most common symptom of disease. Management depends on determining its cause, alleviating triggering and potentiating factors, and providing rapid relief whenever possible. Pain may be of somatic (skin, joints, muscles), visceral, or neuropathic (injury to nerves, spinal cord pathways, or thalamus) origin. Characteristics of each are summarized in Table 6-1.

Neuropathic Pain

Definitions: *neuralgia*: pain in the distribution of a single nerve, as in trigeminal neuralgia; *dysesthesia*: spontaneous, unpleasant, abnormal sensations; *hyperalgesia* and *hyperesthesia*: exaggerated responses to nociceptive or touch stimulus, respectively; *allodynia*: perception of light mechanical stimuli as painful, as when vibration evokes painful sensation. Reduced pain perception is called *hypalgesia* or, when absent, *analgesia*. *Causalgia* is continuous severe burning pain with indistinct boundaries and accompanying sympathetic nervous system dysfunction (sweating; vascular, skin, and hair changes—sympathetic dystrophy) that occurs after injury to a peripheral nerve.

Sensitization refers to a lowered threshold for activating primary nociceptors following repeated stimulation in damaged or inflamed tissues; inflammatory mediators play a role. Sensitization contributes to tenderness, soreness, and hyperalgesia (as in sunburn).

Referred pain results from the convergence of sensory inputs from skin and viscera on single spinal neurons that transmit pain signals to the brain. Because of this convergence, input from deep structures is mislocalized to a region of skin innervated by the same spinal segment.

TABLE 6-1	CHARACTERISTICS OF SOMATIC AND NEUROPATHIC PAIN

Somatic pain
    Nociceptive stimulus usually evident
    Usually well localized
    Similar to other somatic pains in pt's experience
    Relieved by anti-inflammatory or narcotic analgesics
Visceral pain
    Most commonly activated by inflammation
    Pain poorly localized and usually referred
    Associated with diffuse discomfort, e.g., nausea, bloating
    Relieved by narcotic analgesics
Neuropathic pain
    No obvious nociceptive stimulus
    Associated evidence of nerve damage, e.g., sensory impairment, weakness
    Unusual, dissimilar from somatic pain, often shooting or electrical quality
    Only partially relieved by narcotic analgesics, may respond to antidepressants
      or anticonvulsants

Chronic Pain

The problem is often difficult to diagnose, and pts may appear emotionally distraught. Several factors can cause, perpetuate, or exacerbate chronic pain: (1) painful disease for which there is no cure (e.g., arthritis, cancer, migraine headaches, diabetic neuropathy); (2) neural factors initiated by a bodily disease that persist after the disease has resolved (e.g., damaged sensory or sympathetic nerves); (3) psychological conditions. Pay special attention to the medical history and to depression. Major depression is common, treatable, and potentially fatal (suicide).

PATHOPHYSIOLOGY: ORGANIZATION OF PAIN PATHWAYS

Pain-producing (nociceptive) sensory stimuli in skin and viscera activate peripheral nerve endings of primary afferent neurons, which synapse on second-order neurons in spinal cord or medulla (Fig. 6-1). These second-order neurons form crossed ascending pathways that reach the thalamus and are projected to somatosensory cortex. Parallel ascending neurons connect with brainstem nuclei and ventrocaudal and medial thalamic nuclei. These parallel pathways project to the limbic system and underlie the emotional aspect of pain. Pain transmission is

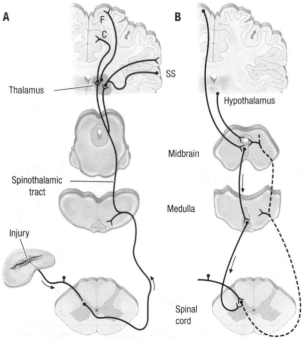

FIGURE 6-1 Pain transmission and modulatory pathways. *A.* Transmission system for nociceptive messages. Noxious stimuli activate the sensitive peripheral ending of the primary afferent nociceptor by the process of transduction. The message is then transmitted over the peripheral nerve to the spinal cord, where it synapses with cells of origin of the major ascending pain pathway, the spinothalamic tract. The message is relayed in the thalamus to the anterior cingulate (C), frontal insular (F), and somatosensory cortex (SS). *B.* Pain-modulation network. Inputs from frontal cortex and hypothalamus activate cells in the midbrain that control spinal pain-transmission cells via cells in the medulla.

TABLE 6-2   DRUGS FOR RELIEF OF PAIN

Generic Name	Dose, mg	Interval
Nonnarcotic Analgesics: Usual Doses and Intervals		
Acetylsalicylic acid	650 PO	q 4 h
Acetaminophen	650 PO	q 4 h
Ibuprofen	400 PO	q 4–6 h
Naproxen	250–500 PO	q 12 h
Fenoprofen	200 PO	q 4–6 h
Indomethacin	25–50 PO	q 8 h
Ketorolac	15–60 IM/IV	q 4–6 h
Celecoxib	100–200 PO	q 12–24 h
Valdecoxib	10–20 PO	q12–24 h

Generic Name	Parenteral Dose, mg	PO Dose, mg
Narcotic Analgesics: Usual Doses and Intervals		
Codeine	30–60 q 4 h	30–60 q 4 h
Oxycodone	—	5–10 q 4–6 h
Morphine	10 q 4 h	60 q 4 h
Morphine sustained release	—	30–200 bid to tid
Hydromorphone	1–2 q 4 h	2–4 q 4 h
Levorphanol	2 q 6–8 h	4 q 6–8 h
Methadone	10 q 6–8 h	20 q 6–8 h
Meperidine	75–100 q 3–4 h	300 q 4 h
Butorphanol	—	1–2 q 4 h
Fentanyl	25–100 µg/h	—
Tramadol	—	50–100 q 4–6 h

Generic Name	Uptake Blockade		Sedative Potency	Anticholinergic Potency
	5-HT	NE		
Antidepressants[a]				
Doxepin	++	+	High	Moderate
Amitriptyline	++++	++	High	Highest
Imipramine	++++	++	Moderate	Moderate
Nortriptyline	+++	++	Moderate	Moderate
Desipramine	+++	++++	Low	Low
Venlafaxine	+++	++	Low	None
Duloxetine	+++	+++	Low	None

Generic Name	PO Dose, mg	Interval
Anticonvulsants and Antiarrhythmics[a]		
Phenytoin	300	daily/qhs
Carbamazepine	200–300	q 6 h
Oxcarbazine	300	bid

[a]Antidepressants, anticonvulsants, and antiarrhythmics have not been approved by the U.S. Food and Drug Administration (FDA) for the treatment of pain.

Comments

Enteric-coated preparations available
Side effects uncommon
Available without prescription
Delayed effects may be due to long half-life
Contraindicated in renal disease
Gastrointestinal side effects common
Available for parenteral use
Useful for arthritis
Removed from U.S. market in 2005

Comments

Nausea common
Usually available with acetaminophen or aspirin

Oral slow-release preparation
Shorter acting than morphine sulfate
Longer acting than morphine sulfate; absorbed well PO
Delayed sedation due to long half-life
Poorly absorbed PO; normeperidine a toxic metabolite
Intranasal spray
72 h Transdermal patch
Mixed opioid/adrenergic action

Orthostatic Hypotension	Cardiac Arrhythmia	Ave. Dose, mg/d	Range, mg/d
Moderate	Less	200	75–400
Moderate	Yes	150	25–300
High	Yes	200	75–400
Low	Yes	100	40–150
Low	Yes	150	50–300
None	No	150	75–400
None	No	40	30–60

Generic Name	PO Dose, mg	Interval
Clonazepam	1	q 6 h
Gabapentin[b]	600–1200	q 8 h
Pregabalin	150–600	bid

[b]Gabapentin in doses up to 1800 mg/d is FDA approved for postherpetic neuralgia.
Note: 5-HT, serotonin; NE, norepinephrine.

regulated at the dorsal horn level by descending bulbospinal pathways that contain serotonin, norepinephrine, and several neuropeptides.

Agents that modify pain perception may act to reduce tissue inflammation (NSAIDs, prostaglandin synthesis inhibitors), to interfere with pain transmission (narcotics), or to enhance descending modulation (narcotics and antidepressants). Anticonvulsants (gabapentin, carbamazepine) may be effective for aberrant pain sensations arising from peripheral nerve injury.

 Pain

ACUTE SOMATIC PAIN

If moderate, it can usually be treated effectively with nonnarcotic analgesics, e.g., aspirin, acetaminophen, and NSAIDs (Table 6-2). All inhibit cyclooxygenase (COX) and, except for acetaminophen, all have anti-inflammatory actions, especially at high dosages. For subacute musculoskeletal pain and arthritis, selective COX-2 inhibitors such as celecoxib are useful but are associated with increased cardiovascular risk. Narcotic analgesics are usually required for relief of severe pain; the dose should be titrated to produce effective analgesia.

CHRONIC PAIN

After evaluation, an explicit treatment plan should be developed, including specific and realistic goals for therapy, e.g., getting a good night's sleep, being able to go shopping, or returning to work. A multidisciplinary approach that utilizes medications, counseling, physical therapy, nerve blocks, and even surgery may be required to improve the pt's quality of life. Psychological evaluation is key; behaviorally based treatment paradigms are frequently helpful. Some pts may require referral to a pain clinic; for others, pharmacologic management alone can provide significant help.

The tricyclic antidepressants are useful in management of chronic pain from many causes, including headache, diabetic neuropathy, postherpetic neuralgia, atypical facial pain, chronic low back pain, and post-stroke pain. Anticonvulsants or antiarrhythmics benefit pts with neuropathic pain and little or no evidence of sympathetic dysfunction (e.g., diabetic neuropathy, trigeminal neuralgia). The combination of the anticonvulsant gabapentin and an antidepressant such as nortriptyline may be effective for chronic neuropathic pain.

The long-term use of opioids is accepted for pain due to malignant disease but is controversial for chronic pain of nonmalignant origin. When other approaches fail, long-acting opioid compounds such as levorphanol, methadone, sustained-release morphine, or transdermal fentanyl may be considered for these pts (Table 6-2).

For a more detailed discussion, see Fields HL, Martin JB: Pain: Pathophysiology and Management, Chap. 12, p. 81, in HPIM-17.

7 Assessment of Nutritional Status

Stability of body weight requires that energy intake and expenditures are balanced over time. The major categories of energy output are resting energy expenditure (REE) and physical activity; minor sources include the energy cost of metabolizing food (thermic effect of food or specific dynamic action) and shivering thermogenesis. The average energy intake is about 2800 kcal/d for men and about 1800 kcal/d for women, though these estimates vary with age, body size, and activity level. Basal energy expenditure (BEE), measured in kcal/d, may be estimated by the Harris and Benedict formula (Fig. 7-1).

Dietary reference intakes (DRI) and recommended dietary allowances (RDA) have been defined for many nutrients, including 9 essential amino acids, 4 fat-soluble and 10 water-soluble vitamins, several minerals, fatty acids, choline, and water (Tables 70-1 and 70-2, pp. 438 and 439, in HPIM-17). The usual water requirements are 1.0–1.5 mL/kcal energy expenditure in adults, with adjustments for excessive losses. The RDA for protein is 0.6 g/kg ideal body weight, representing 15% of total caloric intake. Fat should comprise ≤30% of calories, and saturated fat should be <10% of calories. At least 55% of calories should be derived from carbohydrates.

MALNUTRITION

Malnutrition results from inadequate intake or abnormal gastrointestinal assimilation of dietary calories, excessive energy expenditure, or altered metabolism of energy supplies by an intrinsic disease process.

Both outpatients and inpatients are at risk for malnutrition if they meet one or more of the following criteria:

- Unintentional loss of >10% of usual body weight in the preceding 3 months
- Body weight < 90% of ideal for height (Table 7-1)
- Body mass index (BMI: weight/height^2 in kg/m^2) < 18.5

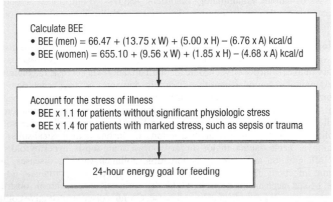

Calculate BEE
- BEE (men) = 66.47 + (13.75 x W) + (5.00 x H) − (6.76 x A) kcal/d
- BEE (women) = 655.10 + (9.56 x W) + (1.85 x H) − (4.68 x A) kcal/d

Account for the stress of illness
- BEE x 1.1 for patients without significant physiologic stress
- BEE x 1.4 for patients with marked stress, such as sepsis or trauma

24-hour energy goal for feeding

FIGURE 7-1 Basal energy expenditure (BEE) calculation in kcal/d, estimated by the Harris and Benedict formula. W, Weight in kg; H, height in cm; A, age in years.

TABLE 7-1	IDEAL WEIGHT FOR HEIGHT						
Men				Women			
Height[a]	Weight[a]	Height	Weight	Height	Weight	Height	Weight
145	51.9	166	64.0	140	44.9	161	56.9
146	52.4	167	64.6	141	45.4	162	57.6
147	52.9	168	65.2	142	45.9	163	58.3
148	53.5	169	65.9	143	46.4	164	58.9
149	54.0	170	66.6	144	47.0	165	59.5
150	54.5	171	67.3	145	47.5	166	60.1
151	55.0	172	68.0	146	48.0	167	60.7
152	55.6	173	68.7	147	48.6	168	61.4
153	56.1	174	69.4	148	49.2	169	62.1
154	56.6	175	70.1	149	49.8		
155	57.2	176	70.8	150	50.4		
156	57.9	177	71.6	151	51.0		
157	58.6	178	72.4	152	51.5		
158	59.3	179	73.3	153	52.0		
159	59.9	180	74.2	154	52.5		
160	60.5	181	75.0	155	53.1		
161	61.1	182	75.8	156	53.7		
162	61.7	183	76.5	157	54.3		
163	62.3	184	77.3	158	54.9		
164	62.9	185	78.1	159	55.5		
165	63.5	186	78.9	160	56.2		

[a]Values are expressed in cm for height and kg for weight. To obtain height in inches, divide by 2.54. To obtain weight in pounds, multiply by 2.2.
Source: Adapted from GL Blackburn et al.: Nutritional and metabolic assessment of the hospitalized patient. J Parenter Enteral Nutr 1:11, 1977; with permission.

Two forms of severe malnutrition can be seen: *marasmus*, which refers to generalized starvation that occurs in the setting of chronically decreased energy intake, and *kwashiorkor*, which refers to selective protein malnutrition due to decreased protein intake and catabolism in the setting of acute, life-threatening illnesses or chronic inflammatory disorders. Aggressive nutritional support is indicated in kwashiorkor to prevent infectious complications and poor wound healing.

Etiology The major etiologies of malnutrition are starvation, stress from surgery or severe illness, and mixed mechanisms. Starvation results from decreased dietary intake (from poverty, chronic alcoholism, anorexia nervosa, fad diets, severe depression, neurodegenerative disorders, dementia, or strict vegetarianism; abdominal pain from intestinal ischemia or pancreatitis; or anorexia associated with AIDS, disseminated cancer, or renal failure) or decreased assimilation of the diet (from pancreatic insufficiency; short bowel syndrome; celiac disease; or esophageal, gastric, or intestinal obstruction). Contributors to physical stress include fever, acute trauma, major surgery, burns, acute sepsis, hyperthyroidism, and inflammation as occurs in pancreatitis, collagen vascular diseases, and chronic infectious diseases such as tuberculosis or AIDS opportunistic infections. Mixed mechanisms occur in AIDS, disseminated cancer, chronic obstructive pulmonary disease, chronic liver disease, Crohn's disease, ulcerative colitis, and renal failure.

Clinical Features

- *General*—weight loss, temporal and proximal muscle wasting, decreased skin-fold thickness
- *Skin, hair, and nails*—easily plucked hair (protein); sparse hair (protein, biotin, zinc); coiled hair, easy bruising, petechiae, and perifollicular hemorrhages (vit. C); "flaky paint" rash of lower extremities (zinc); hyperpigmentation of skin in exposed areas (niacin, tryptophan); spooning of nails (iron)
- *Eyes*—conjunctival pallor (anemia); night blindness, dryness, and Bitot spots (vit. A); ophthalmoplegia (thiamine)
- *Mouth and mucous membranes*—glossitis and/or cheilosis (riboflavin, niacin, vit. B_{12}, pyridoxine, folate), diminished taste (zinc), inflamed and bleeding gums (vit. C)
- *Neurologic*—disorientation (niacin, phosphorus); confabulation, cerebellar gait, or past pointing (thiamine); peripheral neuropathy (thiamine, pyridoxine, vit. E); lost vibratory and position sense (vit. B_{12})
- *Other*—edema (protein, thiamine), heart failure (thiamine, phosphorus), hepatomegaly (protein)

Laboratory findings in protein malnutrition include a low serum albumin, low total iron-binding capacity, and anergy to skin testing. Specific vitamin deficiencies may also be present.

For a more detailed discussion, see Dwyer J: Nutritional Requirements and Dietary Assessment, Chap. 70, p. 437; Heimberger DC: Malnutrition and Nutritional Assessment, Chap. 72, p. 450; and Russell RM and Suter PM: Vitamin and Trace Mineral Deficiency and Excess, Chap. 71, p. 450, in HPIM-17.

8 Enteral and Parenteral Nutrition

Nutritional support should be initiated in pts with malnutrition or in those at risk for malnutrition (e.g., conditions that preclude adequate oral feeding or pts in catabolic states, such as sepsis, burns, or trauma). An approach for deciding when to use various types of specialized nutrition support (SNS) is summarized in Fig. 8-1.

Enteral therapy refers to feeding via the gut, using oral supplements or infusion of formulas via various feeding tubes (nasogastric, nasoduodenal, gastrostomy, jejunostomy, or combined gastrojejunostomy). *Parenteral therapy* refers to the infusion of nutrient solutions into the bloodstream via a peripherally inserted central catheter (PICC), a centrally inserted externalized catheter, or a centrally inserted tunneled catheter or subcutaneous port. When feasible, enteral nutrition is the preferred route because it sustains the digestive, absorptive, and immunologic functions of the GI tract. Parenteral nutrition is often indicated in severe pancreatitis, necrotizing enterocolitis, prolonged ileus, and distal bowel obstruction.

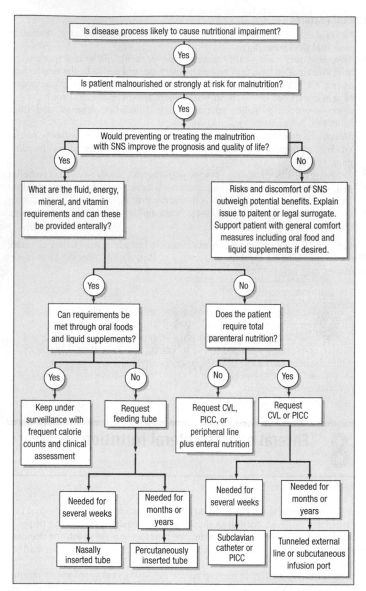

FIGURE 8-1 Decision tree for initiating specialized nutrition support (SNS). CVL, central venous line; PICC, peripherally inserted central catheter.

ENTERAL NUTRITION

The components of a standard enteral formula are as follows:

- Caloric density: 1 kcal/mL
- Protein: ~14% cals; caseinates, soy, lactalbumin

- Fat: ~30% cals; corn, soy, safflower oils
- Carbohydrate: ~60% cals; hydrolyzed corn starch, maltodextrin, sucrose
- Recommended daily intake of all minerals and vitamins in ≥1500 kcal/d
- Osmolality (mosmol/kg): ~300

However, modification of the enteral formula may be required based on various clinical indications and/or associated disease states. After elevation of the head of the bed and confirmation of correct tube placement, continuous gastric infusion is initiated using a half-strength diet at a rate of 25–50 mL/h. This can be advanced to full strength as tolerated to meet the energy target. The major risks of enteral tube feeding are aspiration, diarrhea, electrolyte imbalance, warfarin resistance, sinusitis, and esophagitis.

PARENTERAL NUTRITION

The components of parenteral nutrition include adequate fluid (30 mL/kg body weight for adults, plus any abnormal loss); energy from glucose, amino acids, and lipid solutions; nutrients essential in severely ill pts, such as glutamine, nucleotides, and products of methionine metabolism; electrolytes, vitamins, and minerals. The risks of parenteral therapy include mechanical complications from insertion of the infusion catheter, catheter sepsis, fluid overload, hyperglycemia, hypophosphatemia, hypokalemia, acid-base and electrolyte imbalance, cholestasis, metabolic bone disease, and micronutrient deficiencies.

The following parameters should be monitored in all patients receiving supplemental nutrition, whether enteral or parenteral:

- Fluid balance (weight, intake vs. output)
- Glucose, electrolytes, BUN (daily until stable, then 2× per week)
- Serum creatinine, albumin, phosphorus, calcium, magnesium, Hb/Hct, WBC (baseline, then 2× per week)
- INR (baseline, then weekly)
- Micronutrient tests as indicated

TABLE 8-1	**THERAPY FOR COMMON VITAMIN AND MINERAL DEFICIENCIES**
Nutrient	Therapy
Vitamin A[a,b,c]	60 mg PO, repeated 1 and 14 days later if ocular changes; 30 mg for ages 6–11 mo
	15 mg PO qd × 1 month if chronic malabsorption
Vitamin C	200 mg PO qd
Vitamin E[a]	800–1200 mg PO qd
Vitamin K[a]	10 mg IV × 1
	1–2 mg PO qd or 1–2 mg IV weekly in chronic malabsorption
Thiamine[b]	100 mg IV qd × 7 days, followed by 10 mg PO qd
Niacin	100–200 mg PO tid for 5 days
Pyridoxine	50 mg PO qd, 100–200 mg PO qd if deficiency related to medication
Zinc[b,c]	60 mg PO bid

[a]Associated with fat malabsorption, along with vitamin D deficiency.
[b]Associated with chronic alcoholism; always replete thiamine before carbohydrates in alcoholics to avoid precipitation of acute thiamine deficiency.
[c]Associated with protein-calorie malnutrition.

SPECIFIC MICRONUTRIENT DEFICIENCY

Appropriate therapies for micronutrient deficiencies are outlined in Table 8-1.

 For a more detailed discussion, see Russell RM and Suter PM: Vitamin and Trace Mineral Deficiency and Excess, Chap. 71, p. 441; and Bistrian BR and Driscoll DF: Enteral and Parenteral Nutrition Therapy, Chap. 73, p. 455, HPIM-17.

9 Transfusion and Pheresis Therapy

TRANSFUSIONS

WHOLE BLOOD TRANSFUSION

Indicated when acute blood loss is sufficient to produce hypovolemia, whole blood provides both oxygen-carrying capacity and volume expansion. In acute blood loss, hematocrit may not accurately reflect degree of blood loss for 48 h until fluid shifts occur.

RED BLOOD CELL TRANSFUSION

Indicated for symptomatic anemia unresponsive to specific therapy or requiring urgent correction. Packed red blood cell (RBC) transfusions may be indicated in pts who are symptomatic from cardiovascular or pulmonary disease when Hb is between 70 and 90 g/L (7 and 9 g/dL). Transfusion is usually necessary when Hb is <70 g/L (<7 g/dL). One unit of packed RBCs raises the Hb by approximately 10 g/L (1 g/dL). In the setting of acute hemorrhage, packed RBCs, fresh-frozen plasma (FFP), and platelets in an approximate ratio of 3:1:10 units are an adequate replacement for whole blood. Removal of leukocytes reduces risk of alloimmunization and transmission of cytomegalovirus. Washing to remove donor plasma reduces risk of allergic reactions. Irradiation prevents graft-versus-host disease in immunocompromised recipients by killing alloreactive donor lymphocytes. Avoid related donors.

Other Indications (1) *Hypertransfusion therapy* to block production of defective cells, e.g., thalassemia, sickle cell anemia; (2) *exchange transfusion*—hemolytic disease of newborn, sickle cell crisis; (3) *transplant recipients*—decreases rejection of cadaveric kidney transplants.

Complications (See Table 9-1) (1) *Transfusion reaction*—immediate or delayed, seen in 1–4% of transfusions; IgA-deficient pts at particular risk for severe reaction; (2) *infection*—bacterial (rare); hepatitis C, 1 in 1,600,000 transfusions; HIV transmission, 1 in 1,960,000; (3) *circulatory overload*; (4) *iron overload*—each unit contains 200–250 mg iron; hemochromatosis may develop after 100 U of RBCs (less in children), in absence of blood loss; iron chelation therapy with deferoxamine indicated; (5) *graft-versus-host disease*; (6) *alloimmunization*.

TABLE 9-1	RISKS OF TRANSFUSION COMPLICATIONS

	Frequency, Episodes:Unit
Reactions	
Febrile (FNHTR)	1–4:100
Allergic	1–4:100
Delayed hemolytic	1:1000
TRALI	1:5000
Acute hemolytic	1:12,000
Fatal hemolytic	1:100,000
Anaphylactic	1:150,000
Infections[a]	
Hepatitis B	1:63,000
Hepatitis C	1:1,600,000
HIV-1	1:1,960,000
HIV-2	None reported
HTLV-I and -II	1:641,000
Malaria	1:4,000,000
Other complications	
RBC allosensitization	1:100
HLA allosensitization	1:10
Graft-versus-host disease	Rare

[a]Infectious agents rarely associated with transfusion, theoretically possible, or of unknown risk, include hepatitis A virus, parvovirus B-19, *Babesia microti* (babesiosis), *Borrelia burgdorferi* (Lyme disease), *Trypanosoma cruzi* (Chagas' disease), *Treponema pallidum*, human herpesvirus-8, and hepatitis G virus.
Note: FNHTR, febrile nonhemolytic transfusion reaction; TRALI, transfusion-related acute lung injury; HTLV, human T lymphotropic virus; RBC, red blood cell; HLA, human leukocyte antigen.

AUTOLOGOUS TRANSFUSION

Use of pt's own stored blood avoids hazards of donor blood; also useful in pts with multiple RBC antibodies. Pace of autologous donation may be accelerated using erythropoietin (50–150 U/kg SC three times a week) in the setting of normal iron stores.

PLATELET TRANSFUSION

Prophylactic transfusions usually reserved for platelet count < 10,000/μL (<20,000/μL in acute leukemia). One unit elevates the count by about 10,000/μL if no platelet antibodies are present as a result of prior transfusions. Efficacy assessed by 1-h and 24-h posttransfusion platelet counts. HLA-matched single-donor platelets may be required in pts with platelet alloantibodies.

TRANSFUSION OF PLASMA COMPONENTS

FFP is a source of coagulation factors, fibrinogen, antithrombin, and proteins C and S. It is used to correct coagulation factor deficiencies, rapidly reverse warfarin effects, and treat thrombotic thrombocytopenic purpura (TTP). Cryoprecipitate is a source of fibrinogen, factor VIII, and von Willebrand factor; it may be used when recombinant factor VIII or factor VIII concentrates are not available.

THERAPEUTIC HEMAPHERESIS

Hemapheresis is removal of a cellular or plasma constituent of blood; the specific procedure is referred to by the blood fraction removed.

LEUKAPHERESIS

Removal of WBCs; most often used in acute leukemia, esp. acute myeloid leukemia (AML) in cases complicated by marked elevation (>100,000/μL) of the peripheral blast count, to lower risk of leukostasis (blast-mediated vasoocclusive events resulting in central nervous system or pulmonary infarction, hemorrhage). Leukapheresis is replacing bone marrow aspiration to obtain hematopoietic stem cells. After treatment with a chemotherapeutic agent and granulocyte-macrophage colony-stimulating factor, hematopoietic stem cells are mobilized from marrow to the peripheral blood; such cells are leukapheresed and then used for hematopoietic reconstitution after high-dose myeloablative therapy.

PLATELETPHERESIS

Used in some pts with thrombocytosis associated with myeloproliferative disorders with bleeding and/or thrombotic complications. Other treatments are generally used first. Plateletpheresis also enhances platelet yield from blood donors.

PLASMAPHERESIS

Indications　(1) *Hyperviscosity states*—e.g., Waldenström's macroglobulinemia; (2) *TTP*; (3) *immune-complex* and *autoantibody disorders*—e.g., Goodpasture's syndrome, rapidly progressive glomerulonephritis, myasthenia gravis; possibly Guillain-Barré, systemic lupus erythematosus, idiopathic thrombocytopenic purpura; (4) cold agglutinin disease, cryoglobulinemia.

For a more detailed discussion, see Dzieczkowski JS, Anderson KC: Transfusion Biology and Therapy, Chap. 107, p. 707, in HPIM-17

10 Palliative and End-of-Life Care

In 2006, 2,425,901 people died in the United States; death rates are declining. Heart disease and cancer are the two leading causes of death and together account for nearly half of all deaths. About 70% of deaths occur in people who have a condition that is known to be leading to their death; thus, planning for terminal care is relevant and important. An increasing fraction of deaths are occurring in hospices or at home rather than in the hospital.

Optimal care depends on a comprehensive assessment of pt needs in all four domains affected by illness: physical, psychological, social, and spiritual. A variety of assessment tools are available to assist in the process.

Communication and continuous assessment of management goals are key components to addressing end-of-life care. Physicians must be clear about the likely outcome of the illness(es) and provide an anticipated schedule with goals and landmarks in the care process. When the goals of care have changed from cure to palliation, that transition must be clearly explained and defended. Seven steps are involved in establishing goals:

1. Ensure that the medical information is as complete as possible and understood by all relevant parties.
2. Explore the pt's goals while making sure the goals are achievable.
3. Explain the options.
4. Show empathy as the pt and the family adjust to changing expectations.
5. Make a plan with realistic goals.
6. Follow through with the plan.
7. Review and revise the plan periodically as the pt's situation changes.

Advance Directives   Only 29% of pts (and less than one-third of physicians) have executed advance directives that define the level of intervention the pt is willing to accept. It is useful to have the pt's wishes for level of intervention defined before a medical crisis occurs. Two types of legal documents can be used: the advance directive, in which specific instructions from the pt may be made known, and the durable attorney for health care, in which a person is designated as having the pt's authority to make health decisions on the pt's behalf. Forms are available free of charge from the National Hospice and Palliative Care Organization (www.nhpco.org).

Physical Symptoms and Their Management   The most common physical and psychological symptoms among terminally ill pts are shown in Table 10-1. Studies of pts with advanced cancer have shown that pts experience an average of 11.5 symptoms.

Pain   Pain is noted in 36–90% of terminally ill pts. The various types of pain and their management are discussed in Chap. 6.

TABLE 10-1   COMMON PHYSICAL AND PSYCHOLOGICAL SYMPTOMS OF TERMINALLY ILL PATIENTS

Physical Symptoms	Psychological Symptoms
Pain	Anxiety
Fatigue and weakness	Depression
Dyspnea	Hopelessness
Insomnia	Meaninglessness
Dry mouth	Irritability
Anorexia	Impaired concentration
Nausea and vomiting	Confusion
Constipation	Delirium
Cough	Loss of libido
Swelling of arms or legs	
Itching	
Diarrhea	
Dysphagia	
Dizziness	
Fecal and urinary incontinence	
Numbness/tingling in hands/feet	

Constipation Constipation is noted in up to 90% of terminally ill pts. Medications commonly contribute to constipation, including opioids used to manage pain and dyspnea, and tricyclic antidepressants with their anticholinergic effects. Inactivity, poor diet, and hypercalcemia may contribute. GI tract obstruction also may play a role in some settings.

Interventions Improved physical activity (if possible), adequate hydration; opioid effects can be antagonized by the μ-opioid receptor blocker methylnaltrexone; rule out surgically correctable obstruction; laxatives and stool softeners (Table 10-2).

Nausea Up to 70% of pts with advanced cancer have nausea. Nausea may result from uremia, liver failure, hypercalcemia, bowel obstruction, severe constipation, infection, gastroesophageal reflux disease, vestibular disease, brain metastases, medications (cancer chemotherapy, antibiotics, nonsteroidal anti-inflammatory drugs, opioids, proton pump inhibitors), and radiation therapy.

Interventions Treatment should be tailored to the cause. Offending medications should be stopped. Underlying conditions should be alleviated, if possible. If decreased bowel motility is suspected, metoclopramide may help. Nausea from cancer chemotherapy agents can generally be prevented with glucocorticoids and serotonin receptor blockers like ondansetron or dolasetron. Aprepitant is useful in controlling nausea from highly emetogenic agents like cisplatin. Vestibular nausea may respond to antihistamines (meclizine) or anticholinergics (scopolamine). Anticipatory nausea may be prevented with a benzodiazepine

TABLE 10-2	MEDICATIONS FOR THE MANAGEMENT OF CONSTIPATION	
Intervention	Dose	Comment
Stimulant laxatives		These agents directly stimulate peristalsis and may reduce colonic absorption of water. Work in 6–12 h.
Prune juice	120–240 mL/d	
Senna (Senokot)	2–8 tablets PO bid	
Bisacodyl	5–15 mg/d PO, PR	
Osmotic laxatives		These agents are not absorbed. They attract and retain water in the gastrointestinal tract.
Lactulose	15–30 mL PO q4–8h	
Magnesium hydroxide (Milk of Magnesia)	15–30 mL/d PO	Lactulose may cause flatulence and bloating.
Magnesium citrate	125–250 mL/d PO	Lactulose works in 1 day; magnesium products in 6 h.
Stool softeners		These agents work by increasing water secretion and as detergents increasing water penetration into the stool. Work in 1–3 days.
Sodium docusate (Colace)	300–600 mg/d PO	
Calcium docusate	300–600 mg/d PO	
Suppositories and enemas		
Bisacodyl	10–15 PR qd	Fixed dose, 4.5 oz, Fleet's.
Sodium phosphate enema	PR qd	

such as lorazepam. Haloperidol is sometimes useful when the nausea does not have a single specific cause.

Dyspnea Up to 75% of dying pts experience dyspnea. Dyspnea exerts perhaps the greatest adverse effect on the pt, often even more distressing than pain. It may be caused by parenchymal lung disease, infection, effusions, pulmonary emboli, pulmonary edema, asthma, or compressed airway. While many of the causes may be treated, often the underlying cause cannot be reversed.

Interventions Underlying causes should be reversed, where possible, as long as the intervention is not more unpleasant (e.g. repeated thoracenteses) than the dyspnea. Most often the treatment is symptomatic (Table 10-3).

Fatigue Fatigue is nearly a universal symptom in terminally ill pts. It is often a direct consequence of the disease process (and the cytokines produced in response to that process) and may be complicated by inanition, dehydration, anemia, infection, hypothyroidism, and drug effects. Depression may also contribute to fatigue. Functional assessments include the Karnofsky performance status or the Eastern Cooperative Oncology Group system based on how much time the pt spends in bed each day: 0, normal activity; 1, symptomatic without being bedridden; 2, in bed <50% of the day; 3, in bed >50% of the day; 4, bedbound.

Interventions Modest exercise and physical therapy may reduce muscle wasting and depression and improve mood; discontinue medications that worsen fatigue, if possible; glucocorticoids may increase energy and enhance mood; dextroamphetamine (5–10 mg/d) or methylphenidate (2.5–5 mg/d) in the morning may enhance energy levels but should be avoided at night because they may produce insomnia; modafinil and L-carnitine have shown some early promise.

Depression Up to 75% of terminally ill pts experience depression. The inexperienced physician may feel that depression is an appropriate response to terminal illness; however, in a substantial fraction of pts the depression is more intense and

TABLE 10-3	MEDICATIONS FOR THE MANAGEMENT OF DYSPNEA	
Intervention	Dose	Comments
Weak opioids		For patients with mild
Codeine (or codeine	30 mg PO q4h	dyspnea
with 325 mg aceta-		For opioid-naïve patient
minophen)		
Hydrocodone	5 mg PO q4h	
Strong opioids		For opioid-naïve patients
Morphine	5–10 mg PO q4h	with moderate to se-
	30–50% of baseline	vere dyspnea
	opioid dose q4h	For patients already tak-
Oxycodone	5–10 mg PO q4h	ing opioids for pain or
Hydromorphone	1–2 mg PO q4h	other symptoms
Anxiolytics		Give a dose every hour
Lorazepam	0.5–2.0 mg PO/SL/IV	until the patient
	qh then q4–6h	is relaxed, then provide
Clonazepam	0.25–2.0 mg PO q12h	a dose for maintenance
Midazolam	0.5 mg IV q15min	

disabling than usual. Pts with a previous history of depression are at greater risk. A number of treatable conditions can cause depression-like symptoms including hypothyroidism, Cushing's syndrome, electrolyte abnormalities (e.g., hypercalcemia), and drugs including dopamine blockers, interferon, tamoxifen, interleukin 2, vincristine, and glucocorticoids.

Interventions   Dextroamphetamine or methylphenidate (see above); serotonin reuptake inhibitors such as fluoxetine, paroxetine, and citalopram; modafinil 100 mg/d; pemoline 18.75 mg in the A.M. and at noon.

Delirium   Delirium is a global cerebral dysfunction associated with altered cognition and consciousness; it is frequently preceded by anxiety. Unlike dementia, it is of sudden onset, is characterized by fluctuating consciousness and inattention, and may be reversible. It is generally manifested in the hours before death. It may be caused by metabolic encephalopathy in renal or liver failure, hypoxemia, infection, hypercalcemia, paraneoplastic syndromes, dehydration, constipation, urinary retention, and central nervous system spread of cancer. It is also a common medication side effect; offending agents include those commonly used in dying pts including opioids, glucocorticoids, anticholinergics, antihistamines, antiemetics, and benzodiazepines. Early recognition is key because the pt should be encouraged to use the periods of lucidity for final communication with loved ones. Day-night reversal with changes in mentation may be an early sign.

Interventions   Stop any and all unnecessary medications that may have this side effect; provide a calendar, clock, newspaper, or other orienting signals; gently correct hallucinations or cognitive mistakes; pharmacologic interventions are shown in Table 10-4.

Care during the Last Hours   The clinical course of a dying pt may largely be predictable. Figure 10-1 shows common and uncommon changes during the last days of life. Informing families that these changes might occur can help minimize the distress that they cause. In particular, the physician needs to be sensitive to the sense of guilt and helplessness that family members feel. They should be reassured that the illness is taking its course and their care of the pt is not at fault in any way. The pt stops eating because they are dying; they are not dying because they have stopped eating. Families and caregivers should be encouraged to communicate directly with the dying pt whether or not the pt is unconscious.

TABLE 10-4	MEDICATIONS FOR THE MANAGEMENT OF DELIRIUM
Interventions	**Dose**
Neuroleptics	
Haloperidol	0.5–5 mg q2–12h, PO/IV/SC/IM
Thioridazine	10–75 mg q4–8h, PO
Chlorpromazine	12.5–50 mg q4–12h, PO/IV/IM
Atypical neuroleptics	
Olanzapine	2.5–5 mg qd or bid, PO
Risperidone	1–3 mg q12h, PO
Anxiolytics	
Lorazepam	0.5–2 mg q1–4h, PO/IV/IM
Midazolam	1–5 mg/h continuous infusion, IV/SC
Anesthetics	
Propofol	0.3–2.0 mg/h continuous infusion, IV

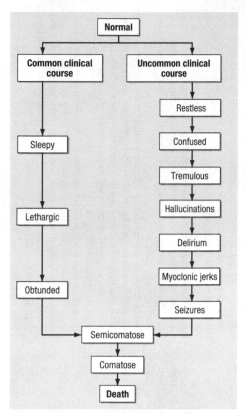

FIGURE 10-1 Common and uncommon clinical courses in the last days of terminally ill patients. (*Adapted from FD Ferris et al: Module 4: Palliative care, in Comprehensive Guide for the Care of Persons with HIV Disease. Toronto: Mt. Sinai Hospital and Casey Hospice, 1995, at www.cp-sonline.info/content/resources/hivmodule4.html.*)

Holding the pt's hand may be a source of comfort to both the pt and the family member/caregiver. Table 10-5 provides a listing of some changes in the pt's condition in the final hours and advice on how to manage the changes.

Additional resources for managing terminally ill pts may be found at the following websites: www.epec.net, www.eperc.mcw.edu, www.capc.org, and www.nhpco.org.

For a more detailed discussion, see Emanuel EJ, Hauser J, Emanuel LL: Palliative and End-of-Life Care, Chap. 11, p. 66, in HPIM-17.

TABLE 10-5   MANAGING CHANGES IN THE PATIENT'S CONDITION DURING THE FINAL DAYS AND HOURS

Changes in the Patient's Condition	Potential Complication	Family's Possible Reaction and Concern	Advice and Intervention
Profound fatigue	Bedbound with development of pressure ulcers that are prone to infection, malodor, and pain, and joint pain	Patient is lazy and giving up.	Reassure family and caregivers that terminal fatigue will not respond to interventions and should not be resisted. Use an air mattress if necessary.
Anorexia	None	Patient is giving up; patient will suffer from hunger and will starve to death.	Reassure family and caregivers that the patient is not eating because he or she is dying; not eating at the end of life does not cause suffering or death. Forced feeding, whether oral, parenteral, or enteral, does not reduce symptoms or prolong life.
Dehydration	Dry mucosal membranes (see below)	Patient will suffer from thirst and die of dehydration.	Reassure family and caregivers that dehydration at the end of life does not cause suffering because patients lose consciousness before any symptom distress. Intravenous hydration can worsen symptoms of dyspnea by pulmonary edema and peripheral edema as well as prolong dying process. Do not force oral intake.
Dysphagia	Inability to swallow oral medications needed for palliative care		Discontinue unnecessary medications that may have been continued including antibiotics, diuretics, anti-depressants, and laxatives. If swallowing pills is difficult, convert essential medications (analgesics, antiemetics, anxiolytics, and psychotropics) to oral solutions, buccal, sublingual, or rectal administration.
"Death rattle"— noisy breathing		Patient is choking and suffocating.	Reassure the family and caregivers that this is caused by secretions in the oropharynx and the patient is not choking. Reduce secretions with scopolamine (0.2–0.4 mg SC q4h or 1–3 patches q3d) Reposition patient to permit drainage of secretions. Do not suction. Suction can cause patient and family discomfort, and is usually ineffective.

Sign/Symptom	Clinical consequence	Family/caregiver perception	Management
Apnea, Cheyne-Stokes respirations, dyspnea		Patient is suffocating.	Reassure family and caregivers that unconscious patients do not experience suffocation or air hunger. Apneic episodes are frequently a premorbid change. Opioids or anxiolytics may be used for dyspnea. Oxygen is unlikely to relieve dyspneic symptoms and may prolong the dying process.
Urinary or fecal incontinence	Skin breakdown if days until death. Potential transmission of infectious agents to caregivers	Patient is dirty, malodorous, and physically repellent.	Remind family and caregivers to use universal precautions. Frequent changes of bedclothes and bedding. Use diapers, urinary catheter, or rectal tube if diarrhea or high urine output.
Agitation or delirium	Day/night reversal. Hurt self or caregivers	Patient is in horrible pain and going to have a horrible death.	Reassure family and caregivers that agitation and delirium do not necessarily connote physical pain. Depending upon the prognosis and goals of treatment, consider evaluating for causes of delirium and modify medications. Manage symptoms with haloperidol, chlorpromazine, diazepam, or midazolam.
Dry mucosal membranes	Cracked lips, mouth sores, and candidiasis can also cause pain. Odor	Patient may be malodorous, physically repellent.	Use baking soda mouthwash or saliva preparation q15–30min. Use topical nystatin for candidiasis. Coat lips and nasal mucosa with petroleum jelly q60–90min. Use ophthalmic lubricants q4h or artificial tears q30min.

11 Cardiovascular Collapse and Sudden Death

Unexpected cardiovascular collapse and death most often result from ventricular fibrillation in pts with underlying coronary artery disease, with or without acute MI. Other common causes are listed in Table 11-1. The arrhythmic causes may be provoked by electrolyte disorders (primarily hypokalemia), hypoxemia, acidosis, or massive sympathetic discharge, as may occur in CNS injury. Immediate institution of cardiopulmonary resuscitation (CPR) followed by advanced life support measures (see below) are mandatory. Ventricular fibrillation, or asystole, without institution of CPR within 4–6 min is usually fatal.

MANAGEMENT OF CARDIAC ARREST

Basic life support (BLS) must commence immediately (Fig. 11-1):

- Phone 911 (or emergency line); Get automated external defibrillator (AED) if quickly available on site.
- Open mouth of patient and remove visible debris or dentures. If there is respiratory stridor, consider aspiration of a foreign body and perform Heimlich maneuver.
- Tilt head backward, lift chin, and begin mouth-to-mouth respiration if rescue equipment is not available (pocket mask is preferable to prevent trans-

TABLE 11-1	DIFFERENTIAL DIAGNOSIS OF CARDIOVASCULAR COLLAPSE AND SUDDEN DEATH

1. Ventricular fibrillation due to:
   Myocardial ischemia (severe coronary artery disease, acute MI)
   Heart failure
   Dilated or hypertrophic cardiomyopathy
   Myocarditis
   Right ventricular dysplasia
   Valvular disease [aortic stenosis, mitral valve prolapse (rare)]
   Cardiac infiltrative diseases
   Preexcitation syndromes (Wolff-Parkinson-White)
   Prolonged QT syndromes (congenital, drug-induced)
   Brugada syndrome
2. Asystole or severe bradycardia
3. Sudden marked decrease in LV stroke volume from:
   Massive pulmonary embolism
   Cardiac tamponade
   Severe aortic stenosis
4. Sudden marked decrease in intravascular volume, e.g.:
   Ruptured aortic aneurysm
   Aortic dissection

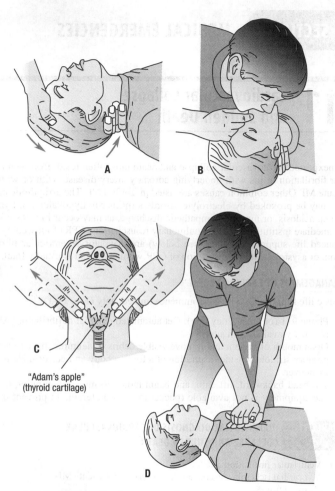

"Adam's apple"
(thyroid cartilage)

FIGURE 11-1 Major steps in cardiopulmonary resuscitation. *A.* Make certain that the victim has an open airway. *B.* Start respiratory resuscitation immediately. *C.* Feel for the carotid pulse in the groove alongside the "Adam's apple" or thyroid cartilage. *D.* If pulse is absent, begin cardiac massage. Use 100 compressions/min with two lung inflations in rapid succession for every 30 compressions. (*From J Henderson, Emergency Medical Guide, 4th ed, New York, McGraw-Hill, 1978.*)

mission of infection). The lungs should be inflated twice in rapid succession for every 30 chest compressions.

- If carotid pulse is absent, perform chest compressions (depressing sternum 4–5 cm) at rate of 100 per min. For one rescuer, 30 compressions are performed before returning to ventilating twice.
- As soon as resuscitation equipment is available, begin advanced life support with continued chest compressions and ventilation.
- Although performed as simultaneously as possible, defibrillation takes highest priority (Fig. 11-2), followed by placement of intravenous access and intubation. 100% O_2 should be administered by endotracheal tube or, if rapid

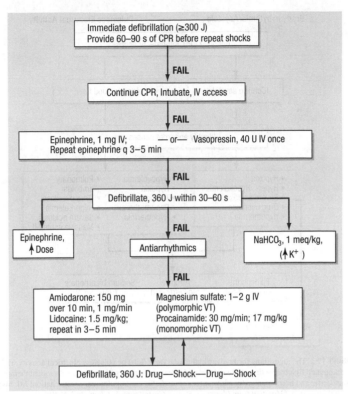

FIGURE 11-2 Management of cardiac arrest. The algorithm of ventricular fibrillation or hypotensive ventricular tachycardia begins with defibrillation attempts. If that fails, it is followed by epinephrine or vasopressin and then antiarrhythmic drugs. CPR, cardiopulmonary resuscitation. (*Modified from Myerburg RJ and Castellanos A, Chap. 267, HPIM-17.*)

intubation cannot be accomplished, by bag-valve-mask device; respirations should not be interrupted for more than 30 s while attempting to intubate.

- Initial intravenous access should be through the antecubital vein, but if drug administration is ineffective, a central line (internal jugular or subclavian) should be placed. Intravenous $NaHCO_3$ should be administered only if there is persistent severe acidosis (pH < 7.15) despite adequate ventilation. Calcium is *not* routinely administered but should be given to pts with known hypocalcemia, those who have received toxic doses of calcium channel antagonists, or if acute hyperkalemia is thought to be the triggering event for resistant ventricular fibrillation.

- The approach to cardiovascular collapse caused by bradyarrhythmias, asystole, or pulseless electrical activity is shown in Fig. 11-3.

FOLLOW-UP

If cardiac arrest was due to ventricular fibrillation in initial hours of an acute MI, follow-up is standard post-MI care (Chap. 126). For other survivors of a ventricular fibrillation arrest, extensive assessment, including evaluation of coronary anatomy, left ventricular function, and invasive electrophysiologic test-

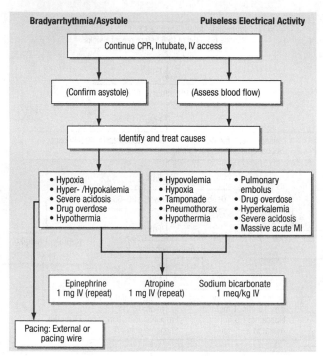

FIGURE 11-3 The algorithms for bradyarrhythmia/asytole (left) or pulseless electrical activity (right) is dominated first by continued life support and a search for reversible causes. Subsequent therapy is nonspecific and accompanied by a low success rate. CPR, cardiopulmonary resuscitation; MI, myocardial infarction. (*Modified from Myerburg RJ and Castellanos A, Chap. 267, HPIM-17.*)

ing, is often recommended. In absence of a transient or reversible cause, placement of an implantable cardioverter defibrillator is usually indicated.

For a more detailed discussion, see Myerburg RJ, Castellanos A: Cardiovascular Collapse, Cardiac Arrest, and Sudden Cardiac Death, Chap. 267, p. 1707, in HPIM-17.

12 Shock

DEFINITION

Condition of severe impairment of tissue perfusion leading to cellular injury and dysfunction. Cell membrane dysfunction is a common end stage for various forms of shock. Rapid recognition and treatment are essential to prevent irreversible organ damage. Common causes are listed in Table 12-1.

| **TABLE 12-1** | **COMMON FORMS OF SHOCK** |

Oligemic shock
   Hemorrhage
   Volume depletion (e.g., vomiting, diarrhea, diuretic over-usage, ketoacidosis)
   Internal sequestration (ascites, pancreatitis, intestinal obstruction)
Cardiogenic shock
   Myopathic (acute MI, dilated cardiomyopathy)
   Mechanical (acute mitral regurgitation, ventricular septal defect, severe aortic
     stenosis)
   Arrhythmic
Extracardiac obstructive shock
   Pericardial tamponade
   Massive pulmonary embolism
   Tension pneumothorax
Distributive shock (profound decrease in systemic vascular tone)
   Sepsis
   Toxic overdoses
   Anaphylaxis
   Neurogenic (e.g., spinal cord injury)
   Endocrinologic (Addison's disease, myxedema)

CLINICAL MANIFESTATIONS

- Hypotension (systolic bp < 90, mean bp < 60), tachycardia, tachypnea, pallor, restlessness, and altered sensorium.
- Signs of intense peripheral vasoconstriction, with weak pulses and cold clammy extremities. In distributive (e.g., septic) shock, vasodilatation predominates and extremities are warm.
- Oliguria (<20 mL/h) and metabolic acidosis common.
- Acute lung injury and acute respiratory distress syndrome (ARDS; see Chap. 15) with noncardiogenic pulmonary edema, hypoxemia, and diffuse pulmonary infiltrates.

APPROACH TO THE PATIENT

Obtain history for underlying cause, including
- Known cardiac disease (coronary disease, CHF, pericarditis)
- Recent fever or infection (leading to sepsis)
- Drugs, e.g., excess diuretics or antihypertensives
- Conditions predisposing for pulmonary embolism (Chap. 140)
- Possible bleeding from any site, particularly GI tract.

PHYSICAL EXAMINATION

- Jugular veins are flat in oligemic or distributive shock; jugular venous distention (JVD) suggests cardiogenic shock; JVD in presence of paradoxical pulse (Chap. 117) may reflect cardiac tamponade (Chap. 123).
- Look for evidence of CHF (Chap. 131), murmurs of aortic stenosis, acute regurgitation (mitral or aortic), ventricular septal defect.
- Check for asymmetry of pulses (aortic dissection) (Chap. 132).
- Tenderness or rebound in abdomen may indicate peritonitis or pancreatitis; high-pitched bowel sounds suggest intestinal obstruction. Perform stool guaiac to rule out GI bleeding.

- Fever and chills usually accompany septic shock. Sepsis may not cause fever in elderly, uremic, or alcoholic patients.
- Skin lesion may suggest specific pathogens in septic shock: petechiae or purpura (*Neisseria meningitidis*), erythyma gangrenosum (*Pseudomonas aeruginosa*), generalized erythroderma (toxic shock due to *Staphylococcus aureus* or *Streptococcus pyogenes*).

LABORATORY

- Obtain hematocrit, WBC, electrolytes. If actively bleeding, check platelet count, PT, PTT, DIC screen.
- Arterial blood gas usually shows metabolic acidosis (in septic shock, respiratory alkalosis precedes metabolic acidosis). If sepsis suspected, draw blood cultures, perform urinalysis, and obtain Gram stain and cultures of sputum, urine, and other suspected sites.
- Obtain ECG (myocardial ischemia or acute arrhythmia), chest x-ray (CHF, tension pneumothorax, aortic dissection, pneumonia). Echocardiogram may be helpful (cardiac tamponade, CHF).
- Central venous pressure or pulmonary capillary wedge (PCW) pressure measurements may be necessary to distinguish between different categories of shock (Table 12-2): Mean PCW < 6 mmHg suggests oligemic or distributive shock; PCW > 20 mmHg suggests left ventricular failure. Cardiac output (thermodilution) is decreased in cardiogenic and oligemic shock, and usually increased initially in septic shock.

℞ Shock See Fig. 12-1.

Aimed at rapid improvement of tissue hypoperfusion and respiratory impairment:

- Serial measurements of bp (intraarterial line preferred), heart rate, continuous ECG monitor, urine output, pulse oximetry, blood studies: Hct, electrolytes, creatinine, BUN, ABGs, pH, calcium, phosphate, lactate, urine Na

| TABLE 12-2 | HEMODYNAMIC PROFILES IN SHOCK STATES |

Diagnosis	PCW Pressure	Cardiac Output (CO)	Systemic Vascular Resistance	Comments
Cardiogenic shock	↑	↓	↑	PCW is normal or ↓ in RV infarction
Cardiac tamponade	↑	↑	↑	Equalization of intra-cardiac diastolic pressures
Massive pulmonary embolus	Normal or ↓	↓	↑	Right-sided cardiac pressures may be elevated
Oligemic shock	↓	↓	↑	
Distributive shock	↓	↑	↓	CO may ↓ later if sepsis results in LV dysfunction or if intravascular volume is inadequate

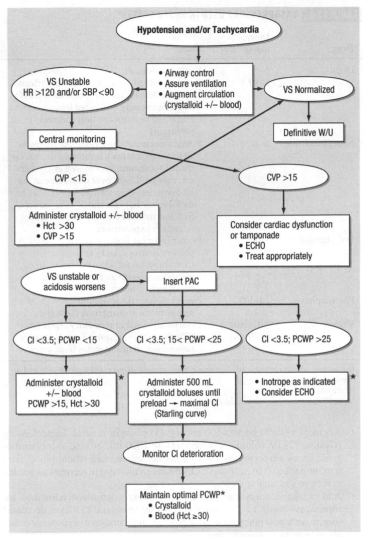

FIGURE 12-1 An algorithm for the resuscitation of the patient in shock. VS, vital signs; HR, heart rate; SBP, systolic blood pressure; W/U, workup; CVP, central venous pressure; Hct, hematocrit; ECHO, echocardiogram; PAC, pulmonary artery catheter; CI, cardiac index in $(L/min)/m^2$; PCWP, pulmonary capillary wedge pressure in mmHg.

*Monitor SV_{O_2}, SVRI, and RVEDVI as additional markers of correction for perfusion and hypovolemia. Consider age-adjusted CI. SV_{O_2}, saturation of hemoglobin with O_2 in venous blood; SVRI, systemic vascular resistance index; RVEDVI, right-ventricular end-diastolic volume index.

concentration (<20 mmol/L suggests volume depletion). Consider continuous monitoring of CVP and/or pulmonary artery pressure, with serial PCW pressures in pts with ongoing blood loss or suspected cardiac dysfunction.

- Insert Foley catheter to monitor urine flow.
- Assess mental status frequently.

TABLE 12-3   **VASOPRESSORS USED IN SHOCK STATES**[a]

Drug	Dose, (μg/kg)/min	Notes
Dopamine	1–5	Facilitates diuresis
	5–10	Positive inotropic and chronotropic effects; may increase O_2 consumption as well as O_2 delivery; use may be limited by tachycardia
	10–20	Generalized vasoconstriction (decrease renal perfusion)
Norepinephrine	2–8	Potent vasoconstrictor; moderate inotropic effect; in septic shock is thought to increase tissue O_2 consumption as well as O_2 delivery; may be chosen over dopamine in sepsis due to less chronotropic effect; may be useful in cardiogenic shock with reduced SVR but should generally be reserved for refractory hypotension
Dobutamine	1–20	Primarily for cardiogenic shock (Chap. 126): positive inotrope; lacks vasoconstrictor activity; most useful when only mild hypotension present and avoidance of tachycardia desired
Phenylephrine	20–200	Potent vasoconstrictor without inotropic effect; may be useful in distributive (septic) shock
Vasopressin	0.01–0.04 U/min[b]	Occasionally used in refractory septic (distributive) shock; restores vascular tone in vasopressin-deficient states (e.g., sepsis)

[a]Isoproterenol not recommended in shock states because of potential hypotension and arrhythmogenic effects.
[b]Dose not based on weight.
Note: SVR, systemic vascular resistance.

- Augment systolic bp to >100 mmHg: (1) place in reverse Trendelenburg position; (2) IV volume infusion (500- to 1000-mL bolus), unless cardiogenic shock suspected (begin with normal saline, then whole blood, dextran, or packed RBCs, if anemic); continue volume replacement as needed to restore vascular volume.
- Add vasoactive drugs after intravascular volume is optimized; administer vasopressors (Table 12-3) if systemic vascular resistance (SVR) is decreased (begin with norepinephrine or dopamine; for persistent hypotension add phenylephrine or vasopressin).
- If CHF present, add inotropic agents (usually dobutamine) (Table 12-3); aim to maintain cardiac index > 2.2(L/m^2)/min [>4.0(L/m^2)/min in septic shock].
- Administer 100% O_2; intubate with mechanical ventilation if P_{O_2} < 70 mmHg.
- If severe metabolic acidosis present (pH < 7.15), administer $NaHCO_3$ (44.6–89.2 mmol).
- Identify and treat underlying cause of shock. Cardiogenic shock in acute MI is discussed in Chap. 126. Emergent coronary revascularization may be lifesaving if persistent ischemia is present. Consider cardiac tamponade (see Chap. 123).

SEPTIC SHOCK   (See Chap. 13)

For a more detailed discussion, see Maier RV: Approach to the Patient with Shock, Chap. 264, p. 1689, in HPIM-17.

13 Sepsis and Septic Shock

DEFINITIONS

Systemic inflammatory response syndrome (SIRS)—Two or more of the following:

- Fever (oral temperature >38°C) or hypothermia (oral temperature <36°C)
- Tachypnea (>24 breaths/min)
- Tachycardia (>90 beats/min)
- Leukocytosis (>12,000/µL), leukopenia (<4000/µL), or >10% bands; may have a noninfectious etiology

Sepsis—SIRS with a proven or suspected microbial etiology
Severe sepsis—Sepsis with one or more signs of organ dysfunction
Septic shock—Sepsis with arterial blood pressure <90 mmHg or 40 mmHg below pt's normal blood pressure for at least 1 h despite fluid resuscitation or need for vasopressors to maintain systolic blood pressure ≥90 mmHg or mean arterial pressure ≥70 mmHg

ETIOLOGY

Blood cultures are positive in 20–40% of sepsis cases and in 40–70% of septic shock cases. Of cases with positive blood cultures, a single gram-positive or gram-negative bacterial species accounts for ~70% of isolates; the remainder are fungi or a mixture of microorganisms.

EPIDEMIOLOGY AND RISK FACTORS

The incidence of severe sepsis and septic shock is increasing in the United States, with >700,000 cases each year. Two-thirds of cases occur in pts with significant underlying disease. Sepsis is a contributing factor in >200,000 deaths each year in the United States.

The higher incidence of sepsis is due to the aging of the population, longer survival of pts with chronic diseases, a relatively high frequency of sepsis among AIDS patients, medical treatments (e.g., with glucocorticoids or antibiotics), invasive procedures (e.g., catheter placement), and mechanical ventilation.

Invasive bacterial infections are a prominent cause of death around the world, especially among young children. In sub-Saharan Africa, at least one-quarter of deaths of children >1 year of age are due to community-acquired bacteremia (e.g., with nontyphoidal *Salmonella* species, *Streptococcus pneumoniae*, *Haemophilus influenzae*, and *Escherichia coli*).

PATHOGENESIS AND PATHOLOGY

Local and Systemic Host Responses

- Cytokines and other mediators that increase blood flow to the infected site, enhance the permeability of local blood vessels, attract neutrophils to the infected site, and elicit pain are released.

- Key features of the systemic immune response include intravascular fibrin deposition, thrombosis, and disseminated intravascular coagulation (DIC); the underlying mechanisms are the activation of intrinsic and extrinsic clotting pathways, impaired function of the protein C–protein S inhibitory pathway, depletion of antithrombin and protein C, and prevention of fibrinolysis by increased plasma levels of plasminogen activator inhibitor 1.

Organ Dysfunction and Shock

- Endothelial injury: Widespread endothelial injury is believed to be the major mechanism for multiorgan dysfunction.
- Septic shock is characterized by a decrease in peripheral vascular resistance despite increased levels of vasopressor catecholamines. Although blood flow to peripheral tissues increases, oxygen utilization by these tissues is greatly impaired.

CLINICAL FEATURES

- Hyperventilation
- Encephalopathy (disorientation, confusion)
- Acrocyanosis, ischemic necrosis of peripheral tissues (e.g., digits) due to DIC
- Skin: hemorrhagic lesions, bullae, cellulitis. Skin lesions may suggest specific pathogens—e.g., petechiae and purpura with *Neisseria meningitidis*, ecthyma gangrenosum in pts with *Pseudomonas aeruginosa*.
- Gastrointestinal: nausea, vomiting, diarrhea, ileus, cholestatic jaundice

Major Complications

- *Cardiopulmonary manifestations*
- Ventilation-perfusion mismatch, increased alveolar capillary permeability, increased pulmonary water content, and decreased pulmonary compliance impede oxygen exchange and lead to acute respiratory distress syndrome (progressive diffuse pulmonary infiltrates and arterial hypoxemia) in ~50% of pts.
- Hypotension: Normal or increased cardiac output and decreased systemic vascular resistance distinguish septic shock from cardiogenic or hypovolemic shock.
- Myocardial function is depressed with decreased ejection fraction.
- *Renal manifestations*: oliguria, azotemia, proteinuria, renal failure due to acute tubular necrosis
- *Coagulopathy*
- *Neurologic manifestations*: polyneuropathy with distal motor weakness in prolonged sepsis

Laboratory Findings

- Leukocytosis with a left shift, thrombocytopenia
- Prolonged thrombin time, decreased fibrinogen, presence of D-dimers, suggestive of DIC. With DIC, platelet counts usually fall below 50,000/μL.
- Hyperbilirubinemia, increase in hepatic aminotransferases, azotemia, proteinuria, hypoalbuminemia
- Metabolic acidosis, elevated anion gap, elevated lactate levels, hypoxemia

DIAGNOSIS

Definitive diagnosis requires isolation of the microorganism from blood or a local site of infection. Culture of infected cutaneous lesions may help establish the diagnosis.

 Sepsis and Septic Shock

Patients in whom sepsis is suspected must be managed expeditiously, if possible within 1 h of presentation.

1. Antibiotic treatment: See Table 13-1.
2. Removal or drainage of a focal source of infection
   a. Remove indwelling intravascular catheters; replace Foley and other drainage catheters; drain local sources of infection.
   b. Rule out sinusitis in pts with nasal intubation.
   c. Perform CT or MRI to rule out abscess.
3. Hemodynamic, respiratory, and metabolic support
   a. Maintain intravascular volume with IV fluids. Initiate treatment with 1–2 L of normal saline administered over 1–2 h, keeping pulmonary capillary wedge pressure at 12–16 mmHg or central venous pressure at 8–12

TABLE 13-1	**INITIAL ANTIMICROBIAL THERAPY FOR SEVERE SEPSIS WITH NO OBVIOUS SOURCE IN ADULTS WITH NORMAL RENAL FUNCTION**
Clinical Condition	**Antimicrobial Regimens (IV Therapy)**
Immunocompetent adult	The many acceptable regimens include (1) ceftriaxone (2 g q24h) *or* ticarcillin-clavulanate (3.1 g q4–6h) *or* piperacillin-tazobactam (3.375 g q4–6h); (2) imipenem-cilastatin (0.5 g q6h) *or* meropenem (1 g q8h) *or* cefepime (2 g q12h). Gentamicin *or* tobramycin (5–7 mg/kg q24h) may be *added* to either regimen. If the pt is allergic to β-lactam agents, use ciprofloxacin (400 mg q12h) *or* levofloxacin (500–750 mg q12h) *plus* clindamycin (600 mg q8h). If the institution has a high incidence of MRSA infections, *add* vancomycin (15 mg/kg q12h) to each of the above regimens.
Neutropenia[a] (<500 neutrophils/μL)	Regimens include (1) imipenem-cilastatin (0.5 g q6h) *or* meropenem (1 g q8h) *or* cefepime (2 g q8h); (2) ticarcillin-clavulanate (3.1 g q4h) *or* piperacillin-tazobactam (3.375 g q4h) *plus* tobramycin (5–7 mg/kg q24h). Vancomycin (15 mg/kg q12h) should be used if the pt has an infected vascular catheter, if staphylococci are suspected, if the pt has received quinolone prophylaxis, if the pt has received intensive chemotherapy that produces mucosal damage, if the institution has a high incidence of MRSA infections, or if MRSA isolates are highly prevalent in the community.
Splenectomy	Cefotaxime (2 g q6–8h) *or* ceftriaxone (2 g q12h) should be used. If the local prevalence of cephalosporin-resistant pneumococci is high, *add* vancomycin. If the pt is allergic to β-lactam drugs, vancomycin (15 mg/kg q12h) *plus* ciprofloxacin (400 mg q12h) *or* levofloxacin (750 mg q12h) *or* aztreonam (2 g q8h) should be used.
IV drug user	Nafcillin *or* oxacillin (2 g q8h) *plus* gentamicin (5–7 mg/kg q24h). If the local prevalence of MRSA is high or if the pt is allergic to β-lactam drugs, vancomycin (15 mg/kg q12h) with gentamicin should be used.
AIDS	Cefepime (2 g q8h), ticarcillin-clavulanate (3.1 g q4h), *or* piperacillin-tazobactam (3.375 g q4h) *plus* tobramycin (5–7 mg/kg q24h) should be used. If the pt is allergic to β-lactam drugs, ciprofloxacin (400 mg q12h) *or* levofloxacin (750 mg q12h) *plus* vancomycin (15 mg/kg q12h) *plus* tobramycin should be used.

[a]Adapted in part from WT Hughes et al: Clin Infect Dis 25:551, 1997.
Note: MRSA, methicillin-resistant *Staphylococcus aureus*.

cmH$_2$O, urine output at >0.5 mL/kg per hour, mean arterial blood pressure at >65 mmHg, and cardiac index at ≥4 (L/min)/m^2. Add vasopressor therapy if needed. A study of early goal-directed therapy (EGDT) found that prompt resuscitation based on maintenance of oxygen saturation at >70% was associated with significant improvement in survival in patients with severe sepsis. Therapy included rapid administration of IV fluids, antibiotics, and vasopressor support; erythrocyte transfusions to maintain hematocrit above 30%; and use of dobutamine if other measures did not result in a central venous oxygen saturation >70%.

b. Maintain oxygenation with ventilator support as indicated. Recent studies favor the use of low tidal volumes.

c. Monitor for adrenal insufficiency or reduced adrenal reserve. Survival rates may be improved among pts with a plasma cortisol level <15 μg/dL if hydrocortisone (50 mg q6h IV) is administered. If clinical improvement results within 24–48 h, most experts would continue hydrocortisone treatment for 5–7 days.

4. Recombinant activated protein C (aPC), given as a constant infusion of 24 μg/kg per hour for 96 h, has been approved for treatment of severe sepsis or septic shock in pts with APACHE II scores of ≥25 prior to aPC infusion and low risk of hemorrhagic complications.

5. General support: Nutritional supplementation should be given to pts with prolonged sepsis (i.e., that lasting >2–3 days). Prophylactic heparin should be administered to prevent deep-venous thrombosis if no active bleeding or coagulopathy is present. Tight control of blood glucose levels in pts who have just undergone major surgery may improve survival rates.

PROGNOSIS

In all, 20–35% of pts with severe sepsis and 40–60% of pts with septic shock die within 30 days, and further deaths occur within the first 6 months. The severity of underlying disease most strongly influences the risk of dying.

PREVENTION

Nosocomial infections cause most episodes of severe sepsis and septic shock in the United States. Measures to reduce those infections could reduce the incidence of sepsis.

For a more detailed discussion, see Munford RS: Severe Sepsis and Septic Shock, Chap. 265, p. 1695, in HPIM-17.

14 Acute Pulmonary Edema

Life-threatening, acute development of alveolar lung edema often due to:

- Elevation of hydrostatic pressure in the pulmonary capillaries (left heart failure, mitral stenosis)

TABLE 14-1	PRECIPITANTS OF ACUTE PULMONARY EDEMA

Acute tachy- or bradyarrhythmia
Infection, fever
Acute MI
Severe hypertension
Acute mitral or aortic regurgitation
Increased circulating volume (Na ingestion, blood transfusion, pregnancy)
Increased metabolic demands (exercise, hyperthyroidism)
Pulmonary embolism
Noncompliance (sudden discontinuation) of chronic CHF medications

- Specific precipitants (Table 14-1), resulting in cardiogenic pulmonary edema in pts with previously compensated CHF or without previous cardiac history
- Increased permeability of pulmonary alveolar-capillary membrane (noncardiogenic pulmonary edema). For common causes, see Table 14-2.

PHYSICAL FINDINGS

Patient appears severely ill, sitting bolt upright, tachypneic, dyspneic, with marked perspiration; cyanosis may be present. Bilateral pulmonary rales; third heart sound may be present. Frothy and blood-tinged sputum.

LABORATORY

Early arterial blood gases show reductions of both Pa_{O_2} and Pa_{CO_2}

- Later, with progressive respiratory failure, hypercapnia develops with progressive acidemia.
- CXR shows pulmonary vascular redistribution, diffuse haziness in lung fields with perihilar "butterfly" appearance.

EVALUATION See Fig. 14-1.

℞ Acute Pulmonary Edema

Immediate, aggressive therapy is mandatory for survival. The following measures should be instituted nearly simultaneously for cardiogenic pulmonary edema:

TABLE 14-2	COMMON CAUSES OF NONCARDIOGENIC PULMONARY EDEMA

Direct Injury to Lung

Chest trauma, pulmonary contusion	Pneumonia
Aspiration	Oxygen toxicity
Smoke inhalation	Pulmonary embolism, reperfusion

Hematogenous Injury to Lung

Sepsis	Multiple transfusions
Pancreatitis	Intravenous drug use, e.g., heroin
Nonthoracic trauma	Cardiopulmonary bypass

Possible Lung Injury Plus Elevated Hydrostatic Pressures

High altitude pulmonary edema	Reexpansion pulmonary edema
Neurogenic pulmonary edema	

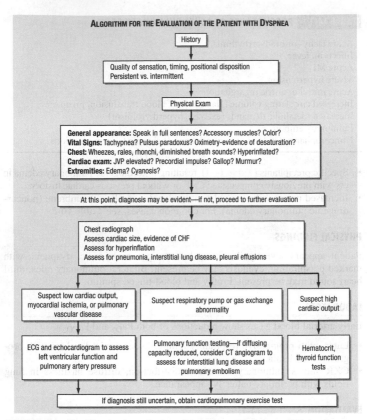

ALGORITHM FOR THE EVALUATION OF THE PATIENT WITH DYSPNEA

History

Quality of sensation, timing, positional disposition
Persistent vs. intermittent

Physical Exam

General appearance: Speak in full sentences? Accessory muscles? Color?
Vital Signs: Tachypnea? Pulsus paradoxus? Oximetry-evidence of desaturation?
Chest: Wheezes, rales, rhonchi, diminished breath sounds? Hyperinflated?
Cardiac exam: JVP elevated? Precordial impulse? Gallop? Murmur?
Extremities: Edema? Cyanosis?

At this point, diagnosis may be evident—if not, proceed to further evaluation

Chest radiograph
Assess cardiac size, evidence of CHF
Assess for hyperinflation
Assess for pneumonia, interstitial lung disease, pleural effusions

Suspect low cardiac output, myocardial ischemia, or pulmonary vascular disease

Suspect respiratory pump or gas exchange abnormality

Suspect high cardiac output

ECG and echocardiogram to assess left ventricular function and pulmonary artery pressure

Pulmonary function testing—if diffusing capacity reduced, consider CT angiogram to assess for interstitial lung disease and pulmonary embolism

Hematocrit, thyroid function tests

If diagnosis still uncertain, obtain cardiopulmonary exercise test

FIGURE 14-1 An algorithm for the evaluation of the patient with dyspnea. JVP, jugular venous pulse; CHF, congestive heart failure; ECG, electrocardiogram; CT, computed tomography. (*From RM Schwartzstein: HPIM-17, p. 224.*)

- Seat pt upright to reduce venous return.
- Administer 100% O_2 by mask to achieve $Pa_{O_2} > 60$ mmHg; in pts who can tolerate it, continuous positive airway pressure (10 cmH$_2$O pressure) by mask improves outcome. Assisted ventilation by mask or endotracheal tube is frequently necessary.
- Intravenous loop diuretic (furosemide, 40–100 mg, or bumetanide, 1 mg); use lower dose if pt does not take diuretics chronically.
- Morphine 2–4 mg IV (repetitively); assess frequently for hypotension or respiratory depression; naloxone should be available to reverse effects of morphine if necessary.

Additional therapy may be required if rapid improvement does not ensue:

- The precipitating cause of cardiogenic pulmonary edema (Table 14-1) should be sought and treated, particularly acute arrhythmias or infection.
- Several noncardiogenic conditions may result in pulmonary edema in the absence of left heart dysfunction; therapy is directed toward the primary condition.
- Inotropic agents, e.g., dobutamine (Chap. 12), in cardiogenic pulmonary edema with shock.

- Reduce intravascular volume by phlebotomy (removal of ~250 mL through antecubital vein) if rapid diuresis does not follow diuretic administration.
- Nitroglycerin (sublingual 0.4 mg × 3 q5min) followed by 5–10 μg/min IV. Alternatively, nesiritide [2-μg/kg bolus IV followed by 0.01 (μg/kg)/min] may be used.
- For refractory pulmonary edema associated with persistent cardiac ischemia, early coronary revascularization may be life-saving.
- For noncardiac pulmonary edema, identify and treat/remove cause (Table 14-2).

For a more detailed discussion, see Schwartzstein RM: Dyspnea and Pulmonary Edema, Chap. 33, p. 221; and Hochman JS, Ingbar D: Cardiogenic Shock and Pulmonary Edema, Chap. 266, p. 1702, in HPIM-17.

15 Acute Respiratory Distress Syndrome

DEFINITION AND ETIOLOGY

Acute respiratory distress syndrome (ARDS) develops rapidly and includes severe dyspnea and hypoxemia; it typically causes respiratory failure. Key diagnostic criteria for ARDS include (1) diffuse bilateral pulmonary infiltrates on chest x-ray (CXR); (2) Pa_{O_2} (arterial partial pressure of oxygen in mmHg) FI_{O_2} (inspired O_2 fraction) ≤ 200 mmHg; and (3) absence of elevated left atrial pressure (pulmonary capillary wedge pressure ≤ 18 mmHg). Acute lung injury is a related but milder syndrome, with less profound hypoxemia ($Pa_{O_2}/FI_{O_2} \leq 300$ mmHg), that can develop into ARDS. Although many medical and surgical conditions can cause ARDS, most cases (>80%) result from sepsis, bacterial pneumonia, trauma, multiple transfusions, gastric acid aspiration, and drug overdose. Individuals with more than one predisposing factor have a greater risk of developing ARDS. Other risk factors include older age, chronic alcohol abuse, metabolic acidosis, and overall severity of critical illness.

CLINICAL COURSE AND PATHOPHYSIOLOGY

There are three phases in the natural history of ARDS:

1. *Exudative phase*—Characterized by alveolar edema and leukocytic inflammation, with subsequent development of hyaline membranes from diffuse alveolar damage. The alveolar edema is most prominent in the dependent portions of the lung; this causes atelectasis and reduced lung compliance. Hypoxemia, tachypnea, and progressive dyspnea develop, and increased pulmonary dead space can also lead to hypercarbia. CXR reveals bilateral, diffuse alveolar and interstitial opacities. The differential diagnosis is broad, but common alternative etiologies to consider are cardiogenic pulmonary edema, pneumonia, and alveolar hemorrhage. Unlike cardiogenic pulmonary edema, the CXR in ARDS rarely shows cardiomegaly, pleural effusions, or pulmo-

nary vascular redistribution. The exudative phase duration is typically up to 7 days in length and usually begins within 12–36 h after the inciting insult.

2. *Proliferative phase*—This phase can last from approximately days 7 to 21 after the inciting insult. Although most pts recover, some will develop progressive lung injury and evidence of pulmonary fibrosis. Even among pts who show rapid improvement, dyspnea and hypoxemia often persist during this phase.

3. *Fibrotic phase*—Although the majority of pts recover within 3–4 weeks of the initial pulmonary injury, some experience progressive fibrosis, necessitating prolonged ventilatory support and/or supplemental O_2.

℞ Acute Respiratory Distress Syndrome

Progress in recent therapy has emphasized the importance of general critical care of pts with ARDS in addition to lung protective ventilator strategies. General care requires treatment of the underlying medical or surgical problem that caused lung injury, minimizing iatrogenic complications (e.g., procedure-related), prophylaxis to prevent venous thromboembolism and GI hemorrhage, prompt treatment of infections, and adequate nutritional support. An algorithm for the initial management of ARDS is presented in Fig. 15-1.

MECHANICAL VENTILATORY SUPPORT

Pts with ARDS typically require mechanical ventilatory support due to hypoxemia and increased work of breathing. A substantial improvement in outcomes from ARDS occurred with the recognition that mechanical ventilator–related overdistention of normal lung units with positive pressure can produce or exacerbate lung injury, causing or worsening ARDS. Currently recommended ventilator strategies limit alveolar distention but maintain adequate tissue oxygenation.

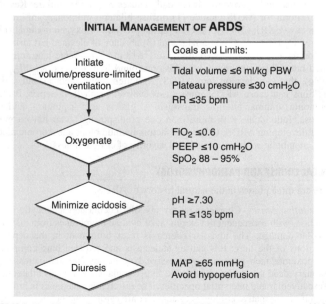

INITIAL MANAGEMENT OF ARDS

Initiate volume/pressure-limited ventilation

Goals and Limits:
Tidal volume ≤6 ml/kg PBW
Plateau pressure ≤30 cmH$_2$O
RR ≤35 bpm

Oxygenate

FiO$_2$ ≤0.6
PEEP ≤10 cmH$_2$O
SpO$_2$ 88 – 95%

Minimize acidosis

pH ≥7.30
RR ≤135 bpm

Diuresis

MAP ≥65 mmHg
Avoid hypoperfusion

FIGURE 15-1 Algorithm for the initial management of ARDS. Clinical trials have provided evidence-based therapeutic goals for a step-wise approach to the early mechanical ventilation, oxygenation, correction of acidosis and diuresis of critically ill patients with ARDS.

It has been clearly shown that low tidal volumes (≤6 mL/kg predicted body weight) provide reduced mortality compared with higher tidal volumes (12 mL/kg predicted body weight). In ARDS, alveolar collapse can occur due to alveolar/interstitial fluid accumulation and loss of surfactant, thus worsening hypoxemia. Therefore, low tidal volumes are combined with the use of positive end-expiratory pressure (PEEP) at levels that strive to minimize alveolar collapse and achieve adequate oxygenation with the lowest FI_{O_2}. Use of PEEP levels higher than required to optimize oxygenation has not been proven to be of benefit. Other techniques that may improve oxygenation while limiting alveolar distention include extending the time of inspiration on the ventilator (inverse ratio ventilation) and placing the pt in the prone position. However, these approaches are not of proven benefit in reducing mortality from ARDS.

ANCILLARY THERAPIES

Pts with ARDS have increased pulmonary vascular permeability leading to interstitial and alveolar edema. Therefore, they should receive IV fluids only as needed to achieve adequate cardiac output and tissue O_2 delivery as assessed by urine output, acid-base status, and arterial pressure. There is not convincing evidence currently to support the use of glucocorticoids or nitric oxide in ARDS.

OUTCOMES

Mortality from ARDS has declined with improvements in general critical care treatment and with the introduction of low tidal volume ventilation. Current mortality from ARDS is 41–65%, with most deaths due to sepsis and nonpulmonary organ failure. Increased risk of mortality from ARDS is associated with advanced age, preexisting organ dysfunction (e.g., chronic liver disease, chronic immunosuppression, chronic renal disease), and direct lung injury (e.g., pneumonia, aspiration) compared with indirect lung injury (e.g., sepsis, trauma, pancreatitis). Most surviving ARDS pts do not have significant long-term pulmonary disability.

 For a more detailed discussion, see Levy BD, Shapiro SD: Acute Respiratory Distress Syndrome, Chap. 262, p. 1680, in HPIM-17.

16 Respiratory Failure

DEFINITION AND CLASSIFICATION OF RESPIRATORY FAILURE

Respiratory failure is defined as inadequate gas exchange due to malfunction of one or more components of the respiratory system.

There are two main types of respiratory failure: hypoxemic and hypercarbic. Hypoxemic respiratory failure is defined by arterial O_2 saturation <90% while receiving an inspired O_2 fraction >0.6. Acute hypoxemic respiratory failure can result from pneumonia, pulmonary edema (cardiogenic or noncardiogenic), and alveolar hemorrhage. Hypoxemia results from ventilation-perfusion mismatch and intrapulmonary shunting.

Hypercarbic respiratory failure is characterized by respiratory acidosis with pH <7.30. Hypercarbic respiratory failure results from decreased minute ventilation and/or increased physiologic dead space. Common conditions associated with hypercarbic respiratory failure include neuromuscular diseases, such as myasthenia gravis, and respiratory diseases associated with respiratory muscle fatigue, such as asthma and chronic obstructive pulmonary disease (COPD). In acute hypercarbic respiratory failure, Pa_{CO_2} is typically >50 mmHg. With acute-on-chronic respiratory failure, as is often seen with COPD exacerbations, considerably higher Pa_{CO_2} values may be observed. The degree of respiratory acidosis, the pt's mental status, and the pt's degree of respiratory distress are better indicators of the need for mechanical ventilation than a specific Pa_{CO_2} level in acute-on-chronic respiratory failure.

MODES OF MECHANICAL VENTILATION

Respiratory failure often requires treatment with mechanical ventilation. Various modes of mechanical ventilation are commonly used; different modes are characterized by a trigger (what the ventilator senses to initiate a machine-delivered breath), a cycle (what determines the end of inspiration), and limiting factors (specified values for key parameters that are monitored by the ventilator and not allowed to be exceeded). Four of the common modes of mechanical ventilation are described below; additional information is provided in Table 16-1:

- Assist-control ventilation: The trigger for a machine delivered breath is the pt's inspiratory effort, which causes a synchronized breath to be delivered. If no effort is detected over a prespecified time interval, a timer-triggered machine breath is delivered. Assist control is volume-cycled with an operator-determined tidal volume. Limiting factors include the minimum respiratory rate, which is specified by the operator; pt efforts can lead to higher rates. Other limiting factors include the airway pressure limit, which is also set by the operator. Because the pt will receive a full tidal breath with each inspiratory effort, tachypnea due to nonrespiratory drive (such as pain) can lead to respiratory alkalosis. In pts with airflow obstruction (e.g., asthma or COPD), auto-PEEP can develop.
- Synchronized intermittent mandatory ventilation (SIMV): As with Assist-control, SIMV is volume-cycled, with similar limiting factors. As with Assist-control, the trigger for a machine-delivered breath can be either pt effort or a specified time interval. However, if the pt's next inspiratory effort occurs before the time interval for another mandatory breath has elapsed, only their spontaneous respiratory effort (without machine support) is delivered. Thus, the number of machine-delivered breaths is limited in SIMV.
- Pressure-control ventilation (PCV): PCV is triggered by a specified time interval, and the inspiratory pressure that is delivered after that time trigger is time-cycled. The level of inspiratory pressure is an operator-specified limiting factor in this mode of ventilation; the achieved tidal volume and inspiratory flow rate result from this prespecified pressure limit, and a specific tidal volume or minute ventilation may not be achieved. For pts in whom limiting airway pressure is desired (e.g., barotrauma), PCV is often used.
- Pressure-support ventilation (PSV): PSV is triggered by the pt's inspiratory effort. The cycle of PSV is determined by the inspiratory flow rate. Because a specific respiratory rate is not provided, this mode of ventilation may be combined with SIMV to ensure that an adequate respiratory rate is achieved in pts with respiratory depression.

MANAGEMENT OF MECHANICALLY VENTILATED PATIENTS

General care of mechanically ventilated pts is reviewed in Chap. 5, along with weaning from mechanical ventilation. A cuffed endotracheal tube is often used

TABLE 16-1 CLINICAL CHARACTERISTICS OF COMMONLY USED MODES OF MECHANICAL VENTILATION

Ventilator Mode	Independent Variables (Set by User)	Dependent Variables (Monitored by User)	Trigger/Cycle Limit	Advantages	Disadvantages	Initial Settings
ACMV[a]	F_{IO_2} Tidal volume Ventilator rate Level of PEEP Inspiratory flow pattern Peak inspiratory flow Pressure limit	Peak airway pressure, Pa_{O_2}, Pa_{CO_2} Mean airway pressure I/E ratio	Patient/timer Pressure limit	Timer backup Patient-vent synchrony Patient controls minute ventilation	Not useful for weaning Potential for dangerous respiratory alkalosis	$F_{IO_2} = 1.0^b$ $V_t = 10\text{–}15$ mL/kg^a $f = 12\text{–}15$/min PEEP = 0–5 cmH$_2$O Inspiratory flow = 60 L/min
SIMV[a]	Same as for ACMV	Same as for ACMV	Same as for ACMV	Timer backup useful for weaning	Potential dyssynchrony	Same as for ACMV^a
PCV[a]	F_{IO_2} Inspiratory pressure level Ventilator rate Level of PEEP Pressure limit I/E ratio	Tidal volume Flow rate, pattern Minute ventilation Pa_{O_2}, Pa_{CO_2}	Timer/patient Timer/pressure limit	System pressures regulated Useful for barotrauma treatment Timer backup	Requires heavy sedation Not useful for weaning	$F_{IO_2} = 1.0^b$ PC = 20–40 cmH$_2$O^a PEEP = 5–10 cmH$_2$O $f = 12\text{–}15$/min I/E = 0.7/1–4/1
PSV[a]	F_{IO_2} Inspiratory pressure level PEEP Pressure limit	Same as for PCV + I/E ratio	Inspiratory flow Pressure limit	Assures synchrony Good for weaning	No timer backup	$F_{IO_2} = 0.5\text{–}1.0^b$ PS = 10–30 cmH$_2$O 5 cmH$_2$O usually the level used PEEP = 0–5 cmH$_2$O

^{a}Open lung ventilation (OLV) involves the use of any of these specific modes with tidal volumes (or applied pressures) to achieve 5–6 mL/kg, and positive end-expiratory pressures achieve maximal alveolar recruitment.

$^b F_{IO_2}$ is usually set to 1.0 initially, unless there is a specific clinical indication to minimize F_{IO_2} such as history of chemotherapy with bleomycin. Once adequate oxygenation is documented by blood gas analysis, F_{IO_2} should be decreased in decrements of 0.1–0.2 as tolerated, until the lowest F_{IO_2} required for an $Sa_{O_2} > 90\%$ is achieved.

Abbreviations: f, frequency; I/E, inspiration/expiration; F_{IO_2}, inspired O$_2$; PEEP, positive end-expiratory pressure; for ventilator modes, see text; V_t, tidal ventilation.

to provide positive pressure ventilation with conditioned gas. After an endotracheal tube has been in place for an extended period of time, tracheostomy should be considered, primarily to improve pt comfort and management of respiratory secretions. No absolute time frame for tracheostomy placement exists, but pts who are likely to require mechanical ventilatory support for >3 weeks should be considered for a tracheostomy.

A variety of complications can result from mechanical ventilation. Barotrauma, overdistention and damage of lung tissue, typically occurs at high airway pressures (>50 cmH$_2$O). Barotrauma can cause pneumomediastinum, subcutaneous emphysema, and pneumothorax; pneumothorax typically requires treatment with tube thoracostomy. Ventilator-associated pneumonia is a major complication of mechanical ventilation; common pathogens include *Pseudomonas aeruginosa* and other gram-negative bacilli, as well as *Staphylococcus aureus*.

In some circumstances, noninvasive positive pressure ventilation (NPPV) delivered through a tightly fitting nasal or full facemask should be considered for treatment of impending respiratory failure. Pressure support ventilation is typically used with noninvasive ventilation, and positive end-expiratory pressure (PEEP) can also be included. NPPV has been used quite successfully in the management of COPD exacerbations (Chap. 139), and it appears to reduce the risk of ventilator-associated pneumonia.

 For a more detailed discussion, see Ingenito EP: Mechanical Ventilatory Support, Chap. 263, p. 1684, in HPIM-17.

17 Confusion, Stupor, and Coma

APPROACH TO THE PATIENT: DISORDERS OF CONSCIOUSNESS

Disorders of consciousness are common; these always signify a disorder of the nervous system. Assessment should determine whether there is a change in level of consciousness (drowsy, stuporous, comatose) and/or content of consciousness (confusion, perseveration, hallucinations). *Confusion* is a lack of clarity in thinking with inattentiveness; *delirium* is used to describe an acute confusional state; *stupor*, a state in which vigorous stimuli are needed to elicit a response; *coma*, a condition of unresponsiveness. Patients in such states are usually seriously ill, and etiologic factors must be assessed (Tables 17-1 and 17-2).

DELIRIUM

Delirium is a clinical diagnosis made at the bedside; a careful history and physical exam are necessary, focusing on common etiologies of delirium, especially toxins and metabolic conditions. Observation will usually reveal an altered level of consciousness or a deficit of attention. Attention can be assessed through a

TABLE 17-1 **COMMON ETIOLOGIES OF DELIRIUM**

Toxins
    Prescription medications: especially those with anticholinergic properties, narcotics and benzodiazepines
    Drugs of abuse: alcohol intoxication and alcohol withdrawal, opiates, ecstasy, LSD, GHB, PCP, ketamine, cocaine
    Poisons: inhalants, carbon monoxide, ethylene glycol, pesticides
Metabolic conditions
    Electrolyte disturbances: hypoglycemia, hyperglycemia, hyponatremia, hypernatremia, hypercalcemia, hypocalcemia, hypomagnesemia
    Hypothermia and hyperthermia
    Pulmonary failure: hypoxemia and hypercarbia
    Liver failure/hepatic encephalopathy
    Renal failure/uremia
    Cardiac failure
    Vitamin deficiencies: B_{12}, thiamine, folate, niacin
    Dehydration and malnutrition
    Anemia
Infections
    Systemic infections: urinary tract infections, pneumonia, skin and soft tissue infections, sepsis
    CNS infections: meningitis, encephalitis, brain abscess
Endocrinologic conditions
    Hyperthyroidism, hypothyroidism
    Hyperparathyroidism
    Adrenal insufficiency
Cerebrovascular disorders
    Global hypoperfusion states
    Hypertensive encephalopathy
    Focal ischemic strokes and hemorrhages: especially nondominant parietal and thalamic lesions
Autoimmune disorders
    CNS vasculitis
    Cerebral lupus
Seizure-related disorders
    Nonconvulsive status epilepticus
    Intermittent seizures with prolonged post-ictal states
Neoplastic disorders
    Diffuse metastases to the brain
    Gliomatosis cerebri
    Carcinomatous meningitis
Hospitalization
Terminal end of life delirium

Abbreviations: LSD, lysergic acid diethylamide; GHB, γ-hydroxybutyrate; PCP, phencyclidine; CNS, central nervous system.

simple bedside test of digits forward—pts are asked to repeat successively longer random strings of digits beginning with two digits in a row; a digit span of four digits or less usually indicates an attentional deficit unless hearing or language barriers are present. Delirium is vastly underrecognized, especially in pts presenting with a quiet, hypoactive state.

A cost-effective approach to the evaluation of delirium allows the history and physical exam to guide tests. No single algorithm will fit all pts due to the

TABLE 17-2   DIFFERENTIAL DIAGNOSIS OF COMA

1. Diseases that cause no focal or lateralizing neurologic signs, usually with normal brainstem functions; CT scan and cellular content of the CSF are normal
   a. Intoxications: alcohol, sedative drugs, opiates, etc.
   b. Metabolic disturbances: anoxia, hyponatremia, hypernatremia, hypercalcemia, diabetic acidosis, nonketotic hyperosmolar hyperglycemia, hypoglycemia, uremia, hepatic coma, hypercarbia, addisonian crisis, hypo- and hyperthyroid states, profound nutritional deficiency
   c. Severe systemic infections: pneumonia, septicemia, typhoid fever, malaria, Waterhouse-Friderichsen syndrome
   d. Shock from any cause
   e. Postseizure states, status epilepticus, subclinical epilepsy
   f. Hypertensive encephalopathy, eclampsia
   g. Severe hyperthermia, hypothermia
   h. Concussion
   i. Acute hydrocephalus
2. Diseases that cause meningeal irritation with or without fever, and with an excess of WBCs or RBCs in the CSF, usually without focal or lateralizing cerebral or brainstem signs; CT or MRI shows no mass lesion
   a. Subarachnoid hemorrhage from ruptured aneurysm, arteriovenous malformation, trauma
   b. Acute bacterial meningitis
   c. Viral encephalitis
   d. Miscellaneous: Fat embolism, cholesterol embolism, carcinomatous and lymphomatous meningitis, etc.
3. Diseases that cause focal brainstem or lateralizing cerebral signs, with or without changes in the CSF; CT and MRI are abnormal
   a. Hemispheral hemorrhage (basal ganglionic, thalamic) or infarction (large middle cerebral artery territory) with secondary brainstem compression
   b. Brainstem infarction due to basilar artery thrombosis or embolism
   c. Brain abscess, subdural empyema
   d. Epidural and subdural hemorrhage, brain contusion
   e. Brain tumor with surrounding edema
   f. Cerebellar and pontine hemorrhage and infarction
   g. Widespread traumatic brain injury
   h. Metabolic coma (see above) with preexisting focal damage
   i. Miscellaneous: cortical vein thrombosis, herpes simplex encephalitis, multiple cerebral emboli due to bacterial endocarditis, acute hemorrhagic leukoencephalitis, acute disseminated (postinfectious) encephalomyelitis, thrombotic thrombocytopenic purpura, cerebral vasculitis, gliomatosis cerebri, pituitary apoplexy, intravascular lymphoma, etc.

Note: CSF, cerebrospinal fluid; WBCs, white blood cells; RBCs, red blood cells.

large number of potential etiologies, but one step-wise approach is shown in Table 17-3.

Management of the delirious pt begins with treatment of the underlying inciting factor (e.g., pts with systemic infections should be given appropriate antibiotics, and electrolyte disturbances judiciously corrected). Relatively simple methods of supportive care can be quite effective, such as frequent reorientation by staff, preservation of sleep-wake cycles, and attempting to mimic the home environment as much as possible. Chemical restraints exacerbate delirium and should be used only when necessary to protect pt or staff from possible injury; antipsychotics at low dose are usually the treatment of choice.

TABLE 17-3	STEP-WISE EVALUATION OF A PATIENT WITH DELIRIUM

Initial evaluation
   History with special attention to medications (including over-the-counter and herbals)
   General physical examination and neurologic examination
   Complete blood count
   Electrolyte panel including calcium, magnesium, phosphorus
   Liver function tests including albumin
   Renal function tests
First-tier further evaluation guided by initial evaluation
   Systemic infection screen
      Urinalysis and culture
      Chest radiograph
      Blood cultures
   Electrocardiogram
   Arterial blood gas
   Serum and/or urine toxicology screen (perform earlier in young persons)
   Brain imaging with MRI with diffusion and gadolinium (preferred) or CT
   Suspected CNS infection: lumbar puncture following brain imaging
   Suspected seizure-related etiology: electroencephalogram (EEG) (if high suspicion should be performed immediately)
Second-tier further evaluation
   Vitamin levels: B_{12}, folate, thiamine
   Endocrinologic laboratories: thyroid-stimulating hormone (TSH) and free T4; cortisol
   Serum ammonia
   Sedimentation rate
   Autoimmune serologies: antinuclear antibodies (ANA), complement levels; p-ANCA, c-ANCA
   Infectious serologies: rapid plasmin reagin (RPR); fungal and viral serologies if high suspicion; HIV antibody
   Lumbar puncture (if not already performed)
   Brain MRI with and without gadolinium (if not already performed)

Note: p-ANCA, perinuclear antineutrophil cytoplasmic antibody; c-ANCA, cytoplasmic antineutrophil cytoplasmic antibody.

COMA

Because coma demands immediate attention, the physician must employ an organized approach. Almost all instances of coma can be traced to widespread abnormalities of the bilateral cerebral hemispheres or to reduced activity of the reticular activating system in the brainstem.

History Pt should be aroused, if possible, and questioned regarding use of insulin, narcotics, anticoagulants, other prescription drugs, suicidal intent, recent trauma, headache, epilepsy, significant medical problems, and preceding symptoms. Witnesses and family members should be interviewed, often by phone. History of sudden headache followed by loss of consciousness suggests intracranial hemorrhage; preceding vertigo, nausea, diplopia, ataxia, hemisensory disorder suggest basilar insufficiency; chest pain, palpitations, and faintness suggest a cardiovascular cause.

Immediate Assessment Acute respiratory and cardiovascular problems should be attended to prior to the neurologic assessment. Vital signs should be evaluated, and appropriate support initiated. Thiamine, glucose, and naloxone should be administered if the etiology of coma is not immediately apparent.

Blood should be drawn for glucose, electrolytes, calcium, and renal (BUN, creatinine) and hepatic (ammonia, transaminases) function; also screen for presence of alcohol and other toxins. Arterial blood-gas analysis is helpful in pts with lung disease and acid-base disorders. Fever, especially with petechial rash, suggests meningitis. Examination of CSF is essential in diagnosis of meningitis and encephalitis; lumbar puncture should not be deferred if meningitis is a possibility, but CT scan should be obtained first to exclude a mass lesion. Empirical antibiotic coverage for meningitis may be instituted until CSF results are available. Fever with dry skin suggests heat shock or intoxication with anticholinergics. Hypothermia suggests myxedema, intoxication, sepsis, exposure, or hypoglycemia. Marked hypertension occurs with increased intracranial pressure (ICP) and hypertensive encephalopathy.

Neurologic Examination Focus on establishing pt's best level of function and uncovering signs that enable a specific diagnosis. Comatose pt's best motor and sensory function should be assessed by testing reflex responses to noxious stimuli; carefully note any asymmetric responses, which suggest a focal lesion. Multifocal myoclonus indicates that a metabolic disorder is likely; intermittent twitching may be the only sign of a seizure.

Responsiveness Stimuli of increasing intensity are applied to gauge the degree of unresponsiveness and any asymmetry in sensory or motor function. Motor responses may be purposeful or reflexive. Spontaneous flexion of elbows with leg extension, termed *decortication*, accompanies severe damage to contralateral hemisphere above midbrain. Internal rotation of the arms with extension of elbows, wrists, and legs, termed *decerebration*, suggests damage to midbrain or diencephalon. These postural reflexes occur in profound encephalopathic states.

Pupillary Signs In comatose pts, equal, round, reactive pupils exclude midbrain damage as cause and suggest a metabolic abnormality. Pinpoint pupils occur in narcotic overdose (except meperidine, which causes midsize pupils), pontine damage, hydrocephalus, or thalamic hemorrhage; the response to naloxone and presence of reflex eye movements (usually intact with drug overdose) can distinguish these. A unilateral, enlarged, often oval, poorly reactive pupil is caused by midbrain lesions or compression of third cranial nerve, as occurs in transtentorial herniation. Bilaterally dilated, unreactive pupils indicate severe bilateral midbrain damage, anticholinergic overdose, or ocular trauma.

Ocular Movements Examine spontaneous and reflex eye movements. Intermittent horizontal divergence is common in drowsiness. Slow, to-and-fro horizontal movements suggest bihemispheric dysfunction. Conjugate eye deviation to one side indicates damage to the pons on the opposite side or a lesion in the frontal lobe on the same side ("*The eyes look toward a hemispheral lesion and away from a brainstem lesion*"). An adducted eye at rest with impaired ability to turn eye laterally indicates an abducens (VI) nerve palsy, common in raised ICP or pontine damage. The eye with a dilated, unreactive pupil is often abducted at rest and cannot adduct fully due to third nerve dysfunction, as occurs with transtentorial herniation. Vertical separation of ocular axes (skew deviation) occurs in pontine or cerebellar lesions. Doll's head maneuver (oculocephalic reflex) and cold caloric–induced eye movements allow diagnosis of gaze or cranial nerve palsies in pts who do not move their eyes purposefully. Doll's head maneuver is tested by observing eye movements in response to lateral rotation of head (this should not be performed in pts with possible neck injury); full conjugate movement of eyes occurs in bihemispheric dysfunction. In comatose pts with intact brainstem function, raising head to 60° above the horizontal and irrigating external auditory canal with cool water causes tonic deviation of gaze to side of irrigated ear ("cold calorics"). In conscious pts, it causes nystagmus, vertigo, and emesis.

Respiratory Patterns Respiratory pattern may suggest site of neurologic damage. Cheyne-Stokes (periodic) breathing occurs in bihemispheric dysfunction and is common in metabolic encephalopathies. Respiratory patterns composed of gasps or other irregular breathing patterns are indicative of lower brainstem damage; such pts usually require intubation and ventilatory assistance.

Radiologic Examination Lesions causing raised ICP commonly cause impaired consciousness. CT or MRI scan of the brain is often abnormal in coma but may not be diagnostic; appropriate therapy should not be postponed while awaiting a CT or MRI scan. Pts with disordered consciousness due to high ICP can deteriorate rapidly; emergent CT study is necessary to confirm presence of mass effect and to guide surgical decompression. CT scan is normal in some pts with subarachnoid hemorrhage; the diagnosis then rests on clinical history combined with RBCs or xanthrochromia in spinal fluid. MR angiography or cerebral angiography may be necessary to establish basilar artery stroke as cause of coma in pts with brainstem signs. The EEG is useful in metabolic or drug-induced states but is rarely diagnostic; exceptions are coma due to seizures or herpesvirus encephalitis.

BRAIN DEATH

This results from total cessation of cerebral function while somatic function is maintained by artificial means and the heart continues to pump. It is legally and ethically equivalent to cardiorespiratory death. The pt is unresponsive to all forms of stimulation (widespread cortical destruction), brainstem reflexes are absent (global brainstem damage), and there is complete apnea (destruction of the medulla). Demonstration of apnea requires that the P_{CO_2} be high enough to stimulate respiration, while P_{O_2} and bp are maintained. EEG is isoelectric at high gain. The absence of deep tendon reflexes is not required because the spinal cord may remain functional. Special care must be taken to exclude drug toxicity and hypothermia prior to making a diagnosis of brain death. Diagnosis should be made only if the state persists for some agreed-upon period, usually 6–24 h.

For a more detailed discussion, see Josephson SA, Miller BL: Confusion and Delirium, Chap. 26, p. 158, in HPIM-17. and Ropper AH: Coma, Chap. 268, p. 1714, in HPIM-17.

18 Stroke

Sudden onset of a neurologic deficit from a vascular mechanism: 85% are ischemic; 15% are primary hemorrhages [subarachnoid (Chap. 19) and intraparenchymal]. An ischemic deficit that resolves rapidly is termed a *transient ischemic attack* (TIA); 24 h is a commonly used boundary between TIA and stroke whether or not a new infarction has occurred, although most TIAs last between 5 and 15 min. Stroke is the leading cause of neurologic disability in adults; 200,000 deaths annually in the United States. Much can be done to limit morbidity and mortality through prevention and acute intervention.

PATHOPHYSIOLOGY

Ischemic stroke is most often due to embolic occlusion of large cerebral vessels; source of emboli may be heart, aortic arch, or other arterial lesions such as the carotid arteries. Small, deep ischemic lesions are most often related to intrinsic small-vessel disease (lacunar strokes). Low-flow strokes are seen with severe proximal stenosis and inadequate collaterals challenged by systemic hypotensive episodes. Hemorrhages most frequently result from rupture of aneurysms or small vessels within brain tissue. Variability in stroke recovery is influenced by collateral vessels, blood pressure, and the specific site and mechanism of vessel occlusion; if blood flow is restored prior to significant cell death, the pt may experience only transient symptoms, i.e., a TIA.

CLINICAL FEATURES

Ischemic Stroke   Abrupt and dramatic onset of focal neurologic symptoms is typical of ischemic stroke. Pts may not seek assistance on their own because they are rarely in pain and may lose appreciation that something is wrong (*anosagnosia*). Symptoms reflect the vascular territory involved (Table 18-1). Transient monocular blindness (amaurosis fugax) is a particular form of TIA due to retinal ischemia; pts describe a shade descending over the visual field.

Lacunar Syndromes (Small-Vessel Strokes)   Most common are:
- Pure motor hemiparesis of face, arm, and leg (internal capsule or pons)
- Pure sensory stroke (ventral thalamus)
- Ataxic hemiparesis (pons or internal capsule)
- Dysarthria—clumsy hand (pons or genu of internal capsule).

Intracranial Hemorrhage   Vomiting and drowsiness occur in some cases, and headache in about one-half. Signs and symptoms are often not confined to a single vascular territory. Etiologies are diverse but hypertension-related is the most common (Table 18-2). Hypertensive hemorrhages typically occur in the following locations:

- Putamen: Contralateral hemiparesis.
- Thalamus: Hemiparesis with prominent sensory deficit.
- Pons: Quadriplegic, "pinpoint" pupils, impaired horizontal eye movements.
- Cerebellum: Headache, vomiting, gait ataxia.

A neurologic deficit that evolves relentlessly over 5–30 min strongly suggests intracerebral bleeding.

Rx Stroke

Principles of management are outlined in Fig. 18-1. Stroke needs to be distinguished from potential mimics, including seizure, migraine, tumor, and metabolic derangements. After initial stabilization, an emergency noncontrast head CT scan is necessary to differentiate ischemic from hemorrhagic stroke. With large ischemic strokes, CT abnormalities are usually evident within the first few hours, but small infarcts can be difficult to visualize by CT. CT or MR angiography (CTA/MRA) and perfusion may help reveal vascular occlusions and tissue at risk for infarction. Diffusion-weighted MRI has a high sensitivity for identifying ischemic stroke even minutes after onset.

TABLE 18-1	ANATOMIC LOCALIZATION IN STROKE

Signs and Symptoms

Cerebral Hemisphere, Lateral Aspect (Middle Cerebral A.)

Hemiparesis
Hemisensory decit
Motor aphasia (Broca's)—hesitant speech with word-nding difculty and pre-
   served comprehension
Central aphasia (Wernicke's)—anomia, poor comprehension, jargon speech
Unilateral neglect, apraxias
Homonymous hemianopia or quadrantanopia
Gaze preference witheyes deviated to side of lesion

Cerebral Hemisphere, Medial Aspect (Anterior Cerebral A.)

Paralysis of foot and leg withor without paresis of arm
Cortical sensory loss over leg
Grasp and sucking reexes
Urinary incontinence
Gait apraxia

Cerebral Hemisphere, Posterior Aspect (Posterior Cerebral A.)

Homonymous hemianopia
Cortical blindness
Memory decit
Dense sensory loss, spontaneous pain, dysesthesias, choreoathetosis

Brainstem, Midbrain (Posterior Cerebral A.)

Third nerve palsy and contralateral hemiplegia
Paralysis/paresis of vertical eye movement
Convergence nystagmus, disorientation

Brainstem, Pontomedullary Junction (Basilar A.)

Facial paralysis
Paresis of abduction of eye
Paresis of conjugate gaze
Hemifacial sensory decit
Horner's syndrome
Diminished pain and thermal sense over half body (with or without face)
Ataxia

Brainstem, Lateral Medulla (Vertebral A.)

Vertigo, nystagmus
Horner's syndrome (miosis, ptosis, decreased sweating)
Ataxia, falling toward side of lesion
Impaired pain and thermal sense over half body with or without face

ACUTE ISCHEMIC STROKE

Patient care in comprehensive stroke centers followed by rehabilitation services improves neurologic outcomes and reduces mortality. Treatments designed to reverse or lessen tissue infarction include: (1) medical support, (2) thrombolysis and endovascular techniques, (3) antiplatelet agents, (4) anticoagulation, and (5) neuroprotection.

TABLE 18-2 CAUSES OF INTRACRANIAL HEMORRHAGE

Cause	Location	Comments
Head trauma	Intraparenchymal: frontal lobes, anterior temporal lobes; subarachnoid	Coup and contracoup injury during brain deceleration
Hypertensive hemorrhage	Putamen, globus pallidus, thalamus, cerebellar hemisphere, pons	Chronic hypertension produces hemorrhage from small (~100 μm) vessels in these regions
Transformation of prior ischemic infarction	Basal ganglion, subcortical regions, lobar	Occurs in 1–6% of ischemic strokes with predilection for large hemispheric infarctions
Metastatic brain tumor	Lobar	Lung, choriocarcinoma, melanoma, renal cell carcinoma, thyroid, atrial myxoma
Coagulopathy	Any	Uncommon cause; often associated with prior stroke or underlying vascular anomaly
Drug	Lobar, subarachnoid	Cocaine, amphetamine, phenylpropanolamine
Arteriovenous malformation	Lobar, intraventricular, subarachnoid	Risk is ~2–4% per year for bleeding
Aneurysm	Subarachnoid, intraparenchymal, rarely subdural	Mycotic and nonmycotic forms of aneurysms
Amyloid angiopathy	Lobar	Degenerative disease of intracranial vessels; linkage to Alzheimer's disease, rare in patients <60
Cavernous angioma	Intraparenchymal	Multiple cavernous angiomas linked to mutations in KRIT1, CCM2, and PDCD10 genes
Dural arteriovenous fistula	Lobar, subarachnoid	Produces bleeding by venous hypertension
Capillary telangiectasias	Usually brainstem	Rare cause of hemorrhage

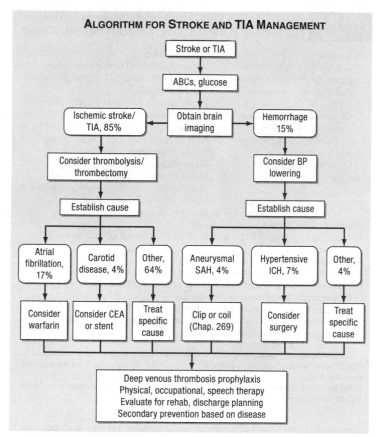

ALGORITHM FOR STROKE AND TIA MANAGEMENT

Stroke or TIA

↓

ABCs, glucose

↓

Obtain brain imaging

→ **Ischemic stroke/ TIA, 85%**

→ **Hemorrhage 15%**

Ischemic stroke/TIA branch:

Consider thrombolysis/ thrombectomy

↓

Establish cause

- **Atrial fibrillation, 17%** → **Consider warfarin**
- **Carotid disease, 4%** → **Consider CEA or stent**
- **Other, 64%** → **Treat specific cause**

Hemorrhage branch:

Consider BP lowering

↓

Establish cause

- **Aneurysmal SAH, 4%** → **Clip or coil (Chap. 269)**
- **Hypertensive ICH, 7%** → **Consider surgery**
- **Other, 4%** → **Treat specific cause**

**Deep venous thrombosis prophylaxis
Physical, occupational, speech therapy
Evaluate for rehab, discharge planning
Secondary prevention based on disease**

FIGURE 18-1 Medical management of stroke and TIA. Rounded boxes are diagnoses; rectangles are interventions. Numbers are percentages of stroke overall. Abbreviations: TIA, transient ischemic attack; ABCs, airway, breathing, circulation; BP, blood pressure; CEA, carotid endarterectomy, SAH, subarachnoid hemorrhage; ICH, intracerebral hemorrhage.

Medical Support

Immediate goal is to optimize perfusion in ischemic penumbra surrounding the infarct. Blood pressure should never be lowered precipitously (exacerbates the underlying ischemia), and only in the most extreme situations should gradual lowering be undertaken (e.g., malignant hypertension with bp > 220/120 or, if thrombolysis planned, bp > 185/110 mmHg). Intravascular volume should be maintained with isotonic fluids as volume restriction is rarely helpful. Osmotic therapy with mannitol may be necessary to control edema in large infarcts, but isotonic volume must be replaced to avoid hypovolemia. In cerebellar infarction (or hemorrhage), rapid deterioration can occur from brainstem compression and hydrocephalus, requiring neurosurgical intervention.

Thrombolysis and Endovascular Techniques

Ischemic deficits of <3 h duration, with no hemorrhage by CT criteria, may benefit from thrombolytic therapy with IV recombinant tissue plasminogen activator (Table 18-3). Ischemic stroke from large-vessel intracranial occlu-

TABLE 18-3	ADMINISTRATION OF INTRAVENOUS RECOMBINANT TISSUE PLASMINOGEN ACTIVATOR (RTPA) FOR ACUTE ISCHEMIC STROKE[a]

Indication	Contraindication
Clinical diagnosis of stroke	Sustained BP >185/110 despite treatment
Onset of symptoms to time of drug administration ≤3 h	Platelets <100,000; HCT <25%; glucose <50 or >400 mg/dL
CT scan showing no hemorrhage or edema of > 1/3 of the MCA territory	Use of heparin within 48 h and prolonged PTT, or elevated INR
	Rapidly improving symptoms
Age ≥18 years	Prior stroke or head injury within 3 months; prior intracranial hemorrhage
Consent by patient or surrogate	Major surgery in preceding 14 days
	Minor stroke symptoms
	Gastrointestinal bleeding in preceding 21 days
	Recent myocardial infarction
	Coma or stupor

Administration of rtPA

Intravenous access with two peripheral IV lines (avoid arterial or central line placement)

Review eligibility for rtPA

Administer 0.9 mg/kg intravenously (maximum 90 mg) IV as 10% of total dose by bolus, followed by remainder of total dose over 1 h

Frequent cuff blood pressure monitoring

No other antithrombotic treatment for 24 h

For decline in neurologic status or uncontrolled blood pressure, stop infusion, give cryoprecipitate, and reimage brain emergently

Avoid urethral catheterization for ≥2 h

[a]See Activase (tissue plasminogen activator) package insert for complete list of contraindications and dosing.
Note: BP, blood pressure; HCT, hematocrit; INR, international normalized ratio; MCA, middle cerebral artery; PTT, partial thromboplastin time.

sion results in high rates of morbidity and mortality; pts with such occlusions may benefit from intraarterial thombolysis (<6 h duration) or embolectomy (<8 h duration) administered at the time of an urgent cerebral angiogram at specialized centers. Only a small percentage of stroke pts are seen early enough to receive treatment with these techniques.

Antiplatelet Agents

Aspirin (up to 325 mg/d) is safe and has a small but definite benefit in acute stroke.

Anticoagulation

Trials do not support the use of heparin or other anticoagulants for pts with acute stroke although some physicians continue to use this treatment in specific situations such as TIA in the setting of atrial fibrillation.

Neuroprotection

Hypothermia is effective in coma following cardiac arrest but has not been adequately studied in pts with stroke. Other neuroprotective agents have shown no benefit in human trials despite promising animal data.

ACUTE INTRACEREBRAL HEMORRHAGE

Noncontrast head CT will confirm diagnosis. Rapidly identify and correct any coagulopathy. Nearly 50% of pts die; prognosis is determined by volume and location of hematoma. Stuporous or comatose patients generally are treated presumptively for elevated ICP. Neurosurgical consultation should be sought for possible urgent evacuation of cerebellar hematoma; in other locations, data do not support surgical intervention. Treatment for edema and mass effect with osmotic agents may be necessary; glucocorticoids not helpful.

EVALUATION: DETERMINING THE CAUSE OF STROKE

Although initial management of acute ischemic stroke or TIA does not depend on the etiology, establishing a cause is essential to reduce risk of recurrence (Table 18-4); particular attention should be on atrial fibrillation and carotid atherosclerosis as these etiologies have proven secondary prevention strategies. Nearly 30% of strokes remain unexplained despite extensive evaluation.

Clinical examination should be focused on the peripheral and cervical vascular system. Routine studies include CXR and ECG, urinalysis, CBC/platelets, electrolytes, glucose, ESR, lipid profile, PT, PTT, and serologic tests for syphilis. If a hypercoagulable state is suspected, further studies of coagulation are indicated.

Imaging evaluation may include brain MRI (compared with CT, increased sensitivity for small infarcts of cortex and brainstem); MR or CT angiography (evaluate patency of intracranial vessels and extracranial carotid and vertebral vessels); noninvasive carotid tests ("duplex" studies, combine ultrasound imaging of the vessel with Doppler evaluation of blood flow characteristics); or cerebral angiography ("gold standard" for evaluation of intracranial and extracranial vascular disease). For suspected cardiogenic source, cardiac echocardiogram with attention to right-to-left shunts, and 24-h Holter or long-term cardiac event monitoring indicated.

PRIMARY AND SECONDARY PREVENTION OF STROKE

Risk Factors   Atherosclerosis is a systemic disease affecting arteries throughout the body. Multiple factors including hypertension, diabetes, hyperlipidemia, and family history influence stroke and TIA risk (Table 18-5). Cardioembolic risk factors include atrial fibrillation, MI, valvular heart disease, and cardiomyopathy. Hypertension and diabetes are also specific risk factors for lacunar stroke and intraparenchymal hemorrhage. Smoking is a potent risk factor for all vascular mechanisms of stroke. *Identification of modifiable risk factors and prophylactic interventions to lower risk is probably the best approach to stroke overall.*

Antiplatelet Agents   Platelet antiaggregation agents can prevent atherothrombotic events, including TIA and stroke, by inhibiting the formation of intraarterial platelet aggregates. Aspirin (50–325 mg/d) inhibits thromboxane A_2, a platelet aggregating and vasoconstricting prostaglandin. Aspirin, clopidogrel (blocks the platelet ADP receptor), and the combination of aspirin plus extended-release dipyrimadole (inhibits platelet uptake of adenosine) are the antiplatelet agents most commonly used. In general, antiplatelet agents reduce new stroke events by 25–30%. Every patient who has experienced an atherothrombotic stroke or TIA and has no contraindication should take an antiplatelet agent regularly because the average annual risk of another stroke is 8–10%.

Embolic Stroke   In pts with atrial fibrillation, the choice between warfarin or aspirin prophylaxis is determined by age and risk factors; the presence of any risk factor tips the balance in favor of anticoagulation (Table 18-6). Anticoagulation reduces the risk of embolism in acute MI; most clinicians recommend a 3-month course of therapy when there is anterior Q-wave infarction or other complica-

TABLE 18-4 CAUSES OF ISCHEMIC STROKE

Common Causes	Uncommon Causes
Thrombosis	Hypercoagulable disorders
Lacunar stroke (small vessel)	Protein C deficiency
Large vessel thrombosis	Protein S deficiency
Dehydration	Antithrombin III deficiency
Embolic occlusion	Antiphospholipid syndrome
Artery-to-artery	Factor V Leiden mutation[a]
Carotid bifurcation	Prothrombin G20210 mutation[a]
Aortic arch	Systemic malignancy
Arterial dissection	Sickle cell anemia
Cardioembolic	β-Thalassemia
Atrial fibrillation	Polycythemia vera
Mural thrombus	Systemic lupus erythematosus
Myocardial infarction	Homocysteinemia
Dilated cardiomyopathy	Thrombotic thrombocytopenic purpura
Valvular lesions	Disseminated intravascular coagulation
Mitral stenosis	Dysproteinemias
Mechanical valve	Nephrotic syndrome
Bacterial endocarditis	Inflammatory bowel disease
Paradoxical embolus	Oral contraceptives
Atrial septal defect	Venous sinus thrombosis[b]
Patent foramen ovale	Fibromuscular dysplasia
Atrial septal aneurysm	Vasculitis
Spontaneous echo contrast	Systemic vasculitis (PAN, Wegener's,
	Takayasu's, giant cell arteritis)
	Primary CNS vasculitis
	Meningitis (syphilis, tuberculosis, fungal,
	bacterial, zoster)
	Cardiogenic
	Mitral valve calcification
	Atrial myxoma
	Intracardiac tumor
	Marantic endocarditis
	Libman-Sacks endocarditis
	Subarachnoid hemorrhage vasospasm
	Drugs: cocaine, amphetamine
	Moyamoya disease
	Eclampsia

[a]Chiefly cause venous sinus thrombosis.
[b]May be associated with any hypercoagulable disorder.
Note: CNS, central nervous system; PAN, polyarteritis nodosa.

tions. For prosthetic heart valve pts, a combination of aspirin and warfarin may be indicated depending on the type and location of the prosthetic valve.

Anticoagulation Therapy for Noncardiogenic Stroke Data do not support the use of long-term warfarin for preventing atherothrombotic stroke for either intracranial or extracranial cerebrovascular disease.

Surgical Therapy Carotid endarterectomy benefits many pts with *symptomatic* severe (>70%) *carotid stenosis*; the relative risk reduction is ~65%. However, if the perioperative stroke rate is >6% for any surgeon, the benefit is lost. Endovascular stenting is an emerging option which has thus far been shown to be

TABLE 18-5 **RISK FACTORS FOR STROKE**

Risk Factor	Relative Risk	Relative Risk Reduction with Treatment	Number Needed to Treat[a]	
			Primary Prevention	Secondary Prevention
Hypertension	2–5	38%	100–300	50–100
Atrial fibrillation	1.8–2.9	68% warfarin, 21% aspirin	20–83	13
Diabetes	1.8–6	No proven effect		
Smoking	1.8	50% at 1 year, baseline risk at 5 years post cessation		
Hyperlipidemia	1.8–2.6	16–30%	560	230
Asymptomatic carotid stenosis	2.0	53%	85	N/A
Symptomatic carotid stenosis (70–99%)		65% at 2 years	N/A	12
Symptomatic carotid stenosis (50–69%)		29% at 5 years	N/A	77

[a]Number needed to treat to prevent one stroke annually. Prevention of other cardiovascular outcomes is not considered here.
Note: N/A, not applicable.

noninferior to endarterectomy only in very high-risk patients. Surgical results in pts with *asymptomatic carotid stenosis* are less robust, and medical therapy for reduction of atherosclerosis risk factors plus antiplatelet medications is generally recommended in this group.

TABLE 18-6 **CONSENSUS RECOMMENDATION FOR ANTITHROMBOTIC PROPHYLAXIS IN ATRIAL FIBRILLATION**

Age	Risk Factors[a]	Recommendation
Age ≤65	≥1	Warfarin INR 2–3
	0	Aspirin
Age 65–75	≥1	Warfarin INR 2–3
	0	Warfarin INR 2–3 or aspirin
Age >75		Warfarin INR 2–3

[a]Risk factors include previous transient ischemic attack or stroke, hypertension, heart failure, diabetes, systemic embolism, mitral stenosis, or prosthetic heart valve.
Source: Modified from DE Singer et al: Antithrombotic therapy in atrial fibrillation. Chest 126:429S, 2004; with permission.

For a more detailed discussion, see Smith WS, English JD, Johnston SC: Cerebrovascular Diseases, Chap. 364, p. 2513, in HPIM-17.

19 Subarachnoid Hemorrhage

Excluding head trauma, most common cause of subarachnoid hemorrhage (SAH) is rupture of an intracranial (saccular) aneurysm; other etiologies include bleeding from a vascular malformation (arteriovenous malformation or dural arterial-venous fistula), infective (mycotic) aneurysms, and extension into the subrachnoid space from a primary intracerebral hemorrhage. Approximately 2% of the population harbor aneurysms, and 25,000–30,000 cases of aneurysmal rupture producing SAH occur each year in the United States; rupture risk for aneurysms ≥10 mm in size is 0.5–1% per year.

Clinical Presentation Sudden, severe headache, often with transient loss of consciousness at onset; vomiting is common. Bleeding may injure adjacent brain tissue and produce focal neurologic deficits. A progressive third nerve palsy, usually involving the pupil, along with headache suggests posterior communicating artery aneurysm. In addition to dramatic presentations, aneurysms can undergo small ruptures with leaks of blood into the subarachnoid space (sentinel bleeds). The initial clinical manifestations of SAH can be graded using established scales (Table 19-1); prognosis for good outcome falls as the grade increases.

Initial Evaluation

- Noncontrast CT is the initial study of choice and usually demonstrates the hemorrhage if obtained within 72 h. LP is required for diagnosis of suspected SAH if the CT is nondiagnostic; xanthrochromia of the spinal fluid is seen within 6–12 h after rupture and lasts for 1–4 weeks.
- Cerebral angiography is necessary to localize and define the anatomic details of the aneurysm and to determine if other unruptured aneurysms exist; angiography should be performed as soon as possible after the diagnosis of SAH is made.

Grade	Hunt-Hess Scale	World Federation of Neurosurgical Societies (WFNS) Scale
TABLE 19-1	**GRADING SCALES FOR SUBARACHNOID HEMORRHAGE**	
1	Mild headache, normal mental status, no cranial nerve or motor findings	Glasgow Coma Scale[a] (GCS) score 15, no motor deficits
2	Severe headache, normal mental status, may have cranial nerve deficit	GCS 13–14, no motor deficits
3	Somnolent, confused, may have cranial nerve or mild motor deficit	GCS 13–14, with motor deficits
4	Stupor, moderate to severe motor deficit, may have intermittent reflex posturing	GCS 7–12, with or without motor deficits
5	Coma, reflex posturing or flaccid	GCS 3–6, with or without motor deficits

[a]Glasgow Coma Scale: See Fig. 373-2, HPIM 17.

- ECG may reveal ST-segment and T-wave changes similar to those associated with cardiac ischemia; caused by circulating catecholamines and excessive discharge of sympathetic neurons. A reversible cardiomyopathy producing shock or congestive heart failure may result.
- Studies of coagulation and platelet count should be obtained, and rapid correction should ensue if SAH is documented.

R$_x$ Subarachnoid Hemorrhage

Aneurysm Repair

Early aneurysm repair prevents rerupture and allows the safe application of techniques used to improve blood flow should symptomatic vasospasm develop. The International Subarachnoid Aneurysm Trial (ISAT) demonstrated improved outcomes with endovascular therapy compared to surgery; however, some aneurysms have a morphology not amenable to endovascular treatment, and therefore surgery is still an important treatment option.

Medical Management

Closely follow serum electrolytes and osmolality; hyponatremia ("cerebral salt wasting") frequently develops several days after SAH, and supplemental oral salt plus IV normal saline or hypertonic saline may be used to overcome renal losses. Anticonvulsants may be begun at diagnosis and continued at least until the aneurysm is treated, although some experts reserve this therapy only for patients in whom a seizure has occurred. Blood pressure should be carefully controlled initially, while preserving cerebral blood flow, in order to decrease the risk of rerupture until the aneurysm is repaired. All patients should have pneumatic compression stockings applied to prevent pulmonary embolism; unfractionated heparin administered subcutaneously for DVT prophylaxis can be initiated immediately following endovascular treatment and within days following craniotomy and surgical clipping.

Hydrocephalus

Severe hydrocephalus may require urgent placement of a ventricular catheter for external CSF drainage; some patients will require permanent shunt placement. Deterioration of a SAH patient in the first hours to days should prompt repeat CT scanning to evaluate ventricular size.

Vasospasm

Symptomatic vasospasm is the leading cause of mortality and morbidity following initial rupture; may occur by day 4 and continue through day 14, leading to focal ischemia and possibly stroke. Medical treatment with the calcium channel antagonist nimodipine (60 mg PO every 4 h) improves outcome, probably by preventing ischemic injury rather than reducing the risk of vasospasm. Cerebral perfusion can be improved in symptomatic vasospasm by increasing mean arterial pressure with vasopressor agents such as phenylephrine or norepinephrine, and intravascular volume can be expanded with crystalloid, augmenting cardiac output and reducing blood viscosity by reducing the hematocrit; this so-called "triple-H" (hypertension, hemodilution, and hypervolemic) therapy is widely used. If symptomatic vasospasm persists despite optimal medical therapy, intra-arterial vasodilators and angioplasty of the cerebral vessels can be effective.

For a more detailed discussion, see Hemphill JC III and Smith WS: Neurologic Critical Care, Including Hypoxic-Ischemic Encephalopathy and Subarachnoid Hemorrhage. Chap. 269, p. 1720, in HPIM-17.

20 Increased Intracranial Pressure and Head Trauma

INCREASED INTRACRANIAL PRESSURE

A limited volume of extra tissue, blood, CSF, or edema can be added to the intracranial contents without raising the intracranial pressure (ICP). Clinical deterioration or death may follow increases in ICP that shift intracranial contents, distort vital brainstem centers, or compromise cerebral perfusion. Cerebral perfusion pressure (CPP), defined as the mean arterial pressure (MAP) minus the ICP, is the driving force for circulation across capillary beds of the brain; decreased CPP is a fundamental mechanism of secondary ischemic brain injury and constitutes an emergency that requires immediate attention. In general, ICP should be maintained at <20 mmHg and CPP should be maintained at ≥60 mmHg.

Clinical Features   Elevated ICP may occur in a wide range of disorders including head trauma, intracerebral hemorrhage, subarachnoid hemorrhage (SAH) with hydrocephalus, and fulminant hepatic failure.

Symptoms of high ICP include drowsiness, headache (especially a constant ache that is worse upon awakening), nausea, emesis, diplopia, and blurred vision. Papilledema and sixth nerve palsies are common. If not controlled, then cerebral hypoperfusion, pupillary dilation, coma, focal neurologic deficits, posturing, abnormal respirations, systemic hypertension, and bradycardia may result.

Masses that cause raised ICP also distort midbrain and diencephalic anatomy, leading to stupor and coma. Brain tissue is pushed away from the mass against fixed intracranial structures and into spaces not normally occupied. Posterior fossa masses, which may initially cause ataxia, stiff neck, and nausea, are especially dangerous because they can both compress vital brainstem structures and cause obstructive hydrocephalus.

Herniation syndromes (Fig. 20-1) include:

- *Uncal*: Medial temporal lobe displaced through the tentorium, compressing the third cranial nerve and pushing the cerebral peduncle against the tentorium, leading to ipsilateral pupillary dilation, contralateral hemiparesis, and posterior cerebral artery occlusion.
- *Central*: Downward displacement of the thalamus through the tentorium; miotic pupils and drowsiness are early signs.
- *Transfalcial*: Cingulate gyrus displaced under the midline falx, leading to anterior cerebral artery occlusion and stroke.
- *Foraminal*: Cerebellar tonsils displaced into the foramen magnum, causing medullary compression and cardiorespiratory collapse.

℞ Increased Intracranial Pressure

A number of different interventions may lower ICP, and ideally the selection of treatment will be based on the underlying mechanism responsible for the elevated ICP (Table 20-1). For example, in hydrocephalus from SAH, the principal cause of elevated ICP is impaired CSF drainage; in this setting, ventricular drainage of CSF is likely to be sufficient. In head trauma and stroke, cytotoxic edema may be most responsible, and the use of osmotic diuretics such as mannitol becomes an appropriate early step. Elevated ICP may cause

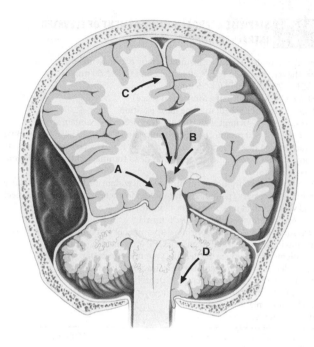

FIGURE 20-1 Types of cerebral herniation. A, uncal; B, central; C, transfalcial; D, foraminal.

tissue ischemia; the resulting vasodilatation can lead to a cycle of worsening ischemia. Paradoxically, administration of vasopressor agents to increase mean arterial pressure may actually lower ICP by increasing perfusion; therefore, hypertension should be treated carefully, if at all. Free water should be restricted, and fever treated aggressively. Hyperventilation is best used for only short periods of time until a more definitive treatment can be instituted. ICP monitoring can be an important tool to guide medical and surgical decisions in selected pts with cerebral edema (Fig. 20-2).

After stabilization and initiation of the above therapies, a CT scan (or MRI, if feasible) is performed to delineate the cause of the elevated ICP. Emergency surgical intervention is sometimes necessary to decompress the intracranial contents. Hydrocephalus, cerebellar stroke with edema, surgically accessible tumor, and subdural or epidural hemorrhage often require lifesaving neurosurgery.

HEAD TRAUMA

Almost 10 million head injuries occur annually in the United States, about 20% of which are serious enough to cause brain damage.

Clinical Features   Head trauma can cause immediate loss of consciousness. If transient and unaccompanied by other serious brain pathology other than a short period of amnesia, it is called *concussion*. Prolonged alterations in consciousness may be due to parenchymal, subdural, or epidural hematoma or to diffuse shearing of axons in the white matter. Skull fracture should be suspected in pts with CSF rhinorrhea, hemotympanum, and periorbital or mastoid ecchymoses.

TABLE 20-1	STEPWISE APPROACH TO TREATMENT OF ELEVATED INTRACRANIAL PRESSURE[a]

Insert ICP monitor—ventriculostomy versus parenchymal device
General goals: maintain ICP < 20 mmHg and CPP ≥ 60 mmHg
For ICP > 20–25 mmHg for >5 min:

1. Drain CSF via ventriculostomy (if in place)
2. Elevate head of the bed; midline head position
3. Osmotherapy—mannitol 25–100 g q4h as needed (maintain serum osmolality < 320 mosmol) or hypertonic saline (30 mL, 23.4% NaCl bolus)
4. Glucocorticoids—dexamethasone 4 mg q6h for vasogenic edema from tumor, abscess (avoid glucocorticoids in head trauma, ischemic and hemorrhagic stroke)
5. Sedation (e.g., morphine, propofol, or midazolam); add neuromuscular paralysis if necessary (patient will require endotracheal intubation and mechanical ventilation at this point, if not before)
6. Hyperventilation—to Pa_{CO_2} 30–35 mmHg
7. Pressor therapy—phenylephrine, dopamine, or norepinephrine to maintain adequate MAP to ensure CPP ≥ 60 mmHg (maintain euvolemia to minimize deleterious systemic effects of pressors)
8. Consider second-tier therapies for refractory elevated ICP
   a. High-dose barbiturate therapy ("pentobarb coma")
   b. Aggressive hyperventilation to Pa_{CO_2} < 30 mmHg
   c. Hypothermia
   d. Hemicraniectomy

[a]Throughout ICP treatment algorithm, consider repeat head CT to identify mass lesions amenable to surgical evacuation.
Note: CPP, cerebral perfusion pressure; CSF, cerebrospinal fluid; MAP, mean arterial pressure; Pa_{CO_2}, arterial partial pressure of carbon dioxide.

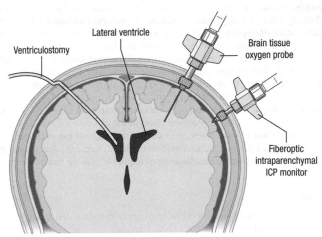

FIGURE 20-2 Intracranial pressure and brain tissue oxygen monitoring. A ventriculostomy allows for drainage of cerebrospinal fluid to treat elevated intracranial pressure (ICP). Fiberoptic ICP and brain tissue oxygen monitors are usually secured using a screwlike skull bolt. Cerebral blood flow and microdialysis probes (not shown) may be placed in a manner similar to the brain tissue oxygen probe.

APPROACH TO THE PATIENT WITH HEAD INJURY

Medical personnel caring for head injury patients should be aware that:

- Spinal injury often accompanies head injury and care must be taken to prevent compression of the spinal cord due to instability of the spinal column.
- Intoxication is a frequent accompaniment of traumatic brain injury and, when appropriate, testing should be carried out for drugs and alcohol.
- Accompanying systemic injuries, including ruptures of abdominal organs, may produce vascular collapse or respiratory compromise requiring immediate attention.

Minor Concussive Injury   The pt with minor head injury who is alert and attentive after a short period of unconsciousness (<1 min) may have headache, dizziness, faintness, nausea, a single episode of emesis, difficulty with concentration, or slight blurring of vision. Such patients have usually sustained a concussion and are expected to have a brief amnestic period. After several hours of observation, pts with this category of injury can be accompanied home and observed for a day by family or friends. Persistent severe headache and repeated vomiting are usually benign if the neurologic exam remains normal, but in such situations radiologic studies should be obtained and hospitalization is justified.

Older age, two or more episodes of vomiting, >30 min of retrograde or persistent anterograde amnesia, seizure, and concurrent drug or alcohol intoxication are sensitive (but not specific) indicators of intracranial hemorrhage that justify CT scanning; it is appropriate to be more liberal in obtaining CT scans in children.

Injury of Intermediate Severity   Pts who are not comatose but who have persistent confusion, behavioral changes, subnormal alertness, extreme dizziness, or focal neurologic signs such as hemiparesis should be admitted to the hospital and soon thereafter have a CT scan. Usually a cerebral contusion or subdural hematoma is found. Pts with intermediate head injury require medical observation to detect increasing drowsiness, respiratory dysfunction, and pupillary enlargement or other changes in the neurologic exam. Abnormalities of attention, intellect, spontaneity, and memory tend to return to normal weeks or months after the injury, although some cognitive deficits may be persistent.

Severe Injury   Patients who are comatose from onset require immediate neurologic attention and often resuscitation. After intubation (with care taken to avoid deforming the cervical spine), the depth of coma, pupillary size and reactivity, limb movements, and Babinski responses are assessed. As soon as vital functions permit and cervical spine x-rays and a CT scan have been obtained, the pt should be transported to a critical care unit. CT scan may be normal in comatose pts with axonal shearing lesions in cerebral white matter.

The finding of an epidural or subdural hematoma or large intracerebral hemorrhage requires prompt decompressive surgery in otherwise salvageable pts. Subsequent treatment is probably best guided by direct measurement of ICP. All potentially exacerbating factors should be eliminated; hypoxia, hyperthermia, hypercarbia, awkward head positions, and high mean airway pressures from mechanical ventilation all increase ICP. Persistently raised ICP after treatment of these factors generally indicates a poor outcome. The use of prophylactic anticonvulsants has been recommended by some neurosurgeons but there are few supportive data.

For a more detailed discussion, see Ropper AH: Coma, Chap. 268, p. 1714; Hemphill JC Smith WS: Neurologic Critical Care, Including Hypoxic-Ischemic Encephalopathy and Subarachnoid Hemorrhage, Chap. 269, p. 1720; and Ropper AH: Concussion and Other Head Injuries, Chap. 373, p. 2596, in HPIM-17.

21 Spinal Cord Compression

APPROACH TO THE PATIENT: SPINAL CORD INJURY

The initial symptoms of spinal cord injury, focal neck or back pain, evolve over days to weeks. These are followed by various combinations of paresthesias, sensory loss, motor weakness, and sphincter disturbance evolving over hours to several days. Partial lesions may selectively involve one or more tracts and may be limited to one side of the cord. In severe or abrupt cases, areflexia reflecting spinal shock may be present, but hyperreflexia supervenes over days to weeks. A sensory level to pain may be present on the trunk, indicating localization to the cord at that dermatomal level.

The first priority is to exclude a treatable compression of the spinal cord by a mass. Compressive disease is more likely to be preceded by warning signs of neck or back pain, bladder disturbances, and sensory symptoms prior to development of weakness; noncompressive etiologies such as infarction and hemorrhage are more likely to produce myelopathy without antecedent symptoms.

MRI with gadolinium, centered on the clinically suspected level, is the initial diagnostic procedure (CT myelography may be helpful in patients who have contraindications to MRI). It may be useful to image the entire spine to search for additional clinically silent lesions. Infectious etiologies, unlike tumor, often cross the disc space to involve adjacent vertebral bodies.

NEOPLASTIC SPINAL CORD COMPRESSION

Occurs in 5–10% of pts with cancer and is the first manifestation of malignancy in about 10% of these pts. Most neoplasms are epidural in origin, resulting from metastases to the adjacent spinal bones. Almost any malignant tumor can metastasize to the spinal column with breast, lung, prostate, kidney, lymphoma, and plasma cell dyscrasia being particularly frequent. The thoracic cord is most commonly involved; exceptions include prostate and ovarian tumors, which preferentially involve the lumbar and sacral segments from spread through veins in the anterior epidural space. The most common presenting symptom is localized back pain and tenderness followed by symptoms of neurologic compromise. Urgent MRI is indicated when the diagnosis is suspected; up to 40% of patients with neoplastic cord compression at one level are found to have asymptomatic epidural disease elsewhere, so the entire spine should be imaged.

℞ Neoplastic Spinal Cord Compression

Management includes glucocorticoids to reduce edema (dexamethasone, up to 40 mg daily), local radiotherapy (initiated as soon as possible), and specific therapy for the underlying tumor type. Glucocorticoids can be administered before the imaging study if the clinical suspicion is high, and continued at a lower dose until radiotherapy (generally 3000 cGy administered in 15 daily fractions) is completed. Biopsy is needed if there is no history of underlying malignancy; a simple workup including chest imaging, mammography, measurement of prostate-specific antigen (PSA), and abdominal CT may reveal the diagnosis. Radiotherapy appears to be as effective as surgical treatments. Surgery, either decompression by laminectomy or vertebral body resection, should be considered when signs of cord compression worsen despite radiotherapy, when the maximum tolerated dose of radiotherapy has been delivered previously to the site, or when a vertebral compression fracture or spinal instability contributes to cord compression. Time is of the essence in treatment; fixed motor deficits (paraplegia or quadriplegia) once established for >12 h do not usually improve, and beyond 48 h the prognosis for substantial motor recovery is poor; those who start treatment while ambulatory, usually (75%) remain so.

SPINAL EPIDURAL ABSCESS

Presents as a triad of pain, fever, and progressive limb weakness. Aching pain is almost always present, either over the spine or in a radicular pattern. The duration of pain prior to presentation is generally <2 weeks but may be several months or longer. Fever is usually present along with elevated white blood cell count and sedimentation rate. Risk factors include an impaired immune status (diabetes mellitus, HIV, renal failure, alcoholism, malignancy), intravenous drug abuse, and infections of the skin or other soft tissues. Most cases are due to *Staphylococcus aureus*; other important causes include gram-negative bacilli, *Streptococcus*, anaerobes, fungi, and tuberculosis (Pott's disease).

MRI localizes the abscess. Lumbar puncture (LP) is only required if encephalopathy or other clinical signs raise the question of associated meningitis, a feature found in <25% of cases. The level of the LP should be planned to minimize risk of meningitis due to passage of the needle through infected tissue.

℞ Spinal Epidural Abcess

Decompressive laminectomy with debridement combined with long-term antibiotic treatment. Surgical evacuation is unlikely to improve deficits of more than several days' duration. Antibiotics should be started empirically before surgery and then modified on the basis of culture results and continued for at least 4 weeks.

SPINAL EPIDURAL HEMATOMA

Hemorrhage into the epidural (or subdural) space causes acute focal or radicular pain followed by variable signs of a spinal cord disorder. Therapeutic anticoagulation, trauma, tumor, or blood dyscrasia are predisposing conditions; rarely complication of LP or epidural anesthesia. Treatment consists of prompt reversal of any underlying bleeding disorder and surgical decompression.

HEMATOMYELIA

Hemorrhage into the substance of the spinal cord is a rare result of trauma, vasculitis, bleeding disorders, spinal cord neoplasm, or intraparenchymal vascular malformation. Usually presents as a painful myelopathy. Diagnosis is by MRI or CT. Therapy is supportive, and surgical intervention is generally not useful; an exception is hematomyelia due to an underlying vascular malformation, for which selective spinal angiography may be indicated, followed by surgery to evacuate the thrombus and remove the underlying vascular lesion.

For a more detailed discussion, see Gucalp R and Dutcher J: Oncologic Emergencies, Chap. 270, p. 1730, in HPIM-17 and Hauser SL and Ropper AH: Diseases of the Spinal Cord, Chap. 372, p. 2588, in HPIM-17.

22 Hypoxic-Ischemic Encephalopathy

Results from lack of delivery of oxygen to the brain because of hypotension or respiratory failure. Most common causes are MI, cardiac arrest, shock, asphyxiation, paralysis of respiration, and carbon monoxide or cyanide poisoning. In some circumstances, hypoxia may predominate. Carbon monoxide and cyanide poisoning are termed *histotoxic hypoxia* since they cause a direct impairment of the respiratory chain.

CLINICAL MANIFESTATIONS

Mild degrees of pure hypoxia (e.g., high altitude) cause impaired judgment, inattentiveness, motor incoordination, and, at times, euphoria. However, with hypoxia-ischemia, such as occurs with circulatory arrest, consciousness is lost within seconds. If circulation is restored within 3–5 min, full recovery may occur, but with longer periods permanent cerebral damage is the rule. It may be difficult to judge the precise degree of hypoxia-ischemia, and some pts make a relatively full recovery even after 8–10 min of global ischemia. The distinction between pure hypoxia and hypoxia-ischemia is important, since a Pa_{O_2} as low as 2.7 kPa (20 mmHg) can be well tolerated if it develops gradually and normal blood pressure is maintained, but short periods of very low or absent cerebral circulation may result in permanent impairment.

Clinical examination at different time points after an insult (especially cardiac arrest) helps to assess prognosis (Fig. 22-1). The prognosis is better for pts with intact brainstem function, as indicated by normal pupillary light responses, intact oculocephalic (doll's eyes) reflexes, and oculovestibular (caloric) and corneal reflexes (Chap. 18). Absence of these reflexes and the presence of persistently dilated pupils that do not react to light are grave prognostic signs. A uniformly dismal prognosis is conveyed by the absence of pupillary light reflex or absence of a motor response to pain on day 3 following the injury. Bilateral absence of the cortical somatosensory evoked potentials (SSEP) in the first sev-

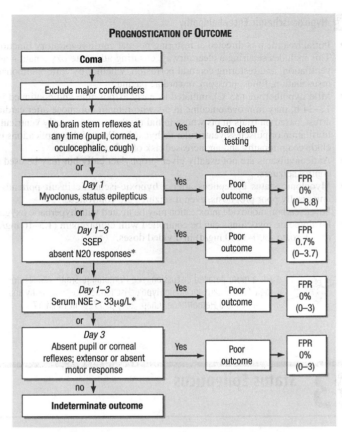

FIGURE 22-1 Prognostication of outcome in comatose survivors of cardiopulmonary resuscitation. Numbers in parentheses are 95% confidence intervals. Confounders could include use of sedatives or neuromuscular blocking agents, hypothermia therapy, organ failure, or shock. Tests denoted with an * may not be available in a timely and standardized manner. SSEP, somatosensory evoked potentials; NSE, neuron-specific enolase; FPR, false-positive rate. [*From EFM Wijdicks et al: Practice parameter: Prediction of outcome in comatose survivors after cardiopulmonary resuscitation (an evidence-based review). Neurology 67:203, 2006; with permission.*]

eral days also conveys a poor prognosis, as does a very elevated serum level (>33 µg/L) of the biochemical marker neuron-specific enolase (NSE); currently these two ancillary tests are limited by the ability to obtain them in a timely fashion along with the need for expert interpretation (SSEP) and lack of standardization in laboratory methods (NSE measurements).

Long-term consequences include persistent coma or vegetative state, dementia, visual agnosia, parkinsonism, choreoathetosis, ataxia, myoclonus, seizures, and an amnestic state. Delayed postanoxic encephalopathy is an uncommon phenomenon where patients appear to make an initial recovery following an insult and then have a relapse with a progressive course often characterized by widespread demeylination on imaging studies.

Rx Hypoxic-Ischemic Encephalopathy

- Initial treatment is directed at restoring normal cardiorespiratory function. This includes securing a clear airway, ensuring adequate oxygenation and ventilation, and restoring cerebral perfusion, whether by cardiopulmonary resuscitation, fluids, pressors, or cardiac pacing.
- Mild hypothermia (33°C), initiated as early as possible and continued for 12–24 h, may improve outcome in pts who remain comatose after cardiac arrest, based on trials in pts whose initial rhythm was primarily ventricular fibrillation or pulseless ventricular tachycardia. Potential complications include coagulopathy and an increased risk of infection.
- Anticonvulsants are not usually given prophylactically but may be used to control seizures.
- Myoclonic status epilepticus after a hypoxic-ischemic insult portends a universally poor prognosis, even if seizures are controlled.
- Severe carbon monoxide intoxication may be treated with hyperbaric oxygen.
- Posthypoxic myoclonus can be controlled with clonazepam (1.5–10 mg/d) or valproate (300–1200 mg/d) in divided doses.

For a more detailed discussion, see Hemphill JC Smith WS: Neurologic Critical Care, Including Hypoxic-Ischemic Encephalopathy and Subarachnoid Hemorrhage, Chap. 269, p. 1720, in HPIM-17.

23 Status Epilepticus

Defined as continuous seizures or repetitive, discrete seizures with impaired consciousness in the interictal period. The duration of seizure activity to meet the definition has traditionally been 15–30 min. A more practical definition is any situation requiring the acute use of anticonvulsants; in generalized convulsive status epilepticus (GCSE), this is typically when seizures last >5 min.

CLINICAL FEATURES

Has numerous subtypes: GCSE (e.g., persistent, generalized electrographic seizures, coma, and tonic-clonic movements), and nonconvulsive status epilepticus (e.g., persistent absence seizures or partial seizures, confusion, or partially impaired consciousness, and minimal motor abnormalities). GCSE is obvious when overt convulsions are present, but after 30–45 min of uninterrupted seizures, the signs may become increasingly subtle (mild clonic movements of the fingers; fine, rapid movements of the eyes; or paroxysmal episodes of tachycardia, pupillary dilatation, and hypertension). EEG may be the only method of diagnosis with these subtle signs; therefore, if a patient remains comatose after a seizure, EEG should be performed to exclude ongoing status epilepticus. GCSE is life-threatening when accompanied by hyperpyrexia, acidosis (from prolonged muscle activity), respiratory or cardiovascular compromise. Irreversible neuronal injury may occur from persistent seizures, even when pt is paralyzed from neuromuscular blockade.

ETIOLOGY

Principal causes of GCSE are antiepileptic drug withdrawal or noncompliance, metabolic disturbances, drug toxicity, CNS infections, CNS tumors, refractory epilepsy, and head trauma.

℞ Status Epilepticus

GCSE is a medical emergency. First attend to any acute cardiorespiratory problems or hyperthermia, perform a brief medical and neurologic exam, establish venous access, and send lab studies to screen for metabolic abnormalities including anticonvulsant levels if pt has a history of epilepsy. Anticonvulsant therapy should then begin without delay (Fig. 23-1). In parallel, it is essential to determine the cause of the seizures to prevent recurrence and treat any underlying abnormalities.

The treatment of nonconvulsive status epilepticus is somewhat less urgent since the ongoing seizures are not accompanied by the severe metabolic disturbances of GCSE; however, evidence points to local cellular injury in the region of the seizure focus, so the condition should be treated as promptly as possible using the general approach for GCSE.

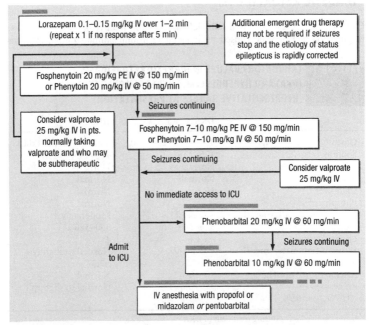

FIGURE 23-1 Pharmacologic treatment of generalized tonic-clonic status epilepticus in adults. The horizontal bars indicate the approximate duration of drug infusions. IV, intravenous; PE, phenytoin equivalents.

PROGNOSIS

The mortality rate is 20% in GCSE, and the incidence of permanent neurologic sequelae is 10–30%.

For a more detailed discussion, see Lowenstein DH: Seizures and Epilepsy, Chap. 363, p. 2498, in HPIM-17.

24 Diabetic Ketoacidosis and Hyperosmolar Coma

Diabetic ketoacidosis (DKA) and hyperglycemic hyperosmolar state (HHS) are acute complications of diabetes mellitus (DM). DKA is seen primarily in individuals with type 1 DM and HHS in individuals with type 2 DM. Both disorders are associated with absolute or relative insulin deficiency, volume depletion, and altered mental status. The metabolic similarities and differences in DKA and HHS are summarized in Table 24-1.

DIABETIC KETOACIDOSIS

Etiology   DKA results from insulin deficiency with a relative or absolute increase in glucagon and may be caused by inadequate insulin administration, infection

TABLE 24-1   LABORATORY VALUES IN DIABETIC KETOACIDOSIS (DKA) AND HYPERGLYCEMIC HYPEROSMOLAR STATE (HHS) (REPRESENTATIVE RANGES AT PRESENTATION)

	DKA	HHS
Glucose,[a] mmol/L (mg/dL)	13.9–33.3 (250–600)	33.3–66.6 (600–1200)
Sodium, meq/L	125–135	135–145
Potassium,[a] meq/L	Normal to ↑[b]	Normal
Magnesium[a]	Normal[b]	Normal
Chloride[a]	Normal	Normal
Phosphate[a]	↓	Normal
Creatinine, μmol/L (mg/dL)	Slightly ↑	Moderately ↑
Osmolality (mOsm/mL)	300–320	330–380
Plasma ketones[a]	++++	±
Serum bicarbonate,[a] meq/L	<15 meq/L	Normal to slightly ↓
Arterial pH	6.8–7.3	>7.3
Arterial P_{CO_2},[a] mmHg	20–30	Normal
Anion gap[a] [Na – (Cl + HCO₃)], meq/L	↑	Normal to slightly ↑

[a]Large changes occur during treatment of DKA.
[b]Although plasma levels may be normal or high at presentation, total-body stores are usually depleted.

(pneumonia, urinary tract infection, gastroenteritis, sepsis), infarction (cerebral, coronary, mesenteric, peripheral), surgery, drugs (cocaine), or pregnancy.

Clinical Features   The initial symptoms of DKA include anorexia, nausea, vomiting, polyuria, and thirst. Abdominal pain, altered mental function, or frank coma may ensue. Classic signs of DKA include Kussmaul respirations and an acetone odor on the pt's breath. Volume depletion can lead to dry mucous membranes, tachycardia, and hypotension. Fever and abdominal tenderness may also be present. Laboratory evaluation reveals hyperglycemia, ketosis (β-hydroxybutyrate > acetoacetate), and metabolic acidosis (arterial pH 6.8–7.3) with an increased anion gap (Table 24-1). The fluid deficit is often 3–5 L. Despite a total-body potassium deficit, the serum potassium at presentation may be normal or mildly high as a result of acidosis. Leukocytosis, hypertriglyceridemia, and hyperlipoproteinemia are common. Hyperamylasemia is usually of salivary origin but may suggest a diagnosis of pancreatitis. The measured serum sodium is reduced as a consequence of hyperglycemia [1.6-meq reduction for each 5.6-mmol/L (100-mg/dL) rise in the serum glucose].

 Diabetic Ketoacidosis

The management of DKA is outlined in Table 24-2.

HYPERGLYCEMIC HYPEROSMOLAR STATE

Etiology   Relative insulin deficiency and inadequate fluid intake are the underlying causes of HHS. Hyperglycemia induces an osmotic diuresis that leads to profound intravascular volume depletion. HHS is often precipitated by a serious, concurrent illness such as myocardial infarction or sepsis and compounded by conditions that impede access to water.

Clinical Features   Presenting symptoms include polyuria, thirst, and altered mental state, ranging from lethargy to coma. Notably absent are symptoms of nausea, vomiting, and abdominal pain and the Kussmaul respirations characteristic of DKA. The prototypical pt is an elderly individual with a several week history of polyuria, weight loss, and diminished oral intake. The laboratory features are summarized in Table 24-1. In contrast to DKA, acidosis and ketonemia are usually not found; however, a small anion gap may be due to lactic acidosis, and moderate ketonuria may occur from starvation. Though the measured serum sodium may be normal or slightly low, the corrected serum sodium is usually increased [add 1.6 meq to measured sodium for each 5.6-mmol/L (100-mg/dL) rise in the serum glucose].

 Hyperglycemic Hyperosmolar State

The precipitating problem should be sought and treated. Sufficient IV fluids (1–3 L of 0.9% normal saline over the first 2–3 h) must be given to stabilize the hemodynamic status. The calculated free water deficit (usually 9–10 L) should be reversed over the next 1–2 days, using 0.45% saline initially then 5% dextrose in water. Potassium repletion is usually necessary. The plasma glucose may drop precipitously with hydration alone, though insulin therapy with an IV bolus of 0.1 units/kg followed by a constant infusion rate (0.1 units/kg per hour) is usually required. If the serum glucose does not fall, the insulin infusion rate should be doubled. Glucose should be added to IV fluid

TABLE 24-2 **MANAGEMENT OF DIABETIC KETOACIDOSIS**

1. Confirm diagnosis ($\uparrow$ plasma glucose, positive serum ketones, metabolic acidosis).
2. Admit to hospital; intensive-care setting may be necessary for frequent monitoring or if pH < 7.00 or unconscious.
3. Assess: Serum electrolytes (K^+, Na^+, Mg^{2+}, Cl^-, bicarbonate, phosphate)
   Acid-base status—pH, HCO_3^-, P_{CO_2}, β-hydroxybutyrate
   Renal function (creatinine, urine output)
4. Replace fluids: 2–3 L of 0.9% saline over first 1–3 h (10–15 mL/kg per hour); subsequently, 0.45% saline at 150–300 mL/h; change to 5% glucose and 0.45% saline at 100–200 mL/h when plasma glucose reaches 14 mmol/L, (250 mg/dL).
5. Administer short-acting insulin: IV (0.1 units/kg) or IM (0.3 units/kg), then 0.1 units/kg per hour by continuous IV infusion; increase 2- to 3-fold if no response by 2–4 h. If initial serum potassium is < 3.3 mmol/L (3.3 meq/L), do not administer insulin until the potassium is corrected to > 3.3 mmol/L (3.3 meq/L).
6. Assess patient: What precipitated the episode (noncompliance, infection, trauma, infarction, cocaine)? Initiate appropriate workup for precipitating event (cultures, CXR, ECG).
7. Measure capillary glucose every 1–2 h; measure electrolytes (especially K^+, bicarbonate, phosphate) and anion gap every 4 h for first 24 h.
8. Monitor blood pressure, pulse, respirations, mental status, fluid intake and output every 1–4 h.
9. Replace K^+: 10 meq/h when plasma K^+ < 5.5 meq/L, ECG normal, urine flow and normal creatinine documented; administer 40–80 meq/h when plasma K^+ <3.5 meq/L or if bicarbonate is given.
10. Continue above until patient is stable, glucose goal is 150–250 mg/dL, and acidosis is resolved. Insulin infusion may be decreased to 0.05–0.1 units/kg per hour.
11. Administer intermediate or long-acting insulin as soon as patient is eating. Allow for overlap in insulin infusion and subcutaneous insulin injection.

Note: CXR, chest x-ray; ECG, electrocardiogram.
Source: Adapted from M Sperling, in *Therapy for Diabetes Mellitus and Related Disorders*, American Diabetes Association, Alexandria, VA, 1998; and AE Kitabchi et al: Diabetes Care 29:2739, 2006.

and the insulin infusion rate decreased when the plasma glucose falls to 13.9 mmol/L (250 mg/dL). The insulin infusion should be continued until the patient has resumed eating and can be transitioned to a subcutaneous insulin regimen.

For a more detailed discussion, see Powers AC: Diabetes Mellitus, Chap. 338, p. 2275, in HPIM-17.

25 Hypoglycemia

Glucose is an obligate metabolic fuel for the brain. Hypoglycemia should be considered in any patient with confusion, altered level of consciousness, or seizures. Counterregulatory responses to hypoglycemia include insulin suppression and the release of catecholamines, glucagon, growth hormone, and cortisol.

The laboratory diagnosis of hypoglycemia is usually defined as a plasma glucose level <2.5–2.8 mmol/L (<45–50 mg/dL), although the absolute glucose level at which symptoms occur varies among individuals. For this reason, *Whipple's triad* should be present: (1) symptoms consistent with hypoglycemia, (2) a low plasma glucose concentration measured by precise method (not a glucose monitor), and (3) relief of symptoms after the plasma glucose level is raised.

ETIOLOGY

Hypoglycemia occurs most commonly as a result of treating patients with diabetes mellitus. Additional factors to be considered in any pt with hypoglycemia are listed below.

1. Drugs: insulin, insulin secretagogues (especially chlorpropamide, repaglinide, nateglinide), alcohol, high doses of salicylates, sulfonamides, pentamidine, quinine, quinolones
2. Critical illness: hepatic, renal, or cardiac failure; sepsis; prolonged starvation
3. Hormone deficiencies: adrenal insufficiency, hypopituitarism
4. Insulinoma: pancreatic β cell tumor, β cell hyperplasia (a.k.a. nesidioblastosis; congenital or after gastric or bariatric surgery)
5. Other rare etiologies: Non-β cell tumors (large mesenchymal or epithelial tumors producing IGF-II, other non-pancreatic tumors), insulin or insulin receptor antibodies, inherited enzymatic defects

CLINICAL FEATURES

Symptoms of hypoglycemia can be divided into autonomic (adrenergic: palpitations, tremor, and anxiety; cholinergic: sweating, hunger, and paresthesia) and neuroglycopenic (behavioral changes, confusion, fatigue, seizure, loss of consciousness, and, if hypoglycemia is severe and prolonged, death). Tachycardia, elevated systolic blood pressure, pallor, and diaphoresis may be present on physical examination.

Recurrent hypoglycemia shifts thresholds for the autonomic symptoms and counterregulatory responses to lower glucose levels, leading to hypoglycemic unawareness. Under these circumstances, the first manifestation of hypoglycemia is neuroglycopenia, placing patients at risk of being unable to treat themselves.

DIAGNOSIS

Diagnosis of the hypoglycemic mechanism is critical for choosing a treatment that prevents recurrent hypoglycemia (Fig. 25-1). Urgent treatment is often necessary in patients with suspected hypoglycemia. Nevertheless, blood should be drawn at the time of symptoms, whenever possible before the administration of glucose, to allow documentation of the glucose level. If the glucose level is low and the cause of hypoglycemia is unknown, additional assays should be

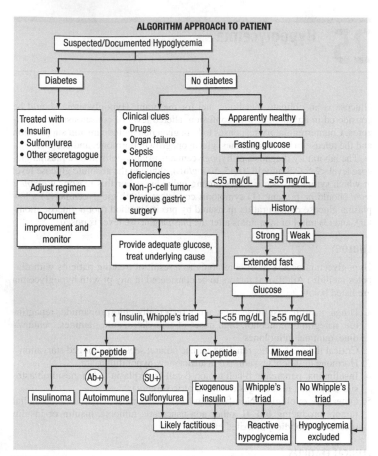

FIGURE 25-1 Diagnostic approach to a patient with suspected hypoglycemia based on a history of symptoms, a low plasma glucose concentration, or both.

performed on blood obtained at the time of a low plasma glucose. These should include insulin, C-peptide, sulfonylurea levels, cortisol, and ethanol. In the absence of documented spontaneous hypoglycemia, overnight fasting or food deprivation during observation in the outpatient setting will sometimes elicit hypoglycemia and allow diagnostic evaluation. An extended (up to 72 h) fast under careful supervision in the hospital may otherwise be required—the test should be terminated if plasma glucose drops below 2.5 mmol/L (45 mg/dL) and the patient has symptoms.

Interpretation of fasting test results is shown in Table 25-1.

℞ **Hypoglycemia**

The syndrome of hypoglycemic unawareness in patients with diabetes mellitus is reversible after as little as 2 weeks of scrupulous avoidance of hypoglycemia. This involves a shift of glycemic thresholds back to higher glucose concentrations.

	TABLE 25-1	**DIAGNOSTIC INTERPRETATION OF HYPOGLYCEMIA**			
Diagnosis	Glucose, mmol/L (mg/dL)	Insulin, μU/mL	C-Peptide, pmol/L	Proinsulin, pmol/L	Urine or Plasma Sulfonylurea
Nonhypogly-cemic	≥2.2 (≥40)	<3	<200	<5	No
Insulinoma	≤2.5 (≤45)	≥3	≥200	≥5	No
Exogenous insulin	≤2.5 (≤45)	≥3[a]	<200	<5	No
Sulfonylurea	≤2.5 (≤45)	≥3	≥200	≥5	Yes
Non-insulin mediated	≤2.5 (≤45)	<3	<200	<5	No

[a]Often very high.

Acute therapy of hypoglycemia requires administration of oral glucose or 25 g of a 50% solution IV followed by a constant infusion of 5 or 10% dextrose if parenteral therapy is necessary. Hypoglycemia from sulfonylureas is often prolonged, requiring treatment and monitoring for 24 h or more. Subcutaneous or intramuscular glucagon can be used in diabetics. Prevention of recurrent hypoglycemia requires treatment of the underlying cause of hypoglycemia, including discontinuation or dose reduction of offending drugs, treatment of critical illnesses, replacement of hormonal deficiencies, and surgery of insulinomas or other tumors. Treatment of other forms of hypoglycemia is dietary, with avoidance of fasting and ingestion of frequent small meals.

For a more detailed discussion, see Cryer PE: Hypoglycemia, Chap. 339, p. 2305, in HPIM-17.

26 Infectious Disease Emergencies

GENERAL CONSIDERATIONS

- Acutely ill infected febrile pts requiring emergent attention must be appropriately evaluated and treated at presentation to improve outcome. A quick assessment of general appearance provides a subjective sense of whether the pt is septic or toxic.
- *History*: The physician should assess:
    Onset and duration of symptoms, changes in severity or rate of progression over time
    Host factors (e.g., alcoholism, IV drug use) and comorbid conditions (e.g., asplenia, diabetcs)
    Potential nidus for invasive infection (e.g., URI or influenza, trauma, burn, foreign body)

Exposure history (e.g., travel, pets, diet, medication use, vaccination history, sick contacts, menstruation history, sexual contacts)
- *Physical examination*
  General appearance (e.g., agitation or lethargy, vital signs)
  Special attention to skin and soft tissue exam, neurologic examination, assessment of mental status
- *Diagnostic workup*
  Bloodwork: cultures, CBC with differential, electrolytes, BUN, creatinine, LFTs, blood smear examination, buffy coat
  CSF cultures if meningitis is possible. With focal neurologic signs, papilledema, or abnormal mental status, obtain blood cultures, begin antibiotics, perform brain imaging, and then consider LP.
  CT or MRI to evaluate focal abscesses; cultures of wounds or scraping of skin lesions as indicated. No diagnostic procedure should delay treatment for more than minutes.
- *Treatment*
  See Table 26-1. Adjunctive therapy (e.g., glucocorticoids or IV immunoglobulin) can decrease morbidity and mortality rates. Dexamethasone for bacterial meningitis must be given before or with the first dose of antibiotic. Urgent surgical attention may be indicated.

SPECIFIC PRESENTATIONS (Table 26-1)

Sepsis without an Obvious Focus of Primary Infection

1. Septic shock: primary site may not be identified initially; bacteremia and shock are evident.
2. Overwhelming infection in asplenic pts
   a. The risk of severe sepsis remains increased throughout life, but 50–70% of cases occur in the first 2 years after splenectomy.
   b. *Streptococcus pneumoniae* is the most common etiologic agent, with mortality rates up to 80%.
3. Babesiosis: history of travel to endemic areas, tick bite 1–4 weeks previously
   a. Asplenia, age >60 years, and infection with the European strain *Babesia divergens* are risk factors for severe disease.
   b. *Babesia microti* is transmitted by the *Ixodes scapularis* tick, which also transmits *Borrelia burgdorferi* (Lyme disease) and ehrlichiae. Co-infections can result in more severe disease.
   c. Nonspecific symptoms can progress to hemolysis, jaundice, and renal and respiratory failure.
4. Tularemia and plague can produce typhoidal or septic syndromes with mortality rates ~30%.

Sepsis with Skin Manifestations

1. Maculopapular rashes: usually not emergent but can occur in early meningococcemia or rickettsial disease
2. Petechiae
   a. Meningococcemia: young children and their household contacts are at greatest risk; outbreaks occur in schools and army barracks. Serogroup A meningococcal disease is endemic in sub-Saharan Africa; epidemic outbreaks occur every 8–12 years.
      Headache, nausea, myalgias, altered mental status, meningismus
      Petechiae begin at ankles, wrists, axillae, and mucosal surfaces and progress to purpura and DIC.

TABLE 26-1 COMMON INFECTIOUS DISEASE EMERGENCIES

Clinical Syndrome	Possible Etiologies	Treatment	Comments
Sepsis without a Clear Focus			
Septic shock	*Pseudomonas* spp., gram-negative enteric bacilli, *Staphylococcus* spp., *Streptococcus* spp.	Vancomycin (1 g q12h) *plus* Gentamicin (5 mg/kg per day) *plus either* Piperacillin/tazobactam (3.375 g q4h) *or* Cefepime (2 g q12h)	Adjust treatment when culture data become available. Drotrecogin alfa (activated)[a] or low-dose hydrocortisone and fludrocortisone[b] may improve outcome in patients with septic shock.
Overwhelming post-splenectomy sepsis	*Streptococcus pneumoniae, Haemophilus influenzae, Neisseria meningitidis*	Ceftriaxone (2 g q12h) *plus* Vancomycin (1 g q12h)	If a β-lactam–sensitive strain is identified, vancomycin can be discontinued.
Babesiosis	*Babesia microti* (U.S.), *B. divergens* (Europe)	**Either:** Clindamycin (600 mg tid) *plus* Quinine (650 mg tid) *or* Atovaquone (750 mg q12h) *plus* Azithromycin (500-mg loading dose, then 250 mg/d)	Atovaquone and azithromycin are as effective as clindamycin and quinine and are associated with fewer side effects. Treatment with doxycycline (100 mg bid[c]) for potential co-infection with *Borrelia burgdorferi* or *Ehrlichia* spp. may be prudent.
Sepsis with Skin Findings			
Meningococcemia	*N. meningitidis*	Penicillin (4 mU q4h) *or* Ceftriaxone (2 g q12h)	Consider protein C replacement in fulminant meningococcemia.

(continued)

TABLE 26-1 COMMON INFECTIOUS DISEASE EMERGENCIES (CONTINUED)

Clinical Syndrome	Possible Etiologies	Treatment	Comments
Rocky Mountain spotted fever (RMSF)	*Rickettsia rickettsii*	Doxycycline (100 mg bid)	If both meningococcemia and RMSF are being considered, use chloramphenicol alone (50–75 mg/kg per day in four divided doses) *or* ceftriaxone (2 g q12h) *plus* doxycycline (100 mg bid[c]) If RMSF is diagnosed, doxycycline is the proven superior agent.
Purpura fulminans	*S. pneumoniae, H. influenzae, N. meningitidis*	Ceftriaxone (2 g q12h) *plus* Vancomycin (1 g q12h)	If a β-lactam–sensitive strain is identified, vancomycin can be discontinued.
Erythroderma: toxic shock syndrome	Group A *Streptococcus, Staphylococcus aureus*	Vancomycin (1 g q12h) *plus* Clindamycin (600 mg q8h)	If a penicillin- or oxacillin-sensitive strain is isolated, those agents are superior to vancomycin (penicillin, 2 mU q4h; or oxacillin, 2 g q4h). The site of toxigenic bacteria should be debrided; IV immunoglobulin can be used in severe cases.[d]
Sepsis with Soft Tissue Findings			
Necrotizing fasciitis	Group A *Streptococcus,* mixed aerobic/anaerobic flora	Penicillin (2 mU q4h) *plus* Clindamycin (600 mg q8h) *plus* Gentamicin (5 mg/kg per day)	Urgent surgical evaluation is critical. If community-acquired methicillin-resistant *S. aureus* is a concern, vancomycin (1 g q12h) can be substituted for penicillin while culture data are pending.
Clostridial myonecrosis	*Clostridium perfringens*	Penicillin (2 mU q4h) *plus* Clindamycin (600 mg q8h)	Urgent surgical evaluation is critical.
Neurologic Infections			
Bacterial meningitis	*S. pneumoniae, N. meningitidis*	Ceftriaxone (2 g q12h) *plus* Vancomycin (1 g q12h)	If a β-lactam–sensitive strain is identified, vancomycin can be discontinued. If the patient is >50 years old or has comorbid disease, add ampicillin (2 g q4h) for *Listeria* coverage. Dexamethasone (10 mg q6h × 4 days) improves outcome in adult patients with meningitis (especially pneumococcal) and cloudy CSF, positive CSF Gram's stain, or a CSF leukocyte count >1000/μL.

Brain abscess, suppurative intracranial infections	Streptococcus spp., Staphylococcus spp., anaerobes, gram-negative bacilli	Vancomycin (1 g q12h) **plus** Metronidazole (500 mg q8h) **plus** Ceftriaxone (2 g q12h)	Urgent surgical evaluation is critical. If a penicillin- or oxacillin-sensitive strain is isolated, those agents are superior to vancomycin (penicillin, 4 mU q4h; or oxacillin, 2 g q4h).
Cerebral malaria	Plasmodium falciparum	Quinine (650 mg tid) **plus** Tetracycline (250 mg tid)	Do not use glucocorticoids.
Spinal epidural abscess	Staphylococcus spp., gram-negative bacilli	Vancomycin (1 g q12h) **plus** Ceftriaxone (2 g q24h)	Surgical evaluation is essential. If a penicillin- or oxacillin-sensitive strain is isolated, those agents are superior to vancomycin (penicillin, 4 mU q4h; or oxacillin, 2 g q4h).
Focal Infections			
Acute bacterial endocarditis	S. aureus, β-hemolytic streptococci, HACEK group,[e] Neisseria spp., S. pneumoniae	Ceftriaxone (2 g q12h) **plus** Vancomycin (1 g q12h)	Adjust treatment when culture data become available. Surgical evaluation is essential.

[a] Drotrecogin alfa (activated) is administered at a dose of 24 µg/kg per hour for 96 h. It has been approved for use in patients with severe sepsis and a high risk of death as defined by an Acute Physiology and Chronic Health Evaluation II (APACHE II) score of ≥25 and/or multiorgan failure.

[b] Hydrocortisone (50-mg IV bolus q6h) with fludrocortisone (50-µg tablet daily for 7 days) may improve outcomes of severe sepsis, particularly in the setting of relative adrenal insufficiency.

[c] Tetracyclines can be antagonistic in action to β-lactam agents. Adjust treatment as soon as the diagnosis is confirmed.

[d] The optimal dose of IV immunoglobulin has not been determined, but the median dose in observational studies is 2 g/kg (total dose administered over 1–5 days).

[e] Haemophilus aphrophilus, H. paraphrophilus, H. parainfluenzae, Actinobacillus actinomycetemcomitans, Cardiobacterium hominis, Eikenella corrodens, and Kingella kingae.

Mortality rates exceed 90% among pts without meningitis who have rash, hypotension, and a normal or low WBC count and ESR.

b. Rocky Mountain spotted fever: history of tick bite and/or travel or outdoor activity

Headache, malaise, myalgias, nausea, vomiting, anorexia

In progressive disease: hypotension, noncardiogenic pulmonary edema, confusion, lethargy, encephalitis, coma

Rash by day 3: blanching macules that become hemorrhagic, starting at wrists and ankles and spreading to legs and trunk, then palms and soles

c. Other rickettsial diseases: Mediterranean spotted fever (Africa) can be severe in the elderly or pts with comorbid illness; mortality rates in these populations approach 50%. Epidemic typhus occurs in louse-infested areas, usually in a setting of poverty, war, or natural disaster; mortality rates are 10–15%. In scrub typhus (Southeast Asia), death occurs in 1–35% of cases.

d. Purpura fulminans: cutaneous manifestation of DIC; large ecchymotic areas and hemorrhagic bullae; associated with CHF, septic shock, acute renal failure, acidosis

3. Ecthyma gangrenosum: hemorrhagic vesicles with central necrosis and ulceration in septic shock with *Pseudomonas aeruginosa* or *Aeromonas hydrophila*

4. Other emergent infections associated with rash

a. *Vibrio vulnificus* and other noncholera vibrios: Bacteremic infections and sepsis with lower-extremity bullous or hemorrhagic lesions develop after contaminated shellfish ingestion, typically in hosts with liver disease.

b. *Capnocytophaga canimorsus*: septic shock in asplenic pts, typically after dog bite. Skin manifestations: exanthem, erythema multiforme, peripheral cyanosis, petechiae

5. Erythroderma and toxic shock syndrome (TSS): diffuse sunburn-like rash that desquamates after 1–2 weeks; hypotension; multiorgan failure; renal failure (may precede hypotension)

a. *Staphylococcus aureus* TSS: colonization of vagina or postoperative wound; usually no primary focal infection; 5–15% mortality

b. Streptococcal TSS: less frequent desquamation, 30–70% mortality

6. Viral hemorrhagic fevers: zoonotic viral illness from animal reservoirs or arthropod vectors—e.g., Lassa fever in Africa, hantavirus hemorrhagic fever with renal syndrome in Asia, Ebola and Marburg virus infections in Africa, and yellow fever in Africa and South America. Dengue is the most common arboviral disease worldwide. Dengue hemorrhagic fever is the more severe form, with a triad of hemorrhagic manifestations, plasma leakage, and platelet counts <100,000/μL. Mortality is 10–20% but approaches 40% if dengue shock syndrome develops. Supportive care and volume replacement therapy are life-saving.

Sepsis with a Soft Tissue/Muscle Primary Focus

1. Necrotizing fasciitis

a. Risk factors: minimal trauma, surgical incision, varicella, comorbid conditions (diabetes, peripheral vascular disease, IV drug use)

b. Bacteremia, hypotension, physical findings minimal compared to degree of pain, fever, toxicity; infected area red, hot, shiny, exquisitely tender

c. Progression to bullae, necrosis; decreased pain due to peripheral nerve destruction an ominous sign

d. Mortality: 100% without surgery, 70% in setting of TSS, 25–30% overall

2. Clostridial myonecrosis
   a. Either secondary to trauma or surgery or spontaneous (associated with *Clostridium septicum* infection and underlying malignancy)
   b. Pain and toxicity are out of proportion to physical findings. Pts are apathetic, tachycardic, and tachypneic, with a sense of impending doom.
   c. Mottled, bronze-colored overlying skin or bullous lesions; crepitus; drainage with mousy or sweet odor; massive necrotizing gangrene, toxicity, shock, death within hours
   d. Mortality: 12% (extremity myonecrosis) to 63–65% (trunk or spontaneous myonecrosis)

Neurologic Infections with or without Septic Shock

1. Bacterial meningitis
   a. Classic triad of headache, meningismus, and fever in one-half to two-thirds of pts
   b. Blood cultures positive in 50–60% of pts
   c. Death associated with coma, respiratory distress, shock, CSF protein >2.5 g/L, peripheral WBC count <5000/μL, serum Na level <135 mmol/L
2. Brain abscess
   a. Often without systemic signs, can present as space-occupying lesion
   b. Headache, focal neurologic signs, papilledema
   c. From contiguous foci or hematogenous infection (e.g., endocarditis)
   d. Prognosis worsens with fulminant course, delayed diagnosis, rupture into ventricles, multiple abscesses, and/or abnormal mental status at presentation.

Focal Syndromes with a Fulminant Course

1. Rhinocerebral mucormycosis
   a. Seen in patients with diabetes, malignancy
   b. Low-grade fever, dull sinus pain, diplopia, decreased mental status, chemosis, proptosis, hard-palate lesions that respect the midline
2. Acute bacterial endocarditis
   a. Seen in patients with malignancy, diabetes, IV drug use, alcoholism
   b. Etiologies include *S. aureus*, *S. pneumoniae*, *Haemophilus* spp., and group A, B, or G streptococci.
   c. Rapid valvular destruction, pulmonary edema, hypotension, myocardial abscesses, conduction abnormalities and arrhythmias, large friable vegetations, major arterial emboli with tissue infarction
   d. Mortality: 10–40%
3. Respiratory illnesses
   a. Inhalational anthrax: mediastinal widening, pulmonary infiltrates, pleural effusions
   b. Avian influenza (H5N1): Southeast Asia; poultry contact; progressive dyspnea and ARDS, multiorgan failure, and ultimately (within 9–10 days) death
   c. Hantavirus pulmonary syndrome: rural U.S., Canada, and South America; rodent exposure. Nonspecific viral prodrome can progress to pulmonary edema, respiratory failure, myocardial depression, and death.

For a more detailed discussion, see Barlam TF, Kasper DL: Approach to the Acutely Ill Infected Febrile Patient, Chap. 115, p. 761, in HPIM-17.

27 Oncologic Emergencies

Emergencies in the cancer pt may be classified into three categories: effects from tumor expansion, metabolic or hormonal effects mediated by tumor products, and treatment complications.

STRUCTURAL/OBSTRUCTIVE ONCOLOGIC EMERGENCIES

The most common problems are superior vena cava syndrome; pericardial effusion/tamponade; spinal cord compression; seizures (Chap. 191) and/or increased intracranial pressure; and intestinal, urinary, or biliary obstruction. The last three conditions are discussed in Chap. 270 in HPIM-17.

SUPERIOR VENA CAVA SYNDROME

Obstruction of the superior vena cava reduces venous return from the head, neck, and upper extremities. About 85% of cases are due to lung cancer; lymphoma and thrombosis of central venous catheters are also causes. Pts often present with facial swelling, dyspnea, and cough. In severe cases, the mediastinal mass lesion may cause tracheal obstruction. Dilated neck veins and increased collateral veins on anterior chest wall are noted on physical exam. Chest x-ray (CXR) documents widening of the superior mediastinum; 25% of pts have a right-sided pleural effusion.

℞ **Superior Vena Cava Syndrome**

Radiation therapy is the treatment of choice for non-small cell lung cancer; addition of chemotherapy to radiation therapy is effective in small cell lung cancer and lymphoma. Symptoms recur in 10–30% and can be palliated by venous stenting. Clotted central catheters producing this syndrome should be removed and anticoagulation therapy initiated. Catheter clots may be prevented with warfarin, 1 mg/d.

PERICARDIAL EFFUSION/TAMPONADE

Accumulation of fluid in the pericardium impairs filling of the heart and decreases cardiac output. Most commonly seen in pts with lung or breast cancers, leukemias, or lymphomas, pericardial tamponade may also develop as a late complication of mediastinal radiation therapy (constrictive pericarditis). Common symptoms are dyspnea, cough, chest pain, orthopnea, and weakness. Pleural effusion, sinus tachycardia, jugular venous distention, hepatomegaly, and cyanosis are frequent physical findings. Paradoxical pulse, decreased heart sounds, pulsus alternans, and friction rub are less common with malignant than nonmalignant pericardial disease. Echocardiography is diagnostic; pericardiocentesis may show serous or bloody exudate, and cytology usually shows malignant cells.

Pericardial Effusion/Tamponade

Drainage of fluid from the pericardial sac may be lifesaving until a definitive surgical procedure (pericardial stripping or window) can be performed.

SPINAL CORD COMPRESSION

Primary spinal cord tumors occur rarely, and cord compression is most commonly due to epidural metastases from vertebral bodies involved with tumor, especially from prostate, lung, breast, lymphoma, and myeloma primaries. Pts present with back pain, worse when recumbent, with local tenderness. Loss of bowel and bladder control may occur. On physical exam, pts have a loss of sensation below a horizontal line on the trunk, called a *sensory level*, that usually corresponds to one or two vertebrae below the site of compression. Weakness and spasticity of the legs and hyperactive reflexes with upgoing toes on Babinski testing are often noted. Spine radiographs may reveal erosion of the pedicles (winking owl sign), lytic or sclerotic vertebral body lesions, and vertebral collapse. Collapse alone is not a reliable indicator of tumor; it is a common manifestation of a more common disease, osteoporosis. MRI can visualize the cord throughout its length and define the extent of tumor involvement.

 Spinal Cord Compression   (See Fig. 27-1)

Radiation therapy plus dexamethasone, 4 mg IV or PO q4h, is successful in arresting and reversing symptoms in about 75% of pts who are diagnosed while still ambulatory. Only 10% of pts made paraplegic by the tumor recover the ability to ambulate.

EMERGENT PARANEOPLASTIC SYNDROMES

Most paraneoplastic syndromes have an insidious onset (Chap. 81). Hypercalcemia, syndrome of inappropriate antidiuretic hormone secretion (SIADH), and adrenal insufficiency may present as emergencies.

HYPERCALCEMIA

The most common paraneoplastic syndrome, it occurs in about 10% of cancer pts, particularly those with lung, breast, head and neck, and kidney cancer and myeloma. Bone resorption mediated by parathormone-related protein is the most common mechanism; interleukin 1 (IL-1), IL-6, tumor necrosis factor, and transforming growth factor β may act locally in tumor-involved bone. Pts usually present with nonspecific symptoms: fatigue, anorexia, constipation, weakness. Hypoalbuminemia associated with malignancy may make symptoms worse for any given serum calcium level because more calcium will be free rather than protein bound.

 Hypercalcemia

Saline hydration, antiresorptive agents (e.g., pamidronate, 60–90 mg IV over 4 h, or zoledronate, 4–8 mg IV), and glucocorticoids usually lower calcium levels significantly within 1–3 days. Treatment effects usually last several weeks. Treatment of the underlying malignancy is also important.

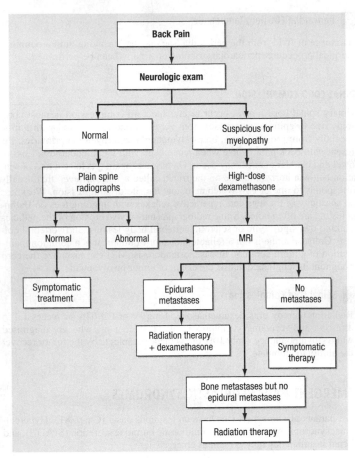

FIGURE 27-1 Management of cancer patients with back pain.

SIADH

Induced by the action of arginine vasopressin produced by certain tumors (especially small cell cancer of the lung), SIADH is characterized by hyponatremia, inappropriately concentrated urine, and high urine sodium excretion in the absence of volume depletion. Most pts with SIADH are asymptomatic. When serum sodium falls to <115 meq/L, pts may experience anorexia, depression, lethargy, irritability, confusion, weakness, and personality changes.

 SIADH

Water restriction controls mild forms. Demeclocycline (150–300 mg PO tid or qid) inhibits the effects of vasopressin on the renal tubule but has a slow onset of action (1 week). Treatment of the underlying malignancy is also important. If the patient has mental status changes with sodium levels <115 meq/L, normal saline infusion plus furosemide to increase free water clearance may provide more rapid improvement. Rate of correction should not exceed 0.5–1 meq/L per h. More rapid change can produce fluid shifts that lead to brain damage.

ADRENAL INSUFFICIENCY

The infiltration of the adrenals by tumor and their destruction by hemorrhage are the two most common causes. Symptoms such as nausea, vomiting, anorexia, and orthostatic hypotension may be attributed to progressive cancer or to treatment side effects. Certain treatments (e.g., ketoconazole, aminoglutethimide) may directly interfere with steroid synthesis in the adrenal.

Rx Adrenal Insufficiency

In emergencies, a bolus of 100 mg IV hydrocortisone is followed by a continuous infusion of 10 mg/h. In nonemergent but stressful circumstances, 100–200 mg/d oral hydrocortisone is the beginning dose, tapered to maintenance of 15–37.5 mg/d. Fludrocortisone (0.1 mg/d) may be required in the presence of hyperkalemia.

TREATMENT COMPLICATIONS

Complications from treatment may occur acutely or emerge only many years after treatment. Toxicity may be either related to the agents used to treat the cancer or from the response of the cancer to the treatment (e.g., leaving a perforation in a hollow viscus or causing metabolic complications such as tumor lysis syndrome). Several treatment complications present as emergencies. Fever and neutropenia and tumor lysis syndrome will be discussed here; others are discussed in Chap. 270 in HPIM-17.

FEVER AND NEUTROPENIA

Many cancer pts are treated with myelotoxic agents. When peripheral blood granulocyte counts are <1000/μL, the risk of infection is substantially increased (48 infections/100 pts). A neutropenic pt who develops a fever (>38°C) should undergo physical exam with special attention to skin lesions, mucous membranes, IV catheter sites, and perirectal area. Two sets of blood cultures from different sites should be drawn and a CXR performed, and any additional tests should be guided by findings from the history and physical exam. Any fluid collections should be tapped, and urine and/or fluids should be examined under the microscope for evidence of infection.

Rx Fever and Neutropenia

After cultures are obtained, all pts should receive IV broad-spectrum antibiotics (e.g., ceftazidime, 1 g q8h). If an obvious infectious site is found, the antibiotic regimen is designed to cover organisms that may cause the infection. Usually therapy should be started with an agent or agents that cover both gram-positive and -negative organisms. If the fever resolves, treatment should continue until neutropenia resolves. Persistence of febrile neutropenia after 7 days should lead to addition of amphotericin B to the antibiotic regimen.

TUMOR LYSIS SYNDROME

When rapidly growing tumors are treated with effective chemotherapy regimens, the dying tumor cells can release large amounts of nucleic acid breakdown products (chiefly uric acid), potassium, phosphate, and lactic acid. The phosphate elevations can lead to hypocalcemia. The increased uric acid, especially in the setting of acidosis, can precipitate in the renal tubules and lead to renal failure. The renal failure can exacerbate the hyperkalemia.

℞ Tumor Lysis Syndrome

Prevention is the best approach. Maintain hydration with 3 L/d of saline, keep urine pH > 7.0 with bicarbonate administration, and start allopurinol, 300 mg/m^2 per day, 24 h before starting chemotherapy. Once chemotherapy is given, monitor serum electrolytes every 6 h. If after 24 h, uric acid (>8 mg/dL) and serum creatinine (>1.6 mg/dL) are elevated, rasburicase (recombinant urate oxidase), 0.2 mg/kg IV daily, may lower uric acid levels. If serum potassium is >6.0 meq/L and renal failure ensues, hemodialysis may be required. Maintain normal calcium levels.

For a more detailed discussion, see Finberg R: Infections in Patients with Cancer, Chap. 82, p. 533; and Gucalp R, Dutcher J: Oncologic Emergencies, Chap. 270, p. 1730, in HPIM-17.

28 Anaphylaxis

DEFINITION

A life-threatening systemic hypersensitivity reaction to contact with an allergen; it may appear within minutes of exposure to the offending substance. Manifestations include respiratory distress, pruritus, urticaria, mucous membrane swelling, gastrointestinal disturbances (including nausea, vomiting, pain, and diarrhea), and vascular collapse. Virtually any allergen may incite an anaphylactic reaction, but among the more common agents are proteins such as antisera, hormones, pollen extracts, Hymenoptera venom, foods; drugs (especially antibiotics); and diagnostic agents. Atopy does not seem to predispose to anaphylaxis from penicillin or venom exposures. Anaphylactic transfusion reactions are covered in Chap. 9.

CLINICAL PRESENTATION

Time to onset is variable, but symptoms usually occur within seconds to minutes of exposure to the offending antigen:

- Respiratory: mucous membrane swelling, hoarseness, stridor, wheezing
- Cardiovascular: tachycardia, hypotension
- Cutaneous: pruritus, urticaria, angioedema

DIAGNOSIS

Made by obtaining history of exposure to offending substance with subsequent development of characteristic complex of symptoms.

℞ Anaphylaxis

Mild symptoms such as pruritus and urticaria can be controlled by administration of 0.3–0.5 mL of 1:1000 (1.0 mg/mL) epinephrine SC or IM, with repeated doses as required at 5- to 20-min intervals for a severe reaction.

An IV infusion should be initiated for administration of 2.5 mL of 1:10,000 epinephrine solution at 5- to 10-min intervals, volume expanders such as normal saline, and vasopressor agents, e.g., dopamine, if intractable hypotension occurs.

Epinephrine provides both α- and β-adrenergic effects, resulting in vasoconstriction and bronchial smooth-muscle relaxation. Beta blockers are relatively contraindicated in persons at risk for anaphylactic reactions.

The following should also be used as necessary:
- Antihistamines such as diphenhydramine 50–100 mg IM or IV
- Aminophylline 0.25–0.5 g IV for bronchospasm
- Oxygen
- Glucocorticoids (medrol 0.5–1.0 mg/kg IV); not useful for acute manifestations but may help control persistent hypotension or bronchospasm
- For antigenic material injected into an extremity consider: use of a tourniquet proximal to the site, 0.2 mL of 1:1000 epinephrine into the site, removal of an insect stinger if present.

PREVENTION

Avoidance of offending antigen, where possible; skin testing and desensitization to materials such as penicillin and Hymenoptera venom, if necessary. Individuals should wear an informational bracelet and have immediate access to an unexpired epinephrine kit.

For a more detailed discussion, see Austen KF: Allergies, Anaphylaxis, and Systemic Mastocytosis, Chap. 311, p. 2061, in HPIM-17.

29 Bites, Venoms, Stings, and Marine Poisonings

MAMMALIAN BITES

Each year, there are ~300 dog and cat bites per 100,000 population in the United States.

DOG BITES

Epidemiology   Of all mammalian bite wounds, 80% are inflicted by dogs, and 15–20% of these wounds become infected.

Etiology   (See Table 29-1.)   In addition to bacterial infections, dog bites may transmit rabies (Chap. 111) and may lead to tetanus (Chap. 99) or tularemia (Chap. 98).

Clinical Features

- Pain, cellulitis, and a purulent, sometimes foul-smelling discharge may develop 8–24 h after the bite.
- Infection is usually localized, but systemic spread (e.g., bacteremia, endocarditis, brain abscess) can occur.
- *Capnocytophaga canimorsus* infection can present as sepsis syndrome, DIC, and renal failure, particularly in pts who are splenectomized, have hepatic dysfunction, or are otherwise immunosuppressed.

CAT BITES

Epidemiology   In >50% of cases, infection occurs as a result of deep tissue penetration of narrow, sharp feline incisors. Cat bites are more likely than dog bites to cause septic arthritis or osteomyelitis.

Etiology   The microflora is usually mixed, although *Pasteurella multocida* is the most important pathogen. Cat bites may transmit rabies or may lead to tetanus. Cat bites and scratches may also transmit *Bartonella henselae*, the agent of cat-scratch disease (Chap. 98), as well as *Francisella tularensis*, the agent of tularemia (Chap. 98).

Clinical Features   *P. multocida* can cause rapidly advancing, painful inflammation within a few hours after the bite as well as purulent discharge. Dissemination may occur.

OTHER NONHUMAN MAMMALIAN BITES

- Bite infections reflect oral flora. Bites from Old World monkeys (*Macaca* spp.) may transmit herpes B virus (*Herpesvirus simiae*), which can cause CNS infections with high mortality rates.
- Small rodents and the animals that prey on them may transmit *rat-bite fever*, caused by *Streptobacillus moniliformis* (in the United States) or *Spirillum minor* (in Asia). Infection with *S. moniliformis* manifests 3–10 days after the bite as fever, chills, myalgias, headache, and migratory arthralgias; these manifestations are followed by a maculopapular rash. Complications can include metastatic abscesses, endocarditis, meningitis, or pneumonia. Diagnosis can be made by culture on enriched media and serologic testing. Infection with *S. minor* causes local pain, purple swelling with lymphangitis, and regional lymphadenopathy 1–4 weeks after the bite, with evolution into a systemic illness. Diagnosis can be made by detection of spirochetes on microscopic examination.

HUMAN BITES

Human bites become infected more frequently than bite wounds from other animals. *Occlusional* injuries are inflicted by actual biting. *Clenched-fist* injuries result when the fist of one individual strikes the teeth of another and are particularly prone to serious infection.

Etiology   See Table 29-1.

TABLE 29-1 **MANAGEMENT OF WOUND INFECTIONS FOLLOWING ANIMAL AND HUMAN BITES**

Biting Species	Commonly Isolated Pathogens	Preferred Antibiotic(s)[a]	Alternative Agent(s) for Penicillin-Allergic Patients	Prophylaxis Advised for Early Uninfected Wounds	Other Considerations
Dog	Staphylococcus aureus, Pasteurella multocida, anaerobes, Capnocytophaga canimorsus	Amoxicillin/clavulanate (250–500 mg PO tid) or ampicillin/sulbactam (1.5–3.0 g IV q6h)	Clindamycin (150–300 mg PO qid) plus either TMP-SMX (1 double-strength tablet bid) or ciprofloxacin (500 mg PO bid)	Sometimes[b]	Consider rabies prophylaxis.
Cat	P. multocida, S. aureus, anaerobes	Amoxicillin/clavulanate or ampicillin/sulbactam, as for dog bite	Clindamycin plus either TMP-SMX (as for dog bite) or a fluoroquinolone	Usually	Consider rabies prophylaxis. Carefully evaluate for joint or bone penetration.
Human, occlusional bite	Viridans streptococci, S. aureus, Haemophilus influenzae, anaerobes	Amoxicillin/clavulanate or ampicillin/sulbactam, as for dog bite	Erythromycin (500 mg PO qid) or a fluoroquinolone	Always	—
Human, clenched-fist injury	As for occlusional plus Eikenella corrodens	Ampicillin/sulbactam, as for dog bite; or imipenem (500 mg q6h)	Cefoxitin[c]	Always	Examine for tendon, nerve, or joint involvement.
Monkey	As for human bite	As for human bite	As for human bite	Always	For macaque monkeys, consider herpes B virus prophylaxis with acyclovir.

(continued)

Biting Species	Commonly Isolated Pathogens	Preferred Antibiotic(s)[a]	Alternative Agent(s) for Penicillin-Allergic Patients	Prophylaxis Advised for Early Uninfected Wounds	Other Considerations
Snake[d]	*Pseudomonas aeruginosa, Proteus* spp., *Bacteroides fragilis, Clostridium* spp.	Ampicillin/sulbactam, as for dog bite	Clindamycin plus either TMP-SMX (as for dog bite) or a fluoroquinolone	Sometimes, especially for venomous snakebites	Antivenom for venomous snakebite
Rodent	*Streptobacillus moniliformis, Leptospira* spp., *P. multocida*	Penicillin VK (500 mg PO qid)	Doxycycline (100 mg PO bid)	Sometimes	—

[a]Antibiotic choices should be based on culture data when available. These are suggestions for empirical therapy and need to be tailored to individual circumstances and local conditions. IV regimens should be used for hospitalized pts. A single IV dose of antibiotic may be given to pts who will be discharged after initial management.

[b]Prophylactic antibiotics are suggested for severe or extensive wounds, facial wounds, and crush injuries; when bone or joint may be involved; or when comorbidity is present.

[c]May be hazardous to pts with immediate-type hypersensitivity reaction to penicillin.

[d]See Chap. 391 in HPIM-17.

Note: TMP-SMX, trimethoprim-sulfamethoxazole.

Mammalian Bites

- *Wound management*: Wound closure is controversial in bite injuries. After thorough cleansing, facial wounds are usually sutured for cosmetic reasons and because the abundant facial blood supply lessens the risk of infection. For wounds elsewhere on the body, many authorities do not attempt primary closure, preferring instead to irrigate the wound copiously, debride devitalized tissue, remove foreign bodies, and approximate the margins. Delayed primary closure may be undertaken after the risk of infection has passed.
- *Antibiotic therapy*: See Table 29-1. If prophylactic antibiotics are given, the course is 3–5 days long.
- *Other prophylaxis*: Rabies prophylaxis (passive immunization with rabies immune globulin and active immunization with rabies vaccine) should be given in consultation with local and regional public health authorities. A tetanus booster for pts immunized previously but not boosted within 5 years should be considered, as should primary immunization and tetanus immune globulin administration for pts not previously immunized.

VENOMOUS SNAKEBITES

Etiology and Epidemiology   Worldwide, >125,000 people die each year from venomous snakebite injuries, most often in temperate and tropical regions. Snake venoms are complex mixtures of enzymes and other substances that promote vascular leaking and bleeding, tissue necrosis, and neurotoxicity and affect the coagulation cascade.

Venomous Snakebites

FIELD MANAGEMENT

- Get the victim to definitive care as soon as possible.
- Keep the victim inactive to minimize the systemic spread of venom.
- Splint a bitten extremity and keep it at heart level.
- Pressure immobilization (wrapping of the entire limb in a bandage at a pressure of 40–70 mmHg and splinting) can be used if the venom is primarily neurotoxic without local tissue effects, if the rescuer is skilled in this technique, and if the victim can be carried to medical care.
- *Avoid* incisions into the bite wound, cooling, consumption of alcoholic beverages by the victim, and electric shock.
- Best first aid: Do it RIGHT: *R*eassure victim, *I*mmobilize extremity, *G*et to the *H*ospital, inform physician of *T*elltale signs and symptoms.

HOSPITAL MANAGEMENT

- Monitor vital signs, cardiac rhythm, and O_2 saturation closely, and watch for evidence of difficulty swallowing or respiratory insufficiency.
- Note the level of erythema and swelling and the limb circumference every 15 min until swelling has stabilized.
- Treat shock initially by crystalloid fluid resuscitation with isotonic saline. If hypotension persists, try 5% albumin and vasopressors.
- Begin the search for appropriate, specific antivenom early in all cases of known venomous snakebite. In the United States, round-the-clock assistance is available from regional poison control centers.

1. Any evidence of systemic envenomation (systemic symptoms or signs, laboratory abnormalities) and (possibly) significant, progressive local finding are indications for antivenom administration.
2. Treating physicians should seek advice from snakebite experts regarding indications and dosing of antivenom. Antivenom administration should be continued until the victim shows definite improvement. However, neurotoxicity from the bite of an elapid (e.g., a cobra) is harder to reverse with antivenom. Once neurotoxicity is established and intubation is required, further antivenom is unlikely to help.
3. CroFab, an antivenom used in the United States against North American pit viper species, has a low risk of allergy elicitation. Worldwide, antivenom quality varies, and rates of anaphylactoid reaction can exceed 50%.
4. If the risk of allergy is significant, pts should be premedicated with IV antihistamines (e.g., diphenhydramine, 1 mg/kg up to a maximum dose of 100 mg; plus cimetidine, 5–10 mg/kg up to a maximum dose of 300 mg) and given IV crystalloids to expand intravascular volume. Epinephrine should be immediately available. The antivenom in dilute solution should be administered slowly by the IV route, with a physician present in case of an acute reaction.
5. Acetylcholinesterase inhibitors may cause neurologic improvement in pts bitten by snakes with postsynaptic neurotoxins.

- Elevate the bitten extremity once antivenom administration has been initiated.
- Update tetanus immunization.
- Observe pt for muscle-compartment syndrome.
- Observe pts with signs of envenomation in the hospital for at least 24 h. Pts with "dry" bites should be watched for at least 8 h because symptoms are commonly delayed.

The overall mortality rate for venomous snakebite is <1% among U.S. victims who receive antivenom. Eastern and western diamondback rattlesnakes are responsible for most deaths from snakebite in the United States.

MARINE ENVENOMATIONS

INVERTEBRATES

Injuries from nematocysts (stinging cells) of hydroids, fire coral, jellyfish, Portuguese man-of-wars, and sea anemones cause similar clinical symptoms that differ in severity.

Clinical Features   Pain (prickling, burning, and throbbing), pruritus, and paresthesia develop immediately at the site of the bite. Neurologic, GI, renal, cardiovascular, respiratory, rheumatologic, and ocular symptoms have been described.

℞   Marine Invertebrate Envenomations

- Decontaminate the skin immediately with vinegar (5% acetic acid) or rubbing alcohol (40–70% isopropanol). Baking soda, unseasoned meat tenderizer (papain), lemon or lime juice, household ammonia, olive oil, or sugar may be effective.
- Shaving the skin may help remove nematocysts.
- After decontamination, topical anesthetics, antihistamines, or steroid lotions may be helpful.

- Narcotics may be necessary for persistent pain.
- Muscle spasms may respond to IV 10% calcium gluconate (5–10 mL) or diazepam (2–5 mg titrated upward as needed).

VERTEBRATES

Marine vertebrates, including stingrays, scorpionfish, and catfish, are capable of envenomating humans.

Clinical Features

- Immediate and intense pain at the site can last up to 48 h.
- Systemic symptoms include weakness, diaphoresis, nausea, vomiting, diarrhea, dysrhythmia, syncope, hypotension, muscle cramps, muscle fasciculations, and paralysis. Fatal cases are rare.
- Stingray wounds can become ischemic and heal poorly.
- The sting of a stonefish is the most serious marine vertebrate envenomation and can be life-threatening.

Rx Marine Vertebrate Envenomations

- Immerse the affected part immediately in nonscalding hot water (113°F/ 45°C) for 30–90 min.
- Explore, debride, and vigorously irrigate the wound.
- Antivenom is available for stonefish and scorpionfish envenomations.
- Leave wounds to heal by secondary intention or to be treated by delayed primary closure.
- Update tetanus immunization.
- Consider empirical antibiotics to cover *Staphylococcus* and *Streptococcus* spp. for serious wounds or envenomations in immunocompromised hosts.

SOURCES OF ANTIVENOMS AND OTHER ASSISTANCE

To locate a specific antivenom in the United States, contact the nearest regional poison control center. Divers Alert Network is a source of helpful information (round-the-clock at 919-684-8111 or *www.diversalertnetwork.org*). Antivenom for stonefish and severe scorpionfish envenomation is made in Australia at the Commonwealth Serum Laboratories (*www.csl.com.au*, 61-3-389-1911).

MARINE POISONINGS

CIGUATERA

Ciguatera poisoning is the most common nonbacterial food poisoning associated with fish in the United States. Tropical and semitropical marine coral reef fish are usually the source; 75% of cases involve barracuda, snapper, jack, or grouper. Toxins may not affect the appearance or taste of the fish and are resistant to heat, cold, freeze-drying, and gastric acid.

Clinical Features   Most victims experience diarrhea, vomiting, and abdominal pain (typically 2–6 h after ingestion of contaminated fish), and symptoms increase in severity over the ensuing 4–6 h. The myriad manifestations include neurologic signs (e.g., paresthesia, weakness, fasciculations, ataxia), maculopapular or vesicular rash, and hemodynamic instability. A pathognomonic symptom—reversal of hot and cold perception—develops within 3–5 days and can last for months. Death is rare. A diagnosis is made on clinical grounds.

R_X Ciguatera Poisoning

Therapy is supportive and based on symptoms. Cool showers, hydroxyzine (25 mg PO q6–8h), or amitriptyline (25 mg PO bid) may ameliorate pruritus and dysesthesias. During recovery, the pt should avoid ingestion of fish, shell-fish, fish oils, fish or shellfish sauces, alcohol, nuts, and nut oils.

PARALYTIC SHELLFISH POISONING (PSP)

PSP is induced by ingestion of contaminated clams, oysters, scallops, mussels, and other species that concentrate water-soluble, heat- and acid-stable chemical toxins. Pts develop oral paresthesias that progress to the neck and extremities and that change to numbness within minutes to hours after ingestion of contam-inated shellfish. Flaccid paralysis and respiratory insufficiency may follow 2–12 h later. Treatment is supportive. If pts present within hours of ingestion, gas-tric lavage and stomach irrigation with 2 L of a 2% sodium bicarbonate solution may help, as may administration of activated charcoal (50–100 g) and a cathar-tic (sorbitol, 20–50 g). The pt should be monitored for respiratory paralysis for at least 24 h.

SCOMBROID

Etiology and Clinical Features   Scombroid poisoning is a histamine intoxica-tion due to inadequately preserved or refrigerated scombroid fish (e.g., tuna, mackerel, saury, needlefish, wahoo, skipjack, and bonito); it can also occur with exposure to nonscombroid fish, including sardines and herring. Within 15–90 min of ingestion, victims present with flushing, pruritus or urticaria, broncho-spasm, GI symptoms, tachycardia, and hypotension. Symptoms generally resolve within 8–12 h.

R_X Scombroid Poisoning

Treatment consists of antihistamine (H_1 or H_2) administration.

ARTHROPOD BITES AND STINGS

TICK BITES AND TICK PARALYSIS

Etiology and Clinical Features

- Ticks are important carriers of vector-borne diseases in the United States.
- Ticks attach and feed painlessly on blood from their hosts, but tick secre-tions may produce local reactions. Tick bites may cause a small area of in-duration and erythema. A necrotic ulcer occasionally develops; chronic nodules or tick granulomas may require surgical excision. Tick-induced fever and malaise resolve within 36 h after tick removal.
- Tick paralysis is an ascending flaccid paralysis due to a toxin in tick saliva that causes neuromuscular block and decreased nerve conduction. Paralysis begins in the lower extremities within 6 days after the tick's attachment and ascends symmetrically, causing complete paralysis of the extremities and cranial nerves. Deep tendon reflexes are decreased or absent, but sensory

examination and LP yield normal findings. Tick removal results in improvement within hours. Failure to remove the tick may lead ultimately to respiratory paralysis and death. The tick is often hidden beneath hair.

℞ Tick Bites and Tick Paralysis

Ticks should be removed with forceps applied close to the point of attachment, and the site of attachment should then be disinfected. Removal within 48 h of attachment usually prevents transmission of the agents of Lyme disease, babesiosis, anaplasmosis, and ehrlichiosis. Protective clothing and DEET application are protective measures that can be effective against ticks.

SPIDER BITES

Recluse Spider Bites Severe necrosis of skin and SC tissue follows a bite by the brown recluse spider. Spiders seek dark, undisturbed spots and bite only if threatened or pressed against the skin. The venoms contain enzymes that produce necrosis and hemolysis.

Clinical Features
- Initially the bite is painless or stings, but within hours the site becomes painful, pruritic, and indurated, with zones of ischemia and erythema.
- Fever and other nonspecific systemic symptoms may develop within 3 days of the bite.
- Lesions typically resolve within 2–3 days, but severe cases can leave a large ulcer and a depressed scar that take months to years to heal. Deaths are rare and are due to hemolysis and renal failure.

℞ Recluse Spider Bites

- Wound care, cold compress application, elevation and loose immobilization of the affected limb, and administration of analgesics, antihistamines, antibiotics, and tetanus prophylaxis should be undertaken as indicated.
- Dapsone administration within 48–72 h (50–100 mg PO bid after G6PD deficiency has been ruled out) may halt progression of necrotic lesions.

Widow Spider Bites **Etiology and Clinical Features** The black widow spider is most abundant in the southeastern United States. It measures up to 1 cm in body length and 5 cm in leg span, is shiny black, and has a red hourglass marking on the ventral abdomen. Female widow spiders produce a potent neurotoxin that binds irreversibly to nerves and causes release and depletion of acetylcholine and other neurotransmitters from presynaptic terminals. Within 60 min, painful cramps spread from the bite site to large muscles of the extremities and trunk. Extreme abdominal muscular rigidity and pain may mimic peritonitis, but the abdomen is nontender. Other features include salivation, diaphoresis, vomiting, hypertension, tachycardia, and myriad neurologic signs. Respiratory arrest, cerebral hemorrhage, or cardiac failure may occur.

℞ Widow Spider Bites

Treatment consists of local cleansing of the wound, application of ice packs to slow the spread of the venom, and tetanus prophylaxis. Analgesics, antispasmodics, and other supportive care should be given. Equine antivenom is available; rapid IV administration relieves pain and can be life-saving. However, because of the risk of anaphylaxis and serum sickness, antivenom use should be reserved for severe cases involving respiratory arrest, refractory hypertension, seizures, or pregnancy.

SCORPION STINGS

Etiology and Clinical Features   Among the venoms of scorpions in the United States, only the venom of the bark scorpion (*Centruroides sculpturatus* or *C. exilicauda*) is potentially lethal. The scorpion's neurotoxin opens sodium channels, and neurons fire repetitively. The sting causes little swelling, but pain, paresthesia, and hyperesthesia are prominent. Cranial nerve dysfunction and skeletal muscle hyperexcitability develop within hours. Symptoms include restlessness, blurred vision, abnormal eye movements, profuse salivation, slurred speech, diaphoresis, nausea, and vomiting. Complications include tachycardia, arrhythmias, hypertension, hyperthermia, rhabdomyolysis, and acidosis. Manifestations peak at 5 h and subside within a day or two, although paresthesias can last for weeks. Outside the United States, scorpion envenomations can cause massive release of endogenous catecholamines with hypertensive crises, arrhythmias, pulmonary edema, and myocardial damage.

 Scorpion Stings

Aggressive supportive care should include pressure dressings and cold packs to decrease the absorption of venom. Continuous IV administration of midazolam to decrease agitation and involuntary muscle movements may be needed. The benefit of scorpion antivenom has not been established in controlled trials.

HYMENOPTERA STINGS

The hymenoptera include apids (bees and bumblebees), vespids (wasps, hornets, and yellow jackets), and ants. About 100 deaths from hymenoptera stings occur annually in the United States, nearly all due to allergic reactions to venoms.

Clinical Features

- Honeybees can sting only once; other bees, vespids, and ants can sting many times in succession.
- Uncomplicated stings cause pain, a wheal-and-flare reaction, and local edema that subsides within hours.
- Multiple stings can lead to vomiting, diarrhea, generalized edema, dyspnea, hypotension, rhabdomyolysis, renal failure, and death.
- Large (>10 cm) local reactions progressing over 1–2 days are not uncommon and resemble cellulitis but are hypersensitivity reactions.
- About 0.4–4% of the U.S. population exhibits immediate-type hypersensitivity to insect stings. Serious reactions occur within 10 min of the sting and include upper airway edema, bronchospasm, hypotension, shock, and death.

 Hymenoptera Stings

- Stingers embedded in skin should be removed promptly by any method.
- The site should be cleansed and ice packs applied. Elevation of the bite site and administration of analgesics, oral antihistamines, and topical calamine lotion may ease symptoms.

- Oral glucocorticoids are indicated for large local reactions.
- Anaphylaxis is treated with epinephrine hydrochloride (0.3–0.5 mL of a 1:1000 solution, given SC q20–30min as needed). For profound shock, epinephrine (2–5 mL of a 1:10,000 solution by slow IV push) is indicated. Pts should be observed for 24 h because of the risk of recurrence.
- Pts with a history of allergy to insect stings should carry a sting kit and seek medical attention immediately after the kit is used. Adults with a history of anaphylaxis should undergo desensitization.

For a more detailed discussion, see Madoff LC, Pereyra F: Infectious Complications of Burns and Bites, Chap. e15 in Harrison's DVD and in Harrison's Online; and Auerbach PS, Norris RL: Disorders Caused by Reptile Bites and Marine Animal Exposures, Chap. 391, p. 2741; and Pollack RJ, Maguire JH: Ectoparasite Infestations and Arthropod Bites and Stings, Chap. 392, p. 2748, in HPIM-17.

30 Hypothermia and Frostbite

HYPOTHERMIA

Hypothermia is defined as a core body temperature of ≤35°C and is classified as mild (32.2°–35°C), moderate (28°–32.2°C), or severe (<28°C).

Etiology Most cases occur during the winter in cold climates, but hypothermia may occur in mild climates and is usually multifactorial. Heat is generated in most tissues of the body and is lost by radiation, conduction, convection, evaporation, and respiration. Factors that impede heat generation and/or increase heat loss lead to hypothermia (Table 30-1).

Clinical Features Acute cold exposure causes tachycardia, increased cardiac output, peripheral vasoconstriction, and increased peripheral vascular resistance. As body temperature drops below 32°C, cardiac conduction becomes impaired, the heart rate slows, and cardiac output decreases. Atrial fibrillation with slow ventricular response is common. Other ECG changes include Osborn (J) waves. Additional manifestations of hypothermia include volume depletion, hypotension, increased blood viscosity (which can lead to thrombosis), coagulopathy, thrombocytopenia, DIC, acid-base disturbances, and bronchospasm. CNS abnormalities are diverse and can include ataxia, amnesia, hallucinations, hyporeflexia, and (in severe hypothermia) an isoelectric EEG. Hypothermia may mask other concurrent disorders, such as an acute abdomen, drug toxicity, or spinal cord injury.

Diagnosis Hypothermia is confirmed by measuring the core temperature, preferably at two sites. Since oral thermometers are usually calibrated only as low as 34.4°C, the exact temperature of a patient whose initial reading is <35°C should be determined with a rectal thermocouple probe inserted to ≥15 cm and not adjacent to cold feces. Simultaneously, an esophageal probe should be placed 24 cm below the larynx.

TABLE 30-1 **RISK FACTORS FOR HYPOTHERMIA**

Age extremes	Neurologic-related
Elderly	Stroke
Neonates	Hypothalamic disorders
Outdoor exposure	Parkinson's disease
Occupational	Spinal cord injury
Sports-related	Multisystem
Inadequate clothing	Malnutrition
Cold-water immersion	Sepsis
Drugs and intoxicants	Shock
Ethanol	Hepatic or renal failure
Phenothiazines	Diabetic ketoacidosis
Barbiturates	Lactic acidosis
Anesthetics	Burns and exfoliative dermatologic disorders
Neuromuscular blockers	Immobility or debilitation
Endocrine-related	
Hypoglycemia	
Hypothyroidism	
Adrenal insufficiency	
Hypopituitarism	

R̲x̲ Hypothermia

Cardiac monitoring and supplemental oxygen should be instituted, along with attempts to limit further heat loss. Mild hypothermia is managed by passive external rewarming and insulation. The pt should be placed in a warm environment and covered with blankets to allow endogenous heat production to restore normal body temperature. With the head also covered, the rate of rewarming is usually 0.5°–2.0°C/h. Active rewarming is necessary for moderate to severe hypothermia, cardiovascular instability, age extremes, CNS dysfunction, endocrine insufficiency, or hypothermia due to complications from systemic disorders. Active rewarming may be external (forced-air heating blankets, radiant heat sources, and hot packs) or internal (by inspiration of heated, humidified oxygen warmed to 40°–45°C, by administration of IV fluids warmed to 40°–42°C, or by peritoneal or pleural lavage with dialysate or saline warmed to 40°–45°C). The most efficient active internal rewarming techniques are extracorporeal rewarming by hemodialysis and cardiopulmonary bypass. External rewarming may cause a fall in blood pressure by relieving peripheral vasoconstriction. Volume should be repleted with warmed isotonic solutions; lactated Ringer's solution should be avoided because of impaired lactate metabolism in hypothermia. If sepsis is a possibility, empirical broad-spectrum antibiotics should be administered after sending blood cultures. Atrial arrhythmias usually require no specific treatment. Ventricular fibrillation is often refractory. Only a single sequence of 3 defibrillation attempts (2 J/kg) should be attempted when the temperature is <30°C. Since it is sometimes difficult to distinguish profound hypothermia from death, cardiopulmonary resuscitation efforts and active internal rewarming should continue until the core temperature is >32°C or cardiovascular status has been stabilized.

FROSTBITE

Frostbite occurs when the tissue temperature drops below 0°C. Clinically, it is most practical to classify frostbite as superficial (involves skin only) or deep

TABLE 30-2	TREATMENT FOR FROSTBITE	
Before Thawing	During Thawing	After Thawing
Remove from environment	Consider parenteral analgesia and ketorolac	Gently dry and protect part; elevate; pledgets between toes, if macerated
Prevent partial thawing and refreezing	Administer ibuprofen, 400 mg PO	If clear vesicles are intact, the fluid will reabsorb in days; if broken, debride and dress with antibiotic or sterile aloe vera ointment
Stabilize core temperature and treat hypothermia	Immerse part in 37°–40°C (thermometer-monitored) circulating water containing an antiseptic soap until distal flush (10–45 min)	Leave hemorrhagic vesicles intact to prevent infection
Protect frozen part—no friction or massage	Encourage patient to gently move part	Continue ibuprofen 400 mg PO (12 mg/kg per day) q8–12h
Address medical or surgical conditions	If pain is refractory, reduce water temperature to 33°–37°C and administer parenteral narcotics	Consider tetanus and streptococcal prophylaxis; elevate part
Hydrotherapy at 37°C

(involves deep tissues, muscle, and bone). Classically, frostbite is retrospectively graded like a burn (first- to fourth-degree) once the resultant pathology is demarcated over time.

Clinical Features   The initial presentation of frostbite can be deceptively benign. The symptoms always include a sensory deficit affecting light touch, pain, and temperature perception. Deep frostbitten tissue can appear waxy, mottled, yellow, or violaceous-white. Favorable presenting signs include some warmth or sensation with normal color. Hemorrhagic vesicles reflect a serious injury to the microvasculature and indicate third-degree frostbite. Differential diagnosis of frostbite includes chilblain and immersion (trench) foot.

℞ Frostbite

A treatment protocol for frostbite is summarized in Table 30-2. Frozen tissue should be rapidly and completely thawed by immersion in circulating water at 37°–40°C. Thawing should not be terminated prematurely due to pain from reperfusion; ibuprofen, 400 mg, should be given, and parenteral narcotics are often required. If cyanosis persists after rewarming, the tissue compartment pressures should be monitored carefully. Patients with parts showing no flow on ^{99m}Tc scintiscan may be candidates for tissue plasminogen activator (tPA)

For a more detailed discussion, see Danzl DF: Hypothermia and Frostbite, Chap. 20, p. 135, in HPIM-17.

31 Poisoning and Drug Overdose

Poisoning refers to the development of harmful effects following exposure to chemicals. *Overdosage* is exposure to excessive amounts of a substance normally intended for consumption and does not necessarily imply poisoning. Chemical exposures result in an estimated 5 million requests in the United States for medical advice or treatment each year, and about 5% of victims of chemical exposure require hospitalization. Suicide attempts account for most serious or fatal poisonings. Up to 30% of psychiatric admissions are prompted by attempted suicide via overdosage.

Carbon monoxide (CO) poisoning is the leading cause of death. Acetaminophen toxicity is the most common pharmaceutical agent causing fatalities. Other drug-related fatalities are commonly due to analgesics, antidepressants, sedative-hypnotics, neuroleptics, stimulants and street drugs, cardiovascular drugs, anticonvulsants, antihistamines, and asthma therapies. Nonpharmaceutical agents implicated in fatal poisoning include alcohols and glycols, gases and fumes, chemicals, cleaning substances, pesticides, and automotive products. The diagnosis of poisoning or drug overdose must be considered in any pt who presents with coma, seizure, or acute renal, hepatic, or bone marrow failure.

DIAGNOSIS

The correct diagnosis can usually be reached by history, physical exam, and routine and toxicologic laboratory evaluation. All available sources should be used to determine the exact nature of the ingestion or exposure. The *history* should include the time, route, duration, and circumstances (location, surrounding events, and intent) of exposure; time of onset, nature, and severity of symptoms; relevant past medical and psychiatric history. The Physicians Desk Reference, regional poison control centers, and local/hospital pharmacies may be useful for identification of ingredients and potential effects of toxins.

The diagnosis of poisoning in cases of unknown etiology primarily relies on pattern recognition. The first step is a *physical exam* with initial focus on the pulse, blood pressure, respiratory rate, temperature, and neurologic status and then characterization of the overall physiologic state as stimulated, depressed, discordant, or normal (Table 31-1).

Examination of the eyes (for nystagmus, pupil size, and reactivity), abdomen (for bowel activity and bladder size), and skin (for burns, bullae, color, warmth, moisture, pressure sores, and puncture marks) may narrow the diagnosis to a particular disorder. The pt should also be examined for evidence of trauma and underlying illnesses. When the history is unclear, all orifices should be examined for the presence of chemical burns and drug packets. The odor of breath or vomitus and the color of nails, skin, or urine may provide diagnostic clues.

Initial laboratory studies should include glucose, serum electrolytes, serum osmolality, BUN/creatinine, LFTs, PT/PTT, and ABGs. An increased anion-gap metabolic acidosis is characteristic of advanced methanol, ethylene glycol, and salicylate intoxication but can occur with other agents and in any poisoning that results in hepatic, renal, or respiratory failure; seizures; or shock. An increased osmolal gap—the difference between the serum osmolality (measured by freezing point depression) and that calculated from the serum sodium, glucose, and

TABLE 31-1 DIFFERENTIAL DIAGNOSIS OF POISONING BASED ON PHYSIOLOGIC STATE

Stimulated	Depressed	Discordant	Normal
Sympathetics	Sympatholytics	Asphyxiants	Nontoxic exposure
Sympathomimetics	α_1-Adrenergic antagonists	Cytochrome oxidase inhibitors	Psychogenic illness
Ergot alkaloids	α_2-Adrenergic agonists	Inert gases	Toxic time-bombs
Methylxanthines	ACE inhibitors	Irritant gases	Slow absorption
MAO inhibitors	Angiotensin receptor blockers	Methemoglobin inducers	Anticholinergics
Thyroid hormones	Antipsychotics	Oxidative phosphorylation inhibitors	Carbamazepine
Anticholinergics	β-Adrenergic blockers	AGMA inducers	Concretion formers
Antihistamines	Calcium channel blockers	Alcohol (ketoacidosis)	Dilantin Kapseals
Antiparkinsonian agents	Cardiac glycosides	Ethylene glycol	Drug packets
Antipsychotics	Cyclic antidepressants	Iron	Enteric-coated pills
Antispasmodics	Cholinergics	Methanol	Lomotil
Belladonna alkaloids	Acetylcholinesterase inhibitors	Salicylate	Opioids
Cyclic antidepressants	Muscarinic agonists	Toluene	Salicylates
Muscle relaxants	Nicotinic agonists	CNS syndromes	Sustained-release pills
Mushrooms and plants	Opioids	Extrapyramidal reactions	Slow distribution
Hallucinogens	Analgesics	Hydrocarbon inhalation	Cardiac glycosides
Cannabinoids (marijuana)	GI antispasmodics	Isoniazid	Lithium
LSD and analogues	Heroin	Lithium	Metals
Mescaline and analogues	Sedative-hypnotics	Neuroleptic malignant syndrome	Salicylate
Mushrooms	Alcohols	Serotonin syndrome	Toxic metabolite
Phencyclidine and analogues	Anticonvulsants	Strychnine	Acetaminophen
Withdrawal syndromes	Barbiturates	Membrane-active agents	Carbon tetrachloride
Barbiturates	Benzodiazepines	Amantidine	Cyanogenic glycosides
Benzodiazepines	GABA precursors	Antiarrhythmics	Ethylene glycol

(continued)

131

TABLE 31-1 DIFFERENTIAL DIAGNOSIS OF POISONING BASED ON PHYSIOLOGIC STATE (CONTINUED)

Stimulated	Depressed	Discordant	Normal
Ethanol	Muscle relaxants	Antihistamines	Methanol
Opioids	Other agents	Antipsychotics	Methemoglobin inducers
Sedative-hypnotics	GHB Products	Carbamazepine	Mushroom toxins
Sympatholytics		Cyclic antidepressants	Organophosphate insecticides
		Local anesthetics	Paraquat
		Opioids (some)	Metabolism disruptors
		Orphenadrine	Antineoplastic agents
		Quinoline antimalarials	Antiviral agents
			Colchicine
			Hypoglycemic agents
			Immunosuppressive agents
			MAO inhibitors
			Metals
			Salicylate
			Warfarins

Note: AGMA, anion-gap metabolic alkalosis; GHB, γ-hydroxybutyric; LSD, lysergic acid diethylamide; GABA, γ-aminobutyric acid; MAO; monoamine oxidase.

BUN of >10 mmol/L—suggests the presence of a low-molecular-weight solute such as an alcohol, glycol, or ketone or an unmeasured electrolyte or sugar. Ketosis suggests acetone, isopropyl alcohol, or salicylate poisoning. Hypoglycemia may be due to poisoning with β-adrenergic blockers, ethanol, insulin, oral hypoglycemic agents, quinine, and salicylates, whereas hyperglycemia can occur in poisoning with acetone, β-adrenergic agonists, calcium channel blockers, iron, theophylline, or Vacor.

Radiologic studies should include a chest x-ray to exclude aspiration or ARDS. Radiopaque densities may be visible on abdominal x-rays. Head CT or MRI is indicated in stuporous or comatose pts to exclude structural lesions or subarachnoid hemorrhage, and LP should be performed when CNS infection is suspected. The *ECG* can be useful to assist with the differential diagnosis and to guide treatment. *Toxicologic analysis* of urine and blood (and occasionally of gastric contents and chemical samples) may be useful to confirm or rule out suspected poisoning. Although rapid screening tests for a limited number of drugs of abuse are available, comprehensive screening tests require 2–6 h for completion, and immediate management must be based on the history, physical exam, and routine ancillary tests. Quantitative analysis is useful for poisoning with acetaminophen, acetone, alcohol (including ethylene glycol), antiarrhythmics, anticonvulsants, barbiturates, digoxin, heavy metals, lithium, salicylate, and theophylline, as well as for carboxyhemoglobin and methemoglobin. Results can often be available within an hour.

The response to antidotes may be useful for diagnostic purposes. Resolution of altered mental status and abnormal vital signs within minutes of intravenous administration of dextrose, naloxone, or flumazenil is virtually diagnostic of hypoglycemia, narcotic poisoning, and benzodiazepine intoxication, respectively. The prompt reversal of acute dystonic (extrapyramidal) reactions following an intravenous dose of benztropine or diphenhydramine confirms a drug etiology. Although physostigmine reversal of both central and peripheral manifestations of anticholinergic poisoning is diagnostic, it may cause arousal in patients with CNS depression of any etiology.

R_X　Poisoning and Drug Overdose

Goals of therapy include support of vital signs, prevention of further absorption, enhancement of elimination, administration of specific antidotes, and prevention of reexposure. Fundamentals of poisoning management are listed in Table 31-2. Treatment is usually initiated before routine and toxicologic data are known. All symptomatic pts need large-bore IV access, supplemental O_2, cardiac monitoring, continuous observation, and, if mental status is altered, 100 mg thiamine (IM or IV), 1 ampule of 50% dextrose in water, and 4 mg of naloxone along with specific antidotes as indicated. Unconscious pts should be intubated. Activated charcoal may be given PO or via a large-bore gastric tube; gastric lavage requires an orogastric tube. Severity of poisoning determines the management. Admission to an ICU is indicated for pts with severe poisoning (coma, respiratory depression, hypotension, cardiac conduction abnormalities, arrhythmias, hypothermia or hyperthermia, seizures); those needing close monitoring, antidotes, or enhanced elimination therapy; and those with progressive clinical deterioration or significant underlying medical problems. Suicidal pts require constant observation by qualified personnel.

Supportive Care
Airway protection is mandatory. Gag reflex alone is not a reliable indicator of the need for intubation. Need for O_2 supplementation and ventilatory support

TABLE 31-2	FUNDAMENTALS OF POISONING MANAGEMENT

Supportive Care

Airway protection	Treatment of seizures
Oxygenation/ventilation	Correction of temperature abnormalities
Treatment of arrhythmias	Correction of metabolic derangements
Hemodynamic support	Prevention of secondary complications

Prevention of Further Poison Absorption

Gastrointestinal decontamination	Decontamination of other sites
Gastric lavage	Eye decontamination
Activated charcoal	Skin decontamination
Whole-bowel irrigation	Body cavity evacuation
Catharsis	
Dilution	
Endoscopic/surgical removal	

Enhancement of Poison Elimination

Multiple-dose activated charcoal	Extracorporeal removal
Diuresis	Peritoneal dialysis
Alteration of urinary pH	Hemodialysis
Chelation	Hemoperfusion
	Hemofiltration
	Plasmapheresis
	Exchange transfusion
	Hyperbaric oxygenation

Administration of Antidotes

Neutralization by antibodies	Metabolic antagonism
Neutralization by chemical binding	Physiologic antagonism

Prevention of Reexposure

Adult education	Notification of regulatory agencies
Child-proofing	Psychiatric referral

can be assessed by measurement of ABGs. Drug-induced pulmonary edema is usually secondary to hypoxia, but myocardial depression may contribute. Measurement of pulmonary artery pressure may be necessary to establish etiology. Electrolyte imbalances should be corrected as soon as possible.

Supraventricular tachycardia (SVT) with hypertension and CNS excitation is almost always due to sympathetic, anticholinergic, or hallucinogenic stimulation or to drug withdrawal. Treatment is indicated if associated with hemodynamic instability, chest pain, or ischemia on ECG. Treatment with combined alpha and beta blockers or combinations of beta blocker and vasodilator is indicated in severe sympathetic hyperactivity. Physostigmine is useful for anticholinergic hyperactivity. SVT without hypertension usually responds to fluid administration.

Ventricular tachycardia (VT) can be caused by sympathetic stimulation, myocardial membrane destabilization, or metabolic derangements. Lidocaine and phenytoin are generally safe. Drugs that prolong the QT interval (quinidine, procainamide) should not be used in VT due to tricyclic antidepressant overdose. Magnesium sulfate and overdrive pacing (by isoproterenol or a pacemaker) may be useful for torsades de pointes. Arrhythmias may be resistant to therapy until underlying acid-base and electrolyte derangements, hypoxia, and hypothermia are corrected. It is acceptable to observe hemodynamically stable pts without pharmacologic intervention.

Seizures are best treated with γ-aminobutyric acid agonists such as benzodiazepines or barbiturates. Barbiturates should be given only after intubation. Seizures caused by isoniazid overdose may respond only to large doses of pyridoxine IV. Seizures from beta blockers or tricyclic antidepressants may require phenytoin and benzodiazepines.

Prevention of Poison Absorption

Whether or not to perform GI decontamination, and which procedure to use, depends on the time since ingestion; the existing and predicted toxicity of the ingestant; the availability, efficacy, and contraindications of the procedure; and the nature, severity, and risk of complications. The efficacy of activated charcoal and gastric lavage decreases with time, and there are insufficient data to support or exclude a beneficial effect when they are used >1 h after ingestion. Activated charcoal has comparable or greater efficacy, fewer contraindications and complications, and is less invasive than gastric lavage and is the preferred method of GI decontamination in most situations.

Activated charcoal is prepared as a suspension in water, either alone or with a cathartic. It is given orally via a nippled bottle (for infants), or via a cup, straw, or small-bore nasogastric tube. The recommended dose is 1 g/kg body weight, using 8 mL of diluent per gram of charcoal if a premixed formulation is not available. Charcoal may inhibit absorption of other orally administered agents and is contraindicated in pts with corrosive ingestion.

When indicated, gastric lavage is performed using a 28F orogastric tube in children and a 40F orogastric tube in adults. Saline or tap water may be used in adults or children (use saline in infants). Place pt in Trendelenburg and left lateral decubitus position to minimize aspiration (occurs in 10% of pts). Lavage is contraindicated with corrosives and petroleum distillate hydrocarbons because of risk of aspiration-induced pneumonia and gastroesophageal perforation.

Whole-bowel irrigation may be useful with ingestions of foreign bodies, drug packets, and slow-release medications. Golytely is given orally or by gastric tube up to a rate of 2 L/h. Cathartic salts (magnesium citrate) and saccharides (sorbitol, mannitol) promote evacuation of the rectum. Dilution of corrosive acids and alkali is accomplished by having pt drink 5 mL water/kg. Endoscopy or surgical intervention may be required in large foreign-body ingestion, heavy metal ingestion, and when ingested drug packets leak or rupture.

Syrup of ipecac, once the most commonly used decontamination procedure, has no role in the hospital setting. The American Academy of Pediatrics (AAP) issued a policy statement in 2003 recommending that ipecac should no longer be routinely considered in poisoning treatment. Some argue it can still be considered for the home management of patients with accidental ingestions, reliable histories, and mild predicted toxicity when transport to a hospital site is prolonged. It is administered orally in doses of 30 mL for adults, 15 mL for children, and 10 mL for infants. Vomiting should occur within 20 min. Ipecac is contraindicated with marginal airway patency, CNS depression, recent GI surgery, seizures, corrosive (lye) ingestion, petroleum hydrocarbon ingestion, and rapidly acting CNS poisons (camphor, cyanide, tricyclic antidepressants, propoxyphene, strychnine).

Skin and eyes are decontaminated by washing with copious amounts of water or saline.

TABLE 31-3 PATHOPHYSIOLOGIC FEATURES AND TREATMENT OF SPECIFIC TOXIC SYNDROMES AND POISONINGS

Physiologic Condition, Causes	Examples	Mechanism of Action	Clinical Features	Specific Treatments
Stimulated				
Sympathetics (see also Chap. 389)				
Sympathomimetics	α₁-Adrenergic agonists (decongestants): phenylephrine, phenylpropanolamine β₂-Adrenergic agonists (bronchodilators): albuterol, terbutaline Nonspecific adrenergic agonists: amphetamines, cocaine, ephedrine	Stimulation of central and peripheral sympathetic receptors directly or indirectly (by promoting the release or inhibiting the reuptake of norepinephrine and sometimes dopamine)	Physiologic stimulation (Table e35-2); reflex bradycardia can occur with selective α₁ agonists; β agonists can cause hypotension and hypokalemia.	Phentolamine, a nonselective α₁-adrenergic receptor antagonist, for severe hypertension due to α₁-adrenergic agonists; propranolol, a nonselective β blocker, for hypotension and tachycardia due to β₂ agonists; labetalol, a β blocker with α-blocking activity, or phentolamine with esmolol, metoprolol, or other cardioselective β blocker for hypertension with tachycardia due to nonselective agents (β blockers, if used alone, can exacerbate hypertension and vasospasm due to unopposed α stimulation); benzodiazepines; propofol.

| Ergot alkaloids | Ergotamine, methysergide, bromocriptine, pergolide | Stimulation and inhibition of serotonergic and α-adrenergic receptors; stimulation of dopamine receptors | Physiologic stimulation (Table e35–2); formication; vasospasm with limb (isolated or generalized), myocardial, and cerebral ischemia progressing to gangrene or infarction; hypotension, bradycardia, and involuntary movements can also occur. | Nitroprusside or nitroglycerine for severe vasospasm; prazocin (an α_1 blocker), captopril, nifedipine, and cyproheptidene (a serotonin receptor antagonist) for mild to moderate limb ischemia; dopamine receptor antagonists (antipsychotics) for hallucinations and movement disorders |
| Methylxanthines | Caffeine, theophylline | Inhibition of adenosine synthesis and adenosine receptor antagonism; stimulation of epinephrine and norepinephrine release; inhibition of phosphodiesterase resulting in increased intracellular cyclic adenosine and quanosine monophosphate | Physiologic stimulation (Table e35–2); pronounced gastrointestinal symptoms and β agonist effects (see above). Toxicity occurs at lower drug levels in chronic poisoning than in acute poisoning. | Propranolol, a nonselective β blocker, for tachycardia with hypotension; any β blocker for supraventricular or ventricular tachycardia without hypotension; elimination enhanced by multiple-dose charcoal, hemoperfusion, and hemodialysis; indications for hemoperfusion or hemodialysis include unstable vital signs, seizures, and a theophylline level of 80–100 µg/mL after acute overdose and 40–60 µg/mL with chronic exposure. |

(continued)

137

TABLE 31-3 PATHOPHYSIOLOGIC FEATURES AND TREATMENT OF SPECIFIC TOXIC SYNDROMES AND POISONINGS (CONTINUED)

Physiologic Condition, Causes	Examples	Mechanism of Action	Clinical Features	Specific Treatments
Monoamine oxidase inhibitors	Phenelzine, tranylcypromine, selegiline	Inhibition of monoamine oxidase resulting in impaired metabolism of endogenous catecholamines and exogenous sympathomimetic agents	Delayed or slowly progressive physiologic stimulation (Table e35-2); terminal hypotension and bradycardia in severe cases.	Short-acting agents (e.g., nitroprusside, esmolol) for severe hypertension and tachycardia; direct-acting sympathomimetics (e.g., norepinephrine, epinephrine) for hypotension and bradycardia
Anticholinergics Antihistamines	Diphenhydramine, doxylamine, pyrilamine	Inhibition of central and postganglionic parasympathetic muscarinic cholinergic receptors. At high doses, amantidine, diphenhydramine, orphenadrine, phenothiazines, and tricyclic antidepressants have additional nonanticholinergic activity (see below).	Physiologic stimulation (Table e35-2); dry skin and mucous membranes, decreased bowel sounds, flushing, and urinary retention; myoclonus and picking activity. Central effects may occur without significant autonomic dysfunction.	Physostigmine, an acetylcholinesterase inhibitor (see below) for delirium, hallucinations, and neuromuscular hyperactivity. Contraindications include nonanticholinergic cardiovascular toxicity (e.g., cardiac conduction abnormalities, hypotension, and ventricular arrhythmias).
Antiparkinsonian agents	Amantidine, trihexiphenydyl			
Antipsychotics	Chlorpromazine, olanzapine, quetiapine, thioridazine			
Antispasmotics	Clinidium, dicyclomine			
Belladonna alkaloids	Atropine, hyoscyamine, scopolamine			
Cyclic antidepressants	Amitriptyline, doxepin, imipramine			
Muscle relaxants	Cyclobenzaprine, orphenadrine			
Mushrooms and plants	Amanita muscaria and A. pantherina, henbane, jimson weed, nightshade			

Depressed

Sympatholytics			
α_2-Adrenergic agonists	Clonidine, guanabenz, tetrahydrozoline and other imidazoline decongestants, tizanidine and other imidazoline muscle relaxants	Stimulation of α_2-adrenergic receptors leading to inhibition of CNS sympathetic outflow; activity at nonadrenergic imidazoline binding sites also contributes to CNS effects.	Physiologic depression (Table e35-2), miosis. Transient initial hypertension may be seen.	Dopamine and norepinephrine for hypotension. Atropine for symptomatic bradycardia. Naloxone for CNS depression (inconsistently effective).
Antipsychotics	Chlorpromazine, clozapine, haloperidol, risperidone, thioridazine	Inhibition of α-adrenergic, dopaminergic, histaminergic, muscarinic, and serotonergic receptors. Some agents also inhibit sodium, potassium, and calcium channels.	Physiologic depression (Table e35-2), miosis, anticholinergic effects (see above), extrapyramidal reactions (see below), tachycardia. Cardiac conduction delays (increased PR, QRS, JT, and QT intervals) with ventricular tachydysrhythmias, including torsades des pointes, can sometimes develop.	Sodium bicarbonate and lidocaine for ventricular tachydysrhythmias associated with QRS prolongation. Magnesium, isoproterenol, and overdrive pacing for torsades de pointes. Avoid class IA, IC, and III antiarrhythmics.

(continued)

139

Physiologic Condition, Causes	Examples	Mechanism of Action	Clinical Features	Specific Treatments
β-Adrenergic blockers	Cardioselective (β₁) blockers: atenolol, esmolol, metoprolol Nonselective (β₁ and β₂) blockers: nadolol, propranolol, timolol Partial β agonists: acebutolol, pindolol α₁ Antagonists: carvedilol, labetalol Membrane-active agents: acebutolol, propranolol, sotalol	Inhibition of β-adrenergic receptors (class II antiarrhythmic effect). Some agents have activity at additional receptors or have membrane effects (see below).	Physiologic depression (Table e35-2), atrioventricular block, hypoglycemia, hyperkalemia, seizures. Partial agonists can cause hypertension and tachycardia. Sotalol can cause increased QT interval and ventricular tachydysrhythmias. Onset may be delayed after sotalol and sustained-release formulation overdose.	Glucagon and calcium for hypotension and symptomatic bradycardia. Atropine, isoproterenol, amrinone, dopamine, dobutamine, epinephrine, and norepinephrine may sometimes be effective. High-dose insulin (with glucose and potassium to maintain euglycemia and normokalemia), electrical pacing, and mechanical cardiovascular support for refractory cases.
Calcium channel blockers	Diltiazem, nifedipine and other dihydropyridine derivatives, verapamil	Inhibition of slow (type L) cardiovascular calcium channels (class IV antiarrhythmic effect).	Physiologic depression (Table e35-2), atrioventricular block, organ ischemia and infarction, hyperglycemia, seizures. Hypotension is usually due to decreased vascular resistance rather than to decreased cardiac output. Onset may be delayed for ≥12 h after overdose of sustained-release formulations.	Calcium and glucagon for hypotension and symptomatic bradycardia. Dopamine, epinephrine, norepinephrine, atropine, and isoproterenol are less often effective but can be used adjunctively. Amrinone, high-dose insulin (with glucose and potassium to maintain euglycemia and normokalemia), electrical pacing, and mechanical cardiovascular support for refractory cases.

	Pharmacologic Effects	Clinical Presentation	Treatment
Cardiac glycosides	Digoxin, endogenous cardioactive steroids, foxglove and other plants, toad skin secretions (*Bufonidae* sp.)	Inhibition of cardiac Na$^+$, K$^+$-ATPase membrane pump.	Physiologic depression (Table e35-2); gastrointestinal, psychiatric, and visual symptoms; atrioventricular block with or without concomitant supraventricular tachyarrhythmia; ventricular tachyarrhythmias. Hyperkalemia in acute poisoning. Toxicity occurs at lower drug levels in chronic poisoning than in acute poisoning.	Digoxin-specific antibody fragments for hemodynamically compromising dysrhythmias, Mobitz II or third-degree atrioventricular block, hyperkalemia (>5.5 meq/L; in acute poisoning only). Temporizing measures include atropine, dopamine, epinephrine, phenytoin, and external cardiac pacing for bradydysrhythmias and magnesium, lidocaine, phenytoin, and bretylium for ventricular tachydysrhythmias. Internal cardiac pacing and cardioversion can increase ventricular irritability and should be reserved for refractory cases.
Cyclic antidepressants	Amitriptyline, doxepin, imipramine	Inhibition of α-adrenergic dopaminergic, GABA-ergic, histaminergic, muscarinic, and serotonergic receptors; inhibition of sodium channels (see membrane-active agents); inhibition of norepinephrine and serotonin reuptake.	Physiologic depression (Table e35-2), seizures, tachycardia, cardiac conduction delays (increased PR, QRS, JT, and QT intervals; terminal QRS right axis deviation) with aberrancy and ventricular tachydysrhythmias. Anticholinergic toxidrome (see above).	Hypertonic sodium bicarbonate (or hypertonic saline) and lidocaine for ventricular tachydysrhythmias associated with QRS prolongation. Use of phenytoin is controversial. Avoid class IA, IC, and III antiarrhythmics.

(continued)

Physiologic Condition, Causes	Examples	Mechanism of Action	Clinical Features	Specific Treatments
Cholinergics				
Acetylcholinesterase inhibitors	Carbamate insecticides (aldicarb, carbaryl, propoxur) and medicinals (neostigmine, physostigmine, tacrine); nerve gases (sarin, soman, tabun, VX) organophosphate insecticides (diazinon, chlopryriphos, malathion)	Inhibition of acetylcholinesterase leading to increased synaptic acetylcholine at muscarinic and nicotinic cholinergic receptor sites	Physiologic depression (Table e35-2). Muscarinic signs and symptoms: seizures, excessive secretions (lacrimation, salivation, bronchorrhea and wheezing, diaphoresis), and increased bowel and bladder activity with nausea, vomiting, diarrhea, abdominal cramps, and incontinence of feces and urine. Nicotinic signs and symptoms: hypertension, tachycardia, muscle cramps, fasciculations, weakness, and paralysis. Death is usually due to respiratory failure. Cholinesterase activity in plasma and red cells <50% of normal in acetylcholinesterase inhibitor poisoning.	Atropine for muscarinic signs and symptoms. Pralidoxime (2-PAM), a cholinesterase reactivator, for nicotinic signs and symptoms due to organophosphates, nerve gases, or an unknown anticholinesterase.
Muscarinic agonists	Bethanecol, mushrooms (*Boletus, Clitocybe, Inocybe* sp.), pilocarpine	Stimulation of CNS and postganglionic parasympathetic cholinergic (muscarinic) receptors		
Nicotinic agonists	Lobeline, nicotine (tobacco)	Stimulation of preganglionic sympathetic and parasympathetic and striated muscle (neuromuscular junction) cholinergic (nicotine) receptors		

Sedative-hypnotics (see also Chap. 388)

	Examples	Mechanism	Clinical features	Treatment
Anticonvulsants	Carbamazepine, ethosuximide, felbamate, gabapentin, lamotrigine, levetiracetam, oxcarbazepine, phenytoin, tiagabine, topiramate, valproate, zonisamide	Ethosuximide, valproate, and zonisamide decrease conduction through T-type calcium channels; valproate	Physiologic depression (Table e35-2), nystagmus. Delayed absorption can occur with carbamazepine, phenytoin, and valproate. Myoclonus, seizures, hypertension, and tachyarrhythmias can occur with baclofen, carbamazepine, and orphenadrine.	Flumazenil for benzodiazepine and zolpidem poisoning. Benzodiazepines and barbiturates for seizures. Elimination of phenobarbital and possibly other long-acting agents enhanced by multiple-dose charcoal. Hemodialysis and hemoperfusion may be indicated for severe poisoning by some agents (see Extracorporeal Removal, in text). See above and below for treatment of anticholinergic and sodium channel (membrane) blocking effects.
Barbiturates	Short-acting: butabarbital, pentobarbital, secobarbital	Potentiation of the inhibitory effects of GABA by binding to the neuronal GABA-A chloride channel receptor complex and increasing the frequency or duration of chloride channel opening in response to GABA stimulation. Baclofen and, to some extent, GHB act at the GABA-B receptor complex; meprobamate, its metabolite carisoprodol, felbamate, and orphenidrine antagonize *N*-methyl-D-aspartate (NDMA) excitatory receptors; ethosuximide,	Tachyarrhythmias can also occur with chloral hydrate. AGMA, hypernatremia, hyperosmolality, hyperammonemia, chemical hepatitis, and hypoglycemia can be seen in valproate poisoning. Carbamazepine and oxcarbazepine may produce hyponatremia from SIADH.	
	Long-acting: phenobarbital, primadone			
Benzodiazepines	Ultrashort-acting: estazolam, midazolam, temazepam, triazolam			
	Short-acting: alprazolam, flunitrazepam, lorazepam, oxazepam			
	Long-acting: chlordiazepoxide, clonazepam, diazepam, flurazepam			
	Pharmacologically related agents: zaleplon, zolpidem			

(continued)

TABLE 31-3 PATHOPHYSIOLOGIC FEATURES AND TREATMENT OF SPECIFIC TOXIC SYNDROMES AND POISONINGS (CONTINUED)

Physiologic Condition, Causes	Examples	Mechanism of Action	Clinical Features	Specific Treatments
GABA precursors	γ-Hydroxybutyrate (sodium oxybate; GHB), γ-butyrolactone (GBL), 1,4-butanediol.	Decreases GABA degradation, and tiagabine blocks GABA reuptake; carbamazepine, lamotrigine, oxcarbazepine, phenytoin, topiramate, valproate, and zonisamide slow the rate of recovery of inactivated sodium channels. Some agents also have α_2 agonist, anticholinergic, and sodium channel blocking activity (see above and below).	Some agents can cause anticholinergic and sodium channel (membrane) blocking effects (see above and below).	
Muscle relaxants	Baclofen, carisoprodol, cyclobenzaprine, etomidate, metaxalone, methocarbamol, orphenadrine, propafol, tizanidine and other imidazoline muscle relaxants.			
Other agents	Chloral hydrate, ethchlorvynol, glutethimide, meprobamate, methaqualone, methyprylon.			

Discordant

Asphyxiants			
Cytochrome oxidase inhibitors	Carbon monoxide, cyanide, hydrogen sulfide	Inhibition of mitochondrial cytochrome oxidase, thereby blocking electron transport and oxidative metabolism. Carbon monoxide also binds to hemoglobin and myoglobin and prevents oxygen binding, transport, and tissue uptake (binding to hemoglobin shifts the oxygen dissociation curve to the left).	Signs and symptoms of hypoxia with initial physiologic stimulation and subsequent depression (Table e35-2); lactic acidosis; normal P_{O_2} and calculated oxygen saturation but decreased oxygen saturation by co-oximetry (that measured by pulse oximetry is falsely elevated but is less than the normal and less than the calculated value). Headache and nausea are common with carbon monoxide. Sudden collapse may occur with cyanide and hydrogen sulfide exposure. A bitter almond breath odor may be noted with cyanide ingestion, and hydrogen sulfide smells like rotten eggs.	High-dose oxygen. Inhaled amyl nitrite and IV sodium nitrite and sodium thiosulfate (Lilly cyanide antidote kit) for coma, metabolic acidosis, and cardiovascular dysfunction in cyanide poisoning. Amyl and sodium nitrite (without thiosulfate) for similar toxicity in hydrogen sulfide poisoning. Hyperbaric oxygen for moderate to severe carbon monoxide poisoning and for cyanide or hydrogen sulfide poisoning unresponsive to other measures.

(continued)

145

TABLE 31-3	**PATHOPHYSIOLOGIC FEATURES AND TREATMENT OF SPECIFIC TOXIC SYNDROMES AND POISONINGS (CONTINUED)**			
Physiologic Condition, Causes	Examples	Mechanism of Action	Clinical Features	Specific Treatments
Methemoglobin inducers	Aniline derivatives, dapsone, local anesthetics, nitrates, nitrites, nitrogen oxides, nitro- and nitrosohydrocarbons, phenazopyridine, primaquine-type antimalarials, sulfonamides.	Oxidation of hemoglobin iron from ferrous (Fe^{2+}) to ferric (Fe^{3+}) state prevents oxygen binding, transport, and tissue uptake (methemoglobinemia shifts oxygen dissociation curve to the left). Oxidation of hemoglobin protein causes hemoglobin precipitation and hemolytic anemia (manifest as Heinz bodies and "bite cells" on peripheral blood smear).	Signs and symptoms of hypoxia with initial physiologic stimulation and subsequent depression (Table e35-2), graybrown cyanosis unresponsive to oxygen at methemoglobin fractions > 15–20%, headache, lactic acidosis (at methemoglobin fractions > 45%), normal P_{O_2} and calculated oxygen saturation but decreased oxygen saturation and increased methemoglobin fraction by co-oximetry (oxygen saturation by pulse oximetry may be falsely increased or decreased but is less than normal and less than the calculated value).	High-dose oxygen. Intravenous methylene blue for methemoglobin fraction > 30%, symptomatic hypoxia, or ischemia (contraindicated in G6PD deficiency). Exchange transfusion and hyperbaric oxygen for severe or refractory cases.

Category	Agent	Mechanism	Clinical Features	Treatment
AGMA inducers	Ethylene glycol	Ethylene glycol causes CNS depression and increased serum osmolality. Metabolites (primarily glycolic acid) cause AGMA, CNS depression, and renal failure. Precipitation of oxalic acid metabolite as calcium salt in tissues and urine results in hypocalcemia, tissue edema, and crystalluria.	Initial ethanol-like intoxication, nausea, vomiting, increased osmolar gap, calcium oxalate crystalluria. Delayed AGMA, back pain, renal failure. Coma, seizures, hypotension, ARDS in severe cases.	Gastric aspiration for recent ingestions. Sodium bicarbonate to correct acidemia. Thiamine, folinic acid, magnesium, and high-dose pyridoxine to facilitate metabolism. Ethanol or fomepizole for AGMA, crystalluria or renal dysfunction, ethylene glycol level > 3 mmol/L (20 mg/dL), and for ethanol-like intoxication or increased osmolal gap if level not readily obtainable. Hemodialysis for persistent AGMA, lack of clinical improvement, and renal dysfunction. Hemodialysis also useful for enhancing ethylene glycol elimination and shortening duration of treatment when ethylene glycol level > 8 mmol/L (50 mg/dL).
AGMA inducers	Iron	Hydration of ferric (Fe^{3+}) ion generates H^+. Non-transferrin-bound iron catalyzes formation of free radicals that cause mitochondrial injury, lipid peroxidation, increased capillary permeability, vasodilation, and organ toxicity.	Initial nausea, vomiting, abdominal pain, diarrhea. AGMA, cardiovascular and CNS depression, hepatitis, coagulopathy, and seizures in severe cases. Radiopaque iron tablets may be seen on abdominal x-ray.	Whole-bowel irrigation for large ingestions. Endoscopy and gastrostomy if clinical toxicity and large number of tablets still visible on x-ray. IV hydration. Sodium bicarbonate for acidemia. IV deferoxamine for systemic toxicity, iron level > 90 μmol/L (500 μg/dL).

(continued)

TABLE 31-3 PATHOPHYSIOLOGIC FEATURES AND TREATMENT OF SPECIFIC TOXIC SYNDROMES AND POISONINGS (CONTINUED)

Physiologic Condition, Causes	Examples	Mechanism of Action	Clinical Features	Specific Treatments
	Methanol	Methanol causes ethanol-like CNS depression and increased serum osmolality. Formic acid metabolite causes AGMA and retinal toxicity.	Initial ethanol-like intoxication, nausea, vomiting, increased osmolar gap. Delayed AGMA, visual (clouding, spots, blindness) and retinal (edema, hyperemia) abnormalities. Coma, seizures, cardiovascular depression in severe cases. Possible pancreatitis.	Gastric aspiration for recent ingestions. Sodium bicarbonate to correct acidemia. High-dose folinic acid or folate to facilitate metabolism. Ethanol or fomepizole for AGMA, visual symptoms, methanol level > 6 mmol/L (20 mg/dL), and for ethanol-like intoxication or increased osmolal gap if level not readily obtainable. Hemodialysis for persistent AGMA, lack of clinical improvement, and renal dysfunction. Hemodialysis also useful for enhancing methanol elimination and shortening duration of treatment when methanol level > 15 mmol/L (50 mg/dL).

Salicylate		Increased sensitivity of CNS respiratory center to changes in P_{O_2} and P_{CO_2} stimulates respiration. Uncoupling of oxidative phosphorylation, inhibition of Kreb's cycle enzymes, and stimulation of carbohydrate and lipid metabolism generate unmeasured endogenous anions and cause AGMA.	Initial nausea, vomiting, hyperventilation, alkalemia, alkaluria. Subsequent alkalemia with both respiratory alkalosis and AGMA, and paradoxical aciduria. Late acidemia with CNS and respiratory depression. Cerebral and pulmonary edema in severe cases. Hypoglycemia, hypocalcemia, hypokalemia, and seizures can occur.	IV hydration and supplemental glucose. Sodium bicarbonate to correct acidemia. Alkaline diuresis for systemic toxicity. Hemodialysis for coma, cerebral edema, seizures, pulmonary edema, renal failure, progressive acid-base disturbances or clinical toxicity, salicylate level > 7 mmol/L (100 mg/dL) following acute overdose.
CNS syndromes Extrapyramidal reactions	Antipsychotics (see above), some cyclic antidepressants and antihistamines.	Decreased CNS dopaminergic activity with relative excess of cholinergic activity.	Akathisia, dystonia, parkinsonism	Oral or parenteral anticholinergic agent such as benztropine or diphenhydramine.

(continued)

Physiologic Condition, Causes	Examples	Mechanism of Action	Clinical Features	Specific Treatments
Isoniazid		Interference with activation and supply of pyridoxal-5-phosphate, a cofactor for glutamic acid decarboxylase, which converts glutamic acid to GABA, results in decreased levels of this inhibitory CNS neurotransmitter; complexation with and depletion of pyridoxine itself; inhibition of nicotine-adenine dinucleotide dependent lactate and hydroxybutyrate dehydrogenases resulting in substrate accumulation.	Nausea, vomiting, agitation, confusion; coma, respiratory depression, seizures, lactic and ketoacidosis in severe cases.	High-dose intravenous pyridoxine (vitamin B_6) for agitation, confusion, coma, and seizures. Diazepam or barbiturates for seizures.

| Lithium | Interference with cell membrane ion transport, adenylate cyclase and Na^+, K^+-ATPase activity, and neurotransmitter release. | Nausea, vomiting, diarrhea, ataxia, choreoathetosis, encephalopathy, hyperreflexia, myoclonus, nystagmus, nephrogenic diabetes insipidus, falsely elevated serum chloride with low anion gap, tachycardia. Coma, seizures, arrhythmias, hyperthermia, and prolonged or permanent encephalopathy and movement disorders in severe cases. Delayed onset after acute overdose, particularly with delayed-release formations. Toxicity occurs at lower drug levels in chronic poisoning than in acute poisoning. | Whole-bowel irrigation for large ingestions. Consider endoscopic removal if high and rising drug level with progressive clinical toxicity. IV hydration. Hemodialysis for coma, seizures, severe, progressive, or persistent encephalopathy or neuromuscular dysfunction, peak lithium level > 8 meq/L (mmol/L) following acute overdose. |

(continued)

TABLE 31-3 PATHOPHYSIOLOGIC FEATURES AND TREATMENT OF SPECIFIC TOXIC SYNDROMES AND POISONINGS (CONTINUED)

Physiologic Condition, Causes	Examples	Mechanism of Action	Clinical Features	Specific Treatments
Serotonin syndrome	Amphetamines, cocaine, dextromethorphan, meperidine, MAO inhibitors, selective serotonin (5HT) reuptake inhibitors, tricyclic antidepressants, tramadol, triptans, tryptophan.	Promotion of serotonin release, inhibition of serotonin reuptake, or direct stimulation of CNS and peripheral serotonin receptors (primarily 5HT-1a and 5HT-2), alone or in combination.	Altered mental status (agitation, confusion, mutism, coma, seizures), neuromuscular hyperactivity (hyperreflexia, myoclonus, rigidity, tremors), and autonomic dysfunction (abdominal pain, diarrhea, diaphoresis, fever, flushing, labile hypertension, mydriasis, tearing, salivation, tachycardia). Complications include hyperthermia, lactic acidosis, rhabdomyolysis, and multisystem organ failure.	Serotonin receptor antagonist such as cyproheptadine or chlorpromazine.

| Membrane-active agents | Amantadine, antiarrhythmics (class I and III agents; some β blockers), antipsychotics (see above), antihistamines (particularly diphenhydramine), carbamazepine, local anesthetics (including cocaine), opioids (meperidine, propoxyphene), orphenadrine, quinoline antimalarials (chloroquine, hydroxychloroquine, quinine), cyclic antidepressants (see above). | Blockade of fast sodium membrane channels prolongs phase 0 (depolarization) of the cardiac action potential, which prolongs the QRS duration and promotes reentrant (monomorphic) ventricular tachycardia. Class Ia, Ic, and III antiarrhythmics also block potassium channels during phases 2 and 3 (repolarization) of the action potential, prolonging the JT interval and promoting early after-depolarizations and polymorphic (torsades des pointes) ventricular tachycardia. Similar effects on neuronal membrane channels cause CNS dysfunction. Some agents also block α-adrenergic and cholinergic receptors or have opioid effects (see above and Chap. 388). | QRS and JT prolongation (or both) with hypotension, ventricular tachyarrhythmias, CNS depression, seizures. Anticholinergic effects with amantadine, antihistamines, carbamazepine, disopyramide, antipsychotics, and cyclic antidepressants (see above). Opioid effects with meperidine and propoxyphene (see Chap. 388). Cinchonism (hearing loss, tinnitus, nausea, vomiting, vertigo, ataxia, headache, flushing, diaphoresis) and blindness with quinoline antimalarials. | Hypertonic sodium bicarbonate (or hypertonic saline) for cardiac conduction delays and monomorphic ventricular tachycardia. Lidocaine for monomorphic ventricular tachycardia (except when due to class Ib antiarrhythmics). Magnesium, isoproterenol, and overdrive pacing for polymorphic ventricular tachycardia. Physostigmine for anticholinergic effects (see above). Naloxone for opioid effects (see Chap. 388). Extracorporeal removal for some agents (see text). |

Note: AGMA, anion-gap metabolic acidosis; ARDS, adult respiratory distress syndrome; dehydrogenase; MAO, monoamine oxidase; SIADH, syndrome of inappropriate antidiuretic hormone.
CNS, central nervous system; GABA, γ-aminobutyric acid; G6PD, glucose-6-phosphate uretic hormone.

TABLE 31-4	HEAVY METALS	
Main Sources	**Metabolism**	**Toxicity**
Arsenic		
Smelting and microelectronics industries; wood preservatives, pesticides, herbicides, fungicides; contaminant of deep-water wells; folk remedies; and coal; incineration of these products	Organic arsenic (arsenobentaine, arsenocholine) is ingested in seafood and fish, but is nontoxic; inorganic arsenic is readily absorbed (lung and GI); sequesters in liver, spleen, kidneys, lungs, and GI tract; residues persist in skin, hair, and nails; biomethylation results in detoxification, but this process saturates.	Acute arsenic poisoning results in necrosis of intestinal mucosa with hemorrhagic gastroenteritis, fluid loss, hypotension, delayed cardiomyopathy, acute tubular necrosis, and hemolysis. Chronic arsenic exposure causes diabetes, vasospasm, peripheral vascular insufficiency and gangrene, peripheral neuropathy, and cancer of skin, lung, liver (angiosarcoma), bladder, kidney. Lethal dose: 120–200 mg (adults); 2 mg/kg (children).
Cadmium		
Metal-plating, pigment, smelting, battery, and plastics industries; tobacco; incineration of these products; ingestion of food that concentrates cadmium (grains, cereals).	Absorbed through ingestion or inhalation; bound by metallothionein, filtered at the glomerulus, but reabsorbed by proximal tubules (thus, poorly excreted). Biologic $1/2$ life: 10–30 y. Binds cellular sulfhydryl groups, competes with zinc, calcium for binding sites. Concentrates in liver and kidneys.	Acute cadmium inhalation causes pneumonitis after 4–24 h; acute ingestion causes gastroenteritis. Chronic exposure causes anosmia, yellowing of teeth, emphysema, minor LFT elevations, microcytic hypochromic anemia unresponsive to iron therapy, proteinuria, increased urinary β_2-microglobulin, calciuria, leading to chronic renal failure, osteomalacia, and fractures.

Diagnosis	Treatment
Nausea, vomiting, diarrhea, abdominal pain, delirium, coma, seizures; garlicky odor on breath; hyperkeratosis, hyperpigmentation, exfoliative dermatitis, and Mees' lines (transverse white striae of the fingernails); sensory and motor polyneuritis, distal weakness. Radiopaque sign on abdominal x-ray; ECG–QRS broadening, QT prolongation, ST depression, T-wave flattening; 24-h urinary arsenic >67 µmol/d or 50 µg/d; (no seafood × 24 h); if recent exposure, serum arsenic >0.9 µmol/L (7 µg/dL). High arsenic in hair or nails.	If acute ingestion, gastric lavage, activated charcoal with a cathartic. Supportive care in ICU. Dimercaprol 3–5 mg/kg IM q4h × 2 days; q6h × 1 day, then q12h × 10 days; alternative: oral succimer.
With inhalation: pleuritic chest pain, dyspnea, cyanosis, fever, tachycardia, nausea, noncardiogenic pulmonary edema. With ingestion: nausea, vomiting, cramps, diarrhea. Bone pain, fractures with osteomalacia. If recent exposure, serum cadmium >500 nmol/L (5 µg/dL). Urinary cadmium >100 nmol/L (10 µg/g creatinine) and/or urinary β_2-microglobulin >750 µg/g creatinine (but urinary β_2-microglobulin also increased in other renal diseases such as pyelonephritis).	There is no effective treatment for cadmium poisoning (chelation not useful; dimercaprol can exacerbate nephrotoxicity). Avoidance of further exposure, supportive therapy, vitamin D for osteomalacia.

(continued)

TABLE 31-4	HEAVY METALS (CONTINUED)	
Main Sources	Metabolism	Toxicity
Lead		

Main Sources	Metabolism	Toxicity
Manufacturing of auto batteries, lead crystal, ceramics, fishing weights, etc.; demolition or sanding of lead-painted houses, bridges; stained glass making, plumbing, soldering; environmental exposure to paint chips, house dust (in home built <1975), firing ranges (from bullet dust), food or water from improperly glazed ceramics, lead pipes; contaminated herbal remedies, candies; exposure to the combustion of leaded fuels.	Absorbed through ingestion or inhalation; organic lead (e.g., tetraethyl lead) absorbed dermally. In blood, 95–99% sequestered in RBCs—thus, must measure lead in whole blood (not serum). Distributed widely in soft tissue, with $1/2$ life ~30 days; 15% of dose sequestered in bone with $1/2$ life of >20 years. Excreted mostly in urine, but also appears in other fluids including breast milk. Interferes with mitochondrial oxidative phosphorylation, ATPases, calcium-dependent messengers; enhances oxidation and cell apoptosis.	Acute exposure with blood lead levels (BPb) of > 60–80 μg/dL can cause impaired neurotransmission and neuronal cell death (with central and peripheral nervous system effects); impaired hematopoiesis and renal tubular dysfunction. At higher levels of exposure (e.g., BPb > 80–120 μg/dL), acute encephalopathy with convulsions, coma, and death may occur. Subclinical exposures in children (BPb 25–60 μg/dL) are associated with anemia; mental retardation; and deficits in language, motor function, balance, hearing, behavior, and school performance. Impairment of IQ appears to occur at even lower levels of exposure with no measurable threshold above the limit of detection in most assays of 1 μg/dL. In adults, chronic subclinical exposures (BPb > 40 μg/dL) are associated with an increased risk of anemia, demyelinating peripheral neuropathy (mainly motor), impairments of reaction time, hypertension, ECG conduction delays, interstitial nephritis and chronic renal failure, diminished sperm counts, spontaneous abortions.

Diagnosis	Treatment

Abdominal pain, irritability, lethargy, anorexia, anemia, Fanconi's syndrome, pyuria, azotemia in children with blood lead level (BPb) >80 µg/dL; may also see epiphyseal plate "lead lines" on long bone x-rays. Convulsions, coma at BPb > 120 µg/dL. Noticeable neurodevelopmental delays at BPb of 40–80 µg/dL; may also see symptoms associated with higher BPb levels. In the U.S., screening of all children when they begin to crawl (~6 months) is recommended by the CDC; source identification and intervention is begun if the BPb > 10 µg/dL. In adults, acute exposure causes similar symptoms as in children as well as headaches, arthralgias, myalgias, depression, impaired short-term memory, loss of libido. Physical exam may reveal a "lead line" at the gingiva-tooth border, pallor, wrist drop, and cognitive dysfunction (e.g., declines on the mini-mental status exam); lab tests may reveal a normocytic, normochromic anemia, basophilic stippling, an elevated blood protoporphyrin level (free erythrocyte or zinc), and motor delays on nerve conduction. In the U.S., OSHA requires regular testing of lead-exposed workers with removal if BPb > 40 µg/dL.

Identification and correction of exposure sources is critical. In some U.S. states, screening and reporting to local health boards of children with BPb > 10 µg/dL and workers with BPb > 40 µg/dL is required. In the highly exposed individual with symptoms, chelation is recommended with oral DMSA (succimer); if acutely toxic, hospitalization and IV or IM chelation with edentate calcium disodium (CaEDTA) may be required, with the addition of dimercaprol to prevent worsening of encephalopathy. It is uncertain whether children with asymptomatic lead exposure (e.g., BPb 20–40 µg/dL) benefit from chelation. Correction of dietary deficiencies in iron, calcium, magnesium, and zinc will lower lead absorption and may also improve toxicity. Vitamin C is a weak but natural chelating agent.

(continued)

TABLE 31-4   HEAVY METALS (CONTINUED)

Main Sources	Metabolism	Toxicity
Mercury		

Main Sources	Metabolism	Toxicity
Metallic, mercurous, and mercuric mercury (Hg°, Hg^+, Hg^{2+}) exposures occur in some chemical, metal-processing, electrical-equipment, automotive industries; they are also in thermometers, dental amalgams, batteries. Mercury is dispersed by waste incineration. Environmental bacteria convert inorganic to organic mercury, which then bioconcentrates up the aquatic food chain to contaminate tuna, swordfish, and other pelagic fish.	Elemental mercury (Hg°) is not well absorbed; however, it will volatilize into highly absorbable vapor. Inorganic mercury is absorbed through the gut and skin. Organic mercury is well absorbed through inhalation and ingestion. Elemental and organic mercury cross the blood-brain barrier and placenta. Mercury is excreted in urine and feces and has a $1/2$ life in blood of ~60 days; however, deposits will remain in the kidney and brain for years. Exposure to mercury stimulates the kidney to produce metallothionein, which provides some detoxification benefit. Mercury binds sulfhydryl groups and interferes with a wide variety of critical enzymatic processes.	Acute inhalation of Hg° vapor causes pneumonitis and noncardiogenic pulmonary edema leading to death, CNS symptoms, and polyneuropathy. Chronic high exposure causes CNS toxicity (mercurial); lower exposures impair renal function, motor speed, memory, coordination. Acute ingestion of inorganic mercury causes gastroenteritis, the nephritic syndrome, or acute renal failure, hypertension, tachycardia, and cardiovascular collapse, with death at a dose of 10–42 mg/kg. Ingestion of organic mercury causes gastroenteritis, arrhythmias, and lesions in the basal ganglia, gray matter, and cerebellum at doses >1.7 mg/kg. High exposure during pregnancy causes derangement of fetal neuronal migration resulting in severe mental retardation. Mild exposures during pregnancy (from fish consumption) are associated with declines in neurobehavioral performance in offspring. Dimethylmercury, a compound only found in research labs, is "supertoxic"—a few drops of exposure via skin absorption or inhaled vapor can cause severe cerebellar degeneration and death.

Note: IQ, intelligence quotient; CDC, Centers for Disease Control and Prevention; OSHA, Occupational Safety and Health Administration; CNS.

Diagnosis	Treatment

Chronic exposure to metallic mercury vapor produces a characteristic intention tremor and mercurial *erethism*: excitability, memory loss, insomnia, timidity, and delirium ("mad as a hatter"). On neurobehavioral tests: decreased motor speed, visual scanning, verbal and visual memory, visuomotor coordination.

Children exposed to mercury in any form may develop *acrodynia* ("pink disease"): flushing, itching, swelling, tachycardia, hypertension, excessive salivation or perspiration, irritability, weakness, morbilliform rashes, desquamation of palms and soles.

Toxicity from elemental or inorganic mercury exposure begins when blood levels >180 nmol/L (3.6 µg/dL) and urine levels >0.7 µmol/L (15 µg/dL). Exposures that ended years ago may result in a >20-µg increase in 24-h urine after a 2-g dose of succimer.

Organic mercury exposure is best measured by levels in blood (if recent) or hair (if chronic); CNS toxicity in children may derive from fetal exposures associated with maternal hair Hg > 30 nmol/g (6 µg/g).

Treat acute ingestion of mercuric salts with induced emesis or gastric lavage and polythiol resins (to bind mercury in the GI tract). Chelate with dimercaprol (up to 24 mg/kg per day IM in divided doses), DMSA (succimer), or penicillamine, with 5-day courses separated by several days of rest. If renal failure occurs, treat with peritoneal dialysis, hemodialysis, or extracorporeal regional complexing hemodialysis and succimer.

Chronic inorganic mercury poisoning is best treated with *N*-acetyl penicillamine.

Enhancement of Elimination

Activated charcoal in repeated doses of 1 g/kg q2–4h is useful for ingestions of drugs with enteral circulation such as carbamazepine, dapsone, diazepam, digoxin, glutethimide, meprobamate, methotrexate, phenobarbital, phenytoin, salicylate, theophylline, and valproic acid.

Forced urinary alkalinization enhances the elimination of chlorphenoxyacetic acid herbicides, chlorpropamide, diflunisal, fluoride, methotrexate, phenobarbital, sulfonamides, and salicylates. Sodium bicarbonate, 1–2 ampules per liter of 0.45% NaCl, is given at a rate sufficient to maintain urine pH ≥ 7.5 and urine output at 3–6 mL/kg per h. Acid diuresis is no longer recommended.

Peritoneal dialysis or hemodialysis may be useful in severe poisoning due to barbiturates, bromide, chloral hydrate, ethanol, ethylene glycol, isopropyl alcohol, lithium, heavy metals, methanol, procainamide, and salicylate. Hemoperfusion may be indicated for chloramphenicol, disopyramide, and hypnotic-sedative overdose. Exchange transfusion removes poisons affecting red blood cells.

The features of specific toxic syndromes and approaches to treatment are summarized in Table 31-3. The features of selected heavy metal toxicity and approaches to treatment are summarized in Table 31-4. Readers are encouraged to contact poison control centers for additional information (*http://www.aapcc.org/DNN/*).

For a more detailed discussion, see Linden CH, Burns MJ: Poisoning and Drug Overdosage, Chap. 377, p. 2580; and Hu H: Heavy Metal Poisoning, Chap. 376, p. 2577, in HPIM-16.

32 Bioterrorism

MICROBIAL BIOTERRORISM

Microbial bioterrorism refers to the use of microbial pathogens as weapons of terror that target civilian populations. A primary goal of bioterrorism is not necessarily to produce mass casualties but to destroy the morale of a society through creating fear and uncertainty. The events of September 11, 2001, followed by the anthrax attacks through the U.S. Postal Service illustrate the vulnerability of the American public to terrorist attacks, including those that use microbes. The key to combating bioterrorist attacks is a highly functioning system of public health surveillance and education that rapidly identifies and effectively contains the attack.

Agents of microbial bioterrorism may be used in their natural form or may be deliberately modified to maximize their deleterious effect. Modifications that increase the deleterious effect of a biologic agent include genetic alteration of microbes to produce antimicrobial resistance, creation of fine-particle aerosols, chemical treatment to stabilize and prolong infectivity, and alteration of the host range through changes in surface protein receptors. Certain of these approaches

---

TABLE 32-1 **KEY FEATURES OF BIOLOGIC AGENTS USED AS BIOWEAPONS**

1. High morbidity and mortality
2. Potential for person-to-person spread
3. Low infective dose and highly infectious by aerosol
4. Lack of rapid diagnostic capability
5. Lack of universally available effective vaccine
6. Potential to cause anxiety
7. Availability of pathogen and feasibility of production
8. Environmental stability
9. Database of prior research and development
10. Potential to be "weaponized"

Source: From L Borio et al: JAMA 287:2391, 2002; with permission.

fall under the category of *weaponization*, a term that describes the processing of microbes or toxins in a manner that enhances their deleterious effect after release. The key features that characterize an effective biologic weapon are summarized in Table 32-1.

The U.S. Centers for Disease Control and Prevention (CDC) has classified microbial agents that could potentially be used in bioterrorism attacks into three categories: A, B, and C (Table 32-2). Category A agents are the highest-priority

---

TABLE 32-2 **CDC CATEGORY A, B, AND C AGENTS**

Category A
  Anthrax (*Bacillus anthracis*)
  Botulism (*Clostridium botulinum* toxin)
  Plague (*Yersinia pestis*)
  Smallpox (Variola major)
  Tularemia (*Francisella tularensis*)
  Viral hemorrhagic fevers
    Arenaviruses: Lassa, New World (Machupo, Junin, Guanarito, and Sabia)
    Bunyaviridae: Crimean Congo, Rift Valley
    Filoviridae: Ebola, Marburg
    Flaviviridae: Yellow fever; Omsk fever; Kyasanur Forest

Category B
  Brucellosis (*Brucella* spp.)
  Epsilon toxin of *Clostridium perfringens*
  Food safety threats (e.g., *Salmonella* spp., *Escherichia coli* 0157:H7, *Shigella*)
  Glanders (*Burkholderia mallei*)
  Melioidosis (*B. pseudomallei*)
  Psittacosis (*Chlamydia psittaci*)
  Q fever (*Coxiella burnetii*)
  Ricin toxin from *Ricinus communis* (castor beans)
  Staphylococcal enterotoxin B
  Typhus fever (*Rickettsia prowazekii*)
  Viral encephalitis [alphaviruses (e.g., Venezuelan, eastern, and western equine encephalitis)]
  Water safety threats (e.g., *Vibrio cholerae*, *Cryptosporidium parvum*)

Category C
  Emerging infectious diseases threats such as Nipah, hantavirus, SARS coronavirus, and pandemic influenza.

Source: Centers for Disease Control and Prevention and the National Institute of Allergy and Infectious Diseases.

pathogens. They pose the greatest risk to national security because they (1) can be easily disseminated or transmitted from person to person, (2) are associated with high case-fatality rates, (3) have potential to cause significant public panic and social disruption, and (4) require special action and public health preparedness.

CATEGORY A AGENTS

Anthrax (*Bacillus anthracis*)   **Anthrax as a Bioweapon**   Anthrax in many ways is the prototypic bioweapon. Although it is only rarely spread by person-to-person contact, it has many of the other features of an ideal biologic weapon listed in Table 32-1. The potential impact of anthrax as a bioweapon is illustrated by the apparent accidental release in 1979 of anthrax spores from a Soviet bioweapons facility in Sverdlosk, Russia. As a result of this atmospheric release of anthrax spores, at least 77 cases of anthrax (of which 66 were fatal) occurred in individuals within an area 4 km downwind of the facility. Deaths were noted in livestock up to 50 km from the facility. The interval between probable exposure and onset of symptoms ranged from 2–43 days, with the majority of cases occurring within 2 weeks. In September of 2001 the American public was exposed to anthrax spores delivered through the U.S. Postal Service. There were 22 confirmed cases: 11 cases of inhaled anthrax (5 died) and 11 cases of cutaneous anthrax (no deaths). Cases occurred in individuals who opened contaminated letters as well as in postal workers involved in processing the mail.

Microbiology and Clinical Features   (See also Chaps. 214 and 131, HPIM-17)

- Anthrax is caused by infections with *B. anthracis*, a gram-positive, nonmotile, spore-forming rod that is found in soil and predominantly causes disease in cattle, goats, and sheep.
- Spores can remain viable for decades in the environment and be difficult to destroy with standard decontamination procedures. These properties make anthrax an ideal bioweapon.
- Naturally occurring human infection generally results from exposure to infected animals or contaminated animal products.

There are three major clinical forms of anthrax:

1. *Gastrointestinal anthrax* is rare and is unlikely to result from a bioterrorism event.
2. *Cutaneous anthrax* follows introduction of spores through an opening in the skin. The lesion begins as a papule followed by the development of a black eschar. Prior to the availability of antibiotics, about 20% of cutaneous anthrax cases were fatal.
3. *Inhalation anthrax* is the form most likely to result in serious illness and death in a bioterrorism attack. It occurs following inhalation of spores that become deposited in the alveolar spaces. The spores are phagocytosed by alveolar macrophages and are transported to regional lymph nodes where they germinate. Following germination, rapid bacterial growth and toxin production occur. Subsequent hematologic dissemination leads to cardiovascular collapse and death. The earliest symptoms are typically those of a viral-like prodrome with fever, malaise, and abdominal/chest symptoms that rapidly progress to a septic shock picture. Widening of the mediastinum and pleural effusions are typical findings on chest radiography. Once considered 100% fatal, experience from the Sverdlosk and U.S. Postal outbreaks indicate that with prompt initiation of appropriate antibiotic therapy, survival may be >50%. Awareness of the possibility of the diagnosis of anthrax is critical to the prompt initiation of therapy.

℞ Anthrax   (See Table 32-3)

Anthrax can be successfully treated if the disease is promptly recognized and appropriate antibiotic therapy is initiated.
- Penicillin, ciprofloxacin, and doxycycline are currently licensed for the treatment of anthrax.
- Clindamycin and rifampin have in vitro activity against the organism and may be used as part of the treatment regimen.
- Patients with inhalation anthrax are not contagious and do not require special isolation procedures.

Vaccination and Prevention
- Currently there is a single vaccine licensed for use; produced from a cell-free culture supernatant of an attenuated strain of *B. anthracis* (Stern strain).
- Current recommendation for postexposure prophylaxis is 60 days of antibiotics (see Table 32-1); recent animal studies have suggested that postexposure vaccination may be of some additional benefit.

Plague (*Yersinia pestis*) (See also Chap. 98)
Plague as a Bioweapon   Although plague lacks the environmental stability of anthrax, the highly contagious nature of the infection and the high mortality rate make it a potentially important agent of bioterrorism. As a bioweapon, plague would likely be delivered via an aerosol leading to primary pneumonic plague. In such an attack, person-to-person transmission of plague via respiratory aerosol could lead to large numbers of secondary cases.

Microbiology and Clinical Features   See Chap. 98.

℞ Plague   See Table 32-3 and Chap. 98.

Smallpox (Variola major and V. minor)   (See also Chap. 176, HPIM-17)
Smallpox as a Bioweapon   Smallpox as a disease was globally eradicated by 1980 through a worldwide vaccination program. However, with the cessation of smallpox immunization programs in the United States in 1972 (and worldwide in 1980), close to half the U.S. population is fully susceptible to smallpox today. Given the infectious nature and the 10–30% mortality of smallpox in unimmunized individuals, the deliberate release of virus could have devastating effects on the population. In the absence of effective containment measures, an initial infection of 50–100 persons in a first generation of cases could expand by a factor of 10 to 20 with each succeeding generation. These considerations make smallpox a formidable bioweapon.

Microbiology and Clinical Features   The disease smallpox is caused by one of two closely related double-strand DNA viruses, V. major and V. minor. Both viruses are members of the Orthopoxvirus genus of the Poxviridae family. Infection with V. minor is generally less severe, with low mortality rates; thus, V. major is the only one considered as a potential bioweapon. Infection with V. major typically occurs following contact with an infected person from the time that a maculopapular rash appears through scabbing of the pustular lesions. Infection is thought to occur from inhalation of virus-containing saliva droplets from oropharyngeal lesions. Contaminated clothing or linen can also spread infection. About 12–14 days following initial exposure the patient develops high fever, malaise, vomiting, headache, back pain, and a maculopapular rash that

TABLE 32-3 TREATMENT STRATEGIES FOR DISEASES CAUSED BY CATEGORY A AGENTS

Agent	Diagnosis	Treatment	Prophylaxis
Bacillus anthracis (anthrax)	Culture, Gram stain, PCR, Wright stain of peripheral smear	*Postexposure:* Ciprofloxacin, 500 mg, PO bid × 60 d *or* Doxycycline, 100 mg PO bid × 60 d (Amoxicillin, 500 mg PO q8h, likely to be effective if strain penicillin sensitive) *Active disease:* Ciprofloxacin, 400 mg IV q12h *or* Doxycycline, 100 mg IV q12 *plus* Clindamycin, 900 mg IV q8h and/or rifampin, 300 mg IV q12h; switch to PO when stable × 60 d total	Anthrax vaccine adsorbed Recombinant protective antigen vaccines are under study
Yersinia pestis (pneumonic plague)	Culture, Gram stain, direct fluorescent antibody, PCR	*Antitoxin strategies:* Neutralizing monoclonal and polyclonal antibodies are under study Gentamicin, 2.0 mg/kg IV loading then 1.7 mg/kg q8h IV *or* Streptomycin, 1.0 g q12h IM or IV Alternatives include doxycycline, 100 mg bid PO or IV; chloramphenicol 500 mg qid PO or IV	Doxycycline, 100 mg PO bid (ciprofloxacin may also be active) Formalin-fixed vaccine (FDA licensed; not available)
Variola major (smallpox)	Culture, PCR, electron microscopy	Supportive measures; consideration for cidofovir, antivaccinia immunoglobulin	Vaccinia immunization

Francisella tularensis (tularemia)	Gram stain, culture, immunohistochemistry, PCR	Streptomycin, 1 g IM bid *or* Gentamicin, 5 mg/kg per day div q8h IV for 14 days Doxycycline, 100 mg IV bid *or* Chloramphenicol, 15 mg/kg IV qid *or* Ciprofloxacin, 400 mg IV bid	Doxycycline, 100 mg PO bid × 14 days *or* Ciprofloxacin, 500 mg PO bid × 14 days
Viral hemorrhagic fevers	RT-PCR, serologic testing for antigen or antibody Viral isolation by CDC or U.S. Army Medical Institute of Infectious Diseases (US-AMRIID)	Supportive measures Ribavirin 30 mg/kg up to 2 g × 1, followed by 16 mg/kg IV up to 1 g q6h for 4 days, followed by 8 mg/kg IV up to 0.5 g q8h × 6 days	No known chemoprophylaxis Consideration for ribavirin in high-risk situations Vaccine exists for yellow fever
Botulinum toxin (*Clostridium botulinum*)	Mouse bioassay, toxin immunoassay	Supportive measures including ventilation 5000–9000 IU equine antitoxin	Administration of antitoxin

Note: CDC, U.S. Centers for Disease Control and Prevention; FDA, U.S. Food and Drug Administration; PCR, polymerase chain reaction; RT-PCR, reverse transcriptase PCR.

begins on the face and extremities and spreads to the trunk. The skin lesions evolve into vesicles that eventually become pustular with scabs. The oral mucosa also develops macular lesions that progress to ulcers. Smallpox is associated with a 10–30% mortality. Historically, about 5–10% of naturally occurring cases manifest as highly virulent atypical forms, classified as *hemorrhagic* and *malignant*. These are difficult to recognize due to their atypical manifestations. Both forms have similar onset of a severe prostrating illness characterized by high fever, severe headache, and abdominal and back pain. In the hemorrhagic form, cutaneous erythema develops followed by petechiae and hemorrhage into the skin and mucous membranes. In the malignant form, confluent skin lesions develop but never progress to the pustular stage. Both of these forms are often fatal, with death occurring in 5–6 days.

 Smallpox

> Treatment is supportive. There is no licensed specific antiviral therapy for smallpox; however, certain candidate drugs look promising in pre-clinical testing in animal models. Smallpox is highly infectious to close contacts; patients who are suspected cases should be handled with strict isolation procedures.

Vaccination and Prevention Smallpox is a preventable disease following immunization with vaccinia. Past and current experience indicates that the smallpox vaccine is associated with a very low incidence of severe complications (see Table 214-4, p. 1349, HPIM-17). The current dilemma facing our society regarding assessment of the risk/benefit of smallpox vaccination is that, while the risks of vaccination are known, the risk of someone deliberately and effectively releasing smallpox into the general population is unknown. Given the rare, but potentially severe complications associated with smallpox vaccination using the currently available vaccine together with the current level of threat, it has been decided by public health authorities that vaccination of the general population is not indicated.

Tularemia (*Francisella tularensis*) (See also Chap. 98)

Tularemia as a Bioweapon Tularemia has been studied as a biologic agent since the mid-twentieth century. Reportedly, both the United States and the former Soviet Union had active programs investigating this organism as a possible bioweapon. It has been suggested that the Soviet program extended into the era of molecular biology and that some strains of *F. tularensis* may have been genetically engineered to be resistant to commonly used antibiotics. *F. tularensis* is extremely infectious and can cause significant morbidity and mortality. These facts make it reasonable to consider this organism as a possible bioweapon that could be disseminated by either aerosol or contamination of food or drinking water.

Microbiology and Clinical Features See Chap. 98.

 Tularemia See Table 32-3 and Chap. 98.

Viral Hemorrhagic Fevers (See also Chap. 111)

Hemorrhagic Fever Viruses as Bioweapons Several of the hemorrhagic fever viruses have been reported to have been weaponized by the former Soviet Union and the United States. Nonhuman primate studies indicate that infection can be established with very few virions and that infectious aerosol preparations can be produced.

Microbiology and Clinical Features   See Chap. 111.

 Viral Hemorrhagic Fevers   See Table 32-3 and Chap. 111.

Botulinum Toxin (*Clostridium botulinum*)   (See also Chap. 99)
Botulinum Toxin as a Bioweapon   In a bioterrorism attack, botulinum toxin would likely be dispersed as an aerosol or used to contaminate food. Contamination of the water supply is possible, but the toxin would likely be degraded by chlorine used to purify drinking water. The toxin can also be inactivated by heating food to >85°C for >5 min. The United States, the former Soviet Union, and Iraq have all acknowledged studying botulinum toxin as a potential bioweapon. Unique among the Category A agents for not being a live organism, botulinum toxin is one of the most potent and lethal toxins known to man. It has been estimated that 1 g of toxin is sufficient to kill 1 million people if adequately dispersed.

Microbiology and Clinical Features   See Chap. 99.

 Botulinum Toxin   See Table 32-3 and Chap. 99.

CATEGORY B AND C AGENTS   (See Table 32-2)

Category B agents are the next highest priority and include agents that are moderately easy to disseminate, produce moderate morbidity and low mortality, and require enhanced diagnostic capacity.

Category C agents are the third highest priority agents in the biodefence agenda. These agents include emerging pathogens, such as SARS (severe acute respiratory syndrome) coronavirus or a pandemic influenza virus, to which the general population lacks immunity. Category C agents could be engineered for mass dissemination in the future. It is important to note that these categories are empirical, and, depending on future circumstances, the priority ratings for a given microbial agent may change.

PREVENTION AND PREPAREDNESS

As indicated above, a diverse array of agents have the potential to be used against a civilian population in a bioterrorism attack. The medical profession must maintain a high index of suspicion that unusual clinical presentations or clustering of rare diseases may not be a chance occurrence, but rather the first sign of a bioterrorism attack. Possible early indicators of a bioterrorism attack could include:

- The occurrence of rare diseases in healthy populations
- The occurrence of unexpectedly large numbers of a rare infection
- The appearance in an urban population of an infectious disease that is usually confined to rural settings

Given the importance of rapid diagnosis and early treatment for many of these diseases, it is important that the medical care team report any suspected cases of bioterrorism immediately to local and state health authorities and/or the CDC (888-246-2675).

CHEMICAL BIOTERRORISM

The use of chemical warfare agents (CWAs) as weapons of terror against civilian populations is a potential threat that must be addressed by public health officials and the medical profession. The use of both nerve agents and sulfur mustard by Iraq against Iranian military and Kurdish civilians and the sarin attacks in 1994–1995 in Japan underscore this threat.

A detailed description of the various CWAs can be found in Chap. 215, HPIM-17, and on the CDC website at *www.bt.cdc.gov/agent/agentlistchem.asp*. In this section only vesicants and nerve agents will be discussed as these are considered the most likely agents to be used in a terrorist attack.

VESICANTS (SULFUR MUSTARD, NITROGEN MUSTARD, LEWISITE)

Sulfur mustard is the prototype for this group of CWAs and was first used on the battlefields of Europe in World War I. This agent constitutes both a vapor and liquid threat to exposed epithelial surfaces. The organs most commonly affected are the skin, eyes, and airways. Exposure to large quantities of sulfur mustard can result in bone marrow toxicity. Sulfur mustard dissolves slowly in aqueous media such as sweat or tears, but once dissolved it forms reactive compounds that react with cellular proteins, membranes, and importantly DNA. Much of the biologic damage from this agent appears to result from DNA alkylation and cross-linking in rapidly dividing cells in the corneal epithelium, skin, bronchial mucosal epithelium, GI epithelium, and bone marrow. Sulfur mustard reacts with tissue within minutes of entering the body.

Clinical Features   The topical effects of sulfur mustard occur in the skin, airways, and eyes. Absorption of the agent may produce effects in the bone marrow and GI tract (direct injury to the GI tract may occur if sulfur mustard is ingested in contaminated food or water).

- *Skin*: erythema is the mildest and earliest manifestation; involved areas of skin then develop vesicles that coalesce to form bullae; high-dose exposure may lead to coagulation necrosis within bullae.
- *Airways*: initial and, with mild exposures, the only airway manifestations are burning of the nares, epistaxis, sinus pain, and pharyngeal pain. With exposure to higher concentrations, damage to the trachea and lower airways may occur, producing laryngitis, cough, and dyspnea. With large exposures, necrosis of the airway mucosa occurs leading to pseudomembrane formation and airway obstruction. Secondary infection may occur due to bacterial invasion of denuded respiratory mucosa.
- *Eyes*: the eyes are the most sensitive organ to injury by sulfur mustard. Exposure to low concentrations may produce only erythema and irritation. Exposure to higher concentrations produces progressively more severe conjunctivitis, photophobia, blepharospasm pain, and corneal damage.
- GI tract manifestations include nausea and vomiting, lasting up to 24 h.
- Bone marrow suppression, with peaks at 7–14 days following exposure, may result in sepsis due to leukopenia.

℞ Sulfur Mustard

Immediate decontamination is essential to minimize damage. Immediately remove clothing and gently wash skin with soap and water. Eyes should be flushed with copious amounts of water or saline. Subsequent medical care is supportive. Cutaneous vesicles should be left intact. Larger bullae should be debrided and treated with topical antibiotic preparations. Intensive care similar to that given to severe burn patients is required for pts with severe exposure. Oxygen may be required for mild/moderate respiratory exposure. Intubation and mechanical ventilation may be necessary for laryngeal spasm and severe lower airway damage. Pseudomembranes should be removed by suctioning; bronchodilators are of benefit for bronchospasm. The use of granulocyte colony-stimulating factor and/or stem cell transplantation may be effective for severe bone marrow suppression.

NERVE AGENTS

The organophosphorus nerve agents are the deadliest of the CWAs and work by inhibiting synaptic acetylcholinesterase, creating an acute cholinergic crisis. The "classic" organophosphorus nerve agents are tabun, sarin, soman, cyclosarin, and VX. All agents are liquid at standard temperature and pressure. With the exception of VX, all these agents are highly volatile, and the spilling of even a small amount of liquid agent represents a serious vapor hazard.

Mechanism Inhibition of acetylcholinesterase accounts for the major life-threatening effects of these agents. At the cholinergic synapse, the enzyme acetylcholinesterase functions as a "turn off" switch to regulate cholinergic synaptic transmission. Inhibition of this enzyme allows released acetylcholine to accumulate, resulting in end-organ overstimulation and leading to what is clinically referred to as *cholinergic crisis.*

Clinical Features The clinical manifestations of nerve agent exposure are identical for vapor and liquid exposure routes. Initial manifestations include miosis, blurred vision, headache, and copious oropharyngeal secretions. Once the agent enters the bloodstream (usually via inhalation of vapors) manifestations of cholinergic overload include nausea, vomiting, abdominal cramping, muscle twitching, difficulty breathing, cardiovascular instability, loss of consciousness, seizures, and central apnea. The onset of symptoms following vapor exposure is rapid (seconds to minutes). Liquid exposure to nerve agents results in differences in speed of onset and order of symptoms. Contact of a nerve agent with intact skin produces localized sweating followed by localized muscle fasciculations. Once in the muscle, the agent enters the circulation and causes the symptoms described above.

Rx Nerve Agents

Since nerve agents have a short circulating half-life, improvement should be rapid if exposure is terminated and supportive care and appropriate antidotes are given. Thus, the treatment of acute nerve agent poisoning involves decontamination, respiratory support, antidotes.
1. *Decontamination*: Procedures are the same as those described above for sulfur mustard.
2. *Respiratory support*: Death from nerve agent exposure is usually due to respiratory failure. Ventilation will be complicated by increased airway resistance and secretions. Atropine should be given before mechanical ventilation is instituted.
3. *Antidotal therapy* (see Table 32-4):
    a. *Atropine*: Generally the preferred anticholinergic agent of choice for treating acute nerve agent poisoning. Atropine rapidly reverses cholin-

TABLE 32-4 ANTIDOTE RECOMMENDATIONS FOLLOWING EXPOSURE TO NERVE AGENTS

Patient Age	Antidotes		Other Treatment
	Mild/Moderate Effects[a]	Severe Effects[b]	
Infants (0–2 yrs)	Atropine: 0.05 mg/kg IM, or 0.02 mg/kg IV; and 2-PAM chloride: 15 mg/kg IM or IV slowly	Atropine: 0.1 mg/kg IM, or 0.02 mg/kg IV; and 2-PAM chloride: 25 mg/kg IM, or 15 mg/kg IV slowly	Assisted ventilation after antidotes for severe exposure. Repeat atropine (2 mg IM, or 1 mg IM for infants) at 5- to 10-min intervals until secretions have diminished and breathing is comfortable or airway resistance has returned to near normal. Phentolamine for 2-PAM-induced hypertension: (5 mg IV for adults; 1 mg IV for children). Diazepam for convulsions: (0.2–0.5 mg IV for infants <5 years; 1 mg IV for children >5 years; 5 mg IV for adults).
Child (2–10 yrs)	Atropine: 1 mg IM, or 0.02 mg/kg IV; and 2-PAM chloride[c]: 15 mg/kg IM or IV slowly	Atropine: 2 mg IM, or 0.02 mg/kg IV; and 2-PAM chloride[c]: 25 mg/kg IM, or 15 mg/kg IV slowly	
Adolescent (>10 yrs)	Atropine: 2 mg IM, or 0.02 mg/kg IV; and 2-PAM chloride[c]: 15 mg/kg IM or IV slowly	Atropine: 4 mg IM, or 0.02 mg/kg IV; and 2-PAM chloride[c]: 25 mg/kg IM, or 15 mg/kg IV slowly	
Adult	Atropine: 2–4 mg IM or IV; and 2-PAM chloride: 600 mg IM, or 15 mg/kg IV slowly	Atropine: 6 mg IM; and 2-PAM chloride: 1800 mg IM, or 15 mg/kg IV slowly	
Elderly, frail	Atropine: 1 mg IM; and 2-PAM chloride: 10 mg/kg IM, or 5–10 mg/kg IV slowly	Atropine: 2–4 mg IM; and 2-PAM chloride: 25 mg/kg IM, or 5–10 mg/kg IV slowly	

[a]Mild/moderate effects include localized sweating, muscle fasciculations, nausea, vomiting, weakness, dyspnea.

[b]Severe effects include unconsciousness, convulsions, apnea, flaccid paralysis.

[c]If calculated dose exceeds the adult IM dose, adjust accordingly.

Note: 2-PAM chloride is pralidoxime chloride or protopam chloride.

Source: State of New York, Department of Health.

170

ergic overload at muscarinic synapses but has little effect at nicotinic synapses. Thus, atropine can rapidly treat the life-threatening respiratory effects of nerve agents but will probably not help neuromuscular effects. The field loading dose is 2–6 mg IM, with repeat doses given every 5–10 min until breathing and secretions improve. In the mildly affected pt with miosis and no systemic symptoms, atropine or homoatropine eye drops may suffice.

b. *Oxime therapy*: Oximes are nucleophiles that help restore normal enzyme function by reactivating the cholinesterase whose active site has been occupied and bound by the nerve agent. The oxime available in the United States is 2-pralidoxime chloride (2-PAM Cl). Treatment with 2-PAM may cause blood pressure elevation.

c. *Anticonvulsant*: Seizures caused by nerve agents do not respond to the usual anticonvulsants such as phenytoin, phenobarbital, carbamazepine, valproate, and lamotrigine. The only class of drugs known to have efficacy in treating nerve agent–induced seizures are the benzodiazepines. Diazepam is the only benzodiazepine approved by the U.S. Food and Drug Administration for the treatment of seizures (although other benzodiazepines have been shown to work well in animal models of nerve agent–induced seizures).

RADIATION BIOTERRORISM

Nuclear or radiation-related devices represent a third category of weapon that could be used in a terrorism attack. There are two major types of attacks that could occur. The first is the use of radiologic dispersal devices that cause the dispersal of radioactive material without detonation of a nuclear explosion. Such devices could use conventional explosives to disperse radionuclides. The second, and less probable, scenario would be the use of actual nuclear weapons by terrorists against a civilian target.

TYPES OF RADIATION

Alpha radiation consists of heavy, positively charged particles containing two protons and two neutrons. Due to their large size, alpha particles have limited penetrating power. Cloth and human skin can usually prevent alpha particles from penetrating into the body. If alpha particles are internalized, they can cause significant cellular damage.

Beta radiation consists of electrons and can travel only short distances in tissue. Plastic layers and clothing can stop most beta particles. Higher energy beta particles can cause injury to the basal stratum of skin similar to a thermal burn.

Gamma radiation and *x-rays* are forms of electromagnetic radiation discharged from the atomic nucleus. Sometimes referred to as *penetrating radiation*, both gamma and x-rays easily penetrate matter and are the principle type of radiation to cause whole-body exposure (see below).

Neutron particles are heavy and uncharged; often emitted during a nuclear detonation. Their ability to penetrate tissues is variable, depending upon their energy. They are less likely to be generated in various scenarios of radiation bioterrorism.

The commonly used units of radiation are the *rad* and the *gray*. The rad is the energy deposited within living matter and is equal to 100 ergs/g of tissue. The rad has been replaced by the SI unit of the gray (Gy). 100 rad = 1 Gy.

TYPES OF EXPOSURE

Whole-body exposure represents deposition of radiation energy over the entire body. Alpha and beta particles have limited penetration power and do not cause significant whole-body exposure unless they are internalized in large amounts. Whole-body exposure from gamma rays, x-rays, or high-energy neutron particles can penetrate the body, causing damage to multiple tissues and organs.

External contamination results from fallout of radioactive particles landing on the body surface, clothing, and hair. This is the dominant form of contamination likely to occur in a terrorist strike that utilizes a dispersal device. The most likely contaminants would emit alpha and beta radiation. Alpha particles do not penetrate the skin and thus would produce minimal systemic damage. Beta emitters can cause significant cutaneous burns. Gamma emitters not only cause cutaneous burns but can also cause significant internal damage.

Internal contamination will occur when radioactive material is inhaled, ingested, or is able to enter the body via a disruption in the skin. The respiratory tract is the main portal of entrance for internal contamination, and the lung is the organ at greatest risk. Radioactive material entering the GI tract will be absorbed according to its chemical structure and solubility. Penetration through the skin usually occurs when wounds or burns have disrupted the cutaneous barrier. Absorbed radioactive materials will travel throughout the body. Liver, kidney, adipose tissue, and bone tend to bind and retain radioactive material more than do other tissues.

Localized exposure results from close contact between highly radioactive material and a part of the body, resulting in discrete damage to the skin and deeper structures.

ACUTE RADIATION SICKNESS

Radiation interactions with atoms can result in ionization and free radical formation that damages tissue by disrupting chemical bonds and molecular structures in the cell, including DNA. Radiation can lead to cell death; cells that recover may have DNA mutations that pose a higher risk for malignant transformation. Cell sensitivity to radiation damage increases as replication rate increases. Bone marrow and mucosal surfaces in the GI tract have high mitotic activity and thus are significantly more prone to radiation damage than slowly dividing tissues such as bone and muscle. Acute radiation sickness (ARS) can develop following exposure of all or most of the human body to ionizing radiation. The clinical manifestation of ARS reflect the dose and type of radiation as well as the parts of the body that are exposed.

Clinical Features   ARS produces signs and symptoms related to damage of three major organ systems: GI tract, bone marrow, and neurovascular. The type and dose of radiation and the part of the body exposed will determine the dominant clinical picture.

- There are four major stages of ARS:
    1. *Prodrome* occurs between hours to 4 days after exposure and lasts from hours to days. Manifestations include: nausea, vomiting, anorexia, and diarrhea.
    2. The *latent stage* follows the prodrome and is associated with minimal or no symptoms. It most commonly lasts up to 2 weeks but can last as long as 6 weeks.
    3. *Illness* follows the latent stage.
    4. *Death or recovery* is the final stage of ARS.

- The higher the radiation dose, the shorter and more severe the stage.
- At low radiation doses (0.7–4 Gy), bone marrow suppression occurs and constitutes the main illness. The pt may develop bleeding or infection secondary to thrombocytopenia and leukopenia. The bone marrow will generally recover in most pts. Care is supportive (transfusion, antibiotics, colony-stimulating factors).
- With exposure to 6–8 Gy, the clinical picture is more complicated; the bone marrow may not recover and death will ensue. Damage to the GI mucosa producing diarrhea, hemorrhage, sepsis, fluid and electrolyte imbalance may occur and complicate the clinical picture.
- Whole-body exposure to >10 Gy is usually fatal. In addition to severe bone marrow and GI tract damage, a neurovascular syndrome characterized by vascular collapse, seizures, and death may occur (especially at doses >20 Gy).

℞ Acute Radiation Sickness

Treatment of ARS is largely supportive (Fig. 32-1).
1. Persons contaminated either externally or internally should be decontaminated as soon as possible. Contaminated clothes should be removed; showering or washing the entire skin and hair is very important. A radiation

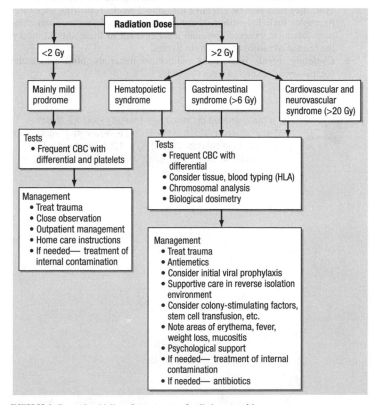

FIGURE 32-1 General guidelines for treatment of radiation casualties.

detector should be used to check for residual contamination. Decontamination of medical personnel should occur following emergency treatment and decontamination of the pt.

2. Treatment for the hematopoietic system includes appropriate therapy for neutropenia and infection, transfusion of blood products as needed, and hematopoietic growth factors. The value of bone marrow transplantation in this situation is unknown.

3. Partial or total parenteral nutrition is appropriate supportive therapy for pts with significant injury to the GI mucosa.

4. Treatment of internal radionuclide contamination is aimed at reducing absorption and enhancing elimination of the ingested material (Table 216-2, HPIM-17).

   a. Clearance of the GI tract may be achieved by gastric lavage, emetics, or purgatives, laxatives, ion exchange resins, and aluminum-containing antacids.

   b. Administration of *blocking agents* is aimed at preventing the entrance of radioactive materials into tissues (e.g., potassium iodide, which blocks the uptake of radioactive iodine by the thyroid).

   c. *Diluting agents* decrease the absorption of the radionuclide (e.g., water in the treatment of tritium contamination).

   d. *Mobilizing agents* are most effective when given immediately; however, they may still be effective for up to 2 weeks following exposure. Examples include antithyroid drugs, glucocorticoids, ammonium chloride, diuretics, expectorants, and inhalants. All of these should induce the release of radionuclides from tissues.

   e. *Chelating agents* bind many radioactive materials, after which the complexes are excreted from the body.

For a more detailed discussion, see Lane HC, Fauci AS: Microbial Bioterrorism, Chap. 214, p. 1343; Hurst CG, Newmark J, Romano JA: Chemical Bioterrorism, Chap. 215, p. 1352; Tochner ZA, Glatstein E: Radiation Bioterrorism, Chap. 216, p. 1358; in HPIM-17.

33 Chest Pain

There is little correlation between the severity of chest pain and the seriousness of its cause. The range of disorders that cause chest discomfort is shown in Table 33-1.

POTENTIALLY SERIOUS CAUSES

The differential diagnosis of chest pain is shown in Figs. 33-1 and 33-2. It is useful to characterize the chest pain as (1) new, acute, and ongoing; (2) recurrent, episodic; and (3) persistent, sometimes for days.

Myocardial Ischemia   Angina Pectoris Substernal pressure, squeezing, constriction, with radiation typically to left arm; usually on exertion, especially after meals or with emotional arousal. Characteristically relieved by rest and nitroglycerin.

Acute Myocardial Infarction (Chaps. 126 and 127) Similar to angina but usually more severe, of longer duration (≥ 30 min), and not immediately relieved by rest or nitroglycerin. S_3 and S_4 common.

TABLE 33-1	DIFFERENTIAL DIAGNOSES OF PATIENTS ADMITTED TO HOSPITAL WITH ACUTE CHEST PAIN RULED NOT MYOCARDIAL INFARCTION

Diagnosis	Percent
Gastroesophageal disease[a]	42
Gastroesophageal reflux	
Esophageal motility disorders	
Peptic ulcer	
Gallstones	
Ischemic heart disease	31
Chest wall syndromes	28
Pericarditis	4
Pleuritis/pneumonia	2
Pulmonary embolism	2
Lung cancer	1.5
Aortic aneurysm	1
Aortic stenosis	1
Herpes zoster	1

[a]In order of frequency.
Source: Fruergaard P et al: Eur Heart J 17:1028, 1996.

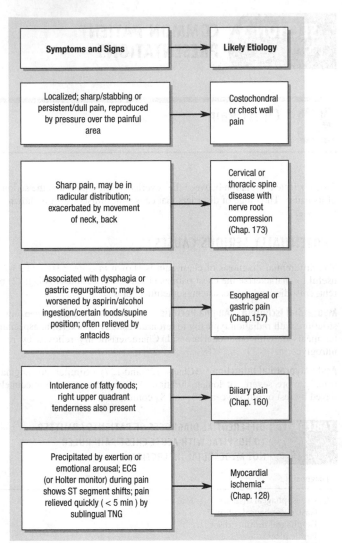

FIGURE 33-1 Differential diagnosis of recurrent chest pain. *If myocardial ischemia suspected, also consider aortic valve disease (Chap. 121) and hypertrophic obstructive cardiomyopathy (Chap. 122) if systolic murmur present.

Pulmonary Embolism   (Chap. 140)   May be substernal or lateral, pleuritic in nature, and associated with hemoptysis, tachycardia, and hypoxemia.

Aortic Dissection   (Chap. 132)   Very severe, in center of chest, a sharp "ripping" quality, radiates to back, not affected by changes in position. May be associated with weak or absent peripheral pulses.

Mediastinal Emphysema   Sharp, intense, localized to substernal region; often associated with audible crepitus.

	Acute myocardial infarction (Chaps. 126 and 127)	Aortic dissection (Chap. 132)	Acute pericarditis (Chap. 123)	Pulmonary embolism (Chap. 140)	Acute pneumothorax (Chap. 142)	Rupture of esophagus
Description of pain	Oppressive, constrictive, or squeezing; may radiate to arm(s), neck, back	"Tearing" or "ripping"; may travel from anterior chest to mid-back	Crushing, sharp, pleuritic; relieved by sitting forward	Pleuritic, sharp; possibly accompanied by cough/hemoptysis	Very sharp, pleuritic	Intense substernal and epigastric; accompanied by vomiting ± hematemesis
Background history	Less severe, similar pain on exertion; + coronary risk factors	Hypertension or Marfan syndrome (Chap. 169)	Recent upper respiratory tract infection, or other conditions which predispose to pericarditis (Chap. 123)	Recent surgery or other immobilization	Recent chest trauma, or history of chronic obstructive lung disease	Recent recurrent vomiting/retching
Key Physical findings	Diaphoresis, pallor; S4 common; S3 less common	Weak, asymmetric peripheral pulses; possible diastolic murmur of aortic insufficiency (Chap. 121)	Pericardial friction rub (usually 3 components, best heard by sitting patient forward)	Tachypnea; possible pleural friction rub	Tachypnea; breath sounds & hyperresonance over affected lung field	Subcutaneous emphysema; audible crepitus adjacent to the sternum
Confirmatory tests	• Serial ECGs • Serial cardiac markers (esp. troponins, CK)	• CXR – widened mediastinal silhouette • MRI, CT, or transesophageal echogram: intimal flap visualized • Aortic angiogram: definitive diagnosis	• ECG: diffuse ST elevation and PR segment depression • Echogram: pericardial effusion often visualized	• Normal d-dimer makes diagnosis unlikely • CT angiography or lung scan: V/Q mismatch • Pulmonary angiogram: arterial luminal filling defects	• CXR: radiolucency within pleural space; poss. collapse of adjacent lung segment; if tension pneumothorax, mediastinum is shifted to opp. side	• CXR – pneumomediastinum • Esophageal endoscopy is diagnostic

FIGURE 33-2 Differential diagnosis of acute chest pain.

Acute Pericarditis (Chap. 123) Usually steady, crushing, substernal; often has pleuritic component aggravated by cough, deep inspiration, supine position, and relieved by sitting upright; one-, two-, or three-component pericardial friction rub often audible.

Pleurisy Due to inflammation; less commonly tumor and pneumothorax. Usually unilateral, knifelike, superficial, aggravated by cough and respiration.

LESS SERIOUS CAUSES

Costochondral Pain In anterior chest, usually sharply localized, may be brief and darting or a persistent dull ache. Can be reproduced by pressure on costochondral and/or chondrosternal junctions. In Tietze's syndrome (costochondritis), joints are swollen, red, and tender.

Chest Wall Pain Due to strain of muscles or ligaments from excessive exercise or rib fracture from trauma; accompanied by local tenderness.

Esophageal Pain Deep thoracic discomfort; may be accompanied by dysphagia and regurgitation.

Emotional Disorders Prolonged ache or dartlike, brief, flashing pain; associated with fatigue, emotional strain.

OTHER CAUSES

(1) Cervical disk; (2) osteoarthritis of cervical or thoracic spine; (3) abdominal disorders: peptic ulcer, hiatus hernia, pancreatitis, biliary colic; (4) tracheobronchitis, pneumonia; (5) diseases of the breast (inflammation, tumor); (6) intercostal neuritis (herpes zoster).

APPROACH TO THE PATIENT WITH CHEST PAIN

A meticulous history of the behavior of pain, what precipitates it and what relieves it, aids diagnosis of recurrent chest pain. Figure 33-2 presents clues to diagnosis and workup of acute, life-threatening chest pain.

An ECG is key to the initial evaluation to rapidly distinguish patients with acute ST elevation MI, who typically warrant immediate reperfusion therapies (Chap. 126).

 For a more detailed discussion, see Lee TH: Chest Discomfort, Chap. 13, p. 87, in HPIM-17.

34 Abdominal Pain

Numerous causes, ranging from acute, life-threatening emergencies to chronic functional disease and disorders of several organ systems, can generate abdominal pain. Evaluation of acute pain requires rapid assessment of likely causes and early initiation of appropriate therapy. A more detailed and time-consuming approach to diagnosis may be followed in less acute situations. Table 34-1 lists the common causes of abdominal pain.

TABLE 34-1   COMMON ETIOLOGIES OF ABDOMINAL PAIN

Mucosal or muscle inflammation in hollow viscera: Peptic disease (ulcers, erosions, inflammation), hemorrhagic gastritis, gastroesophageal reflux, appendicitis, diverticulitis, cholecystitis, cholangitis, inflammatory bowel diseases (Crohn's, ulcerative colitis), infectious gastroenteritis, mesenteric lymphadenitis, colitis, cystitis, or pyelonephritis

Visceral spasm or distention: Intestinal obstruction (adhesions, tumor, intussusception), appendiceal obstruction with appendicitis, strangulation of hernia, irritable bowel syndrome (muscle hypertrophy and spasm), acute biliary obstruction, pancreatic ductal obstruction (chronic pancreatitis, stone), ureteral obstruction (kidney stone, blood clot), fallopian tubes (tubal pregnancy)

Vascular disorders: Mesenteric thromboembolic disease (arterial or venous), arterial dissection or rupture (e.g., aortic aneurysm), occlusion from external pressure or torsion (e.g., volvulus, hernia, tumor, adhesions, intussusception), hemoglobinopathy (esp. sickle cell disease)

Distention or inflammation of visceral surfaces: Hepatic capsule (hepatitis, hemorrhage, tumor, Budd-Chiari syndrome, Fitz-Hugh-Curtis syndrome), renal capsule (tumor, infection, infarction, venous occlusion), splenic capsule (hemorrhage, abscess, infarction), pancreas (pancreatitis, pseudocyst, abscess, tumor), ovary (hemorrhage into cyst, ectopic pregnancy, abscess)

Peritoneal inflammation: Bacterial infection (perforated viscus, pelvic inflammatory disease, infected ascites), intestinal infarction, chemical irritation, pancreatitis, perforated viscus (esp. stomach and duodenum), reactive inflammation (neighboring abscess, incl. diverticulitis, pleuropulmonary infection or inflammation), serositis (collagen-vascular diseases, familial Mediterranean fever), ovulation (mittelschmerz)

Abdominal wall disorders: Trauma, hernias, muscle inflammation or infection, hematoma (trauma, anticoagulant therapy), traction from mesentery (e.g., adhesions)

Toxins: Lead poisoning, black widow spider bite

Metabolic disorders: Uremia, ketoacidosis (diabetic, alcoholic), Addisonian crisis, porphyria, angioedema (C1 esterase deficiency), narcotic withdrawal

Neurologic disorders: Herpes zoster, tabes dorsalis, causalgia, compression or inflammation of spinal roots, (e.g., arthritis, herniated disk, tumor, abscess), psychogenic

Referred pain: From heart, lungs, esophagus, genitalia (e.g., cardiac ischemia, pneumonia, pneumothorax, pulmonary embolism, esophagitis, esophageal spasm, esophageal rupture)

APPROACH TO THE PATIENT: ABDOMINAL PAIN

HISTORY
History is of critical diagnostic importance. Physical exam may be unrevealing or misleading, and laboratory and radiologic exams delayed or unhelpful.

CHARACTERISTIC FEATURES OF ABDOMINAL PAIN
Duration and Pattern
These provide clues to nature and severity, although acute abdominal crisis may occasionally present insidiously or on a background of chronic pain.

Type and location provide a rough guide to nature of disease. *Visceral pain* (due to distention of a hollow viscus) localizes poorly and is often perceived in the midline. Intestinal pain tends to be crampy; when originating proximal to the ileocecal valve, it usually localizes above and around the umbilicus. Pain of colonic origin is perceived in the hypogastrium and lower quadrants. Pain from biliary or ureteral obstruction often causes pts to writhe in discomfort. *Somatic pain* (due to peritoneal inflammation) is usually sharper and more precisely localized to the diseased region (e.g., acute appendicitis; capsular distention of liver, kidney, or spleen), exacerbated by movement, causing pts to remain still. Pattern of radiation may be helpful: right shoulder (hepatobiliary origin), left shoulder (splenic), midback (pancreatic), flank (proximal urinary tract), groin (genital or distal urinary tract).

Factors That Precipitate or Relieve Pain
Ask about its relationship to eating (e.g., upper GI, biliary, pancreatic, ischemic bowel disease), defecation (colorectal), urination (genitourinary or colorectal), respiratory (pleuropulmonary, hepatobiliary), position (pancreatic, gastroesophageal reflux, musculoskeletal), menstrual cycle/menarche (tuboovarian, endometrial, including endometriosis), exertion (coronary/intestinal ischemia, musculoskeletal), medication or specific foods (motility disorders, food intolerance, gastroesophageal reflux, porphyria, adrenal insufficiency, ketoacidosis, toxins), and stress (motility disorders, nonulcer dyspepsia, irritable bowel syndrome).

Associated Symptoms
Look for fevers/chills (infection, inflammatory disease, infarction), weight loss (tumor, inflammatory disease, malabsorption, ischemia), nausea/vomiting (obstruction, infection, inflammatory disease, metabolic disease), dysphagia/odynophagia (esophageal), early satiety (gastric), hematemesis (esophageal, gastric, duodenal), constipation (colorectal, perianal, genitourinary), jaundice (hepatobiliary, hemolytic), diarrhea (inflammatory disease, infection, malabsorption, secretory tumors, ischemia, genitourinary), dysuria/hematuria/vaginal or penile discharge (genitourinary), hematochezia (colorectal or, rarely, urinary), skin/joint/eye disorders (inflammatory disease, bacterial or viral infection).

Predisposing Factors
Inquire about family history (inflammatory disease, tumors, pancreatitis), hypertension and atherosclerotic disease (ischemia), diabetes mellitus (motility disorders, ketoacidosis), connective tissue disease (motility disorders, serositis), depression (motility disorders, tumors), smoking (ischemia), recent smoking cessation (inflammatory disease), ethanol use (motility disorders, hepatobiliary, pancreatic, gastritis, peptic ulcer disease).

PHYSICAL EXAMINATION

Evaluate abdomen for prior trauma or surgery, current trauma; abdominal distention, fluid, or air; direct, rebound, and referred tenderness; liver and spleen size; masses, bruits, altered bowel sounds, hernias, arterial masses. Rectal examination assesses presence and location of tenderness, masses, blood (gross or occult). Pelvic examination in women is essential. *General examination*: evaluate for evidence of hemodynamic instability, acid-base disturbances, nutritional deficiency, coagulopathy, arterial occlusive disease, stigmata of liver disease, cardiac dysfunction, lymphadenopathy, and skin lesions.

ROUTINE LABORATORY AND RADIOLOGIC STUDIES

Choices depend on clinical setting (esp. severity of pain, rapidity of onset) and may include complete blood count, serum electrolytes, coagulation parameters, serum glucose, and biochemical tests of liver, kidney, and pancreatic function; chest x-ray to determine the presence of diseases involving heart, lung, mediastinum, and pleura; electrocardiogram is helpful to exclude referred pain from cardiac disease; plain abdominal radiographs to evaluate bowel displacement, intestinal distention, fluid and gas pattern, free peritoneal air, liver size, and abdominal calcifications (e.g., gallstones, renal stones, chronic pancreatitis).

SPECIAL STUDIES

These include abdominal ultrasonography (to visualize biliary ducts, gallbladder, liver, pancreas, and kidneys); CT to identify masses, abscesses, evidence of inflammation (bowel wall thickening, mesenteric "stranding," lymphadenopathy), aortic aneurysm; barium contrast radiographs (barium swallow, upper GI series, small-bowel follow-through, barium enema); upper GI endoscopy, sigmoidoscopy, or colonoscopy; cholangiography (endoscopic, percutaneous, or via MRI), angiography (direct or via CT or MRI), and radionuclide scanning. In selected cases, percutaneous biopsy, laparoscopy, and exploratory laparotomy may be required.

ACUTE, CATASTROPHIC ABDOMINAL PAIN

Intense abdominal pain of acute onset or pain associated with syncope, hypotension, or toxic appearance necessitates rapid yet orderly evaluation. Consider obstruction, perforation, or rupture of hollow viscus; dissection or rupture of major blood vessels (esp. aortic aneurysm); ulceration; abdominal sepsis; ketoacidosis; and adrenal crisis.

Brief History and Physical Examination   Historic features of importance include age; time of onset of the pain; activity of the pt when the pain began; location and character of the pain; radiation to other sites; presence of nausea, vomiting, or anorexia; temporal changes; changes in bowel habits; and menstrual history. Physical exam should focus on the pt's overall appearance [writhing in pain (ureteral lithiasis) vs. still (peritonitis, perforation)], position (a pt leaning forward may have pancreatitis or gastric perforation into the lesser sac), presence of fever or hypothermia, hyperventilation, cyanosis, bowel sounds, direct or rebound abdominal tenderness, pulsating abdominal mass, abdominal bruits, ascites, rectal blood, rectal or pelvic tenderness, and evidence of coagulopathy. Useful laboratory studies include hematocrit (may be normal with acute hemorrhage or misleadingly high with dehydration), WBC with differential count, arterial blood gases, serum electrolytes, BUN, creatinine, glucose, lipase or amylase, and UA. Females of reproductive age should have a pregnancy test. Radiologic studies should include supine and upright abdominal films (left lateral decubitus view if upright unobtainable) to evaluate bowel caliber and presence of free peritoneal air, cross-table lateral film to assess aortic diameter; CT (when available) to detect evidence of bowel perforation, inflammation, solid organ infarction, retroperitoneal bleeding, abscess, or tumor. Abdominal paracentesis (or peritoneal lavage in cases of trauma) can detect evidence of bleeding or peritonitis. Abdominal ultrasound (when available) reveals evidence of abscess, cholecystitis, biliary or ureteral obstruction, or hematoma and is used to determine aortic diameter.

Diagnostic Strategies The initial decision point is based on whether the pt is hemodynamically stable. If not, one must suspect a vascular catastrophe such as a leaking abdominal aortic aneurysm. Such pts receive limited resuscitation and move immediately to surgical exploration. If the pt is hemodynamically stable, the next decision point is whether the abdomen is rigid. Rigid abdomens are most often due to perforation or obstruction. The diagnosis can generally be made by a chest and plain abdominal radiograph.

If the abdomen is not rigid, the causes may be grouped based on whether the pain is poorly localized or well localized. In the presence of poorly localized pain, one should assess whether an aortic aneurysm is possible. If so, a CT scan can make the diagnosis; if not, early appendicitis, early obstruction, mesenteric ischemia, inflammatory bowel disease, pancreatitis, and metabolic problems are all in the differential diagnosis.

Pain localized to the epigastrium may be of cardiac origin or due to esophageal inflammation or perforation, gastritis, peptic ulcer disease, biliary colic or cholecystitis, or pancreatitis. Pain localized to the right upper quadrant includes those same entities plus pyelonephritis or nephrolithiasis, hepatic abscess, subdiaphragmatic abscess, pulmonary embolus, or pneumonia, or it may be of musculoskeletal origin. Additional considerations with left upper quadrant localization are infarcted or ruptured spleen, splenomegaly, and gastric or peptic ulcer. Right lower quadrant pain may be from appendicitis, Meckel's diverticulum, Crohn's disease, diverticulitis, mesenteric adenitis, rectus sheath hematoma, psoas abscess, ovarian abscess or torsion, ectopic pregnancy, salpingitis, familial fever syndromes, uterolithiasis, or herpes zoster. Left lower quadrant pain may be due to diverticulitis, perforated neoplasm, or other entities previously mentioned.

℞ Acute, Catastrophic Abdominal Pain

IV fluids, correction of life-threatening acid-base disturbances, and assessment of need for emergent surgery are the first priority; careful follow-up with frequent reexamination (when possible, by the same examiner) is essential. Relieve the pain. The use of narcotic analgesia is controversial. Traditionally, narcotic analgesics were withheld pending establishment of diagnosis and therapeutic plan, since masking of diagnostic signs may delay needed intervention. However, evidence that narcotics actually mask a diagnosis is sparse.

For a more detailed discussion, see Silen W: Abdominal Pain, Chap. 14, p. 91, in HPIM-17.

35 Headache

APPROACH TO THE PATIENT: HEADACHE

Headache is among the most common reasons that pts seek medical attention. Headache can be either primary or secondary (Table 35-1). First step—distinguish serious from benign etiologies. Symptoms that raise suspicion for a serious cause are listed in Table 35-2. Intensity of head pain rarely has diagnostic value; most pts who present to emergency ward with worst headache of their lives have migraine. Headache location can suggest involvement of local structures (temporal pain in giant cell arteritis, facial pain in sinusitis). Ruptured aneurysm (instant onset), cluster headache (peak over 3–5 min), and migraine (onset over minutes to hours) differ in time to peak intensity. Provocation by environmental factors suggests a benign cause.

Complete neurologic exam is important in the evaluation of headache. If exam is abnormal or if serious underlying cause is suspected, an imaging study (CT or MRI) is indicated as a first step. Lumbar puncture (LP) is required when meningitis (stiff neck, fever) or subarachnoid hemorrhage (after negative imaging) is a possibility. The psychological state of the patient should also be evaluated since a relationship exists between pain and depression.

MIGRAINE

A benign and recurring syndrome of headache associated with other symptoms of neurologic dysfunction in varying admixtures. The second most common cause of headache; afflicts ~15% of women and 6% of men. Diagnostic criteria for migraine are listed in Table 35-3. Onset usually in childhood, adolescence, or early adulthood; however, initial attack may occur at any age. Family history often positive. Women may have increased sensitivity to attacks during menstrual cycle. Classic triad: premonitory visual (scotoma or scintillations) sensory or motor symptoms, unilateral throbbing headache, nausea and vomiting. Most do not have visual aura and are therefore referred to as having "common migraine." Photo- and phonophobia common. Vertigo may occur. Focal neurologic disturbances without headache or vomiting (migraine equivalents) may also occur. An

TABLE 35-1	COMMON CAUSES OF HEADACHE			
Primary Headache		**Secondary Headache**		
Type	%	Type	%	
Migraine	16	Systemic infection	63	
Tension-type	69	Head injury	4	
Cluster	0.1	Vascular disorders	1	
Idiopathic stabbing	2	Subarachnoid hemorrhage	<1	
Exertional	1	Brain tumor	0.1	

Source: After J Olesen et al: *The Headaches.* Philadelphia, Lippincott, Williams & Wilkins, 2005, with permission.

TABLE 35-2	HEADACHE SYMPTOMS THAT SUGGEST A SERIOUS UNDERLYING DISORDER

"Worst" headache ever
First severe headache
Subacute worsening over days or weeks
Abnormal neurologic examination
Fever or unexplained systemic signs
Vomiting that precedes headache
Pain induced by bending, lifting, cough
Pain that disturbs sleep or presents immediately upon awakening
Known systemic illness
Onset after age 55
Pain associated with local tenderness, e.g., region of temporal artery

attack lasting 4–72 h is typical, as is relief after sleep. Attacks may be triggered by wine, cheese, chocolate, contraceptives, stress, exercise, or travel.

 Migraine

Three approaches to migraine treatment: nonpharmacologic (such as the avoidance of patient-specific triggers; information for pts is available at *www.achenet.org*); drug treatment of acute attacks (Tables 35-4 and 35-5); and prophylaxis (Table 35-6). Drug treatment necessary for most migraine pts, but avoidance or management of environmental triggers is sufficient for some. General principles of pharmacologic treatment: (1) response rates vary from 60–90%; (2) initial drug choice is empirical—influenced by age, coexisting illnesses, and side effect profile; (3) efficacy of prophylactic treatment may take several months to assess with each drug; (4) when an acute attack requires additional medication 60 min after the first dose, then the initial drug dose should be increased for subsequent attacks. Mild-to-moderate acute migraine attacks often respond to over-the-counter (OTC) NSAIDs when taken early in the attack. Triptans are widely used also but many have recurrence of pain after initial relief. There is less frequent headache recurrence when using ergots, but more frequent side effects. For prophylaxis, tricyclic antidepressants are a good first choice for young people with difficulty falling asleep; verapamil is often a first choice for prophylaxis in the elderly.

TABLE 35-3	SIMPLIFIED DIAGNOSTIC CRITERIA FOR MIGRAINE

Repeated attacks of headache lasting 4–72 h in patients with a normal physical examination, no other reasonable cause for the headache, and:

At least 2 of the following features:	Plus at least 1 of the following features:
Unilateral pain	Nausea/vomiting
Throbbing pain	Photophobia and phonophobia
Aggravation by movement	
Moderate or severe intensity	

Source: Adapted from the International Headache Society Classification (Headache Classification Committee of the International Headache Society, 2004).

TABLE 35-4   TREATMENT OF ACUTE MIGRAINE

Drug	Trade Name	Dosage
Simple Analgesics		
Acetaminophen, aspirin, caffeine	Excedrin Migraine	Two tablets or caplets q6h (max 8 per day)
NSAIDs		
Naproxen	Aleve, Anaprox, generic	220–550 mg PO bid
Ibuprofen	Advil, Motrin, Nuprin, generic	400 mg PO q3–4h
Tolfenamic acid	Clotam Rapid	200 mg PO. May repeat x 1 after 1–2 h
5-HT$_1$ Agonists		
Oral		
Ergotamine	Ergomar	One 2 mg sublingual tablet at onset and q^1/$_2$h (max 3 per day, 5 per week)
Ergotamine 1 mg, caffeine 100 mg	Ercaf, Wigraine	One or two tablets at onset, then one tablet q^1/$_2$h (max 6 per day, 10 per week)
Naratriptan	Amerge	2.5 mg tablet at onset; may repeat once after 4 h
Rizatriptan	Maxalt Maxalt-MLT	5–10 mg tablet at onset; may repeat after 2 h (max 30 mg/d)
Sumatriptan	Imitrex	50–100 mg tablet at onset; may repeat after 2 h (max 200 mg/d)
Frovatriptan	Frova	2.5 mg tablet at onset, may repeat after 2 h (max 5 mg/d)
Almotriptan	Axert	12.5 mg tablet at onset, may repeat after 2 h (max 25 mg/d)
Eletriptan	Relpax	40 or 80 mg
Zolmitriptan	Zomig Zomig Rapimelt	2.5 mg tablet at onset; may repeat after 2 h (max 10 mg/d)
Nasal		
Dihydroergotamine	Migranal Nasal Spray	Prior to nasal spray, the pump must be primed 4 times; 1 spray (0.5 mg) is administered, followed in 15 min by a second spray
Sumatriptan	Imitrex Nasal Spray	5–20 mg intranasal spray as 4 sprays of 5 mg or a single 20 mg spray (may repeat once after 2 h, not to exceed a dose of 40 mg/d)
Zolmitriptan	Zomig	5 mg intranasal spray as one spray (may repeat once after 2 h, not to exceed a dose of 10 mg/d)

(continued)

TABLE 35-4	TREATMENT OF ACUTE MIGRAINE (CONTINUED)	
Drug	Trade Name	Dosage
Parenteral		
Dihydroergota-mine	DHE-45	1 mg IV, IM, or SC at onset and q1h (max 3 mg/d, 6 mg per week)
Sumatriptan	Imitrex Injection	6 mg SC at onset (may repeat once after 1 h for max of 2 doses in 24 h)
Dopamine Antagonists		
Oral		
Metoclopramide	Reglan,[a] generic[a]	5–10 mg/d
Prochlorperazine	Compazine,[a] generic[a]	1–25 mg/d
Parenteral		
Chlorpromazine	Generic[a]	0.1 mg/kg IV at 2 mg/min; max 35 mg/d
Metoclopramide	Reglan,[a] generic	10 mg IV
Prochlorperazine	Compazine,[a] generic[a]	10 mg IV
Other		
Oral		
Acetaminophen, 325 mg, *plus* dichloralphena-zone, 100 mg, *plus* isomethep-tene, 65 mg	Midrin, Duradrin, generic	Two capsules at onset followed by 1 capsule q1h (max 5 capsules)
Nasal		
Butorphanol	Stadol[a]	1 mg (1 spray in 1 nostril), may repeat if necessary in 1–2 h
Parenteral		
Narcotics	Generic[a]	Multiple preparations and dosages; see Table 6-2

[a]Not all drugs are specifically indicated by the FDA for migraine. Local regulations and guidelines should be consulted.

Note: Antiemetics (e.g., domperidone 10 mg or ondansetron) or prokinetics (e.g., metoclopramide 10 mg) are sometimes useful adjuncts.

Abbreviations: NSAIDs, nonsteroidal anti-inflammatory drugs; 5-HT, 5-hydroxytryptamine.

Tension Headache Common in all age groups. Pain is holocephalic, described as bilateral pressure or a tight band. May persist for hours or days; usually builds slowly. Pain can be managed generally with simple analgesics such as acetaminophen, aspirin, or NSAIDs. Often related to stress; responds to behavioral approaches including relaxation. Amitriptyline may be helpful for chronic tension-type headache prophylaxis.

Cluster Headache Rare form of primary headache; population frequency 0.1%. Characterized by episodes of recurrent, deep, nocturnal, unilateral, retroorbital searing pain. Typically, a young male (three times more common in males) awakens 2–4 h after sleep onset with severe pain, unilateral lacrimation, and nasal and conjunctival congestion. Visual complaints, nausea, or vomiting are rare. Unlike

TABLE 35-5	CLINICAL STRATIFICATION OF ACUTE SPECIFIC MIGRAINE TREATMENTS
Clinical Situation	Treatment Options

Failed NSAIDS/analgesics	**First tier**
	   Sumatriptan 50 mg or 100 mg PO
	   Almotriptan 12.5 mg PO
	   Rizatriptan 10 mg PO
	   Eletriptan 40 mg PO
	   Zolmitriptan 2.5 mg PO
	Slower effect/better tolerability
	   Naratriptan 2.5 mg PO
	   Frovatriptan 2.5 mg PO
	Infrequent headache
	   Ergotamine 1–2 mg PO
	   Dihydroergotamine nasal spray 2 mg

Early nausea or difficulties taking tablets	Zolmitriptan 5 mg nasal spray Sumatriptan 20 mg nasal spray Rizatriptan 10 mg MLT wafer
Headache recurrence	Ergotamine 2 mg (most effective PR/usually with caffeine) Naratriptan 2.5 mg PO Almotriptan 12.5 mg PO Eletriptan 40 mg
Tolerating acute treatments poorly	Naratriptan 2.5 mg Almotriptan 12.5 mg
Early vomiting	Zolmitriptan 5 mg nasal spray Sumatriptan 25 mg PR Sumatriptan 6 mg SC

Menses-related headache	**Prevention**
	   Ergotamine PO at night
	   Estrogen patches
	Treatment
	   Triptans
	   Dihydroergotamine nasal spray

Very rapidly developing symptoms	Zolmitriptan 5 mg nasal spray Sumatriptan 6 mg SC Dihydroergotamine 1 mg IM

migraine, patients with cluster tend to move about during attacks. A core feature is periodicity. Pain lasts 30–120 min but tends to recur at the same time of night or several times each 24 h over 4–8 weeks (a cluster). A pain-free period of months or years may be followed by another cluster of headaches. Alcohol provokes attacks in 70%. Prophylaxis with verapamil (40–80 mg twice daily to start), lithium (600–900 mg/d), prednisone (60 mg/d for 7 days followed by a rapid taper), or ergotamine (1–2 mg suppository 1–2 h before expected attack). High-flow oxygen (10–12 L/min for 15–20 min) or sumatriptan (6 mg SC or 20-mg nasal spray) is useful for the acute attack. Deep-brain stimulation of the posterior hypothalamic gray matter is successful for refractory cases.

Post-Concussion Headache Common following motor vehicle collisions, other head trauma; severe injury or loss of consciousness often not present. Symptoms of headache, dizziness, vertigo, impaired memory, poor concentration, irritability; typically remits after several weeks to months. Neurologic examina-

TABLE 35-6   PREVENTIVE TREATMENTS IN MIGRAINE[a]

Drug	Dose	Selected Side Effects
Pizotifen[b]	0.5–2 mg qd	Weight gain Drowsiness
Beta blocker		
Propranolol	40–120 mg bid	Reduced energy Tiredness Postural symptoms *Contraindicated in asthma*
Tricyclics		
Amitriptyline	10–75 mg at night	Drowsiness
Dothiepin	25–75 mg at night	
Nortriptyline	25–75 mg at night	*Note:* Some patients may only need a total dose of 10 mg, although generally 1–1.5 mg/kg body weight is required
Anticonvulsants		
Topiramate	25–200 mg/d	Paresthesias Cognitive symptoms Weight loss Glaucoma Caution with nephrolithiasis
Valproate	400–600 mg bid	Drowsiness Weight gain Tremor Hair loss Fetal abnormalities Hematologic or liver abnormalities
Gabapentin	900–3600 mg qd	Dizziness Sedation
Serotonergic drugs		
Methysergide	1–4 mg qd	Drowsiness Leg cramps Hair loss Retroperitoneal fibrosis (1-month drug holiday is required every 6 months)
Flunarizine[b]	5–15 mg qd	Drowsiness Weight gain Depression Parkinsonism
No convincing evidence from controlled trials		
Verapamil		
Controlled trials demonstrate *no effect*		
Nimodipine		
Clonidine		
SSRIs: fluoxetine		

[a]Commonly used preventives are listed with reasonable doses and common side effects. Not all listed medicines are approved by the FDA; local regulations and guidelines should be consulted.

[b]Not available in the United States.

tion and neuroimaging studies normal. Not a functional disorder; cause unknown and treatment usually not satisfactory.

Lumbar Puncture Headache Typical onset 24–48 h after LP; follows 10–30% of LPs. Positional: onset when pt sits or stands, relief by lying flat. Most cases remit spontaneously in ≤1 week. Intravenous caffeine (500 mg IV, repeat in 1 h if dose ineffective) successful in 85%; epidural blood patch effective immediately in refractory cases.

Cough Headache Transient severe head pain with coughing, bending, lifting, sneezing, or stooping; lasts from seconds to several minutes; men > women. Usually benign, but posterior fossa mass lesion in ~25%. Consider brain MRI.

Indomethacin-Responsive Headaches A diverse set of disorders that respond often exquisitely to indomethacin include:

- *Paroxysmal hemicrania*: Frequent unilateral, severe, short-lasting episodes of headache that are often retroorbital and associated with autonomic phenomena such as lacrimation and nasal congestion.
- *Hemicrania continua*: Moderate and continuous unilateral pain associated with fluctuations of severe pain that may be associated with autonomic features.
- *Primary stabbing headache*: Stabbing pain confined to the head or rarely the face lasting from 1 to many seconds or minutes.
- *Primary cough headache*
- *Primary exertional headache*: Has features similar to cough headache and migraine; usually precipitated by any form of exercise.

FACIAL PAIN

Most common cause of facial pain is dental; triggered by hot, cold, or sweet foods. Exposure to cold repeatedly induces dental pain. Trigeminal neuralgia consists of paroxysmal, electric shock–like episodes of pain in the distribution of trigeminal nerve; occipital neuralgia presents as lancinating occipital pain. These disorders are discussed in Chap. 197.

For a more detailed discussion, see Goadsby PJ and Raskin NH: Headache, Chap. 15, p. 95, in HPIM-17.

36 Back and Neck Pain

LOW BACK PAIN

The cost of low back pain (LBP) in the United States is ~$100 billion annually. Back symptoms are the most common cause of disability in those <45 years; ~1% of the United States population is disabled because of back pain.

Types of Low Back Pain

- *Local pain*—caused by stretching of pain-sensitive structures that compress or irritate nerve endings; pain (i.e., tears, stretching) located near the affected part of the back.
- *Pain referred to the back*—abdominal or pelvic origin; back pain unaffected by routine movements.
- *Pain of spine origin*—restricted to the back or referred to lower limbs or buttock. Diseases of upper lumbar spine refer pain to upper lumbar region, groin, or anterior thighs. Diseases of lower lumbar spine refer pain to buttocks or posterior thighs.
- *Radicular back pain*—radiates from spine to leg in specific nerve root territory. Coughing, sneezing, lifting heavy objects, or straining may elicit pain.
- *Pain associated with muscle spasm*—diverse causes; accompanied by taut paraspinal muscles and abnormal posture.

Examination Include abdomen, pelvis, and rectum to search for visceral sources of pain. Inspection may reveal scoliosis or muscle spasm. Palpation may elicit pain over a diseased spine segment. Pain from hip may be confused with spine pain; manual internal/external rotation of leg at hip (knee and hip in flexion) reproduces the hip pain.

Straight leg raising (SLR) sign—elicited by passive flexion of leg at the hip with pt in supine position; maneuver stretches L5/S1 nerve roots and sciatic nerve passing posterior to the hip; SLR sign is positive if maneuver reproduces the pain. Crossed SLR sign—positive when SLR on one leg reproduces symptoms in opposite leg or buttocks; nerve/nerve root lesion is on the painful side. Reverse SLR sign—passive extension of leg backwards with pt standing; maneuver stretches L2–L4 nerve roots and femoral nerve passing anterior to the hip.

Neurologic exam—search for focal atrophy, weakness, reflex loss, diminished sensation in a dermatomal distribution. Findings with radiculopathy are summarized in Table 36-1.

Laboratory Evaluation "Routine" laboratory studies and lumbar spine x-rays are rarely needed for acute LBP (<3 months) but indicated when risk factors for serious underlying disease are present (Table 36-2). MRI and CT-myelography are tests of choice for anatomic definition of spine disease. Electromyography (EMG) and nerve conduction studies useful for functional assessment of peripheral nervous system.

Etiology **Lumbar Disk Disease** Common cause of low back and leg pain; usually at L4-L5 or L5-S1 levels. Dermatomal sensory loss, reduction or loss of deep tendon reflexes, or myotomal pattern of weakness more informative than pain pattern for localization. Usually unilateral; can be bilateral with large central disk herniations compressing multiple nerve roots and causing cauda equina syndrome (Chap. 198). Indications for lumbar disk surgery: (1) progressive motor weakness from nerve root injury, (2) progressive motor impairment by EMG, (3) abnormal bowel or bladder function, (4) incapacitating nerve root pain despite conservative treatment for at least 4 weeks, and (5) recurrent incapacitating pain despite conservative treatment. The latter two criteria are controversial.

Spinal Stenosis A narrowed spinal canal producing neurogenic claudication, i.e., back, buttock, and/or leg pain induced by walking or standing and relieved by sitting. Symptoms are usually bilateral. Unlike vascular claudication, symptoms are provoked by standing without walking. Unlike lumbar disk disease, symptoms are relieved by sitting. Focal neurologic deficits common; severe neurologic deficits (paralysis, incontinence) rare. Stenosis results from acquired

TABLE 36-1 LUMBOSACRAL RADICULOPATHY—NEUROLOGIC FEATURES

Lumbosacral Nerve Roots	Examination Findings			Pain Distribution
	Reflex	Sensory	Motor	
L2[a]	—	Upper anterior thigh	Psoas (hip flexion)	Anterior thigh
L3[a]	—	Lower anterior thigh Anterior knee	Psoas (hip flexion) Quadriceps (knee extension) Thigh adduction	Anterior thigh, knee
L4[a]	Quadriceps (knee)	Medial calf	Quadriceps (knee extension)[b] Thigh adduction Tibialis anterior (foot dorsiflexion)	Knee, medial calf Anterolateral thigh
L5[c]	—	Dorsal surface—foot Lateral calf	Peroneii (foot eversion)[b] Tibialis anterior (foot dorsiflexion) Gluteus medius (hip abduction) Toe dorsiflexors	Lateral calf, dorsal foot, posterolateral thigh, buttocks
S1[c]	Gastrocnemius/soleus (ankle)	Plantar surface—foot Lateral aspect—foot	Gastrocnemius/soleus (foot plantar flexion)[b] Abductor hallucis (toe flexors)[b] Gluteus maximus (hip extension)	Bottom foot, posterior calf, posterior thigh, buttocks

[a]Reverse straight leg–raising sign present—see "Examination of the Back."
[b]These muscles receive the majority of innervation from this root.
[c]Straight leg–raising sign present—see "Examination of the Back."

TABLE 36-2	**ACUTE LOW BACK PAIN: RISK FACTORS FOR AN IMPORTANT STRUCTURAL CAUSE**

History
- Pain worse at rest or at night
- Prior history of cancer
- History of chronic infection (esp. lung, urinary tract, skin)
- History of trauma
- Incontinence
- Age > 50 years
- Intravenous drug use
- Glucocorticoid use
- History of a rapidly progressive neurologic deficit

Examination
- Unexplained fever
- Unexplained weight loss
- Percussion tenderness over the spine
- Abdominal, rectal, or pelvic mass
- Patrick's sign or heel percussion sign
- Straight leg– or reverse straight leg–raising signs
- Progressive focal neurologic deficit

(75%), congenital, or mixed acquired/congenital factors. Symptomatic treatment adequate for mild disease; surgery indicated when pain interferes with activities of daily living or focal neurologic signs present. Most patients treated surgically experience at least 75% relief of back and leg pain; 25% develop recurrent stenosis within 5 years.

Trauma *Low back strain* or *sprain* used to describe minor, self-limited injuries associated with LBP. *Vertebral fractures* from trauma result in anterior wedging or compression of vertebral bodies; burst fractures involving vertebral body and posterior spine elements can occur. Neurologic impairment common with vertebral fractures; early surgical intervention indicated. CT scans are used as a screening tool for spine disease in moderate to severe trauma as they are superior to routine x-rays for bony disease. Most common cause of *nontraumatic fracture* is osteoporosis; others are osteomalacia, hyperparathyroidism, hyperthyroidism, multiple myeloma, or metastatic carcinoma; glucocorticoid use may predispose vertebral body to fracture. Clinical context, exam findings, and imaging establish diagnosis.

Spondylolisthesis Slippage of anterior spine forward, leaving posterior elements behind; L4-L5 > L5-S1 levels; can produce LBP or radiculopathy/cauda equina syndrome (see Chap. 198).

Osteoarthritis Back pain induced by spine movement and associated with stiffness. Increases with age; radiologic findings do not correlate with severity of pain. Facet syndrome—radicular symptoms and signs, nerve root compression by unilateral facet hypertrophy and osteophytes. Loss of intervertebral disk height reduces vertical dimensions of intervertebral foramen; descending pedicle can compress the exiting nerve root.

Vertebral Metastases Back pain most common neurologic symptom in patients with systemic cancer and may be presenting complaint; pain typically unrelieved by rest. Metastatic carcinoma, multiple myeloma, and lymphomas frequently involve spine. MRI or CT-myelography demonstrates vertebral body metastasis; disk space is spared.

TABLE 36-3	VISCERAL CAUSES OF LOW BACK PAIN

Stomach (posterior wall)—gallbladder—gallstones
Pancreas—tumor, cyst, pancreatitis
Retroperitoneal—hemorrhage, tumor, pyelonephritis
Vascular—abdominal aortic aneurysm, renal artery and vein thrombosis
Colon—colitis, diverticulitis, neoplasm
Uterosacral ligaments—endometriosis, carcinoma
Uterine malposition
Menstrual pain
Neoplastic infiltration of nerves
Radiation neurosis of tumors/nerves
Prostate—carcinoma, prostatitis
Kidney—renal stones, inflammatory disease, neoplasm, infection

Vertebral Osteomyelitis   Back pain unrelieved by rest; focal spine tenderness, elevated ESR. Primary source of infection (lung, urinary tract, or skin) found in fewer than half of cases; IV drug abuse a risk factor. Destruction of the vertebral bodies and disk space common. Lumbar spinal epidural abscess presents as back pain and fever; exam may be normal or show radicular findings, spinal cord involvement, or cauda equina syndrome. Extent of abscess best defined by MRI.

Lumbar Arachnoiditis   May follow inflammation within subarachnoid space; fibrosis results in clumping of nerve roots, best seen by MRI; treatment is unsatisfactory.

Immune Disorders   Ankylosing spondylitis, rheumatoid arthritis, Reiter's syndrome, psoriatic arthritis, and chronic inflammatory bowel disease. Ankylosing spondylitis—typically male <40 years with nocturnal back pain and morning stiffness; pain unrelieved by rest but improves with exercise.

Osteoporosis   Loss of bone substance resulting from hyperparathyroidism, chronic glucocorticoid use, immobilization, other medical disorders, or increasing age (particularly in females). Sole manifestation may be back pain exacerbated by movement. Can also occur in the upper back.

Visceral Diseases   (Table 36-3)   Pelvis refers pain to sacral region, lower abdomen to mid-lumbar region, upper abdomen to lower thoracic or upper lumbar region. Local signs are absent; normal movements of the spine are painless. A contained rupture of an abdominal aortic aneurysm may produce isolated back pain.

Other   Chronic LBP with no clear cause; psychiatric disorders, substance abuse may be associated.

 Low Back Pain

ACUTE LOW BACK PAIN (ALBP)

Pain of <3 months' duration; full recovery occurs in 85%. Management controversial; few well-controlled clinical trials exist. Algorithms are presented in Fig. 36-1. If "risk factors" (Table 36-2) are absent, initial treatment is symptomatic and no diagnostic tests necessary. Spine infections, fractures, tumors, or rapidly progressive neurologic deficits require urgent diagnostic evaluation.

   Clinical trials do not show benefit from bed rest >2 days. Possible benefits of early activity—cardiovascular conditioning, disk and cartilage nutrition, bone and muscle strength, increased endorphin levels. Studies of traction or posture

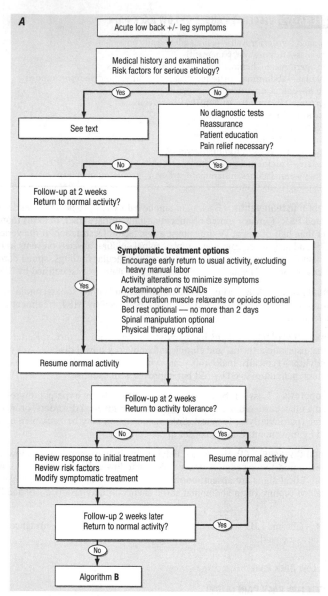

FIGURE 36-1 Algorithms for management of acute low back pain, age ≥ 18 years. *A.* Symptoms <3 months, first 4 weeks. *B.* Management weeks 4–12. ①, entry point from Algorithm *C* postoperatively or if patient declines surgery. *C.* Surgical options. (NSAIDs, nonsteroidal anti-inflammatory drugs; CBC, complete blood count; ESR, erythrocyte sedimentation rate; UA, urinalysis; EMG, electromyography; NCV, nerve conduction velocity studies; MRI, magnetic resonance imaging; CT, computed tomography; CNS, central nervous system.)

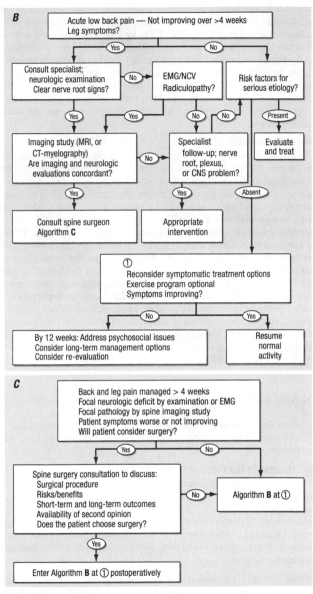

FIGURE 36-1 *(Continued)*

modification fail to show benefit. Proof lacking to support acupuncture, ultrasound, diathermy, transcutaneous electrical nerve stimulation, massage, biofeedback, magnets, or electrical stimulation. Self-application of ice or heat or use of shoe insoles is optional given low cost and risk. A short course of lumbar spinal manipulation or physical therapy is a reasonable option. Temporary suspension of activities known to increase mechanical stress on the spine (heavy lifting, straining at stool, prolonged sitting/bending/twisting) may relieve symptoms. Value of education ("back school") in long-term prevention is unclear.

Pharmacologic treatment of ALBP includes NSAIDs and acetaminophen (Chap 6). Muscle relaxants (cyclobenzaprine) provide short-term benefit (4–7 days), but drowsiness limits use. Opioids are not superior to NSAIDs or acetaminophen for ALBP. Epidural glucocorticoids may occasionally produce short-term pain relief, but proof is lacking for a benefit beyond 1 month. Systemic glucocorticoids, opioids, or tricyclic antidepressants are not indicated as initial treatment.

CHRONIC LOW BACK PAIN (CLBP)

Pain lasting >3 months; differential diagnosis includes most conditions described above. CLBP causes can be clarified by neuroimaging and EMG/nerve conduction studies; diagnosis of radiculopathy secure when results concordant with findings on neurologic exam. Treatment should not be based on neuroimaging alone: up to one-third of asymptomatic young adults have a herniated lumbar disk by CT or MRI.

Management is not amenable to a simple algorithmic approach. Treatment based upon identification of underlying cause; when specific cause not found, conservative management necessary. Pharmacologic and comfort measures similar to those described for ALBP. Exercise ("work hardening") regimens effective in returning some pts to work, diminishing pain, and improving walking distances. Hydrotherapy may be useful. Some pts report short-term pain relief with percutaneous electrical nerve stimulation, which has not been adequately studied. An unblinded study in patients with chronic sciatica found that surgery could hasten relief of symptoms by ~2 months; however, at 1 year there was no advantage of surgery over conservative medical therapy; nearly all (95%) pts in both groups made a full recovery.

NECK AND SHOULDER PAIN

Usually arises from diseases of the cervical spine and soft tissues of the neck; typically precipitated by movement and may be accompanied by focal tenderness and limitation of motion.

Etiology   Trauma to the Cervical Spine   Trauma to the cervical spine (fractures, subluxation) places the spine at risk for compression; immediate immobilization of the neck is essential to minimize movement of unstable cervical spine segments.

Whiplash injury is due to trauma (usually automobile accidents) causing cervical musculoligamental sprain or strain due to hyperflexion or hyperextension. This diagnosis is not applied to pts with fractures, disk herniation, head injury, or altered consciousness.

Cervical Disk Disease   Herniation of a lower cervical disk is a common cause of neck, shoulder, arm, or hand pain or tingling. Neck pain (worse with movement), stiffness, and limited range of neck motion are common. With nerve root compression, pain may radiate into a shoulder or arm. Extension and lateral rotation of the neck narrows the intervertebral foramen and may reproduce radicular symptoms (Spurling's sign). In young individuals, acute radiculopathy from a ruptured disk is often traumatic. *Subacute radiculopathy* is less likely to be related to a specific traumatic incident and may involve both disk disease and spondylosis. Clinical features of cervical nerve root lesions are summarized in Table 36-4.

TABLE 36-4 CERVICAL RADICULOPATHY—NEUROLOGIC FEATURES

Cervical Nerve Roots	Examination Findings			Pain Distribution
	Reflex	Sensory	Motor	
C5	Biceps	Over lateral deltoid	Supraspinatus[a] (initial arm abduction) Infraspinatus[a] (arm external rotation) Deltoid[a] (arm abduction) Biceps (arm flexion)	Lateral arm, medial scapula
C6	Biceps	Thumb, index fingers Radial hand/forearm	Biceps (arm flexion) Pronator teres (internal forearm rotation)	Lateral forearm, thumb, index finger
C7	Triceps	Middle fingers Dorsum forearm	Triceps[a] (arm extension) Wrist extensors[a] Extensor digitorum[a] (finger extension)	Posterior arm, dorsal forearm, lateral hand
C8	Finger flexors	Little finger Medial hand and forearm	Abductor pollicis brevis (abduction D1) First dorsal interosseous (abduction D2) Abductor digiti minimi (abduction D5)	4th and 5th fingers, medial forearm
T1	Finger flexors	Axilla and medial arm	Abductor pollicis brevis (abduction D1) First dorsal interosseous (abduction D2) Abductor digiti minimi (abduction D5)	Medial arm, axilla

[a]These muscles receive the majority of innervation from this root.

Cervical Spondylosis Osteoarthritis of the cervical spine may produce neck pain that radiates into the back of the head, shoulders, or arms; can also be source of headaches in the posterior occipital region. A combined radiculopathy and myelopathy may occur. An electrical sensation elicited by neck flexion and radiating down the spine from the neck (Lhermitte's symptom) usually indicates spinal cord involvement. MRI or CT-myelography can define the anatomic abnormalities, and EMG and nerve conduction studies can quantify the severity and localize the levels of nerve root injury.

Other Causes of Neck Pain Includes *rheumatoid arthritis* of the cervical apophyseal joints, ankylosing spondylitis, *herpes zoster* (shingles), *neoplasms* metastatic to the cervical spine, *infections* (osteomyelitis and epidural abscess), and *metabolic bone diseases*. Neck pain may also be referred from the heart with coronary artery ischemia (cervical angina syndrome).

Thoracic Outlet An anatomic region containing the first rib, the subclavian artery and vein, the brachial plexus, the clavicle, and the lung apex. Injury may result in posture- or task-related pain around the shoulder and supraclavicular region. *True neurogenic thoracic outlet syndrome* results from compression of the lower trunk of the brachial plexus by an anomalous band of tissue; treatment consists of surgical division of the band. *Arterial thoracic outlet syndrome* results from compression of the subclavian artery by a cervical rib; treatment is with thrombolyis or anticoagulation, and surgical excision of the cervical rib. *Disputed thoracic outlet syndrome* includes a large number of patients with chronic arm and shoulder pain of unclear cause; surgery is controversial, and treatment is often unsuccessful.

Brachial Plexus and Nerves Pain from injury to the brachial plexus or peripheral nerves can mimic pain of cervical spine origin. *Neoplastic infiltration* can produce this syndrome, as can *postradiation fibrosis* (pain less often present). *Acute brachial neuritis* consists of acute onset of severe shoulder or scapular pain followed over days by weakness of proximal arm and shoulder girdle muscles innervated by the upper brachial plexus; onset often preceded by an infection or immunization.

Shoulder If signs of radiculopathy are absent, differential diagnosis includes mechanical shoulder pain (tendinitis, bursitis, rotator cuff tear, dislocation, adhesive capsulitis, and cuff impingement under the acromion) and referred pain (subdiaphragmatic irritation, angina, Pancoast tumor). Mechanical pain is often worse at night, associated with shoulder tenderness, and aggravated by abduction, internal rotation, or extension of the arm.

℞ Neck and Shoulder Pain

Symptomatic treatment of neck pain includes analgesic medications and/or a soft cervical collar. Indications for cervical disk and lumbar disk surgery are similar; however, with cervical disease, an aggressive approach is indicated if spinal cord injury is threatened. Surgery of *cervical herniated disks* consists of an anterior approach with diskectomy followed by anterior interbody fusion; a simple posterior partial laminectomy with diskectomy is an acceptable alternative. Another surgical approach involves implantation of an artificial disk, which is not yet approved for use in the United States. The cumulative risk of subsequent radiculopathy or myelopathy at cervical segments adjacent to the fusion is 3% per year. *Nonprogressive cervical radiculopathy* due to a herniated cervical disk may be treated conservatively with a high rate of success. *Cervical spondylosis* with bony, compressive cervical radiculopathy is generally treated with surgical decompression to interrupt the progression of neurologic signs. *Spondylotic myelopathy* is managed with either anterior decompression and fusion or laminectomy because myelopathy progresses in 20–30% of untreated patients. One prospective study comparing surgery versus conservative treatment for mild cervical spondylotic myelopathy showed no difference in outcome after 2 years of follow-up.

 For more detailed discussion, see Engstrom JW: Back and Neck Pain, Chap. 16, p. 107, in HPIM-17.

37 Fever, Hyperthermia, Chills, and Rash

FEVER

Definitions   *Temperature*: Normal body temperature is maintained (≤37.2°C/98.9°F in the morning and ≤37.7°C/99.9°F in the evening) because the hypothalamic thermoregulatory center balances excess heat production from metabolic activity in muscle and liver with heat dissipation from the skin and lungs.

Fever: an elevation of normal body temperature in conjunction with an increase in the hypothalamic set point. Infectious causes are common.

Fever of unknown origin (FUO):

1. *Classic FUO*: three outpt visits or 3 days in the hospital without elucidation of a cause of fever; *or* 1 week of unproductive intelligent and invasive ambulatory investigation, temperatures >38.3°C (>101°F) on several occasions, and duration of fever for >3 weeks
2. *Nosocomial FUO*: at least 3 days of investigation and 2 days of culture incubation failing to elucidate a cause of fever in a hospitalized pt with temperatures >38.3°C (>101°F) on several occasions and no infection on admission
3. *Neutropenic FUO*: at least 3 days of investigation and 2 days of culture incubation failing to elucidate a cause of fever in a pt with temperatures >38.3°C (>101°F) on several occasions whose neutrophil count is <500/μL or is expected to fall to that level within 1–2 days
4. *HIV-associated FUO*: failure of appropriate investigation to reveal a cause of fever in an HIV-infected pt with temperatures >38.3°C (>101°F) on several occasions over a period of >4 weeks for outpts and >3 days for hospitalized pts

Hyperpyrexia: temperatures >41.5°C (>106.7°F) that can occur with severe infections but more commonly occur with CNS hemorrhages

Etiology   Most fevers are associated with self-limited infections (usually viral) and have causes that are easily identified.

• *Classic FUO*: As the duration of fever increases, the likelihood of an infectious etiology decreases. Etiologies to consider include:

1. Infection–e.g., extrapulmonary tuberculosis; EBV, CMV, or HIV infection; occult abscesses; endocarditis; fungal disease
2. Neoplasm–e.g., lymphoma and hematologic malignancies, hepatoma, renal cell carcinoma
3. Miscellaneous noninfectious inflammatory diseases
   a. Systemic rheumatologic disease or vasculitis–e.g., Still's disease, lupus erythematosus
   b. Granulomatous disease–e.g., granulomatous hepatitis, sarcoidosis, Crohn's disease
   c. Miscellaneous diseases–e.g., pulmonary embolism, hereditary fever syndromes, drug fever, factitious fevers

- *Nosocomial FUO*
  Infectious–e.g., infected foreign bodies or catheters, *Clostridium difficile* colitis, sinusitis
  Noninfectious–e.g., drug fever, pulmonary embolism
- *Neutropenic FUO*: Neutropenic pts are susceptible to focal bacterial and fungal infections, bacteremic infections, perianal infections, and catheter-associated infections. More than 50–60% of pts with febrile neutropenia are infected, and 20% are bacteremic.
- *HIV-associated FUO*: More than 80% of pts are infected, but drug fever and lymphoma are also possible etiologies.

Pathogenesis   The hypothalamic set point increases. The pt feels cold as a result of the peripheral vasoconstriction and shivering that are needed to raise body temperature to a new set point. Peripheral vasodilation and sweating commence when the set point is lowered again by resolution or treatment of the fever.

Fever caused by:

- Exogenous pyrogens (e.g., lipopolysaccharide endotoxin)
- Endogenous pyrogens [e.g., interleukin (IL) 1, tumor necrosis factor] induced by exogenous pyrogens
- Prostaglandin E_2 (in CNS, raises hypothalamic set point; in peripheral tissues, causes myalgias and arthralgias)

APPROACH TO THE PATIENT: FEVER

A meticulous history is essential. Attention must be paid to the chronology of events (e.g., in the case of rash: the site of onset and the direction and rate of spread; see below) and the relation of symptoms to medications, pet exposure, sick contacts, sexual contacts, travel, trauma, and the presence of prosthetic materials. A thorough physical examination should be performed. The temperature can be taken orally or rectally, but a consistent site should be used.

Skin examination can be especially revealing in pts with fever. Close attention should be paid to any rash, with a precise definition of its salient features.

1. Type of lesion (e.g., macule, papule, nodule, vesicle, pustule, purpura, ulcer)
2. Classification of rash
   a. Centrally distributed maculopapular eruptions (e.g., measles, rubella)
   b. Peripheral eruptions (e.g., Rocky Mountain spotted fever, secondary syphilis)
   c. Confluent desquamative erythemas (e.g., toxic shock syndrome)
   d. Vesiculobullous eruptions (e.g., varicella, primary herpes simplex infection, rickettsialpox)

e. Urticarial eruptions: Hypersensitivity reactions usually are not associated with fever. The presence of fever suggests serum sickness, connective-tissue disease, or infection (hepatitis B, enteroviral or parasitic infection).

f. Nodular eruptions (e.g., disseminated candidiasis, cryptococcosis, erythema nodosum, Sweet's syndrome)

g. Purpuric eruptions (e.g., acute meningococcemia, echovirus 9 infection, disseminated gonococcemia)

h. Eruptions with ulcers or eschars (e.g., rickettsial diseases, such as scrub typhus; tularemia; anthrax)

Diagnosis   In most cases, initial history, physical examination, and laboratory tests (including CBC with differential, ESR, C-reactive protein) lead to a diagnosis or the pt recovers spontaneously. For the pt with FUO, an approach to diagnosis is found in Fig. 37-1.

℞ Fever

The diagnosed infection should be treated appropriately. In pts with FUO, "shotgun" empirical therapy should be avoided if vital signs are stable and the pt is not neutropenic. Cirrhosis, asplenia, immunosuppressive drug use, or recent exotic travel may be appropriate settings for empirical treatment.

Treatment of fever and its symptoms with antipyretics does no harm and does not slow the resolution of common viral and bacterial infections. Treatment of fever is appropriate to relieve symptoms and reduce oxygen demand in pts with underlying cardiovascular or pulmonary disease and to prevent seizures in children with a history of febrile seizures. Antipyretic treatment should be given on a regular schedule rather than intermittently; otherwise, it will aggravate chills and sweats.

However, withholding antipyretics may be helpful in evaluating the therapeutic effectiveness of a particular antibiotic or in allowing observation of important clinical indicators such as a relapsing pattern in malaria or a reversal of the usual times of peak and trough temperatures in typhoid fever and disseminated tuberculosis.

Aspirin, NSAIDs, and glucocorticoids are effective antipyretics. Acetaminophen is preferred because it does not mask signs of inflammation, does not impair platelet function, and is not associated with Reye's syndrome.

Recurrent fever occurs in most autoimmune and in all autoinflammatory diseases. These fevers respond dramatically to anticytokine therapy that blocks IL-1β activity. However, chronic anticytokine therapy (e.g., for rheumatoid arthritis or Crohn's disease) may reduce the febrile response while increasing susceptibility to certain infections, such as tuberculosis.

Prognosis   Failure of efforts to identify the source of FUO for >6 months is generally associated with a good prognosis. Debilitating symptoms can be treated with antipyretics.

HYPERTHERMIA

Definitions and Etiology   *Hyperthermia*: an unchanged setting of the hypothalamic set point in conjunction with an uncontrolled increase in body temper-

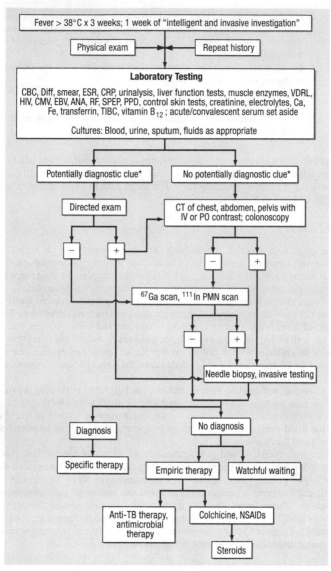

FIGURE 37-1 Approach to the pt with classic FUO. *"Potentially diagnostic clues," as outlined by EMHA DeKleijn and colleagues (Medicine 76:401, 1997), may be key findings in the history, localizing signs, or key symptoms. Abbreviations: CRP, C-reactive protein; Diff, differential; RF, rheumatoid factor; SPEP, serum protein electrophoresis; TB, tuberculosis; TIBC, total iron-binding capacity.

ature that exceeds the body's ability to lose heat. Hyperthermia does not involve pyrogenic molecules.

Heat stroke: thermoregulatory failure in association with a warm environment

• *Exertional*: caused by exercise in high heat or humidity

- *Nonexertional*: typically occurs in either very young or elderly individuals, particularly during heat waves. In the United States, 7000 deaths were attributed to heat injury in 1979–1997. The elderly, the bedridden, persons confined to poorly ventilated or non-air-conditioned areas, and those taking anticholinergic, antiparkinsonian, or diuretic drugs are most susceptible.
- *Drug-induced*: caused by drugs such as monoamine oxidase inhibitors, tricyclic antidepressants, amphetamines, and cocaine and other illicit agents

Malignant hyperthermia: hyperthermic and systemic response to halothane and other inhalational anesthetics in pts with genetic abnormality

Neuroleptic malignant syndrome: syndrome caused by use of neuroleptic agents (e.g., haloperidol) and consisting of lead-pipe muscle rigidity, extrapyramidal side effects, autonomic dysregulation, and hyperthermia

Clinical Features/Diagnosis   High core temperature in association with an appropriate history (heat exposure, certain drug treatments) and dry skin, hallucinations, delirium, pupil dilation, muscle rigidity, and/or elevated levels of creatine phosphokinase. Unlike pts with fever, hyperthermic pts have a history of heat exposure or treatment with drugs that interfere with thermoregulation; their skin is hot but dry; and antipyretic agents do not lower the body temperature. Febrile pts can have cold skin as a result of vasoconstriction or hot, moist skin; antipyretics usually result in some lowering of the body temperature of pts with fever.

℞ Hyperthermia

Physical cooling:
- Sponging, fans, cooling blankets, ice baths
- IV fluids, internal cooling by gastric or peritoneal lavage with iced saline
- In extreme cases, hemodialysis or cardiopulmonary bypass

For malignant hyperthermia: cessation of anesthesia and administration of dantrolene (1–2.5 mg/kg q6h for at least 24–48 h) *plus* procainamide administration because of the risk of ventricular fibrillation. Dantrolene is also useful in neuroleptic malignant syndrome and drug-induced hyperthermia and may be helpful in serotonin syndrome and thyrotoxicosis.

For a more detailed discussion, see Kaye KM, Kaye ET: Atlas of Rashes Associated with Fever, Chap. e5 in *Harrison's* DVD and *Harrison's Online*; and Dinarello CA, Porat R: Fever and Hyperthermia, Chap. 17, p. 117; and Kaye ET, Kaye KM: Fever and Rash, Chap. 18, p. 121; and Gelfand JA, Callahan MV: Fever of Unknown Origin, Chap. 19, p. 130, in HPIM-17.

---

38 Pain and Swelling of Joints

Musculoskeletal complaints are extremely common in outpatient medical practice and are among the leading causes of disability and absenteeism from work. Pain in the joints must be evaluated in a uniform, thorough, and logical fashion to ensure the best chance of accurate diagnosis and to plan appropriate follow-up testing and therapy. Joint pain and swelling may be manifestations of disorders affecting primarily the musculoskeletal system or may reflect systemic disease.

INITIAL ASSESSMENT OF A MUSCULOSKELETAL COMPLAINT (See Fig. 38-1)

1. *Articular versus nonarticular.* Is the pain located in a joint or in a periarticular structure such as soft tissue or muscle?

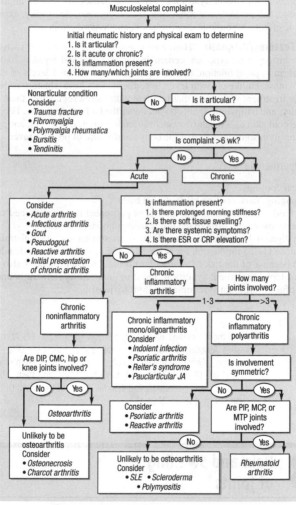

FIGURE 38-1 Algorithm for the diagnosis of musculoskeletal complaints. An approach to formulating a differential diagnosis (shown in italics). ESR, erythrocyte sedimentation rate; CRP, C-reactive protein; DIP, distal interphalangeal; CMC, carpometacarpal; PIP, proximal interphalangeal; MCP, metacarpophalangeal; MTP, metatarsophalangeal; SLE, systemic lupus erythematosus; JA, juvenile arthritis.

2. *Inflammatory versus noninflammatory.* Inflammatory disease is suggested by local signs of inflammation (erythema, warmth, swelling); systemic features (morning stiffness, fatigue, fever, weight loss); or laboratory evidence of inflammation (thrombocytosis, elevated ESR or C-reactive protein).

3. *Acute (≤6 weeks) versus chronic.*

4. *Localized versus systemic.*

HISTORIC FEATURES

- Age, sex, race, and family history
- Symptom onset (abrupt or indolent), evolution (chronic constant, intermittent, migratory, additive), and duration (acute versus chronic)
- Number and distribution of involved structures: monarticular (one joint), oligoarticular (2–3 joints), polyarticular (>3 joints); symmetry
- Other articular features: morning stiffness, effect of movement, features that improve/worsen Sx
- Extraarticular Sx: e.g., fever, rash, weight loss, visual change, dyspnea, diarrhea, dysuria, numbness, weakness
- Recent events: e.g., trauma, drug administration, travel, other illnesses

PHYSICAL EXAMINATION

Complete examination is essential: particular attention to skin, mucous membranes, nails (may reveal characteristic pitting in psoriasis), eyes. Careful and thorough examination of involved and uninvolved joints and periarticular structures; this should proceed in an organized fashion from head to foot or from extremities inward toward axial skeleton; special attention should be paid to identifying the presence or absence of:

- Warmth and/or erythema
- Swelling
- Synovial thickening
- Subluxation, dislocation, joint deformity
- Joint instability
- Limitations to active and passive range of motion
- Crepitus
- Periarticular changes
- Muscular changes including weakness, atrophy

LABORATORY INVESTIGATIONS

Additional evaluation usually indicated for monarticular, traumatic, inflammatory, or chronic conditions or for conditions accompanied by neurologic changes or systemic manifestations.

- For all evaluations: include CBC, ESR, or C-reactive protein
- Where there are suggestive clinical features, include: rheumatoid factor, ANA, antineutrophilic cytoplasmic antibodies (ANCA), antistreptolysin O titer, Lyme antibodies
- Where systemic disease is present or suspected: renal/hepatic function tests, UA
- Uric acid–useful only when gout diagnosed and therapy contemplated
- CPK, aldolase–consider with muscle pain, weakness
- Synovial fluid aspiration and analysis: always indicated for acute monarthritis or when infectious or crystal-induced arthropathy is suspected. Should be examined for (1) appearance, viscosity; (2) cell count and differential (sus-

pect septic joint if WBC count > 50,000/μL); (3) crystals using polarizing microscope; (4) Gram's stain, cultures (Fig. 38-2).

DIAGNOSTIC IMAGING

Conventional radiography using plain x-rays is a valuable tool in the diagnosis and staging of articular disorders (Table 38-1).

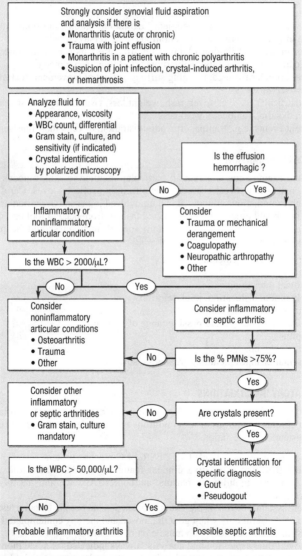

FIGURE 38-2 Algorithmic approach to the use and interpretation of synovial fluid aspiration and analysis.

TABLE 38-1	APPLICATIONS FOR CONVENTIONAL RADIOGRAPHY IN ARTICULAR DISEASE

- Trauma
- Suspected chronic joint or bone infection
- Progressive joint disability
- Monarticular involvement
- Baseline assessment of a chronic articular process
- When therapeutic alterations are considered (such as for rheumatoid arthritis)

Additional imaging procedures, including ultrasound, radionuclide scintigraphy, CT, and MRI, may be helpful in selected clinical settings.

SPECIAL CONSIDERATIONS IN THE ELDERLY PATIENT

The evaluation of joint and musculoskeletal disorders in the elderly pt presents a special challenge given the frequently insidious onset and chronicity of disease in this age group, the confounding effect of other medical conditions, and the increased variability of many diagnostic tests in the geriatric population. Although virtually all musculoskeletal conditions may afflict the elderly, certain disorders are especially frequent. Special attention should be paid to identifying the potential rheumatic consequences of intercurrent medical conditions and therapies when evaluating the geriatric pt with musculoskeletal complaints.

For a more detailed discussion, see Cush JJ, Lipsky PE: Approach to Articular and Musculoskeletal Disorders, Chap. 325, p. 2149, in HPIM-17.

39 Syncope

Syncope is a transient loss of consciousness and postural tone due to reduced cerebral blood flow. It may occur suddenly, without warning, or may be preceded by presyncopal symptoms such as lightheadedness, weakness, nausea, dimming vision, ringing in ears, or sweating. *Faintness* refers to prodromal symptoms that precede the loss of consciousness in syncope. The syncopal pt appears pale, has a faint, rapid, or irregular pulse, and breathing may be almost imperceptible; transient myoclonic or clonic movements may occur. Recovery of consciousness is prompt if the pt is maintained in a horizontal position and cerebral perfusion is restored.

APPROACH TO THE PATIENT WITH SYNCOPE

The cause of syncope may be apparent only at the time of the event, leaving few, if any, clues when the pt is seen by the physician. First consider serious

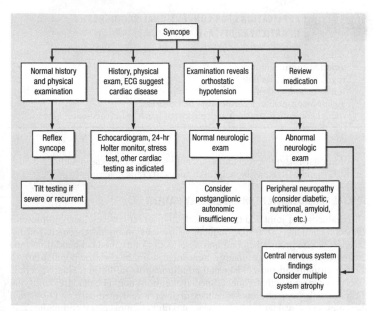

FIGURE 39-1 Approach to the patient with syncope.

underlying etiologies; among these are massive internal hemorrhage or myocardial infarction, which may be painless, and cardiac arrhythmias. In elderly persons, a sudden faint without obvious cause should raise the question of complete heart block or a tachyarrhythmia. Loss of consciousness in particular situations, such as during venipuncture or micturition, suggests a benign abnormality of vascular tone. The position of the pt at the time of the syncopal episode is important; syncope in the supine position is unlikely to be vasovagal and suggests an arrhythmia or a seizure. Medications must be considered, including nonprescription drugs or health store supplements, with particular attention to recent changes. Symptoms of impotence, bowel and bladder difficulties, disturbed sweating, or an abnormal neurologic exam, suggest a primary neurogenic cause. An algorithmic approach to syncope is presented in Fig. 39-1.

ETIOLOGY

Transiently decreased cerebral blood flow is usually due to disorders of vascular tone or blood volume including vasovagal syncope and postural hypotension, cardiovascular disorders including cardiac arrhythmias, or uncommonly cerebrovascular disease (Table 39-1). Not infrequently the cause of syncope is multifactorial.

Neurocardiogenic (Vasovagal and Vasodepressor) Syncope The common faint, experienced by normal persons, accounts for approximately half of all episodes of syncope. It is frequently recurrent and may be provoked by hot or crowded environment, alcohol, fatigue, pain, hunger, prolonged standing, or stressful situations.

| **TABLE 39-1** | **CAUSES OF SYNCOPE** |

I. Disorders of Vascular Tone or Blood Volume
   A. Reflex syncopes
      1. Neurocardiogenic
      2. Situational
         Cough
         Micturition
         Defecation
         Valsalva
         Deglutition
      3. Carotid sinus hypersensitivity
   B. Orthostatic hypotension
      1. Drug-induced (antihypertensive or vasodilator drugs)
      2. Pure autonomic failure (idiopathic orthostatic hypotension)
      3. Multisystem atrophies
      4. Peripheral neuropathy (diabetic, alcoholic, nutritional, amyloid)
      5. Physical deconditioning
      6. Sympathectomy
      7. Decreased blood volume
II. Cardiovascular Disorders
   A. Structural and obstructive causes
      1. Pulmonary embolism
      2. Pulmonary hypertension
      3. Atrial myxoma
      4. Mitral valvular stenosis
      5. Myocardial disease (massive acute myocardial infarction)
      6. Left ventricular myocardial restriction or constriction
      7. Pericardial constriction or tamponade
      8. Aortic outflow tract obstruction
      9. Aortic valvular stenosis
      10. Hypertrophic obstructive cardiomyopathy
   B. Cardiac arrhythmias
      1. Bradyarrhythmias
         a. Sinus bradycardia, sinoatrial block, sinus arrest, sick-sinus syndrome
         b. Atrioventricular block
      2. Tachyarrhythmias
         a. Supraventricular tachycardia with structural cardiovascular disease
         b. Atrial fibrillation with the Wolff-Parkinson-White syndrome
         c. Atrial flutter with 1:1 atrioventricular conduction
         d. Ventricular tachycardia
III. Cerebrovascular Disease
   A. Vertebrobasilar insufficiency
   B. Basilar artery migraine
IV. Other Disorders that May Resemble Syncope
   A. Metabolic
      1. Hypoxia
      2. Anemia
      3. Diminished carbon dioxide due to hyperventilation
      4. Hypoglycemia
   B. Psychogenic
      1. Anxiety attacks
      2. Hysterical fainting
   C. Seizures

Postural (Orthostatic) Hypotension Sudden rising from a recumbent position or standing quietly are precipitating circumstances. Cause of syncope in 30% of elderly; polypharmacy with antihypertensive or antidepressant drugs often a contributor; physical deconditioning may also play a role. Also occurs with autonomic nervous system disorders, either peripheral (diabetes, nutritional, or amyloid polyneuropathy) or central (multiple system atrophy, Parkinson's disease). Some cases are idiopathic.

DIFFERENTIAL DIAGNOSIS

Anxiety Attacks Frequently resembles presyncope although the symptoms are not accompanied by facial pallor and are not relieved by recumbency. Attacks can often be reproduced by hyperventilation and have associated symptoms of panic attacks such as a feeling of impending doom, air hunger, palpitations, and tingling of the fingers and perioral region.

Seizures The differential diagnosis is often between syncope and a generalized seizure. Syncope is more likely if the event was provoked by acute pain or anxiety or occurred immediately after arising from a lying or sitting position. Seizures are typically not related to posture. Pts with syncope often describe a stereotyped transition from consciousness to unconsciousness that develops over a few seconds. Seizures occur either very abruptly without a transition or are preceded by premonitory symptoms such as an epigastric rising sensation, perception of odd odors, or racing thoughts. Pallor is seen during syncope; cyanosis is usually seen during a seizure. The duration of unconsciousness is usually very brief (i.e., seconds) in syncope and more prolonged (i.e., >5 min) in a seizure. Injury from falling and incontinence are common in seizure, rare in syncope. Headache and drowsiness, which with mental confusion are the usual sequelae of a seizure, do not follow a syncopal attack.

Hypoglycemia Severe hypoglycemia is usually due to a serious disease. The glucose level at the time of a spell is diagnostic.

Hysterical Fainting The attack is usually unattended by an outward display of anxiety. Lack of change in pulse and blood pressure or color of the skin distinguishes it from a vasodepressor faint.

℞ Syncope

Therapy is determined by the underlying cause. Pts with vasovagal syncope should be instructed to avoid situations or stimuli that provoke attacks. Episodes associated with intravascular volume depletion may be prevented by salt and fluid preloading prior to provocative events.

Drug therapy may be necessary for resistant vasovagal syncope. β-Adrenergic antagonists (metoprolol 25–50 mg twice daily; atenolol 25–50 m/d; or nadolol 10–20 mg twice daily; all starting doses) are the most widely used agents; serotonin reuptake inhibitors (paroxetine 20–40 mg/d, or sertraline 25–50 mg/d) and bupropion SR (150 mg/d) are also effective. The mineralocorticoid hydrofludrocortisone (0.1–0.2 mg/d) or the α-agonist proamatine (2.5–10 mg twice or three times a day) may be helpful for refractory pts with recurrent vasovagal syncope, but side effects, including increases in resting bp, limit their usefulness. Recent trials suggest that there may be significant age-related differences in response to pharmacologic therapy. Permanent cardiac pacing may be effective for pts whose episodes of vasovagal syncope are frequent or associated with prolonged asystole.

Management of orthostatic hypotension is discussed in Chap. 196.

For a more detailed discussion, see Carlson MD: Syncope, Chap. 21, p. 139, in HPIM-17.

40 Dizziness and Vertigo

APPROACH TO THE PATIENT WITH DIZZINESS OR VERTIGO

The term *dizziness* is used by pts to describe a variety of head sensations or gait unsteadiness. With a careful history, distinguishing between *faintness* (presyncope; Chap. 39) and *vertigo* (an illusory or hallucinatory sense of movement of the body or the environment, most often a feeling of spinning) is usually possible.

When the meaning of "dizziness" is uncertain, provocative tests to reproduce the symptoms may be helpful. Valsalva maneuver, hyperventilation, or postural changes leading to orthostasis may reproduce faintness. Rapid rotation in a swivel chair is a simple provocative test to reproduce vertigo. Benign positional vertigo is identified by positioning the turned head of a recumbent patient in extension over the edge of the bed to elicit vertigo and the characteristic nystagmus. If a central cause for the vertigo is suspected (e.g., signs of peripheral vertigo are absent or other neurologic abnormalities are present), then prompt evaluation for central pathology is required. The initial test is usually an MRI scan of the posterior fossa, and, depending upon the results, vertebrobasilar angiography or evoked potentials may be indicated. Vestibular function tests, including electronystagmography (calorics), can help distinguish between central and peripheral etiologies.

FAINTNESS

Faintness is usually described as light-headedness followed by visual blurring and postural swaying along with a feeling of warmth, diaphoresis, and nausea. It is a symptom of insufficient blood, oxygen, or, rarely, glucose supply to the brain. It can occur prior to a syncopal event of any etiology (Chap. 39) and with hyperventilation or hypoglycemia. Lightheadedness can rarely occur as an aura before a seizure. Chronic lightheadedness is a common somatic complaint in patients with depression.

VERTIGO

Usually due to a disturbance in the vestibular system; abnormalities in the visual or somatosensory systems may also contribute to vertigo. Frequently accompanied by nausea, postural unsteadiness, and gait ataxia; may be provoked or worsened by head movement.

TABLE 40-1	FEATURES OF PERIPHERAL AND CENTRAL VERTIGO	
Sign or Symptom	Peripheral (Labyrinth)	Central (Brainstem or Cerebellum)
Direction of associated nystagmus	Unidirectional; fast phase opposite lesion[a]	Bidirectional or unidirectional
Purely horizontal nystagmus without torsional component	Uncommon	Common
Vertical or purely torsional nystagmus	Never present	May be present
Visual fixation	Inhibits nystagmus and vertigo	No inhibition
Severity of vertigo	Marked	Often mild
Direction of spin	Toward fast phase	Variable
Direction of fall	Toward slow phase	Variable
Duration of symptoms	Finite (minutes, days, weeks) but recurrent	May be chronic
Tinnitus and/or deafness	Often present	Usually absent
Associated CNS abnormalities	None	Extremely common (e.g., diplopia, hiccups, cranial neuropathies, dysarthria)
Common causes	BPPV, infection (labyrinthitis), Ménière's, neuronitis, ischemia, trauma, toxin	Vascular, demyelinating, neoplasm

[a]In Ménière's disease, the direction of the fast phase is variable.

Physiologic vertigo results from unfamiliar head movement (seasickness) or a mismatch between visual-proprioceptive-vestibular system inputs (height vertigo, visual vertigo during motion picture chase scenes). True vertigo almost never occurs as a presyncopal symptom.

Pathologic vertigo may be caused by a peripheral (labyrinth or eighth nerve) or central CNS lesion. Distinguishing between these causes is the essential first step in diagnosis (Table 40-1).

Peripheral Vertigo Usually severe, accompanied by nausea and emesis. Tinnitus, a feeling of ear fullness, or hearing loss may occur. A characteristic jerk nystagmus is almost always present. The nystagmus does not change direction with a change in direction of gaze, it is usually horizontal with a torsional component and has its fast phase away from the side of the lesion. It is inhibited by visual fixation. The pt senses spinning motion away from the lesion and tends to have difficulty walking, with falls towards the side of the lesion, particularly in the darkness or with eyes closed. No other neurologic abnormalities are present.

Acute unilateral labyrinthine dysfunction may be caused by infection, trauma, or ischemia. Often no specific etiology is uncovered, and the nonspecific term *acute labyrinthitis* (or *vestibular neuritis*) is used to describe the event; herpes simplex virus type 1 infection has been implicated. The attacks are brief and leave the patient for some days with a mild vertigo: recurrent episodes may occur. *Acute bilateral labyrinthine dysfunction* is usually due to drugs (ami-

TABLE 40-2	BENIGN PAROXYSMAL POSITIONAL VERTIGO AND CENTRAL POSITIONAL VERTIGO	
Features	BPPV	Central
Latency[a]	3–40 s	None: immediate vertigo and nystagmus
Fatigability[b]	Yes	No
Habituation[c]	Yes	No
Intensity of vertigo	Severe	Mild
Reproducibility[d]	Variable	Good

[a]Time between attaining head position and onset of symptoms.
[b]Disappearance of symptoms with maintenance of offending position.
[c]Lessening of symptoms with repeated trials.
[d]Likelihood of symptom production during any examination session.

noglycoside antibiotics) or alcohol. *Recurrent labyrinthine dysfunction* with signs and symptoms of cochlear disease is usually due to *Ménière's disease* (recurrent vertigo accompanied by tinnitus and deafness). Positional vertigo is usually precipitated by a recumbent head position. *Benign paroxysmal positional vertigo* (BPPV) of the posterior semicircular canal is particularly common; the pattern of nystagmus is distinctive (Table 40-2). BPPV may follow trauma but is usually idiopathic; it generally abates spontaneously after weeks or months. Schwannomas of the eighth cranial nerve (acoustic neuroma) usually present as auditory symptoms of hearing loss and tinnitus, sometimes accompanied by facial weakness and sensory loss due to involvement of cranial nerves VII and V. *Psychogenic vertigo* should be suspected in pts with chronic incapacitating vertigo who also have agoraphobia, panic attacks, a normal neurologic exam, and no nystagmus.

Central Vertigo   Identified by associated abnormal brainstem or cerebellar signs such as dysarthria, diplopia, dysphagia, hiccups, other cranial nerve abnormalities, weakness, or limb ataxia; depending on the cause, headache may be present. The nystagmus can take almost any form (i.e., vertical or multidirectional) but is often purely horizontal without a torsional component and changes direction with different directions of gaze. Central nystagmus is not inhibited by fixation. Central vertigo may be chronic, mild, and is usually unaccompanied by tinnitus or hearing loss. It may be due to vascular, demyelinating, or neoplastic disease. Vertigo may be a manifestation of migraine or, rarely, of temporal lobe epilepsy.

℞ Vertigo

Treatment of acute vertigo consists of bed rest (1–2 days maximum) and vestibular suppressant drugs (Table 40-3). If the vertigo persists more than a few days, most authorities advise ambulation in an attempt to induce central compensatory mechanisms, despite the short-term discomfort to the patient. BPPV may respond dramatically to repositioning exercises such as the Epley procedure designed to empty particulate debris from the posterior semicircular canal (*www.charite.de/ch/neuro/vertigo.html*). Ménière's disease may respond to a low-salt diet (1 g/d) or to a diuretic. Recurrent episodes of migraine-associated vertigo should be treated with antimigraine therapy (Chap. 35). Some data suggest that glucocorticoids improve the likelihood of recovery in vestibular neuritis.

TABLE 40-3	TREATMENT OF VERTIGO
Agent[a]	Dose[b]
Antihistamines	
Meclizine	25–50 mg 3 times/day
Dimenhydrinate	50 mg 1–2 times/day
Promethazine[c]	25–50-mg suppository or IM
Benzodiazepines	
Diazepam	2.5 mg 1–3 times/day
Clonazepam	0.25 mg 1–3 times/day
Phenothiazines	
Prochlorperazine[c]	5 mg IM or 25 mg suppository
Anticholinergic[d]	
Scopolamine transdermal	Patch
Sympathomimetics[d]	
Ephedrine	25 mg/d
Combination preparations[d]	
Ephedrine and promethazine	25 mg/d of each
Exercise therapy	
Repositioning maneuvers[e]	
Vestibular rehabilitation[f]	
Other	
Diuretics or low-salt (1 g/d) diet[g]	
Antimigrainous drugs[h]	
Inner ear surgery[i]	
Glucocorticoids[c]	100 mg/d for 3 days, tapered by 20 mg every 3 days

[a]All listed drugs are U.S. Food and Drug Administration approved, but most are not approved for the treatment of vertigo.
[b]Usual oral (unless otherwise stated) starting dose in adults; maintenance dose can be reached by a gradual increase.
[c]For acute vertigo only.
[d]For motion sickness only.
[e]For benign paroxysmal positional vertigo.
[f]For vertigo other than Ménière's and positional.
[g]For Ménière's disease.
[h]For migraine-associated vertigo (see Chap. 35 for a listing of prophylactic antimigrainous drugs).
[i]For perilymphatic fistula and refractory cases of Ménière's disease.

For a more detailed discussion, see Daroff RB: Dizziness, and Vertigo, Chap. 22, p. 144, in HPIM-17.

41 Acute Visual Loss and Double Vision

APPROACH TO THE PATIENT

Accurate measurement of visual acuity in each eye (with glasses) is of primary importance. Additional assessments include testing of pupils, eye movements, ocular alignment, and visual fields. Slit-lamp examination can exclude corneal infection, trauma, glaucoma, uveitis, and cataract. Ophthalmoscopic exam to inspect the optic disc and retina often requires pupillary dilation using 1% topicamide and 2.5% phenylephrine; risk of provoking an attack of narrow-angle glaucoma is remote.

Visual field mapping by finger confrontation localizes lesions in the visual pathway (Fig. 41-1); formal testing using a perimeter may be necessary. The goal is to determine whether the lesion is anterior, at, or posterior to the optic chiasm. A scotoma confined to one eye is caused by an anterior lesion affecting the optic nerve or globe; swinging flashlight test may reveal an afferent pupil defect. History and ocular exam are usually sufficient for diagnosis. If a bitemporal hemianopia is present, lesion is located at optic chiasm (e.g., pituitary adenoma, meningioma). Homonymous visual field loss signals a retrochiasmal lesion affecting the optic tract, lateral geniculate body, optic radiations, or visual cortex (e.g., stroke, tumor, abscess). Neuroimaging is recommended for any pt with a bitemporal or homonymous hemianopia.

TRANSIENT OR SUDDEN VISUAL LOSS

1. *Amaurosis fugax* (*transient monocular blindness*; a TIA of the retina) usually occurs from a retinal embolus or severe ipsilateral carotid stenosis. Prolonged occlusion of the central retinal artery results in classic fundus appearance of a milky, infarcted retina with cherry-red fovea. Any pt with compromise of the retinal circulation should be evaluated promptly for stroke risk factors (e.g., carotid atheroma, heart disease, atrial fibrillation).

2. *Vertebrobasilar insufficiency* or emboli to the posterior circulation can be confused with amaurosis fugax, because many pts mistakenly ascribe symptoms to their left or right eye, when in fact they are occurring in the left or right hemifield of both eyes. Interruption of blood flow to the visual cortex causes sudden graying of vision, occasionally with flashing lights or other symptoms that mimic *migraine*. The history may be the only guide to the correct diagnosis. Pts should be questioned about the precise pattern and duration of visual loss and other neurologic symptoms such as diplopia, vertigo, numbness, or weakness.

3. *Malignant hypertension* can cause visual loss from exudates, hemorrhages, cotton-wool spots (focal nerve fiber layer infarcts), and optic disc edema.

4. In central or branch *retinal vein occlusion*, the fundus exam reveals engorged, phlebitic veins with extensive retinal hemorrhages.

5. In age-related *macular degeneration*, characterized by extensive drusen and scarring of the pigment epithelium, leakage of blood or fluid from subretinal neovascular membranes can produce sudden central visual loss.

6. Flashing lights and floaters may indicate a fresh *vitreous detachment*. Separation of the vitreous from the retina is a frequent involutional event in

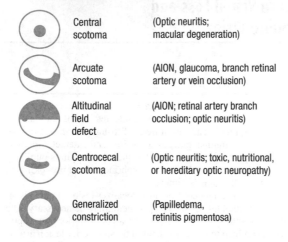

OPTIC NERVE OR RETINA

	Central scotoma	(Optic neuritis; macular degeneration)
	Arcuate scotoma	(AION, glaucoma, branch retinal artery or vein occlusion)
	Altitudinal field defect	(AION; retinal artery branch occlusion; optic neuritis)
	Centrocecal scotoma	(Optic neuritis; toxic, nutritional, or hereditary optic neuropathy)
	Generalized constriction	(Papilledema, retinitis pigmentosa)

OPTIC CHIASM

Left   Right

| | Bitemporal hemianopia | (Optic chiasm compression by pituitary tumor, meningioma) |

RETRO-CHIASMAL PATHWAY

	Right homonymous hemianopia	(Lesion of left optic tract, lateral geniculate body, optic radiations, or visual cortex)
	Superior right quadrantopia ("Pie in the Sky")	(Lesion of left optic radiations in temporal lobe)
	Macular sparing	(Bilateral visual cortex lesions)

FIGURE 41-1 Deficits in visual fields caused by lesions affecting visual pathways.

the elderly. It is not harmful unless it creates sufficient traction to produce a *retinal detachment*.

7. *Vitreous hemorrhage* may occur in diabetic pts from retinal neovascularization.

8. *Papilledema* refers to optic disc edema from raised intracranial pressure. Transient visual obscurations are common, but visual acuity is not affected unless the papilledema is severe, long-standing, or accompanied by macular exudates or hemorrhage. Neuroimaging should be obtained to exclude an intracranial mass. If negative, an LP is required to confirm elevation of the intracranial pressure. *Pseudotumor cerebri* (idiopathic intracranial hy-

pertension) is a diagnosis of exclusion. Most pts are young, female, and obese; some are found to have occult cerebral venous sinus thrombosis. Treatment is with acetazolamide, repeated LPs, and weight loss; some pts require lumboperitoneal shunting or optic nerve sheath fenestration.

9. *Optic neuritis* is a common cause of monocular optic disc swelling and visual loss. If site of inflammation is retrobulbar, fundus will appear normal on initial exam. The typical pt is female, age 15–45, with pain provoked by eye movements. Glucocorticoids, consisting of intravenous methylprednisolone (1 g daily for 3 days) followed by oral prednisone (1 mg/kg daily for 11 days), may hasten recovery in severely affected patients but makes no difference in final acuity (measured 6 months after the attack). If an MR scan shows multiple demyelinating lesions, treatment for multiple sclerosis (Chap. 200) should be considered. Optic neuritis involving both eyes simultaneously or sequentially suggests neuromyelitis optica.

10. *Anterior ischemic optic neuropathy* (AION) is an infarction of the optic nerve head due to inadequate perfusion via the posterior ciliary arteries. Pts have sudden visual loss, often upon awakening, and painless swelling of the optic disc. It is important to differentiate between nonarteritic (idiopathic) AION and arteritic AION. The latter is caused by *giant cell (temporal) arteritis* and requires immediate glucocorticoid therapy to prevent blindness. The ESR should be checked in any elderly pt with acute optic disc swelling or symptoms suggestive of polymyalgia rheumatica.

DOUBLE VISION (DIPLOPIA)

First step—clarify whether diplopia persists in either eye after covering the opposite eye; if it does the diagnosis is monocular diplopia usually caused by disease intrinsic to the eye with no dire implications for the patient.

If pt has diplopia while being examined, motility testing will usually reveal an abnormality in ocular excursions. However, if the degree of angular separation between the double images is small, the limitation of eye movements may be subtle and difficult to detect. In this situation, the cover test is useful. While the pt is fixating upon a distant target, one eye is covered while observing the other eye for a movement of redress as it takes up fixation. If none is seen, the procedure is repeated with the other eye. With genuine diplopia, this test should reveal ocular malalignment, especially if the head is turned or tilted in the position that gives rise to the worst symptoms.

Common causes of diplopia are summarized in Table 41-1. The physical findings in isolated ocular motor nerve palsies are:

- CN III: Ptosis and deviation of the eye down and outwards, causing vertical and horizontal diplopia. A dilated pupil suggests direct compression of the third nerve; if present, the possibility of an aneurysm of the posterior communicating artery must be considered urgently.
- CN IV: Vertical diplopia with cyclotorsion; the affected eye is slightly elevated, and limitation of depression is seen when the eye is held in adduction. The pt may assume a head tilt to the opposite side (e.g., left head tilt in right fourth nerve paresis).
- CN VI: Horizontal diplopia with crossed eyes; the affected eye cannot abduct.

Isolated ocular motor nerve palsies often occur in pts with hypertension or diabetes. They usually resolve spontaneously over several months.

The apparent occurrence of multiple ocular motor nerve palsies, or diffuse ophthalmoplegia, raises the possibility of myasthenia gravis. In this disease, the pupils are always normal. Systemic weakness may be absent. Multiple ocular

TABLE 41-1   **COMMON CAUSES OF DIPLOPIA**

Brainstem stroke (skew deviation, nuclear or fascicular palsy)
Microvascular infarction (III, IV, VI nerve palsy)
Tumor (brainstem, cavernous sinus, superior orbital fissure, orbit)
Multiple sclerosis (internuclear ophthalmoplegia, ocular motor nerve palsy)
Aneurysm (III nerve)
Raised intracranial pressure (VI nerve)
Postviral inflammation
Meningitis (bacterial, fungal, granulomatosis, neoplastic)
Carotid-cavernous fistula or thrombosis
Herpes zoster
Tolosa-Hunt syndrome
Wernicke-Korsakoff syndrome
Botulism
Myasthenia gravis
Guillain-Barré or Fisher syndrome
Graves' disease
Orbital pseudotumor
Orbital myositis
Trauma
Orbital cellulitis

motor nerve palsies should be investigated with neuroimaging focusing on the cavernous sinus, superior orbital fissure, and orbital apex where all three nerves are in close proximity. Diplopia that cannot be explained by a single ocular motor nerve palsy may also be caused by carcinomatous or fungal meningitis, Graves' disease, Guillain-Barré syndrome, Fisher syndrome, or Tolosa-Hunt syndrome.

For a more detailed discussion, see Horton JC: Disorders of the Eye, Chap. 29, p. 180, in HPIM-17.

42   Weakness and Paralysis

APPROACH TO THE PATIENT

Weakness is a reduction of power in one or more muscles. *Paralysis* indicates weakness that is so severe that the muscle cannot be contracted at all, whereas *paresis* refers to weakness that is mild or moderate. The prefix "hemi-" refers to one half of the body, "para-" to both legs, and "quadri-" to all four limbs. The suffix "-plegia" signifies severe weakness or paralysis.

Increased *fatigability* or limitation in function due to pain or articular stiffness is often confused with weakness by pts. Increased time is sometimes required for full power to be exerted, and this *bradykinesia* may be misinterpreted as weakness. Severe proprioceptive sensory loss may also lead to complaints of weakness because adequate feedback information

TABLE 42-1	SIGNS THAT DISTINGUISH ORIGIN OF WEAKNESS		
Sign	Upper Motor Neuron	Lower Motor Neuron	Myopathic
Atrophy	None	Severe	Mild
Fasciculations	None	Common	None
Tone	Spastic	Decreased	Normal/decreased
Distribution of weakness	Pyramidal/ regional	Distal/segmental	Proximal
Tendon reflexes	Hyperactive	Hypoactive/ absent	Normal/ hypoactive
Babinski's sign	Present	Absent	Absent

about the direction and power of movements is lacking. Finally, *apraxia*, a disorder of planning and initiating a skilled or learned movement, is sometimes mistaken for weakness.

The history should focus on the tempo of development of weakness, presence of sensory and other neurologic symptoms, medication history, predisposing medical conditions, and family history.

Weakness or paralysis is typically accompanied by other neurologic abnormalities that help to indicate the site of the responsible lesion (Table 42-1). It

TABLE 42-2	COMMON CAUSES OF WEAKNESS

Upper Motor Neuron

Cortex: ischemia; hemorrhage; intrinsic mass lesion (primary or metastatic cancer, abscess); extrinsic mass lesion (subdural hematoma); degenerative (amyotrophic lateral sclerosis)

Subcortical white matter/internal capsule: ischemia; hemorrhage; intrinsic mass lesion (primary or metastatic cancer, abscess); immunologic (multiple sclerosis); infectious (progressive multifocal leukoencephalopathy)

Brainstem: ischemia; immunologic (multiple sclerosis)

Spinal cord: extrinsic compression (cervical spondylosis, metastatic cancer, epidural abscess); immunologic (multiple sclerosis, transverse myelitis); infectious (AIDS-associated myelopathy, HTLV-I–associated myelopathy, tabes dorsalis); nutritional deficiency (subacute combined degeneration)

Motor Unit

Spinal motor neuron: degenerative (amyotrophic lateral sclerosis); infectious (poliomyelitis)

Spinal root: compressive (degenerative disc disease); immunologic (Guillain-Barré syndrome); infectious (AIDS-associated polyradiculopathy, Lyme disease)

Peripheral nerve: metabolic (diabetes mellitus, uremia, porphyria); toxic (ethanol, heavy metals, many drugs, diphtheria); nutritional (B_{12} deficiency); inflammatory (polyarteritis nodosa); hereditary (Charcot-Marie-Tooth); immunologic (paraneoplastic, paraproteinemia); infectious (AIDS-associated polyneuropathies and mononeuritis multiplex); compressive (entrapment)

Neuromuscular junction: immunologic (myasthenia gravis); toxic (botulism, aminoglycosides)

Muscle: inflammatory (polymyositis, inclusion body myositis); degenerative (muscular dystrophy); toxic (glucocorticoids, ethanol, AZT); infectious (trichinosis); metabolic (hypothyroid, periodic paralyses); congenital (central core disease)

TABLE 42-3   CLINICAL DIFFERENTIATION OF WEAKNESS ARISING FROM DIFFERENT AREAS OF THE NERVOUS SYSTEM

Location of Lesion	Pattern of Weakness	Associated Signs
Upper Motor Neuron		
Cerebral cortex	Hemiparesis (face and arm predominantly, or leg predominantly)	Hemisensory loss, seizures, homonymous hemianopia or quadrantanopia, aphasia, apraxias, gaze preference
Internal capsule	Hemiparesis (face, arm, leg may be equally affected)	Hemisensory deficit; homonymous hemianopia or quadrantanopia
Brainstem	Hemiparesis (arm and leg; face may not be involved at all)	Vertigo, nausea and vomiting, ataxia and dysarthria, eye movement abnormalities, cranial nerve dysfunction, altered level of consciousness, Horner's syndrome
Spinal cord	Quadriparesis if mid-cervical or above Paraparesis if low cervical or thoracic	Sensory level; bowel and bladder dysfunction
	Hemiparesis below level of lesion (Brown-Séquard)	Contralateral pain/temperature loss below level of lesion
Motor Unit		
Spinal motor neuron	Diffuse weakness, may involve control of speech and swallowing	Muscle fasciculations and atrophy; no sensory loss
Spinal root	Radicular pattern of weakness	Dermatomal sensory loss; radicular pain common with compressive lesions
Peripheral nerve		
Polyneuropathy	Distal weakness, usually feet more than hands; usually symmetric	Distal sensory loss, usually feet more than hands
Mononeuropathy	Weakness in distribution of single nerve	Sensory loss in distribution of single nerve
Neuromuscular junction	Fatigable weakness, usually with ocular involvement producing diplopia and ptosis	No sensory loss; no reflex changes
Muscle	Proximal weakness	No sensory loss; diminished reflexes only when severe; may have muscle tenderness

is important to distinguish weakness arising from disorders of upper motor neurons (i.e., motor neurons in the cerebral cortex and their axons that descend through the subcortical white matter, internal capsule, brainstem, and spinal cord) from disorders of the motor unit (i.e., lower motor neurons in the

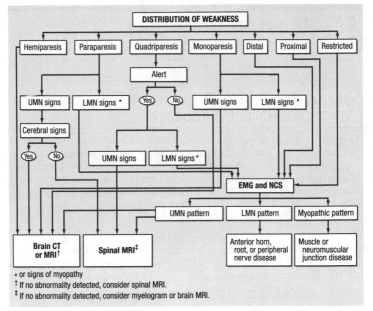

FIGURE 42-1 An algorithm for the initial workup of a patient with weakness. EMG, electromyography; LMN, lower motor neuron; NCS, nerve conduction studies; UMN, upper motor neuron.

ventral horn of the spinal cord and their axons in the spinal roots and peripheral nerves, neuromuscular junction, and skeletal muscle).

Table 42-2 lists common causes of weakness by the primary site of pathology. Table 42-3 summarizes patterns with lesions of different parts of the nervous system.

An algorithm for the initial workup of weakness is shown in Fig. 42-1.

For a more detailed discussion, see Aminoff MA: Weakness and Paralysis, Chap. 23, p. 147, in HPIM-17.

43 Tremor and Movement Disorders

APPROACH TO THE PATIENT WITH TREMOR AND MOVEMENT DISORDERS

Divided into akinetic rigid forms, with muscle rigidity and slowness of movement, and hyperkinetic forms, with involuntary movements. In both types, preservation of strength is the rule. Most movement disorders arise from disruption of basal ganglia circuits; common causes are degenerative diseases (hereditary and idiopathic), drug-induced, organ system failure, CNS infection, and ischemia. Clinical features of the various movement disorders are summarized below.

Bradykinesia   Inability to initiate changes in activity or perform ordinary volitional movements rapidly and easily. There is a slowness of movement and a paucity of automatic motions such as eye blinking and arm swinging while walking. Usually due to Parkinsonism (Chap. 193).

Tremor   Rhythmic oscillation of a part of the body due to intermittent muscle contractions, usually involving the distal limbs and less commonly the head, tongue, or jaw. A coarse tremor at rest, 4–5 beats/s, is usually due to Parkinson's disease. A fine postural tremor of 8–10 beats/s may be an exaggeration of normal physiologic tremor or indicate familial essential tremor. An intention tremor, most pronounced during voluntary movement towards a target, is found with cerebellar pathway disease.

Essential Tremor (ET)   This is the most common involuntary movement disorder. The tremor of ET must be distinguished form that of early Parkinson's disease (Table 43-1). The pathophysiology of ET is unknown. Approximately 50% of cases have a positive family history with an autosomal dominant pattern of inheritance. Many cases are mild and require no treatment. When activities of daily living such as eating and writing are impaired, therapy with primidone (25–100 mg/d) or propranolol (20–80 mg/d) leads to benefit in 50% of patients. Surgical therapies may be effective in refractory cases.

TABLE 43-1   ADVANCED EXAMINATION PEARLS: DIFFERENTIATING ESSENTIAL TREMOR FROM PARKINSONIAN TREMOR

	Essential Tremor	Parkinsonian Tremor
Speed	5–10 Hz	4–6 Hz
Symmetry	Bilateral	Usually asymmetric
Most common component	Postural	Rest
Other Parkinsonian symptoms	Absent	Present
Helped with alcohol	Usually	Rarely
Family history	Present often	Usually absent

Dystonia Consists of sustained or repetitive involuntary muscle contractions, frequently causing twisting movements with abnormal posture. Dystonias may be generalized or focal.

Focal dystonias are common and include blepharospasm of the eyelids; spasmodic dysphonia involving the vocal cords; oromandibular dystonia of the face, lips, tongue, and jaw; cervical dystonia of the neck musculature (torticollis); and limb dystonias that are often task-specific such as writer's cramp, playing a musical instrument, or putting in golf (yips).

Idiopathic torsional dystonia is a predominantly childhood-onset form of generalized dystonia with an autosomal dominant pattern of inheritance that mainly affects Ashkenazi Jewish families; most are linked to a mutation in the *DYT1* gene on chromosome 9. Other generalized dystonias occur as a consequence of drugs such as antiemetics and treatments for Parkinson's disease.

Therapy for focal dystonias usually involves botulinum toxin injections into the affected musculature. All forms of dystonia may respond to anticholinergic medications (e.g., trihexyphenidyl 20–120 mg/d), benzodiazepines, baclofen, or anticonvulsants. Surgical therapies, including deep brain stimulation (DBS), may be effective in refractory cases.

Choreoathetosis A combination of chorea (rapid, jerky movements) and athetosis (slow writhing movements). The two usually exist together, though one may be more prominent. Choreic movements are the predominant involuntary movements in rheumatic (Sydenham's) chorea and Huntington's disease. Systemic lupus erythematosus is the most common systemic disorder that causes chorea, but it can also be seen in patients with hyperthyroidism, various autoimmune disorders, infections including HIV, metabolic alterations, and in association with a wide variety of medications. Hemiballismus is a violent form of chorea that comprises wild, flinging movements on one side of the body; the most common cause is a lesion (often infarct or hemorrhage) of the subthalamic nucleus. Athetosis is prominent in some forms of cerebral palsy. Chronic neuroleptic use may lead to tardive dyskinesia, in which choreoathetotic movements are usually restricted to the buccal, lingual, and mandibular areas.

Huntington's Disease (HD) This is a progressive, fatal, autosomal dominant disorder characterized by motor, behavioral, and cognitive dysfunction. Onset is typically between the ages of 25 and 45 years. Rapid, nonpatterned, semipurposeful, involuntary choriform movements are the hallmark feature with dysarthria, gait disturbance, and oculomotor abnormalities commonly seen. Late stages of the disease feature a reduction in chorea and emergence of dystonia, rigidity, bradykinesia, myoclonus, and spasticity. HD patients eventually develop behavioral and cognitive disturbances that can be a major source of disability. HD is inherited as an autosomal dominant disorder and is caused by an expansion in the number of polyglutamine (CAG) repeats in the coding sequence of the *Huntington* gene on chromosome 4.

Treatment involves a multidisciplinary approach with medical, neuropsychiatric, social, and genetic counseling for patients and their families. Dopamine-blocking agents may control the chorea but may aggravate motor symptoms and often have an unfavorable side-effect profile. Psychosis can be treated with atypical neuroleptic agents. No disease-modifying agents currently exist.

Tics Brief, rapid, recurrent, and seemingly purposeless stereotyped muscle contractions. Gilles de la Tourette syndrome (TS) is a neurobehavioral, multiple tic disorder that may involve motor tics (especially twitches of the face, neck, and shoulders), vocal tics (grunts, words), and "behavioral tics" (coprolalia, echolalia). Patients may experience an irresistible urge to express tics but characteristically can voluntarily suppress them for short periods of time. Onset is usually between 2 and 15 years of age, and tics often lessen or even disappear in adulthood. Drug treatment is only indicated when tics are disabling and interfere with quality of life. Therapy is generally initiated with clonidine, starting at low dose, or guanfacine (0.5–2 mg/d). If these agents are not effective, neuroleptics may be used.

Asterixis Brief, arrhythmic interruptions of sustained voluntary muscle contraction, usually observed as a brief lapse of posture of wrists in dorsiflexion with arms outstretched. This "liver flap" may be seen in any encephalopathy related to drug intoxication, organ system failure, or CNS infection. Therapy is correction of underlying disorder.

Myoclonus Rapid (<100 ms), brief, shocklike, jerky, irregular movements that are usually multifocal. Like asterixis, often indicates a diffuse encephalopathy. Following cardiac arrest, diffuse cerebral hypoxia may produce multifocal myoclonus. Spinal cord injury can also cause myoclonus. Myoclonus occurs in normal individuals when waking up or falling asleep. Treatment of myoclonus, indicated only when function is impaired, consists of treating the underlying condition or removing an offending agent. Drug therapies include valproic acid (1200–3000 mg/d), piracetam (8–20 g/d), clonazepam (2–15 mg/d), or primidone (500–1000 mg/d).

For a more detailed discussion, see Olanow CW: Hyperkinetic Movement Disorders, Chap. 367, p. 2560, in HPIM-17.

44 Aphasias and Related Disorders

Aphasias are disturbances in the comprehension or production of spoken or written language. Clinical examination should assess spontaneous speech (fluency), comprehension, repetition, naming, reading, and writing. A classification scheme is presented in Table 44-1. In nearly all right-handed individuals and many left-handed patients, language localization is in the left hemisphere.

CLINICAL FEATURES

Wernicke's Aphasia Although speech sounds grammatical, melodic, and effortless (fluent), it is virtually incomprehensible due to errors in word usage, structure, and tense and the presence of paraphasic errors and neologisms ("jargon"). Comprehension of written and spoken material is severely impaired, as are reading, writing, and repetition. The pt usually seems unaware of the deficit. Associated symptoms can include parietal lobe sensory deficits and homonymous hemianopia. Motor disturbances are rare.

Lesion is located in posterior perisylvian region. Most common cause is embolism to the inferior division of dominant middle cerebral artery (MCA); less commonly intracerebral hemorrhage, severe head trauma, or tumor is responsible.

TABLE 44-1 **CLINICAL FEATURES OF APHASIAS AND RELATED CONDITIONS**

	Comprehension	Repetition of Spoken Language	Naming	Fluency
Wernicke's	Impaired	Impaired	Impaired	Preserved or increased
Broca's	Preserved (except grammar)	Impaired	Impaired	Decreased
Global	Impaired	Impaired	Impaired	Decreased
Conduction	Preserved	Impaired	Impaired	Preserved
Nonfluent (motor) transcortical	Preserved	Preserved	Impaired	Impaired
Fluent (sensory) transcortical	Impaired	Preserved	Impaired	Preserved
Isolation	Impaired	Echolalia	Impaired	No purposeful speech
Anomic	Preserved	Preserved	Impaired	Preserved except for word-finding pauses
Pure word deafness	Impaired only for spoken language	Impaired	Preserved	Preserved
Pure alexia	Impaired only for reading	Preserved	Preserved	Preserved

Source: M-M Mesulam: HPIM-17, p. 164.

Broca's Aphasia Speech output is sparse (nonfluent), slow, labored, interrupted by many word-finding pauses, and usually dysarthric; output may be reduced to a grunt or single word. Naming and repetition also impaired. Most pts have severe writing impairment. Comprehension of written and spoken language is relatively preserved. Patient is often aware of and visibly frustrated by deficit. With large lesions, a dense hemiparesis may occur, and eyes may deviate toward side of lesion. More commonly, lesser degrees of contralateral face and arm weakness are present. Sensory loss is rarely found, and visual fields are intact.

Lesion involves dominant inferior frontal gyrus (Broca's area), although cortical and subcortical areas along superior sylvian fissure and insula are often involved. Commonly caused by vascular lesions involving the superior division of the MCA; less commonly due to tumor, intracerebral hemorrhage, or abscess.

Global Aphasia All aspects of speech and language are impaired. Pt cannot read, write, or repeat and has poor auditory comprehension. Speech output is minimal and nonfluent. Hemiplegia, hemisensory loss, and homonymous hemianopia are usually present. Syndrome represents the combined dysfunction of Wernicke's and Broca's areas, usually resulting from proximal occlusion of MCA supplying dominant hemisphere (less commonly hemorrhage, trauma, or tumor).

Conduction Aphasia Speech output is fluent but paraphasic, comprehension of spoken language is intact, and repetition is severely impaired, as are naming and writing. Lesion spares, but functionally disconnects, Wernicke's and Broca's areas. Most cases are embolic, involving supramarginal gyrus of dominant parietal lobe, dominant superior temporal lobe, or arcuate fasciculus.

LABORATORY EVALUATION

CT scan or MRI usually identifies the location and nature of the causative lesion.

 Aphasia

Speech therapy may be helpful in treatment of certain types of aphasia. When the lesion is caused by a stroke, recovery of language function generally peaks within 2–6 months, after which time further progress is limited.

 For a more detailed discussion, see Mesulam M-M: Aphasia, Memory Loss, and Other Focal Cerebral Disorders, Chap. 27, p. 162, in HPIM-17.

45 Sleep Disorders

Disorders of sleep are among the most common problems seen by clinicians. More than one-half of adults experience at least intermittent sleep disturbances, and 50–70 million Americans suffer from a chronic sleep disturbance.

APPROACH TO THE PATIENT

Pts may complain of (1) difficulty in initiating and maintaining sleep (insomnia); (2) excessive daytime sleepiness, fatigue, or tiredness; (3) behavioral phenomena occurring during sleep [sleepwalking, rapid eye movement (REM) behavioral disorder, periodic leg movements of sleep, etc.]; or (4) circadian rhythm disorders associated with jet lag, shift work, and delayed sleep phase syndrome. A careful history of sleep habits and reports from the sleep partner (e.g., heavy snoring, falling asleep while driving) are a cornerstone of diagnosis. Pts with excessive sleepiness should be advised to avoid all driving until effective therapy has been achieved. Completion of a day-by-day sleep-work-drug log for at least 2 weeks is often helpful. Work and sleep times (including daytime naps and nocturnal awakenings) as well as drug and alcohol use, including caffeine and hypnotics, should be noted each day. Objective sleep laboratory recording is necessary to evaluate sleep apnea, narcolepsy, REM behavior disorder, periodic leg movements, and other suspected disorders.

INSOMNIA

Insomnia, or the complaint of inadequate sleep, may be subdivided into difficulty falling asleep (*sleep-onset insomnia*), frequent or sustained awakenings (*sleep-offset insomnia*), or persistent sleepiness despite sleep of adequate duration (*nonrestorative sleep*). An insomnia complaint lasting one to several nights is termed *transient insomnia* and is typically due to situational stress or a change in sleep schedule or environment (e.g., jet lag). *Short-term insomnia* lasts from a few days up to 3 weeks; it is often associated with more protracted stress such as recovery from surgery or short-term illness. *Long-term (chronic) insomnia* lasts for months or years and, in contrast to short-term insomnia, requires a thorough evaluation for underlying causes. Chronic insomnia is often a waxing and waning disorder, with spontaneous or stress-induced exacerbations.

Adjustment Insomnia (Acute Insomnia)   *Acute insomnia* can occur after a change in the sleeping environment (e.g., in an unfamiliar hotel or hospital bed) or before or after a significant life event or anxiety-provoking situation. Treatment is symptomatic, with intermittent use of hypnotics and resolution of the underlying stress. *Inadequate sleep hygiene* is characterized by a behavior pattern prior to sleep and/or a bedroom environment that is not conducive to sleep. In preference to hypnotic medications, the pt should attempt to avoid stressful activities before bed, reserve the bedroom environment for sleeping, and maintain regular rising times.

Psychophysiologic Insomnia   These pts are preoccupied with a perceived inability to sleep adequately at night. Rigorous attention should be paid to sleep hygiene and correction of counterproductive, arousing behaviors before bedtime. Behavioral therapies are the treatment of choice.

Drugs and Medications   Caffeine is probably the most common pharmacologic cause of insomnia. Alcohol and nicotine can also interfere with sleep, despite the fact that many pts use these agents to relax and promote sleep. A number of prescribed medications, including antidepressants, sympathomimetics, and glucocorticoids, can produce insomnia. In addition, severe rebound insomnia can result from the acute withdrawal of hypnotics, especially following use of high doses of benzodiazepines with a short half-life. For this reason, doses of hypnotics should be low to moderate and prolonged drug tapering is encouraged.

Movement Disorders   Pts with *restless legs syndrome* complain of creeping dysesthesias deep within the calves or feet associated with an irresistible urge to move the affected limbs; symptoms are typically worse at night. One-third of pts have multiple affected family members. Treatment is with dopaminergic drugs (pramipexole 0.25–1.0 mg daily at 8 P.M. or ropinirole 0.5–4.0 mg daily at 8 P.M.). *Periodic limb movements of sleep* (PLMS) consists of stereotyped extensions of the great toe and dorsiflexion of the foot recurring every 20–40 s during non-REM sleep. Treatment options include dopaminergic medications or benzodiazepines.

Other Neurologic Disorders   A variety of neurologic disorders produce sleep disruption through both indirect, nonspecific mechanisms (e.g., neck or back pain) or by impairment of central neural structures involved in the generation and control of sleep itself. Common disorders to consider include *dementia* from any cause, *epilepsy*, *Parkinson's disease*, and *migraine*.

Psychiatric Disorders   Approximately 80% of pts with mental disorders complain of impaired sleep. The underlying diagnosis may be depression, mania, an anxiety disorder, or schizophrenia.

Medical Disorders   In *asthma*, daily variation in airway resistance results in marked increases in asthmatic symptoms at night, especially during sleep. Treatment of asthma with theophylline-based compounds, adrenergic agonists, or glucocorticoids can independently disrupt sleep. Inhaled glucocorticoids that do not disrupt sleep may provide a useful alternative to oral drugs. *Cardiac ischemia* is also associated with sleep disruption; the ischemia itself may result from increases in sympathetic tone as a result of sleep apnea. Pts may present with complaints of nightmares or vivid dreams. *Paroxysmal nocturnal dyspnea* can also occur from cardiac ischemia that causes pulmonary congestion exacerbated by the recumbent posture. *Chronic obstructive pulmonary disease, cystic fibrosis, hyperthyroidism, menopause, gastroesophageal reflux, chronic renal failure,* and *liver failure* are other causes.

℞ Insomnia

Insomnia without Identifiable Cause

Primary insomnia is a diagnosis of exclusion. Treatment is directed toward behavior therapies for anxiety and negative conditioning; pharmacotherapy and/or psychotherapy for mood/anxiety disorders; an emphasis on good sleep hygiene; and intermittent hypnotics for exacerbations of insomnia. Cognitive therapy emphasizes understanding the nature of normal sleep, the circadian rhythm, the use of light therapy, and visual imagery to block unwanted thought intrusions. Behavioral modification involves bedtime restriction, set schedules, and careful sleep environment practices. Judicious use of benzodiazepine receptor agonists with short half-lives can be effective; options include zaleplon (5–20 mg), zolpidem (5–10 mg), or triazolam (0.125–0.25 mg). Limit use to 2–4 weeks maximum for acute insomnia or intermittent use for chronic. Some pts benefit from low-dose sedating antidepressants.

HYPERSOMNIAS (DISORDERS OF EXCESSIVE DAYTIME SLEEPINESS)

Differentiation of sleepiness from subjective complaints of fatigue may be difficult. Quantification of daytime sleepiness can be performed in a sleep laboratory using a multiple sleep latency test (MSLT), the repeated daytime measurement of sleep latency under standardized conditions. Common causes are summarized in Table 45-1.

Sleep Apnea Syndromes Respiratory dysfunction during sleep is a common cause of excessive daytime sleepiness and/or disturbed nocturnal sleep, affecting an estimated 2–5 million individuals in the United States. Episodes may be due to occlusion of the airway (*obstructive sleep apnea*), absence of respiratory effort (*central sleep apnea*), or a combination of these factors (*mixed sleep apnea*). Obstruction is exacerbated by obesity, supine posture, sedatives (especially alcohol), nasal obstruction, and hypothyroidism. Sleep apnea is particularly prevalent in overweight men and in the elderly and is undiagnosed in 80–90% of affected individuals. Treatment consists of correction of the above factors, positive airway pressure devices, oral appliances, and sometimes surgery (Chap. 142).

Narcolepsy A disorder of excessive daytime sleepiness and intrusion of REM-related sleep phenomena into wakefulness (cataplexy, hypnagogic hallucinations, and sleep paralysis). *Cataplexy*, the abrupt loss of muscle tone in arms, legs, or face, is precipitated by emotional stimuli such as laughter or sadness. Symptoms of narcolepsy (Table 45-2) typically begin in the second decade, although the onset ranges from ages 5–50. The prevalence is 1 in 4000 and narcolepsy has a genetic basis; almost all narcoleptics with cataplexy are positive for HLA DQB1*0602. Hypothalamic neurons containing the neuropeptide hypocre-

TABLE 45-1 EVALUATION OF THE PATIENT WITH THE COMPLAINT OF EXCESSIVE DAYTIME SOMNOLENCE

Findings on History and Physical Examination	Diagnostic Evaluation	Diagnosis	Therapy
Obesity, snoring, hypertension	Polysomnography with respiratory monitoring	Obstructive sleep apnea	Continuous positive airway pressure; ENT surgery (e.g., uvulopalatopharyngoplasty); dental appliance; pharmacologic therapy (e.g., protriptyline); weight loss
Cataplexy, hypnogogic hallucinations, sleep paralysis, family history	Polysomnography with multiple sleep latency testing	Narcolepsy-cataplexy syndrome	Stimulants (e.g., modafinil, methylphenidate); REM-suppressant antidepressants (e.g., protriptyline); genetic counseling
Restless legs, disturbed sleep, predisposing medical condition (e.g., iron deficiency or renal failure)	Assessment for predisposing medical conditions	Restless legs syndrome	Treatment of predisposing condition, if possible; dopamine agonists (e.g., pramipexole, ropinirole)
Disturbed sleep, predisposing medical conditions (e.g., asthma) and/or predisposing medical therapies (e.g., theophylline)	Sleep-wake diary recording	Insomnias (see text)	Treatment of predisposing condition and/or change in therapy, if possible; behavioral therapy; short-acting benzodiazepine receptor agonist (e.g., zolpidem)

Note: ENT, ears, nose, throat; REM, rapid eye movement; EMG, electromyogram.
Source: From CA Czeisler et al: HPIM-17, p. 174.

TABLE 45-2	PREVALENCE OF SYMPTOMS IN NARCOLEPSY
Symptom	Prevalence, %
Excessive daytime somnolence	100
Disturbed sleep	87
Cataplexy	76
Hypnagogic hallucinations	68
Sleep paralysis	64
Memory problems	50

Source: Modified from TA Roth, L Merlotti in SA Burton et al (eds), *Narcolepsy 3rd International Symposium: Selected Symposium Proceedings,* Chicago, Matrix Communications, 1989.

tin (orexin) regulate the sleep/wake cycle and have been implicated in narcolepsy. Sleep studies confirm a short daytime sleep latency and a rapid transition to REM sleep.

℞ Hypersomnias

Somnolence is treated with modafinil, a novel wake-promoting agent; the usual dose is 200–400 mg/d given as a single dose. Older stimulants such as methylphenidate (10 mg twice a day to 20 mg four times a day) or dextroamphetamine are alternatives, particularly in refractory pts. Cataplexy, hypnagogic hallucinations, and sleep paralysis respond to the tricyclic antidepressants protriptyline (10–40 mg/d) and clomipramine (25–50 mg/d) and to the selective serotonin uptake inhibitor fluoxetine (10–20 mg/d). Alternatively, γ-hydroxybutyrate (GHB) given at bedtime, and 4 h later, is effective in reducing daytime cataplectic episodes. Adequate nocturnal sleep time and the use of short naps are other useful preventative measures.

DISORDERS OF CIRCADIAN RHYTHMICITY

Insomnia or hypersomnia may occur in disorders of sleep timing rather than sleep generation. Such conditions may be (1) organic—due to a defect in the hypothalamic circadian pacemaker or its input from entraining stimuli, or (2) environmental—due to a disruption of exposure to entraining stimuli (light/dark cycle). Examples of the latter include jet-lag disorder and shift work. Shift work sleepiness can be treated with modafinil (200 mg, taken 30–60 min before the start of each night shift) as well as properly timed exposure to bright light. Safety programs should promote education about sleep and increase awareness of the hazards associated with night work.

Delayed sleep phase syndrome is characterized by late sleep onset and awakening with otherwise normal sleep architecture. Bright-light phototherapy in the morning hours or melatonin therapy during the evening hours may be effective. *Advanced sleep phase syndrome* moves sleep onset to the early evening hours with early morning awakening. These pts may benefit from bright-light phototherapy during the evening hours.

For a more detailed discussion, see Czeisler CA, Winkleman JW, Richardson GS: Sleep Disorders, Chap. 28, p. 171, in HPIM-17.

46 Dyspnea

DEFINITION

Abnormally uncomfortable awareness of breathing; intensity quantified by establishing the amount of physical exertion necessary to produce the sensation. Dyspnea occurs when work of breathing is excessive.

CAUSES

Heart Disease

- Dyspnea most commonly due to ↑ pulmonary capillary pressure, and sometimes fatigue of respiratory muscles. Vital capacity and lung compliance are ↓ and airway resistance ↑.
- Begins as exertional breathlessness → orthopnea → paroxysmal nocturnal dyspnea and dyspnea at rest.
- Diagnosis depends on recognition of heart disease, e.g., Hx of MI, presence of S_3, S_4, murmurs, cardiomegaly, jugular vein distention, hepatomegaly, and peripheral edema (Chap. 131). Objective quantification of ventricular function (echocardiography, radionuclide ventriculography) is often helpful.

Airway Obstruction   (Chap. 138)

- May occur with obstruction anywhere from extrathoracic airways to lung periphery.
- Acute dyspnea with difficulty *inhaling* suggests *upper* airway obstruction. Physical exam may reveal inspiratory stridor and retraction of supraclavicular fossae.
- Acute intermittent dyspnea with expiratory wheezing suggests reversible intrathoracic obstruction due to asthma.
- Chronic, slowly progressive exertional dyspnea characterizes emphysema and CHF.
- Exertional dyspnea with chronic cough and expectoration is typical of chronic bronchitis and bronchiectasis.

Diffuse Parenchymal Lung Diseases   (Chap. 141)   Many parenchymal lung diseases, from sarcoidosis to pneumoconioses, may cause dyspnea. Dyspnea is usually related to exertion early in the course of the illness. Physical exam typically reveals tachypnea and late inspiratory rales.

Pulmonary Embolism   (Chap. 140)   Dyspnea is most common symptom of pulmonary embolism. Repeated discrete episodes of dyspnea may occur with recurrent pulmonary emboli; tachypnea is frequent.

Disease of the Chest Wall or Respiratory Muscles   (Chap. 142)   Severe kyphoscoliosis may produce chronic dyspnea, often with chronic cor pulmonale. Spinal deformity must be severe before respiratory function is compromised.

Pts with bilateral diaphragmatic paralysis appear normal while standing, but complain of severe orthopnea and display paradoxical abnormal respiratory movement when supine.

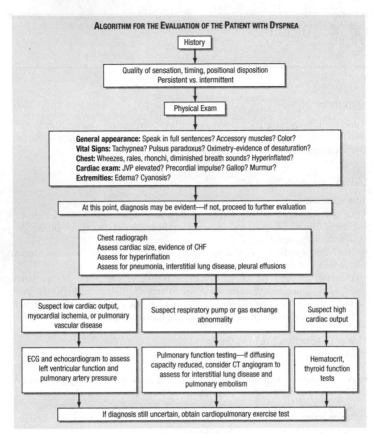

ALGORITHM FOR THE EVALUATION OF THE PATIENT WITH DYSPNEA

History

Quality of sensation, timing, positional disposition
Persistent vs. intermittent

Physical Exam

General appearance: Speak in full sentences? Accessory muscles? Color?
Vital Signs: Tachypnea? Pulsus paradoxus? Oximetry-evidence of desaturation?
Chest: Wheezes, rales, rhonchi, diminished breath sounds? Hyperinflated?
Cardiac exam: JVP elevated? Precordial impulse? Gallop? Murmur?
Extremities: Edema? Cyanosis?

At this point, diagnosis may be evident—if not, proceed to further evaluation

Chest radiograph
Assess cardiac size, evidence of CHF
Assess for hyperinflation
Assess for pneumonia, interstitial lung disease, pleural effusions

Suspect low cardiac output, myocardial ischemia, or pulmonary vascular disease

Suspect respiratory pump or gas exchange abnormality

Suspect high cardiac output

ECG and echocardiogram to assess left ventricular function and pulmonary artery pressure

Pulmonary function testing—if diffusing capacity reduced, consider CT angiogram to assess for interstitial lung disease and pulmonary embolism

Hematocrit, thyroid function tests

If diagnosis still uncertain, obtain cardiopulmonary exercise test

FIGURE 46-1 An algorithm for the evaluation of the patient with dyspnea. JVP, jugular venous pulse; CHF, congestive heart failure; ECG, electrocardiogram. (*Adapted from RM Schwartzstein, D Feller-Kopman. in Primary Cardiology, 2d ed. E Braunwald, L Goldman (eds): Philadelphia; Saunders, 2003.*)

TABLE 46-1 DIFFERENTIATION BETWEEN CARDIAC AND PULMONARY DYSPNEA

- *Careful history*: Dyspnea of lung disease usually more gradual in onset than that of heart disease; nocturnal exacerbations common with each.
- *Examination*: Usually obvious evidence of cardiac or pulmonary disease. Findings may be absent at rest when symptoms are present only with exertion.
- *Brain natriuretic peptide (BNP)*: Elevated in cardiac but not pulmonary dyspnea.
- *Pulmonary function tests*: Pulmonary disease rarely causes dyspnea unless tests of obstructive disease (FEV_1, FEV_1/FVC) or restrictive disease (total lung capacity) are reduced (<80% predicted).
- *Ventricular performance*: LV ejection fraction at rest and/or during exercise usually depressed in cardiac dyspnea.

APPROACH TO THE PATIENT WITH DYSPNEA (See Fig. 46-1)

Elicit a description of the amount of physical exertion necessary to produce the sensation and whether it varies under different conditions.

- If acute upper airway obstruction is suspected, lateral neck films or fiberoptic exam of upper airway may be helpful.
- With chronic upper airway obstruction the respiratory flow-volume curve may show inspiratory cutoff of flow, suggesting variable extrathoracic obstruction.
- Dyspnea due to emphysema is reflected in a reduction in expiratory flow rates (FEV_1), and often by a reduction in diffusing capacity for carbon monoxide (DL_{CO}).
- Pts with intermittent dyspnea due to asthma may have normal pulmonary function if tested when asymptomatic.
- Cardiac dyspnea usually begins as breathlessness on strenuous exertion with gradual (months-to-years) progression to dyspnea at rest.
- Pts with dyspnea due to both cardiac and pulmonary diseases may report orthopnea. Paroxysmal nocturnal dyspnea occurring after awakening from sleep is characteristic of CHF.
- Dyspnea of chronic obstructive lung disease tends to develop more gradually than that of heart disease.
- PFTs should be performed when etiology is not clear. When the diagnosis remains obscure a pulmonary stress test is often useful.
- Management depends on elucidating etiology.

Differentiation between cardiac and pulmonary dyspnea is summarized in Table 46-1.

For a more detailed discussion, see Schwartzstein RM: Dyspnea and Pulmonary Edema, Chap. 33, p. 221, HPIM-17.

47 Cough and Hemoptysis

COUGH

Produced by inflammatory, mechanical, chemical, and thermal stimulation of cough receptors.

Etiology

- *Inflammatory*—edema and hyperemia of airways and alveoli due to laryngitis, tracheitis, bronchitis, bronchiolitis, pneumonitis, lung abscess.
- *Mechanical*—inhalation of particulates (dust) or compression of airways (pulmonary neoplasms, foreign bodies, granulomas, bronchospasm).
- *Chemical*—inhalation of irritant fumes, including cigarette smoke.
- *Thermal*—inhalation of cold or very hot air.

APPROACH TO THE PATIENT WITH COUGH

DIAGNOSIS (Fig. 47-1)

History should consider:

- *Duration*—acute or chronic
- *Presence of fever or wheezing*
- *Sputum quantity and character*—change in sputum character, color, or volume in a smoker with "smoker's cough" necessitates investigation.

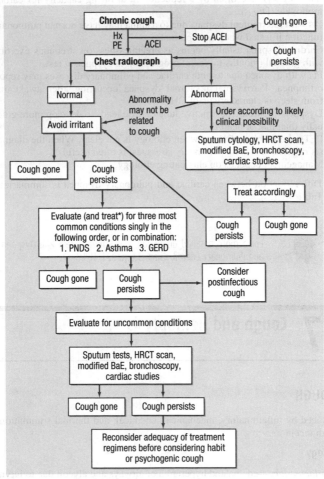

FIGURE 47-1 An algorithm for the evaluation of chronic cough. ACEI, angiotensin-converting enzyme inhibitor; BaE, barium esophagography; GERD, gastroesophageal reflux disease; HRCT, high-resolution CT; PE, physical examination; PNDS, postnasal drip syndrome. *Treatment is either targeted to a presumptive diagnosis or given empirically. [*Adapted from RS Irwin: Chest 114(Suppl):1335, 1998, with permission.*]

- *Temporal or seasonal pattern*—seasonal cough may indicate "cough asthma."
- *Risk factors for underlying disease*—environmental exposures may suggest occupational asthma or interstitial lung disease.
- *Past medical history*—past history of recurrent pneumonias may indicate bronchiectasis, particularly if associated with purulent or copious sputum production. A change in the character of chronic cigarette cough raises suspicion of bronchogenic carcinoma. Chronic CHF causes cough.
- *Drugs*—is pt. on ACE inhibitor? Causes chronic cough in 5–20%.

Short duration with associated fever suggests acute viral or bacterial infection. Persistent cough after viral illness suggests postinflammatory cough. Postnasal drip is common cause of chronic cough. Nocturnal cough may indicate chronic sinus drainage or esophageal reflux.

Physical exam should assess upper and lower airways and lung parenchyma.

- Stridor suggests upper airway obstruction; wheezing suggests bronchospasm as the cause of cough.
- Midinspiratory crackles indicate airways disease (e.g., chronic bronchitis).
- Fine end-inspiratory crackles occur in interstitial fibrosis and heart failure.
- CXR may show neoplasm, infection, interstitial disease, or the hilar adenopathy of sarcoidosis.
- High-resolution CT (HRCT) helpful in unexplained chronic cough.
- PFTs may reveal obstruction or restriction.
- Sputum exam can indicate malignancy or infection.
- Fiberoptic bronchoscopy helpful in defining endobronchial causes.

Complications   (1) Syncope, due to transient decrease in venous return; (2) rupture of an emphysematous bleb with pneumothorax; (3) rib fractures—may occur in otherwise normal individuals.

Rx | Cough (See Fig. 47-2)

- When possible, therapy of cough is that of underlying disease. Eliminate ACE inhibitors and cigarette smoking.
- If no cause can be found, a trial of an inhaled anticholinergic agent (e.g., ipratropium 2–4 puffs four times daily), an inhaled β agonist (e.g., albuterol) or an inhaled steroid (e.g., triamcinolone) can be attempted. Inhaled steroids may take 7–10 days to be effective when used for an irritative cough.
- Cough productive of significant volumes of sputum should generally not be suppressed. Sputum clearance can be facilitated with adequate hydration, expectorants, and mechanical devices. Iodinated glycerol (30 mg four times daily) may be useful in asthma or chronic bronchitis.
- When symptoms from an irritative cough are severe, the cough may be suppressed with a narcotic antitussive agent such as codeine, 15–30 mg up to four times a day, or a nonnarcotic such as dextromethorphan (15 mg four times a day).

HEMOPTYSIS

Includes both streaked sputum and coughing up of gross blood.

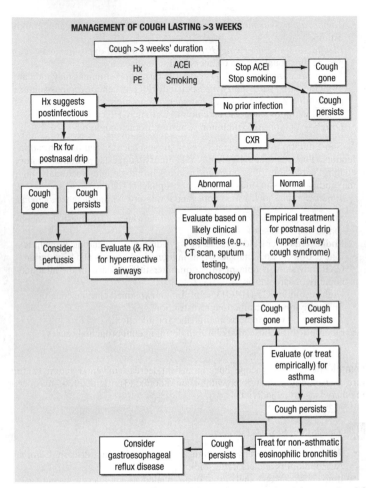

FIGURE 47-2 Algorithm for management of cough lasting >3 weeks. Cough between 3 and 8 weeks is considered subacute; cough >8 weeks is considered chronic. Hx, history, PE, physical examination; ACEI, angiotensin-converting enzyme inhibitor; Rx, treat; CXR, chest x-ray. *(From SE Weinberger, DA Lipson, in HPIM-17, p. 226.)*

Etiology   (Table 47-1)   Bronchitis and pneumonia are common causes. Neoplasm may be the cause, particularly in smokers and when hemoptysis is persistent. Hemoptysis rare in metastatic neoplasm to lung. Pulmonary thromboembolism and infection are other causes. Diffuse hemoptysis may occur with vasculitis involving the lung. Five to 15% of cases with hemoptysis remain undiagnosed.

APPROACH TO THE PATIENT WITH HEMOPTYSIS

DIAGNOSIS   (Fig. 47-3)
Essential to determine that blood is coming from respiratory tract. Often frothy, may be preceded by a desire to cough.

TABLE 47-1   DIFFERENTIAL DIAGNOSIS OF HEMOPTYSIS

Source other than the lower respiratory tract
   Upper airway (nasopharyngeal) bleeding
   Gastrointestinal bleeding
Tracheobronchial source
   Neoplasm (bronchogenic carcinoma, endobronchial metastatic tumor,
     Kaposi's sarcoma, bronchial carcinoid)
   Bronchitis (acute or chronic)
   Bronchiectasis
   Broncholithiasis
   Airway trauma
   Foreign body
Pulmonary parenchymal source
   Lung abscess
   Pneumonia
   Tuberculosis
   Mycetoma ("fungus ball")
   Goodpasture's syndrome
   Idiopathic pulmonary hemosiderosis
   Wegener's granulomatosis
   Lupus pneumonitis
   Lung contusion
Primary vascular source
   Arteriovenous malformation
   Pulmonary embolism
   Elevated pulmonary venous pressure (esp. mitral stenosis)
   Pulmonary artery rupture secondary to balloon-tip pulmonary artery catheter
     manipulation
Miscellaneous/rare causes
   Pulmonary endometriosis
   Systemic coagulopathy or use of anticoagulants or thrombolytic agents

Source: Adapted from SE Weinberger, *Principles of Pulmonary Medicine*, 3d ed, Philadelphia, Saunders, 1998.

- History may suggest diagnosis: chronic hemoptysis in otherwise asymptomatic young woman suggests bronchial adenoma.
- Hemoptysis, weight loss, and anorexia in a smoker suggest carcinoma.
- Hemoptysis with acute pleuritic pain suggests infarction; fever or chills with blood-streaked sputum suggests pneumonia.

Physical exam may also suggest diagnosis: pleural friction rub raises possibility of pulmonary embolism or some other pleural-based lesion (lung abscess, coccidioidomycosis cavity, vasculitis); diastolic rumbling murmur suggests mitral stenosis; localized wheeze suggests bronchogenic carcinoma.

Initial evaluation includes CXR. A normal CXR does not exclude tumor or bronchiectasis as a source of bleeding. The CXR may show an air-fluid level suggesting an abscess or atelectasis distal to an obstructing carcinoma. Follow with chest CT.

Most pts should be assessed by fiberoptic bronchoscopy. Rigid bronchoscopy helpful when bleeding is massive or from proximal airway lesion and when endotracheal intubation is contemplated.

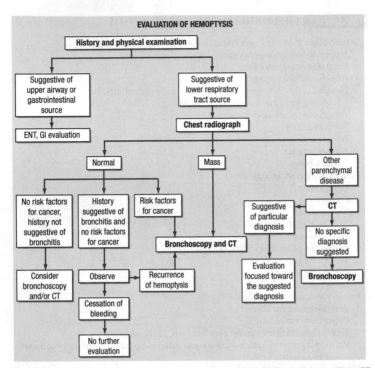

FIGURE 47-3 An algorithm for the evaluation of hemoptysis. ENT, ear, nose and throat. (*From SE Weinberger, DA Lipson, in HPIM-17, p. 228.*)

℞ Hemoptysis

- Treat the underlying condition
- Mainstays are bed rest and cough suppression with an opiate (codeine, 15–30 mg, or hydrocodone, 5 mg q4–6h).
- Pts with massive hemoptysis (>600 mL/d) and pts with respiratory compromise due to aspiration of blood should be monitored intensively with suction and intubation equipment close by so that selective intubation to isolate the bleeding lung can be accomplished. In massive hemoptysis, highest priority is to maintain gas exchange, and this may require intubation with double-lumen endotracheal tubes.
- Choice of medical or surgical therapy often relates to the anatomic site of hemorrhage and the pt's baseline pulmonary function.
- Localized peripheral bleeding sites may be tamponaded by bronchoscopic placement of a balloon catheter in a lobar or segmental airway. Central bleeding sites may be managed with laser coagulation. Pts with severely compromised pulmonary function may be candidates for bronchial artery catherization and embolization.

For a more detailed discussion, see Weinberger SE, Lipson DA: Cough and Hemoptysis, Chap. 34, p. 225, in HPIM-17.

48 Cyanosis

The circulating quantity of reduced hemoglobin is elevated [>50 g/L (>5 g/dL)] resulting in bluish discoloration of the skin and/or mucous membranes.

CENTRAL CYANOSIS

Results from arterial desaturation. Usually evident when arterial saturation is ≤85% or ≤75% in dark-skinned individuals.

- *Impaired pulmonary function:* Poorly ventilated alveoli or impaired oxygen diffusion; most frequent in pneumonia, pulmonary edema, and chronic obstructive pulmonary disease (COPD); in COPD with cyanosis, polycythemia is often present.
- *Anatomic vascular shunting*: Shunting of desaturated venous blood into the arterial circulation may result from congenital heart disease or pulmonary AV fistula.
- *Decreased inspired O_2*: Cyanosis may develop in ascents to altitudes >2400 m (>8000 ft).
- *Abnormal hemoglobins*: Methemoglobinemia, sulfhemoglobinemia, and mutant hemoglobins with low oxygen affinity (see HPIM-17, Chap. 99).

PERIPHERAL CYANOSIS

Occurs with normal arterial O_2 saturation with increased extraction of O_2 from capillary blood caused by decreased localized blood flow. Vasoconstriction due to cold exposure, decreased cardiac output (in shock, Chap. 12), heart failure (Chap. 131), and peripheral vascular disease (Chap. 133) with arterial obstruction or vasospasm (Table 48-1). Local (e.g., thrombophlebitis) or central (e.g., constrictive pericarditis) venous hypertension intensifies cyanosis.

APPROACH TO THE PATIENT WITH CYANOSIS

- Inquire about duration (cyanosis since birth suggests congenital heart disease) and exposures (drugs or chemicals that result in abnormal hemoglobins).
- Differentiate central from peripheral cyanosis by examining nailbeds, lips, and mucous membranes. Peripheral cyanosis most intense in nailbeds and may resolve with gentle warming of extremities.
- Check for clubbing, i.e., selective enlargement of the distal segments of fingers and toes. Clubbing may be hereditary, idiopathic, or acquired and is associated with a variety of disorders, including primary and metastatic lung cancer, infective endocarditis, bronchiectasis, and hepatic cirrhosis. Combination of clubbing and cyanosis is frequent in congenital heart disease and occasionally with pulmonary disease (lung abscess, pulmonary AV shunts but *not* with uncomplicated obstructive lung disease).
- Examine chest for evidence of pulmonary disease, pulmonary edema, or murmurs associated with congenital heart disease.
- If cyanosis is localized to an extremity, evaluate for peripheral vascular obstruction.

TABLE 48-1	CAUSES OF CYANOSIS

Central Cyanosis

Decreased arterial oxygen saturation
    Decreased atmospheric pressure—high altitude
    Impaired pulmonary function
        Alveolar hypoventilation
        Uneven relationships between pulmonary ventilation and perfusion (per-
            fusion of hypoventilated alveoli)
        Impaired oxygen diffusion
        Anatomic shunts
        Certain types of congenital heart disease
        Pulmonary arteriovenous fistulas
        Multiple small intrapulmonary shunts
        Hemoglobin with low affinity for oxygen
Hemoglobin abnormalities
Methemoglobinemia—hereditary, acquired
Sulfhemoglobinemia—acquired
Carboxyhemoglobinemia (not true cyanosis)

Peripheral Cyanosis

Reduced cardiac output
Cold exposure
Redistribution of blood flow from extremities
Arterial obstruction
Venous obstruction

- Obtain arterial blood gas to measure systemic O_2 saturation. Repeat while pt inhales 100% O_2; if saturation fails to increase to >95%, intravascular shunting of blood bypassing the lungs is likely (e.g., right-to-left intracardiac shunts).
- Evaluate abnormal hemoglobins by hemoglobin electrophoresis, spectroscopy, and measurement of methemoglobin level.

For a more detailed discussion, see Braunwald E: Hypoxia and Cyanosis, Chap. 35, p. 229, in HPIM-17.

49   Edema

DEFINITION

Soft tissue swelling due to abnormal expansion of interstitial fluid volume. Edema fluid is a plasma transudate that accumulates when movement of fluid from vascular to interstitial space is favored. Since detectable generalized edema in the adult reflects a gain of ≥ 3 L, renal retention of salt and water is necessary for edema to occur. Distribution of edema can be an important guide to cause.

Localized Edema Limited to a particular organ or vascular bed; easily distinguished from generalized edema. Unilateral extremity edema is usually due to venous or lymphatic obstruction (e.g., deep venous thrombosis, tumor obstruction, primary lymphedema). Stasis edema of a paralyzed lower extremity may also occur. Allergic reactions ("angioedema") and superior vena caval obstruction are causes of localized facial edema. Bilateral lower extremity edema may have localized causes, e.g., inferior vena caval obstruction, compression due to ascites, abdominal mass. Ascites (fluid in peritoneal cavity) and hydrothorax (in pleural space) may also present as isolated localized edema, due to inflammation or neoplasm.

Generalized Edema Soft tissue swelling of most or all regions of the body. Bilateral lower extremity swelling, more pronounced after standing for several hours, and pulmonary edema are usually cardiac in origin. Periorbital edema noted on awakening often results from renal disease and impaired Na excretion. Ascites and edema of lower extremities and scrotum are frequent in cirrhosis or CHF. In *CHF*, diminished cardiac output and effective arterial blood volume result in both decreased renal perfusion and increased venous pressure with resultant renal Na retention due to renal vasoconstriction, intrarenal blood flow redistribution, direct Na-retentive effects of norepinephrine and angiotensin II, and secondary hyperaldosteronism.

In *cirrhosis*, arteriovenous shunts lower renal perfusion, resulting in Na retention. Ascites accumulates when increased intrahepatic vascular resistance produces portal hypertension. Reduced serum albumin and increased abdominal pressure also promote lower extremity edema.

TABLE 49-1	DRUGS ASSOCIATED WITH EDEMA FORMATION

Nonsteroidal anti-inflammatory drugs
Antihypertensive agents
    Direct arterial/arteriolar vasodilators
        Hydralazine
        Clonidine
        Methyldopa
        Guanethidine
        Minoxidil
    Calcium channel antagonists
    α-Adrenergic antagonists
    Thiazolidinediones
Steroid hormones
    Glucocorticoids
    Anabolic steroids
    Estrogens
    Progestins
Cyclosporine
Growth hormone
Immunotherapies
    Interleukin 2
    OKT3 monoclonal antibody

Source: From GM Chertow, in E Braunwald, L Goldman (eds): *Cardiology for the Primary Care Physician,* 2d ed. Philadelphia, Saunders, 2003.

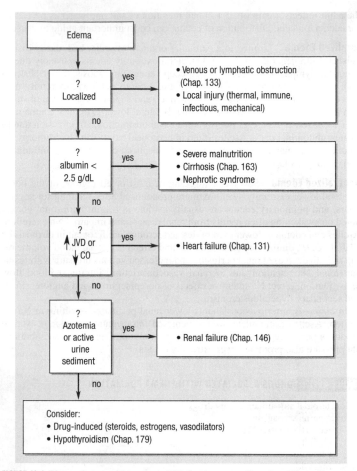

FIGURE 49-1 Diagnostic approach to edema. JVD, jugular venous distention; CO, cardiac output.

In acute or chronic *renal failure*, edema occurs if Na intake exceeds kidney's ability to excrete Na secondary to marked reductions in glomerular filtration. Severe hypoalbuminemia [<25 g/L (2.5 g/dL)] of any cause (e.g., nephrotic syndrome, nutritional deficiency, chronic liver disease) may lower plasma on-cotic pressure, promoting fluid transudation into interstitium; lowering of effective blood volume stimulates renal Na retention, and causes edema.

Less common causes of generalized edema: *idiopathic edema*, a syndrome of recurrent rapid weight gain and edema in women of reproductive age; *hypothyroidism*, in which myxedema is typically located in the pretibial region; *drugs* (see Table 49-1).

 Edema

Primary management is to identify and treat the underlying cause of edema (Fig. 49-1).

TABLE 49-2	DIURETICS FOR EDEMA	
Drug	Usual Dose	Comments
Loop (May Be Administered PO or IV)		
Furosemide	40–120 mg qd or bid	Short-acting; potent; effective with low GFR
Bumetanide	0.5–2 mg qd or bid	May be used if allergic to furosemide
Ethacrynic acid	50–200 mg qd	Longer-acting
Distal, K-Losing		
Hydrochlorothia-zide	25–200 mg qd	First choice; causes hypokalemia; need GFR > 25 mL/min
Chlorthalidone	100 mg qd or qod	Long-acting (up to 72 h); hypokalemia; need GFR > 25 mL/min
Metolazone	1–10 mg qd	Long-acting; hypokalemia; effective with low GFR, especially when combined with a loop diuretic
Distal, K-Sparing		
Spironolactone	25–100 mg qd to qid	Hyperkalemia; acidosis; blocks aldosterone; gynecomastia, impotence, amenorrhea; onset takes 2–3 days; avoid use in renal failure or in combination with ACE inhibitors or potassium supplements
Amiloride	5–10 mg qd or bid	Hyperkalemia; once daily; less potent than spironolactone
Triamterene	100 mg bid	Hyperkalemia; less potent than spironolactone; renal stones

Dietary Na restriction (<500 mg/d) may prevent further edema formation. Bed rest enhances response to salt restriction in CHF and cirrhosis. Supportive stockings and elevation of edematous lower extremities help to mobilize interstitial fluid. If severe hyponatremia (<132 mmol/L) is present, water intake should also be reduced (<1500 mL/d). Diuretics (Table 49-2) are indicated for marked peripheral edema, pulmonary edema, CHF, inadequate dietary salt restriction. Complications are listed in Table 49-3. Weight loss by diuretics should be limited to 1–1.5 kg/d. Distal ("potassium sparing") diuretics or metolazone may be added to loop diuretics for enhanced effect. Note that intestinal edema may impair absorption of oral diuretics and reduce effectiveness. When desired weight is achieved, diuretic doses should be reduced.

In *CHF* (Chap. 131), avoid overdiuresis because it may bring a fall in cardiac output and prerenal azotemia. Avoid diuretic-induced hypokalemia, which predisposes to digitalis toxicity.

In *cirrhosis* and other hepatic causes of edema, spironolactone is the diuretic of choice but may produce acidosis and hyperkalemia. Thiazides or small doses of loop diuretics may also be added. However, renal failure may result from volume depletion. Overdiuresis may result in hyponatremia, hypokalemia, and alkalosis, which may worsen hepatic encephalopathy (Chap. 163).

TABLE 49-3	COMPLICATIONS OF DIURETICS
Common	**Uncommon**
Volume depletion	Interstitial nephritis (thiazides, furosemide)
Prerenal azotemia	Pancreatitis (thiazides)
Potassium depletion	Loss of hearing (loop diuretics)
Hyponatremia (thiazides)	Anemia, leukopenia, thrombocytopenia (thiazides)
Metabolic alkalosis	
Hypercholesterolemia	
Hyperglycemia (thiazides)	
Hyperkalemia (K-sparing)	
Hypomagnesemia	
Hyperuricemia	
Hypercalcemia (thiazides)	
GI complaints	
Rash (thiazides)	

For a more detailed discussion, see Braunwald E, Loscalzo J: Edema, Chap. 36, p. 231, in HPIM-17.

50 Nausea, Vomiting, and Indigestion

NAUSEA AND VOMITING

Nausea refers to the imminent desire to vomit and often precedes or accompanies vomiting. *Vomiting* refers to the forceful expulsion of gastric contents through the mouth. *Retching* refers to labored rhythmic respiratory activity that precedes emesis. *Regurgitation* refers to the gentle expulsion of gastric contents in the absence of nausea and abdominal diaphragmatic muscular contraction. *Rumination* refers to the regurgitation, rechewing, and reswallowing of food from the stomach.

Pathophysiology Gastric contents are propelled into the esophagus when there is relaxation of the gastric fundus and gastroesophageal sphincter followed by a rapid increase in intraabdominal pressure produced by contraction of the abdominal and diaphragmatic musculature. Increased intrathoracic pressure results in further movement of the material to the mouth. Reflex elevation of the soft palate and closure of the glottis protect the nasopharynx and trachea and complete the act of vomiting. Vomiting is controlled by two brainstem areas, the vomiting center and chemoreceptor trigger zone. Activation of the chemoreceptor trigger zone results in impulses to the vomiting center, which controls the physical act of vomiting.

Etiology Nausea and vomiting are manifestations of a large number of disorders (Table 50-1).

TABLE 50-1 CAUSES OF NAUSEA AND VOMITING

Intraperitoneal	Extraperitoneal	Medications/Metabolic Disorders
Obstructing disorders	Cardiopulmonary	Drugs
Pyloric obstruction	disease	Cancer chemotherapy
Small bowel	Cardiomyopathy	Antibiotics
obstruction	Myocardial	Cardiac antiarrhythmics
Colonic obstruction	infarction	Digoxin
Superior mesenteric	Labyrinthine disease	Oral hypoglycemics
artery syndrome	Motion sickness	Oral contraceptives
Enteric infections	Labyrinthitis	Endocrine/metabolic disorders
Viral	Malignancy	Pregnancy
Bacterial	Intracerebral disorders	Uremia
Inflammatory diseases	Malignancy	Ketoacidosis
Cholecystitis	Hemorrhage	Thyroid and parathy-
Pancreatitis	Abscess	roid disease
Appendicitis	Hydrocephalus	Adrenal insufficiency
Hepatitis	Psychiatric illness	Toxins
Impaired motor function	Anorexia and bu-	Liver failure
Gastroparesis	limia nervosa	Ethanol
Intestinal pseudo-	Depression	
obstruction	Psychogenic	
Functional dyspepsia	vomiting	
Gastroesophageal	Postoperative	
reflux	vomiting	
Biliary colic	Cyclic vomiting	
Abdominal irradiation	syndrome	

Evaluation The history, including a careful drug history, and the timing and character of the vomitus can be helpful. For example, vomiting that occurs predominantly in the morning is often seen in pregnancy, uremia, and alcoholic gastritis; feculent emesis implies distal intestinal obstruction or gastrocolic fistula; projectile vomiting suggests increased intracranial pressure; vomiting during or shortly after a meal may be due to psychogenic causes or peptic ulcer disease. Associated symptoms may also be helpful: vertigo and tinnitus in Ménière's disease, relief of abdominal pain with vomiting in peptic ulcer, and early satiety in gastroparesis. Plain radiographs can suggest diagnoses such as intestinal obstruction. The upper GI series assesses motility of the proximal GI tract as well as the mucosa. Other studies may be indicated, such as gastric emptying scans (diabetic gastroparesis) and CT scan of the brain.

Complications Rupture of the esophagus (Boerhaave's syndrome), hematemesis from a mucosal tear (Mallory-Weiss syndrome), dehydration, malnutrition, dental caries and erosions, metabolic alkalosis, hypokalemia, and aspiration pneumonitis.

Rx Nausea and Vomiting

Treatment is aimed at correcting the specific cause. The effectiveness of antiemetic medications depends on etiology of symptoms, pt responsiveness, and side effects. Antihistamines such as meclizine and dimenhydrinate are effective for nausea due to inner ear dysfunction. Anticholinergics such as scopolamine are effective for nausea associated with motion sickness. Haloperidol and phenothiazine derivatives such as prochlorperazine are often effective in controlling mild nausea and vomiting, but sedation, hypotension, and parkinsonian symptoms are common side effects. Selective dopamine antagonists such as metoclopramide may be superior to the phenothiazines in treating severe nausea and vomiting and are particularly useful in treatment of gastroparesis. IV metoclopramide may be effective as prophylaxis against nausea when given before chemotherapy. Ondansetron and granisetron, serotonin receptor blockers, and glucocorticoids are used for treating nausea and vomiting associated with cancer chemotherapy. Aprepitant, a neurokinin receptor blocker, is effective at controlling nausea from highly emetic drugs like cisplatin. Erythromycin is effective in some pts with gastroparesis.

INDIGESTION

Indigestion is a nonspecific term that encompasses a variety of upper abdominal complaints including heartburn, regurgitation, and dyspepsia (upper abdominal discomfort or pain). These symptoms are overwhelmingly due to gastroesophageal reflux disease (GERD).

Pathophysiology   GERD occurs as a consequence of acid reflux into the esophagus from the stomach, gastric motor dysfunction, or visceral afferent hypersensitivity. A wide variety of situations promote GERD: increased gastric contents (from a large meal, gastric stasis, or acid hypersecretion), physical factors (lying down, bending over), increased pressure on the stomach (tight clothes, obesity, ascites, pregnancy), and loss (usually intermittent) of lower esophageal sphincter tone (diseases such as scleroderma, smoking, anticholinergics, calcium antagonists). Hiatal hernia also promotes acid flow into the esophagus.

Natural History   Heartburn is reported once monthly by 40% of Americans and daily by 7%. Functional dyspepsia is defined as >3 months of dyspepsia without an organic cause. Functional dyspepsia is the cause of symptoms in 60% of pts with dyspeptic symptoms. However, peptic ulcer disease from either *Helicobacter pylori* infection or ingestion of nonsteroidal anti-inflammatory drugs (NSAIDs) is present in 15% of cases.

In most cases, the esophagus is not damaged, but 5% of pts develop esophageal ulcers and some form strictures; 8–20% develop glandular epithelial cell metaplasia, termed *Barrett's esophagus*, which can progress to adenocarcinoma.

Extraesophageal manifestations include asthma, laryngitis, chronic cough, aspiration pneumonitis, chronic bronchitis, sleep apnea, dental caries, halitosis, and hiccups.

Evaluation   The presence of dysphagia, odynophagia, unexplained weight loss, recurrent vomiting leading to dehydration, occult or gross bleeding, or a palpable mass or adenopathy are "alarm" signals that demand directed radiographic, endoscopic, and surgical evaluation. Pts without alarm features are generally treated empirically. Individuals >45 years can be tested for the presence of *H. pylori*. Pts positive for the infection are treated to eradicate the organism. Pts who fail to respond to *H. pylori* treatment, those >45 years old, and those with alarm factors generally undergo upper GI endoscopy.

℞ Indigestion

Weight reduction; elevation of the head of the bed; and avoidance of large meals, smoking, caffeine, alcohol, chocolate, fatty food, citrus juices, and

NSAIDs may prevent GERD. Antacids are widely used. Clinical trials suggest that proton pump inhibitors (omeprazole) are more effective than histamine receptor blockers (ranitidine) in patients with or without esophageal erosions. *H. pylori* eradication regimens are discussed in Chap. 156. Motor stimulants like metoclopramide and erythromycin may be useful in a subset of patients with postprandial distress.

Surgical techniques (Nissen fundoplication, Belsey procedure) work best in young individuals whose symptoms have improved on proton pump inhibitors and who otherwise may require lifelong therapy. They can be used in the rare pts who are refractory to medical management. Clinical trials have not documented the superiority of one over another.

For a more detailed discussion, see Hasler WL: Nausea, Vomiting, and Indigestion, Chap. 39, p. 240, in HPIM-17.

51 Weight Loss

Significant unintentional weight loss in a previously healthy individual is often a harbinger of underlying systemic disease. The routine medical history should always include inquiry about changes in weight. Rapid fluctuations of weight over days suggest loss or gain of fluid, whereas long-term changes usually involve loss of tissue mass. Loss of 5% of body weight over 6–12 months should prompt further evaluation.

ETIOLOGY

A list of possible causes of weight loss is extensive (Table 51-1). In older persons the most common causes of weight loss are depression, cancer, and benign gastrointestinal disease. Lung and GI cancers are the most common malignancies in pts presenting with weight loss. In younger individuals diabetes mellitus, hyperthyroidism, anorexia nervosa, and infection, especially with HIV, should be considered.

CLINICAL FEATURES

Before extensive evaluation is undertaken, it is important to confirm that weight loss has occurred. In the absence of documentation, changes in belt notch size or the fit of clothing may help to determine loss of weight.

The *history* should include questions about fever, pain, shortness of breath or cough, palpitations, and evidence of neurologic disease. A history of GI symptoms should be obtained, including difficulty eating, dysphagia, anorexia, nausea, and change in bowel habits. Travel history, use of cigarettes, alcohol, and all medications should be reviewed, and pts should be questioned about previous illness or surgery as well as diseases in family members. Risk factors for HIV should be assessed. Signs of depression, evidence of dementia, and social factors, including financial issues that might affect food intake, should be considered.

TABLE 51-1	CAUSES OF WEIGHT LOSS
Cancer	Medications
Endocrine and metabolic causes	Antibiotics
Hyperthyroidism	Nonsteroidal anti-inflammatory
Diabetes mellitus	drugs
Pheochromocytoma	Serotonin reuptake inhibitors
Adrenal insufficiency	Metformin
Gastrointestinal disorders	Levodopa
Malabsorption	ACE inhibitors
Obstruction	Other drugs
Pernicious anemia	Disorders of the mouth and teeth
Cardiac disorders	Age-related factors
Chronic ischemia	Physiologic changes
Chronic congestive heart failure	Decreased taste and smell
Respiratory disorders	Functional disabilities
Emphysema	Neurologic causes
Chronic obstructive pulmonary	Stroke
disease	Parkinson's disease
Renal insufficiency	Neuromuscular disorders
Rheumatologic disease	Dementia
Infections	Social causes
HIV	Isolation
Tuberculosis	Economic hardship
Parasitic infection	Psychiatric and behavioral causes
Subacute bacterial endocarditis	Depression
	Anxiety
	Bereavement
	Alcoholism
	Eating disorders
	Increased activity or exercise
	Idiopathic

Physical examination should begin with weight determination and documentation of vital signs. The skin should be examined for pallor, jaundice, turgor, surgical scars, and stigmata of systemic disease. Evaluation for oral thrush, dental disease, thyroid gland enlargement, and adenopathy and for respiratory, cardiac, or abdominal abnormalities should be performed. All men should have a rectal examination, including the prostate; all women should have a pelvic examination; and both should have testing of the stool for occult blood. Neurologic examination should include mental status assessment and screening for depression.

Initial *laboratory evaluation* is shown in Table 51-2, with appropriate treatment based on the underlying cause of the weight loss. If an etiology of weight loss is not found, careful clinical follow-up, rather than persistent undirected testing, is reasonable.

℞ Weight Loss

Treatment of weight loss should be directed at correcting the underlying physical cause or social circumstance. In specific situations, nutritional supplements and medications (megastrol acetate, dronabinol, or growth hormone) may be effective for stimulating appetite or increasing weight.

TABLE 51-2	SCREENING TESTS FOR EVALUATION OF INVOLUNTARY WEIGHT LOSS

Initial testing
  CBC
  Electrolytes, calcium, glucose
  Renal and liver function tests
  Urinalysis
  Thyroid-stimulating hormone
  Chest x-ray
  Recommended cancer screening

Additional testing
  HIV test
  Upper and/or lower gastrointestinal
    endoscopy
  Abdominal CT scan or MRI
  Chest CT scan

For a more detailed discussion, see Reife CM: Weight Loss, Chap. 41, p. 255, in HPIM-17.

52 Dysphagia

DYSPHAGIA

Dysphagia is difficulty moving food or liquid through the mouth, pharynx, and esophagus. The pt senses swallowed material sticking along the path. *Odynophagia* is pain on swallowing. *Globus pharyngeus* is the sensation of a lump lodged in the throat, with swallowing unaffected.

Pathophysiology Dysphagia is caused by two main mechanisms: mechanical obstruction or motor dysfunction. Mechanical causes of dysphagia can be luminal (e.g., large food bolus, foreign body), intrinsic to the esophagus (e.g., inflammation, webs and rings, strictures, tumors), or extrinsic to the esophagus (e.g., cervical spondylitis, enlarged thyroid or mediastinal mass, vascular compression). The motor function abnormalities that cause dysphagia may be related to defects in initiating the swallowing reflex (e.g., tongue paralysis, lack of saliva, lesions affecting sensory components of cranial nerves X and XI), disorders of the pharyngeal and esophageal striated muscle (e.g., muscle disorders such as polymyositis and dermatomyositis, neurologic lesions such as myasthenia gravis, polio, or amyotrophic lateral sclerosis), and disorders of the esophageal smooth muscle (e.g., achalasia, scleroderma, myotonic dystrophy).

APPROACH TO THE PATIENT: DYSPHAGIA

History can provide a presumptive diagnosis in about 80% of pts. Difficulty only with solids implies mechanical dysphagia. Difficulty with both solids and liquids may occur late in the course of mechanical dysphagia but is an early sign of motor dysphagia. Pts can sometimes pinpoint the site of food sticking. Weight loss out of proportion to the degree of dysphagia may be a sign of underlying malignancy. Hoarseness may be related to involvement of the larynx in the primary disease process (e.g., neuromuscular disorders), neoplastic disruption of the recurrent laryngeal nerve, or laryngitis from gastroesophageal reflux.

Physical exam may reveal signs of skeletal muscle, neurologic, or oropharyngeal diseases. Neck exam can reveal masses impinging on the esophagus. Skin changes might suggest the systemic nature of the underlying disease (e.g., scleroderma).

Dysphagia is nearly always a symptom of organic disease rather than a functional complaint. If oropharyngeal dysphagia is suspected, videofluoroscopy of swallowing may be diagnostic. Mechanical dysphagia can be evaluated by barium swallow and esophagogastroscopy with endoscopic biopsy. Barium swallow and esophageal motility studies can show the presence of motor dysphagia.

Oropharyngeal Dysphagia Pt has difficulty initiating the swallow; food sticks at the level of the suprasternal notch; nasopharyngeal regurgitation and aspiration may be present.

Causes include the following: for solids only, carcinoma, aberrant vessel, congenital or acquired web (Plummer-Vinson syndrome in iron deficiency), cervical osteophyte; for solids and liquids, cricopharyngeal bar (e.g., hypertensive or hypotensive upper esophageal sphincter), Zenker's diverticulum (outpouching in the posterior midline at the intersection of the pharynx and the cricopharyngeus muscle), myasthenia gravis, glucocorticoid myopathy, hyperthyroidism, hypothyroidism, myotonic dystrophy, amyotrophic lateral sclerosis, multiple sclerosis, Parkinson's disease, stroke, bulbar palsy, pseudobulbar palsy.

Esophageal Dysphagia Food sticks in the mid or lower sternal area; can be associated with regurgitation, aspiration, odynophagia. Causes include the following: for solids only, lower esophageal ring (Schatzki's ring—symptoms are usually intermittent), peptic stricture (heartburn accompanies this), carcinoma, lye stricture; for solids and liquids, diffuse esophageal spasm (occurs with chest pain and is intermittent), scleroderma (progressive and occurs with heartburn), achalasia (progressive and occurs without heartburn).

NONCARDIAC CHEST PAIN

Of pts presenting with chest pain, 30% have an esophageal source rather than angina. History and physical exam often cannot distinguish cardiac from noncardiac pain. Exclude cardiac disease first. Causes include the following: gastroesophageal reflux disease, esophageal motility disorders, peptic ulcer disease, gallstones, psychiatric disease (anxiety, panic attacks, depression).

Evaluation Consider a trial of antireflux therapy (omeprazole); if no response, 24-h ambulatory luminal pH monitoring; if negative, esophageal manometry may show motor disorder. Trial of imipramine, 50 mg PO qhs, may be worthwhile. Consider psychiatric evaluation in selected cases.

ESOPHAGEAL MOTILITY DISORDERS

Pts may have a spectrum of manometric findings ranging from nonspecific abnormalities to defined clinical entities.

Achalasia Motor obstruction caused by hypertensive lower esophageal sphincter (LES), incomplete relaxation of LES, or loss of peristalsis in smooth-muscle portion of esophagus. Causes include the following: primary (idiopathic) or secondary due to Chagas' disease, lymphoma, carcinoma, chronic idiopathic intestinal pseudoobstruction, ischemia, neurotropic viruses, drugs, toxins, radiation therapy, postvagotomy.

Evaluation Chest x-ray shows absence of gastric air bubble. Barium swallow shows dilated esophagus with distal beaklike narrowing and air-fluid level. Endoscopy is done to rule out cancer, particularly in persons >50 years. Manometry shows normal or elevated LES pressure, decreased LES relaxation, absent peristalsis.

℞ Achalasia

Pneumatic balloon dilatation is effective in 85%, with 3–5% risk of perforation or bleeding. Injection of botulinum toxin at endoscopy to relax LES is safe and effective, but effects last only ~12 months. Myotomy of LES (Heller procedure) is effective, but 10–30% of pts develop gastroesophageal reflux. Nifedipine, 10–20 mg, or isosorbide dinitrate, 5–10 mg S/L ac, may avert need for dilatation or surgery. Sildenafil may also augment swallow-induced relaxation of the LES.

Spastic Disorders Diffuse esophageal spasm involves multiple spontaneous and swallow-induced contractions of the esophageal body that are of simultaneous onset and long duration and are recurrent. Causes include the following: primary (idiopathic) or secondary due to gastroesophageal reflux disease, emotional stress, diabetes, alcoholism, neuropathy, radiation therapy, ischemia, or collagen vascular disease.

An important variant is nutcracker esophagus: high-amplitude (>180 mm-Hg) peristaltic contractions; particularly associated with chest pain or dysphagia, but correlation between symptoms and manometry is inconsistent. Condition may resolve over time or evolve into diffuse spasm; associated with increased frequency of depression, anxiety, and somatization.

Evaluation Barium swallow shows corkscrew esophagus, pseudodiverticula, and diffuse spasm. Manometry shows spasm with multiple simultaneous esophageal contractions of high amplitude and long duration. In nutcracker esophagus, the contractions are peristaltic and of high amplitude. If heart disease has been ruled out, edrophonium, ergonovine, or bethanechol can be used to provoke spasm.

℞ Spastic Disorders

Anticholinergics are usually of limited value; nitrates (isosorbide dinitrate, 5–10 mg PO ac) and calcium antagonists (nifedipine, 10–20 mg PO ac) are more effective. Those refractory to medical management may benefit from balloon dilatation. Rare pts require surgical intervention: longitudinal myotomy of esophageal circular muscle. Treatment of concomitant depression or other psychological disturbance may help.

Scleroderma Atrophy of the esophageal smooth muscle and fibrosis can make the esophagus aperistaltic and lead to an incompetent LES with attendant reflux esophagitis and stricture. Treatment of gastroesophageal reflux disease is discussed in Chap. 50.

ESOPHAGEAL INFLAMMATION

Viral Esophagitis Herpesviruses I and II, varicella-zoster virus, and cytomegalovirus (CMV) can all cause esophagitis; particularly common in immunocompromised pts (e.g., AIDS). Odynophagia, dysphagia, fever, and bleeding are symptoms and signs. Diagnosis is made by endoscopy with biopsy, brush cytology, and culture.

R̲x̲ Viral Esophagitis

Disease is usually self-limited in the immunocompetent person; viscous lidocaine can relieve pain; in prolonged cases and in immunocompromised hosts, herpes and varicella esophagitis are treated with acyclovir, 5–10 mg/kg IV q8h for 10–14 d, then 200–400 mg PO 5 times a day. CMV is treated with ganciclovir, 5 mg/kg IV q12h, until healing occurs, which may take weeks. Oral valganciclovir (900 mg bid) is an effective alternative to parenteral treatment. In nonresponders, foscarnet, 60 mg/kg IV q12h for 21 days, may be effective.

Candida Esophagitis

In immunocompromised hosts, or those with malignancy, diabetes, hypoparathyroidism, hemoglobinopathy, systemic lupus erythematosus, corrosive esophageal injury, candidal esophageal infection may present with odynophagia, dysphagia, and oral thrush (50%). Diagnosis is made on endoscopy by identifying yellow-white plaques or nodules on friable red mucosa. Characteristic hyphae are seen on KOH stain. In pts with AIDS, the development of symptoms may prompt an empirical therapeutic trial.

R̲x̲ *Candida* Esophagitis

Oral nystatin (100,000 U/mL), 5 mL q6h, or clotrimazole, 10-mg tablet sucked q6h, is effective. In immunocompromised hosts, fluconazole, 100–200 mg PO daily for 1–3 weeks, is treatment of choice; alternatives include itraconazole, 200 mg PO bid, or ketoconazole, 200–400 mg PO daily; long-term maintenance therapy is often required. Poorly responsive pts may respond to higher doses of fluconazole (400 mg/d) or to amphotericin, 10–15 mg IV q6h for a total dose of 300–500 mg.

Pill-Related Esophagitis Doxycycline, tetracycline, aspirin, nonsteroidal antiinflammatory drugs, KCl, quinidine, ferrous sulfate, clindamycin, alprenolol, and alendronate can induce local inflammation in the esophagus. Predisposing factors include recumbency after swallowing pills with small sips of water and anatomic factors impinging on the esophagus and slowing transit.

R̲x̲ Pill-Related Esophagitis

Withdraw offending drug, use antacids, and dilate any resulting stricture.

Eosinophilic Esophagitis Mucosal inflammation with eosinophils with submucosal fibrosis can be seen especially in pts with food allergies. This diagnosis relies on the presence of symptoms of esophagitis with the appropriate findings on esophageal biopsy. Eotaxin 3, an eosinophil chemokine, has been implicated in its etiology. Treatment involves a 12-week course of swallowed fluticasone (440 μg bid) using a metered-dose inhaler.

Other Causes of Esophagitis in AIDS   *Mycobacteria, Cryptosporidium, Pneumocystis carinii*, idiopathic esophageal ulcers, and giant ulcers (possible cytopathic effect of HIV) can occur. Ulcers may respond to systemic glucocorticoids.

For a more detailed discussion, see Goyal RK: Dysphagia, Chap. 38, p. 237; and Diseases of the Esophagus, Chap. 286, p. 1847, in HPIM-17.

53 Diarrhea, Constipation, and Malabsorption

NORMAL GASTROINTESTINAL FUNCTION

Absorption of Fluid and Electrolytes   Fluid delivery to the GI tract is 8–10 L/d, including 2 L/d ingested; most is absorbed in small bowel. Colonic absorption is normally 0.05–2 L/d, with capacity for 6 L/d if required. Intestinal water absorption passively follows active transport of Na^+, Cl^-, glucose, and bile salts. Additional transport mechanisms include Cl^-/ HCO_3^- exchange, Na^+/H^+ exchange, H^+, K^+, Cl^-, and HCO_3^- secretion, Na^+- glucose cotransport, and active Na^+ transport across the basolateral membrane by Na^+,K^+-ATPase.

Nutrient Absorption

1. *Proximal small intestine*: iron, calcium, folate, fats (after hydrolysis of triglycerides to fatty acids by pancreatic lipase and colipase), proteins (after hydrolysis by pancreatic and intestinal peptidases), carbohydrates (after hydrolysis by amylases and disaccharidases); triglycerides absorbed as micelles after solubilization by bile salts; amino acids and dipeptides absorbed via specific carriers; sugars absorbed by active transport.
2. *Distal small intestine*: vitamin B_{12}, bile salts, water.
3. *Colon*: water, electrolytes.

Intestinal Motility   Allows propulsion of intestinal contents from stomach to anus and separation of components to facilitate nutrient absorption. Propulsion is controlled by neural, myogenic, and hormonal mechanisms; mediated by migrating motor complex, an organized wave of neuromuscular activity that originates in the distal stomach during fasting and migrates slowly down the small intestine. Colonic motility is mediated by local peristalsis to propel feces. Defecation is effected by relaxation of internal anal sphincter in response to rectal distention, with voluntary control by contraction of external anal sphincter.

DIARRHEA

Physiology   Formally defined as fecal output >200 g/d on low-fiber (western) diet; also frequently used to connote loose or watery stools. Mediated by one or more of the following mechanisms:

Osmotic Diarrhea   Nonabsorbed solutes increase intraluminal oncotic pressure, causing outpouring of water; usually ceases with fasting; stool osmolal gap > 40 (see below). Causes include disaccharidase (e.g., lactase) deficiencies, pancreatic insufficiency, bacterial overgrowth, lactulose or sorbitol ingestion, polyvalent laxative abuse, celiac or tropical sprue, and short bowel syndrome. Lactase deficiency can be either primary (more prevalent in blacks and Asians, usually presenting in early adulthood) or secondary (from viral, bacterial, or protozoal gastroenteritis, celiac or tropical sprue, or kwashiorkor).

Secretory Diarrhea   Active ion secretion causes obligatory water loss; diarrhea is usually watery, often profuse, unaffected by fasting; stool Na^+ and K^+ are elevated with osmolal gap < 40. Causes include viral infections (e.g., rotavirus, Norwalk virus), bacterial infections (e.g., cholera, enterotoxigenic *Escherichia coli*, *Staphylococcus aureus*), protozoa (e.g., *Giardia*, *Isospora*, *Cryptosporidium*), AIDS-associated disorders (including mycobacterial and HIV-induced), medications (e.g., theophylline, colchicine, prostaglandins, diuretics), Zollinger-Ellison syndrome (excess gastrin production), vasoactive intestinal peptide (VIP)-producing tumors, carcinoid tumors (histamine and serotonin), medullary thyroid carcinoma (prostaglandins and calcitonin), systemic mastocytosis, basophilic leukemia, distal colonic villous adenomas (direct secretion of potassium-rich fluid), collagenous and microscopic colitis, and cholerrheic diarrhea (from ileal malabsorption of bile salts).

Exudative   Inflammation, necrosis, and sloughing of colonic mucosa; may include component of secretory diarrhea due to prostaglandin release by inflammatory cells; stools usually contain polymorphonuclear leukocytes as well as occult or gross blood. Causes include bacterial infections [e.g., *Campylobacter, Salmonella, Shigella, Yersinia*, invasive or enterotoxigenic *E. coli, Vibrio parahaemolyticus, Clostridium difficile* colitis (frequently antibiotic-induced)], colonic parasites (e.g., *Entamoeba histolytica*), Crohn's disease, ulcerative proctocolitis, idiopathic inflammatory bowel disease, radiation enterocolitis, cancer chemotherapeutic agents, and intestinal ischemia.

Altered Intestinal Motility   Alteration of coordinated control of intestinal propulsion; diarrhea often intermittent or alternating with constipation. Causes include diabetes mellitus, adrenal insufficiency, hyperthyroidism, collagen-vascular diseases, parasitic infestations, gastrin and VIP hypersecretory states, amyloidosis, laxatives (esp. magnesium-containing agents), antibiotics (esp. erythromycin), cholinergic agents, primary neurologic dysfunction (e.g., Parkinson's disease, traumatic neuropathy), fecal impaction, diverticular disease, and irritable bowel syndrome. Blood in intestinal lumen is cathartic, and major upper GI bleeding leads to diarrhea from increased motility.

Decreased Absorptive Surface   Usually arises from surgical manipulation (e.g., extensive bowel resection or rearrangement) that leaves inadequate absorptive surface for fat and carbohydrate digestion and fluid and electrolyte absorption; occurs spontaneously from enteroenteric fistulas (esp. gastrocolic).

Evaluation   History   Diarrhea must be distinguished from fecal incontinence, change in stool caliber, rectal bleeding, and small, frequent, but otherwise nor-

TABLE 53-1	INFECTIOUS CAUSES OF DIARRHEA IN PATIENTS WITH AIDS
Nonopportunistic Pathogens	**Opportunistic Pathogens**
Shigella	Protozoa
Salmonella	Cryptosporidium
Campylobacter	Isospora belli
Entamoeba histolytica	Microsporidia
Chlamydia	Blastocystis hominis
Neisseria gonorrhoeae	Viruses
Treponema pallidum and other spirochetes	Cytomegalovirus
Giardia lamblia	Herpes simplex
	Adenovirus
	HIV
	Bacteria
	Mycobacterium avium complex

mal stools. Careful medication history is essential. Alternating diarrhea and constipation suggests fixed colonic obstruction (e.g., from carcinoma) or irritable bowel syndrome. A sudden, acute course, often with nausea, vomiting, and fever, is typical of viral and bacterial infections, diverticulitis, ischemia, radiation enterocolitis, or drug-induced diarrhea and may be the initial presentation of inflammatory bowel disease. More than 90% of acute diarrheal illnesses are infectious in etiology. A longer (>4 weeks), more insidious course suggests malabsorption, inflammatory bowel disease, metabolic or endocrine disturbance, pancreatic insufficiency, laxative abuse, ischemia, neoplasm (hypersecretory state or partial obstruction), or irritable bowel syndrome. Parasitic and certain forms of bacterial enteritis can also produce chronic symptoms. Particularly foul-smelling or oily stool suggests fat malabsorption. Fecal impaction may cause apparent diarrhea because only liquids pass partial obstruction. Several infectious causes of diarrhea are associated with an immunocompromised state (Table 53-1).

Physical Examination   Signs of dehydration are often prominent in severe, acute diarrhea. Fever and abdominal tenderness suggest infection or inflammatory disease but are often absent in viral enteritis. Evidence of malnutrition suggests chronic course. Certain signs are frequently associated with specific deficiency states secondary to malabsorption (e.g., cheilosis with riboflavin or iron deficiency, glossitis with B_{12}, folate deficiency). Questions to address in patients with chronic diarrhea are shown in Table 53-2.

TABLE 53-2	PHYSICAL EXAMINATION IN PATIENTS WITH CHRONIC DIARRHEA

1. Are there general features to suggest malabsorption or inflammatory bowel disease (IBD) such as anemia, dermatitis herpetiformis, edema, or clubbing?
2. Are there features to suggest underlying autonomic neuropathy or collagen-vascular disease in the pupils, orthostasis, skin, hands, or joints?
3. Is there an abdominal mass or tenderness?
4. Are there any abnormalities of rectal mucosa, rectal defects, or altered anal sphincter functions?
5. Are there any mucocutaneous manifestations of systemic disease such as dermatitis herpetiformis (celiac disease), erythema nodosum (ulcerative colitis), flushing (carcinoid), or oral ulcers for IBD or celiac disease?

Stool Examination Culture for bacterial pathogens, examination for leukocytes, measurement of *C. difficile* toxin, and examination for ova and parasites are important components of evaluation of pts with severe, protracted, or bloody diarrhea. Presence of blood (fecal occult blood test) or leukocytes (Wright's stain) suggests inflammation (e.g., ulcerative colitis, Crohn's disease, infection, or ischemia). Gram's stain of stool can be diagnostic of *Staphylococcus*, *Campylobacter*, or *Candida* infection. Steatorrhea (determined with Sudan III stain of stool sample or 72-h quantitative fecal fat analysis) suggests malabsorption or pancreatic insufficiency. Measurement of Na^+ and K^+ levels in fecal water helps to distinguish osmotic from other types of diarrhea; osmotic diarrhea is implied by stool osmolal gap > 40, where stool osmolal gap = $osmol_{serum}$ [$2 \times (Na^+ + K^+)_{stool}$].

Laboratory Studies Complete blood count may indicate anemia (acute or chronic blood loss or malabsorption of iron, folate, or B_{12}), leukocytosis (inflammation), eosinophilia (parasitic, neoplastic, and inflammatory bowel diseases). Serum levels of calcium, albumin, iron, cholesterol, folate, B_{12}, vitamin D, and carotene; serum iron-binding capacity; and prothrombin time can provide evidence of intestinal malabsorption or maldigestion.

Other Studies D-Xylose absorption test is a convenient screen for small-bowel absorptive function. Small-bowel biopsy is especially useful for evaluating intestinal malabsorption. Specialized studies include Schilling test (B_{12} malabsorption), lactose H_2 breath test (carbohydrate malabsorption), [^{14}C]xylose and lactulose H_2 breath tests (bacterial overgrowth), glycocholic breath test (ileal malabsorption), triolein breath test (fat malabsorption), and bentiromide and secretin tests (pancreatic insufficiency). Sigmoidoscopy or colonoscopy with biopsy is useful in the diagnosis of colitis (esp. pseudomembranous, ischemic, microscopic); it may not allow distinction between infectious and noninfectious (esp. idiopathic ulcerative) colitis. Barium contrast x-ray studies may suggest malabsorption (thickened bowel folds), inflammatory bowel disease (ileitis or colitis), tuberculosis (ileocecal inflammation), neoplasm, intestinal fistula, or motility disorders.

℞ Diarrhea

An approach to the management of acute diarrheal illnesses is shown in Fig. 53-1. Symptomatic therapy includes vigorous rehydration (IV or with oral glucose-electrolyte solutions), electrolyte replacement, binders of osmotically active substances (e.g., kaolin-pectin), and opiates to decrease bowel motility (e.g., loperamide, diphenoxylate); opiates may be contraindicated in infectious or inflammatory causes of diarrhea. An approach to the management of chronic diarrhea is shown in Fig. 53-2.

MALABSORPTION SYNDROMES

Intestinal malabsorption of ingested nutrients may produce osmotic diarrhea, steatorrhea, or specific deficiencies (e.g., iron; folate; B_{12}; vitamins A, D, E, and K). Table 53-3 lists common causes of intestinal malabsorption. Protein-losing enteropathy may result from several causes of malabsorption; it is associated with hypoalbuminemia and can be detected by measuring stool α_1-antitrypsin or radiolabeled albumin levels. Therapy is directed at the underlying disease.

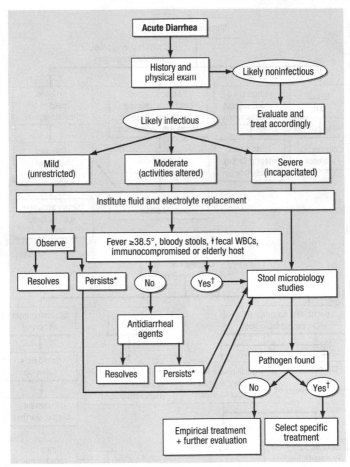

FIGURE 53-1 Algorithm for the management of acute diarrhea. Before evaluation, consider empiric RX with (*) metronidazole and with (†) quinolone.

CONSTIPATION

Defined as decrease in frequency of stools to <1 per week or difficulty in defecation; may result in abdominal pain, distention, and fecal impaction, with consequent obstruction or, rarely, perforation. Constipation is a frequent and often subjective complaint. Contributory factors may include inactivity, low-fiber diet, and inadequate allotment of time for defecation.

Specific Causes Altered colonic motility due to neurologic dysfunction (diabetes mellitus, spinal cord injury, multiple sclerosis, Chagas' disease, Hirschsprung's disease, chronic idiopathic intestinal pseudoobstruction, idiopathic megacolon), scleroderma, drugs (esp. anticholinergic agents, opiates, aluminum- or calcium-based antacids, calcium channel blockers, iron supplements, sucralfate), hypothyroidism, Cushing's syndrome, hypokalemia, hypercalcemia, dehydration, mechanical causes (colorectal tumors, diverticulitis, volvu-

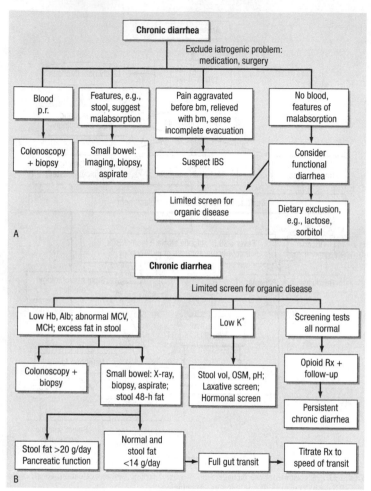

FIGURE 53-2 Algorithm for the management of chronic diarrhea based on accompanying symptoms or features (*A*) or based on a limited screening for organic disease (*B*). p.r., per rectum; bm, bowel movement; IBS, irritable bowel syndrome; Hb, hemoglobin; Alb, albumin; MCV, mean corpuscular volume; MCH, mean corpuscular hemoglobin; OSM, osmolality. (*Reprinted from M Camilleri: Clin Gastrol Hepatol. 2:198, 2004.*)

lus, hernias, intussusception), and anorectal pain (from fissures, hemorrhoids, abscesses, or proctitis) leading to retention, constipation, and fecal impaction.

℞ Constipation

In absence of identifiable cause, constipation may improve with reassurance, exercise, increased dietary fiber, bulking agents (e.g., psyllium), and increased fluid intake. Specific therapies include removal of bowel obstruction (fecalith, tumor), discontinuance of nonessential hypomotility agents (esp. aluminum-

| TABLE 53-3 | COMMON CAUSES OF MALABSORPTION |

Maldigestion: Chronic pancreatitis, cystic fibrosis, pancreatic carcinoma
Bile salt deficiency: Cirrhosis, cholestasis, bacterial overgrowth (blind loop syndromes, intestinal diverticula, hypomotility disorders), impaired ileal reabsorption (resection, Crohn's disease), bile salt binders (cholestyramine, calcium carbonate, neomycin)
Inadequate absorptive surface: Massive intestinal resection, gastrocolic fistula, jejunoileal bypass
Lymphatic obstruction: Lymphoma, Whipple's disease, intestinal lymphangiectasia
Vascular disease: Constrictive pericarditis, right-sided heart failure, mesenteric arterial or venous insufficiency
Mucosal disease: Infection (esp. *Giardia*, Whipple's disease, tropical sprue), inflammatory diseases (esp. Crohn's disease), radiation enteritis, eosinophilic enteritis, ulcerative jejunitis, mastocytosis, tropical sprue, infiltrative disorders (amyloidosis, scleroderma, lymphoma, collagenous sprue, microscopic colitis), biochemical abnormalities (gluten-sensitive enteropathy, disaccharidase deficiency, hypogammaglobulinemia, abetalipoproteinemia, amino acid transport deficiencies), endocrine disorders (diabetes mellitus, hypoparathyroidism, adrenal insufficiency, hyperthyroidism, Zollinger-Ellison syndrome, carcinoid syndrome)

or calcium-containing antacids, opiates), or substitution of magnesium-based antacids for aluminum-based antacids. For symptomatic relief, magnesium-containing agents or other cathartics are occasionally needed. With severe hypo- or dysmotility or in presence of opiates, osmotically active agents (e.g., oral lactulose, intestinal polyethylene glycol–containing lavage solutions) and oral or rectal emollient laxatives (e.g., docusate salts) and mineral oil are most effective.

For a more detailed discussion, see Camilleri M, Murray JA: Diarrhea and Constipation, Chap. 40, p. 245; and Binder HJ: Disorders of Absorption, Chap. 288, p. 1872, in HPIM-17.

54 Gastrointestinal Bleeding

PRESENTATION

1. *Hematemesis*: Vomiting of blood or altered blood ("coffee grounds") indicates bleeding proximal to ligament of Treitz.
2. *Melena*: Altered (black) blood per rectum (>100 mL blood required for one melenic stool) usually indicates bleeding proximal to ligament of Treitz but may be as distal as ascending colon; pseudomelena may be caused by ingestion of iron, bismuth, licorice, beets, blueberries, charcoal.

3. *Hematochezia*: Bright red or maroon rectal bleeding usually implies bleeding beyond ligament of Treitz but may be due to rapid upper GI bleeding (>1000 mL).
4. *Positive fecal occult blood test with or without iron deficiency.*
5. *Symptoms of blood loss*: e.g., light-headedness or shortness of breath.

Hemodynamic Changes Orthostatic drop in BP > 10 mmHg usually indicates >20% reduction in blood volume (± syncope, light-headedness, nausea, sweating, thirst).

Shock BP < 100 mmHg systolic usually indicates <30% reduction in blood volume (± pallor, cool skin).

Laboratory Changes Hematocrit may not reflect extent of blood loss because of delayed equilibration with extravascular fluid. Mild leukocytosis and thrombocytosis. Elevated blood urea nitrogen is common in upper GI bleeding.

Adverse Prognostic Signs Age >60, associated illnesses, coagulopathy, immunosuppression, presentation with shock, rebleeding, onset of bleeding in hospital, variceal bleeding, endoscopic stigmata of recent bleeding [e.g., "visible vessel" in ulcer base (see below)].

UPPER GI BLEEDING

Causes Common Peptic ulcer (accounts for ~50%), gastropathy [alcohol, aspirin, nonsteroidal anti-inflammatory drugs (NSAIDs), stress], esophagitis, Mallory-Weiss tear (mucosal tear at gastroesophageal junction due to retching), gastroesophageal varices.

Less Common Swallowed blood (nosebleed); esophageal, gastric, or intestinal neoplasm; anticoagulant and fibrinolytic therapy; hypertrophic gastropathy (Ménétrier's disease); aortic aneurysm; aortoenteric fistula (from aortic graft); arteriovenous malformation; telangiectases (Osler-Rendu-Weber syndrome); Dieulafoy lesion (ectatic submucosal vessel); vasculitis; connective tissue disease (pseudoxanthoma elasticum, Ehlers-Danlos syndrome); blood dyscrasias; neurofibroma; amyloidosis; hemobilia (biliary origin).

Evaluation After hemodynamic resuscitation (see below and Fig. 54-1).
- History and physical examination: Drugs (increased risk of upper and lower GI tract bleeding with aspirin and NSAIDs), prior ulcer, bleeding history, family history, features of cirrhosis or vasculitis, etc. Hyperactive bowel sounds favor upper GI source.
- Nasogastric aspirate for gross blood, if source (upper versus lower) not clear from history; may be falsely negative in up to 16% of pts if bleeding has ceased or duodenum is the source. Testing aspirate for occult blood is meaningless.
- Upper endoscopy: Accuracy >90%; allows visualization of bleeding site and possibility of therapeutic intervention; mandatory for suspected varices, aortoenteric fistulas; permits identification of "visible vessel" (protruding artery in ulcer crater), which connotes high (~50%) risk of rebleeding.
- Upper GI barium radiography: Accuracy ~80% in identifying a lesion, though does not confirm source of bleeding; acceptable alternative to endoscopy in resolved or chronic low-grade bleeding.
- Selective mesenteric arteriography: When brisk bleeding precludes identification of source at endoscopy.

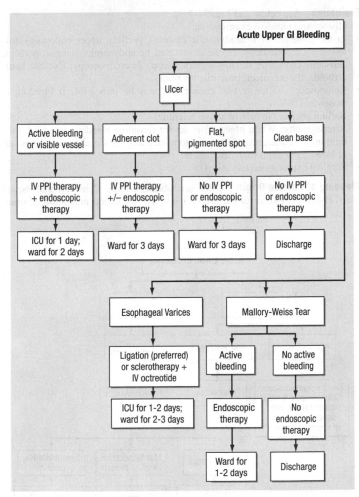

FIGURE 54-1 Suggested algorithm for patients with acute upper GI bleeding. Recommendations on level of care and time of discharge assume patient is stabilized without further bleeding or other concomitant medical problems. PPI, proton pump inhibitor; ICU, intensive care unit.

- Radioisotope scanning (e.g., ^{99}Tc tagged to red blood cells or albumin); used primarily as screening test to confirm bleeding is rapid enough for arteriography to be of value or when bleeding is intermittent and of unclear origin.

LOWER GI BLEEDING

Causes   Anal lesions (hemorrhoids, fissures), rectal trauma, proctitis, colitis (ulcerative colitis, Crohn's disease, infectious colitis, ischemic colitis, radiation), colonic polyps, colonic carcinoma, angiodysplasia (vascular ectasia), diverticulosis, intussusception, solitary ulcer, blood dyscrasias, vasculitis, connective tissue disease, neurofibroma, amyloidosis, anticoagulation.

Evaluation   See below and Fig. 54-2.

- History and physical examination.
- In the presence of hemodynamic changes, perform upper endoscopy followed by colonoscopy. In the absence of hemodynamic changes, perform anoscopy and either flexible sigmoidoscopy or colonoscopy: Exclude hemorrhoids, fissure, ulcer, proctitis, neoplasm.
- Colonoscopy: Often test of choice, but may be impossible if bleeding is massive.
- Barium enema: No role in active bleeding.
- Arteriography: When bleeding is severe (requires bleeding rate >0.5 mL/min; may require prestudy radioisotope bleeding scan as above); defines site of bleeding or abnormal vasculature.
- Surgical exploration (last resort).

Bleeding of Obscure Origin   Often small-bowel source. Consider small-bowel enteroclysis x-ray (careful barium radiography via peroral intubation of small

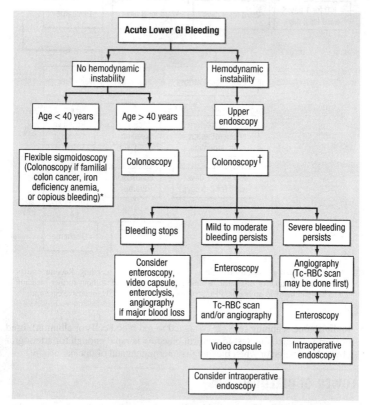

FIGURE 54-2 Suggested algorithm for patients with acute lower GI bleeding. Sequential recommendations under "Hemodynamic instability" assume a test is found to be nondiagnostic before the next test is performed. *Some suggest colonoscopy for any degree of rectal bleeding in patients <40 years as well. †If massive bleeding does not allow time for colonic lavage, proceed to angiography. Tc-RBC, 99mtechnetium-labeled red blood cell.

bowel), Meckel's scan, enteroscopy (small-bowel endoscopy), or exploratory laparotomy with intraoperative enteroscopy.

℞ Upper and Lower GI Bleeding

- Venous access with large-bore IV (14–18 gauge); central venous line for major bleed and pts with cardiac disease; monitor vital signs, urine output, Hct (fall may lag). Gastric lavage of unproven benefit but clears stomach before endoscopy. Iced saline may lyse clots; room-temperature tap water may be preferable. Intubation may be required to protect airway.
- Type and cross-match blood (6 units for major bleed).
- Surgical standby when bleeding is massive.
- Support blood pressure with isotonic fluids (normal saline); albumin and fresh-frozen plasma in cirrhotics. Packed red blood cells when available (whole blood if massive bleeding); maintain Hct >25–30. Fresh-frozen plasma and vitamin K (10 mg SC or IV) in cirrhotics with coagulopathy.
- IV calcium (e.g., up to 10–20 mL 10% calcium gluconate IV over 10–15 min) if serum calcium falls (due to transfusion of citrated blood). Empirical drug therapy (antacids, H_2 receptor blockers, omeprazole) of unproven benefit.
- Specific measures: *Varices*: octreotide (50-μg bolus, 50-μg/h infusion for 2–5 days), Blakemore-Sengstaken tube tamponade, endoscopic sclerosis, or band ligation; propranolol or nadolol in doses sufficient to cause beta blockade reduces risk of recurrent or initial variceal bleeding (do not use in acute bleed) (Chap. 164); *ulcer with visible vessel or active bleeding*: endoscopic bipolar, heater-probe, or laser coagulation or injection of epinephrine; *gastritis*: embolization or vasopressin infusion of left gastric artery; *GI telangiectases*: ethinylestradiol/norethisterone (0.05/1.0 mg PO qd) may prevent recurrent bleeding, particularly in pts with chronic renal failure; *diverticulosis*: mesenteric arteriography with intraarterial vasopressin; *angiodysplasia*: colonoscopic bipolar or laser coagulation, may regress with replacement of stenotic aortic valve.
- Indications for emergency surgery: Uncontrolled or prolonged bleeding, severe rebleeding, aortoenteric fistula. For intractable variceal bleeding, consider transjugular intrahepatic portosystemic shunt (TIPS).

For a more detailed discussion, see Laine L: Gastrointestinal Bleeding, Chap. 42, p. 257, in HPIM-17.

55 Jaundice and Evaluation of Liver Function

JAUNDICE

Definition   Yellow skin pigmentation caused by elevation in serum bilirubin level (also termed *icterus*); often more easily discernible in sclerae. Scleral icterus becomes clinically evident at a serum bilirubin level of ≥51 μmol/L (≥3 mg/dL); yellow skin discoloration also occurs with elevated serum carotene levels but without pigmentation of the sclerae.

Bilirubin Metabolism Bilirubin is the major breakdown product of hemoglobin released from senescent erythrocytes. Initially, it is bound to albumin, transported into the liver, conjugated to a water-soluble form (glucuronide) by glucuronosyl transferase, excreted into the bile, and converted to urobilinogen in the colon. Urobilinogen is mostly excreted in the stool; a small portion is reabsorbed and excreted by the kidney. Bilirubin can be filtered by the kidney only in its conjugated form (measured as the "direct" fraction); thus, increased *direct* serum bilirubin level is associated with bilirubinuria. Increased bilirubin production and excretion (even without hyperbilirubinemia, as in hemolysis) produce elevated urinary urobilinogen levels.

Etiology Hyperbilirubinemia occurs as a result of (1) overproduction; (2) impaired uptake, conjugation, or excretion of bilirubin; (3) regurgitation of unconjugated or conjugated bilirubin from damaged hepatocytes or bile ducts (Table 55-1).

Evaluation The initial steps in evaluating the pt with jaundice are to determine whether (1) hyperbilirubinemia is conjugated or unconjugated, and (2) other biochemical liver tests are abnormal (Figs. 55-1 and 55-2, Tables 55-2 and 55-3). Essential clinical examination includes history (especially duration of jaundice, pruritus, associated pain, risk factors for parenterally transmitted diseases, medications, ethanol use, travel history, surgery, pregnancy, presence of any accompanying symptoms), physical examination (hepatomegaly, tenderness over liver, palpable gallbladder, splenomegaly, gynecomastia, testicular atrophy, other stigmata of chronic liver disease), blood liver tests (see below), and complete blood count.

TABLE 55-1 **CAUSES OF ISOLATED HYPERBILIRUBINEMIA**

I. Indirect hyperbilirubinemia
    A. Hemolytic disorders
        1. Inherited
            a. Spherocytosis, elliptocytosis
            b. Glucose-6-phosphate dehydrogenase and pyruvate kinase deficiencies
            c. Sickle cell anemia
        2. Acquired
            a. Microangiopathic hemolytic anemias
            b. Paroxysmal nocturnal hemoglobinuria
            c. Spur cell anemia
            d. Immune hemolysis
    B. Ineffective erythropoiesis
        1. Cobalamin, folate, thalassemia, and severe iron deficiencies
    C. Drugs
        1. Rifampicin, probenecid, ribavirin
    D. Inherited conditions
        1. Crigler-Najjar types I and II
        2. Gilbert's syndrome
II. Direct hyperbilirubinemia
    A. Inherited conditions
        1. Dubin-Johnson syndrome
        2. Rotor's syndrome

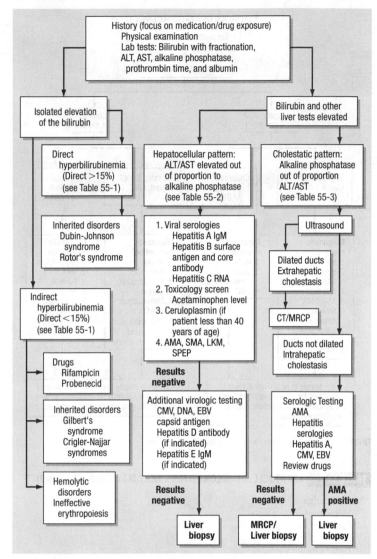

FIGURE 55-1 Evaluation of the patient with jaundice. CT, computed tomography; MRCP, magnetic resonance cholangiopancreatography; ALT, alanine aminotransferase; AST, aspartate aminotransferase; SMA, smooth muscle antibody; AMA, antimitochondrial antibody; LKM; liver-kidney microsomal antibody; SPEP, serum protein electrophoresis; CMV, cytomegalovirus; EBV, Epstein-Barr virus.

Gilbert's Syndrome Impaired conjugation of bilirubin due to reduced bilirubin UDP glucuronosyl transferase activity. Results in mild unconjugated hyperbilirubinemia, almost always <103 μmol/L (<6 mg/dL). Affects 3–7% of the population; males/females 2–7:1.

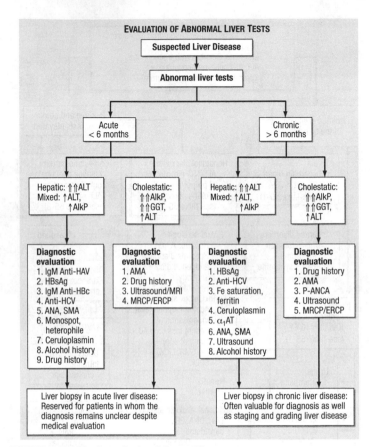

EVALUATION OF ABNORMAL LIVER TESTS

Suspected Liver Disease

Abnormal liver tests

Acute
< 6 months

Chronic
> 6 months

Hepatic: ⇧⇧ALT
Mixed: ↑ALT,
↑AlkP

Cholestatic:
⇧⇧AlkP,
⇧⇧GGT,
↑ALT

Hepatic: ⇧⇧ALT
Mixed: ↑ALT,
↑AlkP

Cholestatic:
⇧⇧AlkP,
⇧⇧GGT,
↑ALT

Diagnostic evaluation
1. IgM Anti-HAV
2. HBsAg
3. IgM Anti-HBc
4. Anti-HCV
5. ANA, SMA
6. Monospot, heterophile
7. Ceruloplasmin
8. Alcohol history
9. Drug history

Diagnostic evaluation
1. AMA
2. Drug history
3. Ultrasound/MRI
4. MRCP/ERCP

Diagnostic evaluation
1. HBsAg
2. Anti-HCV
3. Fe saturation, ferritin
4. Ceruloplasmin
5. α₁AT
6. ANA, SMA
7. Ultrasound
8. Alcohol history

Diagnostic evaluation
1. Drug history
2. AMA
3. P-ANCA
4. Ultrasound
5. MRCP/ERCP

Liver biopsy in acute liver disease: Reserved for patients in whom the diagnosis remains unclear despite medical evaluation

Liver biopsy in chronic liver disease: Often valuable for diagnosis as well as staging and grading liver disease

FIGURE 55-2 Algorithm for evaluation of abnormal liver tests.

TABLE 55-2   HEPATOCELLULAR CONDITIONS THAT MAY PRODUCE JAUNDICE

Viral hepatitis
    Hepatitis A, B, C, D, and E
    Epstein-Barr virus
    Cytomegalovirus
    Herpes simplex
Alcohol
Drug toxicity
    Predictable, dose-dependent, e.g., acetaminophen
    Unpredictable, idiosyncratic, e.g., isoniazid
Environmental toxins
    Vinyl chloride
    Jamaica bush tea—pyrrolizidine alkaloids
    Kava Kava
    Wild mushrooms—*Amanita phalloides* or *A. verna*
Wilson's disease
Autoimmune hepatitis

TABLE 55-3   CHOLESTATIC CONDITIONS THAT MAY PRODUCE JAUNDICE

I. Intrahepatic
   A. Viral hepatitis
      1. Fibrosing cholestatic hepatitis—hepatitis B and C
      2. Hepatitis A, Epstein-Barr virus, cytomegalovirus
   B. Alcoholic hepatitis
   C. Drug toxicity
      1. Pure cholestasis—anabolic and contraceptive steroids
      2. Cholestatic hepatitis—chlorpromazine, erythromycin estolate
      3. Chronic cholestasis—chlorpromazine and prochlorperazine
   D. Primary biliary cirrhosis
   E. Primary sclerosing cholangitis
   F. Vanishing bile duct syndrome
      1. Chronic rejection of liver transplants
      2. Sarcoidosis
      3. Drugs
   G. Inherited
      1. Progressive familial intrahepatic cholestasis
      2. Benign recurrent cholestasis
   H. Cholestasis of pregnancy
   I. Total parenteral nutrition
   J. Nonhepatobiliary sepsis
   K. Benign postoperative cholestasis
   L. Paraneoplastic syndrome
   M. Venoocclusive disease
   N. Graft-versus-host disease
   O. Infiltrative disease
      1. TB
      2. Lymphoma
      3. Amyloidosis
II. Extrahepatic
   A. Malignant
      1. Cholangiocarcinoma
      2. Pancreatic cancer
      3. Gallbladder cancer
      4. Ampullary cancer
      5. Malignant involvement of the porta hepatis lymph nodes
   B. Benign
      1. Choledocholithiasis
      2. Postoperative biliary structures
      3. Primary sclerosing cholangitis
      4. Chronic pancreatitis
      5. AIDS cholangiopathy
      6. Mirizzi syndrome
      7. Parasitic disease (ascariasis)

BLOOD TESTS OF LIVER FUNCTION

Used to detect presence of liver disease (Fig. 55-2), discriminate among different types of liver disease (Table 55-4), gauge the extent of known liver damage, follow response to treatment.

Bilirubin   Provides indication of hepatic uptake, metabolic (conjugation) and excretory functions; conjugated fraction (direct) distinguished from unconjugated by chemical assay (Table 55-1).

TABLE 55-4	LIVER TEST PATTERNS IN HEPATOBILIARY DISORDERS	
Type of Disorder	Bilirubin	Aminotransferases
Hemolysis/Gilbert's syndrome	Normal to 86 µmol/L (5 mg/dL) 85% due to indirect fractions No bilirubinuria	Normal
Acute hepatocellular necrosis (viral and drug hepatitis, hepatotoxins, acute heart failure)	Both fractions may be elevated Peak usually follows aminotransferases Bilirubinuria	Elevated, often >500 IU ALT >AST
Chronic hepatocellular disorders	Both fractions may be elevated Bilirubinuria	Elevated, but usually <300 IU
Alcoholic hepatitis Cirrhosis	Both fractions may be elevated Bilirubinuria	AST:ALT > 2 suggests alcoholic hepatitis or cirrhosis
Intra- and extra-hepatic cholestasis (Obstructive jaundice)	Both fractions may be elevated Bilirubinuria	Normal to moderate elevation Rarely >500 IU
Infiltrative diseases (tumor, granulomata); partial bile duct obstruction	Usually normal	Normal to slight elevation

Aminotransferases (Transaminases)   Aspartate aminotransferase (AST; SGOT) and alanine aminotransferase (ALT; SGPT); sensitive indicators of liver cell injury; greatest elevations seen in hepatocellular necrosis (e.g., viral hepatitis, toxic or ischemic liver injury, acute hepatic vein obstruction), occasionally with sudden, complete biliary obstruction (e.g., from gallstone); milder abnormalities in cholestatic, cirrhotic, and infiltrative disease; poor correlation between degree of liver cell damage and level of aminotransferases; ALT more specific measure of liver injury, since AST also found in striated muscle and other organs; ethanol-induced liver injury usually produces modest increases with more prominent elevation of AST than ALT.

Alkaline Phosphatase   Sensitive indicator of cholestasis, biliary obstruction (enzyme increases more quickly than serum bilirubin), and liver infiltration; mild elevations in other forms of liver disease; limited specificity because of wide tissue distribution; elevations also seen in normal childhood, pregnancy, and bone diseases; tissue-specific isoenzymes can be distinguished by fractionation or by differences in heat stability (liver enzyme activity stable under conditions that destroy bone enzyme activity).

5'-Nucleotidase (5'-NT)   Pattern of elevation in hepatobiliary disease similar to alkaline phosphatase; has greater specificity for liver disorders; used to determine whether liver is source of elevation in serum alkaline phosphatase, esp. in children, pregnant women, pts with possible concomitant bone disease.

Alkaline Phosphatase	Albumin	Prothrombin Time
Normal	Normal	Normal
Normal to <3 times normal elevation	Normal	Usually normal. If >5 × above control and not corrected by parenteral vitamin K, suggests poor prognosis
Normal to <3 times normal elevation	Often decreased	Often prolonged Fails to correct with parenteral vitamin K
Normal to <3 times normal elevation	Often decreased	Often prolonged Fails to correct with parenteral vitamin K
Elevated, often >4 times normal elevation	Normal, unless chronic	Normal If prolonged, will correct with parenteral vitamin K
Elevated, often >4 times normal elevation Fractionate, or confirm liver origin with 5′ nucleo-tidase or γ glutamyl transpeptidase	Normal	Normal

γ-Glutamyltranspeptidase (GGT)   Correlates with serum alkaline phosphatase activity. Elevation is less specific for cholestasis than alkaline phosphatase or 5-NT.

Coagulation Factors   (See also Chap. 68)   Measure of clotting factor activity; prolongation results from clotting factor deficiency or inactivity; all clotting factors except factor VIII are synthesized in the liver, and deficiency can occur rapidly from widespread liver disease as in hepatitis, toxic injury, or cirrhosis; single best acute measure of hepatic synthetic function; helpful in Dx and prognosis of acute liver disease. Clotting factors II, VII, IX, X function only in the presence of the fat-soluble vitamin K; PT prolongation from fat malabsorption distinguished from hepatic disease by rapid and complete response to vitamin K replacement.

Albumin   Decreased serum levels result from decreased hepatic synthesis (chronic liver disease or prolonged malnutrition) or excessive losses in urine or stool; insensitive indicator of acute hepatic dysfunction, since serum half-life is 2–3 weeks; in pts with chronic liver disease, degree of hypoalbuminemia correlates with severity of liver dysfunction.

Globulin   Mild polyclonal hyperglobulinemia often seen in chronic liver diseases; marked elevation frequently seen in *autoimmune* chronic active hepatitis.

Ammonia   Elevated blood levels result from deficiency of hepatic detoxification pathways and portal-systemic shunting, as in fulminant hepatitis, hepatotoxin exposure, and severe portal hypertension (e.g., from cirrhosis); elevation of blood ammonia does not correlate well with hepatic function or the presence or degree of acute encephalopathy.

HEPATOBILIARY IMAGING PROCEDURES

Ultrasonography (US) Rapid, noninvasive examination of abdominal structures; no radiation exposure; relatively low cost, equipment portable; images and interpretation strongly dependent on expertise of examiner; particularly valuable for detecting biliary duct dilatation and gallbladder stones (>95%); much less sensitive for intraductal stones (~60%); most sensitive means of detecting ascites; moderately sensitive for detecting hepatic masses but excellent for discriminating solid from cystic structures; useful in directing percutaneous needle biopsies of suspicious lesions; Doppler US useful to determine patency and flow in portal, hepatic veins and portal-systemic shunts; imaging improved by presence of ascites but severely hindered by bowel gas; endoscopic US less affected by bowel gas and is sensitive for determination of depth of tumor invasion through bowel wall.

CT Particularly useful for detecting, differentiating, and directing percutaneous needle biopsy of abdominal masses, cysts, and lymphadenopathy; imaging enhanced by intestinal or intravenous contrast dye and unaffected by intestinal gas; somewhat less sensitive than US for detecting stones in gallbladder but more sensitive for choledocholithiasis; may be useful in distinguishing certain forms of diffuse hepatic disease (e.g., fatty infiltration, iron overload).

MRI Most sensitive detection of hepatic masses and cysts; allows easy differentiation of hemangiomas from other hepatic tumors; most accurate noninvasive means of assessing hepatic and portal vein patency, vascular invasion by tumor; useful for monitoring iron, copper deposition in liver (e.g., in hemochromatosis, Wilson's disease). Magnetic resonance cholangiography (MRCP) can be useful for visualizing the head of the pancreas and the pancreatic and biliary ducts.

Radionuclide Scanning Using various radiolabeled compounds, different scanning methods allow sensitive assessment of biliary excretion (HIDA, PIPIDA, DISIDA scans), parenchymal changes (technetium sulfur colloid liver/spleen scan), and selected inflammatory and neoplastic processes (gallium scan); HIDA and related scans particularly useful for assessing biliary patency and excluding acute cholecystitis in situations where US is not diagnostic; CT, MRI, and colloid scans have similar sensitivity for detecting liver tumors and metastases; CT and combination of colloidal liver and lung scans sensitive for detecting right subphrenic (suprahepatic) abscesses.

Cholangiography Most sensitive means of detecting biliary ductal calculi, biliary tumors, sclerosing cholangitis, choledochal cysts, fistulas, and bile duct leaks; may be performed via endoscopic (transampullary) or percutaneous (transhepatic) route; allows sampling of bile and ductal epithelium for cytologic analysis and culture; allows placement of biliary drainage catheter and stricture dilatation; endoscopic route (ERCP) permits manometric evaluation of sphincter of Oddi, sphincterotomy, and stone extraction.

Angiography Most accurate means of determining portal pressures and assessing patency and direction of flow in portal and hepatic veins; highly sensitive for detecting small vascular lesions and hepatic tumors (esp. primary hepatocellular carcinoma); "gold standard" for differentiating hemangiomas from solid tumors; most accurate means of studying vascular anatomy in preparation for complicated hepatobiliary surgery (e.g., portal-systemic shunting, biliary reconstruction) and determining resectability of hepatobiliary and pancreatic tumors. Similar anatomic information (but not intravascular pressures) can often be obtained noninvasively by CT- and MR-based techniques.

Percutaneous Liver Biopsy Most accurate in disorders causing diffuse changes throughout the liver; subject to sampling error in focal infiltrative disorders such as metastasis; should not be the initial procedure in the Dx of cholestasis.

> For a more detailed discussion, see Pratt DS, Kaplan MM: Jaundice, Chap. 43, p. 261; Ghany M, Hoofnagle JH: Approach to the Patient with Liver Disease, Chap 295, p. 1918, and Pratt DS, Kaplan MM: Evaluation of Liver Function, Chap. 296, p. 1923, in HPIM-17.

56 Ascites

DEFINITION

Accumulation of fluid within the peritoneal cavity. Small amounts may be asymptomatic; increasing amounts cause abdominal distention and discomfort, anorexia, nausea, early satiety, heartburn, flank pain, and respiratory distress.

DETECTION

Physical Examination Bulging flanks, fluid wave, shifting dullness, "puddle sign" (dullness over dependent abdomen with pt on hands and knees). May be associated with penile or scrotal edema, umbilical or inguinal herniation, pleural effusion. Evaluation should include rectal and pelvic examination, assessment of liver and spleen. Palmar erythema and spider angiomata seen in cirrhosis. Periumbilical nodule (*Sister Mary Joseph's nodule*) suggests metastatic disease from a pelvic or GI tumor.

Ultrasonography/CT Very sensitive; able to distinguish fluid from cystic masses.

EVALUATION

Diagnostic paracentesis (50–100 mL) essential. Routine evaluation includes gross inspection, protein, albumin, glucose, cell count and differential, Gram's and acid-fast stains, culture, cytology; in selected cases check amylase, LDH, triglycerides, culture for tuberculosis (TB). Rarely, laparoscopy or even exploratory laparotomy may be required. Ascites due to CHF (e.g., pericardial constriction) may require evaluation by right-sided heart catheterization.

Differential Diagnosis More than 90% of cases due to cirrhosis, neoplasm, CHF, TB.

Diseases of peritoneum: Infections (bacterial, tuberculous, fungal, parasitic), neoplasms, connective tissue disease, miscellaneous (Whipple's disease, familial Mediterranean fever, endometriosis, starch peritonitis, etc.).

Diseases not involving peritoneum: Cirrhosis, CHF, Budd-Chiari syndrome, hepatic venoocclusive disease, hypoalbuminemia (nephrotic syndrome, protein-losing enteropathy, malnutrition), miscellaneous (myxedema, ovarian diseases, pancreatic disease, chylous ascites).

Pathophysiologic Classification Using Serum-Ascites Albumin Gradient   Difference in albumin concentrations between serum and ascites as a reflection of imbalances in hydrostatic pressures:

1. *Low gradient* (serum-ascites albumin gradient < 1.1): 2° bacterial peritonitis, neoplasm, pancreatitis, vasculitis, nephrotic syndrome.
2. *High gradient* (serum-ascites albumin gradient > 1.1 suggests ascites is due to portal hypertension): cirrhosis, CHF, Budd-Chiari syndrome.

Representative Fluid Characteristics   See Table 56-1.

CIRRHOTIC ASCITES

Pathogenesis   Contributing factors: (1) portal hypertension, (2) hypoalbuminemia, (3) hepatic lymph, (4) renal sodium retention–secondary to hyperaldosteronism, increased sympathetic nervous system activity (renin-angiotensin production). Initiating event may be peripheral arterial vasodilation triggered by endotoxin and cytokines and mediated by nitric oxide.

R̲x̲ Cirrhotic Ascites

Maximum mobilization ~700 mL/d (peripheral edema may be mobilized faster).

1. Rigid salt restriction (<2 g Na/d).
2. For moderate ascites, diuretics usually necessary; spironolactone 100–200 mg/d PO (can be increased to 400–600 mg/d if low-sodium diet is confirmed and fluid not mobilized); furosemide 40–80 mg/d PO or IV may be added if necessary (greater risk of hepatorenal syndrome, encephalopathy), can increase to maximum of 120–160 mg/d until effect achieved or complication occurs.
3. Monitor weight, urinary Na and K, serum electrolytes, and creatinine.

If ascites is still present with the above measures this is defined as *refractory ascites*. Treatment modalities include:

1. Repeated large-volume paracentesis (5 L) with IV infusions of albumin (10 g/L ascites removed).
2. Consider transjugular intrahepatic portosystemic shunt (TIPS). While TIPS manages the ascites, it has not been found to improve survival and is often associated with encephalopathy.

Prognosis for pts with cirrhotic ascites is poor with <50% survival 2 years after onset of ascites. Consider liver transplantation in appropriate candidates with the onset of ascites (Chap. 163).

COMPLICATIONS

Spontaneous Bacterial Peritonitis   Suspect in cirrhotic pt with ascites and fever, abdominal pain, worsening ascites, ileus, hypotension, worsening jaundice, or encephalopathy; low ascitic protein concentration (low opsonic activity) is predisposing factor. Diagnosis suggested by ascitic fluid PMN cell count >250/µL; confirmed by positive culture (usually *Escherichia coli* and other gut bacte-

TABLE 56-1 CHARACTERISTICS OF ASCITIC FLUID IN VARIOUS DISEASE STATES

Condition	Gross Appearance	Protein, g/L	Serum-Ascites Albumin Gradient, g/dL	Red Blood Cells, >10,000/μL	White Blood Cells, per μL	Other Tests
Cirrhosis	Straw-colored or bile-stained	<25 (95%)	>1.1	1%	<250 (90%)[a]; predominantly mesothelial	
Neoplasm	Straw-colored, hemorrhagic, mucinous, or chylous	>25 (75%)	<1.1	20%	>1000 (50%); variable cell types	Cytology, cell block, peritoneal biopsy
Tuberculous peritonitis	Clear, turbid, hemorrhagic, chylous	>25 (50%)	<1.1	7%	>1000 (70%); usually >70% lymphocytes	Peritoneal biopsy, stain and culture for acid-fast bacilli
Pyogenic peritonitis	Turbid or purulent	If purulent, >25	<1.1	Unusual	Predominantly polymorphonuclear leukocytes	Positive Gram's stain, culture
Congestive heart failure	Straw-colored	Variable, 15–53	>1.1	10%	<1000 (90%); usually mesothelial, mononuclear	
Nephrosis	Straw-colored or chylous	<25 (100%)	<1.1	Unusual	<250; mesothelial, mononuclear	If chylous, ether extraction, Sudan staining
Pancreatic ascites (pancreatitis, pseudocyst)	Turbid, hemorrhagic, or chylous	Variable, often >25	<1.1	Variable, may be blood-stained	Variable	Increased amylase in ascitic fluid and serum

[a]Because the conditions of examining fluid and selecting patients were not identical in each series, the percentage figures (in parentheses) should be taken as an indication of the order of magnitude rather than as the precise incidence of any abnormal finding.

ria; however, gram-positive bacteria including *Streptococcus viridans, Staphylococcus aureus,* and *Enterococcus* spp. can also be found). Initial treatment: Cefotaxime 2 g IV q8h. Risk is increased in pts with variceal bleeding and prophylaxis against spontaneous bacterial peritonitis is recommended when a pt presents with upper GI bleeding.

Hepatorenal Syndrome (HRS) Functional renal failure without renal pathology; occurs in 10% of pts with advanced cirrhosis or acute liver failure. Thought to result from altered renal hemodynamics. Two types: type 1 HRS–decrease in renal function within 1–2 weeks of presentation; type 2 HRS–associated with a rise in serum creatinine but is associated with a better outcome. Often seen in pts with refractory ascites. Treatment: midodrine along with octreotide and IV albumin. For either type 1 or 2 HRS, prognosis is poor in the absence of liver transplantation.

> For a more detailed discussion, see Glickman RM, Rajapaksa R: Abdominal Swelling and Ascites, Chap. 44, p. 266; and Bacon BR: Cirrhosis and Its Complications, Chap. 302, p. 1971, in HPIM-17.

57 Azotemia and Urinary Abnormalities

ABNORMALITIES OF RENAL FUNCTION, AZOTEMIA

Azotemia is the retention of nitrogenous waste products excreted by the kidney. Increased levels of blood urea nitrogen (BUN) [>10.7 mmol/L (>30 mg/dL)] and creatinine [>133 μmol/L (>1.5 mg/dL)] are ordinarily indicative of impaired renal function. Renal function can be estimated by determining the clearance of creatinine (CL_{cr}) (normal > 100 mL/min); this can be directly measured from a 24-h urine collection using the following equation:

$$\text{Creatinine Clearance (mL/min)} = (uCr \times uV)/(sCr \times 1440)$$

1. Where uCr is urine creatinine in mg/dL
2. Where sCr is serum creatinine in mg/dL
3. Where uV is 24-h urine volume in mL
4. Where 1440 represents number of minutes in 24 h

The "adequacy" or "completeness" of the collection is estimated by the urinary volume and creatinine content; creatinine is produced from muscle and excreted at a relatively constant rate. For a 20- to 50-year-old man, creatinine excretion should be 18.5–25.0 mg/kg body weight; for a woman of the same age, it should be 16.5–22.4 mg/kg body weight. For example, an 80-kg man should excrete between ~1500 and 2000 mg of creatinine in an "adequate" collection. Creatinine excretion is also influenced by age and muscle mass. Notably, creatinine is an imperfect measure of glomerular filtration rate (GFR), since it is both filtered by glomeruli and secreted by proximal tubular cells; the relative contribution of tubular secretion increases with advancing renal dys-

TABLE 57-1 **THE CLASSIFICATION OF CHRONIC KIDNEY DISEASE (NATIONAL KIDNEY FOUNDATION GUIDELINES)**

Kidney Damage Stage	Description	eGFR (mL/min per 1.73 m^2)
0	With risk factors for CKD[a]	>90
1	With evidence of kidney damage[b]	>90
2	Mild decrease in GFR	60–89
3	Moderate decrease in GFR	30–59
4	Severe decrease in GFR	15–29
5	Kidney failure	<15

[a]Diabetes, high blood pressure, family history, older age, African ancestry.
[b]Abnormal urinalysis, hematuria, proteinuria, albuminuria.
Note: eGFR, estimated glomerular filtration rate; CKD, chronic kidney disease; GFR, glomerular filtration rate.

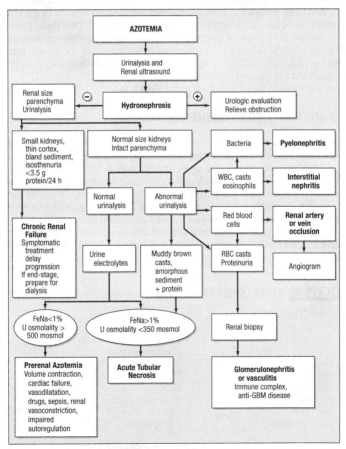

FIGURE 57-1 Approach to the patient with azotemia. WBC, white blood cell; RBC, red blood cell; GBM, glomerular basement membrane. *(From Denker BM, Brenner BM in HPIM-16.)*

function, such that creatinine clearance will provide an overestimate of the "true" GFR in pts with chronic kidney disease. Isotopic markers that are filtered and not secreted (e.g., iothalamate) provide more accurate estimates of GFR.

A formula that allows for an estimate of creatinine clearance in men that accounts for age-related decreases in GFR, body weight, and sex has been derived by Cockcroft-Gault:

$$\text{Creatinine clearance (mL/min)} = (140 - \text{age}) \times \text{lean body weight (kg)}/$$
$$\text{plasma creatinine (mg/dL)} \times 72$$

This value should be multiplied by 0.85 for women.

GFR may also be estimated using serum creatinine–based equations derived from the Modification of Diet in Renal Disease Study. This "eGFR" is now reported with serum creatinine by most clinical laboratories in the United States and is the basis for the National Kidney Foundation classification of chronic kidney disease (Table 57-1).

Manifestations of impaired renal function include volume overload, hypertension, electrolyte abnormalities (e.g., hyperkalemia, hypocalcemia, hyperphosphatemia), metabolic acidosis, and hormonal disturbances (e.g., insulin resistance, functional vitamin D deficiency, secondary hyperparathyroidism). When severe, the symptom complex of "uremia" may develop, encompassing one or more of the following symptoms and signs: anorexia, dysgeusia, nausea, vomiting, lethargy, confusion, asterixis, pleuritis, pericarditis, enteritis, pruritus, sleep and taste disturbance, nitrogenous fetor.

An approach to the pt with azotemia is shown in Fig. 57-1.

ABNORMALITIES OF URINE VOLUME

Oliguria   This refers to reduced urine output, usually defined as <400 mL/d. *Oligoanuria* refers to a more marked reduction in urine output, i.e., <100 mL/d. *Anuria* indicates the complete absence of urine output. Oliguria most often occurs in the setting of volume depletion and/or renal hypoperfusion, resulting in "prerenal azotemia" and acute renal failure (Chap. 146). Anuria can be caused by complete bilateral urinary tract obstruction; a vascular catastrophe (dissection or arterial occlusion); renal vein thrombosis; renal cortical necrosis; severe acute tubular necrosis; nonsteroidal anti-inflammatory drugs, angiotensin-converting enzyme (ACE) inhibitors, and/or angiotensin receptor blockers; and hypovolemic, cardiogenic, or septic shock. Oliguria is never normal, since at least

TABLE 57-2 MAJOR CAUSES OF POLYURIA	
Excessive fluid intake	Nephrogenic diabetes insipidus
Primary polydipsia	Lithium exposure
Iatrogenic (IV fluids)	Urinary tract obstruction
Therapeutic	Papillary necrosis
Diuretic agents	Reflux nephropathy
Osmotic diuresis	Interstitial nephritis
Hyperglycemia	Hypercalcemia
Azotemia	Central diabetes insipidus
Mannitol	Tumor
Radiocontrast	Postoperative
	Head trauma
	Basilar meningitis
	Neurosarcoidosis

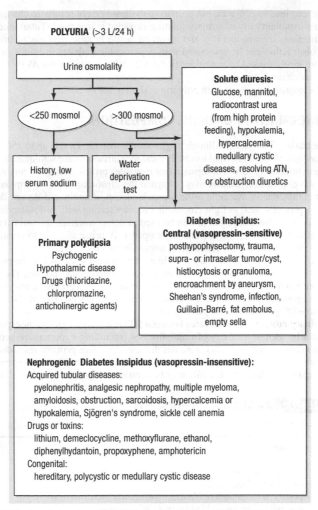

FIGURE 57-2 Approach to the patient with polyuria. OSM, osmolality; ATN, acute tubular necrosis. *(From Denker BM, Brenner BM in HPIM-16.)*

400 mL of maximally concentrated urine must be produced to excrete the obligate daily osmolar load.

Polyuria Polyuria is defined as a urine output >3 L/d. It is often accompanied by nocturia and urinary frequency and must be differentiated from other more common conditions associated with lower urinary tract pathology and urinary urgency or frequency (e.g., cystitis, prostatism). It is often accompanied by hypernatremia (Chap. 2). Polyuria (Table 57-2) can occur as a response to a solute load (e.g., hyperglycemia) or to an abnormality in arginine vasopressin [AVP; also known as antidiuretic hormone (ADH)] action. Diabetes insipidus is termed *central* if due to the insufficient hypothalamic production of AVP and *nephrogenic* if the result of renal insensitivity to the action of AVP. Excess fluid intake can lead to polyuria, but primary polydipsia rarely results in changes in plasma osmolality unless urinary diluting capacity is impaired. Tubulointerstitial diseases, lithium therapy, and resolving acute tubular necrosis or urinary tract obstruction can be associated with nephrogenic diabetes insipidus, which is more rarely caused by mutations in the V2 AVP receptor or the AVP-regulated water channel, aquaporin 2.

The approach to the pt with polyuria is shown in Fig. 57-2.

ABNORMALITIES OF URINE COMPOSITION

Proteinuria   This is the hallmark of glomerular disease. Levels up to 150 mg/d are considered within normal limits. Typical measurements are semiquantitative, using a moderately sensitive dipstick that estimates protein concentration; therefore, the degree of hydration may influence the dipstick protein determination. Most commercially available urine dipsticks detect albumin and do not detect smaller proteins, such as light chains, that require testing with sulfosalicylic acid. More sensitive assays can in turn be used to detect microalbuminuria, an important screening tool for diabetic nephropathy. A urine albumin to creatinine ratio >30 mg/g defines the presence of microalbuminuria.

Formal assessment of urinary protein excretion requires a 24-h urine protein collection (see "Abnormalities of Renal Function, Azotemia," above). The ratio of protein to creatinine in a random, "spot" urine can also provide a rough estimate of protein excretion; for example, a protein/creatinine ratio of 3.0 correlates to ~3.0 g of proteinuria per day.

Urinary protein excretion rates between 500 mg/d and 3 g/d are nonspecific and can be seen in a variety of renal diseases (including hypertensive nephrosclerosis, interstitial nephritis, vascular disease, and other primary renal diseases with little or no glomerular involvement). Transient, lesser degrees of proteinuria (500 mg/d to 1.5 g/d) may be seen after vigorous exercise, changes

TABLE 57-3   MAJOR CAUSES OF HEMATURIA

Lower Urinary Tract

Bacterial cystitis
Interstitial cystitis
Urethritis (infectious or inflammatory)
Passed or passing kidney stone
Transitional cell carcinoma of bladder or structures proximal to it
Squamous cell carcinoma of bladder (e.g., following schistosomiasis)

Upper Urinary Tract

Renal cell carcinoma
Age-related renal cysts
Other neoplasms (e.g., oncocytoma, hamartoma)
Acquired renal cystic disease
Congenital cystic disease, including autosomal dominant form
Glomerular diseases
Interstitial renal diseases, including interstitial nephritis
Nephrolithiasis
Pyelonephritis
Renal infarction
Hypercalciuria
Hyperuricosuria

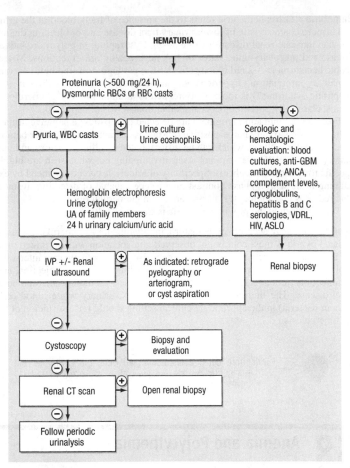

FIGURE 57-3 Approach to the patient with hematuria. RBC, red blood cell; WBC, white blood cell; GBM, glomerular basement membrane; ANCA, antineutrophil cytoplasmic antibody; VDRL, venereal disease research laboratory; ASLO, antistreptolysin O; UA, urinalysis; IVP, intravenous pyelography; CT, computed tomography.

in body position, fever, or congestive heart failure. Protein excretion rates >3 g/d are termed *nephrotic range proteinuria* in that they may be accompanied by hypoalbuminemia, hypercholesterolemia, and edema (the nephrotic syndrome). Nephrotic syndrome can be associated with a variety of extrarenal complications (Chap. 150). Massive degrees of proteinuria (>10 g/d) can be seen with minimal change disease, primary focal segmental sclerosis (FSGS), membranous nephropathy, collapsing glomerulopathy (a subtype of primary FSGS), and HIV-associated nephropathy.

Pharmacologic inhibition of ACE or blockade of angiotensin II should be employed to reduce proteinuria; successful reduction of proteinuria decreases the rate of progression to end-stage renal disease in diabetic nephropathy and other glomerulopathies. Specific therapy for a variety of causes of nephrotic syndrome is discussed in Chap. 150.

Hematuria   Gross hematuria refers to the presence of frank blood in the urine and is more characteristic of lower urinary tract disease and/or bleeding diatheses than intrinsic renal disease (Table 57-3). Cyst rupture in polycystic kidney disease and postpharyngitic flares of IgA nephropathy are exceptions. Microscopic hematuria [>1–2 red blood cells (RBCs) per high-powered field] accompanied by proteinuria, hypertension, and an active urinary sediment (the "nephritic syndrome") is most likely related to an inflammatory glomerulonephritis, classically poststreptococcal glomerulonephritis (Chap. 150).

Free hemoglobin and myoglobin are detected by dipstick; a negative urinary sediment with strongly heme-positive dipstick is characteristic of either hemolysis or rhabdomyolysis, which can be differentiated by clinical history and laboratory testing. RBC casts are not a sensitive finding but when seen are highly specific for glomerulonephritis. Specificity of urinalysis can be enhanced by examining urine with a phase contrast microscope capable of detecting dysmorphic red cells ("acanthocytes") associated with glomerular disease.

The approach to the pt with hematuria is shown in Fig. 57-3.

Pyuria   This may accompany hematuria in inflammatory glomerular diseases. Isolated pyuria is most commonly observed in association with an infection of the upper or lower urinary tract. Pyuria may also occur with allergic interstitial nephritis (often with a preponderance of eosinophils), transplant rejection, and noninfectious, nonallergic tubulointerstitial diseases, including atheroembolic renal disease. The finding of "sterile" pyuria (i.e., urinary white blood cells without bacteria) in the appropriate clinical setting should raise suspicion of renal tuberculosis.

For a more detailed discussion, see Denker BM, Brenner BM: Azotemia and Urinary Abnormalities, Chap. 45, p. 268, in HPIM-17.

58   Anemia and Polycythemia

ANEMIA

According to World Health Organization criteria, anemia is defined as blood hemoglobin (Hb) concentration < 130 g/L (<13 g/dL) or hematocrit (Hct) < 39% in adult males; Hb < 120 g/L (<12 g/dL) or Hct < 37% in adult females.

Signs and symptoms of anemia are varied, depending on the level of anemia and the time course over which it developed. Acute anemia is nearly always due to blood loss or hemolysis. In acute blood loss, hypovolemia dominates the clinical picture; hypotension and decreased organ perfusion are the main issues. Symptoms associated with more chronic onset vary with the age of the pt and the adequacy of blood supply to critical organs. Moderate anemia is associated with fatigue, loss of stamina, breathlessness, and tachycardia. The pt's skin and mucous membranes may appear pale. If the palmar creases are lighter in color than the surrounding skin with the fingers extended, Hb level is often <80 g/L (8 g/dL). In pts with coronary artery disease, anginal episodes may appear or increase in frequency and severity. In pts with carotid artery disease, lightheadedness or dizziness may develop.

A physiologic approach to anemia diagnosis is based on the understanding that a decrease in circulating red blood cells (RBCs) can be related to either inadequate production of RBCs or increased RBC destruction or loss. Within the category of inadequate production, erythropoiesis can be either ineffective, due to an erythrocyte maturation defect (which usually results in RBCs that are too small or too large), or hypoproliferative (which usually results in RBCs of normal size, but too few of them).

Basic evaluations include (1) reticulocyte index (RI), and (2) review of blood smear and RBC indices [chiefly mean corpuscular volume (MCV)] (Fig. 58-1).

The RI is a measure of RBC production. The reticulocyte count is corrected for the Hct level and for early release of marrow reticulocytes into the circulation, which leads to an increase in the lifespan of the circulating reticulocyte beyond the usual 1 day. Thus, RI = (% reticulocytes × pt Hct/45%) × (1/shift correction factor). The shift correction factor varies with the Hct: 1.5 for Hct = 35%, 2 for Hct = 25%, 2.5 for Hct = 15%. RI < 2–2.5% implies inadequate RBC production for the particular level of anemia; RI > 2.5% implies excessive RBC destruction or loss.

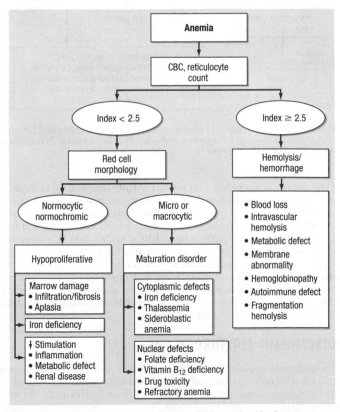

FIGURE 58-1 The physiologic classification of anemia. CBC, complete blood count.

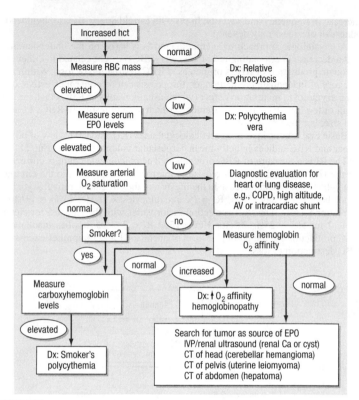

FIGURE 58-2 An approach to diagnosing pts with polycythemia. RBC, red blood cell; EPO, erythropoietin; COPD, chronic obstructive pulmonary disease; AV, atrioventricular; IVP, intravenous pyelogram; CT, computed tomography.

If the anemia is associated with a low RI, RBC morphology helps distinguish a maturation disorder from hypoproliferative marrow states. Cytoplasmic maturation defects such as iron deficiency or Hb synthesis problems produce smaller RBCs, MCV < 80; nuclear maturation defects such as B_{12} and folate deficiency and drug effects produce larger RBCs, MCV > 100. In hypoproliferative marrow states, RBCs are generally normal in morphology but too few are produced. Bone marrow examination is often helpful in the evaluation of anemia but is done most frequently to diagnose hypoproliferative marrow states.

Other laboratory tests indicated to evaluate particular forms of anemia depend on the initial classification based on the pathophysiology of the defect. These are discussed in more detail in Chap. 66.

POLYCYTHEMIA (ERYTHROCYTOSIS)

This is an increase above the normal range of RBCs in the circulation. Concern that the Hb level may be abnormally high should be triggered at a level of 170 g/L (17 g/dL) in men and 150 g/L (15 g/dL) in women. Polycythemia is usually found incidentally at routine blood count. Relative erythrocytosis, due to plasma volume loss (e.g., severe dehydration, burns), does not represent a true increase in total RBC mass. Absolute erythrocytosis is a true increase in total RBC mass.

Causes Polycythemia vera (a clonal myeloproliferative disorder), erythropoietin-producing neoplasms (e.g., renal cancer, cerebellar hemangioma), chronic hypoxemia (e.g., high altitude, pulmonary disease), carboxyhemoglobin excess (e.g., smokers), high-affinity hemoglobin variants, Cushing's syndrome, androgen excess. Polycythemia vera is distinguished from secondary polycythemia by the presence of splenomegaly, leukocytosis, thrombocytosis, and elevated vitamin B_{12} levels, and by decreased erythropoietin levels. An approach to evaluate polycythemic pts is shown in Fig. 58-2.

Complications Hyperviscosity (with diminished O_2 delivery) with risk of ischemic organ injury and thrombosis (venous or arterial) are most common.

℞ Polycythemia

Phlebotomy recommended for Hct $\geq 55\%$, regardless of cause, to low-normal range.

For a more detailed discussion, see Adamson JW, Longo DL: Anemia and Polycythemia, Chap. 58, p. 355, in HPIM-17.

59 Lymphadenopathy and Splenomegaly

LYMPHADENOPATHY

Exposure to antigen through a break in the skin or mucosa results in antigen being taken up by an antigen-presenting cell and carried via lymphatic channels to the nearest lymph node. Lymph channels course throughout the body except for the brain and the bones. Lymph enters the node through the afferent vessel and leaves through an efferent vessel. As antigen-presenting cells pass through lymph nodes, they present antigen to lymphocytes residing there. Lymphocytes in a node are constantly being replaced by antigen-naïve lymphocytes from the blood. They are retained in the node via special homing receptors. B cells populate the lymphoid follicles in the cortex; T cells populate the paracortical regions. When a B cell encounters an antigen to which its surface immunoglobulin can bind, it stays in the follicle for a few days and forms a germinal center where the immunoglobulin gene is mutated in an effort to make an antibody with higher affinity for the antigen. The B cell then migrates to the medullary region, differentiates into a plasma cell, and secretes immunoglobulin into the efferent lymph.

When a T cell in the node encounters an antigen it recognizes, it proliferates and joins the efferent lymph. The efferent lymph laden with antibodies and T cells specific for the inciting antigen passes through several nodes on its way to the thoracic duct, which drains lymph from most of the body. From the thoracic duct, lymph enters the bloodstream at the left subclavian vein. Lymph from the head and neck and the right arm drain into the right subclavian vein. From the bloodstream, the antibody and T cells localize to the site of infection.

Lymphadenopathy may be caused by infections, immunologic diseases, malignancies, lipid storage diseases, or a number of disorders of uncertain etiology (e.g., sarcoidosis, Castleman's disease; Table 59-1). The two major mechanisms of lymphadenopathy are *hyperplasia*, in response to immunologic or in-

---

TABLE 59-1 DISEASES ASSOCIATED WITH LYMPHADENOPATHY

1. Infectious diseases
   a. Viral—infectious mononucleosis syndromes (EBV, CMV), infectious hepatitis, herpes simplex, herpesvirus 6, varicella-zoster virus, rubella, measles, adenovirus, HIV, epidemic keratoconjunctivitis, vaccinia, herpesvirus 8
   b. Bacterial—streptococci, staphylococci, cat-scratch disease, brucellosis, tularemia, plague, chancroid, melioidosis, glanders, tuberculosis, atypical mycobacterial infection, primary and secondary syphilis, diphtheria, leprosy
   c. Fungal—histoplasmosis, coccidioidomycosis, paracoccidioidomycosis
   d. Chlamydial—lymphogranuloma venereum, trachoma
   e. Parasitic—toxoplasmosis, leishmaniasis, trypanosomiasis, filariasis
   f. Rickettsial—scrub typhus, rickettsialpox
2. Immunologic diseases
   a. Rheumatoid arthritis
   b. Juvenile rheumatoid arthritis
   c. Mixed connective tissue disease
   d. Systemic lupus erythematosus
   e. Dermatomyositis
   f. Sjögren's syndrome
   g. Serum sickness
   h. Drug hypersensitivity—diphenylhydantoin, hydralazine, allopurinol, primidone, gold, carbamazepine, etc.
   i. Angioimmunoblastic lymphadenopathy
   j. Primary biliary cirrhosis
   k. Graft-versus-host disease
   l. Silicone-associated
3. Malignant diseases
   a. Hematologic—Hodgkin's disease, non-Hodgkin's lymphomas, acute or chronic lymphocytic leukemia, hairy cell leukemia, malignant histiocytosis, amyloidosis
   b. Metastatic—from numerous primary sites
4. Lipid storage diseases—Gaucher's, Niemann-Pick, Fabry, Tangier
5. Endocrine diseases—hyperthyroidism
6. Other disorders
   a. Castleman's disease (giant lymph node hyperplasia)
   b. Sarcoidosis
   c. Dermatopathic lymphadenitis
   d. Lymphomatoid granulomatosis
   e. Histiocytic necrotizing lymphadenitis (Kikuchi's disease)
   f. Sinus histiocytosis with massive lymphadenopathy (Rosai-Dorfman disease)
   g. Mucocutaneous lymph node syndrome (Kawasaki's disease)
   h. Histiocytosis X
   i. Familial Mediterranean fever
   j. Severe hypertriglyceridemia
   k. Vascular transformation of sinuses
   l. Inflammatory pseudotumor of lymph node

Note: EBV, Epstein-Barr virus; CMV, cytomegalovirus.

fectious stimuli, and *infiltration*, by cancer cells or lipid- or glycoprotein-laden macrophages.

APPROACH TO THE PATIENT: LYMPHADENOPATHY

HISTORY

Age, occupation, animal exposures, sexual orientation, substance abuse history, medication history, and concomitant symptoms influence diagnostic workup. Adenopathy is more commonly malignant in origin in those over age 40. Farmers have an increased incidence of brucellosis and lymphoma. Male homosexuals may have AIDS-associated adenopathy. Alcohol and tobacco abuse increase risk of malignancy. Phenytoin may induce adenopathy. The concomitant presence of cervical adenopathy with sore throat or with fever, night sweats, and weight loss suggests particular diagnoses (mononucleosis in the former instance, Hodgkin's disease in the latter).

PHYSICAL EXAMINATION

Location of adenopathy, size, node texture, and the presence of tenderness are important in differential diagnosis. Generalized adenopathy (three or more anatomic regions) implies systemic infection or lymphoma. Subclavian or scalene adenopathy is always abnormal and should be biopsied. Nodes > 4 cm should be biopsied immediately. Rock-hard nodes fixed to surrounding soft tissue are usually a sign of metastatic carcinoma. Tender nodes are most often benign.

LABORATORY TESTS

Usually lab tests are not required in the setting of localized adenopathy. If generalized adenopathy is noted, an excisional node biopsy should be performed for diagnosis, rather than a panoply of laboratory tests.

℞ Lymphadenopathy

Pts over age 40, those with scalene or supraclavicular adenopathy, those with lymph nodes > 4 cm in diameter, and those with hard nontender nodes should undergo immediate excisional biopsy. In younger pts with smaller nodes that are rubbery in consistency or tender, a period of observation for 7–14 days is reasonable. Empirical antibiotics are not indicated. If the nodes shrink, no further evaluation is necessary. If they enlarge, excisional biopsy is indicated.

SPLENOMEGALY

Just as the lymph nodes are specialized to fight pathogens in the tissues, the spleen is the lymphoid organ specialized to fight bloodborne pathogens. It has no afferent lymphatics. The spleen has specialized areas like the lymph node for making antibodies (follicles) and amplifying antigen-specific T cells (periarteriolar lymphatic sheath, or PALS). In addition, it has a well-developed reticuloendothelial system for removing particles and antibody-coated bacteria. The flow of blood through the spleen permits it to filter pathogens from the blood and to maintain quality control over erythrocytes (RBCs)—those that are old and nondeformable are destroyed, and intracellular inclusions (sometimes including pathogens such as *Babesia* and *Plasmodium* are culled from the cells in

TABLE 59-2 DISEASES ASSOCIATED WITH SPLENOMEGALY GROUPED BY PATHOGENIC MECHANISM

Enlargement Due to Increased Demand for Splenic Function

Reticuloendothelial system hyperplasia (for removal of defective erythrocytes)
    Spherocytosis
    Early sickle cell anemia
    Ovalocytosis
    Thalassemia major
    Hemoglobinopathies
    Paroxysmal nocturnal hemoglobinuria
    Nutritional anemias
Immune hyperplasia
Response to infection (viral, bacterial, fungal, parasitic)
    Infectious mononucleosis
    AIDS
    Viral hepatitis
    Cytomegalovirus
    Subacute bacterial endocarditis
    Bacterial septicemia
    Congenital syphilis
    Splenic abscess
    Tuberculosis
    Histoplasmosis
    Malaria
    Leishmaniasis
    Trypanosomiasis
    Ehrlichiosis
Disordered immunoregulation
    Rheumatoid arthritis (Felty's syndrome)
    Systemic lupus erythematosus
    Collagen vascular diseases
    Serum sickness
    Immune hemolytic anemias
    Immune thrombocytopenias
    Immune neutropenias
    Drug reactions
    Angioimmunoblastic lymphadenopathy
    Sarcoidosis
    Thyrotoxicosis (benign lymphoid hypertrophy)
    Interleukin 2 therapy
Extramedullary hematopoiesis
    Myelofibrosis
    Marrow damage by toxins, radiation, strontium
    Marrow infiltration by tumors, leukemias, Gaucher's disease

Enlargement Due to Abnormal Splenic or Portal Blood Flow

Cirrhosis
Hepatic vein obstruction
Portal vein obstruction, intrahepatic or extrahepatic
Cavernous transformation of the portal vein
Splenic vein obstruction
Splenic artery aneurysm
Hepatic schistosomiasis

(continued)

TABLE 59-2	DISEASES ASSOCIATED WITH SPLENOMEGALY GROUPED BY PATHOGENIC MECHANISM (CONTINUED)

Congestive heart failure
Hepatic echinococcosis
Portal hypertension (any cause including the above): "Banti's disease"

Infiltration of the Spleen

Intracellular or extracellular depositions
　　Amyloidosis
　　Gaucher's disease
　　Niemann-Pick disease
　　Tangier disease
　　Hurler's syndrome and other mucopolysaccharidoses
　　Hyperlipidemias
Benign and malignant cellular infiltrations
　　Leukemias (acute, chronic, lymphoid, myeloid, monocytic)
　　Lymphomas
　　Hodgkin's disease
　　Myeloproliferative syndromes (e.g., polycythemia vera)
　　Angiosarcomas
　　Metastatic tumors (melanoma is most common)
　　Eosinophilic granuloma
　　Histiocytosis X
　　Hamartomas
　　Hemangiomas, fibromas, lymphangiomas
　　Splenic cysts

Unknown Etiology

Idiopathic splenomegaly
Berylliosis
Iron-deficiency anemia

a process called *pitting*. Under certain conditions, the spleen can generate hematopoietic cells in place of the marrow.

The normal spleen is about 12 cm in length and 7 cm in width and is not normally palpable. Dullness from the spleen can be percussed between the ninth and eleventh ribs with the pt lying on the right side. Palpation is best performed with the pt supine with knees flexed. The spleen may be felt as it descends when the pt inspires. Physical diagnosis is not sensitive. CT or ultrasound are superior tests.

Spleen enlargement occurs by three basic mechanisms: (1) hyperplasia or hypertrophy due to an increase in demand for splenic function (e.g., hereditary spherocytosis where demand for removal of defective RBCs is high or immune hyperplasia in response to systemic infection or immune diseases); (2) passive vascular congestion due to portal hypertension; and (3) infiltration with malignant cells, lipid- or glycoprotein-laden macrophages, or amyloid (Table 59-2). Massive enlargement, with spleen palpable >8 cm below the left costal margin, usually signifies a lymphoproliferative or myeloproliferative disorder.

Peripheral blood RBC count, white blood cell count, and platelet count may be normal, decreased, or increased depending on the underlying disorder. Decreases in one or more cell lineages could indicate hypersplenism, increased destruction. In cases with hypersplenism, the spleen is removed and the cytopenia is generally reversed. In the absence of hypersplenism, most causes of splenomegaly are diagnosed on the basis of signs and symptoms and laboratory abnormalities associated with the underlying disorder. Splenectomy is rarely performed for diagnostic purposes.

Individuals who have had splenectomy are at increased risk of sepsis from a variety of organisms including pneumococcus and *Haemophilus influenzae*. Vaccines for these agents should be given before splenectomy is performed. Splenectomy compromises the immune response to these T-independent antigens.

For a more detailed discussion, see Henry PH, Longo DL: Enlargement of Lymph Nodes and Spleen, Chap. 60, p. 370, in HPIM-17.

60 Generalized Fatigue

Fatigue is one of the most common complaints related by pts. It usually refers to nonspecific sense of a low energy level, or the feeling that near exhaustion is reached after relatively little exertion. Fatigue should be distinguished from true neurologic *weakness*, which describes a reduction in the normal power of one or more muscles (Chap. 42). It is not uncommon for pts, especially the elderly, to present with generalized failure to thrive, which may include components of fatigue and weakness, depending on the cause.

CLINICAL MANIFESTATIONS

Because the causes of generalized fatigue are numerous, a thorough history, review of systems (ROS), and physical examination are paramount to narrow the focus to likely causes. The history and ROS should focus on the temporal onset of fatigue and its progression. Has it lasted days, weeks, or months? Activities of daily living, exercise, sexual practices, and sleep habits should be reviewed. Features of depression or dementia should be sought. Travel history and possible exposures to infectious agents should be reviewed, along with the medication list. The ROS may elicit important clues as to organ system involvement. The past medical history may elucidate potential precursors to the current presentation, such as previous malignancy or cardiac problems. The physical exam should specifically assess lymphadenopathy, hepatosplenomegaly, abdominal masses, pallor, rash, heart failure, new murmurs, painful joints or trigger points, and evidence of weakness or neurologic abnormalities. A finding of true weakness or paralysis should prompt consideration of neurologic disorders (Chap. 42).

DIFFERENTIAL DIAGNOSIS

Determining the cause of fatigue can be one of the most challenging diagnostic problems in medicine because the differential diagnosis is very broad, including infection, malignancy, cardiac disease, endocrine disorders, neurologic disease, or serious abnormalities of virtually any organ system, as well as side effects of many medications (Table 60-1). Symptoms of fever and weight loss will focus attention on infectious causes, whereas symptoms of progressive

TABLE 60-1	POTENTIAL CAUSES OF GENERALIZED FATIGUE
Disease Category	Examples
Infection	HIV, TB, Lyme disease, endocarditis, hepatitis, sinusitis, fungal, Epstein-Barr virus (EBV), malaria
Inflammatory disease	RA, polymyalgia rheumatica, chronic fatigue syndrome, fibromyalgia, sarcoidosis
Cancer	Lung, GI, breast, prostate, leukemia, lymphoma, metastases
Psychiatric	Depression, alcoholism, chronic anxiety
Metabolic	Hypothyroidism, hyperthyroidism, diabetes mellitus, Addison's disease, hyperparathyroidism, hypoparathyroidism, McArdle's disease
Electrolyte imbalance	Hypercalcemia, hypokalemia, hyponatremia, hypomagnesesmia,
Nutrition, vitamin deficiency	Starvation, iron deficiency, vitamin B_{12}, folic acid deficiency, vitamin C deficiency (scurvy), thiamine deficiency (beriberi)
Neurologic	Multiple sclerosis, myasthenia gravis, dementia
Cardiac	Heart failure, CAD, valvular disease, cardiomyopathy
Pulmonary	COPD, pulmonary hypertension, chronic pulmonary emboli, sarcoidosis
Sleep disturbances	Sleep apnea, insomnia, restless leg syndrome
Gastroinestinal	Celiac disease, Crohn's, ulcerative colitis, chronic hepatitis, cirrhosis
Hematologic	Anemia
Renal	Renal failure
Medication	Sedatives, antihistamines, narcotics, β blockers, and many other medications

dyspnea might point toward cardiac, pulmonary, or renal causes. A presentation that includes arthralgia suggests the possibility of a rheumatologic disorder. A previous malignancy, thought to be cured or in remission, may have recurred or metastasized widely. A previous history of valvular heart disease or cardiomyopathy may identify a condition that has decompensated. Treatment for Graves' disease may have resulted in hypothyroidism. Changes in medication should always be pursued, whether discontinued or recently started. Almost any new medication has the potential to cause fatigue. However, a temporal association with a new medication should not eliminate other causes, as many patients may have received new medications in an effort to address their complaints. The time course for presentation is also valuable. Indolent presentations over months to years are more likely to be associated with slowly progressive organ failure or endocrinopathies, whereas a more rapid course over weeks to months suggests infection or malignancy.

LABORATORY TESTING

Laboratory testing and imaging should be guided by the history and physical exam. However, a CBC with differential, electrolytes, BUN, creatinine, glucose, calcium, and LFTs are useful in most pts with undifferentiated fatigue, as these tests will rule out many causes and may provide clues to unsuspected disorders. Similarly, a CXR is useful to evaluate many possible disorders rapidly, including heart failure, pulmonary disease, or occult malignancy that may be detected in the lungs or bony structures. Subsequent testing should be based on the initial results and clinical assessment of the likely differential diagnoses. For example, a finding of anemia would dictate the need to assess whether it has features of iron deficiency or hemolysis, thereby narrowing potential causes. Hyponatremia might be caused by SIADH, hypothyroidism, adrenal insufficiency, or medications or by underlying cardiac, pulmonary, liver, or renal dysfunction. An elevated WBC count would raise the possibility of infection or malignancy. Thus, the approach is generally one of gathering information in a serial but cost-effective manner to narrow the differential diagnosis progressively.

℞ Generalized Fatigue

Treatment should be based on the diagnosis, if known. Many conditions, such as metabolic, nutritional, or endocrine disorders, can be corrected quickly by appropriate treatment of the underlying causes. Specific treatment can also be initiated for many infections, such as TB, sinusitis, or endocarditis. Pts with chronic conditions such as COPD, heart failure, renal failure, or liver disease may benefit from interventions that enhance organ function or correct associated metabolic problems, and it may be possible to gradually improve physical conditioning. In patients with cancer, fatigue may be caused by chemotherapy or radiation and may resolve with time; treatment of associated anemia, nutritional deficiency, hyponatremia, or hypercalcemia may increase energy levels. Treatment of depression or sleep disorders, whether a primary cause of fatigue or secondary to a medical disorder, may be beneficial. Withdrawal of medications that potentially contribute to fatigue should be considered, recognizing that other medications may need to be substituted for the underlying condition.

CHRONIC FATIGUE SYNDROME

Chronic fatigue syndrome (CFS) is characterized by debilitating fatigue and several associated physical, constitutional, and neuropsychological complaints. Pts are twice as likely to be women as men and are generally 25–45 years old. The CDC has developed diagnostic criteria for CFS based upon symptoms and the exclusion of other illnesses (Table 60-2). The cause is uncertain, although

TABLE 60-2   CDC[a] CRITERIA FOR DIAGNOSIS OF CHRONIC FATIGUE SYNDROME

A case of chronic fatigue syndrome is defined by the presence of:
1. Clinically evaluated, unexplained, persistent or relapsing fatigue that is of new or definite onset; is not the result of ongoing exertion; is not alleviated by rest; and results in substantial reduction of previous levels of occupational, educational, social, or personal activities; and
2. Four or more of the following symptoms that persist or recur during six or more consecutive months of illness and that do not predate the fatigue:
   • Self-reported impairment in short-term memory or concentration
   • Sore throat
   • Tender cervical or axillary nodes
   • Muscle pain
   • Multijoint pain without redness or swelling
   • Headaches of a new pattern or severity
   • Unrefreshing sleep
   • Postexertional malaise lasting ≥24 h

[a]CDC, U.S. Centers for Disease Control and Prevention.
Source: Adapted from K Fukuda et al: Ann Intern Med 121:953, 1994; with permission.

clinical manifestations often follow a viral illness. Many studies have attempted, without success, to link CFS to infection with EBV, a retrovirus, or an enterovirus. Depression is present in half to two-thirds of pts, and some experts believe that CFS is fundamentally a psychiatric disorder.

CFS remains a diagnosis of exclusion, and no laboratory test can establish the diagnosis or measure its severity. Fortunately, CFS does not appear to progress. On the contrary, many pts experience gradual improvement, and a minority recover fully.

NSAIDs alleviate headache, diffuse pain, and feverishness. Antihistamines or decongestants may be helpful for symptoms of rhinitis and sinusitis. Although the pt may be averse to psychiatric diagnoses, features of depression and anxiety may justify treatment. Nonsedating antidepressants improve mood and disordered sleep and may attenuate the fatigue.

For a more detailed discussion, see Aminoff MJ: Weakness and Paralysis, Chap. 23, p. 147; Czeisler CA, Winkelman JW, Richardson GS: Sleep Disorders, Chap. 28, p. 171; Reife CM: Weight Loss, Chap. 41, p. 255; Straus SE: Chronic Fatigue Syndrome, Chap. 384, p. 2703; Reus VJ: Mental Disorders, Chap. 386, p. 2710, in HPIM-17.

OPHTHALMOLOGY AND OTOLARYNGOLOGY

61 Common Disorders of Vision and Hearing

DISORDERS OF THE EYE

APPROACH TO THE PATIENT WITH EYE DISORDERS

The history and examination permit accurate diagnosis of most eye disorders, without need for laboratory or imaging studies. The essential ocular exam includes assessment of the visual acuity, pupil reactions, eye movements, eye alignment, visual fields, and intraocular pressure. The lids, conjunctiva, cornea, anterior chamber, iris, and lens are examined with a slit lamp. The fundus is viewed with an ophthalmoscope.

Acute visual loss or double vision in a pt with quiet, uninflamed eyes often signifies a serious ocular or neurologic disorder and should be managed emergently (Chap. 41). Ironically, the occurrence of a red eye, even if painful, has less dire implications as long as visual acuity is spared.

SPECIFIC DISORDERS

Red or Painful Eye   Common causes listed in Table 61-1.

Minor Trauma   This may result in corneal abrasion, subconjunctival hemorrhage, or foreign body. The integrity of the corneal epithelium is assessed by placing a drop of fluorescein in the eye and looking with a slit lamp (using cobalt-blue light) or a blue penlight. The conjunctival fornices should be searched carefully for foreign bodies by pulling the lower lid down and everting the upper lid.

TABLE 61-1	CAUSES OF A RED OR PAINFUL EYE
Blunt or penetrating trauma	Dacrocystitis
Chemical exposure	Episcleritis
Corneal abrasion	Scleritis
Foreign body	Anterior uveitis (iritis or iridocyclitis)
Contact lens (overuse or infection)	Endophthalmitis
Corneal exposure (5th, 7th nerve palsy, ectropion)	Acute angle-closure glaucoma
	Medicamentosus
Subconjunctival hemorrhage	Pinguecula
Blepharitis	Pterygium
Conjunctivitis (infectious or allergic)	Proptosis (retrobulbar mass, orbital cellulitis, Graves' ophthalmopathy, orbital pseudotumor, carotid-cavernous fistula)
Corneal ulcer	
Herpes keratitis	
Herpes zoster ophthalmicus	
Keratoconjunctivitis sicca (dry eye)	

Minor Trauma

Chemical splashes and foreign bodies are treated by copious saline irrigation. Corneal abrasions may require application of a topical antibiotic, a mydriatic agent (1% cyclopentolate), and an eye patch.

Infection Infection of the eyelids and conjunctiva (blepharoconjunctivitis) produces redness and irritation but should not cause visual loss or pain. Adenovirus is the most common viral cause of "pink eye." It produces a thin, watery discharge, whereas bacterial infection causes a more mucopurulent exudate. On slit-lamp exam one should confirm that the cornea is not affected, by observing that it remains clear and lustrous. Corneal infection (keratitis) is a more serious condition than blepharoconjunctivitis because it can cause scarring and permanent visual loss. Worldwide, the two leading causes of blindness from keratitis are trachoma from chlamydial infection and Vitamin A deficiency from malnutrition; in the United States, contact lenses play a major role. A dendritic pattern of corneal fluorescein staining is pathognomonic of herpes simplex keratitis but is seen in only a minority of cases.

 Infection

Strict handwashing and broad-spectrum topical antibiotics for blepharoconjunctivitis (sulfacetamide 10%, polymyxin-bacitracin-neomycin, or trimethoprim-polymyxin). Keratitis requires empirical antibiotics (usually topical and subconjunctival) pending culture results from corneal scrapings. Herpes keratitis is treated with topical antiviral agents, cycloplegics, and oral acyclovir.

Inflammation Eye inflammation, without infection, can produce episcleritis, scleritis, or uveitis (iritis or iridocyclitis). Most cases are idiopathic, but some occur in conjunction with autoimmune disease. There is no discharge. A ciliary flush results from injection of deep conjunctival and episcleral vessels near the corneal limbus. The diagnosis of uveitis hinges on the slit-lamp observation of inflammatory cells floating in the aqueous humor of the anterior chamber or deposited on the corneal endothelium (keratic precipitates).

 Inflammation

Mydriatic agents (to reduce pain and prevent the formation of synechiae), NSAIDs, and topical glucocorticoids. (Note: prolonged treatment with ocular glucocorticoids can cause cataract and glaucoma).

Acute Angle-Closure Glaucoma This is a rare but frequently misdiagnosed cause of a red, painful eye. Because the anterior chamber is shallow, aqueous outflow via the anterior chamber angle becomes blocked by the peripheral iris. Intraocular pressure rises abruptly, causing ocular pain, injection, corneal edema, obscurations, headache, nausea, and blurred vision. The key diagnostic step is measurement of the intraocular pressure during an attack.

Acute Angle-Closure Glaucoma

The acute attack is broken by constricting the pupil with a drop of pilocarpine and by lowering the intraocular pressure with acetazolamide (PO or IV), topi-

TABLE 61-2	**CAUSES OF CHRONIC, PROGRESSIVE VISUAL LOSS**
Cataract	Intraocular tumor
Glaucoma	Retinitis pigmentosa
Macular degeneration	Epiretinal membrane
Diabetic retinopathy	Macular hole
Optic nerve or optic chiasm tumor	

cal beta blockers, prostaglandin analogues, and α₂-adrenergic agonists. If these measures fail, laser therapy can be used to create a hole in the peripheral iris to relieve papillary block.

Chronic Visual Loss   Most common causes are listed in Table 61-2.
Cataract   A cloudy lens, due principally to aging. The formation of cataract occurs more rapidly in patients with a history of ocular trauma, uveitis, or diabetes mellitus. Radiation and glucocorticoid treatment can induce a cataract as a side effect. It is treated by surgical extraction and replacement with an artificial intraocular lens.

Glaucoma   An insidious optic neuropathy that leads to slowly progressive visual loss, usually associated with elevated intraocular pressure. Angle closure accounts for only a few cases; most pts have open angles and no identifiable cause for their pressure elevation. The diagnosis is made by documenting arcuate (nerve fiber bundle) scotomas on visual field exam, by observing "cupping" of the optic disc (Fig. 61-1), and measuring intraocular pressure.

℞ Glaucoma

Topical adrenergic agonists, cholinergic agonists, beta blockers, prostaglandin analogues, and oral carbonic anhydrase inhibitors (to lower intraocular pressure) are used for treatment. Laser treatment of the trabecular meshwork in the anterior chamber angle improves aqueous outflow from the eye. If medical and laser treatments fail, a surgical filter (trabeculectomy) or valve must be placed.

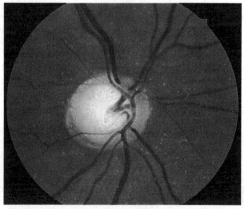

FIGURE 61-1 Glaucoma results in "cupping" as the neural rim is destroyed and the central cup becomes enlarged and excavated. The cup-to-disc ratio is about 0.7/1.0 in this patient. (*From JC Horton, in HPIM-17, p. 190.*)

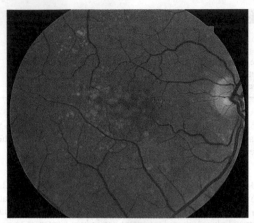

FIGURE 61-2 Age-related macular degeneration begins with the accumulation of drusen within the macula. They appear as scattered yellow subretinal deposits. (*From JC Horton, in HPIM-17, p. 190.*)

Macular Degeneration This occurs in both a "dry" and "wet" form. In the dry form, clumps of extracellular material, called *drusen*, are deposited beneath the retinal pigment epithelium (Fig. 61-2). As they accumulate, vision is slowly lost. In the wet form, neovascular proliferation occurs beneath the retinal pigment epithelium. Bleeding from these neovascular vessels can cause sudden, central visual loss in the elderly, although usually blurring of vision is more gradual. Macular exam shows drusen and subretinal hemorrhage.

 Macular Degeneration

Treatment with vitamins C and E, beta carotene, and zinc may retard dry macular degeneration. Wet macular degeneration can be treated with either photodynamic therapy or intraocular injection of vascular endothelial growth factor antagonists.

Diabetic Retinopathy A leading cause of blindness in the United States. Appears in most pts 10–15 years after onset of diabetes. Background diabetic retinopathy consists of intraretinal hemorrhage, exudates, nerve fiber layer infarcts (cotton-wool spots), and macular edema. Proliferative diabetic retinopathy is characterized by ingrowth of neovascular vessels on the retinal surface, causing blindness from vitreous hemorrhage, retinal detachment, and glaucoma (Fig. 61-3).

 Diabetic Retinopathy

All diabetics should be examined regularly by an ophthalmologist for surveillance of diabetic retinopathy. Macular edema is treated by focal or grid laser application. Neovascularization is treated by panretinal laser photocoagulation.

Tumors Tumors of the optic nerve or chiasm are comparatively rare but often escape detection because they produce insidious visual loss and few physical findings, except for optic disc pallor. Pituitary tumor is the most common lesion. It causes bitemporal or monocular visual loss. Melanoma is the most common primary tumor of the eye itself.

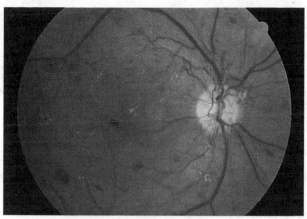

FIGURE 61-3 Diabetic retinopathy results in scattered hemorrhages, yellow exudates, and neovascularization. This patient has neovascular vessels proliferating from the optic disc, requiring urgent pan retinal laser photocoagulation. (*From AC Powers, in HPIM-17, p. 2287.*)

 Tumors

Large pituitary tumors producing chiasm compression are removed transphenoidally. In some cases, small tumors can be observed or controlled pharmacologically (e.g., bromocriptine for prolactinoma).

HEARING DISORDERS

Nearly 10% of the adult population has some hearing loss; up to one-third of individuals over the age of 65 have hearing loss of sufficient magnitude to require a hearing aid. Hearing loss can result from disorders of the auricle, external auditory canal, middle ear, inner ear, or central auditory pathways. *In general, lesions in the auricle, external auditory canal, or middle ear cause conductive hearing losses, while lesions in the inner ear or eighth nerve cause sensorineural hearing losses.*

APPROACH TO THE PATIENT WITH HEARING IMPAIRMENT

The goal is to determine (1) the nature of the hearing impairment (sensorineural vs. conductive vs. mixed), (2) the severity of the impairment, (3) the anatomy of the impairment, and (4) the etiology. Ascertain onset (sudden vs. insidious), progression (rapid vs. slow), and whether symptoms are unilateral or bilateral. Ask about tinnitus, vertigo, imbalance, aural fullness, otorrhea, headache, and facial or other cranial nerve symptoms. Prior head trauma, exposure to ototoxins, occupational or recreational noise exposure, or family history of hearing impairment also important.

Exam should include the auricle, external ear canal, and tympanic membrane. The external ear canal of the elderly is often dry and fragile; it is preferable to clean cerumen with wall-mounted suction and cerumen loops and to avoid irrigation. Inspect the nose, nasopharynx, cranial nerves, and upper respiratory tract. Unilateral serous effusion should prompt a fiberoptic exam of the nasopharynx to exclude neoplasm.

The Weber and Rinne tests differentiate conductive from sensorineural hearing losses. *Rinne test*: the tines of a vibrating tuning fork (512 Hz) are held near the opening of the external auditory canal, and then the stem is placed on the mastoid process. Normally, and with sensorineural hearing loss, air conduction is louder than bone conduction; however, with conductive hearing loss, bone conduction is louder. *Weber test*: the stem of a vibrating tuning fork is placed on the forehead in the midline. With a unilateral conductive hearing loss, the tone is perceived in the affected ear; with a unilateral sensorineural hearing loss, the tone is perceived in the unaffected ear.

LABORATORY EVALUATION

Audiologic Assessment   *Pure tone audiometry* assesses hearing acuity for pure tones. Speech recognition requires greater synchronous neural firing than necessary for appreciation of pure tones; clarity of hearing is tested in *speech audiometry*. *Tympanometry* measures impedance of middle ear to sound; useful in diagnosis of middle-ear effusions. *Otoacoustic emissions* (OAE), measured with microphones inserted in external auditory canal, indicate that outer hair cells of the organ of Corti are intact; useful to assess auditory thresholds and distinguish sensory from neural hearing loss. *Electrocochleography* measures earliest evoked potentials generated in cochlea and auditory nerve; useful in diagnosis of Ménière's disease. *Brainstem auditory evoked responses* (BAER) localize site of sensorineural hearing loss.

Imaging Studies   CT of temporal bone with fine 1-mm cuts can define the caliber of the external auditory canal, integrity of the ossicular chain, presence of middle ear or mastoid disease, inner-ear malformations, and bone erosion (chronic otitis media and cholesteatoma). MRI superior to CT for imaging of retrocochlear structures including cerebellopontine angle (vestibular schwannoma) and brainstem.

CAUSES OF HEARING LOSS   (Fig. 61-4)

Conductive Hearing Loss   May result from obstruction of the external auditory canal by cerumen, debris, and foreign bodies; swelling of the lining of the canal; atresia of the ear canal; neoplasms of the canal; perforations of the tympanic membrane; disruption of the ossicular chain, as occurs with necrosis of the long process of the incus in trauma or infection; otosclerosis; and fluid, scarring, or neoplasms in the middle ear. Hearing loss with otorrhea most likely due to otitis media or cholesteatoma.

Cholesteatoma, i.e., stratified squamous epithelium in the middle ear or mastoid, is a benign, slowly growing lesion that destroys bone and normal ear tissue. A chronically draining ear that fails to respond to appropriate antibiotic therapy suggests cholesteatoma; surgery is required.

Conductive hearing loss with a normal ear canal and intact tympanic membrane suggests ossicular pathology. Fixation of the stapes from *otosclerosis* is a common cause of low-frequency conductive hearing loss; onset is between the late teens to the forties. In women, the hearing loss is often first noticeable during pregnancy. A hearing aid or a surgical stapedectomy can provide auditory rehabilitation.

Eustachian tube dysfunction is common and may predispose to acute otitis media (AOM) or serous otitis media (SOM). Trauma, AOM, or chronic otitis media are the usual factors responsible for tympanic membrane perforation.

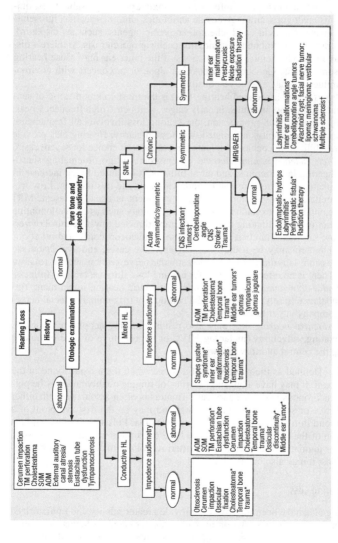

FIGURE 61-4 An algorithm for the approach to hearing loss. HL, hearing loss; TM, tympanic membrane; SNHL, sensorineural hearing loss; SOM, serous otitis media; AOM, acute otitis media; *, CT scan of temporal bone; †, MRI scan. (*From AK Lalwani, in HPIM-17, p. 201.*)

While small perforations often heal spontaneously, larger defects usually require surgical tympanoplasty (>90% effective). Otoscopy is usually sufficient to diagnose AOM, SOM, chronic otitis media, cerumen impaction, tympanic membrane perforation, and eustachian tube dysfunction.

Sensorineural Hearing Loss Damage to hair cells of the organ of Corti may be caused by intense noise, viral infections, ototoxic drugs (e.g., salicylates, quinine and its analogues, aminoglycoside antibiotics, diuretics such as furosemide and ethacrynic acid, and chemotherapeutic agents such as cisplatin), fractures of the temporal bone, meningitis, cochlear otosclerosis, Ménière's disease, and aging. Congenital malformations of the inner ear may cause hearing loss in some adults. Genetic predisposition alone or in concert with environmental influences may also be responsible.

Presbycusis (age-associated hearing loss) is the most common cause of sensorineural hearing loss in adults. In early stages, symmetric high frequency hearing loss is typical; with progression, the hearing loss involves all frequencies. The hearing impairment is associated with loss in clarity. Hearing aids provide limited rehabilitation; cochlear implants are treatment of choice for severe cases.

Ménière's disease is characterized by episodic vertigo, fluctuating sensorineural hearing loss, tinnitus, and aural fullness. It is caused by an increase in endolymphatic fluid pressure due to endolymphatic sac dysfunction. Low-frequency, unilateral sensorineural hearing impairment is usually present. MRI should be obtained to exclude retrocochlear pathology such as cerebellopontine angle tumor or demyelinating disorder. Therapy directed toward control of vertigo; a low-salt diet, diuretics, a short course of glucocorticoids, and intratympanic gentamicin may be useful. For unresponsive cases, endolymphatic sac decompression, labyrinthectomy, and vestibular nerve section abolish rotatory vertigo. There is no effective therapy for hearing loss, tinnitus, or aural fullness.

Vestibular schwannomas present with asymmetric hearing impairment, tinnitus, imbalance (rarely vertigo); cranial neuropathy (trigeminal or facial nerve) may accompany larger tumors.

Sensorineural hearing loss may also result from any neoplastic, vascular, demyelinating, infectious (including HIV), or degenerative disease or trauma affecting the central auditory pathways.

Tinnitus Defined as the perception of a sound when there is no sound in the environment. It may have a buzzing, roaring, or ringing quality and may be pulsatile (synchronous with the heartbeat). Tinnitus is often associated with either a conductive or sensorineural hearing loss and may be the first symptom of a serious condition such as a vestibular schwannoma. Pulsatile tinnitus requires evaluation of the vascular system of the head to exclude vascular tumors such as glomus jugulare tumors, aneurysms, arteriovenous fistulae, and stenotic arterial lesions; it may also occur with SOM.

R̶x̶ Hearing Loss

Hearing aids have been improved to provide greater fidelity and miniaturized so that they can be placed entirely within the ear canal, reducing the stigma associated with their use. Digital hearing aids can be individually programmed, and multiple and directional microphones at the ear level may be helpful in noisy surroundings. If the hearing aid provides inadequate rehabilitation, cochlear implants can be effective.

Treatment of tinnitus is problematic. Relief of the tinnitus may be obtained by masking it with background music. Hearing aids are also helpful in tinnitus suppression, as are tinnitus maskers, devices that present a sound to the affected ear that is more pleasant to listen to than the tinnitus. Antidepressants have also shown some benefit.

Hard-of-hearing individuals often benefit from a reduction in unnecessary noise to enhance the signal-to-noise ratio. Speech comprehension is aided by lip-reading; the face of the speaker should be well-illuminated and easily seen.

PREVENTION

Conductive hearing losses may be prevented by prompt antibiotic therapy for acute otitis media and by ventilation of the middle ear with tympanostomy tubes in middle-ear effusions lasting ≥12 weeks. Loss of vestibular function and deafness due to aminoglycoside antibiotics can largely be prevented by monitoring of serum peak and trough levels.

Ten million Americans have noise-induced hearing loss, and 20 million are exposed to hazardous noise in their employment. Noise-induced hearing loss can be prevented by avoidance of exposure to loud noise or by regular use of ear plugs or fluid-filled muffs to attenuate intense sound.

For a more detailed discussion, see Horton JC: Disorders of the Eye, Chap. 29, p. 180; and Lalwani AK: Disorders of Smell, Taste, and Hearing, Chap. 30, p. 196, in HPIM-17.

62 Sinusitis, Pharyngitis, Otitis, and Other Upper Respiratory Infections

Upper respiratory tract infections (URIs) are common illnesses that are often treated with antibiotics even though bacteria cause only 25% of cases. Inappropriate prescribing of antibiotics for URIs is a leading cause of antibiotic resistance in common community-acquired pathogens such as *Streptococcus pneumoniae*.

NONSPECIFIC URIs

The "common cold" is an acute, mild, catarrhal syndrome that lasts ~1 week and is caused by a wide variety of viruses, including rhinoviruses, coronaviruses, parainfluenza viruses, influenza viruses, adenoviruses, and respiratory syncytial virus. Symptoms include rhinorrhea, nasal congestion, cough, sore throat, hoarseness, malaise, sneezing, and fever. Because secondary bacterial infection complicates only 0.5–2% of colds, antibiotics are not indicated. Only symptom-based treatments should be used.

SINUS INFECTIONS

Sinusitis is an inflammatory condition most commonly involving the maxillary sinus; the next most common sites are the ethmoid, frontal, and sphenoid sinuses.

ACUTE SINUSITIS

Etiology and Epidemiology   Acute sinusitis, defined as disease of <4 weeks' duration, is usually caused by the same viruses that cause nonspecific URIs. *S. pneumoniae*, nontypable *Haemophilus influenzae*, and (in children) *Moraxella catarrhalis* cause acute bacterial sinusitis. Nosocomial cases, which are associated with nasotracheal intubation, are commonly caused by *Staphylococcus aureus* and gram-negative bacilli and are often polymicrobial and highly resistant to antibiotics. Acute fungal sinusitis occurs in compromised hosts (e.g., rhinocerebral mucormycosis in diabetic pts or aspergillosis in neutropenic pts).

Clinical Features   Common manifestations include nasal drainage, congestion, facial pain or pressure, headache, thick purulent nasal discharge, and tooth pain. Pain localizes to the involved sinus and is often worse when the pt bends over or is supine. Rarely, sphenoid or ethmoid sinusitis causes severe frontal or retroorbital pain, cavernous sinus thrombosis, and orbital cellulitis. Advanced frontal sinusitis can present as "Pott's puffy tumor": swelling and edema over the frontal bone. Life-threatening complications include meningitis, epidural abscess, and brain abscess.

Diagnosis   It is difficult to distinguish viral from bacterial sinusitis clinically. Disease of <7 days' duration is considered viral. Of pts with symptoms of >7 days' duration, 40–50% have bacterial sinusitis. If fungal sinusitis is a consideration, biopsies of involved areas should be performed. Nosocomial sinusitis should be confirmed with a CT scan of the sinuses.

Rx   Acute Sinusitis

Most pts improve without therapy. Treatment to facilitate drainage (e.g., oral and topical decongestants) should be used. Pts without improvement or with severe disease at presentation should be given antibiotics. See Table 62-1 for recommended regimens for adults. (Regimens for children can be found in Table 31-1 in HPIM-17.) Lack of response may mandate surgical drainage or lavage. Surgery should be considered for pts with severe disease or intracranial complications. Extensive debridement is usually needed for invasive fungal sinusitis in immunocompromised pts. Nosocomial disease requires agents active against *S. aureus* and gram-negative bacilli, including *Pseudomonas aeruginosa*.

CHRONIC SINUSITIS

Sinusitis of >12 weeks' duration is considered chronic.

- *Chronic bacterial sinusitis*: repeated infections due to impaired mucociliary clearance. Pts have constant nasal congestion and sinus pressure with periods of increased severity. Sinus CT scans can define the extent of disease and response to treatment. Tissue samples for histology and culture should be obtained to guide treatment. Repeated courses of antibiotics are required for 3–4 weeks at a time. Adjunctive treatments include intranasal administration of glucocorticoids, sinus irrigation, and surgical evaluation. Recurrence is common.
- *Chronic fungal sinusitis*: a noninvasive disease in immunocompetent hosts. Mild, indolent disease is usually curable without antifungal agents by endoscopic surgery. Unilateral disease with a mycetoma within the sinus (fungus ball) is treated with surgery and—if bony erosion has occurred—antifungal agents. Allergic fungal sinusitis is seen in pts with nasal polyps and asthma.

TABLE 62-1	GUIDELINES FOR THE DIAGNOSIS AND TREATMENT OF SELECTED UPPER RESPIRATORY TRACT INFECTIONS IN ADULTS[a]

Syndrome, Diagnostic Criteria	Treatment Recommendations
Acute sinusitis[b] 　Moderate symptoms (e.g., nasal purulence/congestion or cough) for >7 d or 　Severe symptoms of any duration, including unilateral/focal facial swelling or tooth pain	*Initial therapy* 　Amoxicillin, 500 mg PO tid or 875 mg PO bid, *or* 　TMP-SMX, 1 DS tablet PO bid for 10–14 d *Exposure to antibiotics within 30 d or >30% prevalence of penicillin-resistant S. pneumoniae* 　Amoxicillin, 1000 mg PO tid, *or* 　Amoxicillin/clavulanate (extended release), 2000 mg PO bid, *or* 　Antipneumococcal fluoroquinolone (e.g., levofloxacin, 500 mg PO qd) *Recent treatment failure[d]* 　Amoxicillin/clavulanate (extended release), 2000 mg PO bid, *or* 　Amoxicillin, 1500 mg bid, plus clindamycin, 300 mg PO qid, *or* 　Antipneumococcal fluoroquinolone (e.g., levofloxacin, 500 mg PO qd)
Acute otitis media[c] 　Fluid in the middle ear, evidenced by decreased tympanic membrane mobility, air/fluid level behind tympanic membrane, bulging tympanic membrane, purulent otorrhea; *and* 　Acute onset of signs and symptoms of middle-ear inflammation, including fever, otalgia, decreased hearing, tinnitus, vertigo, erythematous tympanic membrane	*Initial therapy* 　Observation alone (symptom relief only) *or* 　Amoxicillin, 80–90 mg/kg qd (up 2 g) PO in divided doses (bid or tid), *or* 　Cefdinir, 14 mg/kg qd PO in 1 dose or divided doses (bid), *or* 　Cefuroxime, 30 mg/kg qd PO in divided doses (bid), *or* 　Azithromycin, 10 mg/kg qd PO on day 1 followed by 5 mg/kg qd PO for 4 d *Antibiotic exposure within 30 d,[c] recent treatment failure,[c,d] or severe disease[c,e]* 　Amoxicillin, 90 mg/kg qd (up to 2 g) PO in divided doses (bid), *plus* clavulanate, 6.4 mg/kg qd PO in divided doses (bid), *or* 　Ceftriaxone, 50 mg/kg IV/IM qd for 3 d, *or* 　Clindamycin, 30–40 mg/kg qd PO in divided doses (tid) *or* 　Consider tympanocentesis with culture

(continued)

TABLE 62-1	GUIDELINES FOR THE DIAGNOSIS AND TREATMENT OF SELECTED UPPER RESPIRATORY TRACT INFECTIONS IN ADULTS (CONTINUED)[a]

Syndrome, Diagnostic Criteria	Treatment Recommendations

Acute pharyngitis[b]
  Clinical suspicion of streptococcal pharyngitis (e.g., fever, tonsillar swelling, exudate, enlarged/tender anterior cervical lymph nodes, absence of cough or coryza)[f] with:
  History of rheumatic fever or
  Documented household exposure or
  Positive rapid strep screen
	Penicillin V, 500 mg PO tid, or
	Amoxicillin, 500 mg PO bid, or
	Erythromycin, 250 mg PO qid, or
	Benzathine penicillin G, single dose of 1.2 million units IM

[a]For detailed information on diagnosis and treatment in children, see Tables 31-1, 31-2, and 31-3 in HPIM-17.

[b]Unless otherwise specified, the duration of therapy is generally 10 d, with appropriate follow-up.

[c]The duration of therapy is 5–7 d (10 d for pts with severe disease), with consideration of observation only in previously healthy patients with mild disease.

[d]Failure to improve and/or clinical worsening after 48–72 h of observation or treatment.

[e]As defined to left along with temperature ≥39.0°C or moderate to severe otalgia.

[f]Some organizations support treating adults who have these symptoms and signs without administering a rapid streptococcal antigen test.

Note: TMP-SMX, trimethoprim-sulfamethoxazole; DS, double-strength.

Sources: JM Hickner et al: Ann Intern Med 134:498, 2001; JF Piccirillo: N Engl J Med 351:902, 2004; Sinus and Allergy Health Partnership: Otolaryngol Head Neck Surg 130:1, 2004; SF Dowell et al: Pediatrics 101:165, 1998; RJ Cooper et al: Ann Intern Med 134:509, 2001; and B Schwartz et al: Pediatrics 101:171, 1998.

INFECTIONS OF THE EAR AND MASTOID

EXTERNAL EAR INFECTIONS

Consider noninfectious causes of inflammation—such as trauma, insect bite, autoimmune diseases (e.g., lupus), and vasculitides (e.g., Wegener's granulomatosis)—especially in the absence of local or regional adenopathy.

- *Auricular cellulitis*: Tenderness, erythema, and swelling of the external ear, particularly the lobule, follow minor trauma. Treat with warm compresses, and give antibiotics active against *S. aureus* and streptococci (e.g., dicloxacillin).
- *Perichondritis*: Infection of the perichondrium of the auricular cartilage follows minor trauma (e.g., ear piercing). Treatment should be directed at the most common etiologic agents, *P. aeruginosa* and *S. aureus*, and may consist of an antipseudomonal penicillin or a penicillinase-resistant penicillin (e.g., nafcillin) plus an antipseudomonal quinolone (e.g., ciprofloxacin). Surgical drainage may be needed; resolution can take weeks. If perichondritis fails to respond to adequate therapy, consider noninfectious inflammatory etiologies.
- *Otitis externa*
  1. *Acute localized otitis externa*, furunculosis in the outer third of the ear canal, is usually due to *S. aureus*.
  2. *Acute diffuse otitis externa* is known as "swimmer's ear." *P. aeruginosa* or other gram-negative or gram-positive bacteria cause infection in macerated, irritated canals. Pts have severe pain, erythema and swelling of

the canal and white clumpy discharge from the ear. Treatment includes cleansing of the canal and use of topical antibiotics (e.g., preparations with neomycin and polymyxin), with or without glucocorticoids to reduce inflammation.

3. *Chronic otitis externa* usually arises from persistent drainage from a chronic middle-ear infection, repeated irritation, or rare chronic infections such as tuberculosis or leprosy. Pts have pruritus rather than pain.

4. *Malignant* or *necrotizing otitis externa* is an aggressive, potentially life-threatening disease occurring primarily in elderly diabetic or immunocompromised pts. The disease progresses over weeks to months. Severe otalgia and purulent otorrhea and erythema of the ear and canal are evident. On exam, granulation tissue in the posteroinferior wall of the canal, near the junction of bone and cartilage, is seen. Untreated, this condition has a high mortality rate and can involve the base of the skull, meninges, cranial nerves, and brain. *P. aeruginosa* is the most common etiologic agent, but other gram-negative bacilli, *S. aureus*, *Staphylococcus epidermidis*, and *Aspergillus* can also cause the disease. Biopsy should be performed for diagnostic purposes. IV antipseudomonal agents (e.g., piperacillin, ceftazidime) with an aminoglycoside or fluoroquinolone plus antibiotic drops active against *Pseudomonas* should be given along with glucocorticoids.

MIDDLE EAR INFECTIONS

Eustachian tube dysfunction, often in association with URIs, causes sterile inflammation. Infection results when viral or bacterial superinfection occurs.

- *Acute otitis media*: A viral URI can cause otitis media or predispose to bacterial otitis media. *S. pneumoniae* is the most common bacterial cause; next in frequency are nontypable *H. influenzae* and *M. catarrhalis*. Concern is increasing about community-acquired methicillin-resistant *S. aureus* (MRSA) as an emerging etiologic agent. Pts have fluid in the middle ear. The tympanic membrane is immobile, erythematous, and bulging or retracted and can perforate spontaneously. Other findings include otalgia, otorrhea, decreased hearing, fever, and irritability. Pts with mild to moderate disease will do well if given analgesic and anti-inflammatory agents initially, with antibiotics reserved for pts who do not improve in 2–3 days. Most cases resolve within 1 week without treatment. Amoxicillin remains the drug of choice, despite rising antibiotic resistance. See Table 62-1 for treatment options. (Regimens for children can be found in Table 31-2 in HPIM-17.)
- *Serous otitis media*: Otitis media with effusion can persist for months without signs of infection. Antibiotic therapy or myringotomy with tympanostomy tubes is reserved for pts with bilateral effusions that have persisted for at least 3 months and are associated with bilateral hearing loss.
- *Chronic otitis media*: persistent or recurrent purulent otorrhea with tympanic membrane perforation. Active disease may lead to erosion of bone, meningitis, and brain abscess and is treated surgically. Inactive disease is treated with repeated courses of topical antibiotic drops during periods of drainage.
- *Mastoiditis* has been uncommon in the antibiotic era. Mastoid air cells connect with the middle ear, and purulent exudates can cause erosion of surrounding bone and abscess-like cavities. Pts have pain, erythema, and mastoid process swelling along with the signs and symptoms of otitis media. Rare complications include subperiosteal abscess, deep neck abscess, and septic thrombosis of the lateral sinus. Cultures should be performed and used to direct therapy.

INFECTIONS OF THE PHARYNX AND ORAL CAVITY

ACUTE PHARYNGITIS

- *Viral*: Respiratory viruses typically cause mild disease associated with non-specific URI symptoms, tender cervical adenopathy, and minimal fever. Influenza virus and adenovirus can cause severe exudative pharyngitis with fever. Herpes simplex virus (HSV) causes pharyngeal inflammation and exudates with vesicles and ulcers on the palate. Coxsackievirus A causes small vesicles on the soft palate and uvula that form shallow white ulcers. Epstein-Barr virus and cytomegalovirus cause exudative pharyngitis in association with other signs of infectious mononucleosis. HIV causes fever, myalgias, malaise, and sometimes a maculopapular rash.
- *Bacterial*: Group A *Streptococcus* (GAS) accounts for ~5–15% of cases of pharyngitis in adults but is primarily a disease of children 5–15 years old. Other bacterial causes include streptococci of groups C and G, *Neisseria gonorrhoeae*, *Corynebacterium diphtheriae*, and anaerobic bacteria. Streptococcal pharyngitis ranges from mild disease to profound pharyngeal pain, fever, chills, abdominal pain, and a hyperemic pharyngeal membrane with tonsillar hypertrophy and exudates. Coryzal symptoms are absent. The diagnosis is made by rapid antigen-detection testing for GAS. Most experts recommend that children have a throat culture performed if rapid testing is negative, but this course is not recommended for adults because of the low incidence of disease. For treatment options in adults, see Table 62-1 and Chap. 94. (Regimens for children can be found in Table 31-3 in HPIM-17.)

ORAL INFECTIONS

Oral-labial herpesvirus infections and oral thrush caused by *Candida* are discussed in Chaps. 106 and 113, respectively.

INFECTIONS OF THE LARYNX AND EPIGLOTTIS

- *Laryngitis*: a common syndrome caused by nearly all the major respiratory viruses and only rarely by bacteria (e.g., GAS, *C. diphtheriae*, and *M. catarrhalis*). Pts are hoarse, exhibit reduced vocal pitch or aphonia, and have coryzal symptoms. Treatment consists of humidification, voice rest, and—if GAS is cultured—antibiotic administration.
- *Croup*: viral disease marked by swelling of the subglottic region and primarily affecting children <6 years old
- *Epiglottitis*: acute, rapidly progressive cellulitis of the epiglottis and adjacent structures. Vaccination against *H. influenzae* type b has reduced disease rates among children by >90%, but the incidence among adults is stable. Epiglottitis in adults is caused by GAS, *S. pneumoniae*, *Haemophilus parainfluenzae*, and *S. aureus*. Symptoms include fever, severe sore throat, and systemic toxicity, and pts sometimes drool while sitting forward. Signs of respiratory obstruction may develop and progress rapidly. Adolescents and adults have less acute presentations than children. Examination may reveal respiratory distress, inspiratory stridor, and chest wall retractions. Direct fiberoptic laryngoscopy in a controlled environment (e.g., an operating room) may be performed for diagnosis, procurement of specimens for culture, and placement of an endotracheal tube. Treatment focuses on protection of the airway. Blood and, in some cases, the epiglottis should be cultured; after samples are obtained, IV antibiotics active against *H. influen-*

zae (e.g., ampicillin/sulbactam or a second- or third-generation cephalosporin) should be given for 7–10 days.

INFECTIONS OF DEEP NECK STRUCTURES

These infections, which include Ludwig's angina, Lemierre's syndrome, and retropharyngeal abscess, are discussed in Chap. 99.

For a more detailed discussion, see Rubin MA et al: Pharyngitis, Sinusitis, Otitis, and Other Upper Respiratory Tract Infections, Chap. 31, p. 205, in HPIM-17.

63 General Examination of the Skin

As dermatologic evaluation relies heavily on the objective cutaneous appearance, physical examination is often performed prior to taking a complete history in pts presenting with a skin problem. A differential diagnosis can usually be generated on the basis of a thorough examination with precise descriptions of the skin lesion(s) and narrowed with pertinent facts from the history. Laboratory or diagnostic procedures are then used, when appropriate, to clarify the diagnosis.

PHYSICAL EXAMINATION

Examination of skin should take place in a well-illuminated room with pt completely disrobed. Helpful ancillary equipment includes a hand lens and a pocket flashlight to provide peripheral illumination of lesions. An ideal examination includes evaluation of the skin, hair, nails and mucous membranes. The examination often begins with an assessment of the entire skin viewed at a distance, which is then narrowed down to focus on the individual lesions.

Distribution As illustrated in Fig. 63-1, the distribution of skin lesions can provide valuable clues to the identification of the disorder: Generalized (systemic diseases); sun-exposed (SLE, photoallergic, phototoxic, polymorphous light eruption, porphyria cutanea tarda); dermatomal (herpes zoster); extensor surfaces (elbows and knees in psoriasis); flexural surfaces (antecubital and popliteal fossae in atopic dermatitis).

Arrangement and Shape Can describe individual or multiple lesions: *Linear* (contact dermatitis such as poison ivy); *annular*—"ring-shaped" lesion (erythema chronicum migrans, erythema annulare centrifugum, tinea corporis); *iris* or *target lesion*—two or three concentric circles of differing hue (erythema multiforme); *nummular*—"coin-shaped" (nummular eczema); *morbilliform*—"measles-like" with small confluent papules coalescing into unusual shapes (measles, drug eruption); *herpetiform*—grouped vesicles, papules, or erosions (herpes simplex).

Primary Lesions Cutaneous changes caused directly by disease process (Table 63-1).

Secondary Lesions Changes in area of primary pathology often due to secondary events, e.g., scratching, secondary infection, bleeding (Table 63-2).

Other Descriptive Terms Color, e.g., violaceous, erythematous; physical characteristics, e.g., warm, tender; sharpness of edge, surface contour—flat-topped, pedunculated (on a stalk), verrucous (wartlike), umbilicated (containing a central depression).

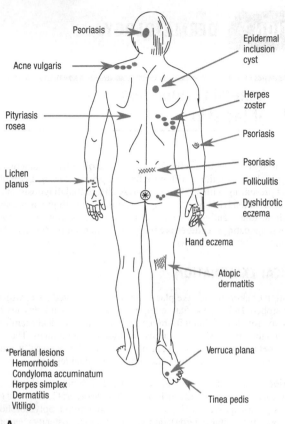

FIGURE 63-1 The distribution of some common dermatologic diseases and lesions.

HISTORY

A complete history should be obtained, with special attention being paid to the following points:

1. Evolution of the lesion—site of onset, manner in which eruption progressed or spread, duration, periods of resolution or improvement in chronic eruptions
2. Symptoms associated with the eruption—itching, burning, pain, numbness; what has relieved symptoms; time of day when symptoms are most severe
3. Current or recent medications—both prescription and over-the-counter
4. Associated systemic symptoms (e.g., malaise, fatigue, arthralgias)
5. Ongoing or previous illnesses
6. History of allergies
7. Presence of photosensitivity
8. Review of systems
9. Family history
10. Social, sexual, or travel history

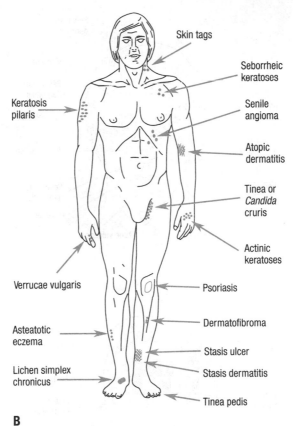

Skin tags

Seborrheic keratoses

Senile angioma

Keratosis pilaris

Atopic dermatitis

Tinea or *Candida* cruris

Actinic keratoses

Verrucae vulgaris

Psoriasis

Dermatofibroma

Asteatotic eczema

Stasis ulcer

Lichen simplex chronicus

Stasis dermatitis

Tinea pedis

B

FIGURE 63-1 *(Continued)*

ADDITIONAL DIAGNOSTIC PROCEDURES

Skin Biopsy   Minor surgical procedure. Choice of site very important.

Potassium Hydroxide Preparation   Useful for detection of dermatophyte or yeast. Scale is collected from advancing edge of a scaling lesion by gently scraping with side of a microscope slide or a scalpel blade. Nail lesions are best sampled by trimming back nail and scraping subungual debris. A drop of 10–20% potassium hydroxide is added to slide, and coverslip is applied. The slide may be gently heated and examined under microscope. This technique can be utilized to identify hyphae in dermatophyte infections, pseudohyphae and budding yeast in *Candida* infections, and "spaghetti and meatballs" yeast forms in tinea versicolor.

Tzanck Preparation   Useful for determining presence of herpes viruses (herpes simplex virus or herpes zoster virus). Optimal lesion to sample is an early vesicle. Lesion is gently unroofed with no. 15 scalpel blade, and base of vesicle is gently scraped with belly of blade (keep blade perpendicular to skin surface to prevent laceration). Scrapings are transferred to slide and stained with Wright's

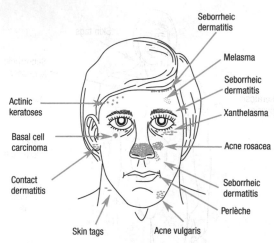

C

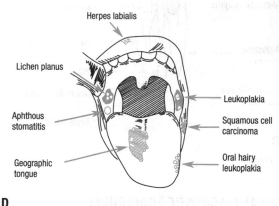

D

FIGURE 63-1 *(Continued)*

or Giemsa stain. A positive preparation has multinuclear giant cells. Culture or immunofluorescence testing must be performed to identify the specific virus.

Diascopy Assesses whether a lesion blanches with pressure. Done by pressing a magnifying lens or microscope slide on lesion and observing changes in vascularity. For example, hemangiomas will usually blanch; purpuric lesions will not.

Wood's Light Examination Useful for detecting bacterial or fungal infection or accentuating features of some skin lesions.

Patch Tests To document cutaneous sensitivity to specific antigens.

TABLE 63-1   DESCRIPTION OF PRIMARY SKIN LESIONS

Macule: A flat, colored lesion, <2 cm in diameter, not raised above the surface of the surrounding skin. A "freckle," or ephelid, is a prototype pigmented macule.

Patch: A large (>2 cm) flat lesion with a color different from the surrounding skin. This differs from a macule only in size.

Papule: A small, solid lesion, <0.5 cm in diameter, raised above the surface of the surrounding skin and hence palpable (e.g., a closed comedone, or whitehead, in acne).

Nodule: A larger (0.5–5.0 cm), firm lesion raised above the surface of the surrounding skin. This differs from a papule only in size (e.g., a dermal nevomelanocytic nevus).

Tumor: A solid, raised growth >5 cm in diameter.

Plaque: A large (>1 cm), flat-topped, raised lesion; edges may either be distinct (e.g., in psoriasis) or gradually blend with surrounding skin (e.g., in eczematous dermatitis).

Vesicle: A small, fluid-filled lesion, <0.5 cm in diameter, raised above the plane of surrounding skin. Fluid is often visible, and the lesions are translucent [e.g., vesicles in allergic contact dermatitis caused by *Toxicodendron* (poison ivy)].

Pustule: A vesicle filled with leukocytes. Note: The presence of pustules does not necessarily signify the existence of an infection.

Bulla: A fluid-filled, raised, often translucent lesion >0.5 cm in diameter.

Wheal: A raised, erythematous, edematous papule or plaque, usually representing short-lived vasodilatation and vasopermeability.

Telangiectasia: A dilated, superficial blood vessel.

TABLE 63-2   DESCRIPTION OF SECONDARY SKIN LESIONS

Lichenification: A distinctive thickening of the skin that is characterized by accentuated skin-fold markings.

Scale: Excessive accumulation of stratum corneum.

Crust: Dried exudate of body fluids that may be either yellow (i.e., serous crust) or red (i.e., hemorrhagic crust).

Erosion: Loss of epidermis without an associated loss of dermis.

Ulcer: Loss of epidermis and at least a portion of the underlying dermis.

Excoriation: Linear, angular erosions that may be covered by crust and are caused by scratching.

Atrophy: An acquired loss of substance. In the skin, this may appear as a depression with intact epidermis (i.e., loss of dermal or subcutaneous tissue) or as sites of shiny, delicate, wrinkled lesions (i.e., epidermal atrophy).

Scar: A change in the skin secondary to trauma or inflammation. Sites may be erythematous, hypopigmented, or hyperpigmented depending on their age or character. Sites on hair-bearing areas may be characterized by destruction of hair follicles.

For a more detailed discussion, see Lawley TJ, Yancey KB: Approach to the Patient with a Skin Disorder, Chap. 52, p. 308, in HPIM-17.

64 Common Skin Conditions

PAPULOSQUAMOUS DISORDERS

Disorders exhibiting papules and scale.

Psoriasis A chronic, recurrent disorder. Classic lesion is a well-marginated, erythematous plaque with silvery-white surface scale. Distribution includes extensor surfaces (i.e., knees, elbows, and buttocks); may also involve palms and scalp (particularly anterior scalp margin). Associated findings include psoriatic arthritis (Chap. 170) and nail changes (onycholysis, pitting or thickening of nail plate with accumulation of subungual debris).

Ṟₓ Psoriasis

Maintain cutaneous hydration; topical glucocorticoids; topical vitamin D analogue (calcipotriol) and retinoid (tazarotene); UV light (PUVA when UV used in combination with psoralens); for severe disease methotrexate or cyclosporine; acitretin can also be used but is teratogenic. Efalizumab (humanized monoclonal antibody directed against CD11a) or alefacept (dimeric fusion protein: LFA-3/Fc human IgG1) can be considered for chronic, moderate to severe plaque psoriasis. Etanercept (dimeric fusion protein: TNF receptor/Fc human IgG1) is approved for psoriatic arthritis and psoriasis.

Pityriasis Rosea A self-limited condition lasting 3–8 weeks. Initially, there is a single 2- to 6-cm annular salmon-colored patch (herald patch) with a peripheral rim of scale, followed in days to weeks by a generalized eruption involving the trunk and proximal extremities. Individual lesions are similar to but smaller than the herald patch and are arranged in symmetric fashion with long axis of each individual lesion along skin lines of cleavage. Appearance may be similar to that of secondary syphilis.

Ṟₓ Pityriasis Rosea

Disorder is self-limited, so treatment is directed at symptoms; oral antihistamines for pruritus; topical glucocorticoids; UV-B phototherapy in some cases.

Lichen Planus Disorder of unknown cause; can follow administration of certain drugs and in chronic graft-versus-host disease; lesions are pruritic, polygonal, flat-topped, and violaceous. Course is variable, but most pts have spontaneous remissions 6–24 months after onset of disease.

Ṟₓ Lichen Planus

Topical glucocorticoids.

ECZEMATOUS DISORDERS

Eczema Eczema, or dermatitis, is a reaction pattern that presents with variable clinical and histologic findings; it is the final common expression for a number of disorders.

Atopic Dermatitis One aspect of atopic triad of hayfever, asthma, and eczema. Usually an intermittent, chronic, severely pruritic, eczematous dermatitis with scaly erythematous patches, vesiculation, crusting, and fissuring. Lesions are most commonly on flexures, with prominent involvement of antecubital and popliteal fossae; generalized erythroderma in severe cases.

℞ Eczema and Atopic Dermatitis

Avoidance of irritants; cutaneous hydration; topical glucocorticoids; treatment of infected lesions [often with *Staphylococcus aureus* (SA)—consider community-acquired methicillin-resistant strains (CA-MRSA)]. Systemic glucocorticoids only for severe exacerbations unresponsive to topical conservative therapy.

Allergic Contact Dermatitis A delayed hypersensitivity reaction that occurs after cutaneous exposure to an antigenic substance. Lesions occur at site of contact and are vesicular, weeping, crusting; linear arrangement of vesicles is common. Most frequent allergens are resin from plants of the genus *Toxicodendron* (poison ivy, oak, sumac), nickel, rubber, and cosmetics.

℞ Allergic Contact Dermatitis

Avoidance of sensitizing agent; topical glucocorticoids; consideration of systemic glucocorticoids over 2–3 weeks for widespread disease.

Irritant Contact Dermatitis Inflammation of the skin due to direct injury by an exogenous agent. The most common area of involvement is the hands, where dermatitis is initiated or aggravated by chronic exposure to water and detergents. Features may include skin dryness, cracking, erythema, edema.

℞ Irritant Contact Dermatitis

Avoidance of irritants; barriers (use of protective gloves); topical glucocorticoids; treatment of secondary bacterial or dermatophyte infection.

Seborrheic Dermatitis A chronic noninfectious process characterized by erythematous patches with greasy yellowish scale. Lesions are generally on scalp, eyebrows, nasolabial folds, axillae, central chest, and posterior auricular area.

℞ Seborrheic Dermatitis

Nonfluorinated topical glucocorticoids; shampoos containing coal tar, salicylic acid, or selenium sulfide.

INFECTIONS

Impetigo   A superficial infection of skin secondary to either *S. aureus* or group A β-hemolytic streptococci. The primary lesion is a superficial pustule that ruptures and forms a "honey-colored" crust. Tense bullae are associated with *S. aureus* infections (bullous impetigo). Lesions may occur anywhere but commonly involve the face. Impetigo and *furunculosis* (painful erythematous nodule, or boil) have gained prominence because of increasing incidence of CA-MRSA.

℞ Impetigo

Gentle debridement of adherent crusts with soaks and topical antibiotics; appropriate oral antibiotics depending on organism (Chap. 84).

Erysipelas   Superficial cellulitis, most commonly on face, characterized by a bright red, sharply demarcated, intensely painful, warm plaque. Because of superficial location of infection and associated edema, surface of plaque may exhibit a *peau d'orange* (orange peel) appearance. Most commonly due to infection with group A β-hemolytic streptococci, occurring at sites of trauma or other breaks in skin.

℞ Erysipelas

Appropriate antibiotics depending on organism (Chap. 84).

Herpes Simplex   (See also Chap. 106)

Recurrent eruption characterized by grouped vesicles on an erythematous base that progress to erosions; often secondarily infected with staphylococci or streptococci. Infections frequently involve mucocutaneous surfaces around the oral cavity, genitals, or anus. Can also cause severe visceral disease including esophagitis, pneumonitis, encephalitis, and disseminated herpes simplex virus infection. Tzanck preparation of an unroofed early vesicle reveals multinuclear giant cells.

℞ Herpes Simplex

Will differ based on disease manifestations and level of immune competence (Chap. 106); appropriate antibiotics for secondary infections, depending on organism.

Herpes Zoster   (See also Chap. 106)

Eruption of grouped vesicles on an erythematous base usually limited to a single dermatome ("shingles"); disseminated lesions can also occur, especially in immunocompromised pts. Tzanck preparation reveals multinucleate giant cells; indistinguishable from herpes simplex except by culture. Postherpetic neuralgia, lasting months to years, may occur, especially in the elderly.

℞ Herpes Zoster

Will differ based on disease manifestations and level of immune competence (Chap. 106).

Dermatophyte Infection   Skin fungus, may involve any area of body; due to infection of stratum corneum, nail plate, or hair. Appearance may vary from mild scaliness to florid inflammatory dermatitis. Common sites of infection include the foot (tinea pedis), nails (tinea unguium), groin (tinea cruris), or scalp (tinea capitis). Classic lesion of tinea corporis ("ringworm") is an erythematous papulosquamous patch, often with central clearing and scale along peripheral advancing border. Hyphae are often seen on KOH preparation, although tinea capitis and tinea corporis may require culture or biopsy.

Dermatophyte Infection

Depends on affected site and type of infection. Topical imidazoles, triazoles, and allylamines may be effective. Haloprogin, undecylenic acid, ciclopiroxolamine, and tolnaftate are also effective, but nystatin is not active against dermatophytes. Griseofulvin, 500 mg/d, if systemic therapy required. Itraconazole or terbinafine may be effective for nail infections.

Candidiasis   Fungal infection caused by a related group of yeasts. Manifestations may be localized to the skin or rarely systemic and life-threatening. Predisposing factors include diabetes mellitus, cellular immune deficiencies, and HIV (Chap. 112). Frequent sites include the oral cavity, chronically wet macerated areas, around nails, intertriginous areas. Diagnosed by clinical pattern and demonstration of yeast on KOH preparation or culture.

℞ Candidiasis

(See also Chap. 113) Removal of predisposing factors; topical nystatin or azoles; systemic therapy reserved for immunosuppressed patients, unresponsive chronic or recurrent disease; vulvovaginal candidiasis may respond to a single dose of fluconazole, 150 mg.

Warts   Cutaneous neoplasms caused by human papilloma viruses (HPVs). Typically dome-shaped lesions with irregular filamentous surface. Propensity for the face, arms, and legs; often spread by shaving. HPVs are also associated with genital or perianal lesions and play a role in the development of cancer of the uterine cervix and external genitalia in females (Chap. 90).

℞ Warts

Cryotherapy with liquid nitrogen, keratinolytic agents (salicylic acid). For genital warts, application of podophyllin solution is effective but can be associated with marked local reactions; topical imiquimod has also been used.

ACNE

Acne Vulgaris   Usually a self-limited disorder of teenagers and young adults. Comedones (small cyst formed in hair follicle) are clinical hallmark; often accompanied by inflammatory lesions of papules, pustules, or nodules. May scar in severe cases.

℞ Acne Vulgaris

Careful cleaning and removal of oils; oral tetracycline or erythromycin; topical antibacterials (e.g., benzoyl peroxide), topical retinoic acid. Systemic isotretinoin only for unresponsive severe nodulocystic acne (risk of severe adverse events including teratogenicity and possible association with depression).

Acne Rosacea Inflammatory disorder affecting predominantly the central face, rarely affecting pts <30 years of age. Tendency toward exaggerated flushing, with eventual superimposition of papules, pustules, and telangiectases. May lead to rhinophyma and ocular problems.

℞ Acne Rosacea

Oral tetracycline, 250–1000 mg/d; topical metronidazole and topical nonfluorinated glucocorticoids may be useful.

VASCULAR DISORDERS

Erythema Nodosum Septal panniculitis characterized by erythematous, warm, tender subcutaneous nodular lesions typically over anterior tibia. Lesions are usually flush with skin surface but are indurated and have appearance of an erythematous/violaceous bruise. Lesions usually resolve spontaneously in 3–6 weeks without scarring. Commonly seen in sarcoidosis, administration of certain drugs (esp. sulfonamides, oral contraceptives, and estrogens), and a wide range of infections including streptococcal and tubercular; may be idiopathic.

℞ Erythema Nodosum

Identification and treatment/removal of underlying cause. NSAID for severe or recurrent lesions; systemic glucocorticoids are effective but dangerous if underlying infection is not appreciated.

Erythema Multiforme A reaction pattern of skin consisting of a variety of lesions but most commonly erythematous papules and bullae. "Target" or "iris" lesion is characteristic and consists of concentric circles of erythema and normal flesh-colored skin, often with a central vesicle or bulla.

Distribution of lesions classically acral, esp. palms and soles. Three most common causes are drug reaction (particularly penicillins and sulfonamides) or concurrent herpetic or *Mycoplasma* infection. Can rarely affect mucosal surfaces and internal organs (erythema multiforme major or Stevens-Johnson syndrome).

℞ Erythema Multiforme

Provocative agent should be sought and eliminated if drug-related. In mild cases limited to skin, only symptomatic treatment is needed (antihistamines, NSAID). For Stevens-Johnson, systemic glucocorticoids have been used, but are controversial; prevention of secondary infection and maintenance of nutrition and fluid/electrolyte balance are critical.

Urticaria A common disorder, either acute or chronic, characterized by evanescent (individual lesions lasting <24 h), pruritic, edematous, pink to erythematous plaques with a whitish halo around margin of individual lesions. Lesions range in size from papules to giant coalescent lesions (10–20 cm in diameter). Often due to drugs, systemic infection, or foods (esp. shellfish). Food additives such as tartrazine dye (FD & C yellow no. 5), benzoate, or salicylates have also been implicated. If individual lesions last >24 h, consider diagnosis of urticarial vasculitis.

 Urticaria

See Chap. 165.

Vasculitis Palpable purpura (nonblanching, elevated lesions) is the cutaneous hallmark of vasculitis. Other lesions include petechiae (esp. early lesions), necrosis with ulceration, bullae, and urticarial lesions (urticarial vasculitis). Lesions usually most prominent on lower extremities. Associations include infections, collagen-vascular disease, primary systemic vasculitides, malignancy, hepatitis B and C, drugs (esp. thiazides), and inflammatory bowel disease. May occur as an idiopathic, predominantly cutaneous vasculitis.

 Vasculitis

Will differ based on cause. Pursue identification and treatment/elimination of an exogenous cause or underlying disease. If part of a systemic vasculitis, treat based on major organ-threatening features (Chap. 168). Immunosuppressive therapy should be avoided in idiopathic, predominantly cutaneous vasculitis as disease frequently does not respond and rarely causes irreversible organ system dysfunction.

CUTANEOUS DRUG REACTIONS

Cutaneous reactions are among the most frequent medication toxicities. These can have a wide range of severity and manifestations including urticaria, photosensitivity, erythema multiforme, fixed drug reactions, erythema nodosum, vasculitis, lichenoid reactions, bullous drug reactions, Stevens-Johnson syndrome, and toxic epidermal necrolysis (TEN). Diagnosis is usually made by appearance and careful medication history.

 Cutaneous Drug Reactions

Withdrawal of the medication. Treatment based on nature and severity of cutaneous pathology.

For a more detailed discussion, see McCall CO, Lawley TJ: Eczema, Psoriasis, Cutaneous Infections, Acne, and Other Common Skin Disorders, Chap. 53, p. 312; Roujeau J-C, Stern RS, Wintroub BU: Cutaneous Drug Reactions, Chap. 56, p. 343; and Bolognia JL, Braverman IM: Skin Manifestations of Internal Disease, Chap. 54, p. 321, in HPIM-17.

65 Examination of Blood Smears and Bone Marrow

BLOOD SMEARS

ERYTHROCYTE (RBC) MORPHOLOGY

- Normal: 7.5-μm diameter. Roughly the size of the nucleus of a small lymphocyte.
- *Reticulocytes* (Wright's stain)—large, grayish-blue, admixed with pink (polychromasia).
- *Anisocytosis*—variation in RBC size; large cells imply delay in erythroid precursor DNA synthesis caused by folate or B_{12} deficiency or drug effect; small cells imply a defect in hemoglobin synthesis caused by iron deficiency or abnormal hemoglobin genes.
- *Poikilocytosis*—abnormal RBC shapes; the following are examples:
  1. *Acanthocytes* (spur cells)—irregularly spiculated; abetalipoproteinemia, severe liver disease, rarely anorexia nervosa.
  2. *Echinocytes* (burr cells)—regularly shaped, uniformly distributed spiny projections; uremia, RBC volume loss.
  3. *Elliptocytes*—elliptical; hereditary elliptocytosis.
  4. *Schistocytes* (schizocytes)—fragmented cells of varying sizes and shapes; microangiopathic or macroangiopathic hemolytic anemia.
  5. *Sickled cells*—elongated, crescentic; sickle cell anemias.
  6. *Spherocytes*—small hyperchromic cells lacking normal central pallor; hereditary spherocytosis, extravascular hemolysis as in autoimmune hemolytic anemia, G6PD deficiency.
  7. *Target cells*—central and outer rim staining with intervening ring of pallor; liver disease, thalassemia, hemoglobin C and sickle C diseases.
  8. *Teardrop cells*—myelofibrosis, other infiltrative processes of marrow (e.g., carcinoma).
  9. *Rouleaux formation*—alignment of RBCs in stacks; may be artifactual or due to paraproteinemia (e.g., multiple myeloma, macroglobulinemia).

RBC INCLUSIONS

- *Howell-Jolly bodies*—1-μm-diameter basophilic cytoplasmic inclusion that represents a residual nuclear fragment, usually single; asplenic pts.
- *Basophilic stippling*—multiple, punctate basophilic cytoplasmic inclusions composed of precipitated mitochondria and ribosomes; lead poisoning, thalassemia, myelofibrosis.
- *Pappenheimer (iron) bodies*—iron-containing granules usually composed of mitochondria and ribosomes resemble basophilic stippling but also stain with Prussian blue; lead poisoning, other sideroblastic anemias.

- *Heinz bodies*—spherical inclusions of precipitated hemoglobin seen only with supravital stains, such as crystal violet; G6PD deficiency (after oxidant stress such as infection, certain drugs), unstable hemoglobin variants.
- *Parasites*—characteristic intracytoplasmic inclusions; malaria, babesiosis.

LEUKOCYTE INCLUSIONS AND NUCLEAR CONTOUR ABNORMALITIES

- *Toxic granulations*—dark cytoplasmic granules; bacterial infection.
- *Döhle bodies*—1- to 2-μm blue, oval cytoplasmic inclusions; bacterial infection, Chédiak-Higashi anomaly.
- *Auer rods*—eosinophilic, rodlike cytoplasmic inclusions; acute myeloid leukemia (some cases).
- *Hypersegmentation*—neutrophil nuclei contain more than the usual 2–4 lobes; usually >5% have ≥5 lobes or a single cell with 7 lobes is adequate to make the diagnosis; folate or B_{12} deficiency, drug effects.
- *Hyposegmentation*—neutrophil nuclei contain fewer lobes than normal, either one or two: Pelger-Hüet anomaly, pseudo-Pelger-Hüet or acquired Pelger-Hüet anomaly in acute leukemia.

PLATELET ABNORMALITIES

Platelet clumping—an in vitro artifact—is often readily detectable on smear; can lead to falsely low platelet count by automated cell counters.

BONE MARROW

Aspiration assesses cell morphology. *Biopsy* assesses overall marrow architecture, including degree of cellularity. Biopsy should precede aspiration to avoid aspiration artifact (mainly hemorrhage) in the specimen.

INDICATIONS

Aspiration Hypoproliferative or unexplained anemia, leukopenia, or thrombocytopenia, suspected leukemia or myeloma or marrow defect, evaluation of iron stores, workup of some cases of fever of unknown origin.

Special Tests Histochemical staining (leukemias), cytogenetic studies (leukemias, lymphomas), microbiology (bacterial, mycobacterial, fungal cultures), Prussian blue (iron) stain (assessment of iron stores, diagnosis of sideroblastic anemias).

Biopsy Performed in addition to aspiration for pancytopenia (aplastic anemia), metastatic tumor, granulomatous infection (e.g., mycobacteria, brucellosis, histoplasmosis), myelofibrosis, lipid storage disease (e.g., Gaucher's, Niemann-Pick), any case with "dry tap" on aspiration; evaluation of marrow cellularity. When biopsy and aspirate are both planned, the biopsy should be performed first because of the risk of bleeding artifact from biopsy of an aspiration site.

Special Tests Histochemical staining (e.g., acid phosphatase for metastatic prostate carcinoma), immunoperoxidase staining (e.g., immunoglobulin or cell surface marker detection in multiple myeloma, leukemia, or lymphoma; lysozyme detection in monocytic leukemia), reticulin staining (increased in myelofibrosis), microbiologic staining (e.g., acid-fast staining for mycobacteria).

INTERPRETATION

Cellularity   Defined as percentage of space occupied by hematopoietic cells. Decreases with age after age 65 years from about 50% to 25–30% with a corresponding increase in fat.

Erythroid:Granulocytic (E:G) Ratio   Normally about 1:2, the E:G ratio is decreased in acute and chronic infection, leukemoid reactions (e.g., chronic inflammation, metastatic tumor), acute and chronic myeloid leukemia, myelodysplastic disorders ("preleukemia"), and pure red cell aplasia; increased in agranulocytosis, anemias with erythroid hyperplasia (megaloblastic, iron-deficiency, thalassemia, hemorrhage, hemolysis, sideroblastic), and erythrocytosis (excessive RBC production); normal in aplastic anemia (though marrow hypocellular), myelofibrosis (marrow hypocellular), multiple myeloma, lymphoma, anemia of chronic disease. Some centers use the term M:E (myeloid to erythroid) ratio; normal value is 2:1 and increases with diseases that promote myeloid activity or inhibit erythroid activity and decreases with diseases that inhibit myeloid activity or promote erythroid activity.

For a more detailed discussion, see Adamson JW, Longo DL: Anemia and Polycythemia, Chap. 58, p. 355; Holland SM, Gallin JI: Disorders of Granulocytes and Monocytes, Chap. 61, p. 375; Longo DL: Atlas of Hematology and Analysis of Peripheral Blood Smears, Chap. e11 in HPIM-17.

66 Red Blood Cell Disorders

Anemia is a common clinical problem in medicine. A physiologic approach (outlined in Chap. 58) provides the most efficient path to diagnosis and management. Anemias arise either because red blood cell (RBC) production is inadequate or because RBC lifespan is shortened through loss from the circulation or destruction.

HYPOPROLIFERATIVE ANEMIAS

These are the most common anemias. Usually the RBC morphology is normal and the reticulocyte index (RI) is low. Marrow damage, early iron deficiency, and decreased erythropoietin production or action may produce anemia of this type.

Marrow damage may be caused by infiltration of the marrow with tumor or fibrosis that crowds out normal erythroid precursors or by the absence of erythroid precursors (aplastic anemia) as a consequence of exposure to drugs, radiation, chemicals, viruses (e.g., hepatitis), autoimmune mechanisms, or genetic factors, either hereditary (e.g., Fanconi's anemia) or acquired (e.g., paroxysmal nocturnal hemoglobinuria). Most cases of aplasia are idiopathic. The tumor or fibrosis that infiltrates the marrow may originate in the marrow (as in leukemia

	Normal	Iron-store depletion	Iron-deficient erythropoiesis	Iron-deficiency anemia
Iron stores				
Erythron iron				
Marrow iron stores	1–3 +	0–1 +	0	0
Serum ferritin (μg/L)	50–200	<20	<15	<15
TIBC (μg/dL)	300–360	>360	>380	>400
SI (μg/dL)	50–150	NL	<50	<30
Saturation (%)	30–50	NL	<30	<10
Marrow sideroblasts (%)	40–60	NL	<10	<10
RBC protoporphyrin (μg/dL)	30–50	NL	>100	>200
RBC morphology	NL	NL	NL	Microcytic/hypochromic

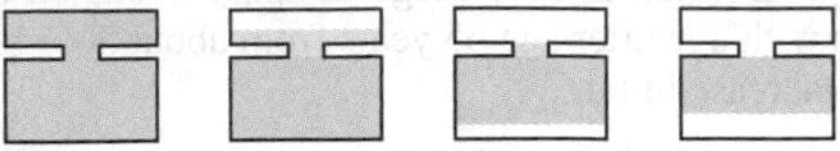

FIGURE 66-1 Laboratory studies in the evolution of iron deficiency. Measurements of marrow iron stores, serum ferritin, and TIBC are sensitive to early iron-store depletion. Iron-deficient erythropoiesis is recognized from additional abnormalities in the SI, percent saturation of transferrin, the pattern of marrow sideroblasts, and the red blood cell protoporphyrin level. Finally, patients with iron-deficiency anemia demonstrate all of these same abnormalities plus an anemia characterized by microcytic hypochromic morphology. (*From RS Hillman, CA Finch: Red Cell Manual, 7th. ed, Philadelphia, Davis, 1996, with permission.*)

or myelofibrosis) or be secondary to processes originating outside the marrow (as in metastatic cancer or myelophthisis).

Early iron-deficiency anemia (or iron-deficient erythropoiesis) is associated with a decrease in serum ferritin levels (<15 μg/L), moderately elevated total iron-binding capacity (TIBC) (>380 μg/dL), serum iron (SI) level <50 μg/dL, and an iron saturation of <30% but >10% (Fig. 66-1). RBC morphology is generally normal until iron deficiency is severe (see below).

Decreased stimulation of erythropoiesis can be a consequence of inadequate erythropoietin production [e.g., renal disease destroying the renal tubular cells that produce it or hypometabolic states (endocrine deficiency or protein starvation) in which insufficient erythropoietin is produced] or of inadequate erythropoietin action. The anemia of chronic disease is a common entity. It is multifactorial in pathogenesis: inhibition of erythropoietin production, inhibition of iron reutilization (which blocks the response to erythropoietin), and inhibition of erythroid colony proliferation by inflammatory cytokines (e.g., tumor necrosis factor, interferon γ). Hepcidin, a small iron-binding molecule produced by the liver during an acute-phase inflammatory response, may bind iron and prevent its reutilization in hemoglobin synthesis. The laboratory tests shown in Table 66-1 may assist in the differential diagnosis of hypoproliferative anemias. Measurement of hepcidin in the urine is not yet practical or widely available.

TABLE 66-1	DIAGNOSIS OF HYPOPROLIFERATIVE ANEMIAS			
Tests	Iron Deficiency	Inflammation	Renal Disease	Hypometabolic States
Anemia	Mild to severe	Mild	Mild to severe	Mild
MCV (fL)	70–90	80–90	90	90
Morphology	Normo-microcytic	Normocytic	Normocytic	Normocytic
SI	<30	<50	Normal	Normal
TIBC	>360	>300	Normal	Normal
Saturation (%)	<10	10–20	Normal	Normal
Serum ferritin (μg/L)	<15	30–200	115–150	Normal
Iron stores	0	2–4+	1–4+	Normal

Note: MCV, mean corpuscular volume; SI, serum iron; TIBC, total iron-binding capacity.

MATURATION DISORDERS

These result from either defective hemoglobin synthesis, leading to cytoplasmic maturation defects and small relatively empty red cells, or abnormally slow DNA replication, leading to nuclear maturation defects and large full red cells. Defects in hemoglobin synthesis usually result from insufficient iron supply (iron deficiency) or decreased globin production (thalassemia) or are idiopathic (sideroblastic anemia). Defects in DNA synthesis are usually due to nutritional problems (vitamin B_{12} and folate deficiency), toxic (methotrexate or other cancer chemotherapeutic agent) exposure, or intrinsic marrow maturation defects (refractory anemia, myelodysplasia).

Laboratory tests useful in the differential diagnosis of the microcytic anemias are shown in Table 66-2. Mean corpuscular volume (MCV) is generally 60–80 fL. Increased lactate dehydrogenase (LDH) and indirect bilirubin levels suggest an increase in RBC destruction and favor a cause other than iron deficiency. Iron status is best assessed by measuring SI, TIBC, and ferritin levels. Macrocytic MCVs are >94 fL. Folate status is best assessed by measuring red blood cell folate levels. Vitamin B_{12} status is best assessed by measuring serum

TABLE 66-2	DIAGNOSIS OF MICROCYTIC ANEMIA		
Tests	Iron Deficiency	Thalassemia	Sideroblastic Anemia
Smear	Micro/hypo	Micro/hypo with targeting	Variable
SI	<30	Normal to high	Normal to high
TIBC	>360	Normal	Normal
Saturation, %	<10	30–80	30–80
Ferritin, μg/L	<15	50–300	50–300
Hemoglobin pattern	Normal	Abnormal	Normal

Note: SI, serum iron; TIBC, total iron-binding capacity.

B_{12}, homocysteine, and methylmalonic acid levels. Homocysteine and methylmalonic acid levels are elevated in the setting of B_{12} deficiency.

ANEMIA DUE TO RBC DESTRUCTION OR ACUTE BLOOD LOSS

Blood Loss Trauma, GI hemorrhage (may be occult) are common causes; less common are genitourinary sources (menorrhagia, gross hematuria), internal bleeding such as intraperitoneal from spleen or organ rupture, retroperitoneal, iliopsoas hemorrhage (e.g., in hip fractures). Acute bleeding is associated with manifestations of hypovolemia, reticulocytosis, macrocytosis; chronic bleeding is associated with iron deficiency, hypochromia, microcytosis.

Hemolysis Causes are listed in Table 66-3.

1. *Intracellular RBC abnormalities*—most are inherited enzyme defects [glucose-6-phosphate dehydrogenase (G6PD) deficiency > pyruvate kinase deficiency], hemoglobinopathies, sickle cell anemia and variants, thalassemia, unstable hemoglobin variants.
2. *G6PD deficiency*—leads to episodes of hemolysis precipitated by ingestion of drugs that induce oxidant stress on RBCs. These include antimalarials (chloroquine), sulfonamides, analgesics (phenacetin), and other miscellaneous drugs (Table 66-4).
3. *Sickle cell anemia*—characterized by a single-amino-acid change in β globin (valine for glutamic acid in the 6th residue) that produces a molecule of decreased solubility, especially in the absence of O_2. Although anemia and chronic hemolysis are present, the major disease manifestations relate to vasoocclusion from misshapen sickled RBCs. Infarcts in lung, bone, spleen, retina, brain, and other organs lead to symptoms and dysfunction (Fig. 66-2).
4. *Membrane abnormalities* (rare)—spur cell anemia (cirrhosis, anorexia nervosa), paroxysmal nocturnal hemoglobinuria, hereditary spherocytosis (increased RBC osmotic fragility, spherocytes), hereditary elliptocytosis (causes mild hemolytic anemia).

TABLE 66-3 **CLASSIFICATION OF HEMOLYTIC ANEMIAS[a]**

	Intracorpuscular Defects	Extracorpuscular Factors
Hereditary	Hemoglobinopathies Enzymopathies Membrane-cytoskeletal defects	Familial hemolytic uremic syndrome (HUS)
Acquired	Paroxysmal nocturnal hemoglobinuria (PNH)	Mechanical destruction (microangiopathic) Toxic agents Drugs Infectious Autoimmune

[a]There is a strong correlation between hereditary causes and intracorpuscular defects, because such defects are due to inherited mutations; the one exception is PNH, because the defect is due to an acquired somatic mutation. There is also a strong correlation between acquired causes and extracorpuscular factors; the one exception is familial HUS, because here an inherited abnormality allows excessive complement activation, with bouts of production of membrane attack complex capable of severely damaging normal cells.

TABLE 66-4	DRUGS THAT CARRY RISK OF CLINICAL HEMOLYSIS IN PERSONS WITH G6PD DEFICIENCY		
	Definite Risk	**Possible Risk**	**Doubtful Risk**
Antimalarials	Primaquine Dapsone/ chlorproguanil	Chloroquine	Quinine
Sulphonamides/ sulphones	Sulfamethoxazole Others Dapsone	Sulfasalazine Sulfadimidine	Sulfisoxazole Sulfadiazine
Antibacterial/ antibiotics	Cotrimoxazole Nalidixic acid Nitrofurantoin Niridazole	Ciprofloxacin Norfloxacin	Chloramphenicol *p*-Aminosalicylic acid

*Antipyretic/
analgesics*
	Acetanilide
	Phenazopyridine
	  (Pyridium)
		Acetylsalicylic
		  acid high dose
		  (>3 g/d)
			Acetylsalicylic acid
			  <3 g/d
			Acetaminophen
			Phenacetin

Other	Naphthalene Methylene blue	Vitamin K analogues Ascorbic acid >1 g Rasburicase	Doxorubicin Probenecid

5. *Immunohemolytic anemia* (positive Coombs' test, spherocytes). Two types: (a) *warm antibody* (usually IgG)—idiopathic, lymphoma, chronic lymphocytic leukemia, systemic lupus erythematosus, drugs (e.g., methyldopa, penicillins, quinine, quinidine, isoniazid, sulfonamides); and (b) *cold antibody*—cold agglutinin disease (IgM) due to *Mycoplasma* infection, infectious mononucleosis, lymphoma, idiopathic; paroxysmal cold hemoglobinuria (IgG) due to syphilis, viral infections.

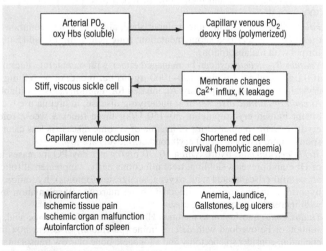

FIGURE 66-2 Pathophysiology of sickle cell crisis.

6. *Mechanical trauma* (macro- and microangiopathic hemolytic anemias; schistocytes)—prosthetic heart valves, vasculitis, malignant hypertension, eclampsia, renal graft rejection, giant hemangioma, scleroderma, thrombotic thrombocytopenic purpura, hemolytic-uremic syndrome, disseminated intravascular coagulation, march hemoglobinuria (e.g., marathon runners, bongo drummers).

7. *Direct toxic effect*—infections (e.g., malaria, *Clostridium perfringens* toxin, toxoplasmosis).

8. *Hypersplenism* (pancytopenia may be present).

Laboratory Abnormalities Elevated reticulocyte index, polychromasia and nucleated RBCs on smear; also spherocytes, elliptocytes, schistocytes, or target, spur, or sickle cells may be present depending on disorder; elevated unconjugated serum bilirubin and LDH, elevated plasma hemoglobin, low or absent haptoglobin; urine hemosiderin present in intravascular but not extravascular hemolysis, Coombs' test (immunohemolytic anemias), osmotic fragility test (hereditary spherocytosis), hemoglobin electrophoresis (sickle cell anemia, thalassemia), G6PD assay (best performed after resolution of hemolytic episode to prevent false-negative result).

 Anemia

General Approaches

The acuteness and severity of the anemia determine whether transfusion therapy with packed RBCs is indicated. Rapid occurrence of severe anemia (e.g., after acute GI hemorrhage resulting in Hct < 25%, following volume repletion) or development of angina or other symptoms is an indication for transfusion. Hct should increase 3–4% [Hb by 10 g/L (1 g/dL)] with each unit of packed RBCs, assuming no ongoing losses. Chronic anemia (e.g., vitamin B_{12} deficiency), even when severe, may not require transfusion therapy if the pt is compensated and specific therapy (e.g., vitamin B_{12}) is instituted.

Specific Disorders

1. *Iron deficiency*: find and treat cause of blood loss, oral iron (e.g., $FeSO_4$ 300 mg tid).

2. *Folate deficiency*: common in malnourished, alcoholics; less common now than before folate food supplementation; folic acid 1 mg PO qd (5 mg qd for pts with malabsorption).

3. *Vitamin B_{12} deficiency*: can be managed either with parenteral vitamin B_{12} 100 μg IM qd for 7 d, then 100–1000 μg IM per month or with 2 mg oral crystalline vitamin B_{12} per day. An inhaled formulation is also available.

4. *Anemia of chronic disease*: treat underlying disease; in uremia use recombinant human erythropoietin, 50–150 U/kg three times a week; role of erythropoietin in other forms of anemia of chronic disease is less clear; response more likely if serum erythropoietin levels are low.

5. *Sickle cell anemia*: hydroxyurea 10–30 mg/kg per day PO increases level of HbF and prevents sickling; treat infections early, supplemental folic acid; painful crises treated with oxygen, analgesics (opioids), hydration, and hypertransfusion; consider allogeneic bone marrow transplantation in pts with increasing frequency of crises.

6. *Thalassemia*: transfusion to maintain Hb > 90 g/L (>9 g/dL), folic acid, prevention of Fe overload with deferoxamine (parenteral) or deferasirox (oral) chelation; consider splenectomy and allogeneic bone marrow transplantation.

7. *Aplastic anemia*: antithymocyte globulin and cyclosporine leads to improvement in 70%, bone marrow transplantation in young pts with a matched donor.
8. *Autoimmune hemolysis*: glucocorticoids, sometimes immunosuppressive agents, danazol, plasmapheresis, rituximab.
9. *G6PD deficiency*: avoid agents known to precipitate hemolysis.

For a more detailed discussion, see Adamson JW, Chap. 98; Benz EJ, Chap. 99; Hoffbrand AV, Chap. 100; Luzzato L, Chap. 101; Young NS, Chap. 102; pp. 628–671, in HPIM-17.

67 Leukocytosis and Leukopenia

LEUKOCYTOSIS

APPROACH

Review smear (? abnormal cells present) and obtain differential count. The normal values for concentration of blood leukocytes are shown in Table 67-1.

NEUTROPHILIA

Absolute neutrophil count (polys and bands) > 10,000/μL. The pathophysiology of neutrophilia involves increased production, increased marrow mobilization, or decreased margination (adherence to vessel walls).

Causes (1) *Exercise, stress*; (2) *infections*—esp. bacterial; smear shows increased numbers of immature neutrophils ("left shift"), toxic granulations, Döhle bodies; (3) *burns*; (4) *tissue necrosis* (e.g., myocardial, pulmonary, renal infarction); (5) *chronic inflammatory disorders* (e.g., gout, vasculitis); (6) *drugs* (e.g., glucocorticoids, epinephrine, lithium); (7) *cytokines* [e.g., granulocyte colony-stimulating factor (G-CSF), granulocyte-macrophage colony-stimulating factor (GM-CSF)]; (8) *myeloproliferative disorders* (Chap. 70); (9) *metabolic* (e.g., ketoacidosis, uremia); (10) *other*—malignant neoplasms, acute hemorrhage or hemolysis, after splenectomy.

TABLE 67-1	NORMAL VALUES FOR LEUKOCYTE CONCENTRATION IN BLOOD		
Cell Type	Mean, cells/μL	95% Confidence Intervals, cells/μL	Total WBC, %
Neutrophil	3650	1830–7250	30–60%
Lymphocyte	2500	1500–4000	20–50%
Monocyte	430	200–950	2–10%
Eosinophil	150	0–700	0.3–5%
Basophil	30	0–150	0.6–1.8%

LEUKEMOID REACTION

Extreme elevation of leukocyte count (>50,000/μL) composed of mature and/or immature neutrophils.

Causes (1) *Infection* (severe, chronic, e.g., tuberculosis), esp. in children; (2) *hemolysis* (severe); (3) *malignant neoplasms* (esp. carcinoma of the breast, lung, kidney); (4) *cytokines* (e.g., G-CSF, GM-CSF). May be distinguished from chronic myeloid leukemia (CML) by measurement of the leukocyte alkaline phosphatase (LAP) level: elevated in leukemoid reactions, depressed in CML.

LEUKOERYTHROBLASTIC REACTION

Similar to leukemoid reaction with addition of nucleated red blood cells (RBCs) and schistocytes on blood smear.

Causes (1) *Myelophthisis*—invasion of the bone marrow by tumor, fibrosis, granulomatous processes; smear shows "teardrop" RBCs; (2) *myelofibrosis*—same pathophysiology as myelophthisis, but the fibrosis is a primary marrow disorder; (3) *hemorrhage* or *hemolysis* (rarely, in severe cases).

LYMPHOCYTOSIS

Absolute lymphocyte count > 5000/μL.

Causes (1) *Infection*—infectious mononucleosis, hepatitis, cytomegalovirus, rubella, pertussis, tuberculosis, brucellosis, syphilis; (2) *endocrine disorders*—thyrotoxicosis, adrenal insufficiency; (3) *neoplasms*—chronic lymphocytic leukemia (CLL), most common cause of lymphocyte count > 10,000/μL.

MONOCYTOSIS

Absolute monocyte count > 800/μL.

Causes (1) *Infection*—subacute bacterial endocarditis, tuberculosis, brucellosis, rickettsial diseases (e.g., Rocky Mountain spotted fever), malaria, leishmaniasis; (2) *granulomatous diseases*—sarcoidosis, Crohn's disease; (3) *collagen vascular diseases*—rheumatoid arthritis, systemic lupus erythematosus (SLE), polyarteritis nodosa, polymyositis, temporal arteritis; (4) *hematologic diseases*—leukemias, lymphoma, myeloproliferative and myelodysplastic syndromes, hemolytic anemia, chronic idiopathic neutropenia; (5) *malignant neoplasms*.

EOSINOPHILIA

Absolute eosinophil count > 500/μL.

Causes (1) *Drugs*, (2) *parasitic infections*, (3) *allergic diseases*, (4) *collagen vascular diseases*, (5) *malignant neoplasms*, (6) *hypereosinophilic syndromes*.

BASOPHILIA

Absolute basophil count > 100/μL.

Causes (1) *Allergic diseases*, (2) *myeloproliferative disorders* (esp. CML), (3) *chronic inflammatory disorders* (rarely).

LEUKOPENIA

Total leukocyte count < 4300/μL.

NEUTROPENIA

Absolute neutrophil count < 2000/μL (increased risk of bacterial infection with count < 1000/μL). The pathophysiology of neutropenia involves decreased production or increased peripheral destruction.

Causes (1) *Drugs*—cancer chemotherapeutic agents are most common cause, also phenytoin, carbamazepine, indomethacin, chloramphenicol, penicillins, sulfonamides, cephalosporins, propylthiouracil, phenothiazines, captopril, methyldopa, procainamide, chlorpropamide, thiazides, cimetidine, allopurinol, colchicine, ethanol, penicillamine, and immunosuppressive agents; (2) *infections*—viral (e.g., influenza, hepatitis, infectious mononucleosis, HIV), bacterial (e.g., typhoid fever, miliary tuberculosis, fulminant sepsis), malaria; (3) *nutritional*—B$_{12}$, folate deficiencies; (4) *benign*—mild cyclic neutropenia common in blacks, no associated risk of infection; (5) *hematologic diseases*—cyclic neutropenia (q21d, with recurrent infections common), leukemia, myelodysplasia (preleukemia), aplastic anemia, bone marrow infiltration (uncommon cause), Chédiak-Higashi syndrome; (6) *hypersplenism*—e.g., Felty's syndrome, congestive splenomegaly, Gaucher's disease; (7) *autoimmune diseases*—idiopathic, SLE, lymphoma (may see positive antineutrophil antibodies).

℞ The Febrile, Neutropenic Patient

(See Chap. 26) In addition to usual sources of infection, consider paranasal sinuses, oral cavity (including teeth and gums), anorectal region; empirical therapy with broad-spectrum antibiotics (e.g., ceftazidime) is indicated after blood and other appropriate cultures are obtained. Prolonged febrile neutropenia (>7 days) leads to increased risk of disseminated fungal infections; requires addition of antifungal chemotherapy (e.g., amphotericin B). The duration of chemotherapy-induced neutropenia may be shortened by a few days by treatment with the cytokines GM-CSF or G-CSF.

LYMPHOPENIA

Absolute lymphocyte count < 1000/μL.

Causes (1) *Acute stressful illness*—e.g., myocardial infarction, pneumonia, sepsis; (2) *glucocorticoid therapy*; (3) *lymphoma* (esp. Hodgkin's disease); (4) *immunodeficiency syndromes*—ataxia telangiectasia and Wiskott-Aldrich and DiGeorge syndromes; (5) *immunosuppressive therapy*—e.g., antilymphocyte globulin, cyclophosphamide; (6) *large-field radiation therapy* (esp. for lymphoma); (7) *intestinal lymphangiectasia* (increased lymphocyte loss); (8) *chronic illness*—e.g., congestive heart failure, uremia, SLE, disseminated malignancies; (9) *bone marrow failure/replacement*—e.g., aplastic anemia, miliary tuberculosis.

MONOCYTOPENIA

Absolute monocyte count < 100/μL.

Causes (1) *Acute stressful illness*, (2) *glucocorticoid therapy*, (3) *aplastic anemia*, (4) *leukemia* (certain types, e.g., hairy cell leukemia), (5) *chemotherapeutic and immunosuppressive agents*.

EOSINOPENIA

Absolute eosinophil count < 50/μL.

Causes   (1) *Acute stressful illness*, (2) *glucocorticoid therapy.*

For a more detailed discussion, see Holland SM, Gallin JI: Disorders of Granulocytes and Monocytes, Chap. 61, p. 375; in HPIM-17.

68 Bleeding and Thrombotic Disorders

BLEEDING DISORDERS

Bleeding may result from abnormalities of (1) platelets, (2) blood vessel walls, or (3) coagulation. Platelet disorders characteristically produce petechial and purpuric skin lesions and bleeding from mucosal surfaces. Defective coagulation results in ecchymoses, hematomas, and mucosal and, in some disorders, recurrent joint bleeding (hemarthroses).

PLATELET DISORDERS

Thrombocytopenia   Normal platelet count is 150,000–350,000/μL. Thrombocytopenia is defined as a platelet count < 100,000/μL. Bleeding time, a measurement of platelet function, is abnormally increased if platelet count < 100,000/μL; injury or surgery may provoke excess bleeding. Spontaneous bleeding is unusual unless count < 20,000/μL; platelet count < 10,000/μL is often associated with serious hemorrhage. Bone marrow examination shows increased number of megakaryocytes in disorders associated with accelerated platelet destruction; decreased number in disorders of platelet production. Evaluation of thrombocytopenia is shown in Fig. 68-1.

Causes   (1) Production defects such as marrow injury (e.g., drugs, irradiation), marrow failure (e.g., aplastic anemia), marrow invasion (e.g., carcinoma, leukemia, fibrosis); (2) sequestration due to splenomegaly; (3) accelerated destruction—causes include:

- *Drugs* such as chemotherapeutic agents, thiazides, ethanol, estrogens, sulfonamides, quinidine, quinine, methyldopa.
- *Heparin-induced thrombocytopenia* is seen in 5% of pts receiving >5 days of therapy and is due to in vivo platelet aggregation often from anti—platelet factor 4 antibodies. Arterial and occasionally venous thromboses may result.
- *Autoimmune destruction* by an antibody mechanism; may be idiopathic or associated with systemic lupus erythematosus (SLE), lymphoma, HIV.
- *Idiopathic thrombocytopenic purpura* (ITP) has two forms: an acute, self-limited disorder of childhood requiring no specific therapy, and a chronic disorder of adults (esp. women 20–40 years). Chronic ITP may be due to autoantibodies to glycoprotein IIb-IIIa or glycoprotein Ib-IX complexes.
- *Disseminated intravascular coagulation* (DIC)—platelet consumption with coagulation factor depletion [prolonged prothrombin time (PT), partial thromboplastin time (PTT)] and stimulation of fibrinolysis [generation of fi-

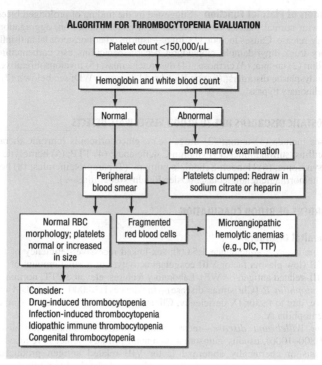

ALGORITHM FOR THROMBOCYTOPENIA EVALUATION

Platelet count <150,000/μL

↓

Hemoglobin and white blood count

↓

Normal → Abnormal

Abnormal ↓

Bone marrow examination

Normal ↓

Peripheral blood smear → Platelets clumped: Redraw in sodium citrate or heparin

Normal RBC morphology; platelets normal or increased in size

Fragmented red blood cells → Microangiopathic hemolytic anemias (e.g., DIC, TTP)

Consider:
Drug-induced thrombocytopenia
Infection-induced thrombocytopenia
Idiopathic immune thrombocytopenia
Congenital thrombocytopenia

FIGURE 68-1 Algorithm for evaluating the thrombocytopenic patient.

brin split products (FSPs)]. Blood smear shows microangiopathic hemolysis (schistocytes). Causes include infection (esp. meningococcal, pneumococcal, gram-negative bacteremias), extensive burns, trauma, or thrombosis; giant hemangioma, retained dead fetus, heat stroke, mismatched blood transfusion, metastatic carcinoma, acute promyelocytic leukemia.

• *Thrombotic thrombocytopenic purpura* (TTP)—rare disorder characterized by microangiopathic hemolytic anemia, fever, thrombocytopenia, renal dysfunction (and/or hematuria), and neurologic dysfunction caused by failure to cleave von Willebrand factor (vWF) normally.

• *Hemorrhage with extensive transfusion.*

Pseudothrombocytopenia   Platelet clumping secondary to collection of blood in EDTA (0.3% of pts). Examination of blood smear establishes diagnosis.

Thrombocytosis   Platelet count > 350,000/μL. Either primary (essential thrombocytosis; Chap. 70) or secondary (reactive); latter secondary to severe hemorrhage, iron deficiency, surgery, after splenectomy (transient), malignant neoplasms (esp. Hodgkin's disease, polycythemia vera), chronic inflammatory diseases (e.g., inflammatory bowel disease), recovery from acute infection, vitamin B_{12} deficiency, drugs (e.g., vincristine, epinephrine). Rebound thrombocytosis may occur after marrow recovery from cytotoxic agents, alcohol. Primary thrombocytosis may be complicated by bleeding and/or thrombosis; secondary rarely causes hemostatic problems.

Disorders of Platelet Function Suggested by the finding of prolonged bleeding time with normal platelet count. Defect is in platelet adhesion, aggregation, or granule release. Causes include (1) drugs—aspirin, other nonsteroidal anti-inflammatory drugs, dipyridamole, clopidogrel, heparin, penicillins, esp. carbenicillin, ticarcillin; (2) uremia; (3) cirrhosis; (4) dysproteinemias; (5) myeloproliferative and myelodysplastic disorders; (6) von Willebrand disease (vWD; see below); (7) cardiopulmonary bypass.

HEMOSTATIC DISORDERS DUE TO BLOOD VESSEL WALL DEFECTS

Causes include (1) aging; (2) drugs—e.g., glucocorticoids (chronic therapy), penicillins, sulfonamides; (3) vitamin C deficiency; (4) TTP; (5) hemolytic uremic syndrome; (6) Henoch-Schönlein purpura; (7) paraproteinemias; (8) hereditary hemorrhagic telangiectasia (Osler-Rendu-Weber disease).

DISORDERS OF BLOOD COAGULATION

Congenital Disorders

1. *Hemophilia A*—incidence 1:5,000; sex-linked recessive deficiency of factor VIII (low plasma factor VIII coagulant activity, but normal amount of factor VIII–related antigen—vWF). Laboratory features: elevated PTT, normal PT.
2. *Hemophilia B* (Christmas disease)—incidence 1:30,000, sex-linked recessive, due to factor IX deficiency. Clinical and laboratory features similar to hemophilia A.
3. *von Willebrand disease*—most common inherited coagulation disorder (1:800–1000), usually autosomal dominant; primary defect is reduced synthesis or chemically abnormal factor VIII–related antigen produced by platelets and endothelium, resulting in abnormal platelet function.

Acquired Disorders

1. *Vitamin K deficiency*—impairs production of factors II (prothrombin), VII, IX, and X; vitamin K is a cofactor in the carboxylation of glutamate residues on prothrombin complex proteins; major source of vitamin K is dietary (esp. green vegetables), with minor production by gut bacteria. Laboratory features: elevated PT and PTT.
2. *Liver disease*—results in deficiencies of all clotting factors except VIII. Laboratory features: elevated PT, normal or elevated PTT.
3. *Other disorders*—DIC, fibrinogen deficiency (liver disease, L-asparaginase therapy, rattlesnake bites), other factor deficiencies, circulating anticoagulants (lymphoma, SLE, idiopathic), massive transfusion (dilutional coagulopathy).

℞ Bleeding Disorders

Thrombocytopenia Caused by Drugs
Discontinue use of possible offending agents; expect recovery in 7–10 days. Platelet transfusions may be needed if platelet count < 10,000/μL.

Heparin-Induced Thrombocytopenia
Discontinue heparin promptly. A direct thrombin inhibitor such as lepirudin (0.4-mg/kg bolus, 0.15-mg/kg per hour infusion; PTT target 1.5–2.5 × baseline) or argatroban (2-μg/kg per min infusion; PTT target 1.5–3 × baseline) should be used for treatment of thromboses. Do not use low-molecular-weight heparin (LMWH), as antibodies often cross-react.

Chronic ITP

Prednisone, initially 1–2 mg/kg per day, then slow taper to keep the platelet count > 60,000/μL. IV immunoglobulin (2 g/kg in divided doses over 2–5 days) to block phagocytic destruction may be useful. Rituximab is effective in pts refractory to glucocorticoids. Splenectomy, danazol (androgen), or other agents (e.g., vincristine, cyclophosphamide, fludarabine) are indicated for refractory pts or those requiring >5–10 mg prednisone daily.

DIC

Control of underlying disease most important; platelets, fresh-frozen plasma (FFP) to correct clotting parameters. Heparin may be beneficial in pts with acute promyelocytic leukemia.

TTP

Plasmapheresis and FFP infusions (plasma exchange), possibly IV IgG; recovery in two-thirds of cases. Plasmapheresis removes inhibitors of the vWF cleavage enzyme (ADAMTS13), and FFP replaces the enzyme.

Disorders of Platelet Function

Remove or reverse underlying cause. Dialysis and/or cryoprecipitate infusions (10 bags/24 h) may be helpful for platelet dysfunction associated with uremia.

Hemostatic Disorders

Withdraw offending drugs, replace vitamin C, plasmapheresis, and plasma infusion for TTP.

Hemophilia A

Factor VIII replacement for bleeding or before surgical procedure; degree and duration of replacement depends on severity of bleeding. Give factor VIII (e.g., Recombinate) to obtain a 15% (for mild bleeding) to 50% (for severe bleeding) factor VIII level. The duration should range from a single dose of factor VIII to therapy bid for up to 2 weeks. Dose is calculated as follows:

$$\text{Factor VIII dose} = (\text{Target level} - \text{baseline level}) \times \text{weight (kg)} \times 0.5 \text{ unit/kg}$$

Hemophilia B

Recombinant factor IX (e.g., Benefix), FFP or factor IX concentrates (e.g., Proplex, Konyne). Because of the longer half-life, once-daily treatment is sufficient. Dose is calculated as follows:

$$\text{Factor IX dose} = (\text{Target level} - \text{baseline level}) \times \text{weight (kg)} \times 1 \text{ unit/kg}$$

von Willebrand Disease

Desmopressin (1-deamino-8-D-arginine vasopressin) increases release of vWF from endothelial stores in type 1 vWD. It is given IV (0.3 μg/kg) or by nasal spray (2 squirts of 1.5-mg/mL fluid in each nostril). For types 2A, 2M, and 3, cryoprecipitate (plasma product rich in factor VIII) or factor VIII concentrate (Humate-P, Koate HS) is used: up to 10 bags bid for 48–72 h, depending on the severity of bleeding.

Vitamin K Deficiency

Vitamin K, 10 mg SC or slow IV.

Liver Disease

Fresh-frozen plasma.

THROMBOTIC DISORDERS

HYPERCOAGULABLE STATE

Consider in pts with recurrent episodes of venous thrombosis [i.e., deep-venous thrombosis (DVT), pulmonary embolism (PE)]. Causes include (1) venous stasis (e.g., pregnancy, immobilization); (2) vasculitis; (3) cancer and myeloproliferative disorders; (4) oral contraceptives; (5) lupus anticoagulant—antibody to platelet phospholipid, stimulates coagulation; (6) heparin-induced thrombocytopenia; (7) deficiencies of endogenous anticoagulant factors—antithrombin III, protein C, protein S; (8) factor V Leiden—mutation in factor V (Arg → Glu at position 506) confers resistance to inactivation by protein C, accounts for 25% of cases of recurrent thrombosis; (9) prothrombin gene mutation—Glu → Arg at position 20210 results in increased prothrombin levels; accounts for about 6% of thromboses; (10) other—paroxysmal nocturnal hemoglobinuria, dysfibrinogenemias (abnormal fibrinogen).

The approach to the diagnosis of the pt with DVT and/or PE is discussed in Chap. 140.

℞ Thrombotic Disorders

Correct underlying disorder whenever possible; long-term warfarin therapy is otherwise indicated.

Anticoagulant Agents

1. *Heparin* (Table 68-1)—enhances activity of antithrombin III; parenteral agent of choice. LMWH is the preparation of choice (enoxaparin or dalteparin). It can be administered SC, monitoring of the PTT is unnecessary, and it is less likely to induce antibodies and thrombocytopenia. The usual dose is 100 U/kg SC bid. Unfractionated heparin should be given only if LMWH is unavailable. In adults, the dose of unfractionated heparin is 25,000–40,000 U continuous IV infusion over 24 h following initial IV bolus of 5000 U; monitor by following PTT; should be maintained between 1.5 and 2 times upper normal limit. Prophylactic anticoagulation to lower risk of venous thrombosis recommended in some pts (e.g., postoperative, immobilized) (Table 68-1). Prophylactic doses of unfractionated heparin are 5000 U SC bid or tid. Major complication of unfractionated heparin therapy is hemorrhage—manage by discontinuing heparin; for severe bleeding, administer protamine (1 mg/100 U heparin); results in rapid neutralization.

2. *Warfarin* (Coumadin)—vitamin K antagonist, decreases levels of factors II, VII, IX, X, and anticoagulant proteins C and S. Administered over 2–3 days; initial load of 5–10 mg PO qd followed by titration of daily dose to keep PT 1.5–2 times control PT or 2–3 times if the International Normalized Ratio method is used. Complications include hemorrhage, warfarin-induced skin necrosis (rare, occurs in persons deficient in protein C), teratogenic effects. Warfarin effect reversed by administration of vitamin K; FFP infused if urgent reversal necessary. Numerous drugs potentiate or antagonize warfarin effect. Potentiating agents include chlorpromazine, chloral hydrate, sulfonamides, chloramphenicol, other broad-spectrum antibiotics, allopurinol, cimetidine, tricyclic antidepressants, disulfiram, laxatives, high-dose salicylates, thyroxine, clofibrate. Some pts who are sensitive to warfarin effects have genetic defects metabolizing the drug. Antagonizing agents include vitamin K, barbiturates, rifampin, cholestyramine, oral contraceptives, thiazides.

TABLE 68-1 **ANTICOAGULANT THERAPY WITH LOW-MOLECULAR-WEIGHT AND UNFRACTIONATED HEPARIN**

Clinical Indication	Heparin Dose and Schedule	Target PTT[a]	LMWH Dose and Schedule[b]
Venous thrombosis pulmonary embolism			
Treatment	5000 U IV bolus; 1000–1500 U/h	2–2.5	100 U/kg SC bid
Prophylaxis	5000 U SC q8–12h	<1.5	100 U/kg SC bid
Acute myocardial infarction			
With thrombolytic therapy	5000 U IV bolus; 1000 U/h	1.5–2.5	100 U/kg SC bid
With mural thrombus	8000 U SC q8h + warfarin	1.5–2.0	100 U /kg SC bid
Unstable angina	5000 U IV bolus; 1000 U/h	1.5–2.5	100 U/kg SC bid
Prophylaxis			
General surgery	5000 U SC bid	<1.5	100 U/kg SC before and bid
Orthopedic surgery	10,000 U SC bid	1.5	100 U/kg SC before and bid
Medical pts with CHF, MI	10,000 U SC bid	1.5	100 U/kg SC bid

[a]Times normal control; assumes PTT has been standardized to heparin levels so that 1.5–2.5 × normal equals 0.2–0.4 U/mL; if PTT is normal (27–35 s), start with 5000 U bolus 1300 U/h infusion monitoring PTT; if PTT at recheck is <50 s, rebolus with 5000 U and increase infusion by 100 U/h; if PTT at recheck is 50–60 s, increase infusion rate by 100 U/h; if PTT at recheck is 60–85 s, no change; if PTT at recheck is 85–100 s, decrease infusion rate 100 U/h; if PTT at recheck is 100–120 s, stop infusion for 30 min and decrease rate 100 U/h at restart; if PTT at recheck is >120 s, stop infusion for 60 min and decrease rate 200 U/h at restart.
[b]LMWH does not affect PTT, and PTT is not used to adjust dosage.
Note: PTT, partial thromboplastin time; LMWH, low-molecular-weight heparin; CHF, congestive heart failure; MI, myocardial infarction.

3. *Fondaparinux*—a pentapeptide that directly inhibits factor Xa. It is given at a dose of 2.5 mg SC daily for prophylaxis and 7.5 mg SC daily for treatment of thrombosis and does not require monitoring. Unlike the heparins, it does not bind to platelet factor 4 and does not elicit the antibodies that produce heparin-induced thrombocytopenia.
4. *Argatroban and lepirudin*—direct thrombin inhibitors. These agents are being compared to LMWH and are commonly used in pts with heparin-induced thrombocytopenia. Both are monitored with the activated PTT.

In-hospital anticoagulation is usually initiated with heparin for 4–10 days, with subsequent maintenance on warfarin after an overlap of 3 days. Duration of therapy depends on underlying condition; calf DVT with clear precipitating cause, 3 months; proximal or idiopathic DVT or PE, 6–12 months; recurrent idiopathic DVT, 12 months minimum; embolic disease with ongoing risk factor, long-term, indefinite.

Fibrinolytic Agents

Tissue plasminogen activators mediate clot lysis by activating plasmin, which degrades fibrin. Currently available versions include streptokinase, urokinase, anistreplase (acylated plasminogen streptokinase activator complex), and three modestly distinct forms of recombinant tissue plasminogen activator (tPA): alteplase, tenecteplase, and reteplase. Indications include treatment of DVT, with lower incidence of postphlebitic syndrome (chronic venous stasis, skin ulceration) than with heparin therapy; massive PE, arterial embolic occlusion of an extremity, treatment of acute myocardial infarction (MI), unstable angina pectoris. Dosages for fibrinolytic agents: (1) tPA—for acute MI and massive PE (adult > 65 kg), 10-mg IV bolus over 1–2 min, then 50 mg IV over 1 h and 40 mg IV over next 2 h (total dose = 100 mg). tPA is slightly more effective but more expensive than streptokinase for treatment of acute MI. (2) Streptokinase—for acute MI, 1.5 million IU IV over 60 min; or 20,000 IU as a bolus intracoronary (IC) infusion, followed by 2000 IU/min for 60 min IC. For PE or arterial or deep-venous thrombosis, 250,000 IU over 30 min, then 100,000 IU/h for 24 h (PE) or 72 h (arterial or deep-venous thrombosis). (3) Urokinase—for PE, 4400 IU/kg IV over 10 min, then 4400 (IU/kg)/h IV for 12 h.

Fibrinolytic therapy is usually followed by a period of anticoagulant therapy with heparin. Fibrinolytic agents are contraindicated in pts with (1) active internal bleeding; (2) recent (<2–3 months) cerebrovascular accident; (3) intracranial neoplasm, aneurysm, or recent head trauma.

Antiplatelet Agents

Aspirin inhibits platelet function by blocking the ability of cyclooxygenase (COX-1) to synthesize thromboxane A2. The thienopyridines (ticlopidine and clopidogrel) inhibit ADP-induced platelet aggregation by blocking its receptor ($P2Y_{12}$). Dipyridamole acts by inhibiting phosphodiesterase, which permits cAMP levels to increase and block activation. Glycoprotein IIb/IIIa (GPIIb/IIIa) antagonists block the integrin receptors on the platelet and prevent platelet aggregation. Three such agents are now in use: abciximab, an Fab antibody fragment that binds to the activated form of GPIIb/IIIa; eptifibatide, a cyclic heptapeptide that includes the KGD tripeptide motif that the GPIIb/IIIa receptor recognizes; and tirofiban, a tyrosine derivative that mimics the KGD motif.

Aspirin (160–325 mg/d) plus clopidogrel (400-mg loading dose then 75 mg/d) may be beneficial in lowering incidence of arterial thrombotic events (stroke, MI) in high-risk pts. Antiplatelet agents are useful in preventing strokes, complications from percutaneous coronary interventions, and progression of unstable angina.

For a more detailed discussion, see Konkle BA: Bleeding and Thrombosis, Chap. 59, p. 363; Konkle BA: Disorders of Platelets and Vessel Wall, Chap. 109, p. 718; Arruda V, High KA: Coagulation Disorders, Chap. 110, p. 725; and Weitz JI: Antiplatelet, Anticoagulant, and Fibrinolytic Drugs, Chap. 112, p. 735, in HPIM-17.

69 Cancer Chemotherapy

BIOLOGY OF TUMOR GROWTH

Two essential features of cancer cells are uncontrolled growth and the ability to metastasize. The malignant phenotype of a cell is the end result of a series of genetic changes that remove safeguards restricting cell growth and induce new features that enable the cell to metastasize, including surface receptors for binding to basement membranes, enzymes to poke holes in anatomic barriers, cytokines to facilitate mobility, and angiogenic factors to develop a new vascular lifeline for nutrients and oxygen. These genetic changes usually involve increased or abnormal expression or activity of certain genes known as *proto-oncogenes* (often growth factors or their receptors, enzymes in growth pathways, or transcription factors), deletion or inactivation of tumor-suppressor genes, and defects in DNA repair enzymes. These genetic changes may occur by point mutation, gene amplification, gene rearrangement, or epigenetic changes such as altered gene methylation.

Once cells are malignant, their growth kinetics are similar to those of normal cells but lack regulation. For unclear reasons, tumor growth kinetics follow a Gompertzian curve: as the tumor mass increases, the fraction of dividing cells declines. Thus, by the time a cancer is large enough to be detected clinically, its growth fraction is often small. Unfortunately, tumor growth usually does not stop altogether before the tumor reaches a lethal tumor burden. Cancer cells proceed through the same cell-cycle stages as normal cycling cells: G_1 (period of preparation for DNA synthesis), S (DNA synthesis), G_2 (tetraploid phase preceding mitosis in which integrity of DNA replication is assessed), and M (mitosis). Some noncycling cells may remain in a G_0, or resting, phase for long periods. Certain chemotherapeutic agents are specific for cells in certain phases of the cell cycle, a fact that is important in designing effective chemotherapeutic regimens.

DEVELOPMENT OF DRUG RESISTANCE

Drug resistance can be divided into de novo resistance or acquired resistance. De novo resistance refers to the tendency of many of the most common solid tumors to be unresponsive to chemotherapeutic agents. In acquired resistance, tumors initially responsive to chemotherapy develop resistance during treatment, usually because resistant clones appear within tumor cell populations (Table 69-1).

Resistance can be specific to single drugs because of (1) defective transport of the drug, (2) decreased activating enzymes, (3) increased drug inactivation, (4) increases in target enzyme levels, or (5) alterations in target molecules. Multiple drug resistance occurs in cells overexpressing the P glycoprotein, a membrane glycoprotein responsible for enhanced efflux of drugs from cells, but there are other mechanisms as well.

CATEGORIES OF CHEMOTHERAPEUTIC AGENTS AND MAJOR TOXICITIES

A partial list of toxicities is shown in Table 69-2; some toxicities may apply only to certain members of a group of drugs.

TABLE 69-1   CURABILITY OF CANCERS WITH CHEMOTHERAPY

Advanced cancers with possible cure

Acute lymphoid and acute myeloid leukemia (pediatric/adult)

Hodgkin's disease (pediatric/adult)

Lymphomas—certain types (pediatric/adult)

Germ cell neoplasms
   Embryonal carcinoma
   Teratocarcinoma
   Seminoma or dysgerminoma
   Choriocarcinoma

Gestational trophoblastic neoplasia

Pediatric neoplasms
   Wilms' tumor
   Embryonal rhabdomyocarcinoma
   Ewing's sarcoma
   Peripheral neuroepithelioma
   Neuroblastoma

Small cell lung carcinoma

Ovarian carcinoma

Advanced cancers possibly cured by chemotherapy and radiation

Squamous carcinoma (head and neck)

Squamous carcinoma (anus)

Breast carcinoma

Carcinoma of the uterine cervix

Non-small cell lung carcinoma (stage III)

Small-cell lung carcinoma

Cancers possibly cured with chemotherapy as adjuvant to surgery

Breast carcinoma

Colorectal carcinoma[a]

Osteogenic sarcoma

Soft tissue sarcoma

Cancers possibly cured with "high-dose" chemotherapy with stem cell support

Relapsed leukemias, lymphoid and myeloid

Relapsed leukemias, lymphoid and myeloid

Relapsed lymphomas, Hodgkin's and non-Hodgkin's

Chronic myeloid leukemia

Multiple myeloma

Cancers responsive with useful palliation, but not cure, by therapy

Bladder carcinoma

Chronic myeloid leukemia

Hairy cell leukemia

Chronic lymphocytic leukemia

Lymphoma—certain types

Multiple myeloma

Gastric carcinoma

Cervix carcinoma

Endometrial carcinoma

Soft tissue sarcoma

Head and neck cancer

Renal carcinoma

Islet-cell neoplasms

Breast carcinoma

Colorectal carcinoma

Tumors poorly responsive in advanced stages to therapy

Pancreatic carcinoma

Biliary-tract neoplasms

Thyroid carcinoma

Carcinoma of the vulva

Non-small cell lung carcinoma

Prostate carcinoma

Melanoma

Hepatocellular carcinoma

Adrenocortical carcinoma

[a]Rectum also receives radiation therapy.

COMPLICATIONS OF THERAPY

While the effects of cancer chemotherapeutic agents may be exerted primarily on the malignant cell population, virtually all currently employed regimens have profound effects on normal tissues as well. Every side effect of treatment must be balanced against potential benefits expected, and pts must always be fully apprised of the toxicities they may encounter. While the duration of certain adverse effects may be short-lived, others, such as sterility and the risk of secondary malignancy, have long-term implications; consideration of these effects is important in the use of regimens as adjuvant therapy. The combined toxicity of regimens involving radiotherapy and chemotherapy is greater than that seen with each modality alone. Teratogenesis is a special concern in treating

TABLE 69-2 TOXICITIES OF CANCER TREATMENTS

Agent	Toxicities
Alkylating agents	
(add alkyl groups to N-7 or O-6 of guanine)	
Busulfan	Nausea, vomiting, myelosuppression,
Chlorambucil	sterility, alopecia, acute leukemia
Cyclophosphamide	(rare), hemorrhagic cystitis, pul-
Ifosfamide	monary fibrosis
Dacarbazine	
Mechlorethamine	
Nitrosoureas	
Melphalan	
Bendamustine	
Antimetabolites	
(inhibit DNA or RNA synthesis)	
5-Fluorouracil	Nausea, vomiting, myelosuppression,
Capecitabine	oral ulceration, hepatic toxicity,
Fludarabine	alopecia, neurologic symptoms
Cladribine	
Cytarabine	
Methotrexate	
Pemetrexed	
Hydroxyurea	
Pentostatin	
Azathioprine	
Thioguanine	
Tubulin poisons	
(block tubule polymerization or depolymerization)	
Vincristine	Nausea, vomiting, myelosuppression,
Vinblastine	vesicant effect, ileus, hypersensitiv-
Vinorelbine	ity reaction, peripheral neuropathy,
Paclitaxel	SIADH
Docetaxel	
Estramustine	
Topoisomerase inhibitors	
(interfere with DNA unwinding/ repair)	
Doxorubicin	Nausea, vomiting, myelosuppression,
Daunorubicin	vesicant effect, cardiac failure,
Idarubicin	acute leukemia (rare)
Epirubicin	
Etoposide	
Irinotecan	
Topotecan	
Mitoxantrone	
Platinum compounds	
(form DNA adducts, disrupt repair)	
Cisplatin	Nausea, vomiting, myelosuppression,
Carboplatin	renal toxicity, neurotoxicity
Oxaliplatin	

(continued)

TABLE 69-2 TOXICITIES OF CANCER TREATMENTS (CONTINUED)

Agent	Toxicities
Antibiotics (diverse mechanisms) Bleomycin Dactinomycin Mithramycin Mitomycin	Nausea, vomiting, myelosuppression, cardiac toxicity, lung fibrosis, hypocalcemia, hypersensitivity reaction
Hormone and nuclear receptor targeting agents Tamoxifen Raloxifene Anastrozole Letrozole Exemestane Tretinoin Bexarotene Flutamide Leuprolide Diethylstilbestrol Medroxyprogesterone	Nausea, vomiting, hot flashes, gynecomastia, impotence
Biologic agents Interferon Interleukin 2 Rituximab Trastuzumab Cetuximab Bevacizumab Gemtuzumab ozogamicin Denileukin diftitox Bortezomib Imatinib Dasatinib Nilotinib Gefitinib Erlotinib Sorafenib Sunitinib Temsirolimus	Nausea, vomiting, fever, chills, vascular leak, respiratory distress, skin rashes, edema
Radiation therapy External beam (teletherapy) Internal implants (brachytherapy) Ibritumomab tiuxetan Tositumomab Samarium-153 EDTMP Strontium-89	Nausea, vomiting, myelosuppression, tissue damage, late second cancers, heart disease, sterility

Note: SIADH, syndrome of inappropriate antidiuretic hormone secretion.

women of childbearing years with radiation or chemotherapy. The most serious late toxicities are sterility (common; from alkylating agents), secondary acute leukemia (rare; from alkylating agents and topoisomerase inhibitors), secondary solid tumors (0.5–1%/year risk for at least 25 years after treatment; from radiation therapy), premature atherosclerosis (3-fold increased risk of fatal

TABLE 69-3   INDICATIONS FOR THE CLINICAL USE OF G-CSF OR GM-CSF

Preventive Uses
With the first cycle of chemotherapy (so-called primary CSF administration)
  Not needed on a routine basis
  Use if the probability of febrile neutropenia is ≥20%
  Use if patient has preexisting neutropenia or active infection
  Age >65 treated for lymphoma with curative intent or other tumor treated by
    similar regimens
  Poor performance status
  Extensive prior chemotherapy
  Dose-dense regimens in a clinical trial or with strong evidence of benefit
With subsequent cycles if febrile neutropenia has previously occurred
  (so-called secondary CSF administration)
  Not needed after short duration neutropenia without fever
  Use if patient had febrile neutropenia in previous cycle
  Use if prolonged neutropenia (even without fever) delays therapy
Therapeutic Uses
Afebrile neutropenic patients
  No evidence of benefit
Febrile neutropenic patients
  No evidence of benefit
  May feel compelled to use in the face of clinical deterioration from sepsis,
    pneumonia, or fungal infection, but benefit unclear
In bone marrow or peripheral blood stem cell transplantation
  Use to mobilize stem cells from marrow
  Use to hasten myeloid recovery
In acute myeloid leukemia
  G-CSF of minor or no benefit
  GM-CSF of no benefit and may be harmful
In myelodysplastic syndromes
  Not routinely beneficial
  Use intermittently in subset with neutropenia and recurrent infection
What Dose and Schedule Should Be Used?
G-CSF: 5 μg/kg per day subcutaneously
GM-CSF: 250 μg/m^2 per day subcutaneously
Peg-filgrastim: one dose of 6 mg 24 h after chemotherapy
When Should Therapy Begin and End?
When indicated, start 24–72 h after chemotherapy
Continue until absolute neutrophil count is 10,000/μL
Do not use concurrently with chemotherapy or radiation therapy

Note: G-CSF, granulocyte colony-stimulating factor; GM-CSF, granulocyte-macrophage colony-stimulating factor.
Source: From the American Society of Clinical Oncology.

myocardial infarction; from radiation therapy that includes the heart), heart failure (rare; from anthracyclines), and pulmonary fibrosis (rare; from bleomycin).

MANAGEMENT OF ACUTE TOXICITIES

Nausea and Vomiting   Mildly to moderately emetogenic agents—prochlorperazine, 5–10 mg PO or 25 mg PR before chemotherapy; effects are enhanced by also administering dexamethasone, 10–20 mg IV. Highly emetogenic agents (such as cisplatin, mechlorethamine, dacarbazine, streptozocin)—ondansetron, 8 mg PO q6h the day before chemotherapy and IV at time of chemotherapy, plus dexamethasone, 20 mg IV at time of chemotherapy. Aprepitant (125 mg PO day 1, 80 mg PO days 2,3 with or without dexamethasone 8 mg), a substance P/neurokinin 1 receptor blocker, decreases the risk of acute and delayed vomiting from cisplatin.

Neutropenia Colony-stimulating factors are often used where they have been shown to have little or no benefit. Specific indications for the use of granulocyte colony-stimulating factor or granulocyte-macrophage colony-stimulating factor are provided in Table 69-3.

Anemia Quality of life is improved by maintaining Hb levels >90 g/L (9 g/dL). This is routinely done with packed red blood cell transfusions. Erythropoietin, 150 U thrice weekly, may improve quality-of-life scores independently of Hb level. Depot forms of erythropoietin may permit less frequent administration. Hb levels may take up to 2 months to increase. Concerns have been raised about the ability of erythropoietin to protect hypoxic cells from dying; studies have found that its use resulted in poorer tumor control.

Thrombocytopenia Rarely, treatment may induce a decline in platelet counts. Platelet transfusions are generally triggered at a platelet count of 10,000/μL in pts with solid tumors and at a platelet count of 20,000/μL in pts with acute leukemia.

For a more detailed discussion, see Sausville EA, Longo DL: Principles of Cancer Treatment, Chap. 81, p. 514, in HPIM-17.

70 Myeloid Leukemias, Myelodysplasia, and Myeloproliferative Syndromes

ACUTE MYELOID LEUKEMIA (AML)

AML is a clonal malignancy of myeloid bone marrow precursors in which poorly differentiated cells accumulate in the bone marrow and circulation.

Signs and symptoms occur because of the absence of mature cells normally produced by the bone marrow, including granulocytes (susceptibility to infection) and platelets (susceptibility to bleeding). In addition, if large numbers of immature malignant myeloblasts circulate, they may invade organs and rarely produce dysfunction. There are distinct morphologic subtypes (Table 70-1) that have largely overlapping clinical features. Of note is the propensity of pts with acute promyelocytic leukemia (APL) (FAB M3) to develop bleeding and disseminated intravascular coagulation, especially during induction chemotherapy, because of the release of procoagulants from their cytoplasmic granules.

Incidence and Etiology In the United States about 13,300 cases occur each year. AML accounts for about 80% of acute leukemias in adults. Etiology is unknown for the vast majority. Three environmental exposures increase the risk: chronic benzene exposure, radiation exposure, and prior treatment with alkylating agents (especially in addition to radiation therapy) and topoisomerase II inhibitors (e.g., doxorubicin and etoposide). Chronic myeloid leukemia (CML),

TABLE 70-1	ACUTE MYELOID LEUKEMIA (AML) CLASSIFICATION SYSTEMS

World Health Organization Classification[a]

I. AML with recurrent genetic abnormalities
   AML with t(8;21)(q22;q22);*RUNX1/RUNX1T1*[b]
   AML with abnormal bone marrow eosinophils [inv(16)(p13q22) or t(16;
      16)(p13;q22);*CBFB/MYH11*][b]
   Acute promyelocytic leukemia [AML with t(15;17)(q22;q12) (*PML/RARA*)
      and variants][b]
   AML with 11q23 (*MLL*) abnormalities

II. AML with multilineage dysplasia
   Following a myelodysplastic syndrome or myelodysplastic syndrome/
      myeloproliferative disorder
   Without antecedent myelodysplastic syndrome

III. AML and myelodysplastic syndromes, therapy-related
   Alkylating agent–related
   Topoisomerase type II inhibitor–related
   Other types

IV. AML not otherwise categorized
   AML minimally differentiated
   AML without maturation
   AML with maturation
   Acute myelomonocytic leukemia
   Acute monoblastic and monocytic leukemia
   Acute erythroid leukemia
   Acute megakaryoblastic leukemia
   Acute basophilic leukemia
   Acute panmyelosis with myelofibrosis
   Myeloid sarcoma

French-American-British (FAB) Classification[c]	Incidence
M0: Minimally differentiated leukemia	5%
M1: Myeloblastic leukemia without maturation	20%
M2: Myeloblastic leukemia with maturation	30%
M3: Hypergranular promyelocytic leukemia	10%
M4: Myelomonocytic leukemia	20%
M4Eo: Variant: Increase in abnormal marrow eosinophils	
M5: Monocytic leukemia	10%
M6: Erythroleukemia (DiGuglielmo's disease)	4%
M7: Megakaryoblastic leukemia	1%

[a]ES Jaffe et al: *World Health Organization Classification of Tumours.* Lyon, IARC Press, 2001.
[b]Diagnosis is AML regardless of blast count.
[c]JM Bennett et al: Ann Intern Med 103:620, 1985.

myelodysplasia, and myeloproliferative syndromes may all evolve into AML. Certain genetic abnormalities are associated with particular morphologic variants: t(15;17) with APL, inv(16) with eosinophilic leukemia; others occur in a number of types. Chromosome 11q23 abnormalities are often seen in leukemias developing after exposure to topoisomerase II inhibitors. Chromosome 5 or 7 deletions are seen in leukemias following radiation plus chemotherapy. The particular genetic abnormality has a strong influence on treatment outcome. Expression of MDR1 (multidrug resistance efflux pump) is common in older pts and adversely affects prognosis.

Clinical and Laboratory Features Initial symptoms of acute leukemia have usually been present for <3 months; a preleukemic syndrome may be present in some 25% of pts with AML. Signs of anemia, pallor, fatigue, weakness, palpitations, and dyspnea on exertion are most common. White blood cell count (WBC) may be low, normal, or markedly elevated; circulating blast cells may or may not be present; with WBC > 100×10^9 blasts per liter, leukostasis in lungs and brain may occur. Minor pyogenic infections of the skin are common. Thrombocytopenia leads to spontaneous bleeding, epistaxis, petechiae, conjunctival hemorrhage, gingival bleeding, and bruising, especially with platelet count <20,000/μL. Anorexia and weight loss are common; fever may be present.

Bacterial and fungal infection are common; risk is heightened with total neutrophil count <5000/μL, and breakdown of mucosal and cutaneous barriers aggravates susceptibility; infections may be clinically occult in presence of severe leukopenia, and prompt recognition requires a high degree of clinical suspicion.

Hepatosplenomegaly occurs in about one-third of pts; leukemic meningitis may present with headache, nausea, seizures, papilledema, cranial nerve palsies.

Metabolic abnormalities may include hyponatremia, hypokalemia, elevated serum lactate dehydrogenase (LDH), hyperuricemia, and (rarely) lactic acidosis. With very high blast cell count in the blood, spurious hyperkalemia and hypoglycemia may occur (potassium released from and glucose consumed by tumor cells after the blood was drawn).

℞ Acute Myeloid Leukemia

Leukemic cell mass at time of presentation may be 10^{11}–10^{12} cells; when total leukemic cell numbers fall below ~10^9, they are no longer detectable in blood or bone marrow and pt appears to be in complete remission (CR). Thus aggressive therapy must continue past the point when initial cell bulk is reduced if leukemia is to be eradicated. Typical phases of chemotherapy include remission induction and postremission therapy, with treatment lasting about 1 year.

Supportive care with transfusions of red cells and platelets [from cytomegalovirus (CMV)-seronegative donors, if pt is a candidate for bone marrow transplantation] is very important, as are aggressive prevention, diagnosis, and treatment of infections. Colony-stimulating factors offer little or no benefit; some recommend their use in older pts and those with active infections. Febrile neutropenia should be treated with broad-spectrum antibiotics (e.g., ceftazidime 1 g q8h); if febrile neutropenia persists beyond 7 days, amphotericin B should be added.

60–80% of pts will achieve initial remission when treated with cytarabine 100–200 (mg/m²)/d by continuous infusion for 7 days, and daunorubicin [45 (mg/m²)/d] or idarubicin [12–13 (mg/m²)/d] for 3 days. Addition of etoposide may improve CR duration. Half of treated pts enter CR with the first cycle of therapy, and another 25% require two cycles. 10–30% of pts achieve 5-year disease-free survival and probable cure. Patients achieving a CR who have low risk of relapse [cells contain t(8;21) or inv(16)] receive 3–4 cycles of cytarabine. Those at high risk of relapse may be considered for allogeneic bone marrow transplantation.

Response to treatment after relapse is short, and prognosis for pts who have relapsed is poor. In APL, addition of *trans*-retinoic acid (tretinoin) to chemotherapy induces differentiation of the leukemic cells and may improve outcome. Arsenic trioxide also induces differentiation in APL cells.

Bone marrow transplantation from identical twin or human leukocyte antigen (HLA)-identical sibling is effective treatment for AML. Typical protocol uses high-dose chemotherapy ± total-body irradiation to ablate host marrow, followed by infusion of marrow from donor. Risks are substantial (unless marrow is from identical twin). Complications include graft-versus-host disease, interstitial pneumonitis, opportunistic infections (especially CMV). Comparison between transplantation and high-dose cytarabine as postremission therapy has not produced a clear advantage for either approach. Up to 30% of otherwise end-stage pts with refractory leukemia achieve probable cure from transplantation; results are better when transplant is performed during remission. Results are best for children and young adults.

CHRONIC MYELOID LEUKEMIA

CML is a clonal malignancy usually characterized by splenomegaly and production of increased numbers of granulocytes; course is initially indolent but eventuates in leukemic phase (blast crisis) that has a poorer prognosis than de novo AML; rate of progression to blast crisis is variable; overall survival averages 4 years from diagnosis.

Incidence and Etiology In the United States, about 4800 cases occur each year. More than 90% of cases have a reciprocal translocation between chromosomes 9 and 22, creating the Philadelphia (Ph) chromosome and a fusion gene product called BCR-ABL (BCR is from 9, ABL from 22). The chromosome abnormality appears in all bone marrow–derived cells except T cells. The protein made by the chimeric gene is 210 kDa in chronic phase and 190 kDa in acute blast transformation. In some pts, the chronic phase is clinically silent and pts present with acute leukemia with the Ph chromosome.

Clinical and Laboratory Features Symptoms develop gradually; easy fatigability, malaise, anorexia, abdominal discomfort and early satiety from the large spleen, excessive sweating. Occasional pts are found incidentally based on elevated leukocyte count. WBC is usually >25,000/μL with the increase accounted for by granulocytes and their precursors back to the myelocyte stage; bands and mature forms predominate. Basophils may account for 10–15% of the cells in the blood. Platelet count is normal or increased. Anemia is often present. Neutrophil alkaline phosphatase score is low. Marrow is hypercellular with granulocytic hyperplasia. Marrow blast cell count is normal or slightly elevated. Serum levels of vitamin B_{12}, B_{12}-binding proteins, and LDH are elevated in proportion to the WBC. With high blood counts, spurious hyperkalemia and hypoglycemia may be seen.

Natural History Chronic phase lasts 2–4 years. Accelerated phase is marked by anemia disproportionate to the disease activity or treatment. Platelet counts fall. Additional cytogenetic abnormalities appear. Blast cell counts increase. Usually within 6–8 months, overt blast crisis develops in which maturation ceases and blasts predominate. The clinical picture is that of acute leukemia. Half of the cases become AML, one-third have morphologic features of acute lymphoid leukemia, 10% are erythroleukemia, and the rest are undifferentiated. Survival in blast crisis is often <4 months.

℞ Chronic Myeloid Leukemia

Criteria for response are provided in Table 70-2. Allogeneic bone marrow transplantation has the potential to cure the disease in chronic phase. However, the first treatment is imatinib, a molecule that inhibits the chimeric gene product's tyrosine kinase activity. A daily oral dose of 400 mg produces complete hematologic remission of >90% and cytogenetic remission in 76%. If a

TABLE 70-2 RESPONSE CRITERIA IN CHRONIC MYELOID LEUKEMIA

Hematologic	
Complete response[a]	White blood cell count <10,000/μL, normal morphology
	Normal hemoglobin and platelet counts
Incomplete response	White blood cell count ≥10,000/μL
Cytogenetic	Percentage of bone marrow metaphases with t(9;22)
Complete response	0
Partial response	≤35
Minor response	36–85[b]
No response	85–100
Molecular	Presence of *BCR/ABL* transcript by RT-PCR
Complete response	None
Incomplete response	Any

[a]Complete hematologic response requires the disappearance of splenomegaly.
[b]Up to 15% normal metaphases are occasionally seen at diagnosis (when 30 metaphases are analyzed).
Note: RT-PCR, reverse transcriptase polymerase chain reaction.

TABLE 70-3 WORLD HEALTH ORGANIZATION CLASSIFICATION OF

Disease	Frequency	Blood Findings
Refractory anemia (RA)	5–10%	Anemia No or rare blasts
Refractory anemia with ringed sideroblasts (RARS)	10–12%	Anemia No blasts
Refractory cytopenia with multilineage dysplasia (RCMD)	24%	Cytopenias (2 or 3 lineages) No or rare blasts No Auer rods <1 × 10⁹/L monocytes
RCMD with ringed sideroblasts (RCMD-RS)	15%	Cytopenias (2 or 3 lineages) No or rare blasts No Auer rods <1 × 10⁹/L monocytes
Refractory anemia with excess blasts-1 (RAEB-1)	40% (RAEB-1 +2)	Cytopenias <5% blasts No Auer rods <1 × 10⁹/L monocytes
Refractory anemia with excess blasts-2 (RAEB-2)		Cytopenias 5–19% blasts ±Auer rods <1 × 10⁹/L monocytes
Myelodysplastic syndrome, unclassified (MDS-U)	Unknown	Cytopenias No or rare blasts No Auer rods
MDS with isolated del(5q)	Unknown	Anemia <5% blasts Platelets nl or increased

Note: BM, bone marrow.
Source: Extracted from Jaffe ES et al (eds): *Pathology and Genetics of Tumors of Haematopoietic and Lymphoid Tissues.* Lyon, IARC Press, 2001.

matched donor is available, it is best to transplant patients in complete remission. Several mechanisms of resistance to imatinib have emerged, and it is unlikely that it leads to permanent remissions when used alone; however, follow-up is not sufficient to draw firm conclusions.

Patients who no longer respond to imatinib may respond to other tyrosine kinase inhibitors such as dasatinib (100 mg PO qd) or nilotinib (400 mg PO bid). The T315I mutation in the *BCR/ABL* gene conveys resistance to all three kinase inhibitors. Allopurinol, 300 mg/d, prevents urate nephropathy. The only curative therapy for the disease is HLA-matched allogeneic bone marrow transplantation. The optimal timing of transplantation is unclear, but transplantation in chronic phase is more effective than transplantation in accelerated phase or blast crisis. Transplantation appears most effective in pts treated within a year of diagnosis. Long-term disease-free survival may be obtained in 50–60% of transplanted pts. Infusion of donor lymphocytes can restore remission in relapsing pts. In pts without a matched donor, autologous transplantation may be helpful using peripheral blood stem cells. Treatment of pts in blast crisis with imatinib can obtain responses, but their durability has not been established.

MYELODYSPLASTIC SYNDROMES

Bone Marrow Findings	Prognosis
Erythroid dysplasia only <5% blasts <15% ringed sideroblasts	Protracted course Leukemic transformation in ~6%
Erythroid dysplasia only ≥15% ringed sideroblasts <5% blasts	Protracted course Leukemia in ~1–2%
Dysplasia in ≥10% of cells in ≥2 lineages <5% blasts No Auer rods <15% ringed sideroblasts	Variable clinical course Leukemia in ~11%
Dysplasia in ≥10% of cells in ≥2 lineages ≥15% ringed sideroblasts <5% blasts No Auer rods	
Unilineage or multilineage dysplasia 5–9% blasts No Auer rods	Progressive BM failure Leukemia in ~25%
Unilineage or multilineage dysplasia 10–19% blasts ±Auer rods	Progressive BM failure Leukemia in ~33%
Dysplasia in myeloid or platelet lineage <5% blasts No Auer rods	Unknown
Nl or increased megakaryocytes with hypolobated nuclei <5% blasts No Auer rods Isolated del(5q)	Long survival

MYELODYSPLASTIC SYNDROMES (MDS)

These are clonal abnormalities of marrow cells characterized by varying degrees of cytopenias affecting one or more cell lines. The World Health Organization classification of myelodysplastic syndromes is shown in Table 70-3. Other terms that have been used to describe one or more of the entities include *preleukemia* and *oligoblastic leukemia*.

Incidence and Etiology About 3000 cases occur each year, mainly in persons >50 years old (median age, 68). As in AML, exposure to benzene, radiation, and chemotherapeutic agents may lead to MDS. Chromosome abnormalities occur in up to 80% of cases, including deletion of part or all of chromosomes 5, 7, and 9 (20 or 21 less commonly) and addition of part or all of chromosome 8.

Clinical and Laboratory Features Symptoms depend on the affected lineages. 85% of pts are anemic, 50% have neutropenia, and about one-third have thrombocytopenia. The pathologic features of MDS are a cellular marrow with varying degrees of cytologic atypia including delayed nuclear maturation, abnormal cytoplasmic maturation, accumulation of ringed sideroblasts (iron-laden mitochondria surrounding the nucleus), uni- or bilobed megakaryocytes, micromegakaryocytes, and increased myeloblasts. Table 70-3 lists features used to identify distinct entities. Prognosis is defined by marrow blast %, karyotype, and lineages affected (Table 70-4).

℞ Myelodysplastic Syndromes

Allogeneic bone marrow transplantation is the only curative therapy and may cure 60% of those so treated. However, the majority of pts with MDS are too old to receive transplantation. 5-Azacitidine (75 mg/m^2 daily × 7, q 4 weeks) can delay transformation to AML by 8–10 months. Decitabine (15 mg/m^2 by continuous IV infusion, q8h daily × 3, q 6 weeks) may induce responses lasting a median of 1 year in 20% of pts. Lenalidomide (10 mg/d), a thalidomide analogue with fewer central nervous system effects, causes a substantial frac-

| TABLE 70-4 | INTERNATIONAL PROGNOSTIC SCORING SYSTEM FOR MYELODYSPLASTIC SYNDROMES |

Prognostic Factors	
% Marrow blasts	<5 = 0 pts; 5–10 = 0.5 pts; 11–20 = 1.5 pts; 21–30 = 2 pts
Karyotype[a]	Good = 0 pts; intermediate = 0.5 pts; poor = 1.5 pts
Cytopenias[b]	0/1 = 0 pts; 2/3 = 0.5 pts

Risk Group	**Low**	**Intermediate-1**	**Intermediate-2**	**High**
Total points	0	0.5–1.0	1.5–2.0	≥2.5
Risk of AML	19%	30%	33%	45%
Median survival, years	5.7	3.5	1.2	0.4

[a]Good karyotypes: normal, Y, del(5q), del(20q)
Poor karyotypes: ≥3 abnormalities, chr 7 abnormalities
Intermediate karyotypes: others
[b]Cytopenias defined as Hb <100 g/L, platelet count <100,000/μL, absolute neutrophil count <1500/μL

tion of patients with the 5q– syndrome to become transfusion-independent. Pts with low erythropoietin levels may respond to erythropoietin, and a minority of pts with neutropenia respond to granulocyte colony-stimulating factor. Supportive care is the cornerstone of treatment.

MYELOPROLIFERATIVE SYNDROMES

The three major myeloproliferative syndromes are polycythemia vera, idiopathic myelofibrosis, and essential thrombocytosis. All are clonal disorders of hematopoietic stem cells and all are associated with a mutation in the *JAK2* kinase (V617F) that results in activation of the kinase. The mutation is seen in 90% of pts with polycythemia vera and ~45% of pts with idiopathic myelofibrosis and essential thrombocytosis.

POLYCYTHEMIA VERA

The most common myeloproliferative syndrome, this is characterized by an increase in red blood cell (RBC) mass, massive splenomegaly, and clinical manifestations related to increased blood viscosity, including neurologic symptoms (vertigo, tinnitus, headache, visual disturbances) and thromboses (myocardial infarction, stroke, peripheral vascular disease; uncommonly, mesenteric and hepatic). It must be distinguished from other causes of increased RBC mass (Chap. 58). This is most readily done by assaying serum erythropoietin levels. Polycythemia vera is associated with very low erythropoietin levels; in other causes of erythrocytosis, erythropoietin levels are high. Pts are effectively managed with phlebotomy. Some pts require splenectomy to control symptoms, and those with severe pruritus may benefit from psoralens and UV light. 20% develop myelofibrosis, <5% acute leukemia.

IDIOPATHIC MYELOFIBROSIS

This rare entity is characterized by marrow fibrosis, myeloid metaplasia with extramedullary hematopoiesis, and splenomegaly. Evaluation of a blood smear reveals teardrop-shaped RBC, nucleated RBC, and some early granulocytic forms, including promyelocytes. However, many entities may lead to marrow fibrosis and extramedullary hematopoiesis, and the diagnosis of primary idiopathic myelofibrosis is made only when the many other potential causes are ruled out. The following diseases are in the differential diagnosis: CML, polycythemia vera, Hodgkin's disease, cancer metastatic to the marrow (especially from breast and prostate), infection (particularly granulomatous infections), and hairy cell leukemia. Supportive therapy is generally used; no specific therapy is known.

ESSENTIAL THROMBOCYTOSIS

This is usually noted incidentally upon routine platelet count done in an asymptomatic person. Like myelofibrosis, many conditions can produce elevated platelet counts; thus, the diagnosis is one of exclusion. Platelet count must be >500,000/μL, and known causes of thrombocytosis must be ruled out including CML, iron deficiency, splenectomy, malignancy, infection, hemorrhage, polycythemia vera, myelodysplasia, and recovery from vitamin B_{12} deficiency. Although usually asymptomatic, pts should be treated if they develop migraine headache, transient ischemic attack, or other bleeding or thrombotic disease manifestations. Interferon α is effective therapy, as are anagrelide and hydroxyurea. Treatment should not be given just because the absolute platelet count is high in the absence of other symptoms.

For a more detailed discussion, see Young NS: Aplastic Anemia, Myelodysplasia, and Related Bone Marrow Failure Syndromes, Chap. 102, p. 663; Spivak JL: Polycythemia Vera and Other Myeloproliferative Diseases, Chap. 103, p. 671; and Wetzler M et al: Acute and Chronic Myeloid Leukemia, Chap. 104, p. 677, in HPIM-17.

71 Lymphoid Malignancies

Definition Neoplasms of lymphocytes usually represent malignant counterparts of cells at discrete stages of normal lymphocyte differentiation. When bone marrow and peripheral blood involvement dominate the clinical picture, the disease is classified as a *lymphoid leukemia*. When lymph nodes and/or other extranodal sites of disease are the dominant site(s) of involvement, the tumor is called a *lymphoma*. The distinction between lymphoma and leukemia is sometimes blurred; for example, small lymphocytic lymphoma and chronic lymphoid leukemia are tumors of the same cell type and are distinguished arbitrarily on the basis of the absolute number of peripheral blood lymphocytes ($>5 \times 10^9$/L defines leukemia).

Classification Historically, lymphoid tumors have had separate pathologic classifications based on the clinical syndrome—lymphomas according to the Rappaport, Kiel, or Working Formulation systems; acute leukemias according to the French-American-British (FAB) system; Hodgkin's disease according to the Rye classification. Myelomas have generally not been subclassified by pathologic features of the neoplastic cells. The World Health Organization (WHO) has proposed a unifying classification system that brings together all lymphoid neoplasms into a single framework. Although the new system bases the definitions of disease entities on histology, genetic abnormalities, immunophenotype, and clinical features, its organization is based on cell of origin (B cell vs. T cell) and maturation stage (precursor vs. mature) of the tumor, features that are of limited value to the clinician. Table 71-1 lists the disease entities according to a more clinically useful schema based on the clinical manifestations and natural history of the diseases.

Incidence Lymphoid tumors are increasing in incidence. Nearly 115,000 cases were diagnosed in 2008 in the United States (Fig. 71-1).

Etiology The cause(s) for the vast majority of lymphoid neoplasms is unknown. The malignant cells are monoclonal and often contain numerous genetic abnormalities. Some genetic alterations are characteristic of particular histologic entities: t(8;14) in Burkitt's lymphoma, t(14;18) in follicular lymphoma, t(11;14) in mantle cell lymphoma, t(2;5) in anaplastic large cell lymphoma, translocations or mutations involving *bcl*-6 on 3q27 in diffuse large cell lymphoma, and others. In most cases, translocations involve insertion of a distant chromosome segment into the antigen receptor genes (either immunoglob-

TABLE 71-1 **CLINICAL SCHEMA OF LYMPHOID NEOPLASMS**

Chronic lymphoid leukemias/lymphomas
  Chronic lymphocytic leukemia/small lymphocytic lymphoma (99% B cell, 1% T cell)
  Prolymphocytic leukemia (90% B cell, 10% T cell)
  Large granular lymphocyte leukemia [80% natural killer (NK) cell, 20% T cell]
  Hairy cell leukemia (99–100% B cell)
Indolent lymphoma
  Follicular center cell lymphoma, grades I and II (100% B cell)
  Lymphoplasmacytic lymphoma/Waldenström's macroglobulinemia (100% B cell)
  Marginal zone lymphoma (100% B cell)
    Extranodal [mucosa-associated lymphatic tissue (MALT) lymphoma]
    Nodal (monocytoid B cell lymphoma)
    Splenic marginal zone lymphoma
  Cutaneous T cell lymphoma (mycosis fungoides) (100% T cell)
Aggressive lymphoma
  Diffuse large cell lymphoma (85% B cell, 15% T cell), includes immunoblastic
  Follicular center cell lymphoma, grade III (100% B cell)
  Mantle cell lymphoma (100% B cell)
  Primary mediastinal (thymic) large B cell lymphoma (100% B cell)
  Burkitt-like lymphoma (100% B cell)
  Peripheral T cell lymphoma (100% T cell)
  Angioimmunoblastic lymphoma (100% T cell)
  Angiocentric lymphoma (80% T cell, 20% NK cell)
  Intestinal T cell lymphoma (100% T cell)
  Anaplastic large cell lymphoma (70% T cell, 30% null cell)
Acute lymphoid leukemias/lymphomas
  Precursor lymphoblastic leukemia/lymphoma (80% T cell, 20% B cell)
  Burkitt's leukemia/lymphoma (100% B cell)
  Adult T cell leukemia/lymphoma (100% T cell)
Plasma cell disorders (100% B cell)
  Monoclonal gammopathy of uncertain significance
  Solitary plasmacytoma
  Extramedullary plasmacytoma
  Multiple myeloma
  Plasma cell leukemia
Hodgkin's disease (cell of origin mainly B cell)
  Lymphocyte predominant
  Nodular sclerosis
  Mixed cellularity
  Lymphocyte depleted

ulin or T cell receptor) during the rearrangement of the gene segments that form the receptors.

Three viruses—Epstein-Barr virus (EBV), human herpesvirus 8 (HHV-8) (both herpes family viruses), and human T-lymphotropic virus type I (HTLV-I, a retrovirus)—may cause some lymphoid tumors. EBV has been strongly associated with African Burkitt's lymphoma and the lymphomas that complicate immunodeficiencies (disease-related or iatrogenic). EBV has an uncertain relationship to mixed cellularity Hodgkin's disease and angiocentric lymphoma. HHV-8 causes a rare entity, body cavity lymphoma, mainly in pts with AIDS. HTLV-I is associated with adult T cell leukemia/lymphoma. Both the virus and the disease are endemic to southwestern Japan and the Caribbean.

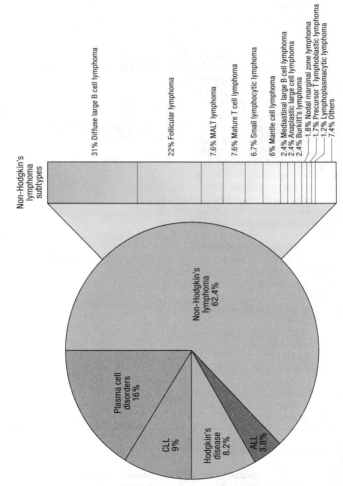

FIGURE 71-1 Relative frequency of lymphoid malignancies.

Non-Hodgkin's lymphoma subtypes

31% Diffuse large B cell lymphoma
22% Follicular lymphoma
7.6% MALT lymphoma
7.6% Mature T cell lymphoma
6.7% Small lymphocytic lymphoma
6% Mantle cell lymphoma
2.4% Mediastinal large B cell lymphoma
2.4% Anaplastic large cell lymphoma
2.4% Burkitt's lymphoma
1.8% Nodal marginal zone lymphoma
1.7% Precursor T lymphoblastic lymphoma
1.2% Lymphoplasmacytic lymphoma
7.4% Others

Non-Hodgkin's lymphoma 62.4%

Plasma cell disorders 16%

CLL 9%

Hodgkin's disease 8.2%

ALL 3.8%

354

Gastric *Helicobacter pylori* infection is associated with gastric mucosa-associated lymphoid tissue (MALT) lymphoma and perhaps gastric large cell lymphoma. Eradication of the infection produces durable remissions in about half of pts with gastric MALT lymphoma. MALT lymphomas of other sites are associated with either infection (ocular adnexae, *Chlamydia psittaci*; small intestine, *Campylobacter jejuni*; skin, *Borrelia*) or autoimmunity (salivary gland, Sjögren's syndrome; thyroid gland, Hashimoto's thyroiditis).

Inherited or acquired immunodeficiencies and autoimmune disorders predispose individuals to lymphoma. Lymphoma is 17 times more common in HIV-infected than in HIV-noninfected people. Lymphoma occurs with increased incidence in farmers and meat workers; Hodgkin's disease is increased in wood workers.

Diagnosis and Staging   Excisional biopsy is the standard diagnostic procedure; adequate tissue must be obtained. Tissue undergoes three kinds of studies: (1) light microscopy to discern the pattern of growth and the morphologic features of the malignant cells, (2) flow cytometry for assessment of immunophenotype, and (3) genetic studies (cytogenetics, DNA extraction). Needle aspirates of nodal or extranodal masses are not adequate diagnostic procedures. Leukemia diagnosis and lymphoma staging include generous bilateral iliac crest bone marrow biopsies. Differential diagnosis of adenopathy is reviewed in Chap. 59.

Staging varies with the diagnosis. In acute leukemia, peripheral blood blast counts are most significant in assessing prognosis. In chronic leukemia, peripheral blood red blood cell (RBC) and platelet counts are most significant in assessing prognosis. Non-Hodgkin's lymphomas have five clinical prognostic factors; indolent and aggressive lymphomas share three of these, advanced stage, high lactate dehydrogenase (LDH) levels, and age >60. In follicular lymphoma, the last two factors are Hb <120 g/L (<12 g/dL) and more than four nodal sites of involvement. In aggressive lymphoma, more than one extranodal site and performance status predict outcome. In myeloma, serum levels of paraprotein, creatinine, and β_2-microglobulin levels predict survival.

CHRONIC LYMPHOID LEUKEMIAS/LYMPHOMAS

Most of these entities have a natural history measured in years. (Prolymphocytic leukemia is very rare and can be very aggressive.) Chronic lymphocytic leukemia is the most common entity in this group (~15,000 cases/year) and the most common leukemia in the Western world.

Chronic Lymphocytic Leukemia (CLL)   Usually presents as asymptomatic lymphocytosis in pts >60 years. The malignant cell is a CD5+ B cell that looks like a normal small lymphocyte. Trisomy 12 is the most common genetic abnormality. Prognosis is related to stage; stage is determined mainly by the degree to which the tumor cells crowd out normal hematopoietic elements from the marrow (Table 71-2). Cells may infiltrate nodes and spleen as well as marrow. Nodal involvement may be related to the expression of an adhesion molecule that allows the cells to remain in the node rather than recirculate. Pts often have hypogammaglobulinemia. Up to 20% have autoimmune antibodies that may produce autoimmune hemolytic anemia, thrombocytopenia, or red cell aplasia. Death is from infection, marrow failure, or intercurrent illnesses. In 5%, the disease evolves to aggressive lymphoma (Richter's syndrome) that is refractory to treatment.

Subsets of CLL may exist based on whether the immunoglobulin expressed by the tumor cell contains mutations (more indolent course, good prognosis) or

TABLE 71-2	STAGING OF B CELL CLL AND RELATION TO SURVIVAL	
Stage	Clinical Features	Median Survival, Years
RAI		
0	Lymphocytosis	12
I	Lymphocytosis + adenopathy	9
II	Lymphocytosis + splenomegaly	7
III	Anemia	1–2
IV	Thrombocytopenia	1–2
BINET		
A	No anemia/thrombocytopenia, <3 involved sites	>10
B	No anemia/thrombocytopenia, >3 involved sites	5
C	Anemia and/or thrombocytopenia	2

retains the germ-line sequence (more aggressive course, poor response to therapy). Methods to distinguish the two subsets clinically are not well defined; CD38+ tumors may have poorer prognosis. The expression of ZAP-70, an intracellular tyrosine kinase normally present in T cells and aberrantly expressed in about 45% of CLL cases, may be a better way to define prognostic subsets. ZAP-70+ cases usually need treatment within about 3–4 years from diagnosis; ZAP-70-negative cases usually don't require treatment for 8–11 years.

℞ Chronic Lymphocytic Leukemia

Supportive care is generally given until anemia or thrombocytopenia develop. At that time, tests are indicated to assess the cause of the anemia or thrombocytopenia. Decreased RBC and/or platelet counts related to peripheral destruction may be treated with splenectomy or glucocorticoids without cytotoxic therapy in many cases. If marrow replacement is the mechanism, cytotoxic therapy is indicated. Fludarabine, 25 (mg/m^2)/d IV × 5 days every 4 weeks, induces responses in about 75% of pts, complete responses in half. Rituximab (375–500 mg/m^2 day 1), fludarabine (25 mg/m^2 days 2–4 on cycle 1 and 1–3 in subsequent cycles), plus cyclophosphamide (250 mg/m^2 with fludarabine) induces complete responses in nearly 70% of pts but the regimen is associated with significant myelotoxicity. Glucocorticoids increase the risk of infection without adding a substantial antitumor benefit. Monthly IV immunoglobulin (IVIg) significantly reduces risk of serious infection but is expensive and usually reserved for pts who have had a serious infection. Alkylating agents are also active against the tumor. Therapeutic intent is palliative in most pts. Young pts may be candidates for high-dose therapy and autologous or allogeneic hematopoietic cell transplantation; long-term disease-free survival has been noted. Mini-transplant, in which the preparative regimen is immunosuppressive but not myeloablative, may be less toxic and as active or more active in disease treatment than high-dose therapy. Monoclonal antibodies alemtuzumab (anti-CD52) and rituximab (anti-CD20) also are active as single agents.

See Chap. 105 in HPIM-17 for discussion of the rarer entities.

INDOLENT LYMPHOMAS

These entities have a natural history measured in years. Median survival is about 10 years. Follicular lymphoma is the most common indolent lymphoma, accounting for about one-third of all lymphoid malignancies.

Follicular Lymphoma Usually presents with painless peripheral lymphadenopathy, often involving several nodal regions. "B symptoms" (fever, sweats, weight loss) occur in 10%, less common than with Hodgkin's disease. In about 25%, nodes wax and wane before the pt seeks medical attention. Median age is 55 years. Disease is widespread at diagnosis in 85%. Liver and bone marrow are commonly involved extranodal sites.

The tumor has a follicular or nodular growth pattern reflecting the follicular center origin of the malignant cell. The t(14;18) is present in 85% of cases, resulting in the overexpression of bcl-2, a protein involved in prevention of programmed cell death. The normal follicular center B cell is undergoing active mutation of the immunoglobulin variable regions in an effort to generate antibody of higher affinity for the selecting antigen. Follicular lymphoma cells also have a high rate of mutation that leads to the accumulation of genetic damage. Over time, follicular lymphomas acquire sufficient genetic damage (e.g., mutated p53) to accelerate their growth and evolve into diffuse large B cell lymphomas that are often refractory to treatment. The majority of pts dying from follicular lymphoma have undergone histologic transformation. This transformation occurs at a rate of about 7% per year and is an attribute of the disease, not the treatment.

℞ Follicular Lymphoma

Only 15% of pts have localized disease, but the majority of these pts are curable with radiation therapy. Although many forms of treatment induce tumor regression in advanced-stage pts, it is not clear that treatment of any kind alters the natural history of disease. No therapy, single-agent alkylators, nucleoside analogues (fludarabine, cladribine), combination chemotherapy, radiation therapy, and biologic agents [interferon (IFN) α, monoclonal antibodies such as rituximab, anti-CD20] are all considered appropriate. More than 90% of pts are responsive to treatment; complete responses are seen in about 50–75% of pts treated aggressively. The median duration of remission of pts treated with cyclophosphamide, doxorubicin, vincristine, and prednisone (CHOP) + rituximab exceeds 6 years. Younger pts are being treated experimentally with high-dose therapy and autologous hematopoietic stem cells or mini-transplant. It is not yet clear whether this is curative. Radioimmunotherapy with isotopes guided by anti-CD20 antibody (ibritumomab tiuxetan, In-111; tositumomab, I-131) may produce durable responses. Combination chemotherapy with or without IFN maintenance may prolong survival and delay or prevent histologic progression, especially in pts with poor prognostic features. Remissions appear to last longer with chemotherapy plus rituximab; some data suggest that the longer remissions are leading to improved survival.

See Chap. 105 in HPIM-17 for discussion of the other indolent lymphomas.

AGGRESSIVE LYMPHOMAS

A large number of pathologic entities share an aggressive natural history; median survival untreated is 6 months, and nearly all untreated pts are dead within 1 year. Pts may present with asymptomatic adenopathy or symptoms referable to involvement of practically any nodal or extranodal site: mediastinal involvement may produce superior vena cava syndrome or pericardial tamponade; retroperitoneal nodes may obstruct ureters; abdominal masses may produce pain, ascites, or GI obstruction or perforation; central nervous system (CNS) involvement may produce confusion, cranial nerve signs, headache, seizures, and/or spinal cord compression; bone involvement may produce pain or pathologic fracture. About 45% of pts have B symptoms.

Diffuse large B cell lymphoma is the most common histologic diagnosis among the aggressive lymphomas, accounting for 35–45% of all lymphomas. Aggressive lymphomas together account for ~60% of all lymphoid tumors. About 85% of aggressive lymphomas are of mature B cell origin; 15% are derived from peripheral (postthymic) T cells.

APPROACH TO THE PATIENT: AGGRESSIVE LYMPHOMA

Early diagnostic biopsy is critical. Pt workup is directed by symptoms and known patterns of disease. Pts with Waldeyer's ring involvement should undergo careful evaluation of the GI tract. Pts with bone or bone marrow involvement should have a lumbar puncture to evaluate meningeal CNS involvement.

℞ Aggressive Lymphomas

Localized aggressive lymphomas are usually treated with four cycles of CHOP combination chemotherapy ± involved-field radiation therapy. About 85% of these pts are cured. CHOP + rituximab appears to be even more effective than CHOP + radiation therapy. The specific therapy used for pts with more advanced disease is controversial. Six cycles of CHOP + rituximab is the treatment of choice for advanced-stage disease. Outcome is influenced by tumor bulk (usually measured by LDH levels, stage, and number of extranodal sites) and physiologic reserve (usually measured by age and Karnofsky status) (Table 71-3). CHOP + rituximab cures about two-thirds of pts. The use of a sequential high-dose chemotherapy regimen in pts with high-intermediate- and

TABLE 71-3	**INTERNATIONAL PROGNOSTIC INDEX FOR NHL**

Five clinical risk factors:
    Age ≥ 60 years
    Serum lactate dehydrogenase levels elevated
    Performance status ≥2 (ECOG) or ≤ 70 (Karnofsky)
    Ann Arbor stage III or IV
    >1 site of extranodal involvement
Patients are assigned a number for each risk factor they have
Patients are grouped differently based upon the type of lymphoma
For diffuse large B cell lymphoma:

0, 1 factor = low risk:	35% of cases; 5-year survival, 73%
2 factors = low-intermediate risk:	27% of cases; 5-year survival, 51%
3 factors = high-intermediate risk:	22% of cases; 5-year survival, 43%
4, 5 factors = high risk:	16% of cases; 5-year survival, 26%

For diffuse large B cell lymphoma treated with R-CHOP:

0 factor = very good:	10% of cases; 5-year survival, 94%
1, 2 factors = good:	45% of cases; 5-year survival, 79%
3, 4, 5 factors = poor:	45% of cases; 5-year survival, 55%

high-risk disease has yielded long-term survival in about 75% of pts in some institutions. Other studies fail to confirm a role for high-dose therapy.

About 30–45% of pts not cured with initial standard combination chemotherapy may be salvaged with high-dose therapy and autologous hematopoietic stem cell transplantation.

Specialized approaches are required for lymphomas involving certain sites (e.g., CNS, stomach) or under certain complicating clinical circumstances (e.g., concurrent illness, AIDS). Lymphomas occurring in iatrogenically immunosuppressed pts may regress when immunosuppressive medication is withheld. Lymphomas occurring post-allogeneic marrow transplant may regress with infusions of donor leukocytes.

Pts with rapidly growing bulky aggressive lymphoma may experience tumor lysis syndrome when treated (Chap. 27); prophylactic measures (hydration, urine alkalinization, allopurinol, rasburicase) may be lifesaving.

ACUTE LYMPHOID LEUKEMIAS/LYMPHOMAS

Acute Lymphoblastic Leukemia and Lymphoblastic Lymphoma These are more common in children than adults (~5400 total cases/year). The majority of cases have tumor cells that appear to be of thymic origin, and pts may have mediastinal masses. Pts usually present with recent onset of signs of marrow failure (pallor, fatigue, bleeding, fever, infection). Hepatosplenomegaly and adenopathy are common. Males may have testicular enlargement reflecting leukemic involvement. Meningeal involvement may be present at diagnosis or develop later. Elevated LDH, hyponatremia, and hypokalemia may be present, in addition to anemia, thrombocytopenia, and high peripheral blood blast counts. The leukemic cells are more often FAB type L2 in adults than in children, where L1 predominates. Leukemia diagnosis requires at least 20% lymphoblasts in the marrow. Prognosis is adversely affected by high presenting white count, age >35 years, and the presence of t(9;22), t(1;19), and t(4;11) translocations. HOX11 expression identifies a more favorable subset of T cell acute lymphoblastic leukemia.

℞ Acute Lymphoblastic Leukemia and Lymphoblastic Lymphoma

Successful treatment requires intensive induction phase, CNS prophylaxis, and maintenance chemotherapy that extends for about 2 years. Vincristine, L-asparaginase, cytarabine, daunorubicin, and prednisone are particularly effective agents. Intrathecal or high-dose systemic methotrexate is effective CNS prophylaxis. Long-term survival of 60–65% of pts may be achieved. The role and timing of bone marrow transplantation in primary therapy is debated, but up to 30% of relapsed pts may be cured with salvage transplantation.

Burkitt's Lymphoma/Leukemia This is also more common in children. It is associated with translocations involving the c-*myc* gene on chromosome 8 rearranging with immunoglobulin heavy or light chain genes. Pts often have disseminated disease with large abdominal masses, hepatomegaly, and adenopathy. If a leukemic picture predominates, it is classified as FAB L3.

℞ Burkitt's Lymphoma/Leukemia

Resection of large abdominal masses improves treatment outcome. Aggressive leukemia regimens that include vincristine, cyclophosphamide, 6-mercaptopurine, doxorubicin, and prednisone are active. CODOX-M and the BFM regimen are the most effective regimens. Cure may be achieved in 50–60%. The need for maintenance therapy is unclear. Prophylaxis against tumor lysis syndrome is important (Chap. 27).

Adult T Cell Leukemia/Lymphoma (ATL)   This is very rare; only a small fraction (~2%) of persons infected with HTLV-I go on to develop the disease. Some HTLV-I-infected pts develop spastic paraplegia from spinal cord involvement without developing cancer. The characteristic clinical syndrome of ATL includes high white count without severe anemia or thrombocytopenia, skin infiltration, hepatomegaly, pulmonary infiltrates, meningeal involvement, and opportunistic infections. The tumor cells are CD4+ T cells with cloven hoof– or flower-shaped nuclei. Hypercalcemia occurs in nearly all pts and is related to cytokines produced by the tumor cells.

℞ Adult T Cell Leukemia/Lymphoma

Aggressive therapy is associated with serious toxicity related to the underlying immunodeficiency. Glucocorticoids relieve hypercalcemia. The tumor is responsive to therapy, but responses are generally short-lived. Zidovudine and IFN may be palliative in some pts.

PLASMA CELL DISORDERS

The hallmark of plasma cell disorders is the production of immunoglobulin molecules or fragments from abnormal plasma cells. The intact immunoglobulin molecule, or the heavy chain or light chain produced by the abnormal plasma cell clone, is detectable in the serum and/or urine and is called the M (for monoclonal) component. The amount of the M component in any given pt reflects the tumor burden in that pt. In some, the presence of a clonal light chain in the urine (Bence Jones protein) is the only tumor product that is detectable. M components may be seen in pts with other lymphoid tumors, nonlymphoid cancers, and noncancerous conditions such as cirrhosis, sarcoidosis, parasitic infestations, and autoimmune diseases.

Multiple Myeloma   A malignant proliferation of plasma cells in the bone marrow (notably not in lymph nodes). Nearly 20,000 new cases are diagnosed each year. Disease manifestations result from tumor expansion, local and remote actions of tumor products, and the host response to the tumor. About 70% of pts have bone pain, usually involving the back and ribs, precipitated by movement. Bone lesions are multiple, lytic, and rarely accompanied by an osteoblastic response. Thus, bone scans are less useful than radiographs. The production of osteoclast-activating cytokines by tumor cells leads to substantial calcium mobilization, hypercalcemia, and symptoms related to it. Decreased synthesis and increased catabolism of normal immunoglobulins leads to hypogammaglobulinemia, and a poorly defined tumor product inhibits granulocyte migration. These changes create a susceptibility to bacterial infections, especially the pneumococcus, *Klebsiella pneumoniae*, and *Staphylococcus aureus* affecting the lung and *Escherichia coli* and other gram-negative pathogens affecting the urinary tract. Infections affect at least 75% of pts at some time in their course. Renal failure may affect 25% of pts; its pathogenesis is multifactorial—hypercalcemia, infection, toxic effects of light chains, urate nephropathy, dehydration. Neurologic symptoms may result from hyperviscosity, cryoglobulins, and rarely amyloid deposition in nerves. Anemia occurs in 80% related to myelophthisis and inhibition of erythropoiesis by tumor products. Clotting abnormalities may produce bleeding.

Diagnosis Marrow plasmacytosis >10%, lytic bone lesions, and a serum and/or urine M component are the classic triad. Monoclonal gammopathy of uncertain significance (MGUS) is much more common than myeloma, affecting about 6% of people over age 70; in general, MGUS is associated with a level of M component <20 g/L, low serum β_2-microglobulin, <10% marrow plasma cells, and no bone lesions. Lifetime risk of progression of MGUS to myeloma is about 25%.

Staging Disease stage influences survival (Table 71-4).

℞ Multiple Myeloma

About 10% of pts have very slowly progressive disease and do not require treatment until the paraprotein levels rise above 50 g/L or progressive bone disease occurs. Pts with solitary plasmacytoma and extramedullary plasmacytoma are usually cured with localized radiation therapy. Supportive care includes early treatment of infections; control of hypercalcemia with glucocorticoids, hydration, and natriuresis; chronic administration of bisphosphonates to antagonize skeletal destruction; and prophylaxis against urate nephropathy and dehydration. Therapy aimed at the tumor is usually palliative. Initial therapy is usually one of several approaches, based on whether the pt is a candidate for high-dose therapy and autologous stem cell transplant. Transplant-eligible (avoid alkylating agents): thalidomide, 400 mg/d PO or 200 mg qhs, plus dexamethasone, 40 mg/d on days 1–4 each month, with or without chemotherapy such as liposomal doxorubicin; addition of bortezomib may be even more effective. Transplant-ineligible: melphalan, 8 mg/m^2 orally for 4–7 days every 4–6 weeks, plus prednisone. About 60% of pts have significant symptomatic improvement plus a 75% decline in the M component. Bortezomib also appears to improve response rates to melphalan. Experimental approaches using sequential high-dose pulses of melphalan plus two successive autologous stem cell transplants have produced complete responses in about 50% of pts <65 years. Long-term follow-up is required to see whether survival is enhanced. Palliatively treated pts generally follow a chronic course for 2–5 years, followed by an acceleration characterized by organ infiltration with myeloma cells and marrow failure. More aggressive treatment may produce median survival of 6 years. New approaches to salvage treatment include bortezomib, 1.3 mg/m^2 on days 1, 4, 8, and 11 every 3 weeks, often used with dexamethasone, vincristine, and/or liposomal doxorubicin. Lenalidomide is also active.

Hodgkin's Disease About 8000 new cases are diagnosed each year. Hodgkin's disease (HD) is a tumor of Reed-Sternberg cells, aneuploid cells that usually express CD30 and CD15 but may also express other B or T cell markers. Most tumors are derived from B cells in that immunoglobulin genes are rearranged but not expressed. Most of the cells in an enlarged node are normal lymphoid, plasma cells, monocytes, and eosinophils. The etiology is unknown, but the incidence in both identical twins is 99-fold increased over the expected concordance, suggesting a genetic susceptibility. Distribution of histologic subtypes is 75% nodular sclerosis, 20% mixed cellularity, with lymphocyte predominant and lymphocyte depleted representing about 5%.

TABLE 71-4 MYELOMA STAGING SYSTEMS

Durie-Salmon Staging System

Stage	Criteria	Estimated Tumor Burden, $\times 10^{12}$ cells/m^2

I	All of the following:
	1. Hemoglobin >100 g/L (>10 g/dL)
	2. Serum calcium <3 mmol/L (<12 mg/dL)
	3. Normal bone x-ray or solitary lesion
	4. Low M-component production
	  a. IgG level <50 g/L (<5 g/dL)
	  b. IgA level <30 g/L (<3 g/dL)
	  c. Urine light chain <4 g/24 h
		<0.6 (low)

II	Fitting neither I nor III	0.6–1.20 (intermediate)

III	One or more of the following:
	1. Hemoglobin <85 g/L (<8.5 g/dL)
	2. Serum calcium >3 mmol/L (>12 mg/dL)
	3. Advanced lytic bone lesions
	4. High M-component production
	  a. IgG level >70 g/L (>7 g/dL)
	  b. IgA level >50 g/L (>5 g/dL)
	  c. Urine light chains >12 g/24 h
		>1.20 (high)

Level	Stage	Median Survival, Months
Subclassification based on serum creatinine levels		
A < 177 µmol/L (<2 mg/dL)	IA	61
B > 177 µmol/L (>2 mg/dL)	IIA, B	55
	IIIA	30
	IIIB	15
International Staging System		
β_2M < 3.5, alb ≥ 3.5	I (28%)	62
β_2M < 3.5, alb < 3.5 *or* β_2M = 3.5–5.5	II (39%)	44
β_2M > 5.5	III (33%)	29

Note: β_2M, serum β_2-microglobulin in mg/L; alb, serum albumin in g/dL; (#), % patients presenting at each stage.

Clinical Manifestations Usually presents with asymptomatic lymph node enlargement or with adenopathy associated with fever, night sweats, weight loss, and sometimes pruritus. Mediastinal adenopathy (common in nodular sclerosing HD) may produce cough. Spread of disease tends to be to contiguous lymph node groups. Superior vena cava obstruction or spinal cord compression may be presenting manifestation. Involvement of bone marrow and liver is rare.

Differential Diagnosis
• Infection—mononucleosis, viral syndromes, toxoplasma, histoplasma, primary tuberculosis

TABLE 71-5	THE ANN ARBOR STAGING SYSTEM FOR HODGKIN'S DISEASE

Stage	Definition
I	Involvement of a single lymph node region or lymphoid structure (e.g., spleen, thymus, Waldeyer's ring)
II	Involvement of two or more lymph node regions on the same side of the diaphragm (the mediastinum is a single site; hilar lymph nodes should be considered "lateralized" and, when involved on both sides, constitute stage II disease)
III	Involvement of lymph node regions or lymphoid structures on both sides of the diaphragm
III_1	Subdiaphragmatic involvement limited to spleen, splenic hilar nodes, celiac nodes, or portal nodes
III_2	Subdiaphragmatic involvement includes paraaortic, iliac, or mesenteric nodes plus structures in III_1
IV	Involvement of extranodal site(s) beyond that designated as "E" More than one extranodal deposit at any location Any involvement of liver or bone marrow
A	No symptoms
B	Unexplained weight loss of >10% of the body weight during the 6 months before staging investigation Unexplained, persistent, or recurrent fever with temperatures >38°C during the previous month Recurrent drenching night sweats during the previous month
E	Localized, solitary involvement of extralymphatic tissue, excluding liver and bone marrow

- Other malignancies—especially head and neck cancers
- Sarcoidosis—mediastinal and hilar adenopathy

Immunologic and Hematologic Abnormalities

- Defects in cell-mediated immunity (remains even after successful treatment of lymphoma); cutaneous anergy; diminished antibody production to capsular antigens of *Haemophilus* and pneumococcus
- Anemia; elevated erythrocyte sedimentation rate; leukemoid reaction; eosinophilia; lymphocytopenia; fibrosis and granulomas in marrow

Staging The Ann Arbor staging classification is shown in Table 71-5. Disease is staged by performing physical exam, chest x-ray, thoracoabdominal CT, bone marrow biopsy; ultrasound examinations, lymphangiogram. Staging laparotomy should be used, especially to evaluate the spleen, if pt has early-stage disease on clinical grounds and radiation therapy is being contemplated. Pathologic staging is unnecessary if the pt is treated with chemotherapy.

Rx Hodgkin's Disease

About 85% of pts are curable. Therapy should be performed by experienced clinicians in centers with appropriate facilities. Most pts are clinically staged and treated with chemotherapy alone or combined-modality therapy. Those with localized disease may be treated with radiation therapy alone. Those with stage II disease often receive either four cycles of ABVD plus involved-field radiation therapy or Stanford V, a combined-modality program using lower doses of chemotherapy. Those with stage III or IV disease receive six cycles of combination chemotherapy, usually either ABVD or MOPP-ABV hybrid therapy or MOPP/ABVD alternating therapy. Pts with any stage disease accompanied by a large mediastinal mass (greater than one-third the greatest chest diameter) should receive combined-modality therapy with MOPP/ABVD or MOPP-ABV hybrid followed by mantle field radiation therapy. (Radiation plus ABVD is too toxic to the lung.) A persistently positive midtreatment positron emission tomography scan may be an index of risk of relapse and need for additional therapy. About one-half of pts (or more) not cured by their initial chemotherapy regimen may be rescued by high-dose therapy and autologous stem cell transplant.

With long-term follow-up, it has become clear that more pts are dying of late fatal toxicities related to radiation therapy (myocardial infarction, stroke, second cancers) than from HD. It may be possible to avoid radiation exposure by using combination chemotherapy in early-stage disease as well as in advanced-stage disease.

For a more detailed discussion, see Longo DL: Malignancies of Lymphoid Cells, Chap. 105, p. 687; Munshi NC et al: Plasma Cell Disorders, Chap. 106, p. 700, in HPIM-17.

72 Skin Cancer

MALIGNANT MELANOMA

Most dangerous cutaneous malignancy; high metastatic potential; poor prognosis with metastatic spread.

Incidence Melanoma was diagnosed in 62,480 people in the United States in 2008 and caused 8420 deaths.

Predisposing Factors (Table 72-1)

Fair complexion, sun exposure, family history of melanoma, dysplastic nevus syndrome (autosomal dominant disorder with multiple nevi of distinctive appearance and cutaneous melanoma, may be associated with 9p deletion), and presence of a giant congenital nevus. Blacks have a low incidence.

Prevention Sun avoidance lowers risk. Sunscreens are not proven effective.

Types

1. *Superficial spreading melanoma*: Most common; begins with initial radial growth phase before invasion.
2. *Lentigo maligna melanoma*: Very long radial growth phase before invasion, lentigo maligna (Hutchinson's melanotic freckle) is precursor lesion, most common in elderly and in sun-exposed areas (esp. face).
3. *Acral lentiginous*: Most common form in darkly pigmented pts; occurs on palms and soles, mucosal surfaces, in nail beds and mucocutaneous junc-

TABLE 72-1	RISK FACTORS FOR CUTANEOUS MELANOMA

High risk (>50-fold increase in risk)
    Persistently changing mole
    Clinically atypical moles in patient with two family members with melanoma
    Adulthood (vs. childhood)
    >50 nevi ≥2 mm in diameter
Intermediate risk (~10-fold increase in risk)
    Family history of melanoma
    Sporadic clinically atypical moles
    Congenital nevi (?)
    White ethnicity (vs. black or East Asian ethnicity)
    Personal history of prior melanoma
Low risk (2- to 4-fold increase in risk)
    Immunosuppression
    Sun sensitivity or excess exposure to sun

Source: Adapted from AR Rhodes et al: JAMA 258:3146, 1987.

tions; similar to lentigo maligna melanoma but with more aggressive biologic behavior.
4. *Nodular*: Generally poor prognosis because of invasive growth from onset.

Clinical Appearance   Generally pigmented (rarely amelanotic); color of lesions varies, but red, white, and/or blue are common, in addition to brown and/or black. Suspicion should be raised by a pigmented skin lesion that is >6 mm in diameter, asymmetric, has an irregular surface or border, or has variation in color.

Prognosis   Best with thin lesions without evidence of metastatic spread; with increasing thickness or evidence of spread, prognosis worsens. Stage I and II (primary tumor without spread) have 85% 5-year survival. Stage III (palpable regional nodes with tumor) has a 50% 5-year survival when only one node is involved and 15–20% when four or more are involved. Stage IV (disseminated disease) has <5% 5-year survival.

℞ Malignant Melanoma

Early recognition and local excision for localized disease is best; 1- to 2-cm margins are as effective as 4- to 5-cm margins and do not usually require skin grafting. Elective lymph node dissection offers no advantage in overall survival compared with deferral of surgery until clinical recurrence. Pts with stage II disease may have improved disease-free survival with adjuvant interferon (IFN) α 3 million units three times weekly for 12–18 months; no overall survival advantage has been shown. In one study, pts with stage III disease had improved survival with adjuvant IFN, 20 million units IV daily × 5 for 4 weeks, then 10 million units SC three times weekly for 11 months. This result was not confirmed in a second study. Metastatic disease may be treated with chemotherapy or immunotherapy. Dacarbazine (250 mg/m^2 IV daily × 5 q3w) plus tamoxifen (20 mg/m^2 PO daily) may induce partial responses in one-third of patients. IFN and interleukin 2 (IL-2) at maximum tolerated doses induce partial responses in 15% of pts. Rare long remissions occur with IL-2. Temozolomide is an oral agent related to dacarbazine that has some activity. It can enter the central nervous system (CNS) and is being evaluated with radiation therapy for CNS metastases. No therapy for metastatic disease is curative. Vaccines and adoptive cellular therapies are being tested.

BASAL CELL CARCINOMA (BCC)

Most common form of skin cancer; most frequently on sun-exposed skin, esp. face.

Predisposing Factors Fair complexion, chronic UV exposure, exposure to inorganic arsenic (i.e., Fowler's solution or insecticides such as Paris green), or exposure to ionizing radiation.

Prevention Avoidance of sun exposure and use of sunscreens lower risk.

Types Five general types: noduloulcerative (most common), superficial (mimics eczema), pigmented (may be mistaken for melanoma), morpheaform (plaquelike lesion with telangiectasia—with keratotic is most aggressive), keratotic (basosquamous carcinoma).

Clinical Appearance Classically a pearly, translucent, smooth papule with rolled edges and surface telangiectasia.

> **Rx** Basal Cell Carcinoma
>
> Local removal with electrodesiccation and curettage, excision, cryosurgery, or radiation therapy; metastases are rare but may spread locally. Exceedingly unusual for BCC to cause death.

SQUAMOUS CELL CARCINOMA (SCC)

Less common than basal cell but more likely to metastasize.

Predisposing Factors Fair complexion, chronic UV exposure, previous burn or other scar (i.e., scar carcinoma), exposure to inorganic arsenic or ionizing radiation. Actinic keratosis is a premalignant lesion.

Types Most commonly occurs as an ulcerated nodule or a superficial erosion on the skin. Variants include:

1. *Bowen's disease*: Erythematous patch or plaque, often with scale; noninvasive; involvement limited to epidermis and epidermal appendages (i.e., SCC in situ).
2. *Scar carcinoma*: Suggested by sudden change in previously stable scar, esp. if ulceration or nodules appear.
3. *Verrucous carcinoma*: Most commonly on plantar aspect of foot; low-grade malignancy but may be mistaken for a common wart.

Clinical Appearance Hyperkeratotic papule or nodule or erosion; nodule may be ulcerated.

> **Rx** Squamous Cell Carcinoma
>
> Local excision and Moh's micrographic surgery are most common; radiation therapy in selected cases. Metastatic disease may be treated with radiation therapy or with combination biologic therapy; 13-*cis*-retinoic acid 1 mg/d PO plus IFN 3 million units/d SC.

Prognosis Favorable if secondary to UV exposure; less favorable if in sun-protected areas or associated with ionizing radiation.

SKIN CANCER PREVENTION

Most skin cancer is related to sun exposure. Encourage pts to avoid the sun and use sunscreen.

For a more detailed discussion, see Sober AJ et al: Cancer of the Skin, Chap. 83, p. 541, in HPIM-17.

73 Head and Neck Cancer

Epithelial cancers may arise from the mucosal surfaces of the head and neck including the sinuses, oral cavity, nasopharynx, oropharynx, hypopharynx, and larynx. These tumors are usually squamous cell cancers. Thyroid cancer is discussed in Chap. 179.

INCIDENCE AND EPIDEMIOLOGY

About 48,000 cases are diagnosed each year. Oral cavity, oropharynx, and larynx are the most frequent sites of primary lesions in the United States; nasopharyngeal primaries are more common in the Far East and Mediterranean countries. Alcohol and tobacco (including smokeless) abuse are risk factors. Human papillomavirus is associated with some of these cancers.

PATHOLOGY

Nasopharyngeal cancer in the Far East has a distinct histology, nonkeratinizing undifferentiated carcinoma with infiltrating lymphocytes called *lymphoepithelioma*, and a distinct etiology, Epstein-Barr virus. Squamous cell head and neck cancer may develop from premalignant lesions (erythroplakia, leukoplakia), and the histologic grade affects prognosis. Pts who have survived head and neck cancer commonly develop a second cancer of the head and neck, lung, or esophagus, presumably reflecting the exposure of the upper aerodigestive mucosa to similar carcinogenic stimuli.

GENETIC ALTERATIONS

Chromosomal deletions and mutations have been found in chromosomes 3p, 9p, 17p, and 13q; mutations in p53 have been reported. Cyclin D1 may be overexpressed. Epidermal growth factor receptor is commonly overexpressed.

CLINICAL PRESENTATION

Most occur in persons > 50 years. Symptoms vary with the primary site. Nasopharynx lesions do not usually cause symptoms until late in the course and then cause unilateral serous otitis media or nasal obstruction or epistaxis. Oral cavity cancers present as nonhealing ulcers, sometimes painful. Oropharyngeal lesions also present late with sore throat or otalgia. Hoarseness may be an early sign of laryngeal cancer. Rare pts present with painless, rock-hard cervical or supraclavicular lymph node enlargement. Staging is based on size of primary tumor and involvement of lymph nodes. Distant metastases occur in <10% of pts.

℞ Treatment

Three categories of disease are common: localized, locally or regionally advanced, and recurrent or metastatic. *Local disease* occurs in about one-third of pts and is treated with curative intent by surgery or radiation therapy. Radiation therapy is preferred for localized larynx cancer to preserve organ function; surgery is used more commonly for oral cavity lesions. Overall 5-year survival is 60–90%, and most recurrences occur within 2 years. *Locally advanced disease* is the most common presentation (>50%). Combined-modality therapy using induction chemotherapy, then surgery followed by concomitant chemotherapy and radiation therapy, is most effective. The use of three cycles of cisplatin (100 mg/m^2 IV day 1) plus 5-fluorouracil (5FU) [1000 (mg/m^2)/d by 96- to 120-h continuous infusion] before or during radiation therapy is more effective than surgery plus radiation therapy, though mucositis is also more severe; 5-year survival is 34–50%. Cetuximab plus radiation therapy may be more effective than radiation therapy alone. Head and neck cancer pts are frequently malnourished and often have intercurrent illness. Pts with *recurrent* or *metastatic disease* (about 10% of pts) are treated palliatively with cisplatin plus 5FU or paclitaxel (200–250 mg/m^2 with granulocyte colony-stimulating factor support) or with single-agent chemotherapy (a taxane, methotrexate, cisplatin, or carboplatin). Response rates are usually 30–50% and median survival about 3 months.

PREVENTION

The most important intervention is to get the pts to stop smoking. Long-term survival is significantly better in those who stop smoking. Chemopreventive therapy with *cis*-retinoic acid [3 months of 1.5 (mg/kg)/d followed by 9 months of 0.5 (mg/kg)/d PO] may cause regression of leukoplakia but has no consistent effect on development of cancer.

For a more detailed discussion, see Vokes EE: Head and Neck Cancer, Chap. 84, p. 548, in HPIM-17.

74 Lung Cancer

INCIDENCE

Lung cancer was diagnosed in about 114,700 men and 100,300 women in the United States in 2008, and 86% of pts die within 5 years. Lung cancer, the leading cause of cancer death, accounts for 31% of all cancer deaths in men and 26% in women. Peak incidence occurs between ages 55 and 65 years. Incidence is decreasing in men and increasing in women.

HISTOLOGIC CLASSIFICATION

Four major types account for 88% of primary lung cancers: epidermoid (squamous), 29%; adenocarcinoma (including bronchioloalveolar), 35%; large cell, 9%; and small cell (or oat cell), 18%. Histology (small cell versus non-small cell types) is a major determinant of treatment approach. Small cell is usually widely disseminated at presentation, while non-small cell may be localized. Epidermoid and small cell typically present as central masses, while adenocarcinomas and large cell usually present as peripheral nodules or masses. Epidermoid and large cell cavitate in 20–30% of pts.

ETIOLOGY

The major cause of lung cancer is tobacco use, particularly cigarette smoking. Lung cancer cells may have ≥10 acquired genetic lesions, most commonly point mutations in *ras* oncogenes; amplification, rearrangement, or transcriptional activation of *myc* family oncogenes; overexpression of *bcl-2*, *Her2/neu*, and telomerase; and deletions involving chromosomes 1p, 1q, 3p12-13, 3p14 (FHIT gene region), 3p21, 3p24-25, 3q, 5q, 9p (p16 and p15 cyclin-dependent kinase inhibitors), 11p13, 11p15, 13q14 (*rb* gene), 16q, and 17p13 (*p53* gene). Loss of 3p and 9p are the earliest events, detectable even in hyperplastic bronchial epithelium; *p53* abnormalities and *ras* point mutations are usually found only in invasive cancers.

CLINICAL MANIFESTATIONS

Only 5–15% are detected while asymptomatic. Central endobronchial tumors cause cough, hemoptysis, wheeze, stridor, dyspnea, pneumonitis. Peripheral lesions cause pain, cough, dyspnea, symptoms of lung abscess resulting from cavitation. Metastatic spread of primary lung cancer may cause tracheal obstruction, dysphagia, hoarseness, Horner's syndrome. Other problems of regional spread include superior vena cava syndrome, pleural effusion, respiratory failure. Extrathoracic metastatic disease affects 50% of pts with epidermoid cancer, 80% with adenocarcinoma and large cell, and >95% with small cell. Clinical problems result from brain metastases, pathologic fractures, liver invasion, and spinal cord compression. Paraneoplastic syndromes may be a presenting finding of lung cancer or first sign of recurrence (Chap. 81). Systemic symptoms occur in 30% and include weight loss, anorexia, fever. Endocrine syndromes occur in 12% and include hypercalcemia (epidermoid), syndrome of inappropriate antidiuretic hormone secretion (small cell), gynecomastia (large cell). Skeletal connective tissue syndromes include clubbing in 30% (most often non-small cell) and hypertrophic pulmonary osteoarthropathy in 1–10% (most often adenocarcinomas), with clubbing, pain, and swelling.

STAGING   See Table 74-1.

Two parts to staging are (1) determination of location (anatomic staging) and (2) assessment of pt's ability to withstand antitumor treatment (physiologic staging). Non-small cell tumors are staged by the TNM/International Staging System (ISS). The T (tumor), N (regional node involvement), and M (presence or absence of distant metastasis) factors are taken together to define different stage groups. Small cell tumors are staged by two-stage system: limited stage disease—confined to one hemithorax and regional lymph nodes; extensive disease—involvement beyond this. General staging procedures include careful ear, nose, and throat examination; chest x-ray (CXR); chest and abdominal CT scanning; and positron emission tomography scan. CT scans may suggest me-

| TABLE 74-1 | **TUMOR, NODE, METASTASIS INTERNATIONAL STAGING SYSTEM FOR LUNG CANCER** |

| | | 5-Year Survival Rate, % | |
Stage	TNM Descriptors	Clinical Stage	Surgical-Pathologic Stage
IA	T1 N0 M0	61	67
IB	T2 N0 M0	38	57
IIA	T1 N1 M0	34	55
IIB	T2 N1 M0	24	39
IIB	T3 N0 M0	22	38
IIIA	T3 N1 M0	9	25
	T1–2–3 N2 M0	13	23
IIIB	T4 N0–1–2 M0	7	<5
	T1–2–3–4 N3 M0	3	<3
IV	Any T any N M1	1	<1

Tumor (T) Status Descriptor

T0	No evidence of a primary tumor
TX	Primary tumor cannot be assessed, or tumor proven by the presence of malignant cells in sputum or bronchial washings but not visualized by imaging or bronchoscopy
TIS	Carcinoma in situ
T1	Tumor <3 cm in greatest dimension, surrounded by lung or visceral pleura, without bronchoscopic evidence of invasion more proximal than lobar bronchus (i.e., not in main bronchus)
T2	Tumor with any of following: >3 cm in greatest dimension; involves main bronchus, ≥2 cm distal to the carina; invades visceral pleura; associated with atelectasis or obstructive pneumonitis extending to hilum but does not involve entire lung
T3	Tumor of any size that directly invades any of the following: chest wall (including superior sulcus tumors), diaphragm, mediastinal pleura, parietal pericardium; or tumor in main bronchus <2 cm distal to carina but without involvement of carina; or associated atelectasis or obstructive pneumonitis of entire lung
T4	Tumor of any size that invades any of the following: mediastinum, heart, great vessels, trachea, esophagus, vertebral body, carina; or tumor with a malignant pleural or pericardial effusion,[a] or with satellite tumor nodule(s) within the ipsilateral primary-tumor lobe of the lung.

Lymph Node (N) Involvement Descriptor

NX	Regional lymph nodes cannot be assessed
N0	No regional lymph node metastasis
N1	Metastasis to ipsilateral peribronchial and/or ipsilateral hilar lymph nodes, and intrapulmonary nodes involved by direct extension of the primary tumor
N2	Metastasis to ipsilateral mediastinal and/or subcarinal lymph nodes(s)
N3	Metastasis to contralateral mediastinal, contralateral hilar, ipsilateral or contralateral scalene, or supraclavicular lymph node(s)

(continued)

TABLE 74-1	TUMOR, NODE, METASTASIS INTERNATIONAL STAGING SYSTEM FOR LUNG CANCER (CONTINUED)

Distant Metastasis (M) Descriptor

MX	Presence of distant metastasis cannot be assessed
M0	No distant metastasis
M1	Distant metastasis present[b]

[a]Most pleural effusions associated with lung cancer are due to tumor. However, in a few pts with multiple negative cytopathologic exams of a nonbloody, non-exudative pleural or pericardial effusion that clinical judgment dictates is not related to the tumor, the effusion should be excluded as a staging element and the pt's disease staged as T1, T2, or T3.
[b]Separate metastatic pulmonary tumor nodule(s) in the ipsilateral nonprimary tumor lobe(s) of the lung are classified as M1.
Source: Adapted from CF Mountain: Chest 111:1710, 1997, with permission.

diastinal lymph node involvement and pleural extension in non-small cell lung cancer, but definitive evaluation of mediastinal spread requires histologic examination. Routine radionuclide scans are not obtained in asymptomatic pts. If a mass lesion is on CXR and no obvious contraindications to curative surgical approach are noted, the mediastinum should be investigated. Major contraindications to curative surgery include extrathoracic metastases, superior vena cava syndrome, vocal cord and phrenic nerve paralysis, malignant pleural effusions, metastases to contralateral lung, and histologic diagnosis of small cell cancer.

Rx Lung Cancer   See Table 74-2.

1. Surgery in pts with localized disease and non-small cell cancer; however, majority initially thought to have curative resection ultimately succumb to metastatic disease. Adjuvant chemotherapy [cisplatin, four cycles at 100 mg/m² plus a second active agent (etoposide, vinblastine, vinorelbine, vindesine, a taxane)] in pts with total resection of stage IIA and IIB disease may modestly extend survival.

2. Solitary pulmonary nodule: factors suggesting resection include cigarette smoking, age ≥35, relatively large (>2 cm) lesion, lack of calcification, chest symptoms, and growth of lesion compared with old CXR. See Fig. 74-1.

3. For unresectable stage II non-small cell lung cancer, combined thoracic radiation therapy and cisplatin-based chemotherapy reduces mortality by about 25% at 1 year.

4. For unresectable non-small cell cancer, metastatic disease, or refusal of surgery: consider for radiation therapy; addition of cisplatin/taxane-based chemotherapy may reduce death risk by 13% at 2 years and improve quality of life. Pemetrexed has activity in pts with progressive disease.

5. Small cell cancer: combination chemotherapy is standard mode of therapy; response after 6–12 weeks predicts median- and long-term survival.

6. Addition of radiation therapy to chemotherapy in limited-stage small cell lung cancer can increase 5-year survival from about 11% to 20%.

7. Prophylactic cranial irradiation improves survival of limited-stage small cell lung cancer by another 5%.

8. Laser obliteration of tumor through bronchoscopy in presence of bronchial obstruction.

9. Radiation therapy for brain metastases, spinal cord compression, symptomatic masses, bone lesions.

TABLE 74-2   SUMMARY OF TREATMENT APPROACH TO PATIENTS WITH LUNG CANCER

Non-Small Cell Lung Cancer

Stages IA, IB, IIA, IIB, and some IIIA:
    Surgical resection for stages IA, IB, IIA, and IIB
    Surgical resection with complete-mediastinal lymph node dissection and con-
       sideration of neoadjuvant CRx for stage IIIA disease with "minimal N2 in-
       volvement" (discovered at thoracotomy or mediastinoscopy)
    Consider postoperative RT for patients found to have N2 disease
    Stage IB: discussion of risk/benefits of adjuvant CRx; not routinely given
    Stage II: Adjuvant CRx
Curative potential RT for "nonoperable" patients
Stage IIIA with selected types of stage T3 tumors:
    Tumors with chest wall invasion (T3): en bloc resection of tumor with in-
       volved chest wall and consideration of postoperative RT
    Superior sulcus (Pancoast's) (T3) tumors: preoperative RT (30–45 Gy) and
       CRx followed by en bloc resection of involved lung and chest wall with
       postoperative RT
    Proximal airway involvement (<2 cm from carina) without mediastinal
       nodes: sleeve resection if possible preserving distal normal lung or
       pneumonectomy
Stages IIIA "advanced, bulky, clinically evident N2 disease" (discovered preoper-
    atively) and IIIB disease that can be included in a tolerable RT port:
    Curative potential concurrent RT + CRx if performance status and general
       medical condition are reasonable; otherwise, sequential CRx followed by
       RT, or RT alone
Stage IIIB disease with carinal invasion (T4) but without N2 involvement:
    Consider pneumonectomy with tracheal sleeve resection with direct reanasto-
       mosis to contralateral mainstem bronchus
Stage IV and more advanced IIIB disease:
    RT to symptomatic local sites
    CRx for ambulatory patients; consider CRx and bevacizumab for selected
       patients
    Chest tube drainage of large malignant pleural effusions
    Consider resection of primary tumor and metastasis for isolated brain or ad-
       renal metastases

Small Cell Lung Cancer

Limited stage (good performance status): combination CRx + concurrent chest
    RT
Extensive stage (good performance status): combination CRx
Complete tumor responders (all stages): consider prophylactic cranial RT
Poor-performance-status patients (all stages):
    Modified-dose combination CRx
    Palliative RT

Broncholoalveolar or Adenocarcinoma with EGF Receptor Mutations

Gefitinib or erlotinib, inhibitors of EGF receptor kinase activity

(continued)

TABLE 74-2	**SUMMARY OF TREATMENT APPROACH TO PATIENTS WITH LUNG CANCER (CONTINUED)**

All Patients

RT for brain metastases, spinal cord compression, weight-bearing lytic bony lesions, symptomatic local lesions (nerve paralyses, obstructed airway, hemoptysis, intrathoracic large venous obstruction, in non-small cell lung cancer and in small cell cancer not responding to CRx)

Appropriate diagnosis and treatment of other medical problems and supportive care during CRx

Encouragement to stop smoking

Entrance into clinical trial, if eligible

Abbreviations: CRx, chemotherapy; EGF, epidermal growth factor; RT, radiotherapy.

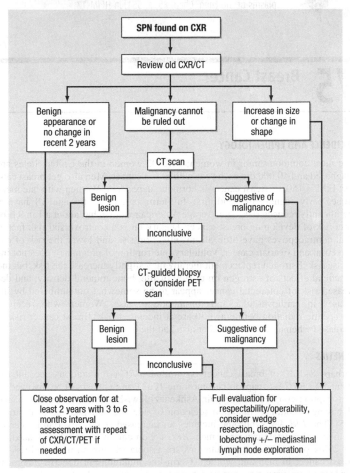

FIGURE 74-1 Algorithm for evaluation of a solitary pulmonary nodule (SPN). CXR, chest x-ray; CT, computed tomography scan; PET, positron emission tomography.

10. Encourage cessation of smoking.
11. Pts with broncholoalveolar carcinoma (3% of all pts with lung cancer) often have activating mutations in the epidermal growth factor (EGF) receptor. These pts often respond to gefitinib or erlotinib, EGF receptor inhibitors.

PROGNOSIS

At time of diagnosis, only 20% of pts have localized disease. Overall 5-year survival is 30% for males and 50% for females with localized disease and 5% for pts with advanced disease.

For a more detailed discussion, see Minna JD, Schiller JH: Neoplasms of the Lung, Chap. 85, p. 551, in HPIM-17.

75 Breast Cancer

INCIDENCE AND EPIDEMIOLOGY

The most common tumor in women; 183,000 women in the United States are diagnosed and 40,000 die each year with breast cancer. Men also get breast cancer; F:M is 150:1. Breast cancer is hormone-dependent. Women with late menarche, early menopause, and first full-term pregnancy by age 18 have a significantly reduced risk. The average American woman has about a 1 in 9 lifetime risk of developing breast cancer. Dietary fat is a controversial risk factor. Oral contraceptives have little, if any, effect on risk and lower the risk of endometrial and ovarian cancer. Voluntary interruption of pregnancy does not increase risk. Estrogen replacement therapy may slightly increase the risk, but the beneficial effects of estrogen on quality of life, bone mineral density, and decreased risk of colorectal cancer appear to be somewhat outnumbered by increases in cardiovascular and thrombotic disease. Women who received therapeutic radiation before age 30 are at increased risk. Breast cancer risk is increased when a sister and mother also had the disease.

GENETICS

Perhaps 8–10% of breast cancer is familial. *BRCA-1* mutations account for about 5%. *BRCA-1* maps to chromosome 17q21 and appears to be involved in transcription-coupled DNA repair. Ashkenazi Jewish women have a 1% chance of having a common mutation (deletion of adenine and guanine at position 185). The *BRCA-1* syndrome includes an increased risk of ovarian cancer in women and prostate cancer in men. *BRCA-2* on chromosome 11 may account for 2–3% of breast cancer. Mutations are associated with an increased risk of breast cancer in men and women. Germ-line mutations in p53 (Li-Fraumeni syndrome) are very rare, but breast cancer, sarcomas, and other malignancies occur in such families. Germ-line mutations in *hCHK2* and *PTEN* may account for some familial breast cancer. Sporadic breast cancers show many genetic alterations, including overexpression of *HER2/neu* in 25% of cases, p53 mutations in 40%, and loss of heterozygosity at other loci.

DIAGNOSIS

Breast cancer is usually diagnosed by biopsy of a nodule detected by mammogram or by palpation. Women should be strongly encouraged to examine their breasts monthly. In premenopausal women, questionable or nonsuspicious (small) masses should be reexamined in 2–4 weeks (Fig. 75-1). A mass in a premenopausal woman that persists throughout her cycle and any mass in a postmenopausal woman should be aspirated. If the mass is a cyst filled with non-bloody fluid that goes away with aspiration, the pt is returned to routine screening. If the cyst aspiration leaves a residual mass or reveals bloody fluid, the pt should have a mammogram and excisional biopsy. If the mass is solid, the pt should undergo a mammogram and excisional biopsy. Screening mammograms performed every other year beginning at age 50 have been shown to save lives. The controversy regarding screening mammograms beginning at age 40 relates to the following facts: (1) the disease is much less common in the 40- to 49-year age group, and screening is generally less successful for less common problems; (2) workup of mammographic abnormalities in the 40- to 49-year age group less commonly diagnoses cancer; and (3) about 50% of women

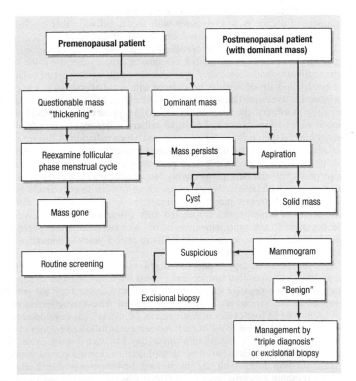

FIGURE 75-1 Approach to a palpable breast mass.

who are screened annually during their forties have an abnormality at some point that requires a diagnostic procedure (usually a biopsy), yet very few evaluations reveal cancer. However, many believe in the value of screening mammography beginning at age 40. After 13–15 years of follow-up, women who start screening at age 40 have a small survival benefit. Women with familial breast cancer more often have false-negative mammograms. MRI is a better screening tool in these women.

STAGING

Therapy and prognosis are dictated by stage of disease (Table 75-1). Unless the breast mass is large or fixed to the chest wall, staging of the ipsilateral axilla is performed at the time of lumpectomy (see below). Within pts of a given stage, individual characteristics of the tumor may influence prognosis: expression of estrogen receptor improves prognosis, while overexpression of *HER-2/neu*, mutations in p53, high growth fraction, and aneuploidy worsen the prognosis. Breast cancer can spread almost anywhere but commonly goes to bone, lungs, liver, soft tissue, and brain.

℞ Breast Cancer

Five-year survival rate by stage is shown in Table 75-2. Treatment varies with stage of disease.

Ductal carcinoma in situ is noninvasive tumor present in the breast ducts. Treatment of choice is wide excision with breast radiation therapy. In one study, adjuvant tamoxifen further reduced the risk of recurrence.

Invasive breast cancer can be classified as operable, locally advanced, and metastatic. In operable breast cancer, outcome of primary therapy is the same with modified radical mastectomy or lumpectomy followed by breast radiation therapy. Axillary dissection may be replaced with sentinel node biopsy to evaluate node involvement. The sentinel node is identified by injecting a dye in the tumor site at surgery; the first node in which dye appears is the sentinel node. Women with tumors <1 cm and negative axillary nodes require no additional therapy beyond their primary lumpectomy and breast radiation. Adjuvant combination chemotherapy for 6 months appears to benefit premenopausal women with positive lymph nodes, pre- and postmenopausal women with negative lymph nodes but with large tumors or poor prognostic features, and postmenopausal women with positive lymph nodes whose tumors do not express estrogen receptors. Estrogen receptor–positive tumors >1 cm with or without involvement of lymph nodes are treated with aromatase inhibitors. Women who began treatment with tamoxifen before aromatase inhibitors were approved should switch to an aromatase inhibitor after 5 years of tamoxifen and continue for another 5 years.

Adjuvant chemotherapy is added to hormonal therapy in estrogen receptor–positive, node-positive women and is used without hormonal therapy in estrogen receptor–negative node-positive women, whether they are pre- or postmenopausal. Various regimens have been used. The most effective regimen appears to be four cycles of doxorubicin, 60 mg/m^2, plus cyclophosphamide, 600 mg/m^2, IV on day 1 of each 3-week cycle followed by four cycles of paclitaxel, 175 mg/m^2, by 3-h infusion on day 1 of each 3-week cycle. The activity of other combinations is being explored. In premenopausal women, ovarian ablation [e.g., with the luteinizing hormone–releasing hormone (LHRH) inhibitor goserelin] may be as effective as adjuvant chemotherapy.

TABLE 75-1	STAGING OF BREAST CANCER

Primary Tumor (T)

T0	No evidence of primary tumor
TIS	Carcinoma in situ
T1	Tumor ≤2 cm
T1a	Tumor >0.1 cm but ≤0.5 cm
T1b	Tumor >0.5 but ≤1 cm
T1c	Tumor >1 cm but ≤2 cm
T2	Tumor >2 cm but ≤5 cm
T3	Tumor >5 cm
T4	Extension to chest wall, inflammation, satellite lesions, ulcerations

Regional Lymph Nodes (N)

PN0(i-)	No regional lymph node metastasis histologically, negative IHC
PN0(i+)	No regional lymph node metastasis histologically, positive IHC, no IHC cluster greater than 0.2 mm
PN0(mol-)	No regional lymph node metastasis histologically, negative molecular findings (RT-PCR)[a]
PN0(mol+)	No regional lymph node metastasis histologically, positive molecular findings (RT-PCR)[a]
PN1	Metastasis in one to three axillary lymph nodes, or in internal mammary nodes with microscopic disease detected by sentinal lymph node dissection but not clinically apparent
PN1mi	Micrometastasis (>0.2mm, none >2.0 mm)
PN1a	Metastasis in one to three axillary lymph nodes
PN1b	Metastasis in internal mammary nodes with microscopic disease detected by sentinel lymph node dissection but not *clinically apparent*[b]
PN1c	Metastasis in one to three axillary lymph nodes and in internal mammary lymph nodes with microscopic disease detected by sentinel lymph node dissection but not clinically apparent.[b] (If associated with greater than three positive axillary lymph nodes, the internal mammary nodes are classified as pN3b to reflect increased tumor burden.)
pN2	Metastasis in four to nine axillary lymph nodes, or in clinically apparent internal mammary lymph nodes in the *absence* of axillary lymph node metastasis
pN3	Metastasis in ten or more axillary lymph nodes, or in infraclavicular lymph nodes, or in clinically apparent[c] ipsilateral internal mammary lymph nodes in the *presence* of 1 or more positive axillary lymph nodes; or in more than 3 axillary lymph nodes with clinically negative microscopic metastasis in internal mammary lymph nodes; or in ipsilateral SCLNs

Distant Metastasis (M)

M0	No distant metastasis
M1	Distant metastasis (includes spread to ipsilateral supraclavicular nodes)

(continued)

TABLE 75-1   STAGING OF BREAST CANCER (CONTINUED)

Stage Grouping

Stage 0	TIS	N0	M0
Stage I	T1	N0	M0
Stage IIA	T0	N1	M0
	T1	N1	M0
	T2	N0	M0
Stage IIB	T2	N1	M0
	T3	N0	M0
Stage IIIA	T0	N2	M0
	T1	N2	M0
	T2	N2	M0
	T3	N1, N2	M0
Stage IIIB	T4	Any N	M0
	Any T	N3	M0
Stage IIIC	Any T	N3	M0
Stage IV	Any T	Any N	M1

[a] RT-PCR, reverse transcriptase/polymerase chain reaction.
[b] Clinically apparent is defined as detected by imaging studies (excluding lymphoscintigraphy) or by clinical examination.
[c] T1 includes T1mic.
Source: Used with permission of the American Joint Committee on Cancer (AJCC), Chicago, Illinois. The original source for this material is the AJCC Cancer Staging Manual, Sixth Edition (2002) published by Springer-New York, *www.springeronline.com.*

Tamoxifen adjuvant therapy (20 mg/d for 5 years) or an aromatase inhibitor (anastrozole, letrozole, exemestane) is used for pre- or postmenopausal women with tumors expressing estrogen receptors whose nodes are positive or whose nodes are negative but with large tumors or poor prognostic features. Breast cancer will recur in about half of pts with localized disease. High-dose adjuvant therapy with marrow support does not appear to benefit even women with high risk of recurrence.

Pts with locally advanced breast cancer benefit from neoadjuvant combination chemotherapy (e.g., CAF: cyclophosphamide 500 mg/m^2, doxorubicin 50 mg/m^2, and 5-fluorouracil 500 mg/m^2 all given IV on days 1 and 8 of a monthly cycle for 6 cycles) followed by surgery plus breast radiation therapy.

Treatment for metastatic disease depends on estrogen receptor status and treatment philosophy. No therapy is known to cure pts with metastatic dis-

TABLE 75-2   5-YEAR SURVIVAL RATE FOR BREAST CANCER BY STAGE

Stage	5-Year Survival (Percentage of Patients)
0	99
I	92
IIA	82
IIB	65
IIIA	47
IIIB	44
IV	14

Source: Modified from data of the National Cancer Institute—Surveillance, Epidemiology, and End Results (SEER).

ease. Randomized trials do not show that the use of high-dose therapy with hematopoietic stem cell support improves survival. Median survival is about 16 months with conventional treatment: aromatase inhibitors for estrogen receptor–positive tumors and combination chemotherapy for receptor-negative tumors. Pts whose tumors express *HER2/neu* have higher response rates by adding trastuzumab (anti-*HER2/neu*) to chemotherapy. Some advocate sequential use of active single agents in the setting of metastatic disease. Active agents in anthracycline- and taxane-resistant disease include capecitabine, vinorelbine, gemcitabine, irinotecan, and platinum agents. Pts progressing on adjuvant tamoxifen may benefit from an aromatase inhibitor such as letrozole or anastrozole. Half of patients who respond to one endocrine therapy will respond to another. Bisphosphonates reduce skeletal complications and may promote antitumor effects of other therapy. Radiation therapy is useful for palliation of symptoms.

Breast Cancer Prevention

Women with breast cancer have a 0.5% per year risk of developing a second breast cancer. Women at increased risk of breast cancer can reduce their risk by 49% by taking tamoxifen for 5 years. Aromatase inhibitors are probably at least as effective as tamoxifen and are under study. Women with *BRCA-1* mutations can reduce the risk by 90% with simple mastectomy.

For a more detailed discussion, see Lippman ME: Breast Cancer, Chap. 86, p. 563, in HPIM-17.

76 Tumors of the Gastrointestinal Tract

ESOPHAGEAL CARCINOMA

In 2008 in the United States, 16,470 cases and 14,280 deaths; less frequent in women than men. Highest incidence in focal regions of China, Iran, Afghanistan, Siberia, Mongolia. In the United States, blacks more frequently affected than whites; usually presents sixth decade or later; 5-year survival <5% because most pts present with advanced disease.

Pathology   60% squamous cell carcinoma, most commonly in upper two-thirds; <40% adenocarcinoma, usually in distal third, arising in region of columnar metaplasia (Barrett's esophagus), glandular tissue, or as direct extension of proximal gastric adenocarcinoma; lymphoma and melanoma rare.

Risk Factors   Major risk factors for squamous cell carcinoma: ethanol abuse, smoking (combination is synergistic); other risks: lye ingestion and esophageal stricture, radiation exposure, head and neck cancer, achalasia, smoked opiates, Plummer-Vinson syndrome, tylosis, chronic ingestion of extremely hot tea, deficiency of vitamin A, zinc, molybdenum. Barrett's esophagus is a risk for adenocarcinoma.

Clinical Features Progressive dysphagia (first with solids, then liquids), rapid weight loss common, chest pain (from mediastinal spread), odynophagia, pulmonary aspiration (obstruction, tracheoesophageal fistula), hoarseness (laryngeal nerve palsy), hypercalcemia (parathyroid hormone–related peptide hypersecretion by squamous carcinomas); bleeding infrequent, occasionally severe; examination often unremarkable.

Diagnosis Double-contrast barium swallow useful as initial test in dysphagia; flexible esophagogastroscopy most sensitive and specific test; pathologic confirmation by combining endoscopic biopsy and cytologic examination of mucosal brushings (neither alone sufficiently sensitive); CT and endoscopic ultrasonography valuable to assess local and nodal spread.

℞ Esophageal Carcinoma

Surgical resection feasible in only 40% of pts; associated with high complication rate (fistula, abscess, aspiration). *Squamous cell carcinoma*: Surgical resection after chemotherapy [5-fluorouracil (5FU), cisplatin] plus radiation therapy prolongs survival and may provide improved cure rate. *Adenocarcinoma*: Curative resection rarely possible; <20% of pts with resectable tumors survive 5 years. Palliative measures include laser ablation, mechanical dilatation, radiotherapy, and a luminal prosthesis to bypass the tumor. Gastrostomy or jejunostomy are frequently required for nutritional support.

GASTRIC CARCINOMA

Highest incidence in Japan, China, Chile, Ireland; incidence decreasing worldwide, eightfold in the United States over past 60 years; in 2008, 21,500 new cases and 10,880 deaths. Male:female = 2:1; peak incidence sixth and seventh decades; overall 5-year survival <15%.

Risk Factors Increased incidence in lower socioeconomic groups; environmental component is suggested by studies of migrants and their offspring. Several dietary factors correlated with increased incidence: nitrates, smoked foods, heavily salted foods; genetic component suggested by increased incidence in first-degree relatives of affected pts; other risk factors: atrophic gastritis, *Helicobacter pylori* infection, Billroth II gastrectomy, gastrojejunostomy, adenomatous gastric polyps, pernicious anemia, hyperplastic gastric polyps (latter two associated with atrophic gastritis), Ménétrier's disease, slight increased risk with blood group A.

Pathology Adenocarcinoma in 85%; usually focal (polypoid, ulcerative), two-thirds arising in antrum or lesser curvature, frequently ulcerative ("intestinal type"); less commonly diffuse infiltrative (linitis plastica) or superficial spreading (diffuse lesions more prevalent in younger pts; exhibit less geographic variation; have extremely poor prognosis); spreads primarily to local nodes, liver, peritoneum; systemic spread uncommon; lymphoma accounts for 15% (most frequent extranodal site in immunocompetent pts), either low-grade tumor of mucosa-associated lymphoid tissue (MALT) or aggressive diffuse large B cell lymphoma; leiomyosarcoma or gastrointestinal stromal tumor (GIST) is rare.

Clinical Features Most commonly presents with progressive upper abdominal discomfort, frequently with weight loss, anorexia, nausea; acute or chronic GI bleeding (mucosal ulceration) common; dysphagia (location in cardia); vomiting (pyloric and widespread disease); early satiety; examination often unrevealing early in course; later, abdominal tenderness, pallor, and cachexia most common signs; palpable mass uncommon; metastatic spread may be manifest by hepatomegaly, ascites, left supraclavicular or scalene adenopathy, periumbilical, ovarian, or prerectal mass (Blumer's shelf), low-grade fever, skin abnormalities (nodules, dermatomyositis, acanthosis nigricans, or multiple seborrheic keratoses). Laboratory findings: iron-deficiency anemia in two-thirds of pts; fecal occult blood in 80%; rarely associated with pancytopenia and microangiopathic hemolytic anemia (from marrow infiltration), leukemoid reaction, migratory thrombophlebitis, or acanthosis nigricans.

Diagnosis Double-contrast barium swallow useful; gastroscopy most sensitive and specific test; pathologic confirmation by biopsy and cytologic examination of mucosal brushings; superficial biopsies less sensitive for lymphomas (frequently submucosal); important to differentiate benign from malignant gastric ulcers with multiple biopsies and follow-up examinations to demonstrate ulcer healing.

℞ Gastric Carcinoma

Adenocarcinoma: Gastrectomy offers only chance of cure (only possible in less than one-third); the rare tumors limited to mucosa are resectable for cure in 80%; deeper invasion, nodal metastases decrease 5-year survival to 20% of pts with resectable tumors in absence of obvious metastatic spread (Table 76-1); CT and endoscopic ultrasonography may aid in determining tumor resectability. Subtotal gastrectomy has similar efficacy to total gastrectomy for distal stomach lesions, but with less morbidity; no clear benefit for resection of spleen and a portion of the pancreas, or for radical lymph node removal. Adjuvant chemotherapy (5FU/leucovorin) plus radiation therapy following primary surgery leads to a 7-month increase in median survival. Neoadjuvant chemotherapy with epirubicin, cisplatin, and 5FU may downstage tumors and increase the efficacy of surgery. Palliative therapy for pain, obstruction, and bleeding includes surgery, endoscopic dilatation, radiation therapy, chemotherapy.

Lymphoma: Low-grade MALT lymphoma is caused by *H. pylori* infection, and eradication of the infection causes complete remissions in 50% of pts; rest are responsive to combination chemotherapy including cyclophosphamide, doxorubicin, vincristine, prednisone (CHOP) plus rituximab. Diffuse large B cell lymphoma may be treated with either CHOP plus rituximab or subtotal gastrectomy followed by chemotherapy; 50–60% 5-year survival.

Leiomyosarcoma: Surgical resection curative in most pts. Tumors expressing the *c-kit* tyrosine kinase (CD117)—GIST—respond to imatinib mesylate in a substantial fraction of cases.

BENIGN GASTRIC TUMORS

Much less common than malignant gastric tumors; hyperplastic polyps most common, with adenomas, hamartomas, and leiomyomas rare; 30% of adenomas and occasional hyperplastic polyps are associated with gastric malignancy; polyposis syndromes include Peutz-Jeghers and familial polyposis (hamartomas and adenomas), Gardner's (adenomas), and Cronkhite-Canada (cystic polyps). See "Colonic Polyps," below.

Clinical Features Usually asymptomatic; occasionally present with bleeding or vague epigastric discomfort.

TABLE 76-1 STAGING SYSTEM FOR GASTRIC CARCINOMA

Stage	TNM	Features	Data from American College of Surgeons Number of Cases, %	Data from American College of Surgeons 5-Year Survival, %
0	TisN0M0	Node negative; limited to mucosa	1	90
IA	T1N0M0	Node negative; invasion of lamina propria or sub-mucosa	7	59
IB	T2N0M0	Node negative; invasion of muscularis propria	10	44
II	T1N2M0 T2N1M0	Node positive; invasion beyond mucosa but within wall *or*		
	T3N0M0	Node negative; extension through wall	17	29
IIIA	T2N2M0 T3N1–2M0	Node positive; invasion of muscularis propria or through wall	21	15
IIIB	T4N0–1M0	Node negative; adherence to surrounding tissue	14	9
IV	T4N2M0	Node positive; adherence to surrounding tissue *or*		
	T1–4N0–2M1	Distant metastases	30	3

Note: TNM, tumor, node, metastasis.

 Benign Gastric Tumors

Endoscopic or surgical excision.

SMALL-BOWEL TUMORS

Clinical Features Uncommon tumors (~5% of all GI neoplasms); usually present with bleeding, abdominal pain, weight loss, fever, or intestinal obstruction (intermittent or fixed); increased incidence of lymphomas in pts with gluten-sensitive enteropathy, Crohn's disease involving small bowel, AIDS, prior organ transplantation, autoimmune disorders.

Pathology Usually benign; most common are adenomas (usually duodenal), leiomyomas (intramural), and lipomas (usually ileal); 50% of malignant tumors are adenocarcinoma, usually in duodenum (at or near ampulla of Vater) or proximal jejunum, commonly coexisting with benign adenomas; primary intestinal lymphomas (non-Hodgkin's) account for 25% and occur as focal mass (Western type), which is usually a T cell lymphoma associated with prior celiac disease, or diffuse infiltration (Mediterranean type), which is usually immunoproliferative small-intestinal disease (IPSID; α-heavy chain disease), a B cell MALT lymphoma associated with *Campylobacter jejuni* infection, which can present as intestinal malabsorption; carcinoid tumors (usually asymptomatic) occasionally produce bleeding or intussusception (see below).

Diagnosis Endoscopy and biopsy most useful for tumors of duodenum and proximal jejunum; otherwise barium x-ray examination best diagnostic test; direct small-bowel instillation of contrast (enteroclysis) occasionally reveals tumors not seen with routine small-bowel radiography; angiography (to detect plexus of tumor vessels) or laparotomy often required for diagnosis; CT useful to evaluate extent of tumor (esp. lymphomas).

℞ Small-Bowel Tumors

Surgical excision; adjuvant chemotherapy appears helpful for focal lymphoma; IPSID appears to be curable with combination chemotherapy used in aggressive lymphoma plus oral antibiotics (e.g., tetracycline); no proven role for chemotherapy or radiation therapy for other small-bowel tumors.

COLONIC POLYPS

TUBULAR ADENOMAS

Present in ~30% of adults; pedunculated or sessile; usually asymptomatic; ~5% cause occult blood in stool; may cause obstruction; overall risk of malignant degeneration correlates with size (<2% if <1.5 cm diam; >10% if >2.5 cm diam) and is higher in sessile polyps; 65% found in rectosigmoid colon; diagnosis by barium enema, sigmoidoscopy, or colonoscopy. *Treatment*: Full colonoscopy to detect synchronous lesions (present in 30%); endoscopic resection (surgery if polyp large or inaccessible by colonoscopy); follow-up surveillance by colonoscopy every 2–3 years.

VILLOUS ADENOMAS

Generally larger than tubular adenomas at diagnosis; often sessile; high risk of malignancy (up to 30% when >2 cm); more prevalent in left colon; occasionally associated with potassium-rich secretory diarrhea. *Treatment*: As for tubular adenomas.

HYPERPLASTIC POLYPS

Asymptomatic; usually incidental finding at colonoscopy; rarely >5 mm; no malignant potential. No treatment required.

HEREDITARY POLYPOSIS SYNDROMES

See Table 76-2.

1. *Familial polyposis coli* (FPC): Diffuse pancolonic adenomatous polyposis (up to several thousand polyps); autosomal dominant inheritance associated with deletion in adenomatous polyposis coli (APC) gene on chromosome 5; colon carcinoma from malignant degeneration of polyp in 100% by age 40. *Treatment*: Prophylactic total colectomy or subtotal colectomy with ileoproctostomy before age 30; subtotal resection avoids ileostomy but necessitates frequent proctoscopic surveillance; periodic colonoscopic or annual radiologic screening of siblings and offspring of pts with FPC until age 35; sulindac and other nonsteroidal anti-inflammatory drugs (NSAIDs) cause regression of polyps and inhibit their development.

TABLE 76-2   HEREDITABLE (AUTOSOMAL DOMINANT) GASTROINTESTINAL POLYPOSIS SYNDROMES

Syndrome	Distribution of Polyps	Histologic Type	Malignant Potential	Associated Lesions
Familial adenomatous polyposis	Large intestine	Adenoma	Common	None
Gardner's syndrome	Large and small intestine	Adenoma	Common	Osteomas, fibromas, lipomas, epidermoid cysts, ampullary cancers, congenital hypertrophy of retinal pigment epithelium
Turcot's syndrome	Large intestine	Adenoma	Common	Brain tumors
Nonpolyposis syndrome (Lynch syndrome)	Large intestine (often proximal)	Adenoma	Common	Endometrial and ovarian tumors
Peutz-Jeghers syndrome	Small and large intestines, stomach	Hamartoma	Rare	Mucocutaneous pigmentation; tumors of the ovary, breast, pancreas, endometrium
Juvenile polyposis	Large and small intestines, stomach	Hamartoma, rarely progressing to adenoma	Rare	Various congenital abnormalities

2. *Gardner's syndrome*: Variant of FPC with associated soft tissue tumors (epidermoid cysts, osteomas, lipomas, fibromas, desmoids); higher incidence of gastroduodenal polyps, ampullary adenocarcinoma. *Treatment*: As for FPC; surveillance for small-bowel disease with fecal occult blood testing after colectomy.

3. *Turcot's syndrome*: Rare variant of FPC with associated malignant brain tumors. *Treatment*: As for FPC.

4. *Nonpolyposis syndrome*: Familial syndrome with up to 50% risk of colon carcinoma; peak incidence in fifth decade; associated with multiple primary cancers (esp. endometrial); autosomal dominant; due to defective DNA mismatch repair.

5. *Juvenile polyposis*: Multiple benign colonic and small-bowel hamartomas; intestinal bleeding common. Other symptoms: abdominal pain, diarrhea; occasional intussusception. Rarely recur after excision; low risk of colon cancer from malignant degeneration of interspersed adenomatous polyps. Prophylactic colectomy controversial.

6. *Peutz-Jeghers syndrome*: Numerous hamartomatous polyps of entire GI tract, though denser in small bowel than colon; GI bleeding common; somewhat increased risk for the development of cancer at GI and non-GI sites. Prophylactic surgery not recommended.

COLORECTAL CANCER

Second most common internal cancer in humans; accounts for 10% of cancer-related deaths in United States; incidence increases dramatically above age 50, nearly equal in men and women. In 2008, 148,810 new cases, 49,960 deaths.

Etiology and Risk Factors Most colon cancers arise from adenomatous polyps. Genetic steps from polyp to dysplasia to carcinoma in situ to invasive cancer have been defined, including point mutation in K-*ras* proto-oncogene, hypomethylation of DNA leading to enhanced gene expression, allelic loss at the *APC* gene (a tumor suppressor), allelic loss at the *DCC* (deleted in colon cancer) gene on chromosome 18, and loss and mutation of p53 on chromosome 17. Hereditary nonpolyposis colon cancer arises from mutations in the DNA mismatch repair genes, *hMSH2* gene on chromosome 2 and *hMLH1* gene on chromosome 3. Mutations lead to colon and other cancers. Diagnosis requires three or more relatives with colon cancer, one of whom is a first-degree relative; one or more cases diagnosed before age 50; and involvement of at least two generations. Environmental factors also play a role; increased prevalence in developed countries, urban areas, advantaged socioeconomic groups; increased risk in pts with hypercholesterolemia, coronary artery disease; correlation of risk with low-fiber, high-animal-fat diets, although direct effect of diet remains unproven; decreased risk with long-term dietary calcium supplementation and, possibly, daily aspirin ingestion. Risk increased in first-degree relatives of pts; families with increased prevalence of cancer; and pts with history of breast or gynecologic cancer, familial polyposis syndromes, >10-year history of ulcerative colitis or Crohn's colitis, >15-year history of ureterosigmoidostomy. Tumors in pts with strong family history of malignancy are frequently located in right colon and commonly present before age 50; high prevalence in pts with *Streptococcus bovis* bacteremia.

Pathology Nearly always adenocarcinoma; 75% located distal to the splenic flexure (except in association with polyposis or hereditary cancer syndromes); may be polypoid, sessile, fungating, or constricting; subtype and degree of differentiation do not correlate with course. Degree of invasiveness at surgery (Dukes' classification) is single best predictor of prognosis (Fig. 76-1). Rectosigmoid tumors may spread to lungs early because of systemic paravertebral venous drainage of this area. Other predictors of poor prognosis: preoperative serum carcinoembryonic antigen (CEA) >5 ng/mL (>5 μg/L), poorly differentiated histology, bowel perforation, venous invasion, adherence to adjacent organs, aneuploidy, specific deletions in chromosomes 5, 17, 18, and mutation of *ras* proto-oncogene. 15% have defects in DNA repair.

Clinical Features Left-sided colon cancers present most commonly with rectal bleeding, altered bowel habits (narrowing, constipation, intermittent diarrhea, tenesmus), and abdominal or back pain; cecal and ascending colon cancers more frequently present with symptoms of anemia, occult blood in stool, or weight loss; other complications: perforation, fistula, volvulus, inguinal hernia; laboratory findings: anemia in 50% of right-sided lesions.

Diagnosis Early diagnosis aided by screening asymptomatic persons with fecal occult blood testing (see below); >50% of all colon cancers are within reach of a

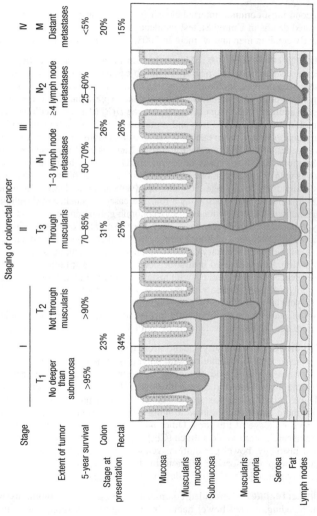

FIGURE 76-1 Staging and prognosis for patients with colorectal cancer.

Stage	I		II	III		IV
	T_1 No deeper than submucosa	T_2 Not through muscularis	T_3 Through muscularis	N_1 1–3 lymph node metastases	N_2 ≥4 lymph node metastases	M Distant metastases
Extent of tumor						
5-year survival	>95%	>90%	70–85%	50–70%	25–60%	<5%
Stage at presentation Colon	23%		31%	26%		20%
Stage at presentation Rectal	34%		25%	26%		15%

Mucosa
Muscularis mucosa
Submucosa
Muscularis propria
Serosa
Fat
Lymph nodes

Staging of colorectal cancer

60-cm flexible sigmoidoscope; air-contrast barium enema will diagnose ~85% of colon cancers not within reach of sigmoidoscope; colonoscopy most sensitive and specific, permits tumor biopsy and removal of synchronous polyps (thus preventing neoplastic conversion), but is more expensive. Radiographic or virtual colonoscopy has not been shown to be a better diagnostic method than colonoscopy.

℞ Colorectal Cancer

Local disease: Surgical resection of colonic segment containing tumor; preoperative evaluation to assess prognosis and surgical approach includes full colonoscopy, chest films, biochemical liver tests, plasma CEA level, and possible abdominal CT. Resection of isolated hepatic metastases possible in selected cases. Adjuvant radiation therapy to pelvis (with or without concomitant 5FU chemotherapy) decreases local recurrence rate of rectal carcinoma (no apparent effect on survival); radiation therapy without benefit on colon tumors; preoperative radiation therapy may improve resectability and local control in pts with rectal cancer. Total mesorectal excision is more effective than conventional anteroposterior resection in rectal cancer. Adjuvant chemotherapy (5FU/leucovorin plus oxaliplatin, or FOLFOX plus bevacizumab, or 5FU/leucovorin plus irinotecan, or FOLFIRI) decreases recurrence rate and improves survival of stage C (III); survival benefit from adjuvant therapy is not so clear in stage B (II) tumors; periodic determination of serum CEA level useful to follow therapy and assess recurrence. *Follow-up after curative resection*: Yearly liver tests, complete blood count, follow-up radiologic or colonoscopic evaluation at 1 year—if normal, repeat every 3 years, with routine screening interim (see below); if polyps detected, repeat 1 year after resection. *Advanced tumor* (locally unresectable or metastatic): Systemic chemotherapy (5FU/leucovorin plus oxaliplatin plus bevacizumab), irinotecan usually used in second treatment; antibodies to the EGF receptor (cetuximab, panitumumab) appear to enhance the effect of chemotherapy; intraarterial chemotherapy [floxuridine (FUDR)] and/or radiation therapy may palliate symptoms from hepatic metastases.

Prevention   Early detection of colon carcinoma may be facilitated by routine screening of stool for occult blood (Hemoccult II, ColonCare, Hemosure); however, sensitivity only ~50% for carcinoma; specificity for tumor or polyp ~25–40%. False positives: ingestion of red meat, iron, aspirin; upper GI bleeding. False negatives: vitamin C ingestion, intermittent bleeding. Annual digital rectal exam and fecal occult blood testing recommended for pts over age 40, screening by flexible sigmoidoscopy every 3 years after age 50, earlier in pts at increased risk (see above); careful evaluation of all pts with positive fecal occult blood tests (flexible sigmoidoscopy and air-contrast barium enema or colonoscopy alone) reveals polyps in 20–40% and carcinoma in ~5%; screening of asymptomatic persons allows earlier detection of colon cancer (i.e., earlier Dukes' stage) and achieves greater resectability rate; decreased overall mortality from colon carcinoma seen only after 13 years of follow-up. More intensive evaluation of first-degree relatives of pts with colon carcinoma frequently includes screening air-contrast barium enema or colonoscopy after age 40. NSAIDs and cyclooxygenase 2 inhibitors appear to prevent polyp development and induce regression in high-risk groups but have not been recommended for average-risk pts at this time.

ANAL CANCER

Accounts for 1–2% of large-bowel cancer, 5070 cases and 680 deaths in 2008; associated with chronic irritation, e.g., from condyloma acuminata, perianal fissures/fistulae, chronic hemorrhoids, leukoplakia, trauma from anal intercourse. Women are more commonly affected than men. Homosexual men are at increased risk. Human papillomavirus may be etiologic. Presents with bleeding, pain, and perianal mass. Radiation therapy plus chemotherapy (5FU and mitomycin) leads to complete response in 80% when the primary lesion is <3 cm. Abdominoperineal resection with permanent colostomy is reserved for those with large lesions or whose disease recurs after chemoradiotherapy.

BENIGN LIVER TUMORS

Hepatocellular adenomas occur most commonly in women in the third or fourth decades who take birth control pills. Most are found incidentally but may cause pain; intratumoral hemorrhage may cause circulatory collapse. 10% may become malignant. Women with these adenomas should stop taking birth control pills. Large tumors near the liver surface may be resected. Focal nodular hyperplasia is also more common in women but seems not to be caused by birth control pills. Lesions are vascular on angiography and have septae and are usually asymptomatic.

HEPATOCELLULAR CARCINOMA

About 21,370 cases in the United States in 2008, but worldwide this may be the most common tumor. Male:female = 4:1; tumor usually develops in cirrhotic liver in persons in fifth or sixth decade. High incidence in Asia and Africa is related to etiologic relationship between this cancer and hepatitis B and C infections. Aflatoxin exposure contributes to etiology and leaves a molecular signature, a mutation in codon 249 of the gene for p53.

Modes of Presentation   A patient with known liver disease develops an abnormality on ultrasound or rising α fetoprotein (AFP) or des-gamma-carboxy prothrombin (DCP) due to absence of vitamin K; abnormal liver function tests; cachexia, abdominal pain, fever.

Physical Findings   Jaundice, asthenia, itching, tremors, disorientation, hepatomegaly, splenomegaly, ascites, peripheral edema.

℞ Hepatocellular Carcinoma

Surgical resection or liver transplantation is therapeutic option but rarely successful. Radiofrequency ablation can cause regression of small tumors. Sorafenib may produce partial responses lasting a few months.

Screening and Prevention   Screening populations at risk has given conflicting results. Hepatitis B vaccine prevents the disease. Interferon α (IFN-α) may prevent liver cancer in persons with chronic active hepatitis C disease and possibly in those with hepatitis B. Ribavirin $\pm$ IFN-α is most effective treatment of chronic hepatitis C.

PANCREATIC CANCER

In 2008 in the United States, about 37,680 new cases and 34,290 deaths. The incidence is decreasing somewhat, but nearly all diagnosed cases are fatal. The tumors are ductal adenocarcinomas and are not usually detected until the disease has spread. About 70% of tumors are in the pancreatic head, 20% in the body, and 10% in the tail. Mutations in K-*ras* have been found in 85% of tumors, and the p16 cyclin-dependent kinase inhibitor on chromosome 9 may also be implicated. Long-standing diabetes, chronic pancreatitis, and smoking increase the risk; coffee-drinking, alcoholism, and cholelithiasis do not. Pts present with pain and weight loss, the pain often relieved by bending forward. Jaundice commonly complicates tumors of the head, due to biliary obstruction. Curative surgical resections are feasible in about 10%. Adjuvant chemotherapy (5FU) may benefit some patients after resection. Gemcitabine plus erlotinib or capecitabine may palliate symptoms in pts with advanced disease.

ENDOCRINE TUMORS OF THE GI TRACT AND PANCREAS

CARCINOID TUMOR

Carcinoid tumor accounts for 75% of GI endocrine tumors; incidence is about 15 cases per million population. 90% originate in Kulchitsky cells of the GI tract, most commonly the appendix, ileum, and rectum. Carcinoid tumors of the small bowel and bronchus have a more malignant course than tumors of other sites. About 5% of pts with carcinoid tumors develop symptoms of the carcinoid syndrome, the classic triad being cutaneous flushing, diarrhea, and valvular heart disease. For tumors of GI tract origin, symptoms imply metastases to liver.

Diagnosis can be made by detecting the site of tumor or documenting production of >15 mg/d of the serotonin metabolite 5-hydroxyindoleacetic acid (5-HIAA) in the urine. Octreotide scintigraphy identifies sites of primary and metastatic tumor in about two-thirds of cases.

℞ Carcinoid Tumor

Surgical resection where feasible. Symptoms may be controlled with histamine blockers and octreotide, 150–1500 mg/d in three doses. Hepatic artery embolization and chemotherapy (5FU plus streptozocin or doxorubicin) have been used for metastatic disease. IFN-α at 3–10 million units SC three times a week may relieve symptoms. Prognosis ranges from 95% 5-year survival for localized disease to 20% 5-year survival for those with liver metastases. Median survival of pts with carcinoid syndrome is 2.5 years from the first episode of flushing.

PANCREATIC ISLET-CELL TUMORS

Gastrinoma, insulinoma, VIPoma, glucagonoma, and somatostatinoma account for the vast majority of pancreatic islet-cell tumors; their characteristics are shown in Table 76-3. The tumors are named for the dominant hormone they produce. They are generally slow-growing and produce symptoms related to hormone production. *Gastrinomas* and *peptic ulcer disease* constitute the Zollinger-Ellison syndrome. Gastrinomas are rare (4 cases per 10 million population), and in 25–50%, the tumor is a component of a multiple endocrine neoplasia type 1 (MEN 1) syndrome (Chap. 186).

Insulinoma may present with Whipple's triad: fasting hypoglycemia, symptoms of hypoglycemia, and relief after IV glucose. Normal or elevated serum insulin levels in the presence of fasting hypoglycemia are diagnostic. Insulinomas may also be associated with MEN 1.

Verner and Morrison described a syndrome of watery diarrhea, hypokalemia, achlorhydria, and renal failure associated with pancreatic islet tumors that

TABLE 76-3 GASTROINTESTINAL ENDOCRINE TUMOR SYNDROMES

Syndrome	Cell Type	Clinical Features	Percentage Malignant	Major Products
Carcinoid syndrome	Enterochromaffin, entero-chromaffin-like	Flushing, diarrhea, wheezing, hypotension	~100	Serotonin, histamine, miscellaneous peptides
Zollinger-Ellison, gastrinoma	Non-β islet cell, duodenal G cell	Peptic ulcers, diarrhea	~70	Gastrin
Insulinoma	Islet β cell	Hypoglycemia	~10	Insulin
VIPoma (Verner-Morrison, WDHA)	Islet D_1 cell	Diarrhea, hypokalemia, hypochlorhydria	~60	Vasoactive intestinal peptide
Glucagonoma	Islet A cell	Mild diabetes mellitus, erythema necrolytica migrans, glossitis	>75	Glucagon
Somatostatinoma	Islet D cell	Diabetes mellitus, diarrhea, steatorrhea, gallstones	~70	Somatostatin

Note: WDHA, watery diarrhea, hypokalemia, achlorhydria.

produce vasoactive intestinal polypeptide (VIP). *VIPomas* are rare (1 case per 10 million) but often grow to a large size before producing symptoms.

Glucagonoma is associated with diabetes mellitus and necrolytic migratory erythema, a characteristic red, raised, scaly rash usually located on the face, abdomen, perineum, and distal extremities. Glucagon levels >1000 ng/L not suppressed by glucose are diagnostic.

The classic triad of *somatostatinoma* is diabetes mellitus, steatorrhea, and cholelithiasis.

Provocative tests may facilitate diagnosis of functional endocrine tumors: tolbutamide enhances somatostatin secretion by somatostatinomas; pentagastrin enhances calcitonin secretion from medullary thyroid (C cell) tumors; secretin enhances gastrin secretion from gastrinomas. If imaging techniques fail to detect tumor masses, angiography or selective venous sampling for hormone determination may reveal the site of tumor. Metastases to nodes and liver should be sought by CT or MRI.

℞ Pancreatic Islet-Cell Tumors

Tumor is surgically removed, if possible. Octreotide inhibits hormone secretion in the majority of cases. IFN-α may reduce symptoms. Streptozotocin plus doxorubicin combination chemotherapy may produce responses in 60–90% of cases. Embolization or chemoembolization of hepatic metastases may be palliative.

> For a more detailed discussion, see Mayer RJ: Gastrointestinal Tract Cancer, Chap. 87, p. 570; Carr BI: Tumors of the Liver and Biliary Tree, Chap. 88, p. 580; Chua YJ, Cunningham D: Pancreatic Cancer, Chap. 89, p. 586; and Jensen RT: Endocrine Tumors of the Gastrointestinal Tract and Pancreas, Chap. 344, p. 2347, in HPIM-17.

77 Genitourinary Tract Cancer

BLADDER CANCER

Incidence and Epidemiology   Annual incidence in the United States is about 69,810 cases with 14,100 deaths. Median age is 65 years. Smoking accounts for 50% of the risk. Exposure to polycyclic aromatic hydrocarbons increases the risk, especially in slow acetylators. Risk is increased in chimney sweeps, dry cleaners, and those involved in aluminum manufacturing. Chronic cyclophosphamide exposure increases risk ninefold. *Schistosoma haematobium* infection also increases risk, especially of squamous histology.

Etiology   Lesions involving chromosome 9q are an early event. Deletions in 17p (p53), 18q (the DCC locus), 13q (RB), 3p, and 5q are characteristic of invasive lesions. Overexpression of epidermal growth factor receptors and *HER2/neu* receptors is common.

Pathology   Over 90% of tumors are derived from transitional epithelium; 3% are squamous, 2% are adenocarcinomas, and <1% are neuroendocrine small cell tumors. Field effects are seen that place all sites lined by transitional epithelium at risk including the renal pelvis, ureter, bladder, and proximal two-thirds of the urethra. 90% of tumors are in the bladder, 8% in the renal pelvis, and 2% in the ureter or urethra. Histologic grade influences survival. Lesion recurrence is influenced by size, number, and growth pattern of the primary tumor.

Clinical Presentation   Hematuria is the initial sign in 80–90%; however, cystitis is a more common cause of hematuria (22% of all hematuria) than is bladder cancer (15%). Pts are initially staged and treated by endoscopy. Superficial tumors are removed at endoscopy; muscle invasion requires more extensive surgery.

Rx Bladder Cancer

Management is based on extent of disease: superficial, invasive, or metastatic. Frequency of presentation is 75% superficial, 20% invasive, and 5% metastatic. Superficial lesions are resected at endoscopy. Although complete resection is possible in 80%, 30–80% of cases recur; grade and stage progression occur in 30%. Intravesical instillation of bacille Calmette-Guérin (BCG) reduces the risk of recurrence by 40–45%. Recurrence is monitored every 3 months.

The standard management of muscle-invasive disease is radical cystectomy. 5-year survival is 70% for those without invasion of perivesicular fat or lymph nodes, 50% for those with invasion of fat but not lymph nodes, 35% for those with one node involved, and 10% for those with six or more involved nodes. Pts who cannot withstand radical surgery may have 30–35% 5-year survival with 5000- to 7000-cGy external beam radiation therapy. Bladder sparing may be possible in up to 45% of pts with two cycles of chemotherapy with CMV (methotrexate, 30 mg/m^2 days 1 and 8, vinblastine, 4 mg/m^2 days 1 and 8, cisplatin, 100 mg/m^2 day 2, q21d) followed by 4000-cGy radiation therapy given concurrently with cisplatin.

Metastatic disease is treated with combination chemotherapy. Useful regimens include CMV (see above), M-VAC (methotrexate, 30 mg/m^2 days 1, 15, 22; vinblastine, 3 mg/m^2 days 2, 15, 22; doxorubicin, 30 mg/m^2 day 2; cisplatin, 70 mg/m^2 day 2; q28d) or cisplatin (70 mg/m^2 day 2) plus gemcitabine (1000 mg/m^2 days 1, 8, 15 of a 28-day cycle) or carboplatin plus paclitaxel. About 70% of pts respond to treatment, and 20% have a complete response; 10–15% have long-term disease-free survival.

RENAL CANCER

Incidence and Epidemiology   Annual incidence in the United States is about 54,390 cases with 13,010 deaths. Cigarette smoking accounts for 20–30% of cases. Risk is increased in acquired renal cystic disease. There are two familial forms: a rare autosomal dominant syndrome and von Hippel–Lindau disease. About 35% of pts with von Hippel–Lindau disease develop renal cancer. Incidence is also increased in those with tuberous sclerosis and polycystic kidney disease.

Etiology   Most cases are sporadic; however, the most frequent chromosomal abnormality (occurs in 60%) is deletion or rearrangement of 3p21-26. The von Hippel–Lindau gene has been mapped to that region and appears to have novel activities, regulation of speed of transcription, and participation in turnover of damaged proteins. It is unclear how lesions in the gene lead to cancer.

Pathology Five variants are recognized: clear cell tumors (75%), chromophilic tumors (15%), chromophobic tumors (5%), oncocytic tumors (3%), and collecting duct tumors (2%). Clear cell tumors arise from cells of the proximal convoluted tubules. Chromophilic tumors tend to be bilateral and multifocal and often show trisomy 7 and/or trisomy 17. Chromophobic and eosinophilic tumors less frequently have chromosomal aberrations and follow a more indolent course.

Clinical Presentation The classic triad of hematuria, flank pain, and flank mass is seen in only 10–20% of pts; hematuria (40%), flank pain (40%), palpable mass (33%), and weight loss (33%) are the most common individual symptoms. Paraneoplastic syndromes of erythrocytosis (3%), hypercalcemia (5%), and nonmetastatic hepatic dysfunction (Stauffer's syndrome) (15%) may also occur. Workup should include IV pyelography, renal ultrasonography, CT of abdomen and pelvis, chest x-ray (CXR), urinalysis, and urine cytology. Stage I is disease restricted to the kidney, stage II is disease contained within Gerota's fascia, stage III is locally invasive disease involving nodes and/or inferior vena cava, stage IV is invasion of adjacent organs or metastatic sites. Prognosis is related to stage: 66% 5-year survival for I, 64% for II, 42% for III, and 11% for IV.

Rx **Renal Cancer**

Radical nephrectomy is standard for stages I, II, and most stage III pts. Surgery may also be indicated in the setting of metastatic disease for intractable local symptoms (bleeding, pain). Response rates of 40–48% have been noted with three different single agents, sunitinib, sorafenib, and temsirolimus. Sunitinib and sorafenib are thought to be antiangiogenic through inhibition of kinases in tumor cells. Temsirolimus is an inhibitor of mTOR. About 10–15% of pts with advanced-stage disease may benefit from interleukin 2 and/or interferon α (IFN-α). Addition of bevacizumab to IFN-α improves the response rate. Some remissions are durable. Chemotherapy is of little or no benefit.

TESTICULAR CANCER

Incidence and Epidemiology Annual incidence is about 8090 cases with 380 deaths. Peak age incidence is 20–40. Occurs 4–5 times more frequently in white than black men. Cryptorchid testes are at increased risk. Early orchiopexy may protect against testis cancer. Risk is also increased in testicular feminization syndromes, and Klinefelter syndrome is associated with mediastinal germ cell tumor.

Etiology The cause is unknown. Disease is associated with a characteristic cytogenetic defect, isochromosome 12p.

Pathology Two main subtypes are noted: seminoma and nonseminoma. Each accounts for ~50% of cases. Seminoma has a more indolent natural history and is highly sensitive to radiation therapy. Four subtypes of nonseminoma are defined: embryonal carcinoma, teratoma, choriocarcinoma, and endodermal sinus (yolk sac) tumor.

Clinical Presentation Painless testicular mass is the classic initial sign. In the presence of pain, differential diagnosis includes epididymitis or orchitis; a brief trial of antibiotics may be undertaken. Staging evaluation includes measurement of serum tumor markers α fetoprotein (AFP) and β-human chorionic gonadotropin (hCG), CXR, and CT scan of abdomen and pelvis. Lymph nodes are

| TABLE 77-1 | GERM CELL TUMOR STAGING AND TREATMENT | | |

| | | Treatment | |
Stage	Extent of Disease	Seminoma	Nonseminoma
IA	Testis only, no vascular/ lymphatic invasion (T1)	Radiation therapy	RPLND or observation
IB	Testis only, with vascular/ lymphatic invasion (T2), or extension through tunica albuginea (T2), or involvement of spermatic cord (T3) or scrotum (T4)	Radiation therapy	RPLND
IIA	Nodes < 2 cm	Radiation therapy	RPLND or chemotherapy often followed by RPLND
IIB	Nodes 2–5 cm	Radiation therapy	RPLND ± adjuvant chemotherapy or chemotherapy followed by RPLND
IIC	Nodes > 5 cm	Chemotherapy	Chemotherapy, often followed by RPLND
III	Distant metastases	Chemotherapy	Chemotherapy, often followed by surgery (biopsy or resection)

Note: RPLND, retroperitoneal lymph node dissection.

staged at resection of the primary tumor through an inguinal approach. Stage I disease is limited to the testis, epididymis, or spermatic cord; stage II involves retroperitoneal nodes; and stage III is disease outside the retroperitoneum. Among seminoma pts, 70% are stage I, 20% are stage II, and 10% are stage III. Among nonseminoma germ cell tumor pts, 33% are found in each stage. hCG may be elevated in either seminoma or nonseminoma, but AFP is elevated only in nonseminoma. 95% of pts are cured if treated appropriately. Primary nonseminoma in the mediastinum is associated with acute leukemia or other hematologic disorders and has a poorer prognosis than testicular primaries (~33%).

℞ Testicular Cancer   Table 77-1

For stages I and II seminoma, inguinal orchiectomy followed by retroperitoneal radiation therapy to 2500–3000 cGy is effective. For stages I and II nonseminoma germ cell tumors, inguinal orchiectomy followed by retroperitoneal lymph node dissection is effective. For pts of either histology with bulky nodes or stage III disease, chemotherapy is given. Cisplatin (20 mg/m^2 days 1–5), etoposide (100 mg/m^2 days 1–5), and bleomycin (30 U days 2, 9, 16) given every 21 days for four cycles is the standard therapy. If tumor markers return to zero, residual masses are resected. Most are necrotic debris or teratomas. Salvage therapy rescues about 25% of those not cured with primary therapy.

For a more detailed discussion, see Scher HI, Motzer RJ: Bladder and Renal Cell Carcinomas, Chap. 90, p. 589; and Motzer RJ, Bosl GJ: Testicular Cancer, Chap. 92, p. 601, in HPIM-17.

78   Gynecologic Cancer

OVARIAN CANCER

Incidence and Epidemiology   Annually in the United States, about 22,000 new cases are found and 15,500 women die of ovarian cancer. Incidence begins to rise in the fifth decade, peaking in the eighth decade. Risk is increased in nulliparous women and reduced by pregnancy (risk decreased about 10% per pregnancy) and oral contraceptives. About 5% of cases are familial.

Genetics   Mutations in *BRCA-1* predispose women to both breast and ovarian cancer. Cytogenetic analysis of epithelial ovarian cancers that are not familial often reveals complex karyotypic abnormalities including structural lesions on chromosomes 1 and 11 and loss of heterozygosity for loci on chromosomes 3q, 6q, 11q, 13q, and 17. C-*myc*, H-*ras*, K-*ras*, and *HER2/neu* are often mutated or overexpressed. Unlike in colon cancer, a stepwise pathway to ovarian carcinoma is not apparent.

Screening   No benefit has been seen from screening women of average risk. Hereditary ovarian cancer accounts for 10% of all cases. Women with *BRCA-1* or -*2* mutations should consider prophylactic bilateral salpingo-oophorectomy by age 40.

Clinical Presentation   Most pts present with abdominal pain, bloating, urinary symptoms, and weight gain indicative of disease spread beyond the true pelvis. Localized ovarian cancer is usually asymptomatic and detected on routine pelvic examination as a palpable nontender adnexal mass. Most ovarian masses detected incidentally in ovulating women are ovarian cysts that resolve over one to three menstrual cycles. Adnexal masses in postmenopausal women are more often pathologic and should be surgically removed. CA-125 serum levels are ≥35 U/mL in 80–85% of women with ovarian cancer, but other conditions may also cause elevations.

Pathology   Half of ovarian tumors are benign, one-third are malignant, and the rest are tumors of low malignant potential. These borderline lesions have cytologic features of malignancy but do not invade. Malignant epithelial tumors may be of five different types: serous (50%), mucinous (25%), endometrioid (15%), clear cell (5%), and Brenner tumors (1%, derived from urothelial or transitional epithelium). The remaining 4% of ovarian tumors are stromal or germ cell tumors, which are managed like testicular cancer in men (Chap. 77). Histologic grade is an important prognostic factor for the epithelial varieties.

Staging   Extent of disease is ascertained by a surgical procedure that permits visual and manual inspection of all peritoneal surfaces and the diaphragm. Total abdominal hysterectomy, bilateral salpingo-oophorectomy, partial omentectomy, pelvic and paraaortic lymph node sampling, and peritoneal washings should be performed. The staging system and its influence on survival are shown in Table 78-1. About 23% of pts are stage I, 13% are stage II, 47% are stage III, and 16% are stage IV.

TABLE 78-1 STAGING AND SURVIVAL IN GYNECOLOGIC MALIGNANCIES

Stage	Ovarian	5-Year Survival, %	Endometrial	5-Year Survival, %	Cervical	5-Year Survival, %
0	—		—		Carcinoma in situ	100
I	Confined to ovary	90–95	Confined to corpus	89	Confined to uterus	85
II	Confined to pelvis	70–80	Involves corpus and cervix	73	Invades beyond uterus but not pelvic wall	65
III	Intraabdominal spread	25–50	Extends outside the uterus but not outside the true pelvis	52	Extends to pelvic wall and/or lower third of vagina, or hydronephrosis	35
IV	Spread outside abdomen	1–5	Extends outside the true pelvis or involves the bladder or rectum	17	Invades mucosa of bladder or rectum or extends beyond the true pelvis	7

Rx **Ovarian Cancer**

Pts with stage I disease, no residual tumor after surgery, and well- or moderately differentiated tumors need no further treatment after surgery and have a 5-year survival of >95%. For stage II pts totally resected and stage I pts with poor histologic grade, adjuvant therapy with single-agent cisplatin or cisplatin plus paclitaxel produces 5-year survival of 80%. Advanced-stage pts should receive paclitaxel, 175 mg/m^2 by 3-h infusion, followed by carboplatin dosed to an area under the curve (AUC) of 7.5 every 3 or 4 weeks. Carboplatin dose is calculated by the Calvert formula: dose = target AUC × (glomerular filtration rate + 25). The complete response rate is about 55%, and median survival is 38 months.

ENDOMETRIAL CANCER

Incidence and Epidemiology The most common gynecologic cancer—40,000 cases are diagnosed in the United States and 7500 pts die annually. It is primarily a disease of postmenopausal women. Obesity, altered menstrual cycles, infertility, late menopause, and postmenopausal bleeding are commonly encountered in women with endometrial cancer. Women taking tamoxifen to prevent breast cancer recurrence and those taking estrogen replacement therapy are at a modestly increased risk. Peak incidence is in the sixth and seventh decades.

Clinical Presentation Abnormal vaginal discharge (90%), abnormal vaginal bleeding (80%), and leukorrhea (10%) are the most common symptoms.

Pathology Endometrial cancers are adenocarcinomas in 75–80% of cases. The remaining cases include mucinous carcinoma; papillary serous carcinoma; and secretory, ciliate, and clear cell varieties. Prognosis depends on stage, histologic grade, and degree of myometrial invasion.

Staging Total abdominal hysterectomy and bilateral salpingo-oophorectomy comprise both the staging procedure and the treatment of choice. The staging scheme and its influence on prognosis are shown in Table 78-1. About 75% of pts are stage I, 13% are stage II, 9% are stage III, and 3% are stage IV.

Rx **Endometrial Cancer**

In women with poor histologic grade, deep myometrial invasion, or extensive involvement of the lower uterine segment or cervix, intracavitary or external beam radiation therapy is given. If cervical invasion is deep, preoperative radiation therapy may improve the resectability of the tumor. Stage III disease is managed with surgery and radiation therapy. Stage IV disease is usually treated palliatively. Progestational agents such as hydroxyprogesterone or megestrol and the antiestrogen tamoxifen may produce responses in 20% of pts. Doxorubicin, 60 mg/m^2 IV day 1, and cisplatin, 50 mg/m^2 IV day 1, every 3 weeks for 8 cycles produces a 45% response rate.

CERVICAL CANCER

Incidence and Epidemiology In the United States about 11,000 cases of invasive cervical cancer are diagnosed each year and 50,000 cases of carcinoma in situ are detected by Pap smear. Cervical cancer kills 3900 women a year, 85% of whom never had a Pap smear. It is a major cause of disease in underdeveloped countries and is more common in lower socioeconomic groups, in women with early sexual activity and/or multiple sexual partners, and in smokers. Human papilloma virus (HPV) types 16 and 18 are the major types associated with cervical cancer. The virus attacks the G_1 checkpoint of the cell cycle; its E7 protein binds and inactivates Rb protein, and E6 induces the degradation of p53.

Screening Women should begin screening when they begin sexual activity or at age 20. After two consecutive negative annual Pap smears, the test should be repeated every 3 years. Abnormal smears dictate the need for a cervical biopsy, usually under colposcopy, with the cervix painted with 3% acetic acid, which shows abnormal areas as white patches. If there is evidence of carcinoma in situ, a cone biopsy is performed, which is therapeutic.

Prevention Women and children age 9–26 should consider vaccination with Gardasil to prevent infection with two serotypes of virus that cause 70% of the cervical cancer in the United States.

Clinical Presentation Pts present with abnormal bleeding or postcoital spotting or menometrorrhagia or intermenstrual bleeding. Vaginal discharge, low back pain, and urinary symptoms may also be present.

Staging Staging is clinical and consists of a pelvic exam under anesthesia with cystoscopy and proctoscopy. Chest x-ray, IV pyelography, and abdominal CT are used to search for metastases. The staging system and its influence on prognosis are shown in Table 78-1. At presentation, 47% of pts are stage I, 28% are stage II, 21% are stage III, and 4% are stage IV.

℞ Cervical Cancer

Carcinoma in situ is cured with cone biopsy. Stage I disease may be treated with radical hysterectomy or radiation therapy. Stages II–IV disease are usually treated with radiation therapy, often with both brachytherapy and teletherapy, or combined-modality therapy. Pelvic exenteration is used uncommonly to control the disease, especially in the setting of centrally recurrent or persistent disease. Women with locally advanced (stage IIB to IVA) disease usually receive concurrent chemotherapy and radiation therapy. The chemotherapy acts as a radiosensitizer. Hydroxyurea, 5-fluorouracil (5FU), and cisplatin have all shown promising results given concurrently with radiation therapy. Cisplatin, 75 mg/m^2 IV over 4 h on day 1, and 5FU, 4 g given by 96-h infusion on days 1–5 of radiation therapy, is a common regimen. Relapse rates are reduced 30–50% by such therapy. Advanced-stage disease is treated palliatively with single agents (cisplatin, irinotecan, ifosfamide).

For a more detailed discussion, see Young RC: Gynecologic Malignancies, Chap. 93, p. 604, in HPIM-17.

79 Prostate Hyperplasia and Carcinoma

PROSTATE HYPERPLASIA

Enlargement of the prostate is nearly universal in aging men. Hyperplasia usually begins by age 45 years, occurs in the area of the prostate gland surrounding the urethra, and produces urinary outflow obstruction. Symptoms develop on average by age 65 in whites and 60 in blacks. Symptoms develop late because hypertrophy of the bladder detrusor compensates for ureteral compression. As obstruction progresses, urinary stream caliber and force diminish, hesitancy in stream initiation develops, and postvoid dribbling occurs. Dysuria and urgency are signs of bladder irritation (perhaps due to inflammation or tumor) and are usually not seen in prostate hyperplasia. As the postvoid residual increases, nocturia and overflow incontinence may develop. Common medications such as tranquilizing drugs and decongestants, infections, or alcohol may precipitate urinary retention. Because of the prevalence of hyperplasia, the relationship to neoplasia is unclear.

On digital rectal exam (DRE), a hyperplastic prostate is smooth, firm, and rubbery in consistency; the median groove may be lost. Prostate-specific antigen (PSA) levels may be elevated but are ≤10 ng/mL unless cancer is also present (see below). Cancer may also be present at lower levels of PSA.

Rx Prostate Hyperplasia

Asymptomatic pts do not require treatment, and those with complications of urethral obstruction such as inability to urinate, renal failure, recurrent urinary tract infection, hematuria, or bladder stones clearly require surgical extirpation of the prostate, usually by transurethral resection (TURP). However, the approach to the remaining pts should be based on the degree of incapacity or discomfort from the disease and the likely side effects of any intervention. If the pt has only mild symptoms, watchful waiting is not harmful and permits an assessment of the rate of symptom progression. If therapy is desired by the pt, two medical approaches may be helpful: terazosin, an α_1-adrenergic blocker (1 mg at bedtime, titrated to symptoms up to 20 mg/d), relaxes the smooth muscle of the bladder neck and increases urine flow; finasteride (5 mg/d), an inhibitor of 5α-reductase, blocks the conversion of testosterone to dihydrotestosterone and causes an average decrease in prostate size of ~24%. TURP has the greatest success rate but also the greatest risk of complications. Transurethral microwave thermotherapy (TUMT) may be comparably effective to TURP. Direct comparison has not been made between medical and surgical management.

PROSTATE CARCINOMA

Prostate cancer was diagnosed in 186,320 men in 2008 in the United States—an incidence comparable to that of breast cancer. About 28,660 men died of prostate cancer in 2008. The early diagnosis of cancers in mildly symptomatic men found on screening to have elevated serum levels of PSA has complicated management. Like most other cancers, incidence is age-related. The disease is more common in blacks than whites. Symptoms are generally similar to and in-

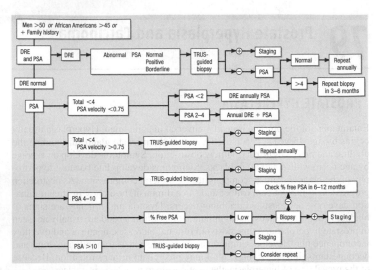

FIGURE 79-1 The use of the annual digital rectal examination (DRE) and measurement of prostate-specific antigen (PSA) as guides for deciding which men should have transrectal ultrasound (TRUS)-guided prostate biopsy. There are at least three schools of thought about what to do if the DRE is negative and the PSA is equivocal (4.1 to 10 ng/mL).

distinguishable from those of prostate hyperplasia, but those with cancer more often have dysuria and back or hip pain. On histology, 95% are adenocarcinomas. Biologic behavior is affected by histologic grade (Gleason score).

In contrast to hyperplasia, prostate cancer generally originates in the periphery of the gland and may be detectable on DRE as one or more nodules on the posterior surface of the gland, hard in consistency and irregular in shape. An approach to diagnosis is shown in Fig. 79-1. Those with a negative DRE and PSA ≤4 ng/mL may be followed annually. Those with an abnormal DRE or a PSA >10 ng/mL should undergo transrectal ultrasound (TRUS)-guided biopsy. Those with normal DRE and PSA of 4.1–10 ng/mL may be handled differently in different centers. Some would perform TRUS and biopsy any abnormality or follow if no abnormality were found. Some would repeat the PSA in a year and biopsy if the increase over that period were >0.75 ng/mL. Other methods of using PSA to distinguish early cancer from hyperplasia include quantitating bound and free PSA and relating the PSA to the size of the prostate (PSA density). Perhaps one-third of persons with prostate cancer do not have PSA elevations.

Lymphatic spread is assessed surgically; it is present in only 10% of those with Gleason grade 5 or lower and in 70% of those with grade 9 or 10. PSA level also correlates with spread; only 10% of those with PSA <10 ng/mL have lymphatic spread. Bone is the most common site of distant metastasis. Whitmore-Jewett staging includes A: tumor not palpable but detected at TURP; B: palpable tumor in one (B1) or both (B2) lobes; C: palpable tumor outside capsule; and D: metastatic disease.

℞ Prostate Carcinoma

For pts with stages A through C disease, surgery (radical retropubic prostatectomy) and radiation therapy (conformal 3-dimensional fields) are said to have similar outcomes; however, most pts are treated surgically. Both modalities are associated with impotence. Surgery is more likely to lead to incontinence. Radiation therapy is more likely to produce proctitis, perhaps with bleeding or stricture. Addition of hormonal therapy (goserelin) to radiation therapy of patients with localized disease appears to improve results. Patients usually must have a 5-year life expectancy to undergo radical prostatectomy. Stage A pts have survival identical to age-matched controls without cancer. Stage B and C pts have a 10-year survival of 82% and 42%, respectively.

Pts treated surgically for localized disease who develop rising PSA may undergo Prostascint scanning (antibody to a prostate-specific membrane antigen). If no uptake is seen, the pt is observed. If uptake is seen in the prostate bed, local recurrence is implied and external beam radiation therapy is delivered to the site. (If the pt was initially treated with radiation therapy, this local recurrence may be treated with surgery.) However, in most cases, a rising PSA after local therapy indicates systemic disease. It is not clear when to intervene in such patients.

For pts with metastatic disease, androgen deprivation is the treatment of choice. Surgical castration is effective, but most pts prefer to take leuprolide, 7.5 mg depot form IM monthly (to inhibit pituitary gonadotropin production), plus flutamide, 250 mg PO tid (an androgen receptor blocker). The value of added flutamide is debated. Alternative approaches include adrenalectomy, hypophysectomy, estrogen administration, and medical adrenalectomy with aminoglutethimide. The median survival of stage D pts is 33 months. Pts occasionally respond to withdrawal of hormonal therapy with tumor shrinkage. Rarely a second hormonal manipulation will work, but most pts who progress on hormonal therapy have androgen-independent tumors, often associated with genetic changes in the androgen receptor and new expression of *bcl*-2, which may contribute to chemotherapy resistance. Chemotherapy is used for palliation in prostate cancer. Mitoxantrone, estramustine, and taxanes appear to be active single agents, and combinations of drugs are being tested. Chemotherapy-treated pts are more likely to have pain relief than those receiving supportive care alone. Bone pain from metastases may be palliated with strontium-89 or samarium-153. Bisphosphonates have not been adequately evaluated.

Prostate Cancer Prevention
Finasteride has been shown to reduce the incidence of prostate cancer by 25%, but no effect on overall survival has been seen with limited follow-up.

For a more detailed discussion, see Scher HI: Benign and Malignant Diseases of the Prostate, Chap. 91, p. 593, in HPIM-17.

80 Cancer of Unknown Primary Site

Cancer of unknown primary site (CUPS) is defined as follows: biopsy-proven malignancy; primary site unapparent after history, physical exam, chest x-ray, abdominal and pelvic CT, complete blood count, chemistry survey, mammography (women), β-human chorionic gonadotropin (hCG) levels (men), α-fetoprotein (AFP) levels (men), and prostate-specific antigen (PSA) levels (men); and histologic evaluation not consistent with a primary tumor at the biopsy site.

CUPS incidence is declining, probably because of better pathology diagnostic criteria; they account for about 3% of all cancers today, down from 10–15% 15 years ago. Most pts are over age 60. The tumors are often aneuploid. Cell lines derived from such tumors frequently have abnormalities in chromosome 1.

Clinical Presentation Pts may present with fatigue, weight loss, pain, bleeding, abdominal swelling, subcutaneous masses, and lymphadenopathy. Once metastatic malignancy is confirmed, diagnostic efforts should be confined to evaluating the presence of potentially curable tumors, such as lymphoma, Hodgkin's disease, germ cell tumor, ovarian cancer, head and neck cancer, and primitive neuroectodermal tumor, or tumors for which therapy may be of significant palliative value such as breast cancer or prostate cancer. In general, efforts to evaluate the presence of these tumor types depend more on the pathologist than on expensive clinical diagnostic testing. Localizing symptoms, a history of carcinogen exposure, or a history of fulguration of skin lesion may direct some clinical testing; however, the careful light microscopic, ultrastructural, immunologic, karyotypic, and molecular biologic examination of adequate volumes of tumor tissue is the most important feature of the diagnostic workup in the absence of suspicious findings on history and physical exam (Table 80-1).

Histology About 60% of CUPS tumors are adenocarcinomas, 5% are squamous cell carcinomas, and 30% are poorly differentiated neoplasms not further classified on light microscopy. Expression of cytokeratin subtypes may narrow the range of possible diagnoses (Fig. 80-1).

Prognosis Pts with squamous cell carcinoma have a median survival of 9 months; those with adenocarcinoma or unclassifiable tumors have a median survival of 4–6 months. Pts in whom a primary site is identified usually have a better prognosis. Limited sites of involvement and neuroendocrine histology are favorable prognostic factors. Pts without a primary diagnosis should be treated palliatively with radiation therapy to symptomatic lesions. All-purpose chemotherapy regimens rarely produce responses but always produce toxicity. Certain clinical features may permit individualized therapy.

SYNDROME OF UNRECOGNIZED EXTRAGONADAL GERM CELL CANCER

In pts <50 years with tumor involving midline structures, lung parenchyma, or lymph nodes and evidence of rapid tumor growth, germ cell tumor is a possible diagnosis. Serum tumor markers may or may not be elevated. Cisplatin, etoposide, and bleomycin (Chap. 77) chemotherapy may induce complete responses in ≥25%, and ~15% may be cured. A trial of such therapy should probably also be undertaken in pts whose tumors have abnormalities in chromosome 12.

PERITONEAL CARCINOMATOSIS IN WOMEN

Women who present with pelvic mass or pain and an adenocarcinoma diffusely throughout the peritoneal cavity, but without a clear site of origin, have primary peritoneal papillary serous carcinoma. The presence of psammoma bodies in the tumor or elevated CA-125 levels may favor ovarian origin. Such pts should undergo debulking surgery followed by paclitaxel plus cisplatin or carboplatin combination chemotherapy (Chap. 78). About 20% of pts will respond, and 10% will survive at least 2 years.

CARCINOMA IN AN AXILLARY LYMPH NODE IN WOMEN

Such women should receive adjuvant breast cancer therapy appropriate for their menopausal status even in the absence of a breast mass on physical examination

TABLE 80-1	**POSSIBLE PATHOLOGIC EVALUATION OF BIOPSY SPECIMENS FROM PATIENTS WITH METASTATIC CANCER OF UNKNOWN PRIMARY SITE**

Evaluation/Findings	Suggested Primary Site or Neoplasm
HISTOLOGY (HEMATOXYLIN AND EOSIN STAINING)	
Psammoma bodies, papillary configuration	Ovary, thyroid
Signet ring cells	Stomach
IMMUNOHISTOLOGY	
Leukocyte common antigen (LCA, CD45)	Lymphoid neoplasm
Leu-M1	Hodgkin's disease
Epithelial membrane antigen	Carcinoma
Cytokeratin	Carcinoma
CEA	Carcinoma
HMB45	Melanoma
Desmin	Sarcoma
Thyroglobulin	Thyroid carcinoma
Calcitonin	Medullary carcinoma of the thyroid
Myoglobin	Rhabdomyosarcoma
PSA/prostatic acid phosphatase	Prostate
AFP	Liver, stomach, germ cell
Placental alkaline phosphatase	Germ cell
B, T cell markers	Lymphoid neoplasm
S-100 protein	Neuroendocrine tumor, melanoma
Gross cystic fluid protein	Breast, sweat gland
Factor VIII	Kaposi's sarcoma, angiosarcoma
Thyroid transcription factor 1 (TTF-1)	Lung adenocarcinoma, thyroid
FLOW CYTOMETRY	
B, T cell markers	Lymphoid neoplasm
ULTRASTRUCTURE	
Actin-myosin filaments	Rhabdomyosarcoma
Secretory granules	Neuroendocrine tumors
Desmosomes	Carcinoma
Premelanosomes	Melanoma
CYTOGENETICS	
Isochromosome 12p; 12q(−)	Germ cell
t(11;22)	Ewing's sarcoma, primitive neuro-ectodermal tumor
t(8;14)[a]	Lymphoid neoplasm
3p(−)	Small cell lung carcinoma; renal cell carcinoma, mesothelioma
t(X;18)	Synovial sarcoma
t(12;16)	Myxoid liposarcoma
t(12;22)	Clear cell sarcoma (melanoma of soft parts)
t(2;13)	Alveolar rhabdomyosarcoma
1p(−)	Neuroblastoma

(continued)

TABLE 80-1	POSSIBLE PATHOLOGIC EVALUATION OF BIOPSY SPECIMENS FROM PATIENTS WITH METASTATIC CANCER OF UNKNOWN PRIMARY SITE (CONTINUED)
Evaluation/Findings	Suggested Primary Site or Neoplasm
RECEPTOR ANALYSIS	
Estrogen/progesterone receptor	Breast
MOLECULAR BIOLOGIC STUDIES	
Immunoglobulin, *bcl*-2, T cell receptor gene rearrangement	Lymphoid neoplasm

*a*Or any other rearrangement involving an antigen-receptor gene.
Note: CEA, carcinoembryonic antigen; PSA, prostate-specific antigen; AFP, α-fetoprotein.

or mammography and undetermined or negative estrogen and progesterone receptors on the tumor (Chap. 75). Unless the ipsilateral breast is radiated, up to 50% of these pts will later develop a breast mass. Although this is a rare clinical situation, long-term survival similar to women with stage II breast cancer is possible.

OSTEOBLASTIC BONE METASTASES IN MEN

The probability of prostate cancer is high; a trial of empirical hormonal therapy (leuprolide and flutamide) is warranted (Chap. 79).

CERVICAL LYMPH NODE METASTASES

Even if panendoscopy fails to reveal a head and neck primary, treatment of such pts with cisplatin and 5-fluorouracil chemotherapy may produce a response; some responses are long-lived (Chap. 73).

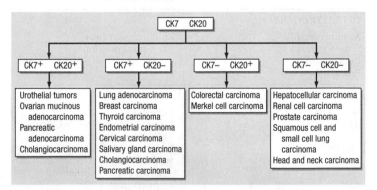

FIGURE 80-1 Approach to cytokeratin (CK7 and CK20) markers used in CUP.

For a more detailed discussion, see Varadhachary GR, Abbruzzese JL: Carcinoma of Unknown Primary, Chap. 95, p. 614, in HPIM-17.

81 Paraneoplastic Endocrine Syndromes

Both benign and malignant tumors of nonendocrine tissue can secrete a variety of hormones, principally peptide hormones, and many tumors produce more than one hormone (Table 81-1). At the clinical level, ectopic hormone production is important for two reasons.

First, endocrine syndromes that result may either be the presenting manifestations of the neoplasm or occur late in the course. The endocrine manifestations in some instances are of greater significance than the tumor itself, as in pts with benign or slowly growing malignancies that secrete corticotropin-releasing hormone and cause fulminant Cushing's syndrome. The frequency with which ectopic hormone production is recognized varies with the criteria used for diagnosis. The most common syndromes of clinical import are those of adrenocorticotropic hormone (ACTH) hypersecretion, hypercalcemia, and hypoglycemia. Indeed, ectopic ACTH secretion is responsible for 15–20% of pts with Cushing's syndrome, and ~50% of pts with persistent hypercalcemia have a malignancy rather than hyperparathyroidism. Because of the rapidity of development of hormone secretion in some rapidly growing tumors, diagnosis may require a high index of suspicion, and hormone levels may be elevated out of proportion to the manifestations.

TABLE 81-1   COMMON PARANEOPLASTIC ENDOCRINE SYNDROMES

Syndrome	Proteins	Tumors Typically Associated with Syndrome
Hypercalcemia of malignancy	Parathyroid hormone–related peptide (PTHrP)	Non–small cell lung cancer Breast cancer Renal cell carcinoma
	Parathyroid hormone (PTH)	Head and neck cancer Bladder cancer Myeloma
Syndrome of inappropriate antidiuretic hormone secretion (SIADH)	Arginine vasopressin (AVP)	Small cell lung cancer Head and neck cancer
	Atrial natriuretic peptide	Non–small cell lung cancer
Cushing's syndrome	Adrenocorticotropic hormone (ACTH) Corticotropin-releasing hormone (CRH)	Small cell lung cancer Carcinoid tumors
Acromegaly	Growth hormone–releasing hormone (GHRH) Growth hormone (GH)	Carcinoid Small cell lung cancer Pancreatic islet cell tumors
Gynecomastia	Human chorionic gonadotropin (hCG)	Testicular cancer Lung cancer Carcinoid tumors of the lung and gastrointestinal tract
Non–islet cell tumor hypoglycemia	Insulin-like growth factor 2 (IGF-2)	Sarcomas

Second, ectopic hormones serve as valuable peripheral markers for neoplasia. Because of the broad spectrum of ectopic hormone secretion, screening measurements of plasma hormone levels for diagnostic purposes are not cost-effective. However, in pts with malignancies that are known to secrete hormones, serial measurements of circulating hormone levels can serve as markers for completeness of tumor excision and for effectiveness of radiation therapy or chemotherapy. Likewise, tumor recurrence may be heralded by reappearance of elevated plasma hormone levels before mass effects of the tumor are evident. However, some tumors at recurrence do not secrete hormones, so hormone measurements cannot be relied on as the sole evidence of tumor activity.

℞ Paraneoplastic Endocrine Syndromes

Therapy of ectopic hormone-secreting tumors should be directed when possible toward removal of the tumor. When the tumor cannot be removed or is incurable, specific therapy can be directed toward inhibiting hormone secretion (octreotide for ectopic acromegaly or mitotane to inhibit adrenal steroidogenesis in the ectopic ACTH syndrome) or blocking the action of the hormone at the tissue level (demeclocycline for inappropriate vasopressin secretion).

HYPERCALCEMIA

The most common paraneoplastic syndrome, hypercalcemia of malignancy accounts for 40% of all hypercalcemia. Of cancer pts with hypercalcemia, 80% have humoral hypercalcemia mediated by parathyroid hormone–related peptide; 20% have local osteolytic hypercalcemia mediated by cytokines such as interleukin 1 and tumor necrosis factor. Many tumor types may produce hypercalcemia (Table 81-1). Pts may have malaise, fatigue, confusion, anorexia, bone pain, polyuria, weakness, constipation, nausea, and vomiting. At high calcium levels, confusion, lethargy, coma, and death may ensue. Median survival of hypercalcemic cancer pts is 1–3 months. Treatment with saline hydration, furosemide diuresis, and pamidronate (60–90 mg IV) or zoledronate (4–8 mg IV) controls calcium levels within 2 days and suppresses calcium release for several weeks. Oral bisphosphonates can be used for chronic treatment.

HYPONATREMIA

Most commonly discovered in asymptomatic individuals as a result of serum electrolyte measurements, hyponatremia is usually due to tumor secretion of arginine vasopressin, a condition called *syndrome of inappropriate antidiuretic hormone secretion* (SIADH). Atrial natriuretic hormone also may produce hyponatremia. SIADH occurs most commonly in small cell lung cancer (15%) and head and neck cancer (3%). A number of drugs may produce the syndrome. Symptoms of fatigue, poor attention span, nausea, weakness, anorexia, and headache may be controlled by restricting fluid intake to 500 mL/d or blocking the effects of the hormone with 600–1200 mg demeclocycline a day. With severe hyponatremia (<115 meq/L) or in the setting of mental status changes, normal saline infusion plus furosemide may be required; rate of correction should be <1 meq/L per hour to prevent complications.

ECTOPIC ACTH SYNDROME

When pro-opiomelanocortin mRNA in the tumor is processed into ACTH, excessive secretion of glucocorticoids and mineralocorticoids may ensue. Pts develop

Cushing's syndrome with hypokalemic alkalosis, weakness, hypertension, and hyperglycemia. About half the cases occur in small cell lung cancer. ACTH production adversely affects prognosis. Ketoconazole (400–1200 mg/d) or metyrapone (1–4 g/d) may be used to inhibit adrenal steroid synthesis.

For a more detailed discussion, see Jameson JL, Johnson BE: Paraneoplastic Syndromes: Endocrinologic/Hematologic, Chap. 96, p. 617, in HPIM-17.

82 Neurologic Paraneoplastic Syndromes

Paraneoplastic neurologic disorders (PNDs) are cancer-related syndromes that can affect any part of the nervous system; caused by mechanisms other than metastasis or by complications of cancer such as coagulopathy, stroke, metabolic and nutritional conditions, infections, and side effects of cancer therapy. In 60% of pts the neurologic symptoms precede cancer diagnosis. PNDs occur in 0.5–1% of all cancer pts, but they occur in 2–3% of pts with neuroblastoma or small cell lung cancer (SCLC), and in 30–50% of pts with thymoma or sclerotic myeloma.

CLINICAL FEATURES

Recognition of a distinctive paraneoplastic syndrome (Table 82-1); should prompt a search for cancer, as prompt treatment of tumor may improve the course of PNDs; many of these disorders also occur without cancer. Diagnosis is based upon the clinical pattern, exclusion of other cancer-related disorders, confirmatory serum or CSF antibodies (Table 82-2), or electrodiagnostic testing. For any type of PND, if antineuronal antibodies are negative, the diagnosis rests on the demonstration of cancer and the exclusion of other cancer-related or independent disorders. Whole-body positron emission tomographic scans often uncover tumors undetected by other tests.

PNDs of the Central Nervous System and Dorsal Root Ganglia
MRI and CSF studies are important to rule out neurologic complications due to the direct spread of cancer. In most PNDs the MRI findings are nonspecific. CSF findings typically consist of mild to moderate pleocytosis (<200 mononuclear cells, predominantly lymphocytes), an increase in the protein concentration, intrathecal synthesis of IgG, and a variable presence of oligoclonal bands. A biopsy of affected nervous system tissue may be useful to rule out other disorders (e.g., metastasis, infection); neuropathologic findings are not specific for PNDs.

- *Limbic encephalitis* is characterized by confusion, depression, agitation, anxiety, severe short-term memory deficits, partial complex seizures, and dementia; the MRI usually shows unilateral or bilateral medial temporal lobe abnormalities.
- *Paraneoplastic cerebellar degeneration* begins as dizziness, oscillopsia, blurry or double vision, nausea, and vomiting; a few days or weeks later, dysarthria, gait and limb ataxia, and variable dysphagia can appear.

TABLE 82-1	PARANEOPLASTIC SYNDROMES OF THE NERVOUS SYSTEM

Syndromes of the brain, brainstem, and cerebellum
    Focal encephalitis
        Cortical encephalitis
        Limbic encephalitis
        Brainstem encephalitis
        Cerebellar dysfunction
        Autonomic dysfunction
    Paraneoplastic cerebellar degeneration
    Opsoclonus-myoclonus
Syndromes of the spinal cord
    Subacute necrotizing myelopathy
    Motor neuron dysfunction
    Myelitis
    Stiff-person syndrome
Syndromes of dorsal root ganglia
    Sensory neuronopathy
Multiple levels of involvement
    Encephalomyelitis,[a] sensory neuronopathy, autonomic dysfunction
Syndromes of peripheral nerve
    Chronic and subacute sensorimotor peripheral neuropathy
    Vasculitis of nerve and muscle
    Neuropathy associated with malignant monoclonal gammopathies
    Peripheral nerve hyperexcitability
    Autonomic neuropathy
Syndromes of the neuromuscular junction
    Lambert-Eaton myasthenic syndrome
    Myasthenia gravis
Syndromes of the muscle
    Polymyositis/dermatomyositis
    Acute necrotizing myopathy
Syndromes affecting the visual system
    Cancer-associated retinopathy (CAR)
    Melanoma-associated retinopathy (MAR)
    Uveitis (usually in association with encephalomyelitis)

[a]Includes cortical, limbic, or brainstem encephalitis, cerebellar dysfunction, myelitis.

- *Opsoclonus-myoclonus syndrome* consists of involuntary, chaotic eye movements in all directions of gaze plus myoclonus; it is frequently associated with ataxia.
- *Acute necrotizing myelopathy.* Reports of paraneoplastic spinal cord syndromes have decreased in recent years; it is unclear if this is due to improved oncological interventions or better detection of nonparaneoplastic etiologies.
- *Paraneoplastic retinopathies* involve cone and rod dysfunction characterized by photosensitivity, progressive loss of vision and color perception, central or ring scotomas, night blindness, and attenuation of photopic and scotopic responses in the electroretinogram (ERG).
- *Dorsal root ganglionopathy* (sensory neuronopathy) is characterized by sensory deficits that may be symmetric or asymmetric, painful dysesthesias, radicular pain, and decreased or absent reflexes; all modalities of sensation can be involved.

PNDs of Nerve and Muscle   These disorders may develop anytime during the course of the neoplastic disease. Serum and urine immunofixation studies

TABLE 82-2   PARANEOPLASTIC ANTINEURONAL ANTIBODIES, ASSOCIATED SYNDROMES AND CANCERS

Antibody	Syndrome	Associated Cancers
Anti-Hu (ANNA-1)	PEM (including cortical, limbic, brainstem encephalitis, cerebellar dysfunction, myelitis), PSN, autonomic dysfunction	SCLC, other neuroendocrine tumors
Anti-Yo (PCA-1)	PCD	Ovary and other gynecologic cancers, breast
Anti-Ri (ANNA-2)	PCD, brainstem encephalitis, opsoclonus-myoclonus	Breast, gynecological, SCLC
Anti-Tr	PCD	Hodgkin's lymphoma
Anti-Zic	PCD, encephalomyelitis	SCLC and other neuroendocrine tumors
Anti-CV$_2$/CRMP5	PEM, PCD, chorea, peripheral neuropathy, uveitis	SCLC, thymoma, other
Anti-Ma proteins[a]	Limbic, hypothalamic, brainstem encephalitis (infrequently PCD)	Germ-cell tumors of testis, lung cancer, other solid tumors
Anti-NR1/NR2 subunits of NMDA receptor	Encephalitis with prominent psychiatric symptoms, seizures, hypoventilation	Ovarian teratoma
Anti-amphiphysin	Stiff-person syndrome, PEM	Breast, SCLC
Anti-VGCC[b]	LEMS, PCD	SCLC, lymphoma
Anti-AChR[b]	MG	Thymoma
Anti-VGKC[b]	Peripheral nerve hyperexcitability (neuromyotonia), limbic encephalitis	Thymoma, SCLC, others
Anti-recoverin	Cancer-associated retinopathy (CAR)	SCLC and other
Anti-bipolar cells of the retina	Melanoma-associated retinopathy (MAR)	Melanoma

[a]Patients with antibodies to Ma2 are usually men with testicular cancer. Patients with additional antibodies to other Ma proteins are men or women with a variety of solid tumors.
[b]These antibodies can occur with or without a cancer association.
Note: PEM: paraneoplastic encephalomyelitis; PCD, paraneoplastic cerebellar degeneration; PSN, paraneoplastic sensory neuronopathy; LEMS, Lambert-Eaton myasthenic syndrome; MG, myasthenia gravis; VGCC, voltage-gated calcium channel; AChR, acetylcholine receptor; VGKC, voltage-gated potassium channel; SCLC, small-cell lung cancer; NMDA, *N*-methyl-D-aspartate.

should be considered in patients with peripheral neuropathy of unknown cause; detection of a monoclonal gammopathy suggests the need for additional studies to uncover a B cell or plasma cell malignancy.

Neuropathies occurring at late stages of cancer or with lymphoma are usually due to axonal degeneration of unclear etiology. These neuropathies are often masked by concurrent neurotoxicity from chemotherapy and other cancer therapies. Neuropathies that develop in the early stages of cancer often show a rapid progression, sometimes with a relapsing and remitting course, and evidence of inflammatory infiltrates and axonal loss or demyelination in biopsy studies. If demyelinating features predominate, IVIg or glucocorticoids may improve symptoms. Myasthenia gravis is discussed in Chap. 204, and dermatomyositis in Chap. 205.

PATHOPHYSIOLOGY

Most PNDs are mediated by immune responses triggered by neuronal proteins (onconeuronal antigens) expressed by tumors. Many specific antibody-associated immune responses have been identified. Target onconeuronal antigens are usually intracellular proteins with roles in neuronal development and function.

℞ Paraneoplastic Neurologic Disorders

These disorders in general respond poorly to therapy. Treatment of PNDs focuses mainly on recognition and control of the underlying malignancy; a stabilization or improvement of symptoms has been reported in some patients with successful tumor control. Variable responses have been described following treatment with glucocorticoids and other immunosuppressive agents as well as IVIg and plasma exchange.

For a more detailed discussion, see Dalmau J, Rosenfeld MR: Paraneoplastic Neurologic Syndromes, Chap. 97, p. 623, in HPIM-17.

83 Diagnosis of Infectious Diseases

The laboratory diagnosis of infection requires the demonstration—either direct or indirect—of viral, bacterial, fungal, or parasitic agents in tissues, fluids, or excreta of the host. The traditional detection methods of microscopy and culture are time-consuming and are increasingly being replaced by nucleic acid probe assays.

BACTERIA, FUNGI, AND VIRUSES

MICROSCOPY

- Wet mounts: The examination of wet mounts does not require fixation of the specimen before microscopy. Wet mounts are useful for certain large and/or motile organisms; e.g., with dark-field illumination, *Treponema* can be detected in genital lesions. Fungal elements may be identified in skin scrapings with 10% KOH wet mount preparations. Some wet mounts use staining to enhance detection—e.g., india ink to visualize encapsulated cryptococci in cerebrospinal fluid (CSF).
- Stains: Without staining, bacteria are difficult to visualize. *Gram's stain* differentiates between organisms with thick peptidoglycan cell walls (gram-positive) and those with thin peptidoglycan cell walls and outer membranes that can be dissolved with alcohol or acetone (gram-negative). This stain is particularly useful for sputum samples that have ≥ 25 polymorphonuclear leukocytes (PMNs) and <10 epithelial cells. In normally sterile fluids (e.g., CSF), the detection of bacteria suggests the infectious etiology (Fig. 83-1) and correlates with the presence of $>10^4$ bacteria/mL. Sensitivity is increased by centrifugation of the sample. *Acid-fast stains* are useful for organisms that retain carbol fuchsin dye after acid/organic solvation (e.g., *Mycobacterium* spp.). Modification of this procedure permits the detection of weakly acid-fast organisms such as *Nocardia*. *Immunofluorescent stains* (antibody coupled directly or indirectly to a fluorescing compound) can detect viral antigens [e.g., cytomegalovirus (CMV), herpes simplex virus, and respiratory viruses] within cultured cells or can reveal difficult-to-grow bacteria such as *Legionella*.

MACROSCOPIC ANTIGEN DETECTION

Latex agglutination assays and enzyme immunoassays (EIAs) are rapid and inexpensive tests that identify bacteria, viruses, or extracellular bacterial toxins by means of their protein or polysaccharide antigens. The assays are performed either directly on clinical specimens or after growth of the organisms in the laboratory.

CULTURE

The success of efforts to culture a specific pathogen often depends on the use of appropriate collection and transport procedures in conjunction with a laboratory-

411

Gram-Negative Organisms

	GRx only	Oxidase +	Oxidase –	Fastidious	Anaerobic	Curved
Rod		*Pseudomonas* *Aeromonas* *Pasteurella* Others	Enterobacteriaceae Others	*Haemophilus* *Legionella* *Bordetella* *Brucella* *Francisella* Others	*Bacteroides* *Prevotella* *Fusobacterium* Others	*Vibrio* *Campylobacter*
Coccus	*Neisseria* *Branhamella*				*Veillonella* *Acidaminococcus* *Megasphaera*	

Gram-Positive Organisms

	Branching	Spores	Acid-Fast	Catalase +	Catalase –
Rod	*Nocardia* *Actinomyces* *Bifidobacterium*	*Clostridium* *Bacillus*	*Mycobacterium*	*Corynebacterium* *Listeria* Others	*Lactobacillus* Others
Coccus				*Staphylococcus* *Micrococcus* Others	*Streptococcus*

FIGURE 83-1 Interpretation of Gram's stain.

processing algorithm suitable for the specimen. Instructions for collection are listed in Table 83-1. Bacterial isolation relies on the use of artificial media that support bacterial growth in vitro. Once bacteria are isolated, different methods are used to characterize specific isolates (e.g., phenotyping, gas-liquid chromatography, nucleic acid tests). Viruses are grown on a monolayer of cultured cells sensitive to infection with the suspected virus. After proliferation of viral particles, cells are examined for cytopathic effects or immunofluorescent studies are performed to detect viral antigens.

SEROLOGY

The measurement of serum antibody provides an indirect marker for past or current infection with a specific viral agent or other pathogen. Quantitative assays detect increases in antibody titers, most often using paired serum samples obtained at illness onset and 10–14 days later (i.e., acute- and convalescent-phase samples). Serology can also be used to document protective levels of antibody, particularly in diseases for which vaccines are available (e.g., rubella, varicella-zoster virus infections).

NUCLEIC ACID PROBES

Techniques for the detection and quantitation of specific DNA and RNA base sequences in clinical specimens have become powerful tools for the diagnosis of infection and are useful in four settings:

1. To detect and/or quantify specific pathogens in clinical specimens
2. To identify organisms that are difficult to identify by conventional methods
3. To determine whether two or more isolates are closely related (e.g., belong to the same clone or strain)
4. To predict sensitivity (typically of viruses) to chemotherapeutic agents

Probes are available for directly detecting various pathogens (e.g., *Chlamydia trachomatis*, *Neisseria gonorrhoeae*) in clinical specimens and for confirming the identity of cultured pathogens (e.g., *Mycobacterium* spp., *Streptococcus* spp., and *Staphylococcus aureus*). The sensitivity and specificity of probe assays for direct detection are comparable to those of more traditional assays, including EIA and culture. Hybrid capture, an alternative assay that anneals an RNA probe to a DNA target, is available for *C. trachomatis, N. gonorrhoeae*, CMV, and human papillomavirus.

- Amplification strategies [e.g., polymerase chain reaction (PCR), ligase chain reaction] enhance the sensitivity of RNA or DNA assays, but false-positive findings can result from even low levels of contamination.

SUSCEPTIBILITY TESTING

Susceptibility testing allows the clinician to choose the optimal antimicrobial agents and to identify potential infection-control problems (e.g., the level of methicillin-resistant *S. aureus* in a hospital). Susceptibility testing for fungi has only recently been standardized; several systems have now been approved.

PARASITES

Table 83-2 summarizes the diagnosis of some common parasitic infections. The cornerstone for the diagnosis of parasitic diseases, as for that of many other infections, is the elicitation of a thorough history of the illness and of epidemiologic factors such as travel, recreational activities, and occupation.

TABLE 83-1 INSTRUCTIONS FOR COLLECTION AND TRANSPORT OF SPECIMENS FOR CULTURE*

Type of Culture (Synonyms)	Specimen	Minimum Volume	Container	Other Considerations
Blood				
Blood, routine (blood culture for aerobes, anaerobes, and yeasts)	Whole blood	10 mL in each of 2 bottles for adults and children; 5 mL, if possible, in aerobic bottles for infants; less for neonates	See below.[a]	See below.[b]
Blood for fungi/*Mycobacterium* spp.	Whole blood	10 mL in each of 2 bottles, as for routine blood cultures, or in Isolator tube requested from laboratory	Same as for routine blood culture	Specify "hold for extended incubation," since fungal agents may require ≥4 weeks to grow.
Blood, Isolator (lysis centrifugation)	Whole blood	10 mL	Isolator tubes	Use mainly for isolation of fungi, *Mycobacterium*, or other fastidious aerobes and for elimination of antibiotics from cultured blood in which organisms are concentrated by centrifugation.
Respiratory Tract				
Nose	Swab from nares	1 swab	Sterile culturette or similar transport system containing holding medium	Swabs made of calcium alginate may be used.
Throat	Swab of posterior pharynx, ulcerations, or areas of suspected purulence	1 swab	Sterile culturette or similar swab collection system containing holding medium	See below.[c]

414

Sputum	Fresh sputum (not saliva)	2 mL	Commercially available sputum collection system or similar sterile container with screw cap	*Cause for rejection:* Care must be taken to ensure that the specimen is sputum and not saliva. Examination of Gram's stain, with number of epithelial cells and PMNs noted, can be an important part of the evaluation process. Induced sputum specimens should not be rejected.
Bronchial aspirates	Transtracheal aspirate, bronchoscopy specimen, or bronchial aspirate	1 mL of aspirate or brush in transport medium	Sterile aspirate or bronchoscopy tube, bronchoscopy brush in a separate sterile container	Special precautions may be required, depending on diagnostic considerations (e.g., *Pneumocystis*).
Stool				
Stool for routine culture; stool for *Salmonella*, *Shigella*, and *Campylobacter*	Rectal swab or (preferably) fresh, randomly collected stool	1 g of stool or 2 rectal swabs	Plastic-coated cardboard cup or plastic cup with tight-fitting lid. Other leak-proof containers are also acceptable.	If *Vibrio* spp. are suspected, the laboratory must be notified, and appropriate collection/transport methods should be used.
Stool for *Yersinia*, *Escherichia coli* O157	Fresh, randomly collected stool	1 g	Plastic-coated cardboard cup or plastic cup with tight-fitting lid	*Limitations:* Procedure requires enrichment techniques.
Stool for *Aeromonas* and *Plesiomonas*	Fresh, randomly collected stool	1 g	Plastic-coated cardboard cup or plastic cup with tight-fitting lid	*Limitations:* Stool should not be cultured for these organisms unless also cultured for other enteric pathogens. *(continued)*

TABLE 83-1 INSTRUCTIONS FOR COLLECTION AND TRANSPORT OF SPECIMENS FOR CULTURE* (CONTINUED)

Type of Culture (Synonyms)	Specimen	Minimum Volume	Container	Other Considerations
Urogenital Tract				
Urine	Clean-voided urine specimen or urine collected by catheter	0.5 mL	Sterile, leak-proof container with screw cap or special urine transfer tube	See below.[d]
Urogenital secretions	Vaginal or urethral secretions, cervical swabs, uterine fluid, prostatic fluid, etc.	1 swab or 0.5 mL of fluid	Vaginal and rectal swabs transported in Amies transport medium or similar holding medium for group B Streptococcus; direct inoculation preferred for Neisseria gonorrhoeae	Vaginal swab samples for "routine culture" should be discouraged whenever possible unless a particular pathogen is suspected. For detection of multiple organisms (e.g., group B Streptococcus, Trichomonas, Chlamydia, or Candida spp.), 1 swab per test should be obtained.
Body Fluids, Aspirates, and Tissues				
Cerebrospinal fluid (lumbar puncture)	Spinal fluid	1 mL for routine cultures; ≥5 mL for Mycobacterium	Sterile tube with tight-fitting cap	Do not refrigerate; transfer to laboratory as soon as possible.
Body fluids	Aseptically aspirated body fluids	1 mL for routine cultures	Sterile tube with tight-fitting cap. Specimen may be left in syringe used for collection if the syringe is capped before transport.	For some body fluids (e.g., peritoneal lavage samples), increased volumes are helpful for isolation of small numbers of bacteria.

Biopsy and aspirated materials	Tissue removed at surgery, bone, anticoagulated bone marrow, biopsy samples, or other specimens from normally sterile areas	1 mL of fluid or a 1-g piece of tissue	Sterile culturette-type swab or similar transport system containing holding medium. Sterile bottle or jar should be used for tissue specimens.	Accurate identification of specimen and source is critical. Enough tissue should be collected for both microbiologic and histopathologic evaluations.
Wounds	Purulent material or abscess contents obtained from wound or abscess without contamination by normal microflora	2 swabs or 0.5 mL of aspirated pus	Culturette swab or similar transport system or sterile tube with tight-fitting screw cap. For simultaneous anaerobic cultures, send specimen in anaerobic transport device or closed syringe.	*Collection:* Abscess contents or other fluids should be collected in a syringe (rather than with a swab) when possible to provide an adequate sample volume and an anaerobic environment.
Special Recommendations				
Fungi	Specimen types listed above may be used. When urine or sputum is cultured for fungi, a first morning specimen is usually preferred.	1 mL or as specified above for individual listing of specimens. Large volumes may be useful for urinary fungi.	Sterile, leak-proof container with tight-fitting cap	*Collection:* Specimen should be transported to microbiology laboratory within 1 h of collection. Contamination with normal flora from skin, rectum, vaginal tract, or other body surfaces should be avoided.
Mycobacterium (acid-fast bacilli)	Sputum, tissue, urine, body fluids	10 mL of fluid or small piece of tissue. Swabs should not be used.	Sterile container with tight-fitting cap	Detection of *Mycobacterium* spp. is improved by use of concentration techniques. Smears and cultures of pleural, peritoneal, and pericardial fluids often have low yields. Multiple cultures from the same pt are encouraged. Culturing in liquid media shortens the time to detection.

(*continued*)

Type of Culture (Synonyms)	Specimen	Minimum Volume	Container	Other Considerations
Legionella	Pleural fluid, lung biopsy, bronchoalveolar lavage fluid, bronchial/transbronchial biopsy. Rapid transport to laboratory is critical.	1 mL of fluid; any size tissue sample, although a 0.5-g sample should be obtained when possible	—	—
Anaerobic organisms	Aspirated specimens from abscesses or body fluids	1 mL of aspirated fluid, 1 g of tissue or 2 swabs	An appropriate anaerobic transport device is required.[e]	Specimens cultured for obligate anaerobes should be cultured for facultative bacteria as well. Fluid or tissue is preferred to swabs.
Viruses[f]	Respiratory secretions, wash aspirates from respiratory tract, nasal swabs, blood samples (including buffy coats), vaginal and rectal swabs, swab specimens from suspicious skin lesions, stool samples (in some cases)	1 mL of fluid, 1 swab, or 1 g of stool in each appropriate transport medium	Fluid or stool samples in sterile containers or swab samples in viral culturette devices (kept on ice but not frozen) are generally suitable. Plasma samples and buffy coats in sterile collection tubes should be kept at 4–8°C. If specimens are to be shipped or kept for a long time, freezing at −80°C is usually adequate.	Most samples for culture are transported in holding medium containing antibiotics to prevent bacterial overgrowth and viral inactivation. Many specimens should be kept cool but not frozen, provided they are transported promptly to the laboratory. Procedures and transport media vary with the agent to be cultured and the duration of transport.

*Note: It is absolutely essential that the microbiology laboratory be informed of the site of origin of the sample to be cultured and of the infections that are suspected. This information determines the selection of culture media and the length of culture time.

[a]For samples from adults and children, two bottles (smaller for pediatric samples) should be used; one with dextrose phosphate, tryptic soy, or another appropriate broth and the other with thioglycollate or another broth containing reducing agents appropriate for isolation of obligate anaerobes. For children, from whom only limited volumes of blood can be obtained, only an aerobic culture should be done unless there is specific concern about anaerobic sepsis (e.g., with abdominal infections). For special situations (e.g., suspected fungal infection, culture-negative endocarditis, or mycobacteremia), different blood collection systems may be used (Isolator systems; see table).

[b]Collection: An appropriate disinfecting technique should be used on both the bottle septum and the pt. Do not allow air bubbles to get into anaerobic broth bottles. Special considerations: There is no more important clinical microbiology test than the detection of blood-borne pathogens. The rapid identification of bacterial and fungal agents is a major determinant of pts' survival. Bacteria may be present in blood either continuously (as in endocarditis, overwhelming sepsis, and the early stages of salmonellosis and brucellosis) or intermittently (as in most other bacterial infections, in which bacteria are shed into the blood on a sporadic basis). Most blood culture systems employ two separate bottles containing broth medium: one that is vented in the laboratory for the growth of facultative and aerobic organisms and a second that is maintained under anaerobic conditions. In cases of suspected continuous bacteremia/fungemia, two or three samples should be drawn before the start of therapy, with additional sets obtained if fastidious organisms are thought to be involved. For intermittent bacteremia, two or three samples should be obtained at least 1 h apart during the first 24 h.

[c]Normal microflora includes α-hemolytic streptococci, saprophytic Neisseria spp, diphtheroids, and Staphylococcus spp. Aerobic culture of the throat ("routine") includes screening for and identification of β-hemolytic Streptococcus spp. and other potentially pathogenic organisms. Although considered components of the normal microflora, organisms such as Staphylococcus aureus, Haemophilus influenzae, and Streptococcus pneumoniae will be identified by most laboratories, if requested. When Neisseria gonorrhoeae or Corynebacterium diphtheriae is suspected, a special culture request is recommended.

[d](1) Clean-voided specimens, midvoid specimens, and Foley or indwelling catheter specimens that yield ≥50,000 organisms/mL and from which no more than three species are isolated should have organisms identified. Neither indwelling catheter tips nor urine from the bag of a catheterized pt should be cultured. (2) Straight-catheterized, bladder-tap, and similar urine specimens should undergo a complete workup (identification and susceptibility testing) for all potentially pathogenic organisms, regardless of colony count. (3) Certain clinical problems (e.g., acute dysuria in women) may warrant identification and susceptibility testing of isolates present at concentrations of <50,000 organisms/mL.

[e]Aspirated specimens in capped syringes or other transport devices designed to limit oxygen exposure are suitable for the cultivation of obligate anaerobes. A variety of commercially available transport devices may be used. Contamination of specimens with normal microflora from the skin, rectum, vaginal vault, or another body site should be avoided. Collection containers for aerobic culture (such as dry swabs) and inappropriate specimens (such as refrigerated samples; expectorated sputum; stool; gastric aspirates; and vaginal, throat, nose, and rectal swabs) should be rejected as unsuitable.

[f]Laboratories generally use diverse methods to detect viral agents, and the specific requirements for each specimen should be checked before a sample is sent.

TABLE 83-2 DIAGNOSIS OF SOME COMMON PARASITIC INFECTIONS

Parasite	Geographic Distribution	Parasite Stage	Body Fluid or Tissue	Serologic Tests	Other
Blood flukes					
Schistosoma mansoni	Africa, Central and South America, West Indies	Ova, adults	Feces	EIA, WB	Rectal snips, liver biopsy
S. haematobium	Africa	Ova, adults	Urine	WB	Liver, urine, or bladder biopsy
S. japonicum	Far East	Ova, adults	Feces	WB	Liver biopsy
Intestinal roundworms					
Strongyloides stercoralis (strongyloidiasis)	Moist tropics and subtropics	Larvae	Feces, sputum, duodenal fluid	EIA	Dissemination in immuno-deficiency
Intestinal protozoans					
Entamoeba histolytica (amebiasis)	Worldwide, especially tropics	Troph, cyst	Feces, liver	EIA, antigen detection	Ultrasound, liver CT, PCR
Giardia lamblia (giardiasis)	Worldwide	Troph, cyst	Feces	Antigen detection	String test, DFA, PCR
Isospora belli	Worldwide	Oocyst	Feces	—	Acid-fast[a]
Cryptosporidium	Worldwide	Oocyst	Feces	Antigen detection	Acid-fast,[a] DFA, biopsy, PCR
Blood and tissue protozoans					
Plasmodium spp. (malaria)	Subtropics and tropics	Asexual	Blood	Limited use	PCR
Babesia microti (babesiosis)	U.S., especially New England	Asexual	Blood	IIF	Animal spp.; in asplenia, PCR
Toxoplasma gondii (toxoplasmosis)	Worldwide	Cyst, troph	CNS, eye, muscles, other	EIA, IIF	PCR

[a]Acid-fastness is best demonstrated by auramine fluorescence or modified acid-fast stain.

Note: WB, western blot; CT, computed tomography; CNS, central nervous system; EIA, enzyme immunoassay; troph, trophozoite; DFA, direct fluorescent antibody; IIF, indirect immunofluorescence; PCR, polymerase chain reaction.

Source: Adapted from Reed SL, Davis CE: Chap. e16, *Harrison's Online.*

INTESTINAL PARASITES

Most helminths and protozoa exit the body in the fecal stream. Feces should be collected in a clean cardboard container, with the time of collection recorded. Contamination with urine or water should be avoided. Fecal samples should be collected before the ingestion of barium or other contrast agents and before treatment with antidiarrheal agents or antacids; these substances alter fecal consistency and interfere with microscopic detection of parasites. The collection of three samples on alternate days is recommended because of the cyclic shedding of most parasites in the feces. Macroscopic examination involves a search for adult worms or tapeworm segments. Microscopic examination is not complete until direct wet mounts have been evaluated and concentration techniques as well as permanent stains applied. Sampling of duodenal contents may be needed to detect *Giardia lamblia*, *Cryptosporidium*, and *Strongyloides* larvae. "Cellophane tape" methods may be needed to detect pinworm ova or *Taenia saginata*.

BLOOD AND TISSUE PARASITES

Invasion of tissue by parasites may direct the evaluation of other samples—e.g., examination of urine sediment is the appropriate way to detect *Schistosoma haematobium*. The laboratory procedures for detection of parasites in other body fluids are similar to those used in the examination of feces. Wet mounts, concentration techniques, and permanent stains should all be used. The parasites most commonly detected in Giemsa-stained blood smears are the plasmodia, microfilariae, and African trypanosomes; however, wet mounts may be more sensitive for microfilariae and African trypanosomes. The timing of blood collection is crucial—e.g., to diagnose *Wuchereria bancrofti*, blood must be drawn near midnight, when the nocturnal microfilariae are active. Diagnosis of malaria and distinctions among *Plasmodium* species are made by microscopic examination of thick and thin blood films.

ANTIBODY AND ANTIGEN DETECTION

In addition to direct detection techniques, antibody assays for many of the important tissue parasites are available. PCR is useful for the diagnosis of many protozoan infections but should be used only as an adjunct to conventional techniques for parasite detection.

For a more detailed discussion, see McAdam AJ, Onderdonk AB: Laboratory Diagnosis of Infectious Diseases, Chap. e14; and Reed SL, Davis CE: Laboratory Diagnosis of Parasitic Infections, Chap. e16, in Harrison's Online.

84   Antibacterial Therapy

The development of vaccines and drugs that prevent and cure bacterial infections was one of the twentieth century's major contributions to human longevity and quality of life. Antibacterial agents are among the most commonly prescribed drugs worldwide.

MECHANISMS OF DRUG ACTION

Antibacterial agents act on unique targets not found in mammalian cells.

- Inhibition of cell-wall synthesis: Drugs that inhibit cell-wall synthesis are almost always bactericidal. Bacterial autolysins (cell-wall recycling enzymes) contribute to cell lysis in the presence of these agents.
    β-lactam antibiotics
    Glycopeptides (vancomycin)
- Inhibition of protein synthesis: Typically, inhibition takes place through interaction with bacterial ribosomes. Except for aminoglycosides, these drugs are bacteriostatic.
    Aminoglycosides
    Macrolides (erythromycin, clarithromycin, azithromycin), ketolides (telithromycin), and lincosamides (clindamycin)
    Streptogramins [quinupristin/dalfopristin (Synercid)]
    Oxazolidinone (linezolid)
    Tetracyclines (tetracycline, doxycycline, minocycline) and glycylcyclines (tigecycline)
- Inhibition of bacterial metabolism: Drugs interfere with bacterial folic acid synthesis.
    Sulfonamides
    Trimethoprim
- Inhibition of nucleic acid synthesis or activity
    Fluoroquinolones (ciprofloxacin, levofloxacin, moxifloxacin)
    Rifampin
    Metronidazole
- Alteration of cell-membrane permeability
    Polymyxins (polymyxin B, colistin)
    Daptomycin

MECHANISMS OF ANTIBACTERIAL RESISTANCE

Bacteria can either be intrinsically resistant to an agent (e.g., anaerobic bacteria are resistant to aminoglycosides) or acquire resistance through mutation of resident genes or acquisition of new genes. The major mechanisms of resistance used by bacteria are drug inactivation, alteration or overproduction of the antibacterial target, acquisition of a new drug-insensitive target, decreased permeability to the agent, failure to convert an inactive prodrug to its active derivative, and active efflux of the agent.

PHARMACOKINETICS OF ANTIBIOTICS

The pharmacokinetic profile refers to drug concentrations in serum and tissue versus time and reflects the processes of absorption, distribution, metabolism, and elimination.

- Absorption: bioavailability after oral, IM, or IV administration. The IM and IV routes offer 100% bioavailability; bioavailability after oral administration ranges from 10% (e.g., penicillin G) to nearly 100% (e.g., amoxicillin, clindamycin, metronidazole, fluoroquinolones).
- Distribution: The concentration of an antibiotic must exceed the minimal inhibitory concentration (MIC) at the site of infection to be effective.
- Metabolism and elimination: Antibacterial agents are disposed of by hepatic elimination (metabolism or biliary elimination), renal excretion of the unchanged or metabolized form, or a combination of the two. The mode of excretion is important in adjusting dosage if elimination is impaired.

PRINCIPLES OF ANTIBACTERIAL CHEMOTHERAPY

- When possible, obtain specimens to identify the etiologic agent prior to treatment.
- Use local susceptibility patterns to help direct empirical treatment.
    Bacteria are considered susceptible to an antibacterial drug if the achievable peak serum concentration exceeds the MIC by ~4-fold.
    The pharmacodynamic profile refers to the quantitative relationships among (1) the time course of antibiotic concentrations in serum and tissue, (2) the MIC, and (3) the microbial response (inhibition of growth or rate of killing). Antibiotic classes are either:
        Concentration dependent (e.g., fluoroquinolones, aminoglycosides): Increases in antibiotic concentration lead to a more rapid rate of bacterial death.
        Time dependent (e.g., β-lactam antibiotics): The reduction in bacterial density is proportional to the duration of the period during which concentrations exceed the MIC.
- Once etiology and susceptibility are known, change the therapeutic regimen to one that has the narrowest effective spectrum and (if possible) is least costly. Although combination chemotherapy usually is not indicated, it is used for certain purposes:
    To prevent emergence of resistance
    For synergistic or additive activity
    For therapy directed against multiple potential pathogens
- Choose a therapeutic agent on the basis of:
    Pharmacologic data
    Adverse reaction profile
    Site of infection (e.g., is it a protected site such as CSF or heart valve vegetation?)
    Host immune status (e.g., does the host have impaired humoral or cellular immune function? is the pt pregnant?)
    Evidence of efficacy in clinical trials
- Check for drug interactions and contraindications before prescribing antibiotics.

CHOICE OF ANTIBACTERIAL AGENTS

Table 84-1 lists infections for which specific antibacterial agents are among the drugs of choice as well as common pathogen resistance rates for those agents. For current and practical information regarding antimicrobial drugs and treatment regimens, consult relevant chapters in HPIM-17. In addition, online references such as the Johns Hopkins antibiotic guide (*www.Hopkins-abxguide.org*) are available. Evidence-based practice guidelines for most infections are available from the Infectious Diseases Society of America (*www.idsociety.org*).

ADVERSE REACTIONS

Adverse reactions are classified as either dose-related (e.g., aminoglycoside-induced nephrotoxicity) or unpredictable. Unpredictable reactions are idiosyncratic or allergic. The most clinically relevant adverse reactions to common antibacterial drugs are listed below.

β-Lactam Drugs
- Allergies in ~1–4% of treatment courses. Cephalosporins cause allergy in 2–4% of penicillin-allergic pts. Aztreonam is safe in β-lactam–allergic pts. Nonallergic skin reactions: Ampicillin "rash" is common among pts with Epstein-Barr virus infection.
- Diarrhea, including *Clostridium difficile* colitis

Vancomycin
- Anaphylactoid reaction ("red man syndrome"). Avoid by giving vancomycin as a 1- to 2-h infusion.
- Nephrotoxicity, ototoxicity, allergy, neutropenia

Daptomycin
- Distal muscle pain or weakness; weekly creatine phosphokinase measurements, especially in pts also receiving statins

Aminoglycosides
- Nephrotoxicity (generally reversible); greatest with prolonged therapy in the elderly or with preexisting renal insufficiency. Monitor serum creatinine every 2–3 days.
- Ototoxicity: often irreversible; risk factors similar to those for nephrotoxicity; both vestibular and hearing toxicities

Macrolides/Ketolides
- GI distress (e.g., erythromycin)
- Ototoxicity (e.g., high-dose IV erythromycin)
- Cardiac toxicity (QTc prolongation and torsades de pointes, especially when inhibitors of erythromycin metabolism are given simultaneously)
- Hepatic toxicity (telithromycin)
- Respiratory failure in pts with myasthenia gravis (telithromycin)

Clindamycin
- Diarrhea, including *C. difficile* colitis

Tetracyclines/Glycylcyclines
- GI distress: up to 20% with tigecycline
- Esophageal ulceration: doxycycline (take in the morning with fluids)

TABLE 84-1 INFECTIONS FOR WHICH SPECIFIC ANTIBACTERIAL AGENTS ARE AMONG THE DRUGS OF CHOICE

Agent	Infections	Common Pathogen(s) (Resistance Rate, %)[a]
Penicillin G	Syphilis, yaws, leptospirosis, groups A and B streptococcal infections, pneumococcal infections, actinomycosis, oral and periodontal infections, meningococcemia, meningococcal meningitis and meningococcemia, viridans streptococcal endocarditis, clostridial myonecrosis, tetanus, anthrax, rat-bite fever, Pasteurella multocida infections, and erysipeloid (Erysipelothrix rhusiopathiae)	Neisseria meningitidis[b] (intermediate,[c] 15–30; resistant, 0; geographic variation) Viridans streptococci (intermediate, 15–30; resistant, 5–10) Streptococcus pneumoniae (intermediate, 23; resistant, 17)
Ampicillin, amoxicillin	Salmonellosis, acute otitis media, Haemophilus influenzae meningitis and epiglottitis, Listeria monocytogenes meningitis, Enterococcus faecalis UTI	Escherichia coli (37) H. influenzae (35) Salmonella spp.[b] (30–50; geographic variation) Enterococcus spp. (24)
Nafcillin, oxacillin	Staphylococcus aureus (non-MRSA) bacteremia and endocarditis	S. aureus (46; MRSA) Staphylococcus epidermidis (78; MRSE)
Piperacillin plus tazobactam	Intraabdominal infections (facultative enteric gram-negative bacilli plus obligate anaerobes); infections caused by mixed flora (aspiration pneumonia, diabetic foot ulcers); infections caused by Pseudomonas aeruginosa	P. aeruginosa (6)
Cefazolin	E. coli UTI, surgical prophylaxis, S. aureus (non-MRSA) bacteremia and endocarditis	E. coli (7) S. aureus (46; MRSA)
Cefoxitin, cefotetan	Intraabdominal infections and pelvic inflammatory disease	Bacteroides fragilis (12)
Ceftriaxone	Gonococcal infections, pneumococcal meningitis, viridans streptococcal endocarditis, salmonellosis and typhoid fever, hospital-acquired infections caused by non-pseudomonal facultative gram-negative enteric bacilli	S. pneumoniae (intermediate, 16; resistant, 0) E. coli and Klebsiella pneumoniae (1; ESBL producers)
Ceftazidime, cefepime	Hospital-acquired infections caused by facultative gram-negative enteric bacilli and Pseudomonas	P. aeruginosa (16) (See ceftriaxone for ESBL producers)
Imipenem, meropenem	Intraabdominal infections, hospital-acquired infections (non-MRSA), infections caused by Enterobacter spp. and ESBL-producing gram-negative bacilli	P. aeruginosa (6) Acinetobacter spp. (35)

(continued)

TABLE 84-1 INFECTIONS FOR WHICH SPECIFIC ANTIBACTERIAL AGENTS ARE AMONG THE DRUGS OF CHOICE (CONTINUED)

Agent	Infections	Common Pathogen(s) (Resistance Rate, %)[a]
Aztreonam	Hospital-acquired infections caused by facultative gram-negative bacilli and Pseudomonas in penicillin-allergic patients	P. aeruginosa (16)
Vancomycin	Bacteremia, endocarditis, and other serious infections due to MRSA; pneumococcal meningitis; antibiotic-associated pseudomembranous colitis[d]	Enterococcus spp. (24)
Daptomycin	VRE infections; MRSA bacteremia	UNK
Gentamicin, amikacin, tobramycin	Combined with a penicillin for staphylococcal, enterococcal, or viridans streptococcal endocarditis; combined with a β-lactam antibiotic for gram-negative bacteremia; pyelonephritis	Gentamicin: E. coli (6) P. aeruginosa (17) Acinetobacter spp. (32)
Erythromycin, clarithromycin, azithromycin	Legionella, Campylobacter, and Mycoplasma infections; CAP; group A streptococcal pharyngitis in penicillin-allergic pts; bacillary angiomatosis (Bartonella henselae); gastric infections due to Helicobacter pylori; Mycobacterium avium-intracellulare infections	S. pneumoniae (28) Streptococcus pyogenes[b] (0–10; geographic variation) H. pylori[b] (2–20; geographic variation)
Clindamycin	Severe, invasive group A streptococcal infections; infections caused by obligate anaerobes; infections caused by susceptible staphylococci	S. aureus (nosocomial = 58; CA-MRSA = 10[b])
Doxycycline, minocycline	Acute bacterial exacerbations of chronic bronchitis, granuloma inguinale, brucellosis (with streptomycin), tularemia, glanders, melioidosis, spirochetal infections caused by Borrelia (Lyme disease and relapsing fever; doxycycline), infections caused by Vibrio vulnificus, some Aeromonas infections, infections due to Stenotrophomonas (minocycline), plague, ehrlichiosis, chlamydial infections (doxycycline), granulomatous skin infections due to Mycobacterium marinum (minocycline), rickettsial infections, mild CAP, skin and soft tissue infections caused by gram-positive cocci (CA-MRSA infections, leptospirosis, syphilis, actinomycosis in the penicillin-allergic pt)	S. pneumoniae (17) MRSA (5)
Trimethoprim-sulfamethoxazole	Community-acquired UTI; S. aureus skin and soft tissue infections (CA-MRSA)	E. coli (19) MRSA (3)
Sulfonamides	Nocardial infections, leprosy (dapsone, a sulfone), and toxoplasmosis (sulfadiazine)	UNK

426

Drug	Clinical uses	Resistant organisms (% resistance)
Ciprofloxacin, levofloxacin, moxifloxacin	CAP (levofloxacin and moxifloxacin); UTI; bacterial gastroenteritis; hospital-acquired gram-negative enteric infections; *Pseudomonas* infections (ciprofloxacin and levofloxacin)	*S. pneumoniae* (1) *E. coli* (13) *P. aeruginosa* (23) *Salmonella* spp. (10–50; geographic variation) *Neisseria gonorrhoeae*[b] (0–5, non–West Coast U.S.; 10–15, California and Hawaii; 20–70, Asia, England, Wales)
Rifampin	Staphylococcal foreign body infections, in combination with other antistaphylococcal agents; *Legionella* pneumonia	Staphylococci rapidly develop resistance during rifampin monotherapy.
Metronidazole	Obligate anaerobic gram-negative bacteria (*Bacteroides* spp.): abscess in lung, brain, or abdomen; bacterial vaginosis; antibiotic-associated *Clostridium difficile* disease	UNK
Linezolid	VRE; staphylococcal skin and soft tissue infection (CA-MRSA)	UNK
Polymyxin E (colistin)	Hospital-acquired infection due to gram-negative bacilli resistant to all other chemotherapy: *P. aeruginosa, Acinetobacter* spp., *Stenotrophomonas maltophilia*	UNK
Quinupristin/dalfopristin	VRE	Vancomycin-resistant *E. faecalis*[b] (100) Vancomycin-resistant *E. faecium* (10)
Mupirocin	Topical application to nares to eradicate *S. aureus* carriage	UNK

[a]Unless otherwise noted, resistance rates are based on all isolates tested in 2005 in the clinical microbiology laboratory at Virginia Commonwealth University Medical Center. The rates are consistent with those reported by the National Nosocomial Infections Surveillance System (Am J Infect Control 32:470, 2004).

[b]Data from recent literature sources.

[c]Intermediate resistance.

[d]Drug is given orally for this indication.

Abbreviations: CA-MRSA, community-acquired methicillin-resistant *S. aureus*; CAP, community-acquired pneumonia; MRSA, methicillin-resistant *S. aureus*; methicillin-resistant *S. epidermidis*; UTI, urinary tract infection; VRE, vancomycin-resistant enterococci; ESBL, extended-spectrum β-lactamase; UNK, resistance rates unknown.

Sulfonamides and Trimethoprim
- Allergic reactions: rash (more common in HIV-infected pts), erythema multiforme, Stevens-Johnson syndrome, toxic epidermal necrolysis
- Hematologic reactions: uncommon; include agranulocytosis and granulocytopenia (more common in HIV-infected pts), hemolytic and megaloblastic anemia, thrombocytopenia
- Renal insufficiency: crystalluria with sulfadiazine

Fluoroquinolones
- Diarrhea, including *C. difficile* colitis
- Contraindicated for general use in pts <18 years old and pregnant women; appear safe in treatment of pulmonary infections in children with cystic fibrosis
- CNS adverse effects (e.g., insomnia)
- Miscellaneous allergies, tendon rupture, dysglycemias, QTc prolongation

Rifampin
- Hepatotoxicity; rare
- Turns secretions such as urine and tears orange
- Intermittent administration can be associated with flulike symptoms, hemolysis, and renal insufficiency.

Metronidazole
- Metallic taste is common.

Linezolid
- Myelosuppression follows long-term treatment.
- Ocular and peripheral neuritis follows long-term treatment.

For a more detailed discussion, see Archer GL, Polk RE: Treatment and Prophylaxis of Bacterial Infections, Chap. 127, p. 851, in HPIM-17. For a discussion of antifungal therapy, see Chap. 114 in this manual; for antimycobacterial therapy, see Chap. 102; for antiviral therapy, see Chaps. 107 through 112; and for antiparasitic therapy, see Chaps. 116 and 117.

85 Health Care–Associated Infections

Hospital-acquired (nosocomial) infections (defined as those not present or incubating at the time of admission to the hospital) and other health care–associated infections are estimated to affect >2 million pts, cost $4.5 billion, and contribute to 88,000 deaths in U.S. hospitals each year. Efforts to lower infection risks have been challenged by the growing numbers of immunocompromised pts, antibiotic-resistant bacteria, fungal and viral superinfections, and invasive procedures and devices.

PREVENTION OF HOSPITAL-ACQUIRED INFECTIONS

Hospital infection-control programs use several mechanisms to prevent nosocomial infections.

- Surveillance: review of microbiology laboratory results, surveys of nursing wards, and use of other mechanisms to keep track of infections acquired after hospital admission. Hospital infection-control programs focus primarily on infections associated with the greatest morbidity or the highest costs.
- Prevention and control measures: Hand hygiene is the single most important measure to prevent cross-infection. Other measures include identifying and eradicating reservoirs of infection and minimizing use of invasive procedures and catheters.
- Isolation techniques to limit the spread of infection
  1. Standard precautions are used for all pts when there is a potential for contact with blood, other body fluids, nonintact skin, or mucous membranes. Hand hygiene and use of gloves are central components of standard precautions; in certain cases, masks, eye protection, and gowns are used as well.
  2. Transmission-based guidelines: Airborne precautions, droplet precautions, and contact precautions are used to prevent transmission of disease from infected pts. More than one precaution can be combined for diseases that have more than one mode of transmission (e.g., varicella). Because antibiotic-resistant bacteria can be present on intact skin of infected pts, any contact with sick pts who may be harboring those bacteria should involve hand hygiene and use of gloves. Gowns are frequently used as well, although their importance in preventing cross-infection is less clear.

NOSOCOMIAL AND DEVICE-RELATED INFECTIONS

Nosocomial infections are due to the combined effect of the pt's own flora and the presence of invasive devices in 25–50% of cases. Intensive education and "bundling" of evidence-based interventions reduce infection rates (see Table 85-1).

Urinary Tract Infections Up to 40–45% of nosocomial infections are UTIs. Most nosocomial UTIs are associated with prior instrumentation or indwelling bladder catheterization. The 3–10% risk of infection for each day a catheter remains in place is due to the ascent of bacteria from the periurethral area or via intraluminal contamination of the catheter. The pt should be assessed for symptoms of upper tract disease, such as flank pain, fever, and leukocytosis. Lower tract symptoms, such as dysuria, are unreliable as markers of infection in catheterized pts. If infection is suspected, the catheter should be replaced and a freshly voided urine specimen obtained for culture; repeat cultures should confirm the persistence of infection at the time therapy is initiated. Urinary sediment should be examined for evidence of infection (e.g., pyuria). See Table 85-1 for interventions to prevent catheter-associated UTIs. In men, condom catheters—unless carefully maintained—are as strongly associated with infection as indwelling catheters.

Pneumonia Accounting for 15–20% of nosocomial infections, pneumonia increases the duration of hospital stay and costs and is associated with more deaths than are infections at any other body site. Pts aspirate endogenous or hospital-acquired flora. Risk factors include events that increase colonization with potential pathogens, such as prior antibiotic use, contaminated ventilator equipment, or increased gastric pH; events that increase risk of aspiration, such as nasogastric or endotracheal intubation or decreased level of consciousness; and conditions that compromise host defense mechanisms in the lung, such as chronic obstructive pulmonary disease. Diagnosis depends on clinical criteria such as fever, leukocytosis, purulent secretions, and new or changing pulmonary infiltrates on chest x-ray. An etiology should be sought by studies of lower

TABLE 85-1	EXAMPLES OF "BUNDLED INTERVENTIONS" TO PREVENT COMMON HEALTH CARE–ASSOCIATED INFECTIONS AND OTHER ADVERSE EVENTS

Prevention of Central Venous Catheter Infections

Educate personnel about catheter insertion and care.
Use chlorhexidine to prepare the insertion site.
Use maximum barrier precautions during catheter insertion.
Ask daily: Is the catheter needed?

Prevention of Ventilator-Associated Pneumonia and Complications

Elevate head of bed to 30–45 degrees.
Give "sedation vacation" and assess readiness to extubate daily.
Use peptic ulcer disease prophylaxis.
Use deep-vein thrombosis prophylaxis (unless contraindicated).

Prevention of Surgical-Site Infections

Administer prophylactic antibiotics within 1 h before surgery; discontinue within 24 h.
Limit any hair removal to the time of surgery; use clippers or do not remove hair at all.
Maintain normal perioperative glucose levels (cardiac surgery patients).[a]
Maintain perioperative normothermia (colorectal surgery patients).[a]

Prevention of Urinary Tract Infections

Place bladder catheters only when absolutely needed (e.g., to relieve obstruction), not solely for the provider's convenience.
Use aseptic technique for catheter insertion and urinary tract instrumentation.
Minimize manipulation or opening of drainage systems.
Remove bladder catheters as soon as is feasible.

[a]These components of care are supported by clinical trials and experimental evidence in the specified populations; they may prove valuable for other surgical patients as well.
Source: Adapted from information presented at the following websites: *www.cdc.gov/ncidod/ dhqp/gl_intravascular.html*; *www.cdc.gov/ncidod/dhqp/gl_hcpneumonia.html*; *www.cdc.gov/ ncidod/dhqp/gl_surgicalsite.html*; *www.cdc.gov/ncidod/dhqp/gl_catheter_assoc.html*; *www.ihi.org*; *www.medqic.org/scip*.

respiratory tract samples protected from upper-tract contamination; quantitative cultures have diagnostic sensitivities in the range of 80%. Febrile pts with naso-gastric tubes should also have sinusitis or otitis media ruled out. Etiologic organisms (some of which are more common among critically ill pts in ICUs) include *Streptococcus pneumoniae* and *Haemophilus influenzae* early during hospitalization and *Staphylococcus aureus*, *Pseudomonas aeruginosa*, *Klebsiella*, *Enterobacter*, *Acinetobacter*, and other gram-negative bacilli later in the hospital stay. Efforts at prevention should focus on meticulous aseptic care of respirator equipment and the interventions listed in Table 85-1.

Surgical Wound Infections   Making up 20–30% of nosocomial infections, surgical wound infections increase the length of hospital stay as well as costs. These infections often become evident after pts have left the hospital; thus it is difficult to assess the true incidence. Common risk factors include deficits in the surgeon's technical skill, the pt's underlying conditions (e.g., diabetes mellitus or obesity), and inappropriate timing of antibiotic prophylaxis. Other factors include the presence of drains, prolonged preoperative hospital stays, shaving of the operative site the day before surgery (rather than just before the procedure), long duration of surgery, and infection at remote sites.

Diagnosis begins with a careful assessment of the surgical site in the febrile postoperative pt. *S. aureus*, coagulase-negative staphylococci, and enteric and anaerobic bacteria are the most common pathogens. In rapidly progressing postoperative infections, group A streptococcal or clostridial etiologies should be considered. Treatment includes administration of appropriate antibiotics and drainage or excision of infected or necrotic material. See Table 85-1 for interventions to prevent surgical wound infections. Other interventions include attention to technical surgical issues, operating room asepsis, and preoperative treatment of active infections.

Intravascular Device Infections   Infections of intravascular devices cause up to 50% of nosocomial bacteremias; central vascular catheters account for 80–90% of these infections. As many as 200,000 bloodstream infections associated with central vascular catheters occur each year in the United States, with attributable mortality rates of 12–25% and a cost of $25,000 per episode. In pts with vascular catheters, infection is suspected on the basis of the appearance of the catheter site and/or the presence of fever or bacteremia without another source. Coagulase-negative staphylococci, *S. aureus* (including methicillin-resistant isolates), enterococci, nosocomial gram-negative bacilli, and *Candida* are the pathogens most frequently associated with these bacteremias. The diagnosis is confirmed by isolation of the same bacteria from peripheral blood cultures and from semiquantitative or quantitative cultures of samples from the vascular catheter tip. In addition to the initiation of appropriate antibiotic treatment, other considerations include the level of risk for endocarditis (relatively high in pts with *S. aureus* bacteremia) and the decision regarding catheter removal, which is usually necessary to cure infection. If salvage of the catheter is attempted, the "antibiotic lock" technique (instillation of concentrated antibiotic solution into the catheter lumen along with systemic antibiotic administration) may be used. If the catheter is changed over a guidewire and cultures of the removed catheter tip are positive, the catheter should be moved to a new site. See Table 85-1 for interventions that have been highly effective in reducing rates of central venous catheter infections. Femoral insertion sites should be avoided.

EPIDEMIC AND EMERGING PROBLEMS

- *Influenza*: Vaccination of pts and health care workers, early use of antiviral agents for control of outbreaks, and adherence to surveillance and droplet precautions for symptomatic pts are the main components of infection control.
- *Nosocomial diarrhea*
    Infection with *Clostridium difficile* is increasing in frequency and severity. Important infection-control components include judicious antibiotic use; heightened suspicion in cases with atypical presentations; and early diagnosis, treatment, and implementation of contact precautions.
    Norovirus causes nosocomial outbreaks of diarrheal syndromes in which nausea and vomiting are prominent aspects. Contact precautions may need to be augmented by environmental cleaning and active exclusion of ill staff and visitors.
- *Chickenpox*: If varicella-zoster virus (VZV) exposure occurs, postexposure prophylaxis with varicella-zoster immune globulin (VZIg) is considered for

immunocompromised or pregnant contacts (with preemptive administration of acyclovir an alternative for some susceptible persons), and susceptible employees are furloughed for 8–21 days (or for 28 days if VZIg has been given). Although VZIg is no longer manufactured in the United States, a new product is awaiting FDA approval. Vaccine should be offered routinely to VZV-susceptible employees.

- *Tuberculosis*: Prompt recognition and isolation of cases, use of negative-pressure private rooms with 100% exhaust and 6–12 air changes per hour, use of approved N95 "respirators," and follow-up skin testing of exposed personnel are required.
- *Aspergillosis*: Linked to hospital renovations and disturbance of dusty surfaces
- *Antibiotic-resistant bacterial infection*: Close laboratory surveillance, strict infection-control practices, and aggressive antibiotic-control policies are the cornerstones of resistance-control efforts.
- *Bioterrorism preparedness*: Education, effective systems of internal and external communication, and risk assessment capabilities are key features.

For a more detailed discussion, see Weinstein RA: Health Care–Associated Infections, Chap. 125, p. 835, in HPIM-17.

86 Infections in the Immunocompromised Host

The immunocompromised pt is at increased risk for infection with both common and opportunistic pathogens.

INFECTIONS IN CANCER PTS

Table 86-1 lists the normal barriers to infection whose disruption may permit infections in cancer pts. Infection-associated mortality rates among cancer pts have decreased as a result of an evolving approach entailing early use of empirical broad-spectrum antibiotics; empirical antifungal therapy in neutropenic pts who, after 4–7 days of antibiotic treatment, remain febrile without positive cultures; and use of antibiotics for afebrile neutropenic pts as broad-spectrum prophylaxis against infections.

System-Specific Syndromes

- Skin infections
  1. Cellulitis caused by streptococci, staphylococci, *Escherichia coli*, *Pseudomonas*, or fungi
  2. Macules or papules due to bacteria (e.g., *Pseudomonas aeruginosa* causing ecthyma gangrenosum) or fungi (*Candida*)
  3. Sweet's syndrome or febrile neutrophilic dermatosis: most often seen in neutropenic leukemic pts; red or bluish-red papules or nodules that form sharply bordered plaques

TABLE 86-1 DISRUPTION OF NORMAL BARRIERS THAT MAY PREDISPOSE TO INFECTIONS IN PTS WITH CANCER

Type of Defense	Specific Lesion	Cells Involved	Organism	Cancer Association	Disease
Physical barrier	Breaks in skin	Skin epithelial cells	Staphylococci, streptococci	Head and neck, squamous cell carcinoma	Cellulitis, extensive skin infection
Emptying of fluid collections	Occlusion of orifices: ureters, bile duct, colon	Luminal epithelial cells	Gram-negative bacilli	Renal, ovarian, biliary tree, metastatic diseases of many cancers	Rapid, overwhelming bacteremia; urinary tract infection
Lymphatic function	Node dissection	Lymph nodes	Staphylococci, streptococci	Breast cancer surgery	Cellulitis
Splenic clearance of microorganisms	Splenectomy	Splenic reticuloendothelial cells	*Streptococcus pneumoniae, Haemophilus influenzae, Neisseria meningitidis, Babesia, Capnocytophaga canimorsus*	Hodgkin's disease, leukemia, idiopathic thrombocytopenic purpura	Rapid, overwhelming sepsis
Phagocytosis	Lack of granulocytes	Granulocytes (neutrophils)	Staphylococci, streptococci, enteric organisms, fungi	Hairy cell, acute myelocytic, and acute lymphocytic leukemias	Bacteremia
Humoral immunity	Lack of antibody	B cells	*S. pneumoniae, H. influenzae, N. meningitidis*	Chronic lymphocytic leukemia, multiple myeloma	Infections with encapsulated organisms, sinusitis, pneumonia
Cellular immunity	Lack of T cells	T cells and macrophages	*Mycobacterium tuberculosis, Listeria,* herpesviruses, fungi, other intracellular parasites	Hodgkin's disease, leukemia, T cell lymphoma	Infections with intracellular bacteria, fungi, parasites

433

    4. Erythema multiforme with mucous membrane involvement due to herpes simplex virus (HSV)

    5. Drug-associated Stevens-Johnson syndrome

- Catheter-related infections: If a red streak develops over the SC part of a "tunneled" catheter, the device must be removed to prevent extensive cellulitis and tissue necrosis. Exit-site infections caused by coagulase-negative staphylococci can be treated with vancomycin without catheter removal. Infections caused by other organisms, including *Staphylococcus aureus*, *P. aeruginosa*, *Candida*, *Stenotrophomonas*, or *Bacillus*, usually require catheter removal.

- Upper GI infections: mouth ulcerations (viridans streptococci, anaerobic bacteria, and HSV); thrush (*Candida albicans*); and esophagitis (*C. albicans* and HSV)

- Lower GI infections

    1. Hepatic candidiasis results from seeding of the liver during neutropenia in pts with hematologic malignancy but presents when neutropenia resolves. Pts have fever, abdominal pain, nausea, and increased alkaline phosphatase levels. CT may reveal bull's-eye lesions. MRI is also helpful in the diagnosis. Amphotericin B is usually prescribed initially, but fluconazole may be useful for outpatient treatment.

    2. Typhlitis/neutropenic colitis is more common among children than among adults and among pts with acute myelocytic leukemia or acute lymphocytic leukemia (ALL) than among pts with other forms of cancer. Pts have fever, right lower quadrant tenderness, and diarrhea that is often bloody. The diagnosis is confirmed by the documentation of a thickened cecal wall via CT, MRI, or ultrasound. Treatment should be directed against gram-negative bacteria and bowel flora.

- CNS infections

    1. Meningitis: Consider *Cryptococcus* or *Listeria*. Splenectomized pts and those with hypogammaglobulinemia are also at risk for infection with encapsulated bacteria such as *Streptococcus pneumoniae*, *Haemophilus influenzae*, and *Neisseria meningitidis*.

    2. Encephalitis can develop in pts receiving high-dose cytotoxic treatment or chemotherapy that affects T cell function. Consider varicella-zoster virus (VZV), JC virus (progressive multifocal leukoencephalopathy), cytomegalovirus (CMV), *Listeria*, HSV, and human herpesvirus 6 (HHV-6).

    3. Brain masses: Consider *Nocardia*, *Cryptococcus*, *Aspergillus*, and *Toxoplasma gondii*. Epstein-Barr virus–associated lymphoproliferative disease (EBV-LPD) may present as a mass lesion.

- Pulmonary infections

    1. Localized: Bacterial pneumonia, *Legionella*, mycobacteria

    2. Nodular: Suggests fungal etiology (e.g., *Mucor*, *Aspergillus*). *Aspergillus* causes invasive disease in neutropenic pts, presenting as a thrombotic event due to blood vessel invasion, pleuritic chest pain, and fever. Hemoptysis is an ominous sign. *Nocardia* can also cause nodular lesions.

    3. Diffuse: Consider viruses (e.g., CMV), *Chlamydophila*, *Pneumocystis*, mycobacteria, and *T. gondii*. Viruses that cause upper respiratory infections in normal hosts (e.g., influenza, respiratory syncytial) may cause fatal pneumonitis.

- Renal and ureteral infections: Usually associated with obstructing tumor masses. *Candida* has a predilection for the kidneys, reaching this site via either hematogenous seeding or retrograde spread from the bladder. Adenovirus can cause hemorrhagic cystitis.

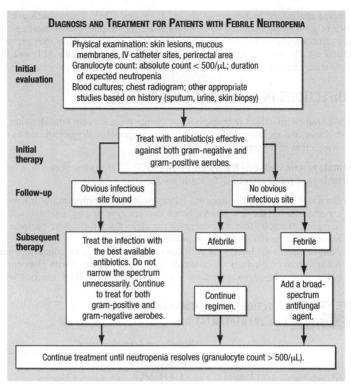

DIAGNOSIS AND TREATMENT FOR PATIENTS WITH FEBRILE NEUTROPENIA

Initial evaluation
Physical examination: skin lesions, mucous membranes, IV catheter sites, perirectal area
Granulocyte count: absolute count < 500/μL; duration of expected neutropenia
Blood cultures; chest radiogram; other appropriate studies based on history (sputum, urine, skin biopsy)

Initial therapy
Treat with antibiotic(s) effective against both gram-negative and gram-positive aerobes.

Follow-up
Obvious infectious site found | No obvious infectious site

Subsequent therapy
Treat the infection with the best available antibiotics. Do not narrow the spectrum unnecessarily. Continue to treat for both gram-positive and gram-negative aerobes.

Afebrile → Continue regimen.

Febrile → Add a broad-spectrum antifungal agent.

Continue treatment until neutropenia resolves (granulocyte count > 500/μL).

FIGURE 86-1 Algorithm for the diagnosis and treatment of febrile neutropenic pts. Several general guidelines are useful in the initial treatment of these pts: (1) It is necessary to use antibiotics active against both gram-negative and gram-positive bacteria in the initial regimen. (2) An aminoglycoside or an antibiotic without good activity against gram-positive organisms (e.g., ciprofloxacin or aztreonam) alone is not adequate in this setting. (3) The agents used should reflect both the epidemiology and the antibiotic resistance pattern of the hospital. (4) A single third-generation cephalosporin constitutes an appropriate initial regimen in many hospitals (if the pattern of resistance justifies its use). (5) Most standard regimens are designed for pts who have not previously received prophylactic antibiotics. The development of fever in a pt receiving antibiotics affects the choice of subsequent therapy (which should target resistant organisms and organisms known to cause infections in pts being treated with the antibiotics already administered). (6) Randomized trials have indicated that it is safe to use oral antibiotic regimens to treat "low-risk" pts with fever and neutropenia. Outpatients who are expected to remain neutropenic for <10 days and who have no concurrent medical problems (such as hypotension, pulmonary compromise, or abdominal pain) can be classified as low-risk and treated with a broad-spectrum oral regimen. (7) Several large-scale studies indicate that prophylaxis with a fluoroquinolone (ciprofloxacin or levofloxacin) decreases morbidity and mortality rates among afebrile patients who are anticipated to have neutropenia of long duration.

Approach to Diagnosis and Treatment of Febrile Neutropenic Pts Figure 86-1 presents an algorithm for the diagnosis and treatment of febrile neutropenic pts. The initial regimen can be refined on the basis of culture data. Adding antibiotics to the initial regimen is not appropriate unless there is a clinical or microbiologic reason to do so. For antifungal treatment, amphotericin B is being supplanted by newer azoles (e.g., voriconazole or posaconazole) or echinocandins (e.g., caspofungin). Echinocandins are useful against infections with azole-resistant *Candida*. Antiviral agents may be appropriate, particularly those directed against the herpes group viruses HSV and CMV. Prophylactic antibiotics (e.g., fluoroquinolones) in severely neutropenic pts or antifungal agents (e.g., fluconazole) in pts with hematopoietic stem cell transplants may prevent infections. *Pneumocystis* prophylaxis is mandatory for pts with ALL and for those receiving glucocorticoid-containing regimens.

INFECTIONS IN TRANSPLANT RECIPIENTS

Evaluation of infections in transplant recipients must involve consideration of both donor and recipient and of the immunosuppressive drugs required to reduce rejection of the transplanted organ.

Hematopoietic Stem Cell Transplantation (HSCT) Infections occur in a predictable time frame after HSCT (Table 86-2).

- *Bacterial infections*: Neutropenia-related infectious complications are most common during the first month. Some centers give prophylactic antibiotics (e.g., levofloxacin) that may decrease the risk of gram-negative bacteremia but increase the risk of *Clostridium difficile* colitis.
- *Fungal infections*: Infections with resistant fungi are more common when pts are given prophylactic fluconazole. Prolonged treatment with glucocorticoids or other immunosuppressive agents increases the risk of infection with

TABLE 86-2 INFECTIONS AFTER HEMATOPOIETIC STEM CELL TRANSPLANTATION

	Period after Transplantation		
Infection Site	Early (<1 Month)	Middle (1–4 Months)	Late (>6 Months)
Disseminated	Aerobic gram-negative, gram-positive bacteria	*Nocardia* *Candida*, *Aspergillus*	Encapsulated bacteria (*Streptococcus pneumoniae, Haemophilus influenzae, Neisseria meningitidis*)
Skin and mucous membranes	HSV	HHV-6	VZV
Lungs	Aerobic gram-negative, gram-positive bacteria *Candida, Aspergillus* HSV	CMV, seasonal respiratory viruses *Pneumocystis* *Toxoplasma*	*Pneumocystis*
Gastrointestinal tract		CMV	
Kidney		BK virus, adenovirus	BK virus
Brain	HHV-6	HHV-6 *Toxoplasma*	*Toxoplasma* JC virus
Bone marrow	HHV-6		

Note: CMV, cytomegalovirus; HHV-6, human herpesvirus 6; HSV, herpes simplex virus; VZV, varicella-zoster virus.

Candida or *Aspergillus* and of reactivation of endemic fungi. Maintenance prophylaxis with trimethoprim-sulfamethoxazole (TMP-SMX; 160/800 mg/d starting 1 month after engraftment and continuing for at least 1 year) is recommended to prevent *Pneumocystis* pneumonia (PcP).

- *Parasitic infections*: PcP prophylaxis with TMP-SMX is also protective against disease caused by *Toxoplasma* as well as against infections caused by certain bacteria, including *Nocardia*, *Listeria*, *S. pneumoniae*, and *H. influenzae*.
- *Viral infections*: Prophylactic acyclovir or valacyclovir for HSV-seropositive pts reduces rates of mucositis and prevents pneumonia and other HSV manifestations. Zoster is usually managed readily with acyclovir. HHV-6 delays monocyte and platelet engraftment and may be linked to encephalitis or pneumonitis. CMV causes interstitial pneumonia, bone marrow suppression, colitis, and graft failure. The risk is highest with a CMV-seropositive donor and a CMV-seronegative recipient. Severe disease is more common among allogeneic transplant recipients and is often associated with graft-versus-host disease. Many centers give prophylactic IV ganciclovir or oral valganciclovir from engraftment to day 120 after allogeneic HSCT. In addition, preemptive therapy is given when CMV is detected in blood by an antigen or DNA test. EBV-LPD as well as infections caused by respiratory syncytial virus, parainfluenza virus, metapneumovirus, influenza virus, and adenovirus can occur. BK virus (a polyomavirus) has been found in the urine of pts after HSCT.

Solid Organ Transplantation   After solid organ transplantation, pts do not go through a stage of neutropenia like that seen after HSCT; thus the infections in these two groups of pts differ. However, solid organ transplant recipients are immunosuppressed for longer periods with agents that chronically impair T cell immunity.

1. Infection risk depends on the interval since transplantation.
   a. Early infections (<1 month): Infections are related to surgery and wounds.
   b. Middle-period infections (1–6 months): Infections are the same as those seen in pts with chronically impaired T cell immunity. CMV causes severe systemic disease or infection of transplanted organs; the latter increases the risk of organ rejection, prompting increased immunosuppression that, in turn, increases CMV replication. Diagnosis, treatment, and prophylaxis of CMV infection are the keys to interrupting this cycle. Late-onset disease may occur when prophylaxis is stopped. However, the transplant recipient is often better equipped to combat late infection as a result of improved graft function and, in many cases, less intense immunosuppression.
   c. Late infections (>6 months): *Listeria*, *Nocardia*, various fungi, and other intracellular organisms associated with defects in cell-mediated immunity may pose problems. When EBV-LPD occurs (often within the transplanted organ), immunosuppression should be decreased or discontinued, if possible.
2. Kidney transplantation: TMP-SMX prophylaxis for the first 4 months decreases infection rates. Valacyclovir or valganciclovir may be considered for prophylactic treatment of high-risk pts to prevent primary or reactivation CMV infection and other herpesvirus disease. BK virus replication is associated with ureteral strictures, nephropathy, and vasculopathy. Reduction of the degree of immunosuppression is critical to reduce rates of graft loss.
3. Heart transplantation
   a. Early period: Sternal wound infection and mediastinitis due to common skin organisms, gram-negative bacteria, fungi, and *Mycoplasma hominis*

TABLE 86-3 VACCINATION OF CANCER PTS RECEIVING CHEMOTHERAPY, PTS WITH HODGKIN'S DISEASE, AND HEMATOPOIETIC STEM CELL TRANSPLANT RECIPIENTS

	Use in Indicated Patients		
Vaccine	Intensive Chemotherapy	Hodgkin's Disease	Hematopoietic Stem Cell Transplantation
Diphtheria-tetanus[a]	Primary series and boosters as necessary	No special recommendation	12, 14, and 24 months after transplantation
Poliomyelitis[b]	Complete primary series and boosters	No special recommendation	12, 14, and 24 months after transplantation
Haemophilus influenzae type b conjugate	Primary series and booster for children	Immunization before treatment and booster 3 months afterward	12, 14, and 24 months after transplantation
Hepatitis A	Not routinely recommended	Not routinely recommended	Not routinely recommended
Hepatitis B	Complete series	No special recommendation	12, 14, and 24 months after transplantation
23-Valent pneumococcal polysaccharide[c]	Every 5 years	Immunization before treatment and booster 3 months afterward	12 and 24 months after transplantation
4-Valent meningococcal conjugate[d]	Should be administered to splenectomized pts and pts living in endemic areas, including college students in dormitories	Should be administered to splenectomized pts and pts living in endemic areas, including college students in dormitories	Should be administered to splenectomized pts and pts living in endemic areas, including college students in dormitories
Influenza	Seasonal immunization	Seasonal immunization	Seasonal immunization
Measles/mumps/rubella	Contraindicated	Contraindicated	After 24 months in pts without graft-versus-host disease
Varicella-zoster virus	Contraindicated[e]	Contraindicated	Contraindicated

[a]The Td (tetanus-diphtheria) combination is currently recommended for adults. Pertussis vaccines have not been recommended for people >6 years of age in the past. However, recent data indicate that the Tdap (tetanus-diphtheria-acellular pertussis) product is both safe and efficacious in adults.

[b]Live-virus vaccine is contraindicated; inactivated vaccine should be used.

[c]The seven-serotype pneumococcal conjugate vaccine is currently recommended only for children. It is anticipated that future vaccines will include more serotypes and will be recommended for adults.

[d]Currently licensed for people 11–55 years of age.

[e]Contact the manufacturer for more information on use in children with acute lymphocytic leukemia.

b. Middle period: The risk of *T. gondii* infection is high. TMP-SMX prophylaxis, which also protects the pt against *Pneumocystis*, *Nocardia*, and other organisms, is warranted. CMV disease due to reactivation or primary infection is associated with poor outcomes.

c. Late period: EBV-LPD, PcP

4. Lung transplantation

a. Early period: Pneumonia, mediastinitis

b. Middle period: CMV disease is most severe in lung or heart-lung transplant recipients; it is very common if either the donor or the recipient is seropositive. Prophylaxis is indicated.

c. Late period: EBV-LPD, PcP. Prophylaxis is given for 1 year.

5. Liver transplantation

a. Early period: Peritonitis, intraabdominal abscesses. Biliary leaks are particularly common in live-donor liver transplants (LDLTs). Fungal infections are common and correlate with preoperative glucocorticoid use or long-term antimicrobial use.

b. Middle period: Cholangitis, especially in LDLTs; viral hepatitis due to reactivation of hepatitis B and C infections. High-dose IV hepatitis B immune globulin is given; other agents are being studied for hepatitis B and C. CMV infection occurs in seronegative recipients of organs from seropositive donors; disease is not usually as severe as in other types of transplantation.

6. Within the first 12 months after solid organ transplantation, tuberculosis occurs at rates higher than those observed after HSCT. The incidence reflects the prevalence of tuberculosis in local populations.

IMMUNIZATIONS IN IMMUNOSUPPRESSED PTS

Recommendations for vaccination of cancer pts receiving chemotherapy, pts with Hodgkin's disease, and hematopoietic stem cell transplant recipients are listed in Table 86-3. In solid organ transplant recipients, the usual vaccines and boosters should be given before immunosuppression. Pneumococcal vaccination should be repeated every 5 years; this vaccine can be given with meningococcal vaccine. Solid organ transplant recipients receiving immunosuppressive agents should not receive live vaccines.

For a more detailed discussion, see Finberg R: Infections in Patients with Cancer, Chap. 82, p. 533; Madoff LC, Kasper DL: Introduction to Infectious Diseases: Host-Pathogen Interactions, Chap. 113, p. 749; and Finberg R, Fingeroth J: Infections in Transplant Recipients, Chap. 126, p. 842, in HPIM-17.

87 Infective Endocarditis

Acute endocarditis is a febrile illness that rapidly damages cardiac structures, seeds extracardiac sites hematogenously, and can progress to death within weeks. *Subacute* endocarditis follows an indolent course, rarely causes metastatic infection, and progresses gradually unless complicated by a major embolic event or a ruptured mycotic aneurysm.

EPIDEMIOLOGY

In developed countries, the incidence of endocarditis ranges from 2.6 to 7.0 cases per 100,000 population per year. Predisposing conditions include congenital heart disease, illicit IV drug use, degenerative valve disease, intracardiac devices, and health care–associated infections. The incidence of endocarditis is increased among the elderly and among pts with prosthetic heart valves. The risk of endocarditis is greatest during the first 6 months after valve replacement.

ETIOLOGY

The causative microorganisms vary, in part because of different portals of entry. In native valve endocarditis (NVE), viridans streptococci, staphylococci, and HACEK organisms (*Haemophilus* spp., *Actinobacillus actinomycetemcomitans*, *Cardiobacterium hominis*, *Eikenella corrodens*, *Kingella kingae*) enter the bloodstream from oral, skin, and upper respiratory tract portals, respectively. *Streptococcus bovis* originates from the gut and is associated with colon polyps or cancer. Enterococci originate from the genitourinary tract. Nosocomial endocarditis, frequently due to *Staphylococcus aureus*, arises most often from bacteremia related to intravascular devices. Prosthetic valve endocarditis (PVE) developing within 2 months of surgery is due to intraoperative contamination or a bacteremic postoperative complication and is typically caused by coagulase-negative staphylococci (CoNS), *S. aureus*, facultative gram-negative bacilli, diphtheroids, or fungi. At 1 year after valve surgery, endocarditis is caused by the same organisms that cause community-acquired NVE. IV drug users are particularly prone to tricuspid valve endocarditis caused by *S. aureus* (often a methicillin-resistant strain); they are also at risk for left-sided endocarditis caused by *S. aureus*, *Pseudomonas aeruginosa*, or *Candida* spp. Fastidious organisms such as the nutritionally variant bacteria *Granulicatella* and *Abiotrophia*, HACEK bacteria, *Bartonella* spp., *Coxiella burnetii*, *Brucella* spp., and *Tropheryma whipplei* can cause culture-negative endocarditis. β-Hemolytic streptococci, *S. aureus*, and pneumococci typically cause acute endocarditis, while viridans streptococci, enterococci, CoNS, and HACEK organisms usually cause subacute disease.

PATHOGENESIS

If endothelial injury occurs, direct infection by pathogens such as *S. aureus* can result, or an uninfected platelet-fibrin thrombus may develop and become infected during transient bacteremia. The vegetation (Fig. 87-1) is the prototypic lesion at the site of infection: a mass of platelets, fibrin, and microcolonies of organisms, with scant inflammatory cells.

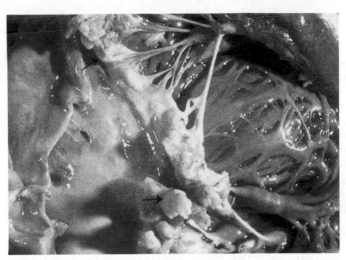

FIGURE 87-1 Vegetations (*arrows*) due to viridans streptococcal endocarditis involving the mitral valve.

CLINICAL FEATURES

The clinical syndrome is variable and spans a continuum between acute and subacute presentations.

Cardiac Manifestations
- Heart murmurs, particularly new or worsened regurgitant murmurs, are ultimately heard in 85% of pts with acute NVE.
- Congestive heart failure (CHF) develops in 30–40% of pts and is usually due to valvular dysfunction.
- Extension of infection can result in perivalvular abscesses, which in turn may cause fistulae from the aortic root into cardiac chambers or may burrow through epicardium and cause pericarditis.
- Heart block may result when infection extends into the conduction system.
- Emboli to a coronary artery may result in myocardial infarcts.

Noncardiac Manifestations
- Hematogenous bacterial seeding (e.g., to the spleen, kidneys, and meninges) can cause abscesses in noncardiac tissues.
- Arterial emboli of vegetation fragments lead to infection or infarction of remote tissues such as the extremities, spleen, kidneys, bowel, or brain. Emboli most commonly arise from vegetations >10 mm in diameter and from those located on the mitral valve. With antibiotic treatment, the frequency of emboli decreases from 13 per 1000 pt-days during the first week of infection to 1.2 per 1000 pt-days during the third week.
- Neurologic complications are seen in up to 40% of pts and include embolic stroke, aseptic or purulent meningitis, intracranial hemorrhage due to ruptured mycotic aneurysms (focal dilations of arteries at points in the artery wall that have been weakened by infection or where septic emboli have lodged) or hemorrhagic infarcts, seizures, encephalopathy, and microabscesses.
- Renal infarcts cause flank pain and hematuria without renal dysfunction.
- Immune complex deposition causes glomerulonephritis and renal dysfunction.

- Peripheral manifestations such as Osler's nodes, subungual hemorrhages, Janeway lesions, and Roth's spots are nonsuppurative complications seen in prolonged infection and are now rare because of early diagnosis and treatment.

Tricuspid Valve Endocarditis   This condition is associated with fever, faint or no heart murmur, and prominent pulmonary findings such as cough, pleuritic chest pain, and nodular pulmonary infiltrates.

Health Care–Associated Endocarditis   Manifestations depend on the presence or absence of a retained intracardiac device. For example, transvenous pacemaker lead–related endocarditis may be associated with generator pocket infection and results in fever, minimal murmur, and pulmonary symptoms due to septic emboli.

Paravalvular Infection   This condition is common in PVE, resulting in partial valve dehiscence, regurgitant murmurs, CHF, or disruption of the conduction system.

DIAGNOSIS

- The Duke criteria (Table 87-1) constitute a sensitive and specific diagnostic schema. *Definite* endocarditis is defined by 2 major, 1 major plus 3 minor, or 5 minor criteria. *Possible* endocarditis is defined by 1 major plus 1 minor criterion or by 3 minor criteria.
- If blood cultures are negative after 48–72 h, 2 or 3 additional cultures should be performed, and the laboratory should be asked for advice regarding optimal culture techniques.
- Serology is helpful in the diagnosis of *Brucella, Bartonella, Legionella*, or *C. burnetii* endocarditis.
- Echocardiography should be performed to confirm the diagnosis, to verify the size of vegetations, to detect intracardiac complications, and to assess cardiac function. Transthoracic echocardiography (TTE) does not detect vegetations <2 mm in diameter and is not adequate to evaluate prosthetic valves or to detect intracardiac complications; however, TTE may be used in pts with a low pretest likelihood of endocarditis (<5%). In other pts, transesophageal echocardiography (TEE) is indicated. TEE detects vegetations in >90% of cases of definite endocarditis and is optimal for evaluation of prosthetic valves and detection of abscesses, valve perforation, or intracardiac fistulas.
- Other laboratory studies should be performed—e.g., a complete blood count, creatinine measurement, liver function tests, chest radiography, and electrocardiography. The erythrocyte sedimentation rate, C-reactive protein level, and circulating immune complex titer are typically elevated.

 Endocarditis

ANTIMICROBIAL THERAPY

Antimicrobial therapy must be bactericidal and prolonged. See Table 87-2 for organism-specific regimens. Most pts defervesce within 5–7 days. Blood cultures should be repeated until sterile, and results should be rechecked if there is recrudescent fever and at 4–6 weeks after therapy to document cure. If pts are febrile for 7 days despite antibiotic therapy, an evaluation for paravalvular or extracardiac abscesses should be performed.

- Pts with acute endocarditis require antibiotic treatment as soon as three sets of blood culture samples are obtained, but stable pts with subacute dis-

TABLE 87-1   THE DUKE CRITERIA FOR THE CLINICAL DIAGNOSIS OF INFECTIVE ENDOCARDITIS

Major Criteria

1. Positive blood culture

   Typical microorganism for infective endocarditis from two separate blood cultures

       Viridans streptococci, *Streptococcus bovis*, HACEK group, *Staphylococcus aureus*, *or*

       Community-acquired enterococci in the absence of a primary focus, *or*

   Persistently positive blood culture, defined as recovery of a microorganism consistent with infective endocarditis from:

       Blood cultures drawn >12 h apart; *or*

       All of three or a majority of four or more separate blood cultures, with first and last drawn at least 1 h apart

   Single positive blood culture for *Coxiella burnetii* or phase I IgG antibody titer of >1:800

2. Evidence of endocardial involvement

   Positive echocardiogram[a]

       Oscillating intracardiac mass on valve or supporting structures or in the path of regurgitant jets or in implanted material, in the absence of an alternative anatomic explanation, *or*

       Abscess, *or*

       New partial dehiscence of prosthetic valve, *or*

   New valvular regurgitation (increase or change in preexisting murmur not sufficient)

Minor Criteria

1. Predisposition: predisposing heart condition or injection drug use
2. Fever ≥38.0°C (≥100.4°F)
3. Vascular phenomena: major arterial emboli, septic pulmonary infarcts, mycotic aneurysm, intracranial hemorrhage, conjunctival hemorrhages, Janeway lesions
4. Immunologic phenomena: glomerulonephritis, Osler's nodes, Roth's spots, rheumatoid factor
5. Microbiologic evidence: positive blood culture but not meeting major criterion as noted previously[b] or serologic evidence of active infection with organism consistent with infective endocarditis

[a] Transesophageal echocardiography is recommended for assessing possible prosthetic valve endocarditis or complicated endocarditis.

[b] Excluding single positive cultures for coagulase-negative staphylococci and diphtheroids, which are common culture contaminants, and organisms that do not cause endocarditis frequently, such as gram-negative bacilli.

Note: HACEK, *Haemophilus* spp., *Actinobacillus actinomycetemcomitans*, *Cardiobacterium hominis*, *Eikenella corrodens*, *Kingella kingae*.

Source: Adapted from JS Li et al: Clin Infect Dis 30:633, 2000, with permission from the University of Chicago Press.

ease should have antibiotics withheld until a diagnosis is made. Pts treated with vancomycin or an aminoglycoside should have serum drug levels monitored. Tests to detect renal, hepatic, and/or hematologic toxicity should be performed periodically.

- Selection of optimal treatment for streptococcal endocarditis requires determination of the minimal inhibitory concentration (MIC) of penicillin for the causative isolate. Two-week regimens should not be used for compli-

TABLE 87-2 ANTIBIOTIC TREATMENT FOR INFECTIVE ENDOCARDITIS CAUSED BY COMMON ORGANISMS^a

Organism	Drug, Dose, Duration	Comments
Streptococci		
Penicillin-susceptible^b streptococci, *S. bovis*	Penicillin G (2–3 mU IV q4h for 4 weeks)	—
	Ceftriaxone (2 g/d IV as a single dose for 4 weeks)	Can use ceftriaxone in pts with nonimmediate penicillin allergy
	Vancomycin^c (15 mg/kg IV q12h for 4 weeks)	Use vancomycin in pts with severe or immediate β-lactam allergy
	Penicillin G (2–3 mU IV q4h) *or* ceftriaxone (2 g IV qd) for 2 weeks	Avoid 2-week regimen when risk of aminoglycoside toxicity is increased and in prosthetic valve or complicated endocarditis
	plus gentamicin^d (3 mg/kg qd IV or IM as a single dose^e or divided into equal doses q8h for 2 weeks)	
Relatively penicillin-resistant^f streptococci	Penicillin G (4 mU IV q4h) *or* ceftriaxone (2 g IV qd) for 4 weeks	Penicillin alone at this dose for 6 weeks or with gentamicin during initial 2 weeks preferred for prosthetic valve endocarditis caused by streptococci with penicillin MICs of ≤0.1 μg/mL
	plus gentamicin^d (3 mg/kg qd IV or IM as a single dose^e or divided into equal doses q8h for 2 weeks)	
	Vancomycin^c as noted above for 4 weeks	
Moderately penicillin-resistant^g streptococci, nutritionally variant organisms, or *Gemella morbillorum*	Penicillin G (4–5 mU IV q4h) *or* ceftriaxone (2 g IV qd) for 6 weeks	Preferred for prosthetic valve endocarditis caused by streptococci with penicillin MICs of >0.1 μg/mL
	plus gentamicin^d (3 mg/kg qd IV or IM as a single dose^e or divided into equal doses q8h for 6 weeks)	
	Vancomycin^c as noted above for 4 weeks	
Enterococci^h	Penicillin G (4–5 mU IV q4h) *plus* gentamicin^d (1 mg/kg IV q8h), both for 4–6 weeks	Can use streptomycin (7.5 mg/kg q12h) in lieu of gentamicin if there is not high-level resistance to streptomycin
	Ampicillin (2 g IV q4h) *plus* gentamicin^d (1 mg/kg IV q8h), both for 4–6 weeks	—
	Vancomycin^c (15 mg/kg IV q12h) *plus* gentamicin^d (1 mg/kg IV q8h), both for 4–6 weeks	Use vancomycin plus gentamicin for penicillin-allergic pts, or desensitize these pts to penicillin

Staphylococci

Methicillin-susceptible, infecting native valves (no foreign devices)	Nafcillin or oxacillin (2 g IV q4h for 4–6 weeks) *plus* (optional) gentamicin[d] (1 mg/kg IM or IV q8h for 3–5 days)	Can use penicillin (4 mU q4h) if isolate is penicillin-susceptible (does not produce β-lactamase)
	Cefazolin (2 g IV q8h for 4–6 weeks) *plus* (optional) gentamicin[d] (1 mg/kg IM or IV q8h for 3–5 days)	Can use cefazolin regimen for pts with nonimmediate penicillin allergy
	Vancomycin[c] (15 mg/kg IV q12h for 4–6 weeks)	Use vancomycin for pts with immediate (urticarial) or severe penicillin allergy
Methicillin-resistant, infecting native valves (no foreign devices)	Vancomycin[c] (15 mg/kg IV q12h for 4–6 weeks)	No role for routine use of rifampin
Methicillin-susceptible, infecting prosthetic valves	Nafcillin or oxacillin (2 g IV q4h for 6–8 weeks) *plus* gentamicin[d] (1 mg/kg IM or IV q8h for 2 weeks) *plus* rifampin[i] (300 mg PO q8h for 6–8 weeks)	Use gentamicin during initial 2 weeks; determine susceptibility to gentamicin before initiating rifampin; if pt is highly allergic to penicillin, use regimen for methicillin-resistant staphylococci; if β-lactam allergy is of the minor, nonimmediate type, can substitute cefazolin for oxacillin/nafcillin
Methicillin-resistant, infecting prosthetic valves	Vancomycin[c] (15 mg/kg IV q12h for 6–8 weeks) *plus* gentamicin[d] (1 mg/kg IM or IV q8h for 2 weeks) *plus* rifampin[i] (300 mg PO q8h for 6–8 weeks)	Use gentamicin during initial 2 weeks; determine gentamicin susceptibility before initiating rifampin
HACEK organisms	Ceftriaxone (2 g/d IV as single dose for 4 weeks)	Can use another third-generation cephalosporin at comparable dosage
	Ampicillin/sulbactam (3 g IV q6h for 4 weeks)	—

[a]Doses are for adults with normal renal function. Doses of gentamicin, streptomycin, and vancomycin must be adjusted for reduced renal function. Ideal body weight is used to calculate doses of gentamicin and streptomycin per kilogram (men = 50 kg + 2.3 kg per inch over 5 feet; women = 45.5 kg + 2.3 kg per inch over 5 feet).

[b]MIC, ≤0.1 μg/mL.

[c]Desirable peak vancomycin level 1 h after completion of a 1-h infusion is 30–45 μg/mL.

[d]Aminoglycosides should not be administered as single daily doses for enterococcal endocarditis and should be introduced as part of the initial treatment. Target peak and trough serum concentrations of divided-dose gentamicin 1 h after a 20- to 30-min infusion or IM injection are ~3–5 μg/mL and ≤1 μg/mL, respectively; target peak and trough serum concentrations of streptomycin (timing as with gentamicin) are 20–35 μg/mL and <10 μg/mL, respectively.

[e]Netilmicin (4 mg/kg qd, as a single dose) can be used in lieu of gentamicin.

[f]MIC, >0.1 μg/mL and <0.5 μg/mL.

[g]MIC, ≥0.5 μg/mL and <8.0 μg/mL.

[h]Antimicrobial susceptibility must be evaluated.

[i]Rifampin increases warfarin and dicumarol requirements for anticoagulation.

cated NVE or for PVE. Groups B, C, and G streptococcal endocarditis should be treated with the regimen recommended for relatively penicillin-resistant streptococci (Table 87-2).

- Enterococci require the synergistic activity of a cell wall–active agent and an aminoglycoside for killing. Enterococci must be tested for high-level resistance to streptomycin and gentamicin; if resistance is detected, the addition of an aminoglycoside will not produce a synergistic effect, and the cell wall–active agent should be given alone for periods of 8–12 weeks or—for *Enterococcus faecalis*—high-dose ampicillin plus ceftriaxone can be given. If treatment fails or the isolate is resistant to commonly used agents, surgical therapy is advised (see below and Table 87-3). The aminoglycoside can be discontinued in those pts who have responded satisfactorily to therapy if toxicity develops after 2–3 weeks of treatment.

- Staphylococcal PVE is treated for 6–8 weeks with a multidrug regimen. Rifampin is important because it kills organisms adherent to foreign material. Two other agents in addition to rifampin help prevent the emergence of rifampin resistance in vivo. Susceptibility testing for gentamicin should be performed before rifampin is given; if the strain is resistant, another aminoglycoside or a fluoroquinolone should be substituted.

- Pts with negative blood cultures and without confounding prior antibiotic treatment should receive ceftriaxone plus gentamicin. If the pt has a prosthetic valve, those two drugs plus vancomycin should be given.

SURGICAL TREATMENT

Surgery should be considered early in the course of illness in pts with the indications listed in Table 87-3, although most of these indications are not absolute. However, pts who develop acute aortic regurgitation with preclosure of the mitral valve or a sinus of Valsalva abscess rupture into the right heart require emergent surgery. Likewise, surgery should not be delayed when severe valvular dysfunction with progressive CHF or uncontrolled or perivalvular infection is present. Cardiac surgery should be delayed for 2–3 weeks if

TABLE 87-3	INDICATIONS FOR CARDIAC SURGICAL INTERVENTION IN PTS WITH ENDOCARDITIS

Surgery required for optimal outcome
    Moderate to severe CHF due to valve dysfunction
    Partially dehisced unstable prosthetic valve
    Persistent bacteremia despite optimal antimicrobial therapy
    Lack of effective microbicidal therapy (e.g., fungal or *Brucella* endocarditis)
    S. aureus PVE with an intracardiac complication
    Relapse of PVE after optimal antimicrobial therapy
Surgery to be strongly considered for improved outcome[a]
    Perivalvular extension of infection
    Poorly responsive *S. aureus* endocarditis involving the aortic or mitral valve
    Large (>10-mm diameter) hypermobile vegetations with increased risk of embolism
    Persistent unexplained fever (≥10 days) in culture-negative NVE
    Poorly responsive or relapsed endocarditis due to highly antibiotic-resistant enterococci or gram-negative bacilli

[a]Surgery must be carefully considered; findings are often combined with other indications to prompt surgery.
Note: CHF, congestive heart failure; NVE, native valve endocarditis; PVE, prosthetic valve endocarditis.

TABLE 87-4	HIGH-RISK CARDIAC LESIONS FOR WHICH ENDOCARDITIS PROPHYLAXIS IS ADVISED BEFORE DENTAL PROCEDURES

Prosthetic heart valves
Prior endocarditis
Unrepaired cyanotic congenital heart disease, including palliative shunts or conduits
Completely repaired congenital heart defects during the 6 months after repair
Incompletely repaired congenital heart disease with residual defects adjacent to
    prosthetic material
Valvulopathy developing after cardiac transplantation

Source: W Wilson et al: *Circulation*, 116:1736, 2007.

possible when the pt has had a nonhemorrhagic embolic stroke and for 4 weeks when the pt has had a hemorrhagic embolic stroke. Ruptured mycotic aneurysms should be clipped and cerebral edema allowed to resolve prior to cardiac surgery.

ANTIBIOTIC THERAPY AFTER CARDIAC SURGERY

- Uncomplicated NVE caused by susceptible organisms, with negative valve cultures at surgery: The duration of pre- and postoperative treatment should equal the total duration of recommended therapy, with ~2 weeks of treatment given postoperatively.
- Endocarditis with paravalvular abscess, partially treated PVE, or culture-positive valves: Pts should receive a full course of therapy postoperatively.

PREVENTION

The American Heart Association has dramatically restricted recommendations for antibiotic prophylaxis, advising prophylaxis only for pts at highest risk of severe morbidity and death from endocarditis. Prophylaxis is recommended

TABLE 87-5	ANTIBIOTIC REGIMENS FOR PROPHYLAXIS OF ENDOCARDITIS IN ADULTS WITH HIGH-RISK CARDIAC LESIONS[a,b]

A. Standard oral regimen
    1. Amoxicillin 2.0 g PO 1 h before procedure
B. Inability to take oral medication
    1. Ampicillin 2.0 g IV or IM within 1 h before procedure
C. Penicillin allergy
    1. Clarithromycin or azithromycin 500 mg PO 1 h before procedure
    2. Cephalexin[c] 2.0 g PO 1 h before procedure
    3. Clindamycin 600 mg PO 1 h before procedure
D. Penicillin allergy, inability to take oral medication
    1. Cefazolin[c] or ceftriaxone 1.0 g IV or IM 30 min before procedure
    2. Clindamycin 600 mg IV or IM 1h before procedure

[a]Dosing for children: For amoxicillin, ampicillin, cephalexin, or cefadroxil, use 50 mg/kg PO; cefazolin, 25 mg/kg IV; clindamycin, 20 mg/kg PO, 25 mg/kg IV; clarithromycin, 15 mg/kg PO; and vancomycin, 20 mg/kg IV.
[b]For high-risk lesions, see Table 87-4. Prophylaxis is not advised for other lesions.
[c]Do not use cephalosporins in pts with immediate hypersensitivity (urticaria, angioedema, anaphylaxis) to penicillin.
Source: W Wilson et al: *Circulation*, 116:1736, 2007.

only for those dental procedures involving manipulation of gingival tissue or the periapical region of the teeth or perforation of the oral mucosa (including respiratory tract surgery). Table 87-4 lists the high-risk cardiac lesions for which prophylaxis is advised, and Table 87-5 lists the recommended antibiotic regimens for this purpose.

For a more detailed discussion, see Karchmer AW: Infective Endocarditis, Chap. 118, p. 789, in HPIM-17.

88 Intraabdominal Infections

Intraperitoneal infections result when normal anatomic barriers are disrupted. Organisms contained within the bowel or an intraabdominal organ enter the sterile peritoneal cavity, causing peritonitis and—if the infection goes untreated and the pt survives—abscesses.

PERITONITIS

Peritonitis is a life-threatening event that is often accompanied by bacteremia and sepsis. Primary peritonitis has no apparent source, whereas secondary peritonitis is caused by spillage from an intraabdominal viscus.

PRIMARY (SPONTANEOUS) BACTERIAL PERITONITIS (PBP)

PBP is most common among pts with cirrhosis (usually due to alcoholism) and preexisting ascites, although it is also described in other settings (e.g., malignancy, hepatitis). PBP is due to hematogenous spread of organisms to ascitic fluid in pts in whom a diseased liver and altered portal circulation compromise the liver's filtration function.

Clinical Features   Fever is common. Although some pts experience an acute onset of abdominal pain or signs of peritoneal irritation, other pts have only nonspecific and nonlocalizing manifestations (e.g., malaise, fatigue, encephalopathy). PBP is diagnosed if peritoneal fluid is sampled and contains >250 polymorphonuclear leukocytes/μL. Enteric gram-negative bacilli such as *Escherichia coli* or gram-positive organisms such as streptococci, enterococci, and pneumococci are the most common etiologic agents; a single organism is typically isolated. Culture yield is improved if 10 mL of peritoneal fluid is placed directly into blood culture bottles. Blood cultures should be performed because bacteremia is common.

℞ Primary (Spontaneous) Bacterial Peritonitis

Ceftriaxone (2 g/d IV) or piperacillin/tazobactam (3.375 g qid IV) constitutes appropriate empirical treatment. The regimen should be narrowed after the etiology is identified. Treatment should continue for 5–14 days, depending on how quickly the pt's condition improves.

Prevention   Up to 70% of pts have a recurrence of PBP within 1 year. Fluoro-quinolones (e.g., ciprofloxacin, 750 mg weekly) or trimethoprim-sulfamethoxazole (TMP-SMX; one double-strength tablet daily) provides effective prophylaxis but increases the risk of serious staphylococcal infections over time.

SECONDARY PERITONITIS

Secondary peritonitis develops when bacteria contaminate the peritoneum as a result of spillage from an intraabdominal viscus. Infection almost always involves a mixed aerobic and anaerobic flora, especially when the contaminating source is colonic.

Clinical Features   Initial symptoms may be localized or vague and depend on the primary organ involved. Once infection has spread to the peritoneal cavity, pain increases; pts lie motionless, often with knees drawn up to avoid stretching the nerve fibers of the peritoneal cavity. Coughing or sneezing causes severe, sharp pain. There is marked voluntary and involuntary guarding of anterior abdominal musculature, tenderness (often with rebound), and fever.

Diagnosis and Treatment   There is marked leukocytosis with a left shift. Studies to find the source of peritonitis are central to treatment. Abdominal taps are done only to exclude hemoperitoneum in trauma cases. The selected antibiotics are aimed at aerobic gram-negative bacilli and anaerobes—e.g., penicillin/β-lactamase inhibitor combinations or, in critically ill pts in the ICU, imipenem (500 mg q6h IV) or drug combinations such as ampicillin plus metronidazole plus ciprofloxacin. Surgical intervention is often needed.

PERITONITIS IN PTS UNDERGOING CHRONIC AMBULATORY PERITONEAL DIALYSIS

Common etiologic agents include *Staphylococcus* spp. such as coagulase-negative staphylococci and *Staphylococcus aureus* (~45% of cases), gram-negative bacilli, and fungi such as *Candida* spp. Several hundred milliliters of removed dialysis fluid should be centrifuged and sent for culture, preferably in blood culture bottles to improve the diagnostic yield. Empirical therapy should be directed against staphylococcal species and gram-negative bacilli (e.g., cefazolin plus a fluoroquinolone or a third-generation cephalosporin such as ceftazidime). Vancomycin should be used instead of cefazolin if methicillin resistance is prevalent, if the pt has an overt exit-site infection, or if the pt appears toxic. Antibiotics are given either continuously (e.g., with each exchange) or intermittently (e.g., once daily with the dose allowed to remain in the peritoneal cavity for 6 h). Severely ill pts should be given the same regimen IV. Catheter removal should be considered if the pt's condition does not improve within 48 h.

INTRAABDOMINAL ABSCESSES

INTRAPERITONEAL ABSCESSES

Seventy-four percent of intraabdominal abscesses are intraperitoneal or retroperitoneal and not visceral. Most abscesses arise from colonic sources. Abscesses develop in untreated peritonitis as an extension of the disease process and as an attempt by the host's defenses to contain the infection. *Bacteroides fragilis* accounts for only 0.5% of the normal colonic flora, but it is the anaerobe most frequently isolated from intraabdominal abscesses and from blood. Scanning procedures facilitate the diagnosis; abdominal CT has the highest yield. Ultrasonography is useful for the right upper quadrant (RUQ), the kidneys, and the pelvis. Indium-labeled white blood cells and gallium localize in abscesses; however, because the bowel takes up gallium, the indium scan may be preferable. Occasionally, exploratory laparotomy is still needed to identify an abscess.

Antimicrobial therapy is adjunctive to drainage and/or surgical correction of an underlying lesion or process, although diverticular abscesses usually wall off locally and surgical intervention is not routinely needed. Antimicrobial agents with activity against gram-negative bacilli and anaerobic organisms are indicated (see "Secondary Peritonitis," above).

VISCERAL ABSCESSES

Liver Abscess   Liver abscesses account for up to half of visceral intraabdominal abscesses and are caused most commonly by biliary tract disease (due to aerobic gram-negative bacilli, enterococci) and less often by local spread from other contiguous sites of infection (mixed aerobic and anaerobic infection) or hematogenous seeding (infection with a single species, usually staphylococci or streptococci). Pts have fever, anorexia, weight loss, nausea, and vomiting, but only ~50% have signs localized to the RUQ, such as pain, tenderness, hepatomegaly, and jaundice. Serum levels of alkaline phosphatase are elevated in ~70% of pts, and leukocytosis is common. About one-third of pts are bacteremic. Amebic liver abscesses are not uncommon; amebic serology has yielded positive results in >95% of affected pts. Drainage remains the mainstay of treatment, but medical management with long courses of antibiotics can be successful. Percutaneous drainage tends to fail when there are multiple, sizable abscesses; viscous abscess contents that plug the pigtail catheter; associated disease (e.g., of the biliary tract); or lack of response in 4–7 days.

Splenic Abscess   Splenic abscesses usually develop by hematogenous spread of infection (e.g., due to endocarditis). Abdominal pain or splenomegaly occurs in ~50% of cases and pain localized to the left upper quadrant in ~25%. Fever and leukocytosis are common. Chest x-ray may show infiltrates or left-sided pleural effusions. Splenic abscesses are most often caused by streptococci; *S. aureus* is the next most common cause. Gram-negative bacilli can cause splenic abscess in pts with urinary tract foci, and *Salmonella* can be responsible in pts with sickle cell disease. The diagnosis is often made only after the pt's death; the condition is frequently fatal if left untreated. Pts with multiple or complex multilocular abscesses should undergo splenectomy, receive adjunctive antibiotics, and be vaccinated against encapsulated organisms (*Streptococcus pneumoniae*, *Haemophilus influenzae*, and *Neisseria meningitidis*). Percutaneous drainage has been successful for single, small (<3-cm) abscesses and may also be useful for pts at high surgical risk.

Perinephric and Renal Abscesses   More than 75% of these abscesses are due to ascending infection and are preceded by pyelonephritis. Areas of abscess within the renal parenchyma may rupture into the perinephric space. The most important risk factor is the presence of renal calculi that produce local obstruction to urinary flow. Other risk factors include structural abnormalities of the urinary tract, a history of urologic surgery, trauma, or diabetes. *E. coli*, *Proteus* spp. (associated with struvite stones), and *Klebsiella* spp. are the most common etiologic agents. Clinical signs are nonspecific and include flank pain, abdominal pain, and fever. The diagnosis should be considered if pts with pyelonephritis have persistent fever after 4 or 5 days of treatment, if a urine culture yields a polymicrobial flora in pts with known renal stone disease, or if fever and pyuria occur in conjunction with a sterile urine culture. Treatment includes drainage and the administration of antibiotics active against the organisms recovered. Percutaneous drainage is usually successful.

Psoas Abscess   Psoas abscesses arise from hematogenous seeding or from contiguous spread from an intraabdominal or pelvic source or from nearby bony structures (e.g., vertebral bodies). *S. aureus* is most common when the source is hematogenous or bony; a mixed enteric flora is likely with an abdominal source. Pts have fever, lower abdominal or back pain, or pain referred to the hip or knee.

> For a more detailed discussion, see Baron MJ, Kasper DL: Intraabdominal Infections and Abscesses, Chap. 121, p. 807, in HPIM-17.

89 Infectious Diarrheas

Infectious diarrheas are the second most common group of diseases worldwide and are a significant cause of morbidity and mortality in developing countries. Disease is mediated by toxins and/or direct invasion of the GI mucosa. The wide range of clinical manifestations is matched by the wide variety of infectious agents involved (Table 89-1).

APPROACH TO THE PATIENT: INFECTIOUS DIARRHEA

The history should include inquiries about fever (which may suggest invasive disease), abdominal pain, nausea, vomiting, frequency and character of stools, duration of diarrhea, food recently ingested (seafood; possible common food sources, such as a picnic), travel (location, duration, and nature of trip), sexual exposures, and general medical history (immunosuppression, treatment with antibiotics or gastric-acid inhibitors). On physical examination, particular attention to signs of dehydration and abdominal findings is warranted. Stool specimens should be examined grossly (e.g., grossly visible blood or mucus in stools suggests an inflammatory process) and microscopically. A fecal leukocyte test can be done but has an unclear predictive value; fecal lactoferrin, a marker for fecal leukocytes, is more sensitive. Whether stool cultures and other tests should be performed depends on the clinical circumstances.

NONINFLAMMATORY DIARRHEA

TRAVELER'S DIARRHEA

Of people traveling to Asia, Africa, or Central or South America, 20–50% experience the sudden onset of abdominal cramps, anorexia, and watery diarrhea. Disease usually begins within 3–5 days of arrival, is associated with ingestion of contaminated food or water, lasts 1–5 days, and is most often due to enterotoxigenic and enteroaggregative *Escherichia coli* (ETEC). Bismuth subsalicylate [2 tablets (525 mg) every 30–60 min, up to 8 doses] can be used prophylactically. Hydration usually constitutes adequate treatment, but, if desired, a 1- to 3-day course of a fluoroquinolone (or azithromycin in children or

TABLE 89-1 GASTROINTESTINAL PATHOGENS CAUSING ACUTE DIARRHEA

Mechanism	Location	Illness	Stool Findings	Examples of Pathogens Involved
Noninflammatory (enterotoxin)	Proximal small bowel	Watery diarrhea	No fecal leukocytes; mild or no increase in fecal lactoferrin	*Vibrio cholerae*, enterotoxigenic *Escherichia coli* (LT and/or ST), enteroaggregative *E. coli*, *Clostridium perfringens*, *Bacillus cereus*, *Staphylococcus aureus*, *Aeromonas hydrophila*, *Plesiomonas shigelloides*, rotavirus, norovirus, enteric adenoviruses, *Giardia lamblia*, *Cryptosporidium* spp., *Cyclospora* spp., microsporidia
Inflammatory (invasion or cytotoxin)	Colon or distal small bowel	Dysentery or inflammatory diarrhea	Fecal polymorphonuclear leukocytes; substantial increase in fecal lactoferrin	*Shigella* spp., *Salmonella* spp., *Campylobacter jejuni*, enterohemorrhagic *E. coli*, enteroinvasive *E. coli*, *Yersinia enterocolitica*, *Vibrio parahaemolyticus*, *Clostridium difficile*, ?*A. hydrophila*, ?*P. shigelloides*, *Entamoeba histolytica*
Penetrating	Distal small bowel	Enteric fever	Fecal mononuclear leukocytes	*Salmonella typhi*, *Y. enterocolitica*, ?*Campylobacter fetus*

Abbreviations: LT, heat-labile enterotoxin; ST, heat-stable enterotoxin.
Source: After RL Guerrant, TS Steiner: Mandell, Douglas and Bennett's *Principles and Practice of Infectious Diseases*, 5th ed, GL Mandell et al (eds). Philadelphia, Churchill Livingstone, 2000, Chap 81.

in travelers to Thailand) can decrease the duration of illness to 24–36 h. Antimotility agents (e.g., loperamide, 4 mg at onset, then 2 mg after each loose stool, to 16 mg in a 24-h period) can control diarrhea.

BACTERIAL FOOD POISONING

Evidence of a common-source outbreak is often found.

1. *Staphylococcus aureus*: Enterotoxin is elaborated in food left at room temperature (e.g., at picnics). The incubation period is 1–6 h. Disease lasts <12 h and consists of diarrhea, nausea, vomiting, and abdominal cramping, usually without fever.
2. *Bacillus cereus*
   a. Emetic form: presents like *S. aureus* food poisoning, is associated with contaminated fried rice
   b. Diarrheal form: incubation period of 8–16 h; diarrhea, cramps, no vomiting
3. *Clostridium perfringens*: Heat-resistant spores in undercooked meat, poultry, or legumes; incubation period, 8–14 h; 24-h illness of diarrhea and abdominal cramps, without vomiting or fever

CHOLERA

Cholera is caused by *Vibrio cholerae* serogroups O1 (classic and El Tor biotypes) and O139. It is native to the Ganges delta on the Indian subcontinent, but currently >90% of cases reported to the World Health Organization (WHO) are from Africa. Spread is by fecal contamination of water and food sources. Infection requires ingestion of a relatively large inoculum (compared with other pathogens). Toxin production causes disease manifestations.

Clinical Manifestations

- Incubation period of 24–48 h followed by painless watery diarrhea and vomiting that can cause profound, rapidly progressive dehydration and death within hours
- "Rice-water" stool: gray, cloudy fluid with flecks of mucus

Diagnosis Stool cultures on selective medium (e.g., TCBS agar)

 Cholera

Rapid fluid replacement, preferably with WHO's oral rehydration solution (ORS), which contains (per liter of water) Na$^+$, 75 mmol; K$^+$, 20 mmol; Cl$^-$, 65 mmol; citrate, 10 mmol; and glucose, 75 mmol. If available, rice-based ORS is considered superior to standard ORS for cholera. Severely dehydrated pts should be managed initially with IV hydration; Ringer's lactate is the best choice. A single dose of an antibiotic can be used in conjunction: doxycycline (300 mg), ciprofloxacin (30 mg/kg, not to exceed 1 g), or azithromycin (1 g).

VIBRIO PARAHAEMOLYTICUS AND NON-O1 *V. CHOLERAE*

These infections are linked to ingestion of seawater or contaminated, undercooked seafood. After an incubation period of 4 h to 4 days, watery diarrhea, abdominal cramps, nausea, vomiting, and occasionally fever and chills develop. The disease lasts a median of 3 days. Dysentery is a less common presentation. Pts with comorbid disease (e.g., liver disease) sometimes have extraintestinal infections that require antibiotics.

NOROVIRUSES AND RELATED HUMAN CALICIVIRUSES

These viruses are common causes of traveler's diarrhea and of viral gastroenteritis in pts of all ages as well as of epidemics worldwide, with a higher prevalence in cold-weather months. In the United States, >90% of outbreaks of nonbacterial gastroenteritis are caused by noroviruses. Very small inocula are required for infection. Thus, although the fecal-oral route is the primary mode of transmission, aerosolization, fomite contact, and person-to-person contact can also result in infection.

Clinical Manifestations After a 24-h incubation period (range, 12–72 h), pts experience the sudden onset of nausea, vomiting, diarrhea, and/or abdominal cramps with constitutional symptoms. Stools are loose, watery, and without blood, mucus, or leukocytes. Disease lasts 12–60 h.

 Infections with Noroviruses and Related Human Caliciviruses

Only supportive measures are required.

ROTAVIRUSES

Most rotavirus infections occur by 3–5 years of age, but adults can become infected if exposed. Reinfections are progressively less severe. Large quantities of virus are shed in the stool during the first week of infection, and transmission takes place both via the fecal-oral route and from person to person. Disease incidence peaks in the cooler fall and winter months. Rotavirus is common in both industrialized and developing nations.

Clinical Manifestations After an incubation period of 1–3 days, disease onset is abrupt. Vomiting often precedes diarrhea (loose, watery stools without blood or fecal leukocytes), and about one-third of pts are febrile. Symptoms resolve within 3–7 days, but life-threatening dehydration is more common than with most other types of gastroenteritis.

Diagnosis Enzyme immunoassays (EIAs) or viral RNA detection techniques, such as polymerase chain reaction, can identify rotavirus in stool samples.

 Rotavirus Infections

Only supportive treatment is needed. Dehydration can be severe, and IV hydration may be needed in pts with frequent vomiting. Avoid antibiotics and antimotility agents.

Prevention A rotavirus vaccine was recommended for routine administration to U.S. infants in 2006; an earlier vaccine had been withdrawn by the U.S. Food and Drug Administration (FDA) because it was causally linked to intussusception. Disease in developing countries occurs in younger children and is more severe than in industrialized countries; further study is needed before global recommendations for vaccine use can be issued.

GIARDIASIS

Giardia lamblia inhabits the small intestines of humans and other mammals. Cysts are ingested from the environment, excyst in the small intestine, and release flagellated trophozoites. Infection results from as few as 10 cysts. Transmission occurs via the fecal-oral route, by ingestion of contaminated food and water, or from person to person in settings with poor fecal hygiene (e.g., day-care centers, institutional settings) or via sexual contact. Standard chlorination techniques used to control bacteria do not destroy cysts. People at the extremes of age, those newly exposed, and pts with hypogammaglobulinemia are at increased risk—a pattern suggesting a role for humoral immunity in resistance.

Clinical Manifestations

- The incubation period lasts 5 days to 3 weeks. Disease ranges from asymptomatic carriage (most common) to fulminant diarrhea and malabsorption.
- Diarrhea, abdominal pain, bloating, belching, flatus, nausea, and vomiting last >1 week. Fever is rare, as is blood or mucus in stool.
- Chronic disease is often dominated by symptoms of malabsorption.

Diagnosis Giardiasis can be diagnosed by parasite antigen detection in feces and/or examination of several samples from freshly collected stool specimens, with concentration methods used to identify cysts (oval, with four nuclei) or trophozoites (pear-shaped, flattened parasites with two nuclei and four pairs of flagella).

℞ Giardiasis

1. Metronidazole (250 mg tid for 5 days) or tinidazole (2 g once)
2. Nitazoxanide (500 mg bid for 3 days)
3. In cases of treatment failure, document continued infection before re-treatment, and seek possible sources of reinfection. Repeat therapy for up to 21 days at higher doses (e.g., metronidazole at 750 mg tid).

CRYPTOSPORIDIOSIS

Cryptosporidial infection is acquired by ingestion of oocysts that subsequently excyst, enter intestinal cells, and generate oocysts that are excreted in feces. Person-to-person transmission of infectious oocysts can occur among close contacts and in day-care settings. Waterborne transmission is common. Oocysts are not killed by routine chlorination.

Clinical Manifestations

- Incubation period: ~1 week
- Asymptomatic infection or watery, nonbloody diarrhea, occasionally with abdominal pain, nausea, anorexia, fever, and/or weight loss lasting 1–2 weeks
- Immunocompromised hosts, especially HIV-infected pts: Disease can be chronic and can cause severe dehydration, weight loss, and wasting, with biliary tract involvement.

Diagnosis On multiple days, examine fecal samples for oocysts (4–5 μm in diameter, smaller than most parasites). Modified acid-fast staining, direct immunofluorescent techniques, and EIAs can enhance diagnosis.

℞ Cryptosporidiosis

- Nitazoxanide: FDA-approved in tablet form for adults (500 mg bid for 3 days) and as an elixir for children. However, this drug is not effective in HIV-infected pts; improved immune status due to antiretroviral therapy can alleviate symptoms in those pts.

- Supportive measures include replacement of fluid and electrolytes and use of antidiarrheal agents.

ISOSPORIASIS

Isospora belli infection is acquired by oocyst ingestion and is most common in tropical and subtropical countries. Acute infection can begin suddenly with fever, abdominal pain, and watery, nonbloody diarrhea and can last for weeks to months. Eosinophilia may occur. Compromised (e.g., HIV-infected) pts may have chronic disease.

Diagnosis   Detection of large oocysts in stool by modified acid-fast staining

 Isosporiasis

Responds to trimethoprim-sulfamethoxazole (TMP-SMX; 160/800 mg qid for 10 days, then tid for 3 weeks). Pyrimethamine (50–75 mg/d) can be given to pts intolerant of TMP-SMX. Pts with AIDS may need suppressive maintenance therapy to prevent relapses.

CYCLOSPORIASIS

Cyclospora cayetanensis can be transmitted through water or food (e.g., basil, raspberries). Clinical symptoms include diarrhea, flulike symptoms, flatulence, and burping. Disease can be self-limited or can persist for >1 month.

Diagnosis   Detection of oocysts in stool (studies must be specifically requested)

 Cyclosporiasis

TMP-SMX (160/800 mg bid for 1 week). Pts with AIDS may need suppressive maintenance therapy to prevent relapses.

INFLAMMATORY DIARRHEA

SALMONELLOSIS

Etiology and Pathogenesis   Salmonellae cause infection when 10^3–10^6 organisms are ingested. Conditions that reduce gastric acidity or decrease intestinal integrity increase susceptibility to infection. Organisms penetrate the small-intestinal mucosa and traverse the intestinal layer through cells within Peyer's patches. *S. typhi* and *S. paratyphi* survive within macrophages, then disseminate throughout the body via lymphatics, and ultimately colonize reticuloendothelial tissues. Nontyphoidal salmonellae most commonly cause gastroenteritis, invading the large- and small-intestinal mucosa and resulting in massive polymorphonuclear leukocyte infiltration.

Epidemiology and Clinical Manifestations

1. *Typhoid (enteric) fever:* Humans are the only hosts for *S. typhi* and *S. paratyphi* (enteric fever, typhoid fever). Disease results from ingestion of contaminated food or water and is rare in developed nations. After an incubation period of 3–21 days, prolonged fever is the most prominent symptom. Additional nonspecific symptoms include chills, headache, sweating,

cough, malaise, and arthralgias. GI symptoms are variable and can include anorexia, nausea, vomiting, and diarrhea or, less often, constipation. Abdominal pain occurs in 30–40% of pts. Physical findings include rash ("rose spots"), hepatosplenomegaly, epistaxis, and relative bradycardia. Late complications include intestinal perforation and/or GI hemorrhage due to ulceration and necrosis of infiltrated Peyer's patches. Long-term *Salmonella* carriage in urine or stool develops in 1–4% of pts, usually in association with disease in the bladder or the biliary and GI tracts.

2. *Nontyphoidal salmonellosis:* The incidence of nontyphoidal salmonellosis in the United States is 14.7 cases per 100,000 persons, with 1.4 million cases and 400 deaths each year. Most disease is caused by *S. typhimurium* or *S. enteritidis.* Disease is acquired from multiple animal reservoirs. The main mode of transmission is from contaminated food products, such as eggs (*S. enteritidis*), poultry, undercooked meat, unpasteurized dairy products, seafood, and fresh produce. Infection is also acquired during exposure to pets, especially reptiles.

a. *Gastroenteritis:* Nausea, vomiting, diarrhea, abdominal cramping, and fever occur 6–48 h after exposure. Diarrhea is usually loose, nonbloody, and moderate in volume, but stools are sometimes bloody. Diarrhea is usually self-limited, abating within 3–7 days, and fever resolves within 72 h in most cases. Stool cultures may remain positive for ≥4–5 weeks.

b. *Extraintestinal infections:* Up to 5% of pts are bacteremic, and 5–10% of bacteremic pts may develop localized infections, particularly in vascular sites (e.g., aortic aneurysms). *S. choleraesuis* and *S. dublin* are unusual serotypes that cause high rates of bacteremia and invasive infection. Localized infections caused by nontyphoidal salmonellae are rare and include abscesses, meningitis, pneumonia, UTIs, and osteomyelitis (particularly in pts with sickle cell disease, hemoglobinopathies, or preexisting bone disease).

c. *Reactive arthritis* (Reiter's syndrome) can follow *Salmonella* gastroenteritis in persons with the HLA-B27 histocompatibility antigen.

Diagnosis Positive cultures of blood, stool, or other specimens are required for diagnosis. If blood cultures are positive for nontyphoidal salmonellae, high-grade bacteremia should be ruled out by obtaining multiple blood cultures.

℞ Salmonellosis

1. *Typhoid fever:* A fluoroquinolone (e.g., ciprofloxacin, 500 mg PO bid) or a third-generation cephalosporin (e.g., ceftriaxone, 1–2 g/d IV or IM) for 10–14 days is recommended. For susceptible strains, a fluoroquinolone is more efficacious than a β-lactam. Dexamethasone may be of benefit in severe cases.

2. *Nontyphoidal salmonellosis:* Antibiotic treatment is not recommended in most cases. However, infants, the elderly, the immunosuppressed, and pts with cardiac, valvular, or endovascular abnormalities may require antibiotic treatment. Fluoroquinolones or third-generation cephalosporins are given until defervescence (if the pt is immunocompetent) or for 1–2 weeks (if the pt is immunocompromised). HIV-infected pts are at high risk for *Salmonella* bacteremia and should receive 4 weeks of oral quinolone therapy after 1–2 weeks of IV treatment. In cases of relapse, long-term suppression with a quinolone or TMP-SMX should be considered. Pts with endovascular infections or endocarditis should receive 6 weeks of treatment with a third-generation cephalosporin. Infected aneurysms or endovascular lesions may require surgical resection.

CAMPYLOBACTERIOSIS

Etiology Campylobacters are a common bacterial cause of gastroenteritis in the United States. Most cases are caused by *C. jejuni*.

Epidemiology Campylobacters are common commensals in the GI tract of many food animals and household pets. In the United States, ingestion of contaminated poultry accounts for 30–70% of cases. Transmission to humans occurs via contact with or ingestion of raw or undercooked food products or direct contact with infected animals.

Clinical Manifestations

1. *Gastroenteritis:* An incubation period of 2–4 days (range, 1–7 days) is followed by a prodrome of fever, headache, myalgia, and/or malaise. Within the next 12–48 h, diarrhea (with stools containing blood, mucus, and leukocytes), cramping abdominal pain, and fever develop. Most cases are self-limited, but illness persists for >1 week in 10–20% of pts and may be confused with inflammatory bowel disease.
2. *Extraintestinal infections:* Other species (e.g., *C. fetus*) can cause a similar illness or prolonged relapsing systemic disease without a primary focus in compromised pts. The course may be fulminant, with bacterial seeding of many organs, particularly vascular sites. Fetal death can result from infection in a pregnant pt.
3. Complications
   a. Severe, persistent, disseminated disease in pts with AIDS or hypogammaglobulinemia
   b. Local suppurative complications (e.g., cholecystitis)
   c. Reactive arthritis in persons with the HLA-B27 phenotype
   d. Guillain-Barré syndrome (campylobacters are associated with 20–40% of cases)

Diagnosis Confirmation of diagnosis is based on cultures of stool, blood, or other specimens on special media and/or with selective techniques (e.g., growth at 42°C).

℞ Campylobacteriosis

1. Fluid and electrolyte replacement
2. Avoidance of antimotility agents, which may prolong symptoms and are associated with toxic megacolon
3. Antibiotic treatment does not benefit all pts but is indicated in cases with high fever, bloody and/or severe diarrhea, disease persistence for >1 week, or worsening symptoms.
   a. Erythromycin (250 mg qid for 5–7 days) or newer macrolides
   b. Ciprofloxacin (500 mg bid) or another fluoroquinolone for 5–7 days (although resistance is increasing)

SHIGELLOSIS AND INFECTION WITH SHIGA TOXIN-PRODUCING/ ENTEROHEMORRHAGIC *ESCHERICHIA COLI* (STEC/EHEC)

Etiology Shigellae are small, gram-negative, nonmotile bacilli that are very closely related to *E. coli*. The four most common *Shigella* serotypes are *S. dysenteriae* type 1, *S. flexneri*, *S. boydii*, and *S. sonnei* (the cause of most shigellosis cases in the United States). There are no animal reservoirs other than higher primates. These bacteria are transmitted from person to person via the fecal-oral route and occasionally via intermediate vectors such as food, water, flies, and fomites. Shigellosis is associated with a high rate of secondary household transmission. Shigellae survive the low pH of the gastric acid barrier, and as few as 100 organisms can cause infection. Shiga toxin and Shiga-like toxins produced by some strains of *E. coli* (including O157:H7) are important factors in disease severity. The toxins target endothelial cells and play a significant role in the microangiopathic complications of *Shigella* and *E. coli* infections, such as hemolytic-uremic syndrome (HUS) and thrombotic thrombocytopenic purpura (TTP). *Shigella* causes extensive ulceration of the epithelial surface of the colonic mucosa.

Clinical Manifestations

1. Pts can remain asymptomatic, develop fever with or without watery diarrhea, or experience a progression to bloody diarrhea and dysentery characterized by small volumes of bloody, mucopurulent stools with associated severe abdominal cramping and tenesmus.
2. Without treatment, most episodes resolve in 1 week.
3. Complications
   a. Severe cases occur most often in children <5 years of age; disease may progress to toxic dilatation, colonic perforation, rectal prolapse, and death.
   b. HUS has been linked to Shiga toxin produced by *S. dysenteriae* type 1 in developing countries but is rare in industrialized countries, where *E. coli* O157:H7 is a more common cause. The syndrome is defined by a triad of microangiopathic, Coombs-negative hemolytic anemia; thrombocytopenia; and acute renal failure due to glomerular capillary thromboses.

Diagnosis

- Shigellosis is diagnosed directly by stool culture. STEC/EHEC infection is diagnosed by screening of stool cultures for *E. coli* strains that do not ferment sorbitol, with subsequent serotyping for O157. The yield is increased if stools contain leukocytes or blood. Most cases of bloody diarrhea in the United States are due to *E. coli* O157:H7 or *C. jejuni*.
- Tests to detect Shiga toxins or toxin genes are sensitive, specific, and rapid. This approach detects non-O157 STEC/EHEC and sorbitol-fermenting strains of O157:H7.

℞ Shigellosis and Infection with STEC/EHEC

1. In the United States, because of the ready transmissibility of *Shigella*, antibiotics are recommended. Fluoroquinolones are effective (e.g., ciprofloxacin, 500 mg bid), as are ceftriaxone, azithromycin, and pivmecillinam. *S. dysenteriae* infection should be treated for 5 days and non-*dysenteriae Shigella* infection for 3 days. Immunocompromised pts should receive 7–10 days of treatment.
2. Antibiotic treatment for STEC/EHEC infections is controversial and may increase the incidence of HUS.
3. Rehydration usually is not needed; *Shigella* infection rarely causes significant dehydration. If required, rehydration should be oral, and nutrition should be started as soon as possible. Use of antimotility agents may prolong fever and increase the risk of HUS and toxic megacolon.

YERSINIOSIS

Etiology and Clinical Manifestations   *Y. enterocolitica* and *Y. pseudotuberculosis* are nonmotile gram-negative rods that cause enteritis or enterocolitis with self-limited diarrhea that lasts an average of 2 weeks (especially common with *Y. en-*

terocolitica) as well as mesenteric adenitis and terminal ileitis that can resemble acute appendicitis (especially common with *Y. pseudotuberculosis*). Septicemia and metastatic focal infections can occur in pts with chronic liver disease, malignancy, diabetes mellitus, and other underlying illnesses. Infection has been linked to reactive arthritis in HLA-B27-positive pts.

Diagnosis Stool culture studies for *Yersinia* must be specifically requested and require the use of special media.

 Yersiniosis

Antibiotics are not indicated for diarrhea caused by yersiniae; supportive measures suffice.

AMEBIASIS

Amebiasis is caused by *Entamoeba histolytica* and is the third most common cause of death from parasitic disease worldwide. The incidence is high in developing countries and among travelers, recent immigrants, men who have sex with men, and inmates of institutions in developed nations. Infection follows ingestion of cysts from fecally contaminated water, food, or hands. Motile trophozoites are released from cysts in the small intestine and then cause infection in the large bowel. Trophozoites may be shed in stool (in active dysentery) or encyst. Excreted cysts survive for weeks in a moist environment.

Clinical Manifestations
- *Asymptomatic infection*: 90% of cases
- *Colitis*: Develops in 10% of pts 2–6 weeks after ingestion of infectious cysts, with lower abdominal pain, mild diarrhea, malaise, weight loss, and diffuse lower abdominal or back pain. Dysentery may develop, with daily passage of 10–12 small stools consisting mostly of blood and mucus. Fewer than 40% of pts have fever. Toxic megacolon is a rare complication. Pts taking glucocorticoids are at greater risk for severe disease. Chronic amebiasis may be confused with inflammatory bowel disease. Amebomas—inflammatory mass lesions—may develop in chronic amebic intestinal disease.
- *Extraintestinal infection*: Liver abscess is the most common type of extraintestinal infection; trophozoites invade veins to reach the liver through the portal venous system. Most pts are febrile and have right upper quadrant pain that can radiate to the shoulder, point tenderness over the liver, and right-sided pleural effusion. Fewer than one-third of pts have active diarrhea. Abscesses can also occur elsewhere (e.g., lung, brain).

Diagnosis Barium rapidly kills trophozoites. At least three fresh stool specimens should be examined for amebic cysts or trophozoites. Sigmoidoscopy with biopsy of ulcers (often flask-shaped) may aid in the diagnosis but poses a risk of perforation. Serologic assays (enzyme-linked immunosorbent assay and agar gel diffusion) are positive in >90% of pts with colitis, amebomas, or liver abscess. Serology reverts to negative within 6–12 months after active disease resolves. Imaging of the liver may assist in the diagnosis of liver abscess.

 Amebiasis

Iodoquinol (650 mg tid for 20 days) and paromomycin (500 mg tid for 10 days) are luminal agents that eradicate cysts in pts with colitis or liver abscess and in asymptomatic carriers. Tissue amebicides include nitroimidazole compounds—e.g., metronidazole (750 mg PO or IV tid for 5–10 days) or tinidazole (2 g PO once)—and should be given with a luminal agent for colitis or liver abscess. A clinical response occurs within 72 h in >90% of pts with liver abscess. Aspiration of liver abscesses usually does not accelerate healing. Indications for aspiration include the need to rule out pyogenic abscess, a lack of response to treatment after 3–5 days, an imminent threat of liver-abscess rupture, or the need to prevent left-lobe abscess rupture into the pericardium.

CLOSTRIDIUM DIFFICILE-ASSOCIATED DISEASE (CDAD)

CDAD is the diarrheal illness most commonly diagnosed in the hospital. The disease is acquired almost exclusively in association with antimicrobial treatment, but use of proton pump inhibitors may also be a risk factor; virtually all antibiotics carry a risk of CDAD. After *C. difficile* colonizes the gut, its spores vegetate, multiply, and secrete toxin A (an enterotoxin) and toxin B (a cytotoxin), causing diarrhea and pseudomembranous colitis. Spores can persist on environmental hospital surfaces for months and on the hands of hospital personnel who do not practice adequate hand hygiene. Rates and severity of CDAD in the United States, Canada, and Europe have increased markedly in the past decade. An epidemic strain accounts for much of the increase and is characterized by production of 16–23 times as much toxin A and toxin B as is documented for control strains, by the presence of a third toxin (binary toxin), and by high-level resistance to fluoroquinolones.

Clinical Manifestations

- Diarrhea, with up to 20 bowel movements per day. Stools usually are not grossly bloody and are soft to watery, with a characteristic odor.
- Fever, abdominal pain, and leukocytosis are common. Pts with unexplained leukocytosis, particularly in the presence of adynamic colon, should be evaluated for CDAD.
- CDAD may become fulminant, and toxic megacolon or sepsis may develop.

Diagnosis If clinically suspected, CDAD should be diagnosed by means of stool studies. Stool culture for toxin-producing *C. difficile* is most sensitive; if the isolate tests positive for toxin, this test is also specific. However, the test takes at least 48 h. The cell culture cytotoxin test is specific but less sensitive and also takes 48 h. EIAs for toxin A, toxins A and B, or *C. difficile* common antigen more rapidly yield results that are moderately sensitive and specific.

 C. difficile-Associated Disease

Primary CDAD
- Discontinue ongoing antimicrobial treatment if possible.
- Promptly initiate specific treatment for CDAD.
    Mild to moderate CDAD: metronidazole (500 mg tid for 10 days), with extension of therapy if the clinical response is slow
    Severe CDAD (e.g., >15,000 WBCs/μL) or failure to respond to metronidazole: vancomycin (125 mg qid PO for 10 days)

Recurrent CDAD
- Occurs in 15–30% of pts, especially affecting the elderly, pts who remain hospitalized, and pts who have already had a CDAD relapse. The first recurrence should be re-treated with metronidazole or vancomycin.

- For multiple recurrences, consider a course of vancomycin treatment followed by *Saccharomyces boulardii* administration, synthetic fecal bacterial enema, or intentional colonization with a nontoxigenic strain of *C. difficile*. Alternative regimens that are sometimes successful are (1) vancomycin given in tapering doses or with pulsed dosing for 4–6 weeks and (2) sequential treatment with vancomycin followed by rifaximin (400 mg bid for 14 days). IV immunoglobulin has also been used with some success.

Fulminant CDAD
- Presentation of acute abdomen: ileus, marked leukocytosis
- Vancomycin, given via nasogastric tube and retention enema, plus IV metronidazole
- Surgical colectomy can be life-saving.

For a more detailed discussion, see Butterton JR, Calderwood SB: Acute Infectious Diarrheal Diseases and Bacterial Food Poisoning, Chap. 122, p. 813; Gerding DN, Johnson S: *Clostridium difficile*–Associated Disease, Including Pseudomembranous Colitis, Chap. 123, p. 818; Russo TA, Johnson JR: Diseases Caused by Gram-Negative Enteric Bacilli, Chap. 143, p. 937; Pegues DA, Miller SI: Salmonellosis, Chap. 146, p. 956; Sansonetti P, Bergounioux J: Shigellosis, Chap. 147, p. 962; Blaser MJ: Infections Due to *Campylobacter* and Related Species, Chap. 148, p. 965; Waldor MK, Keusch GT: Cholera and Other Vibrioses, Chap. 149, p. 968; Dennis DT, Campbell GL: Plague and Other *Yersinia* Infections, Chap. 152, p. 980; Parashar UD, Glass RI: Viral Gastroenteritis, Chap. 183, p. 1204; Reed SL: Amebiasis and Infection with Free-Living Amebas, Chap. 202, p. 1275; and Weller PF: Protozoal Intestinal Infections and Trichomoniasis, Chap. 208, p. 1311, in HPIM-17.

90 Sexually Transmitted Diseases and Reproductive Tract Infections

GENERAL CLINICAL APPROACH

- Assess risk factors and obtain basic demographic data.
- Assess specific symptoms and signs, and perform confirmatory diagnostic tests.
- Institute syndrome-based treatment to cover most likely causes.
- Prevention and control ("4 C's"): contact tracing, compliance with treatment, counseling on risk reduction, condom promotion and provision

SPECIFIC SYNDROMES

Etiology and Epidemiology

- Most cases are caused by either *Neisseria gonorrhoeae* or *Chlamydia trachomatis*. Other causative organisms include *Ureaplasma urealyticum*, *Mycoplasma genitalium*, *Trichomonas vaginalis*, and herpes simplex virus (HSV).
- *Chlamydia* causes 30–40% of nongonococcal urethritis (NGU) cases. *M. genitalium* is the probable cause in many *Chlamydia*-negative cases of NGU.

Clinical Considerations

- Pts present with mucopurulent urethral discharge that can usually be expressed by milking the urethra.
- Exclude both local and systemic complications (e.g., epididymitis and disseminated gonorrhea, respectively).
- A Gram's-stained smear of urethral exudates containing ≥5 polymorphonuclear leukocytes (PMNs)/1000× field is diagnostic of *N. gonorrhoeae* if positive for intracellular gram-negative diplococci. Centrifuged sediment of the day's first 20–30 mL of voided urine can be examined instead.
- Perform tests for *N. gonorrhoeae* and *C. trachomatis* using "multiplex" nucleic acid amplification tests (NAATs) of early-morning, first-voided urine.
- Treat urethritis while test results are pending.

℞ Urethritis in Men

- Treat gonorrhea (unless excluded) with a single dose of ceftriaxone (125 mg IM), cefpodoxime (400 mg PO), or cefixime (400 mg PO), plus treat *Chlamydia* with azithromycin (1 g PO once) or doxycycline (100 mg bid for 7 days); azithromycin may be more effective for *M. genitalium*.
- For recurrent symptoms: With reexposure, re-treat pt and partner. If no reexposure, exclude *T. vaginalis* (with culture or NAATs of urethral swab and early-morning, first-voided urine). Treat with metronidazole or tinidazole (2 g PO once) plus azithromycin (1 g PO once).

Etiology

- In sexually active young men, epididymitis is caused by *C. trachomatis* and, less commonly, by *N. gonorrhoeae*.
- In older men or after urinary tract instrumentation, consider urinary pathogens.
- In men who practice insertive rectal intercourse, consider Enterobacteriaceae.

Clinical Considerations

- Usually unilateral testicular pain of acute onset, intrascrotal swelling, tenderness, and fever
- Rule out testicular torsion, tumor, and trauma.
- If symptoms persist after treatment, rule out testicular tumor and chronic granulomatous disease.

℞ Epididymitis

- Ceftriaxone (250 mg IM once) followed by doxycycline (100 mg PO bid for 10 days)

- Fluoroquinolones are no longer recommended because of increasing resistance in *N. gonorrhoeae*.

URETHRITIS (THE URETHRAL SYNDROME) IN WOMEN

- Caused by *C. trachomatis*, *N. gonorrhoeae*, occasionally HSV
- Internal vs. external dysuria (the latter seen with vulvovaginitis)
- Usually no urinary urgency or frequency, distinct from bacterial cystitis
- Pyuria with culture demonstrating <100 uropathogens/mL of urine supports a diagnosis of urethral syndrome rather than cystitis.
- Evaluate *N. gonorrhoeae* or *C. trachomatis* with specific tests (e.g., NAATs on the first 10 mL of voided urine).

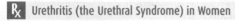

R𝗑 Urethritis (the Urethral Syndrome) in Women

See "Urethritis in Men," above.

VULVOVAGINAL INFECTIONS

- Unsolicited reporting of abnormal vaginal discharge suggests trichomoniasis or bacterial vaginosis (BV).

  Trichomoniasis is characterized by vulvar irritation and a profuse, yellow, purulent, homogeneous vaginal discharge with a pH typically ≥5.0.

  BV is characterized by vaginal malodor and a slight to moderate increase in white, homogeneous vaginal discharge with a pH typically >4.5.

  Genital herpes, which can cause vulvar pruritus, burning, irritation, and lesions as well as external dysuria and vulvar dyspareunia, must be considered in the diagnosis.
- Vulvovaginal infections are associated with increased risk of HIV acquisition.
- Vaginal trichomoniasis and BV early in pregnancy are associated with premature onset of labor.
- Vulvovaginal candidiasis develops with increased frequency among women with systemic illnesses (e.g., diabetes, HIV disease).
- Examine abnormal vaginal discharge for pH, a fishy odor after mixing with 10% KOH (BV), evidence on microscopy of motile trichomonads and/or clue cells of BV (vaginal epithelial cells coated with coccobacillary organisms) when mixed with saline, or hyphae or pseudohyphae on microscopy when 10% KOH is added (vaginal candidiasis).
- A new DNA probe test (the Affirm test) can detect *T. vaginalis*, *Candida albicans*, and increased concentrations of *Gardnerella vaginalis*.

R𝗑 Vulvovaginal Infections

- Vulvovaginal candidiasis: miconazole (100-mg vaginal suppository) or clotrimazole (100-mg vaginal tablet) once daily for 7 days; or fluconazole (150 mg PO once)
- Trichomoniasis: metronidazole or tinidazole (2 g PO once) or metronidazole (500 mg PO bid for 7 days)
- BV: metronidazole (500 mg PO bid for 7 days) or clindamycin 2% cream (one full applicator vaginally each night for 7 days)
- Antenatal treatment of *T. vaginalis* or BV has not reduced rates of perinatal morbidity or preterm delivery.

MUCOPURULENT CERVICITIS

- Inflammation of the columnar epithelium and subepithelium of the endocervix
- "Silent partner" of urethritis in men
- Major etiologies: *N. gonorrhoeae*, *C. trachomatis*, *M. genitalium*. Many cases are idiopathic. HSV cervicitis produces ulcerative lesions on the exocervix.
- Yellow mucopurulent discharge from cervical os, with ≥20 PMNs/1000× field on Gram's stain of cervical mucus
- Intracellular gram-negative diplococci on Gram's stain of cervical mucus are specific but <50% sensitive for gonorrhea.

 Mucopurulent Cervicitis

See "Urethritis in Men," above.

PELVIC INFLAMMATORY DISEASE (PID)

Definition   Infection ascending from the cervix or vagina to the endometrium and/or fallopian tubes (or beyond) to cause peritonitis, perihepatitis, or pelvic abscess

Etiology   *N. gonorrhoeae*, *C. trachomatis*, *M. genitalium*, anaerobic and facultative organisms such as *Prevotella* spp., group B streptococci

Epidemiology
- Each year in the United States, PID accounts for 70,000–100,000 hospitalizations and ~176,000 visits to physicians' offices.
- Risk factors: cervicitis, BV, vaginal douching, menstruation, intrauterine contraceptive device (IUD) use. Oral contraceptive pills decrease risk.
- *N. gonorrhoeae* presentation is usually more acute than that of *C. trachomatis*.

Clinical Manifestations
1. Endometritis: pain and vaginal bleeding; lower quadrant, adnexal, and cervical motion pain not severe if this is the only manifestation of PID
2. Salpingitis: bilateral lower abdominal and pelvic pain, nausea, vomiting, peritoneal signs
   a. Mucopurulent cervicitis with discharge; cervical motion, uterine, and adnexal tenderness or swelling on examination
   b. Fever (one-third of cases), elevated erythrocyte sedimentation rate (75%), elevated peripheral white blood cell count (60%)
3. Perihepatitis and periappendicitis
   a. Fitz-Hugh–Curtis syndrome: perihepatitis associated with salpingitis in 3–10% of PID cases. *Chlamydia* is the most common etiologic agent, but this syndrome is also caused by *N. gonorrhoeae*; right or bilateral upper quadrant pain, occasional hepatic friction rub
   b. Periappendicitis in ~5% of pts with PID due to gonococci or chlamydiae

Diagnosis
- Predictors of PID: pelvic pain, tenderness, endocervical discharge with increased PMNs, onset with menses, history of abnormal menstrual bleeding preceding or coincident with pain in ~40% of women, presence of an IUD, sexual partner with urethritis
- Perform ultrasonography or MRI if tuboovarian or pelvic abscess is a concern.
- Evaluate for pregnancy with human β-chorionic gonadotropin test.
- Unilateral pain or a pelvic mass is an indication for laparoscopy, as are atypical clinical findings or poor responses to appropriate treatment.

- Gram's staining of endocervical swabs for PMNs and gram-negative diplococci; NAATs for *N. gonorrhoeae* and *C. trachomatis*; aerobic and anaerobic cultures

---

℞ Pelvic Inflammatory Disease

Initiate empirical treatment for PID in sexually active young women and other women who are at risk for PID and who have pelvic or lower abdominal pain with no other explanation as well as cervical motion, uterine, or adnexal tenderness.

Recommendations per 2006 CDC guidelines:

1. Parenteral regimens
   a. Cefotetan (2 g IV q12h) or cefoxitin (2 g IV q6h) plus doxycycline (100 mg IV or PO q12h) until 48 h after improvement; then doxycycline (100 mg PO bid) to complete a 14-day course
   b. Alternative: clindamycin (900 mg IV q8h) plus gentamicin (2.0 mg/kg IV or IM load followed by 1.5 mg/kg q8h) until 48 h after improvement; then complete a 14-day course with either oral doxycycline (100 mg bid) or oral clindamycin (450 mg qid). Once-daily aminoglycoside dosing may be used instead.
2. Outpatient regimens: (1) ofloxacin (400 mg PO bid for 14 days) or levofloxacin (500 mg PO once daily for 14 days) plus metronidazole (500 mg PO bid for 14 days); or (2) ceftriaxone (250 mg IM once) plus doxycycline (100 mg PO bid) and metronidazole (500 mg PO bid) for 14 days. Regimen 2 is preferred because of increasing fluoroquinolone resistance in *N. gonorrhoeae*.
3. Consider hospitalization if the diagnosis is uncertain, the pt is pregnant, an abscess is suspected, the illness is severe, nausea and vomiting preclude outpatient treatment, or the pt is infected with HIV, is unlikely to follow an outpatient regimen, or has already had an unsuccessful course of outpatient treatment.
4. Evaluate in 72 h for treatment response.

Prognosis Late sequelae include infertility (11% after one episode of PID, 23% after two, and 54% after three or more); ectopic pregnancy (sevenfold increase in risk); chronic pelvic pain (eightfold increase in rate of hysterectomy); and recurrent salpingitis.

Prevention Risk-based chlamydial screening of young women can reduce PID incidence.

ULCERATIVE GENITAL LESIONS

- See Table 90-1 and sections on individual pathogens below.
- The most common etiologies in the United States are genital herpes, syphilitic ulcers, and chancroid.
- All pts with genital ulcerations should undergo HIV serologic testing.
- Immediate treatment (before all test results are available) is often appropriate to improve response, reduce transmission, and cover pts who might not return for follow-up visits.

PROCTITIS, PROCTOCOLITIS, ENTEROCOLITIS, ENTERITIS

Definitions

- *Proctitis*: inflammation limited to rectal mucosa from direct inoculation of typical sexually transmitted disease (STD) pathogens; associated with pain, mucopurulent discharge, tenesmus, and constipation

TABLE 90-1 CLINICAL FEATURES OF GENITAL ULCERS

Feature	Syphilis	Herpes	Chancroid	Lymphogranuloma Venereum	Donovanosis
Incubation period	9–90 days	2–7 days	1–14 days	3 days–6 weeks	1–4 weeks (up to 6 months)
Early primary lesions	Papule	Vesicle	Pustule	Papule, pustule, or vesicle	Papule
No. of lesions	Usually one	Multiple	Usually multiple, may coalesce	Usually one; often not detected, despite lymphadenopathy	Variable
Diameter	5–15 mm	1–2 mm	Variable	2–10 mm	Variable
Edges	Sharply demarcated, elevated, round, or oval	Erythematous	Undermined, ragged, irregular	Elevated, round, or oval	Elevated, irregular
Depth	Superficial or deep	Superficial	Excavated	Superficial or deep	Elevated
Base	Smooth, nonpurulent, relatively nonvascular	Serous, erythematous, nonvascular	Purulent, bleeds easily	Variable, nonvascular	Red and velvety, bleeds readily
Induration	Firm	None	Soft	Occasionally firm	Firm
Pain	Uncommon	Frequently tender	Usually very tender	Variable	Uncommon
Lymphadenopathy	Firm, nontender, bilateral	Firm, tender, often bilateral with initial episode	Tender, may suppurate, loculated, usually unilateral	Tender, may suppurate, loculated, usually unilateral	None; pseudobuboes

Source: From RM Ballard, in KK Holmes et al (eds): *Sexually Transmitted Diseases,* 4th ed. New York, McGraw-Hill, 2008.

- Ingestion of typical intestinal pathogens through oral-anal exposure during sexual contact can result in the following syndromes, often associated with diarrhea: (1) *proctocolitis*: inflammation from rectum to colon, (2) *enterocolitis*: inflammation involving both large and small intestine, and (3) *enteritis*: inflammation of small intestine alone.

Etiology and Epidemiology

- *N. gonorrhoeae*, HSV, and *C. trachomatis* are the chief causes of proctitis; symptoms are minimal and localized.
- HSV proctitis and lymphogranuloma venereum (LGV) proctocolitis can cause severe pain, fever, and systemic manifestations. Sacral nerve root radiculopathy, with urinary retention or anal sphincter dysfunction, is associated with primary HSV.
- LGV and syphilis can be associated with granulomata and inflammation.
- *Giardia lamblia* is a common cause of enteritis in men who have sex with men (MSM).
- *Campylobacter* or *Shigella* spp. can cause sexually acquired proctocolitis.

℞ Proctitis, Proctocolitis, Enterocolitis, Enteritis

1. Anoscopy to examine mucosa and obtain specimens for diagnosis
2. Ceftriaxone (125 mg IM once) followed by doxycycline (100 mg bid for 7 days) if gonorrhea or chlamydial infection is suspected; syphilis or herpes therapy as indicated

---

INDIVIDUAL PATHOGENS

GONORRHEA

Etiology   *N. gonorrhoeae*: gram-negative, nonmotile, non-spore-forming organisms that grow in pairs and are shaped like coffee beans

Epidemiology

- ~325,000 cases reported in the United States in 2006; actual case numbers higher
- U.S. incidence: 120 cases per 100,000 population—the highest among industrialized nations
- Attack rates are highest among sexually active 15- to 19-year-old women and 20- to 24-year-old men; rates are highest among African Americans.
- Efficient male-to-female transmission; 40–60% rate with a single unprotected encounter; 20% rate to women who practice fellatio with infected partners; chance of HIV acquisition increased if infected person also has gonorrhea
- Drug-resistant strains are widespread. Penicillin, ampicillin, and tetracycline are no longer reliable agents. Third-generation cephalosporins remain effective. Fluoroquinolone-containing regimens are no longer routinely recommended.

Clinical Syndromes

1. *Urethritis* (see above): incubation period, 2–7 days. Uncommon complications include epididymitis, prostatitis, penile edema, abscesses or fistulas, seminal vesiculitis, and balanitis if uncircumcised.
2. *Cervicitis* (see above): incubation period, ~10 days. Co-infection with *N. gonorrhoeae* and *C. trachomatis* is documented in up to 40% of genital gonococcal infections.

3. *Anorectal gonorrhea*: spreads from cervical exudates in women; rarely the sole site of infection or the cause of symptomatic proctitis; recent resurgence in MSM. Anorectal strains in the latter population tend to be more resistant to antibiotics than isolates from other sites.

4. *Pharyngeal gonorrhea*: usually asymptomatic infection resulting from oral-genital sexual exposure; transmission from the pharynx rare; almost always coexists with genital infection. Rate may increase during pregnancy because of altered sexual practices. Most cases resolve spontaneously. If symptomatic, pharyngeal gonorrhea is harder to eradicate than genital disease. Follow-up cultures are needed.

5. *Ocular gonorrhea*: caused by autoinoculation; swollen eyelid, hyperemia, chemosis, profuse purulent discharge, occasional corneal ulceration and perforation. Rule out associated genital infection.

6. *Gonorrhea in pregnancy*: Salpingitis and PID in the first trimester can cause fetal loss. Other STDs must be ruled out. Third-trimester disease can cause prolonged rupture of membranes, premature delivery, chorioamnionitis, funisitis, neonatal sepsis, and perinatal distress and death. Ophthalmia neonatorum, the most common form of gonorrhea in neonates, is preventable by prophylactic 1% silver nitrate drops, but treatment requires systemic antibiotics.

7. *Gonococcal arthritis and disseminated gonococcal infection* (DGI)
   a. DGI strains resist bactericidal action of human serum and often do not elicit inflammation at genital sites.
   b. Up to 13% of pts with DGI have terminal complement deficiencies.
   c. Menstruation is a risk factor for dissemination; two-thirds of pts with DGI are women.
   d. A bacteremic phase, often not clinically recognized, precedes arthritis.
   e. Arthritis presents as painful joints in conjunction with tenosynovitis, skin lesions, and polyarthralgias of knees, elbows, and distal joints. Skin lesions develop in 75% of pts and include papules and pustules, often with hemorrhage. Suppurative arthritis affects one or two joints, most often knees, wrists, ankles, and elbows.

Laboratory Diagnosis

- Intracellular gram-negative cocci in urethral discharge collected from a male pt with Dacron or rayon swabs
- Culture on Thayer-Martin or other media selective for gonococci. Process immediately or store in candle extinction jars prior to incubation. Use special transport systems or culture media with CO_2-generating systems.
- A single culture of endocervical discharge has a sensitivity of 80–90%.
- A DNA probe that hybridizes gonococcal 16S ribosomal RNA has good sensitivity, particularly in high-risk men, but provides no susceptibility information.

 Gonorrhea

See Table 90-2.

INFECTIONS WITH *CHLAMYDIA TRACHOMATIS*

Etiology

- Obligate intracellular bacteria in their own order, Chlamydiales
- Serovars D through K are associated with STDs. Serovars L1, L2, and L3 produce LGV. LGV strains are unique: they are unusually invasive, produce disease in lymphatic tissue, and grow in cell culture systems and macrophages.

TABLE 90-2	**RECOMMENDED TREATMENT FOR GONOCOCCAL INFECTIONS: 2006 GUIDELINES OF THE CENTERS FOR DISEASE CONTROL AND PREVENTION (UPDATED IN 2007)**

Diagnosis	Treatment of Choice
Uncomplicated gonococcal infection of the cervix, urethra, pharynx, or rectum[a]	
First-line regimens	Ceftriaxone (125 mg IM, single dose) *or* Cefixime (400 mg PO, single dose) *plus* If chlamydial infection is not ruled out: Azithromycin (1 g PO, single dose) *or* Doxycycline (100 mg PO bid for 7 days)
Alternative regimens	Ceftizoxime (500 mg IM, single dose) *or* Cefotaxime (500 mg IM, single dose) *or* Spectinomycin (2 g IM, single dose)[b,c] *or* Cefotetan (1 g IM, single dose) plus probenecid (1 g PO, single dose)[b] *or* Cefoxitin (2 g IM, single dose) plus probenecid (1 g PO, single dose)[b]
Epididymitis	See text and Chap. 124, HPIM-17
Pelvic inflammatory disease	See text and Chap. 124, HPIM-17
Gonococcal conjunctivitis in an adult	Ceftriaxone (1 g IM, single dose)[d]
Ophthalmia neonatorum[e]	Ceftriaxone (25–50 mg/kg IV, single dose, not to exceed 125 mg)
Disseminated gonococcal infection[f]	
Initial therapy[g]	
Patients tolerant of β-lactam drugs	Ceftriaxone (1 g IM or IV q24h; recommended) *or* Cefotaxime (1 g IV q8h) *or* Ceftizoxime (1 g IV q8h)
Patients allergic to β-lactam drugs	Spectinomycin (2 g IM q12h)[c]
Continuation therapy	Cefixime (400 mg PO bid)
Meningitis or endocarditis	See Chap. 137, HPIM-17[h]

[a]True failure of treatment with a recommended regimen is rare and should prompt an evaluation for reinfection or consideration of an alternative diagnosis.

[b]Spectinomycin, cefotetan, and cefoxitin, which are alternative agents, currently are unavailable or in short supply in the United States.

[c]Spectinomycin may be ineffective for the treatment of pharyngeal gonorrhea.

[d]Plus lavage of the infected eye with saline solution (once).

[e]Prophylactic regimens are discussed in Chap. 137, HPIM-17.

[f]Hospitalization is indicated if the diagnosis is uncertain, if the pt has frank arthritis with an effusion, or if the pt cannot be relied on to adhere to treatment.

[g]All initial regimens should be continued for 24–48 h after clinical improvement begins, at which time therapy may be switched to one of the continuation regimens to complete a full week of antimicrobial treatment. Treatment for chlamydial infection (as above) should be given if this infection has not been ruled out.

[h]Hospitalization is indicated to exclude suspected meningitis or endocarditis.

Epidemiology

- Most common STDs in the United States; ~4 million cases per year
- Clinical spectrum paralleling that of *N. gonorrhoeae* infections
- Asymptomatic or mild clinical disease more common, but morbidity greater with *Chlamydia* than with *N. gonorrhoeae*
- *C. trachomatis* has been identified in the fallopian tubes or endometrium of up to half of women with PID. Infertility due to fallopian tube scarring has been strongly linked to antecedent *C. trachomatis* infection.

Clinical Syndromes

1. Urethritis, epididymitis, cervicitis, salpingitis, PID, and proctitis (discussed above)
2. Associated with Reiter's syndrome (conjunctivitis, urethritis or cervicitis, arthritis, mucocutaneous lesions). *C. trachomatis* is recovered from the urethra of up to 70% of men with nondiarrheal Reiter's and associated urethritis. More than 80% of pts have the HLA-B27 phenotype.
3. LGV: The primary genital lesion is noted in about one-third of heterosexual men and occasionally in women. See Table 90-1 for clinical details. LGV is associated with systemic symptoms. Painful adenopathy above and below the inguinal ligament presents with the "sign of the groove."

Diagnosis   Four laboratory procedures are available for diagnosis:

- Direct microscopic examination of tissue scrapings (low sensitivity except in conjunctivitis and frequent false-positive results)
- Isolation of the organism in cell culture: low sensitivity, high cost
- Nonculture techniques: direct immunofluorescent antibody (DFA) slide tests; enzyme-linked immunosorbent assay; NAATs using polymerase chain reaction (PCR), ligase chain reaction (LCR), or transcription-mediated amplification (TMA). Tests surpass culture in sensitivity and allow use of urine specimens rather than urethral or cervical swabs.
- Detection of antibody in serum or in local secretions: of limited usefulness except in LGV

℞   Infections with *Chlamydia trachomatis*

- See "Specific Syndromes," above.
- LGV: doxycycline (100 mg PO bid) or erythromycin base (500 mg PO qid) for at least 3 weeks

INFECTIONS DUE TO MYCOPLASMAS

Etiology and Epidemiology

- Smallest free-living organisms known; lack a cell wall; resist in vitro cultivation
- *M. genitalium* and ureaplasmas *(U. parvum* and *U. urealyticum)* cause urethritis and other genital conditions; *M. hominis* and ureaplasmas are part of the complex flora of BV.
- Higher colonization rates in disadvantaged populations

Clinical Syndromes and Diagnosis

- Cause NGU and BV; associated with PID and tubal factor infertility
- Can be associated with reactive arthritis and Reiter's syndrome, which are usually due to *C. trachomatis*

- The ubiquity of the organisms in the lower genital tract makes isolation attempts unnecessary in most cases. Microbiologic diagnosis is beyond the capability of most laboratories. NAATs have been developed.

R_x **Infections Due to Mycoplasmas**

Current recommendations for treatment of NGU and PID are appropriate for genital mycoplasmas.

SYPHILIS

Etiology and Epidemiology

- Caused by *Treponema pallidum* subspecies *pallidum*, a thin, delicate organism with 6–14 spirals and tapered ends (6–15 μm long, 0.2 μm wide)
- Cases acquired by sexual contact with infectious lesions (chancre, mucous patch, skin rash, condyloma latum); nonsexual acquisition through close personal contact, infection in utero, blood transfusion, organ transplantation
- 33,278 reported cases in the United States in 2005
- High-risk populations include MSM, many of whom are co-infected with HIV. Rates among heterosexual African Americans in urban areas peaked in 1990, are now declining, but remain higher than for other racial/ethnic groups.
- One-half of sexual contacts of persons with infectious syphilis become infected. All recently exposed sexual contacts are treated.

Pathogenesis Untreated syphilis penetrates intact mucous membranes or microscopic abrasions, entering lymphatics and blood within hours. Systemic infection and metastatic foci result. The primary lesion appears at the site of inoculation within 4–6 weeks and heals spontaneously. Generalized parenchymal [central nervous system (CNS), liver, lymph node], constitutional, and mucocutaneous manifestations of secondary syphilis appear 6–8 weeks later despite high antibody titers, subsiding in 2–6 weeks. A latent period follows. One-third of pts eventually develop tertiary disease (syphilitic gummas, cardiovascular disease, neurologic disease); one-quarter of those pts die.

Clinical Manifestations

1. *Primary*: chancre at site of inoculation (penis, rectum or anal canal, mouth, cervix, labia). See Table 90-1 for clinical details. Adenopathy can persist long after the chancre heals. Serology can be negative; tests should be repeated in 1–2 weeks.
2. *Secondary*: diffuse mucocutaneous lesions of variable morphologies, generalized nontender lymphadenopathy. Primary chancre may still be present. Initial lesions are bilaterally symmetric, pale red or pink, nonpruritic macules that progress to papules and may become necrotic. Lesions are widely distributed over the trunk and extremities, including the palms and soles. In moist intertriginous areas, papules can enlarge and erode to produce broad, highly infectious lesions called *condylomata lata*. Superficial mucosal erosions are called *mucous patches*. Constitutional symptoms are often present. The CNS is seeded by organisms in ≥30% of cases, although no clinical meningitis is evident. Less common findings include hepatitis, nephropathy, arthritis, optic neuritis, and anterior uveitis.
3. *Latent*: positive syphilis serology without clinical manifestations. Early latent syphilis develops within the first year of infection. Late latent syphilis, which develops >1 year after infection, is unlikely to cause infectious relapse. However, women with latent syphilis can infect the fetus in utero.

4. *Late*
   a. *CNS disease*: a continuum throughout syphilis. Asymptomatic cerebrospinal fluid (CSF) abnormalities exist in up to 40% of pts with primary or secondary syphilis and in 25% of those with latent disease. Symptomatic neurosyphilis develops only in this subset. Meningeal findings, including headache, nausea, vomiting, change in mental status, and neck stiffness, often with associated uveitis or iritis, present within 1 year of infection. Meningovascular involvement (5–10 years after infection) usually presents as a subacute encephalitic prodrome and is followed by a gradually progressive vascular syndrome. Parenchymatous involvement presents at 20 years for general paresis and 25–30 years for tabes dorsalis. A general mnemonic for paresis is *p*ersonality, *a*ffect, *r*eflexes (hyperactive), *e*ye (Argyll Robertson pupils, which react to accommodation but not to light), *s*ensorium (illusions, delusions, hallucinations), *i*ntellect (decrease in recent memory and orientation, judgment, calculations, insight), and *s*peech. Tabes dorsalis is a demyelination of posterior columns, dorsal roots, and dorsal root ganglia, with ataxic, wide-based gait and footslap; paresthesia; bladder disturbances; impotence; areflexia; and loss of position, deep pain, and temperature sensations. Trophic joint degeneration (Charcot's joints), optic atrophy, and Argyll Robertson pupils are also present.
   b. *Cardiovascular syphilis*: About 10% of pts with untreated late latent syphilis develop cardiovascular symptoms 10–40 years later. Endarteritis obliterans of the vasa vasorum providing the blood supply to large vessels results in aortitis, aortic regurgitation, saccular aneurysm, and coronary ostial stenosis.
   c. *Late benign syphilis (gumma)*: usually solitary lesions showing granulomatous inflammation with central necrosis; found most often in the skin and skeletal system, mouth, upper respiratory tract, liver, and stomach
5. *Congenital*: Syphilis can be transmitted throughout pregnancy. Lesions begin to be manifest in the fetus at ~4 months of gestation. All pregnant women should be tested for syphilis early in pregnancy.

Diagnosis

- Dark-field microscopy or immunofluorescence antibody staining of exudates from most lesions (e.g., chancres or condylomata lata) is rarely available today.
- Nontreponemal serologic tests that measure IgG and IgM directed against a cardiolipin-lecithin-cholesterol antigen complex [e.g., rapid plasma reagin (RPR), Venereal Disease Research Laboratory (VDRL)]
- Treponemal serologic tests: agglutination assay (e.g., the Serodia TP-PA test) and the fluorescent treponemal antibody–absorbed (FTA-ABS) test. Results remain positive even after successful treatment.
- Three uses of serology: screening or diagnosis, quantitation of titers (e.g., with RPR) to monitor response to treatment, and confirmation of the diagnosis in a pt with a positive nontreponemal test
- Lumbar puncture (LP) is recommended for pts with syphilis and neurologic signs or symptoms, other late syphilis manifestations, or suspected treatment failure and for HIV-infected pts with untreated syphilis of unknown or >1 year's duration. CSF exam demonstrates pleocytosis and increased protein. A positive CSF VDRL test is specific but not sensitive; an unabsorbed FTA test is sensitive but not specific. A negative unabsorbed FTA test excludes neurosyphilis.
- Pts with syphilis should be evaluated for HIV disease.

	TABLE 90-3	RECOMMENDATIONS FOR THE TREATMENT OF SYPHILIS[a]

Stage of Syphilis	Patients without Penicillin Allergy	Patients with Confirmed Penicillin Allergy
Primary, secondary, or early latent	Penicillin G benzathine (single dose of 2.4 mU IM)	Tetracycline hydrochloride (500 mg PO qid) or doxycycline (100 mg PO bid) for 2 weeks
Late latent (or latent of uncertain duration), cardiovascular, or benign tertiary	Lumbar puncture CSF normal: Penicillin G benzathine (2.4 mU IM weekly for 3 weeks) CSF abnormal: Treat as neurosyphilis	Lumbar puncture CSF normal and pt not infected with HIV: Tetracycline hydrochloride (500 mg PO qid) or doxycycline (100 mg PO bid) for 4 weeks CSF normal and pt infected with HIV: Desensitization and treatment with penicillin if compliance cannot be ensured CSF abnormal: Treat as neurosyphilis
Neurosyphilis (asymptomatic or symptomatic)	Aqueous penicillin G (18–24 mU/d IV, given as 3–4 mU q4h or continuous infusion) for 10–14 days or Aqueous penicillin G procaine (2.4 mU/d IM) plus oral probenecid (500 mg qid), both for 10–14 days	Desensitization and treatment with penicillin
Syphilis in pregnancy	According to stage	Desensitization and treatment with penicillin

[a]See Chap. 162, HPIM-17, for full discussion of syphilis therapy in HIV-infected individuals.
Note: mU, million units; CSF, cerebrospinal fluid.
Source: These recommendations are based on those issued by the Centers for Disease Control and Prevention in 2006.

 Syphilis

See Table 90-3.

- Jarisch-Herxheimer reaction: a dramatic reaction to treatment most commonly seen with initiation of therapy for primary (~50% of pts) or secondary (~90%) syphilis. The reaction is associated with fever, chills, myalgias, tachycardia, headache, tachypnea, and vasodilation. Symptoms subside within 12–24 h without treatment.
- Response to treatment should be monitored with RPR or VDRL titers at 6 and 12 months (every 3 months in HIV-infected persons) in early syphilis and at 6, 12, and 24 months in late or latent syphilis. If the titer rises fourfold or fails to fall fourfold in primary or secondary syphilis or in pts with

latent or late syphilis whose initial titers are ≥1:32, or if symptoms persist or recur, the pt should be re-treated and evaluated with LP to exclude neurosyphilis. In treated neurosyphilis, CSF cell counts should be monitored every 6 months for 2 years or until normal, and quantitative RPR or VDRL should be monitored every 6 months for 2 years.

HERPES SIMPLEX VIRUS INFECTIONS

Etiology and Epidemiology

- HSV is a linear, double-strand DNA virus.
- More than 90% of adults in the United States have antibodies to HSV-1 by age 50; ~20% of the U.S. population has antibodies to HSV-2.
- Unrecognized carriage of HSV-2 and frequent asymptomatic reactivations of virus from the genital tract foster the continued spread of HSV disease.
- Genital lesions caused by HSV-1 have lower recurrence rates in the first year (~55%) than those caused by HSV-2 (~90%).

Clinical Manifestations   See Table 90-1 for clinical details. First episodes of genital herpes can be associated with fever, headache, malaise, and myalgias. More than 80% of women with primary genital herpes have cervical or urethral involvement. Local symptoms include pain, dysuria, vaginal and urethral discharge, and tender inguinal lymphadenopathy.

Diagnosis

- Staining of scrapings with Wright's or Giemsa's (Tzanck preparation) to detect giant cells or intranuclear inclusions is well described, but most clinicians are not skilled in these techniques, which furthermore do not differentiate between HSV and varicella-zoster virus.
- Isolation of HSV in tissue culture or demonstration of HSV antigens or DNA in scrapings from lesions is the most accurate diagnostic method. PCR is increasingly being used for detection of HSV DNA and is more sensitive than culture at mucosal sites.

℞ Herpes Simplex Virus Infections

- *First episodes*: acyclovir (400 mg tid), valacyclovir (1 g bid), or famciclovir (250 mg bid) for 7–14 days
- *Recurrent episodes*: acyclovir (800 mg tid for 2 days), valacyclovir (500 mg bid for 3 days), or famciclovir (750 or 1000 mg bid for 1 day, 1500 mg once, or 500 mg stat followed by 250 mg q12h for 3 days); alternatively, acyclovir (200 mg 5 times per day), valacyclovir (500 mg bid), or famciclovir (125 mg bid) for 5 days
- *Suppression*: acyclovir (400 mg bid or 800 mg qd), famciclovir (250 mg bid), or valacyclovir (500 mg qd for pts with <9 episodes per year; otherwise, 1 g qd or 500 mg bid)
- Once-daily valacyclovir reduces transmission of HSV-2 between sexual partners and is more effective than famciclovir at reducing subclinical shedding.

CHANCROID (*HAEMOPHILUS DUCREYI* INFECTION)

Epidemiology   Significant problem in developing countries, increasing incidence in the United States, associated with HIV infection because of genital ulcerations

Clinical Manifestations   See Table 90-1 for clinical details.

Diagnosis   PCR or culture for *H. ducreyi*

 Chancroid (*Haemophilus ducreyi* Infection)

Azithromycin (1 g PO once), ciprofloxacin (500 mg PO bid for 3 days), ceftriaxone (250 mg IM once), or erythromycin base (500 mg tid for 1 week)

DONOVANOSIS (*KLEBSIELLA GRANULOMATIS* INFECTION)

Etiology and Epidemiology   Also known as *granuloma inguinale* and *granuloma venereum*, donovanosis is caused by *Klebsiella granulomatis*. The infection is endemic in the Caribbean, southern Africa, and southeastern India and among Aborigines in Australia. Fewer than 20 cases are reported annually in the United States.

Clinical Manifestations, Diagnosis, and Treatment   See Table 90-1 for clinical manifestations. Lesions slowly enlarge, causing genital swelling (especially of the labia), with occasional progression to pseudoelephantiasis. Extragenital lesions occur in 6% of pts. Diagnosis is based on identification of typical intracellular Donovan bodies within large mononuclear cells in smears from lesions or biopsy specimens. PCR and serology are also available. Pts should be treated with azithromycin (500 mg/d or 1 g weekly until healing of lesions—usually 3–5 weeks). Doxycycline (100 mg bid) is an alternative.

HUMAN PAPILLOMAVIRUS (HPV) INFECTIONS

Etiology   Papillomaviruses are nonenveloped, double-strand DNA viruses with icosahedral capsids composed of 72 capsomers. HPV-6 and HPV-11 are associated with anogenital warts (condylomata acuminata). HPV types 16, 18, 31, 33, and 45 have been most strongly associated with cervical cancers. Most infections, including those with oncogenic types, are self-limited.

Clinical Manifestations
- Incubation period of 3–4 months (range, 1 month to 2 years)
- Common warts and plantar warts
- Anogenital warts on the skin and mucosal surfaces of genitalia and perianal areas

Diagnosis
- Direct visualization (may be aided by application of 3–5% acetic acid solution to lesions)
- Papanicolaou smears from cervical or anal scrapings show cytologic evidence of HPV infection.
- PCR or hybrid-capture assay of lesions

 Human Papillomavirus Infections

Many lesions resolve spontaneously. Current treatment is not completely effective, and some agents have significant side effects. Provider-administered therapy can include cryotherapy, podophyllin resin (10–25%), trichloroacetic acid or bichloroacetic acid (80–90%), surgical excision, intralesionally administered interferon, or laser surgery. Pt-administered therapy consists of podofilox (0.5% solution or gel) or imiquimod (topically applied interferon inducer; 5% cream).

Prevention   A quadrivalent vaccine containing HPV types 6, 11, 16, and 18 is recommended for administration to girls and young women 9–26 years of age. HPV types 6 and 11 cause 90% of anogenital warts, and HPV types 16 and 18 cause 70% of cervical cancers. Because 30% of cervical cancers are caused by HPV types not included in the vaccine, no changes in clinical cancer-screening programs are currently recommended.

For a more detailed discussion, see Holmes KK: Sexually Transmitted Infections: Overview and Clinical Approach, Chap. 124, p. 821; Ram S, Rice PA: Gonococcal Infections, Chap. 137, p. 914; Murphy TF: *Haemophilus* Infections, Chap. 139, p. 923; Hart G: Donovanosis, Chap. 154, p. 991; Lukehart SA: Syphilis, Chap. 162, p. 1038; McCormack WM: Infections Due to Mycoplasmas, Chap. 168, p. 1068; Stamm WE: Chlamydial Infections, Chap. 169, p. 1070; Corey L: Herpes Simplex Viruses, Chap. 172, p. 1095; and Reichman RC: Human Papillomavirus Infections, Chap. 178, p. 1117, in HPIM-17.

91 Infections of the Skin, Soft Tissues, Joints, and Bones

SKIN AND SOFT TISSUE INFECTIONS

Skin and soft tissue infections are diagnosed principally by a careful history (e.g., temporal progression, travel, animal exposure, bites, trauma, underlying medical conditions) and physical examination (appearance of lesions and distribution). Types of skin and soft tissue manifestations include the following:

1. *Vesicles*: Due to proliferation of organisms, usually viruses, within the epidermis (e.g., varicella; herpes simplex; infections with coxsackievirus, poxviruses, *Rickettsia akari*). Molluscum contagiosum is a poxvirus infection transmitted by close contact, including sexual intercourse. This virus causes distinctive proliferative skin lesions that are 2–5 mm in diameter, pearly, flesh-colored, and umbilicated with a dimple at the center. Lack of inflammation and necrosis distinguishes these lesions from other poxvirus lesions.
2. *Bullae*: Caused by toxin-producing organisms. Different entities affect different skin levels; for example, staphylococcal scalded-skin syndrome and toxic epidermal necrolysis cause cleavage of the stratum corneum and the stratum germinativum, respectively. Bullae are also seen in necrotizing fasciitis, gas gangrene, and *Vibrio vulnificus* infection in pts with cirrhosis who have ingested contaminated raw seafood or been exposed to Gulf of Mexico or Atlantic seaboard waters.
3. *Crusted lesions*: Impetigo caused by either *Streptococcus pyogenes* (impetigo contagiosa) or *Staphylococcus aureus* (bullous impetigo) usually starts with a bullous phase before crusting. Epidemics of impetigo caused by methicillin-resistant *S. aureus* (MRSA) have been reported. It is important to recognize impetigo contagiosa because of its relation to poststreptococcal

glomerulonephritis. Crusted lesions are also seen in some systemic fungal infections, dermatophytic infections, and cutaneous mycobacterial infection.

4. *Folliculitis*: Localized infection of hair follicles is usually due to *S. aureus*. "Hot-tub folliculitis" is a diffuse condition caused by *Pseudomonas aeruginosa*. Freshwater avian schistosomes cause swimmer's itch.

5. *Papular and nodular lesions*: Can be caused by *Bartonella* (cat-scratch disease), *Treponema pallidum*, papillomavirus, mycobacteria, and helminths

6. *Ulcers, with or without eschars*: Can be caused by cutaneous anthrax, ulceroglandular tularemia, plague, mycobacterial infection, and (in the case of genital lesions) chancroid or syphilis

7. *Erysipelas*: Lymphangitis of the dermis, with abrupt onset of fiery red swelling of the face or extremities, well-defined indurated margins, intense pain, and rapid progression. *S. pyogenes* is the exclusive cause (see Chap. 94).

CELLULITIS

Definition Cellulitis, an acute inflammatory condition of the skin, is characterized by localized pain, erythema, swelling, and heat.

Etiology

- May be caused by indigenous skin flora (e.g., *S. aureus*, *S. pyogenes*). *S. aureus* cellulitis spreads from a central localized infection site. *S. pyogenes* can cause a rapidly spreading, diffuse process, often with fever and lymphangitis; recurrent episodes occur in association with chronic venous stasis and lymphedema. Group B streptococcal cellulitis is associated with older age, diabetes, and peripheral vascular disease.

- May also be caused by exogenous bacteria. A thorough history and epidemiologic data may help identify the cause—e.g., *Pasteurella multocida* after a cat or dog bite; *Capnocytophaga canimorsus* after a dog bite; *Eikenella corrodens* after a human bite; *P. aeruginosa* in association with ecthyma gangrenosum in neutropenic pts, a penetrating injury (stepping on a nail), or "hot-tub" folliculitis; *Aeromonas hydrophila* after a laceration sustained in fresh water; or *Erysipelothrix rhusiopathiae* after contact with domestic swine and fish.

Diagnosis If there is a wound or portal of entry, Gram's staining and culture may identify the etiology. If both a wound and a portal of entry are lacking, aspiration or biopsy of the leading edge of the cellulitis tissue yields a diagnosis in only about one-fifth of cases.

℞ Cellulitis

See Table 91-1. A typical course is 2 weeks long. IV therapy is usually given until inflammation and systemic signs and symptoms have improved.

NECROTIZING FASCIITIS

Definition Necrotizing fasciitis is caused by either *S. pyogenes* or mixed aerobic and anaerobic bacteria, usually of GI or genitourinary origin. Strains of MRSA have been implicated as a cause of necrotizing fasciitis. Infection, either apparent or inapparent, results from a breach in integrity of skin or mucous membrane barriers.

Clinical Features

- Onset of severe pain and fever, with minimal physical findings; rapid progression to swelling; brawny edema; dark red induration; bullae; friable, necrotic skin.

TABLE 91-1   TREATMENT OF COMMON INFECTIONS OF THE SKIN

Diagnosis/Condition	Primary Treatment	Alternative Treatment	See Also HPIM-17 Chap(s).
Animal bite (prophylaxis or early infection)[a]	Amoxicillin/clavulanate, 875/125 mg PO bid	Doxycycline, 100 mg PO bid	e15
Animal bite[a] (established infection)	Ampicillin/sulbactam, 1.5–3.0 g IV q6h	Clindamycin, 600–900 mg IV q8h *plus* Ciprofloxacin, 400 mg IV q12h *or* Cefoxitin, 2 g IV q6h	e15
Bacillary angiomatosis	Erythromycin, 500 mg PO qid	Doxycycline, 100 mg PO bid	153
Herpes simplex (primary genital)	Acyclovir, 400 mg PO tid for 10 days	Famciclovir, 250 mg PO tid for 5–10 days *or* Valacyclovir, 1000 mg PO bid for 10 days	172
Herpes zoster (immunocompetent host >50 years of age)	Acyclovir, 800 mg PO 5 times daily for 7–10 days	Famciclovir, 500 mg PO tid for 7–10 days *or* Valacyclovir, 1000 mg PO tid for 7 days	173
Cellulitis (staphylococcal or streptococcal[b,c])	Nafcillin or oxacillin, 2 g IV q4–6h	Cefazolin, 1–2 g q8h *or* Ampicillin/sulbactam, 1.5–3.0 g IV q6h *or* Erythromycin, 0.5–1.0 g IV q6h *or* Clindamycin, 600–900 mg IV q8h	129, 130
MRSA skin infection[d]	Vancomycin, 1 g IV q12h	Linezolid, 600 mg IV q12h	129
Necrotizing fasciitis (group A streptococcal[b])	Clindamycin, 600–900 mg IV q6–8h *plus* Penicillin G, 4 million units IV q4h	Clindamycin, 600–900 mg IV q6–8h *plus* Cephalosporin (first- or second-generation)	130

(continued)

TABLE 91-1   TREATMENT OF COMMON INFECTIONS OF THE SKIN (CONTINUED)

Diagnosis/Condition	Primary Treatment	Alternative Treatment	See Also HPIM-17 Chap(s).
Necrotizing fasciitis (mixed aerobes and anaerobes)	Ampicillin, 2 g IV q4h *plus* Clindamycin, 600–900 mg IV q6–8h *plus* Ciprofloxacin, 400 mg IV q6–8h	Vancomycin, 1 g IV q6h *plus* Metronidazole, 500 mg IV q6h *plus* Ciprofloxacin, 400 mg IV q6–8h	157
Gas gangrene	Clindamycin, 600–900 mg IV q6–8h *plus* Penicillin G, 4 million units IV q4–6h	Clindamycin, 600–900 mg IV q6–8h *plus* Cefoxitin, 2 g IV q6h	135

[a]*Pasteurella multocida*, a species commonly associated with both dog and cat bites, is resistant to cephalexin, dicloxacillin, clindamycin, and erythromycin. *Eikenella corrodens*, a bacterium commonly associated with human bites, is resistant to clindamycin, penicillinase-resistant penicillins, and metronidazole but is sensitive to trimethoprim-sulfamethoxazole and fluoroquinolones.

[b]The frequency of erythromycin resistance in group A *Streptococcus* is currently ~5% in the United States but has reached 70–100% in some other countries. Most, but not all, erythromycin-resistant group A streptococci are susceptible to clindamycin. Approximately 90–95% of *Staphylococcus aureus* strains are sensitive to clindamycin.

[c]Severe hospital-acquired *S. aureus* infections or community-acquired *S. aureus* infections that are not responding to the β-lactam antibiotics recommended in this table may be caused by methicillin-resistant strains, requiring a switch to vancomycin or linezolid.

[d]Some strains of methicillin-resistant *S. aureus* (MRSA) remain sensitive to tetracycline and trimethoprim-sulfamethoxazole. Daptomycin (4 mg/kg IV q24h) or tigecycline (100-mg loading dose followed by 50 mg IV q12h) are alternative treatments for MRSA.

- Thrombosis of blood vessels in dermal papillae leads to ischemia of peripheral nerves and anesthesia of the affected area.
- Infection spreads to deep fascia and along fascial planes through venous channels and lymphatics.
- Pts are toxic and develop shock and multiorgan failure.

Diagnosis   Diagnosis is based on clinical presentation. Other findings may include (1) renal failure, often preceding shock and hypotension; (2) gas in tissue (in mixed infections but rarely with *S. pyogenes*); and (3) markedly elevated serum creatine phosphokinase levels.

℞ Necrotizing Fasciitis

- Emergent surgical exploration to deep fascia and muscle, with removal of necrotic tissue.
- For antibiotic choices, see Table 91-1.

MYOSITIS/MYONECROSIS

Definitions

- *Myositis*: can be caused by viruses (influenza virus, dengue virus, coxsackievirus), parasites (*Trichinella*, cysticerci, *Toxoplasma*), or bacteria (clostridia, streptococci). This condition usually manifests with myalgias, but pain can be severe in coxsackievirus, *Trichinella*, and bacterial infections.
- *Pyomyositis*: localized muscle infection, usually due to *S. aureus.*
- *Myonecrosis*: caused by clostridial species (*C. perfringens, C. septicum, C. histolyticum*) or by mixed aerobic and anaerobic bacteria. Myonecrosis is usually related to trauma; however, spontaneous gangrene—usually due to *C. septicum*—can occur in pts with neutropenia, GI malignancy, or diverticulosis. Myonecrosis occurs with necrotizing fasciitis in ~50% of cases.

Diagnosis and Treatment

- Emergent surgical intervention to remove necrotic tissue, visualize deep structures, obtain materials for culture and sensitivity testing, and reduce compartment pressure.
- Empirical antibiotic treatment should target likely etiologies—e.g., vancomycin (1 g IV every 12 h) for pyomyositis and ampicillin/sulbactam (2–3 g IV every 6 h) for mixed aerobic-anaerobic infections. For treatment of clostridial myonecrosis (gas gangrene), see Table 91-1.

INFECTIOUS ARTHRITIS

Joints become infected by hematogenous seeding (the most common route), by spread from a contiguous site of infection, or by direct inoculation (e.g., during trauma or surgery).

Etiology and Clinical Features

- Children <5 years: *S. aureus, S. pyogenes, Kingella kingae*
- Young adults: *Neisseria gonorrhoeae, S. aureus*
- Adults: *S. aureus, N. gonorrhoeae*, gram-negative bacilli, pneumococci, streptococci (groups A, B, C, F, and G)

Nongonococcal Bacterial Arthritis   Risk is increased in pts with rheumatoid arthritis, diabetes mellitus, glucocorticoid therapy, hemodialysis, malignancy, and IV drug use. An extraarticular focus is found in ~25% of pts.

In 90% of pts, one joint is involved—most often the knee, which is followed in frequency by the hip, shoulder, wrist, and elbow. IV drug users often have spinal, sacroiliac, or sternoclavicular joint involvement. Pts have moderate to severe pain, effusion, decreased range of motion, and fever. Gram-positive cocci (most commonly *S. aureus*, followed by streptococci of groups A and G) cause 75% of cases.

Gonococcal Arthritis   Women are more likely than men to develop disseminated gonococcal disease, particularly during menses and during pregnancy (see Chap. 90). True gonococcal arthritis usually affects a single joint: hip, knee, ankle, or wrist.

Prosthetic Joint Infection

- Complicates 1–4% of joint replacements
- Usually acquired intra- or perioperatively
- Acute presentations are seen in infections caused by *S. aureus*, pyogenic streptococci, and enteric bacilli.
- Indolent presentations are seen in infections caused by coagulase-negative staphylococci and diphtheroids.

Miscellaneous Etiologies Other causes of septic arthritis include Lyme disease, tuberculosis and other mycobacterial infections, fungal infections (coccidioido-mycosis, histoplasmosis), and viral infections (rubella, mumps, hepatitis B, parvovirus infection).

Reiter's Arthritis Reiter's arthritis follows ~1% of cases of nongonococcal ure-thritis and 2% of enteric infections due to *Yersinia enterocolitica, Shigella flex-neri, Campylobacter jejuni*, and *Salmonella* species in genetically susceptible pts.

Diagnosis Infection of the joint is evidenced by clinical signs and symptoms. Examination of synovial fluid from the affected joint is essential. *Normal* synovial fluid contains <180 cells (mostly mononuclear)/μL. *Acute bacterial infection* of joints results in synovial fluid cell counts averaging 100,000/μL (range, 25,000–250,000/μL), with >90% polymorphonuclear leukocytes (PMNs). Synovial fluid in *gonococcal arthritis* contains >50,000 cells/μL, but results of Gram's staining are usually negative, and cultures of synovial fluid are positive in <40% of cases. Other mucosal sites should be cultured to diagnose gonorrhea. Pts with septic arthritis due to *mycobacteria* or *fungi* can have 10,000–30,000 cells/μL in synovial fluid, with 50–70% PMNs. Synovial fluid cell counts in *noninfectious inflammatory arthritides* are typically 30,000–50,000/μL.

Gram's staining of synovial fluid should be performed, and injection into blood culture bottles can increase the yield of synovial fluid cultures. Fluid should be examined for crystals to rule out gout or pseudogout, and an attempt should be made to identify the extraarticular source of hematogenous seeding.

Blood for cultures should be taken before initiation of antibiotic therapy. Blood cultures are positive in up to 50% of cases due to *S. aureus* but are less commonly positive with other organisms.

Plain radiographs show soft tissue swelling, joint space widening, and displacement of tissue planes by distended capsule. Narrowing of the joint space and bony erosions suggest advanced disease.

℞ Infectious Arthritis

Drainage of pus and necrotic debris is needed to cure infection and to prevent destruction of cartilage, postinfectious degenerative arthritis, and joint deformity or instability.

Empirical antibiotics can include oxacillin (2 g every 4 h) if gram-positive cocci are seen in synovial fluid; vancomycin (1 g every 12 h) if MRSA is a concern; or ceftriaxone (1 g q24h) if no organism is evident (to cover community-acquired organisms). In IV drug users, treatment for gram-negative organisms such as *P. aeruginosa* should be considered. After definitive diagnosis, treatment should be adjusted. Treatment for *S. aureus* should be given for 4 weeks, that for enteric gram-negative bacilli for 3–4 weeks, and that for pneumococci or streptococci for 2 weeks. Treatment of gonococcal arthritis should commence with ceftriaxone (1 g/d) until improvement and can be completed with an oral fluoroquinolone (e.g., ciprofloxacin, 500 mg bid). If fluoroquinolone resistance is not prevalent, a fluoroquinolone can be given for the entire course.

Prosthetic joint infections should be treated with surgery and high-dose IV antibiotics for 4–6 weeks. The prosthesis often has to be removed; to avoid joint removal, antibiotic suppression of infection may be tried. A 3- to 6-month course of ciprofloxacin and rifampin has been successful in *S. aureus* prosthetic joint infections of relatively short duration.

OSTEOMYELITIS

Definitions

1. *Osteomyelitis*: infection of bone caused by pyogenic bacteria and mycobacteria that gain access to bone by the hematogenous route (20% of cases, primarily in children), via direct spread from a contiguous focus of infection, or by a penetrating wound
2. *Sequestra*: ischemic necrosis of bone resulting in the separation of large devascularized bone fragments; caused when pus spreads into vascular channels
3. *Involucrum*: elevated periosteal deposits of new bone around a sequestrum

Clinical Features   Acute Hematogenous Osteomyelitis   This condition usually involves a single bone (long bones in children), presenting as an acute febrile illness with localized pain and tenderness. Restriction of movement or difficulty bearing weight is often evident. Infection may extend to joint spaces. In adults, vertebral bodies are most often involved. Organisms seed the end plate and extend into the disk space and thence to adjacent vertebral bodies. A prior history of degenerative disease or trauma is common. Diabetic pts, pts undergoing hemodialysis, and IV drug users are at increased risk. Bacteremic infections or UTIs are common sources in older men. The lumbar and cervical spine is often involved in pyogenic infections and the thoracic spine in tuberculosis. Pts can present either acutely, with ongoing bacteremia, or indolently, with vague dull pain that increases over weeks and low-grade or no fever.

Spinal epidural abscess may complicate vertebral osteomyelitis, presenting as spinal pain and progressing to radicular pain and/or weakness; it is best diagnosed by MRI and must be treated urgently to prevent neurologic complications.

Usually, a single organism causes acute hematogenous osteomyelitis; *S. aureus* accounts for ~50% of cases. Other common pathogens include gram-negative bacilli. Less common causes include *Mycobacterium tuberculosis*, *Brucella*, and fungi.

Osteomyelitis from a Contiguous Focus of Infection

- Accounts for ~80% of all cases
- Includes osteomyelitis in the setting of bites, puncture wounds, open fractures, peripheral vascular disease (particularly in diabetic adults), and foreign bodies
- Although *S. aureus* is one of the pathogens in more than half of cases, infections are often polymicrobial and involve gram-negative and anaerobic bacteria as well.

Chronic Osteomyelitis

- More likely to develop after infection from a contiguous source of infection than is acute hematogenous osteomyelitis.
- The presence of a foreign body also increases risk.
- The clinical course is prolonged and is characterized by quiescent periods with acute exacerbations, lack of fever, and development of sinus tracts that can occasionally drain pus or bits of necrotic bone.

Diagnosis   Erythrocyte sedimentation rate (ESR) and C-reactive protein levels are usually increased in acute infection and can be used to monitor the response to treatment.

Imaging studies are important in the diagnosis of osteomyelitis, but there is a lack of consensus about their optimal use (see Table 91-2). Conditions due to noninfectious etiologies can be distinguished from osteomyelitis by imaging studies because the former do not usually cross the disk space.

TABLE 91-2   DIAGNOSTIC IMAGING STUDIES FOR OSTEOMYELITIS

Type of Study	Comments
Plain radiographs	Insensitive, especially in early osteomyelitis. May show periosteal elevation after 10 days, lytic changes after 2–6 weeks. Useful to look for anatomic abnormalities (e.g., fractures, bony variants, or deformities), foreign bodies, and soft tissue gas.
Three-phase bone scan (^{99m}Tc-MDP)	Characteristic finding in osteomyelitis: increased uptake in all three phases of scan. Highly sensitive (~95%) in acute infection; somewhat less sensitive if blood flow to bone is poor. Specificity moderate if plain films are normal, but poor in presence of neuropathic arthropathy, fractures, tumor, infarction.
Other radionuclide scans	Examples: ^{67}Ga-citrate, ^{111}In-labeled WBCs. ^{111}In-WBCs more specific than gallium but not always available. Often used in conjunction with bone scan because its greater specificity for inflammation than ^{99m}Tc-MDP helps to distinguish infectious from noninfectious processes. Lack of consensus over role; often supplanted by MRI when the latter is available.
Ultrasound	May detect subperiosteal fluid collection or soft tissue abscess adjacent to bone, but largely supplanted by CT and MRI.
CT	Limited role in acute osteomyelitis. In chronic osteomyelitis, excellent for detection of sequestra, cortical destruction, soft tissue abscesses, and sinus tracts. Use limited in the presence of a metallic foreign body.
MRI	As sensitive as ^{99m}Tc-MDP bone scan for acute osteomyelitis (~95%); detects changes in water content of marrow before disruption of cortical bone. High specificity (~87%), with better anatomic detail than nuclear studies. Procedure of choice for vertebral osteomyelitis because of high sensitivity for epidural abscess. Use may be limited by a metallic foreign body.

Note: WBCs, white blood cells; MDP, monodiphosphonate.

If at all possible, appropriate samples for microbiologic studies should be obtained before antibiotic treatment. Blood should be cultured in acute hematogenous osteomyelitis. The results of cultures from sinus tracts do not correlate well with organisms infecting the bone; thus bone samples for cultures must be obtained either percutaneously or intraoperatively.

℞ Osteomyelitis

Antibiotics used for therapy (see Table 91-3) should be bactericidal and given at high doses, usually commencing with IV administration.

1. *Acute hematogenous osteomyelitis in children*: 4–6 weeks of treatment. After 5–10 days, high-dose oral treatment can be used.
2. *Vertebral osteomyelitis*: 6–8 weeks of treatment. Consider a longer course if the ESR does not decline by at least two-thirds. The majority of epidural abscesses require surgical intervention.

TABLE 91-3 SELECTION OF ANTIBIOTICS FOR TREATMENT OF ACUTE OSTEOMYELITIS

Organism	Primary	Suggested Regimen[a] Alternatives[b]
Staphylococcus aureus		
Penicillin-resistant, methicillin-sensitive (MSSA)	Nafcillin or oxacillin, 2 g IV q4h	Cefazolin, 1 g IV q8h; ceftriaxone, 1 g IV q24h; clindamycin, 900 mg IV q8h[c]
Penicillin-sensitive	Penicillin, 3–4 million U IV q4h	Cefazolin, ceftriaxone, clindamycin (as above)
Methicillin-resistant (MRSA)	Vancomycin, 15 mg/kg IV q12h; rifampin, 300 mg PO q12h	Clindamycin[c] (as above); linezolid, 600 mg IV or PO q12h[d]; daptomycin, 4–6 mg/kg IV q24h[d]
Streptococci (including S. *milleri*, β-hemolytic streptococci)	Penicillin (as above)	Cefazolin, ceftriaxone, clindamycin (as above)
Gram-negative aerobic bacilli		
Escherichia coli, other "sensitive" species	Ampicillin, 2 g IV q4h; cefazolin, 1 g IV q8h	Ceftriaxone, 1 g IV q24h; parenteral or oral fluoroquinolone (e.g., ciprofloxacin, 400 mg IV or 750 mg PO q12h)[e]
Pseudomonas aeruginosa	Extended-spectrum β-lactam agent (e.g., piperacillin, 3–4 g IV q4–6h; or ceftazidime, 2 g IV q12h) *plus* tobramycin, 5–7 mg/kg q24h[f]	May substitute parenteral or oral fluoroquinolone for β-lactam agents (if pt is allergic) or for tobramycin (in relation to nephrotoxicity)
Enterobacter spp., other "resistant" species	Extended-spectrum β-lactam agent IV or fluoroquinolone IV or PO[e] (as above)	
Mixed infections possibly involving anaerobic bacteria	Ampicillin/sulbactam, 1.5–3 g IV q6h; piperacillin/tazobactam, 3.375 g IV q6h	Carbapenem antibiotic or a combination of a fluoroquinolone plus clindamycin (as above) or metronidazole, 500 mg PO tid

[a]Duration of treatment is discussed in the text.
[b]Cephalosporins may be used for the treatment of pts allergic to penicillin whose reaction did not consist of anaphylaxis or urticaria (immediate-type hypersensitivity).
[c]Because of the possibility of inducible resistance, clindamycin must be used with caution for the treatment of strains resistant to erythromycin. Consult clinical microbiology laboratory.

[d]Experience is limited; there are anecdotal reports of efficacy.
[e]Oral fluoroquinolones must not be coadministered with divalent cations (calcium, magnesium, iron, aluminum), which block the drugs' absorption.
[f]Tobramycin levels and renal function must be monitored closely to minimize the risks of nephro- and ototoxicity.

3. *Contiguous-focus osteomyelitis*: surgical debridement and 4–6 weeks of treatment unless only the outer cortex of bone is involved. In the latter situation, a 2-week course of antibiotic treatment after thorough debridement has had excellent success.
4. *Chronic osteomyelitis*: It should be decided whether aggressive treatment is warranted or intermittent antibiotic therapy to suppress exacerbations is adequate. Otherwise, surgery and 4–6 weeks of antibiotic therapy can be tried. The value of further suppressive antibiotic treatment remains unproven.

For a more detailed discussion, see Stevens DL: Infections of the Skin, Muscle, and Soft Tissues, Chap. 119, p. 798; Parsonnet J: Osteomyelitis, Chap. 120, p. 803; Wang F: Molluscum Contagiosum, Monkeypox, and Other Poxviruses, Excluding Smallpox Virus, Chap. 176, p. 1113; and Madoff LC et al: Infectious Arthritis, Chap. 328, p. 2169, in HPIM-17.

92 Pneumococcal Infections

ETIOLOGY

Streptococcus pneumoniae (the pneumococcus) is a gram-positive coccus that grows in chains and causes α-hemolysis on blood agar. Nearly every clinical isolate has a polysaccharide capsule. Ninety distinct capsules have been identified.

EPIDEMIOLOGY

S. pneumoniae colonizes the nasopharynx of 5–10% of healthy adults and 20–40% of healthy children on any single occasion. Once colonization takes place, pneumococci usually persist in adults for 4–6 weeks but can persist for up to 6 months. The organisms are spread by direct or droplet transmission as a result of close contact, and their spread is enhanced by crowding or poor ventilation. Outbreaks among adults have occurred in military barracks, prisons, homeless shelters, and nursing homes. Rates of bacteremic infection are highest among children <2 years of age and drop to low levels until age 55, when incidence again begins to increase. Pneumococcal pneumonia occurs annually in an estimated 20 young adults per 100,000 and in 280 persons >70 years of age per 100,000. Native Americans, Native Alaskans, and African Americans are unusually susceptible to invasive disease.

PATHOGENESIS

Once the nasopharynx has been colonized, infection can result if pneumococci are carried into contiguous areas (e.g., the sinuses) or are inhaled or aspirated into the bronchioles or alveoli. Spread to meninges, joints, and other sites through the bloodstream usually arises from a respiratory tract focus of infection. Pneumococci cause an inflammatory response, but—in the absence of anticapsular antibodies, which provide the best specific protection against pneumococcal infection—the polysaccharide capsule renders the organisms resistant to phagocytosis and killing. Many conditions predispose to pneumococcal infection. Risk factors for disease include increased exposure to pneumococci (e.g., in day-care centers, military barracks, prisons, or homeless shelters); antecedent respiratory insult with inflammation (e.g., influenza or upper respiratory viral infection, cigarette smoking, or chronic obstructive pulmonary disease); anatomic disruption (e.g., dural tear); defects in antibody production (e.g., in pts with multiple myeloma or lymphoma); defects in splenic function (e.g., asplenia, sickle cell disease); and other, multifactorial conditions (e.g., infancy or aging, HIV infection, glucocorticoid treatment, cirrhosis, diabetes). The absence of a spleen predisposes to fulminant pneumococcal disease.

SPECIFIC INFECTIONS

Otitis Media and Sinusitis   *S. pneumoniae* is the most common bacterial isolate from middle-ear fluid in acute otitis media and from paranasal sinus fluid during acute sinusitis. See Chap. 62 for more detail.

Pneumonia   Pts usually present with fever, cough, and sputum production. Nausea and vomiting or diarrhea may be prominent. A small subset of pts present with an acute onset of a shaking chill, fever, and cough productive of blood-tinged sputum. On examination, pts usually appear ill and anxious, with fever, tachypnea, and tachycardia. Dullness to percussion, increased vocal fremitus, and bronchial or tubular breath sounds or crackles can be heard on pulmonary examination. Pleural effusions are common and may cause dullness to percussion, decreased breath sounds, and lack of fremitus. Hypoxemia may cause confusion, but meningitis should be considered as well. Empyema complicates ~2% of cases. On chest x-ray, air-space consolidation is the predominant finding; disease is multilobar in about half of pts. Air bronchograms are evident in fewer than half of cases but are more common in bacteremic disease. Leukocytosis [>12,000 white blood cells (WBCs)/μL] is usually present; WBC counts of <6000/μL may be associated with a poor prognosis. Pneumococcal pneumonia is strongly suggested by a sputum Gram's stain with >25 polymorphonuclear leukocytes (PMNs) and <10 squamous epithelial cells per low-power field along with slightly elongated gram-positive cocci in pairs and chains. When a sputum sample of good quality can be obtained prior to antibiotic treatment (which rapidly clears pneumococci from the sputum), Gram's stain and culture are >80% and >90% sensitive, respectively. Blood cultures are positive in ~25% of cases.

Meningitis   *S. pneumoniae* is the most common cause of meningitis in adults; the incidence among children has been dramatically reduced by the use of pediatric pneumococcal conjugate vaccine. Infection usually results from hematogenous spread but can also be the result of drainage from colonized nasopharyngeal lymphatics or veins or of contiguous spread (e.g., dural tear). Clinical and laboratory features resemble those of meningitis due to other bacteria. Pts have fever, headache, and neck stiffness, and disease progresses over 24–48 h to confusion and obtundation. On examination, the pt is acutely ill with a rigid neck. Cerebrospinal fluid (CSF) findings consist of pleocytosis with ≥85% PMNs, elevated protein levels (100–500 mg/dL), and decreased glucose content (<30 mg/dL). Organisms can be seen on a gram-stained specimen of CSF if antibiotics have not yet been given.

Other Syndromes   Pneumococcal endocarditis (an acute infection that results in rapid destruction of heart valves), pericarditis, septic arthritis, osteomyelitis, peritonitis, salpingitis, epidural and brain abscesses, and cellulitis have been described. Unusual manifestations of pneumococcal infection should prompt consideration of testing for HIV infection.

℞ Pneumococcal Infections

Penicillin has been the cornerstone of treatment, but resistance has been slowly increasing. Resistance to other antibiotics is often documented as well. In the United States, ~20% of pneumococcal isolates are intermediately susceptible to penicillin [minimum inhibitory concentration (MIC), 0.1–1.0 μg/mL], and 15% are resistant (MIC, ≥2.0 μg/mL). These definitions are based on levels achievable in the CSF to treat meningitis. Pneumonia caused by a penicillin-resistant strain often still responds to conventional doses of penicillin. Most penicillin-intermediate strains are susceptible to ceftriaxone, cefotaxime, cefepime, and cefpodoxime, but penicillin-resistant pneumococci are often resistant to those cephalosporins as well. One-quarter of pneumococcal isolates in the United States are resistant to macrolides, with particularly high rates among strains that are also resistant to penicillin; doxycycline resistance rates are similar to rates of macrolide resistance. However, >90% of isolates retain sensitivity to clindamycin. The newer quinolones exhibit excellent activity against pneumococci, but resistance is emerging because of the widespread use of these agents.

Pneumonia

- Outpatient treatment: Amoxicillin (1 g q8h) should be effective except against strains highly resistant to penicillin. In those cases, a newer fluoroquinolone (e.g., levofloxacin, 750 mg/d) can be used.
- Inpatient treatment: For strains susceptible or intermediately resistant to penicillin, β-lactam antibiotics are recommended—e.g., penicillin (3–4 mU q4h), ampicillin (1–2 g q6h), or ceftriaxone (1 g q12–24h). Pneumonia that is likely to be due to highly antibiotic-resistant pneumococci should be treated with either vancomycin (1 g q12h) or a quinolone together with a third-generation cephalosporin. Treatment should initially be given by the IV route in most cases, and therapy should continue until at least 5 days after the pt becomes afebrile.

Meningitis

Initial treatment should include ceftriaxone (2 g q12h) plus vancomycin (1 g q12h). Both drugs are used because the cephalosporin is likely to be effective in most cases and penetrates well into the CSF, while vancomycin covers all isolates (including those resistant to penicillin and cephalosporins) but displays unpredictable CSF penetration. If the isolate is susceptible or intermediately resistant to ceftriaxone, vancomycin should be discontinued; if it is resistant to ceftriaxone, both agents should be continued. Treatment for 10 days is recommended. Glucocorticoids should be given before or in conjunction with the first dose of antibiotics.

Endocarditis

Treatment with ceftriaxone and vancomycin, pending susceptibility testing, is indicated. Aminoglycosides can be used for synergy, but rifampin and fluoroquinolones are antagonistic with β-lactam antibiotics against pneumococci.

PREVENTION

Pneumococcal polysaccharide vaccine contains capsular polysaccharide from the 23 most prevalent serotypes of *S. pneumoniae*. One case-control study showed a protection rate of 85% for ≥5 years among persons <55 years of age, but the level and duration of protection decrease with advancing age. Pts at high risk for pneumococcal disease may not respond well to the vaccine. However, because of the safety and low cost of the vaccine, its administration is still recommended. Candidates for the vaccine include pts >2 years of age who are at risk for a serious complication of pneumococcal infection (c.g., asplenic pts; pts >65 years of age; pts with CSF leak, diabetes, alcoholism, cirrhosis, chronic renal insufficiency, chronic pulmonary disease, or advanced cardiovascular disease); pts who have an immunocompromising condition associated with increased risk of pneumococcal disease, such as multiple myeloma or HIV infection; pts who are at genetically increased risk, such as Native Americans and Native Alaskans; and pts who live in environments where outbreaks are likely, such as nursing homes. Recommendations for revaccination are less clear; most experts recommend at least one revaccination 5 years after initial vaccination.

Children <2 years of age should receive the conjugate pneumococcal vaccine, which reduces invasive pneumococcal illness in this age group (and, through a herd effect, in the population as a whole) as well as nasopharyngeal colonization. The conjugate vaccine has also reduced the proportion of cases of pneumococcal disease caused by antibiotic-resistant strains. However, serotypes not contained in the vaccine, which are often antibiotic resistant, have caused an increased number of infections since the commencement of widespread vaccination; this trend is being closely monitored.

For a more detailed discussion, see Musher DM: Pneumococcal Infections, Chap. 128, p. 865, in HPIM-17.

93 Staphylococcal Infections

ETIOLOGY

Staphylococci are gram-positive cocci that form grapelike clusters on Gram's stain and are catalase positive (unlike streptococci), nonmotile, aerobic, and facultatively anaerobic. *Staphylococcus aureus*, which is distinguished from other staphylococci by its production of coagulase, is the most virulent species, causing disease through both toxin-mediated and non-toxin-mediated mechanisms.

S. AUREUS INFECTIONS

Epidemiology   *S. aureus* is a component of the normal human flora, most frequently colonizing the anterior nares but also colonizing the skin (particularly damaged skin), vagina, axilla, perineum, and oropharynx. Of healthy persons, 25–50% may be persistently or transiently colonized with *S. aureus*, and the rate is especially high among insulin-dependent diabetics, HIV-infected persons, injection drug users, hemodialysis pts, and pts with skin damage. Sites of colonization are reservoirs for future infection. *S. aureus* is an important cause of nosocomial as well as community-acquired infections. Methicillin-resistant *S. aureus* (MRSA) is common in hospitals, and its prevalence is increasing dramatically in community settings among individuals without prior medical exposure. In the United States, strain USA300 causes most community-acquired MRSA (CA-MRSA) infections. Outbreaks of CA-MRSA occur among diverse groups, including prisoners, athletes, and drug users. Common risk factors include poor hygienic conditions, close contact, contaminated materials, and damaged skin. CA-MRSA can cause serious disease in immunocompetent individuals.

Pathogenesis   Invasive *S. aureus* Disease   *S. aureus* is a pyogenic pathogen known for its capacity to induce abscess formation. For invasive *S. aureus* infection to occur, some or all of the following steps are necessary.

- Local colonization of tissue surfaces or inoculation directly into tissue—e.g., as a result of minor abrasions or via IV access catheters. The bacteria adhere to different tissue surfaces and can form a biofilm similar to that formed by coagulase-negative staphylococci.
- Invasion: Bacteria replicate at the site of infection and elaborate enzymes that facilitate survival and local spread. CA-MRSA has been linked with the Panton-Valentine leukocidin toxin, which may contribute to more serious infections.
- Evasion of the host response and metastatic spread: *S. aureus* possesses an antiphagocytic polysaccharide microcapsule that facilitates evasion of host defenses and plays a role in abscess formation. In addition, *S. aureus* can survive intracellularly. Recurrences are relatively frequent because the organisms can survive in a quiescent state in various tissues and then cause recrudescent infections when conditions are suitable.

Host Response to *S. aureus* Infection   Polymorphonuclear leukocytes (PMNs) constitute the primary host response to *S. aureus* infection.

Groups at Increased Risk of *S. aureus* Infection   Hosts at increased risk for *S. aureus* infection include those with skin abnormalities, congenital or acquired qualitative or quantitative PMN defects (e.g., neutropenia, chronic granulomatous disease), or indwelling foreign bodies. At-risk populations often have multiple factors that increase susceptibility to *S. aureus* infections. For example, diabetic pts have increased rates of colonization; use injectable insulin, which can introduce the organism into tissue; and may have impaired leukocyte function.

Toxin-Mediated Disease   *S. aureus* produces three types of toxins: cytotoxins, pyrogenic toxins, and exfoliative toxins. Antitoxin antibodies are protective against toxin-mediated staphylococcal illness. Enterotoxins and toxic shock syndrome toxin 1 (TSST-1) act as "superantigens" or T cell mitogens and cause the release of large amounts of inflammatory mediators, producing multisystem disease that includes fever, rash, and hypotension.

Diagnosis   *S. aureus* infections are readily diagnosed by Gram's stain and microscopic examination of infected tissue. The organisms appear as large gram-positive cocci in pairs or clusters. Routine cultures are usually positive. Polymerase chain reaction assays have been developed for rapid testing.

Clinical Syndromes   Skin and Soft Tissue Infections   Predisposing factors include skin disease, skin damage, injections, and poor personal hygiene. These infections are characterized by pus-containing blisters.

- *Folliculitis* involves hair follicles.
- *Furuncles* (boils) extend from follicles to cause true abscesses and more extensive, painful lesions.

- *Carbuncles* are often located in the lower neck, are even more severe and painful, and are due to coalesced lesions extending to deeper SC tissue.
- *Mastitis* occurs in nursing mothers.
- *S. aureus* also causes impetigo, cellulitis, hidradenitis suppurativa, and surgical wound infections (see Chap. 91).

Musculoskeletal Infections

- *S. aureus* is the most common cause of *osteomyelitis* arising from either hematogenous dissemination or contiguous spread from a soft tissue site (e.g., diabetic or vascular ulcers). Hematogenous osteomyelitis in children involves long bones and presents with fever, bone pain, and reluctance to bear weight. Leukocytosis, increased erythrocyte sedimentation rate, and positive blood cultures are typical. Hematogenous osteomyelitis in adults is often vertebral and occurs in pts with endocarditis, pts undergoing hemodialysis, injection drug users, or diabetics. Intense back pain and fever can occur. *Epidural abscess* is a serious complication that can present as trouble voiding or walking or as radicular pain in addition to symptoms of osteomyelitis; neurologic compromise can develop in the absence of timely treatment. Osteomyelitis from contiguous soft tissue infections is suggested by exposure of bone, a draining fistulous tract, failure to heal, or continued drainage.
- *S. aureus* is also the most common cause of *septic arthritis*. *S. aureus* septic arthritis in adults is associated with trauma or surgery or is due to hematogenous dissemination.
- *Pyomyositis*, an infection of skeletal muscles that is seen in tropical climates and in seriously compromised pts (including HIV-infected pts), causes fever, swelling, and pain overlying involved muscle and is usually due to *S. aureus*.

Respiratory Tract Infections

- Infections in newborns and infants: serious infections characterized by fever, dyspnea, and respiratory failure. Pneumatoceles may develop, and pneumothorax and empyema may occur.
- Nosocomial pneumonia: occurs primarily in intubated pts in intensive care units. Clinical presentations resemble those of other nosocomial pneumonias. Pts have an increased volume of purulent sputum, fever, and new pulmonary infiltrates and can develop respiratory distress.
- Community-acquired pneumonia: usually postviral (e.g., after influenza). Pts may present with fever, bloody sputum production, and midlung-field pneumatoceles or multiple patchy pulmonary infiltrates.

Bacteremia and Sepsis   The incidence of metastatic seeding during bacteremia has been estimated to be as high as 31%. Bones, joints, kidneys, and lungs are most commonly infected. Diabetes, HIV infection, and renal insufficiency are often seen in association with *S. aureus* bacteremia and increase the risk of complications.

Infective Endocarditis   (See also Chap. 87) *S. aureus* accounts for 25–35% of cases of bacterial endocarditis. The incidence is increasing as a result of injection drug use, hemodialysis, intravascular prosthetic devices, and immunosuppression. Mortality rates range from 20 to 40% despite the availability of effective antibiotics. There are four clinical settings in which *S. aureus* endocarditis is encountered.

- Right-sided endocarditis in association with injection drug use: Pts have high fever, a toxic appearance, and pleuritic chest pain and produce purulent sputum that is sometimes bloody. Chest x-ray can reveal septic emboli: small, peripheral, circular lesions that may cavitate.

- Left-sided native-valve endocarditis: Compared with pts with right-sided disease, those with left-sided native-valve endocarditis tend to be older, to have a worse prognosis, and to have a higher incidence of complications, including peripheral emboli, cardiac decompensation, and metastatic seeding.
- Prosthetic-valve endocarditis: This infection, which is particularly fulminant if it occurs in the early postoperative period, is associated with a high mortality rate. Valve replacement is usually an urgent priority. Pts are prone to develop valvular insufficiency and myocardial abscesses.
- Nosocomial endocarditis: makes up 15–30% of *S. aureus* endocarditis cases and is related to the increased use of intravascular devices. Pts are often critically ill before the infection, with many comorbid conditions, and the disease can be difficult to recognize.

Urinary Tract Infections (UTIs) UTIs are infrequently caused by *S. aureus*. Unlike UTIs caused by other urinary pathogens, those caused by *S. aureus* are most often due to hematogenous dissemination.

Prosthetic Device–Related Infections In contrast with coagulase-negative staphylococci, *S. aureus* causes more acute disease with localized and systemic manifestations that tend to be rapidly progressive. Successful treatment usually involves removal of the prosthetic device.

Community-Acquired MRSA Infections CA-MRSA infections can have many unusual presentations (e.g., necrotizing fasciitis, necrotic pneumonia, sepsis, purpura fulminans) that reflect the increased virulence of CA-MRSA strains.

Toxin-Mediated Disease

- Toxic shock syndrome (TSS): Pts with staphylococcal TSS may not have a clinically evident staphylococcal infection. TSS results from elaboration of an enterotoxin (many nonmenstrual TSS cases) or TSST-1 (some nonmenstrual cases and >90% of menstrual cases). Menstrual cases occur 2–3 days after menses begin. Diagnosis is based on a constellation of clinical findings. The case definition includes a fever ≥38.9°C (≥102°F); hypotension; a diffuse macular rash that involves the palms and soles, with subsequent desquamation 1–2 weeks after disease onset; multisystem involvement—e.g., hepatic (bilirubin or aminotransferase levels ≥2 times normal), hematologic (platelet count ≤100,000/µL), renal (blood urea nitrogen or creatinine ≥2 times normal), mucous membrane (vaginal, oropharyngeal, or conjunctival hyperemia), GI (vomiting or diarrhea at the onset of illness), muscular (myalgias or serum creatine phosphokinase ≥2 times normal), or central nervous (disorientation or altered consciousness without focal findings); and no evidence of other illnesses.
- Food poisoning: results from inoculation of toxin-producing *S. aureus* into food by colonized food handlers. Toxin is then elaborated in growth-promoting foods, such as custard, potato salad, or processed meat. The heat-stable toxin is not destroyed even if heating kills the bacteria. Disease onset is rapid and explosive, occurring within 1–6 h of ingestion of contaminated food. The chief signs and symptoms are nausea and vomiting, but diarrhea, hypotension, and dehydration may occur. Fever is absent. Symptoms resolve within 8–10 h.
- Staphylococcal scalded-skin syndrome (SSSS): most often affects newborns and children. Disease ranges from localized blisters to exfoliation of most of the skin surface. The skin is fragile, with tender, thick-walled, fluid-filled bullae. Nikolsky's sign is diagnosed when gentle pressure of bullae causes rupture of lesions and leaves denuded underlying skin.

Prevention   Hand washing and careful attention to appropriate isolation procedures prevent the spread of *S. aureus* infection. Mupirocin treatment to eliminate nasal carriage of *S. aureus* has reduced rates of infection among hemodialysis and peritoneal dialysis pts. Reduction in rates of wound infection among pts undergoing surgery is less evident.

INFECTIONS CAUSED BY COAGULASE-NEGATIVE STAPHYLOCOCCI (CoNS)

CoNS are less virulent than *S. aureus* but are important and common causes of prosthetic-device infections. Of CoNS species, *S. epidermidis* most often causes disease. This organism is a normal component of the skin, oropharyngeal, and vaginal flora. *S. saprophyticus* is a cause of UTIs. Two other species of CoNS, *S. lugdunensis* and *S. schleiferi*, are more virulent and cause serious infections such as native-valve endocarditis and osteomyelitis.

Pathogenesis   CoNS are uniquely adapted to cause prosthetic-device infections because they can elaborate extracellular polysaccharide (glycocalyx or slime) that forms a biofilm on the device surface, protecting bacteria from host defenses as well as from antibiotic treatment while allowing bacterial survival.

Clinical Syndromes   CoNS cause diverse prosthetic device–related infections. Signs of localized infection are usually subtle, disease progression is slow, and systemic findings are limited. Fever and mild leukocytosis may be documented. Infections not associated with prosthetic devices are infrequent, but up to 5% of native-valve endocarditis cases have been due to CoNS in some series.

Diagnosis   CoNS are readily detected by standard methods, but distinguishing infection from colonization is often problematic because CoNS are common contaminants of cultures of blood and other sites.

℞ Staphylococcal Infections

Suppurative collections should be surgically drained. The emergence of CA-MRSA has increased the importance of culturing material from all collections to identify the pathogen and determine its antimicrobial susceptibility. In most cases of prosthetic-device infection, the device should be removed, although some CoNS infections can be managed medically. Antibiotic therapy for *S. aureus* infection is generally prolonged (i.e., 4–8 weeks), particularly if blood cultures remain positive 48–96 h after initiation of therapy, if the infection was acquired in the community, if a removable focus of infection is not removed, or if cutaneous or embolic manifestations of infection occur. Antimicrobial therapy for serious *S. aureus* infections is summarized in Table 93-1. Penicillinase-resistant penicillins, such as nafcillin or first-generation cephalosporins, are highly effective against penicillin-resistant strains. The incidence of MRSA is high in hospital settings, and strains intermediately or fully resistant to vancomycin have been described. In general, vancomycin is less bactericidal than the β-lactams and should be used only when absolutely indicated. Among newer antistaphylococcal agents, quinupristin/dalfopristin is typically bactericidal but is only bacteriostatic against isolates resistant to erythromycin or clindamycin; linezolid is bacteriostatic and has not yet been established as efficacious in deep-seated infections such as osteomyelitis; and daptomycin is bactericidal. Tigecycline, a broad-spectrum minocycline analogue, has bacteriostatic activity against MRSA. Other alternatives include the quinolones, but resistance to these drugs is increasing, especially among MRSA strains. Trimethoprim-sulfamethoxazole (TMP-SMX) and minocycline have been successfully used to

TABLE 93-1 ANTIMICROBIAL THERAPY FOR SERIOUS STAPHYLOCOCCAL INFECTIONS[a]

Sensitivity/Resistance of Isolate	Drug of Choice	Alternative(s)	Comments
Sensitive to penicillin	Penicillin G (4 mU q4h)	Nafcillin (2 g q4h) or oxacillin (2 g q4h), cefazolin (2 g q8h), vancomycin (1 g q12h[b])	Fewer than 5% of isolates are sensitive to penicillin.
Sensitive to methicillin	Nafcillin or oxacillin (2 g q4h)	Cefazolin (2 g q8h[b]), vancomycin (1 g q12h[b])	Patients with penicillin allergy can be treated with a cephalosporin if the allergy does not involve an anaphylactic or accelerated reaction; vancomycin is the alternative. Desensitization to β-lactams may be indicated in selected cases of serious infection where maximal bactericidal activity is needed (e.g., prosthetic-valve endocarditis[c]). Type A β-lactamase may rapidly hydrolyze cefazolin and reduce its efficacy in endocarditis.
Resistant to methicillin	Vancomycin (1 g q12h[b])	TMP-SMX (TMP, 5 mg/kg q12h[b]), minocycline or doxycycline (100 mg PO q12h[b]), ciprofloxacin (400 mg q12h[b]), levofloxacin (500 mg q24h[b]), quinupristin/dalfopristin (7.5 mg/kg q8h), linezolid (600 mg q12h except: 400 mg q12h for uncomplicated skin infections); daptomycin (4-6 mg/kg q24h[b,d]) for bacteremia, endocarditis, and complicated skin infections; tigecycline (100 mg IV once, then 50 mg q12h) for skin and soft tissue infections; investigational drugs: oritavancin, dalbavancin, telavancin	Sensitivity testing is necessary before an alternative drug is used. Adjunctive drugs (those that should be used only in combination with other antimicrobial agents) include gentamicin (1 mg/kg q8h[b]), rifampin (300 mg PO q8h), and fusidic acid (500 mg q8h; not readily available in the United States). Quinupristin/dalfopristin is bactericidal against methicillin-resistant isolates unless the strain is resistant to erythromycin or clindamycin. The newer quinolones may retain in vitro activity against ciprofloxacin-resistant isolates; resistance may develop during therapy. The efficacy of adjunctive therapy is not well established in many settings. Both linezolid and quinupristin/dalfopristin have had in vitro activity against most VISA and VRSA strains. See footnote for treatment of prosthetic-valve endocarditis.[c]

| Resistant to methicillin with intermediate or complete resistance to vancomycin[e] | Uncertain | Same as for methicillin-resistant strains; check antibiotic susceptibilities | Same as for methicillin-resistant strains; check antibiotic susceptibilities |
| Not yet known (i.e., empirical therapy) | Vancomycin (1 g q12h) | — | Empirical therapy is given when the susceptibility of the isolate is not known. Vancomycin with or without an aminoglycoside is recommended for suspected community- or hospital-acquired *S. aureus* infections because of the increased frequency of methicillin-resistant strains in the community. |

[a]Recommended dosages are for adults with normal renal and hepatic function. The route of administration is IV unless otherwise indicated.

[b]The dosage must be adjusted in patients with reduced creatinine clearance.

[c]For the treatment of prosthetic-valve endocarditis, the addition of gentamicin (1 mg/kg q8h) and rifampin (300 mg PO q8h) is recommended, with adjustment of the gentamicin dosage if the creatinine clearance rate is reduced.

[d]Daptomycin cannot be used for pneumonia.

[e]Vancomycin-resistant *S. aureus* isolates from clinical infections have been reported.

Note: TMP-SMX, trimethoprim-sulfamethoxazole; VISA, vancomycin-intermediate *S. aureus*; VRSA, vancomycin-resistant *S. aureus*.

Source: Modified with permission of the *New England Journal of Medicine* (Lowy, 1998).

treat MRSA infections in cases of vancomycin toxicity or intolerance. Synergy has been demonstrated for certain antimicrobial combinations: β-lactams and aminoglycosides; vancomycin and gentamicin; vancomycin, gentamicin, and rifampin (against CoNS); and vancomycin and rifampin.

Special considerations for treatment include:

- Uncomplicated skin and soft tissue infections: Oral agents are usually adequate.
- Native-valve endocarditis: A β-lactam for 6 weeks plus gentamicin (1 mg/kg every 8 h) for 3–5 days. (Addition of gentamicin does not alter clinical outcome but reduces the duration of bacteremia.) If infection is due to MRSA, vancomycin (1 g every 12 h) is recommended. Treatment should continue for 6 weeks.
- Prosthetic-valve endocarditis: Surgery is often needed in addition to antibiotics. A β-lactam (or vancomycin if MRSA is involved) with gentamicin and rifampin is indicated.
- Hematogenous osteomyelitis or septic arthritis: A 4-week treatment course is adequate for children, but adults require longer courses. Joint infections require repeated aspiration or arthroscopy to prevent damage from inflammatory cells.
- Chronic osteomyelitis: Surgical debridement is needed in most cases.
- Prosthetic-joint infections: Ciprofloxacin and rifampin have been used successfully in combination, particularly when the prosthesis cannot be removed.
- CA-MRSA infections: Initiation of appropriate empirical therapy is important in skin and soft tissue infections due to CA-MRSA. Oral agents effective against these isolates include clindamycin, TMP-SMX, doxycycline, and linezolid. Susceptibility varies in different geographic regions.
- TSS: Supportive therapy and removal of tampons or other packing material or debridement of an infected site are most important. The role of antibiotics is less clear, but a clindamycin/semisynthetic penicillin combination is recommended. Clindamycin is used because it is a protein synthesis inhibitor and has been shown to decrease toxin synthesis in vitro. IV immunoglobulin may be helpful. The role of glucocorticoids is uncertain.

For a more detailed discussion, see Lowy FD: Staphylococcal Infections, Chap. 129, p. 872, in HPIM-17.

---

94 Streptococcal/Enterococcal Infections, Diphtheria, and Other Infections Caused by Corynebacteria and Related Species

STREPTOCOCCAL/ENTEROCOCCAL INFECTIONS

Streptococci and enterococci are part of the normal human flora, colonizing the respiratory, GI, and genitourinary tracts. These gram-positive cocci form chains when grown in liquid media. Culture on blood agar reveals three hemolytic patterns.

- β-Hemolysis: complete hemolysis around a colony. This pattern is seen with streptococci of Lancefield groups A, B, C, and G. Lancefield grouping is based on cell-wall carbohydrate antigens.
- α-Hemolysis: partial hemolysis imparting a greenish appearance to agar. This pattern is seen with *S. pneumoniae* and viridans streptococci.
- γ-Hemolysis: no hemolysis. This pattern is typical of enterococci, *S. bovis*, and anaerobic streptococci.

GROUP A *STREPTOCOCCUS* (GAS)

Etiology and Pathogenesis GAS causes suppurative infections and is associated with postinfectious syndromes such as acute rheumatic fever (ARF) and poststreptococcal glomerulonephritis (PSGN). Worldwide, GAS contributes to ~500,000 deaths per year. The major surface protein, M protein, and the hyaluronic acid polysaccharide capsule protect against phagocytic ingestion and killing. GAS produces a large number of extracellular products that may contribute to local and systemic toxicity; these include streptolysins S and O, streptokinase, DNases, and pyrogenic toxins that cause the rash of scarlet fever and contribute to the pathogenesis of toxic shock syndrome (TSS) and necrotizing fasciitis.

Clinical Features **Pharyngitis** GAS accounts for 20–40% of all cases of exudative pharyngitis in children >3 years of age. Respiratory droplets spread infection. After an incubation period of 1–4 days, pts develop sore throat, fever, chills, malaise, and GI manifestations. Examination reveals an erythematous pharyngeal mucosa, swelling, purulent exudates over the posterior pharynx and tonsillar pillars, and tender anterior cervical adenopathy. Viral pharyngitis is the more likely diagnosis when patients have coryza, hoarseness, conjunctivitis, or mucosal ulcers. Rapid diagnosis by latex agglutination or enzyme immunoassay is variably sensitive but highly specific. Throat culture is the gold standard for diagnosis. Serologic tests (e.g., antistreptolysin O) confirm past infection in pts with suspected ARF but are not useful for the acute diagnosis of pharyngitis. Symptoms resolve spontaneously in most pts after 3–5 days.

℞ Group A Streptococcal Pharyngitis

The primary goal of treatment is to prevent suppurative complications (e.g., lymphadenitis, abscess, sinusitis, bacteremia, pneumonia) and ARF; therapy does not seem to prevent PSGN. See Table 94-1 for recommended treatments. Macrolides such as erythromycin may be used, but resistance to these agents is increasing. Asymptomatic pharyngeal GAS carriage usually is not treated; however, when the pt is the source of infection in others, penicillin V (500 mg qid for 10 days) with rifampin (600 mg bid for the final 4 days) is used.

Scarlet Fever Scarlet fever is the designation for GAS pharyngitis associated with a characteristic rash. The rash typically appears in the first 2 days of illness over the upper trunk and spreads to the extremities but not to the palms and soles. The skin has a sandpaper feel. Other findings include strawberry tongue (enlarged papillae on a coated tongue) and Pastia's lines (accentuation of rash in skin folds). Rash improves in 6–9 days with desquamation on palms and soles. Scarlet fever is much less common than in the past.

Skin and Soft Tissue Infections See Chap. 91 for further discussion of clinical manifestations and treatment.

TABLE 94-1 TREATMENT OF GROUP A STREPTOCOCCAL INFECTIONS

Infection	Treatment[a]
Pharyngitis	Benzathine penicillin G, 1.2 mU IM; *or* penicillin V, 250 mg PO tid or 500 mg PO bid × 10 days (Children <27 kg: Benzathine penicillin G, 600,000 units IM; *or* penicillin V, 250 mg PO bid or tid × 10 days)
Impetigo	Same as pharyngitis
Erysipelas/cellulitis	Severe: Penicillin G, 1–2 mU IV q4h Mild to moderate: Procaine penicillin, 1.2 mU IM bid
Necrotizing fasciitis/ myositis	Surgical debridement; *plus* penicillin G, 2–4 mU IV q4h; *plus* clindamycin,[b] 600–900 mg q8h
Pneumonia/empyema	Penicillin G, 2–4 mU IV q4h; *plus* drainage of empyema
Streptococcal toxic shock syndrome	Penicillin G, 2–4 mU IV q4h; *plus* clindamycin,[b] 600–900 mg q8h; *plus* intravenous immunoglobulin,[b] 2 g/kg as a single dose

[a]Penicillin allergy: Erythromycin (10 mg/kg PO qid up to a maximum of 250 mg per dose) may be substituted for oral penicillin. Alternative agents for parenteral therapy include first-generation cephalosporins—if the nature of the allergy is not an immediate hypersensitivity reaction (anaphylaxis or urticaria) or another potentially life-threatening manifestation (e.g., severe rash and fever)—or vancomycin.
[b]Efficacy unproven, but recommended by several experts.

1. *Impetigo*: A superficial skin infection, impetigo is also occasionally caused by *Staphylococcus aureus*. The disease is most often seen in young children in warmer months or climates and under poor hygienic conditions. The facial areas around the nose and mouth and the legs are the sites most commonly involved. Red papular lesions evolve into pustules that crust. Pts are usually afebrile. For treatment, see Table 94-1. Empirical antibiotic therapy should cover GAS and *S. aureus*; thus dicloxacillin or cephalexin (250 mg qid for 10 days) is used. Topical mupirocin ointment is also effective. GAS impetigo is associated with PSGN.
2. *Cellulitis*: GAS cellulitis develops at anatomic sites where normal lymphatic drainage has been disrupted (e.g., areas of prior cellulitis, the ipsilateral arm after mastectomy and axillary node dissection). Organisms may enter at sites distant from the area of cellulitis where there is a breach of skin integrity. GAS may cause rapidly developing postoperative wound infection. *Erysipelas*, a form of cellulitis that usually involves the malar facial area or the lower extremities, is caused almost exclusively by GAS. Pts experience an acute onset of bright red swelling that is sharply demarcated from normal skin as well as pain and fever. The illness develops over hours, and blebs or bullae may form after 2 or 3 days. Empirical treatment for cellulitis is directed against GAS and *S. aureus*. For treatment of erysipelas or cellulitis known to be due to GAS, see Table 94-1.
3. *Necrotizing fasciitis*: GAS causes ~60% of cases of necrotizing fasciitis. For treatment, see Table 94-1.

Pneumonia and Empyema GAS occasionally causes pneumonia. The onset can be gradual or abrupt. Pts have pleuritic chest pain, fever, chills, and dyspnea; ~50% have accompanying pleural effusions that are almost always infected and should be drained quickly to avoid loculation. For treatment, see Table 94-1.

Bacteremia In most cases of bacteremia, a focus is readily identifiable. Bacteremia occurs occasionally with cellulitis and frequently with necrotizing fascii-

TABLE 94-2	PROPOSED CASE DEFINITION FOR THE STREPTOCOCCAL TOXIC SHOCK SYNDROME[a]

I. Isolation of group A streptococci (*Streptococcus pyogenes*)
   A. From a normally sterile site
   B. From a nonsterile site
II. Clinical signs of severity
   A. Hypotension *and*
   B. ≥2 of the following signs:
      1. Renal impairment
      2. Coagulopathy
      3. Liver function impairment
      4. Adult respiratory distress syndrome
      5. A generalized erythematous macular rash that may desquamate
      6. Soft tissue necrosis, including necrotizing fasciitis or myositis; *or* gangrene

[a]An illness fulfilling criteria IA, IIA, and IIB is defined as a *definite* case. An illness fulfilling criteria IB, IIA, and IIB is defined as a *probable* case if no other etiology for the illness is identified.
Source: Modified from Working Group on Severe Streptococcal Infections, JAMA 269:390, 1993.

tis. If no focus is evident, a diagnosis of endocarditis, occult abscess, or osteomyelitis should be considered.

Puerperal Sepsis   Common in the preantibiotic era, puerperal sepsis is now rare. Outbreaks are associated with asymptomatic carriage of GAS by delivery room personnel.

Toxic Shock Syndrome   Table 94-2 presents a proposed case definition for streptococcal TSS. Unlike TSS due to *S. aureus*, streptococcal TSS includes bacteremia in most pts, does not usually cause the development of a rash, and commonly includes a soft tissue infection (cellulitis, necrotizing fasciitis, or myositis). The mortality rate for streptococcal TSS is ~30%, with most deaths due to shock and respiratory failure. For treatment, see Table 94-1.

Prevention   Household contacts of individuals with invasive GAS infection are at increased risk of infection; asymptomatic colonization with GAS is detected in up to 25% of persons with >4 h/d of same-room exposure to an index case. However, antibiotic prophylaxis is not routinely recommended.

STREPTOCOCCI OF GROUPS C AND G

Streptococci of groups C and G cause infections similar to those caused by GAS. Strains that form small colonies on blood agar (<0.5 mm) are generally of the *S. milleri* group; large-colony group C and G streptococci are now considered a single species. These organisms cause cellulitis, bacteremia, and septic arthritis. Bacteremia occurs more frequently in elderly or chronically ill pts. Some distinct zoonotic group C species can also cause human infection. Treatment is the same as for GAS infection. Bacteremia or septic arthritis should be treated with penicillin (2–4 mU IV every 4 h). Although it has not been shown to be superior, gentamicin (1 mg/kg every 8 h) is recommended by some experts for endocarditis or septic arthritis due to group C or G streptococci because of a poor clinical response to penicillin alone. Joint infections can require repeated aspiration or open drainage for cure.

GROUP B *STREPTOCOCCUS* (GBS)

GBS is a major cause of meningitis and sepsis in neonates and a frequent cause of peripartum fever in women.

Neonatal Infection *Early-onset infection* occurs within the first week of life (median age, 20 h). The infection is acquired within the maternal genital tract during birth. Neonates have respiratory distress, lethargy, hypotension, bacteremia, pneumonia (one-third to one-half of cases), and meningitis (one-third of cases).

Late-onset infection develops between 1 week and 3 months of age (mean age, 3–4 weeks). Meningitis is the most common manifestation. Infants are lethargic, febrile, and irritable; feed poorly; and may have seizures.

R_x Group B Streptococcal Infections in Neonates

Penicillin or ampicillin is the agent of choice for GBS infections and is administered with gentamicin while cultures are pending. Pts with bacteremia or soft tissue infection should receive penicillin at a dosage of 200,000 units/kg per day in divided doses; those with meningitis should receive 400,000 units/kg per day in divided doses for 14 days. Many physicians continue to give gentamicin until the pt improves clinically.

Prevention About half of the infants delivered vaginally to mothers colonized with GBS (5–40% of women) become colonized, but only 1–2% develop infection. With maternal colonization, the risk of neonatal GBS infection is high if delivery is preterm or if the mother has an early rupture of membranes (>24 h before delivery), prolonged labor, fever, or chorioamnionitis. Identification of high-risk mothers and prophylactic administration of ampicillin or penicillin during delivery reduce the risk of neonatal infection. Screening for anogenital colonization with GBS at 35–37 weeks of pregnancy is currently recommended. Women who have previously given birth to an infant with GBS disease, who have a history of GBS bacteriuria during pregnancy, or who have an unknown culture status but risk factors noted above should receive intrapartum prophylaxis (usually 5 mU of penicillin G followed by 2.5 mU every 4 h until delivery). Cefazolin can be used as well. If the mother is at risk for anaphylaxis and the GBS isolate is known to be susceptible, clindamycin or erythromycin can be used; otherwise, vancomycin is indicated.

Adult Infection Most GBS infections in adults are related to pregnancy and parturition. Other GBS infections are seen in the elderly, especially those with underlying conditions such as diabetes mellitus or cancer. Cellulitis and soft tissue infection, urinary tract infection (UTI), pneumonia, endocarditis, and septic arthritis are most common. Penicillin (12 mU/d for localized infections and 18–24 mU/d for endocarditis or meningitis, in divided doses) is recommended. Vancomycin is an acceptable alternative for penicillin-allergic pts. Relapse or recurrent invasive infection occurs in ~4% of cases.

ENTEROCOCCI AND NONENTEROCOCCAL GROUP D STREPTOCOCCI

Enterococci **Epidemiology** *E. faecalis* and *E. faecium* are significant pathogens that tend to produce infection in elderly or debilitated pts and in those whose mucosal or epithelial barriers are disrupted or whose normal flora is perturbed by antibiotic treatment.

Clinical Features Enterococci cause UTIs, especially in pts who have received antibiotics or have undergone instrumentation; bacteremia related to intravascular catheters; bacterial endocarditis of both native and prosthetic valves (10–20% of cases, usually with a subacute presentation but sometimes with an acute presentation and rapidly progressive valve destruction); biliary tract infections; and mixed infections, including those arising from bowel flora (e.g., abdominal surgical wounds and diabetic foot ulcers).

℞ Enterococcal Infections

Therapy is complicated by the fact that penicillin alone does not reliably kill enterococci except in UTIs as well as by increasing drug resistance.

- Endocarditis and meningitis: penicillin (3–4 mU every 4 h) or ampicillin (2 g every 4 h) *plus* gentamicin (1 mg/kg every 8 h) for 4–6 weeks. Vancomycin may be substituted in penicillin-allergic pts.
- Gentamicin resistance (minimum inhibitory concentration > 2000 μg/mL) is increasingly common. If gentamicin-resistant strains are susceptible to streptomycin, the latter agent should be substituted.
- Penicillin or ampicillin resistance: If resistance is due to β-lactamase production, then β-lactam/β-lactamase inhibitor combinations, carbapenems (e.g., imipenem), or vancomycin may be used along with gentamicin.
- Vancomycin and penicillin resistance: Quinupristin/dalfopristin is effective against *E. faecium* with this resistance pattern. Linezolid, daptomycin, and tigecycline have activity against *E. faecalis* and *E. faecium* with such resistance.

Other Group D Streptococci *S. bovis* has been associated with GI malignancies and other bowel lesions, which are found in ≥60% of pts presenting with *S. bovis* endocarditis. Penicillin alone constitutes adequate therapy.

VIRIDANS STREPTOCOCCI

Many viridans streptococcal species are part of the normal oral flora, residing in close association with the teeth and gingiva. Minor trauma such as flossing or brushing teeth can cause transient bacteremia. Viridans streptococci have a predilection to cause endocarditis. Moreover, they are often part of a mixed flora in sinus infections and brain and liver abscesses. Bacteremia is common in neutropenic pts, who can develop a sepsis syndrome with high fever and shock. Risk factors in these pts include trimethoprim-sulfamethoxazole (TMP-SMX) or fluoroquinolone prophylaxis, mucositis, or antacid or histamine-antagonist therapy. *S. milleri* (also known as *S. intermedius* or *S. anginosus*) differs from other viridans streptococci in both hemolytic pattern and clinical syndromes; this organism commonly causes suppurative infections, especially abscesses of brain and viscera, as well as respiratory tract infections such as pneumonia, empyema, and lung abscess. Neutropenic pts should receive vancomycin pending susceptibility testing; other pts may be treated with penicillin.

ABIOTROPHIA SPECIES (NUTRITIONALLY VARIANT STREPTOCOCCI)

The organisms formerly known as nutritionally variant streptococci are now classified as the separate genus *Abiotrophia*. These fastidious organisms require media that are enriched (e.g., with vitamin B_6) for growth. They are associated with more frequent treatment failure and relapse in cases of endocarditis than are viridans streptococci. Addition of gentamicin (1 mg/kg every 8 h) to the penicillin regimen is recommended when *Abiotrophia* is present.

DIPHTHERIA

Definition Diphtheria is a nasopharyngeal and skin infection caused by *Corynebacterium diphtheriae*. Some strains produce diphtheria toxin, which can cause myocarditis, polyneuropathy, and other systemic toxicities. The toxin is associated with the formation of pseudomembranes in the pharynx during respiratory infection.

Etiology   *C. diphtheriae* is a club-shaped, gram-positive, unencapsulated, non-motile, nonsporulating rod. The bacteria often form clusters of parallel arrays (palisades) in culture, referred to as Chinese characters.

Epidemiology   *C. diphtheriae* is transmitted via the aerosol route, primarily during close contact. Fewer than five cases due to routine immunization are diagnosed per year in the United States. Disease in the United States occurs in elderly and alcoholic individuals—often those of low socioeconomic status—as well as in Native Americans.

Clinical Features   Respiratory Diphtheria   Upper respiratory tract illness due to *C. diphtheriae* typically has a 2- to 5-day incubation period. Clinical diagnosis is based on the constellation of sore throat; low-grade fever; and a tonsillar, pharyngeal, or nasal pseudomembrane. Unlike that of GAS pharyngitis, the pseudomembrane of diphtheria is tightly adherent; dislodging the membrane usually causes bleeding. Occasionally, weakness, dysphagia, headache, and voice change are the initial manifestations. Massive swelling of the tonsils and "bull-neck" diphtheria resulting from submandibular and paratracheal edema can develop. This illness is further characterized by foul breath, thick speech, and stridorous breathing.

Complications

- Respiratory tract obstruction due to swelling and sloughing of pseudomembrane
- Myocarditis (dysrhythmia, dilated cardiomyopathy) is seen in almost one-quarter of hospitalized pts; those who die usually do so within 4 or 5 days.
- Neurologic manifestations may appear during the first 2 weeks of illness. They begin with dysphagia and nasal dysarthria and progress to cranial nerve involvement, including weakness of the tongue and facial numbness. Respiratory and abdominal muscle weakness may follow. Several weeks later, a generalized sensorimotor polyneuropathy with prominent autonomic dysfunction (including hypotension) may occur. Most survivors improve gradually.

Diagnosis   A definitive diagnosis is based on compatible clinical findings and isolation of *C. diphtheriae* from local lesions or its identification by histopathology. Nonselective media and appropriate selective media must be used.

℞ Diphtheria

Diphtheria antitoxin is the most important component of treatment and should be given as soon as possible. Because antitoxin is produced in horses, current protocol includes a test dose to rule out immediate-type hypersensitivity. Pts who exhibit hypersensitivity should be desensitized before receiving a full dose. To obtain antitoxin, contact the National Immunization Program at the CDC (404-639-8257 during the day; 770-488-7100 at other times). See *www.cdc.gov/nip/vaccine/dat/default.htm* for further information. Treatment to prevent transmission to contacts is administered for 14 days; the recommended options are (1) procaine penicillin G (600,000 U IM every 12 h in adults; 12,500–25,000 U/kg IM every 12 h in children) until the pt can take oral penicillin V (125–250 mg qid); or (2) erythromycin (500 mg IV every 6 h in adults; 40–50 mg/kg per day IV in 2–4 divided doses in children) until the pt can take oral erythromycin (500 mg qid). Rifampin and clindamycin are other options. Cultures should document eradication of the organism 1 and 14 days after completion of antibiotic therapy. Supportive care and isolation should be instituted.

Prognosis Risk factors for death include bull-neck diphtheria, myocarditis with ventricular tachycardia, atrial fibrillation, complete heart block, an age of >60 years or <6 months, alcoholism, extensive pseudomembrane elongation, and laryngeal, tracheal, or bronchial involvement. The interval between onset of local disease and antitoxin administration also predicts outcome.

Prevention DTaP (diphtheria and tetanus toxoids and acellular pertussis vaccine adsorbed) is recommended for primary immunization of children up to age 7 years. Tdap (tetanus toxoid with reduced diphtheria toxoid and acellular pertussis) is recommended as the booster vaccine for children 11–12 years old and as the catch-up vaccine for children 7–10 and 13–18 years old. Td (tetanus and diphtheria toxoids) is recommended for routine booster use in adults at 10-year intervals or for tetanus-prone wounds. When >10 years have elapsed since the last Td dose, adults 19–64 years old should receive a single dose of Tdap. Close contacts of pts with respiratory diphtheria should have throat specimens cultured for *C. diphtheriae*, should receive a 7- to 10-day course of oral erythromycin or one dose of benzathine penicillin (1.2 mU for persons ≥6 years old; 600,000 U for children <6 years old), and should receive vaccine if immunization status is uncertain.

INFECTIONS WITH OTHER CORYNEBACTERIA AND RELATED ORGANISMS

Nondiphtherial *Corynebacterium* species and related organisms are common components of the normal human flora. Although frequently considered contaminants, these bacteria are associated with invasive disease in immunocompromised hosts.

- *C. ulcerans* infection is a zoonosis that causes diphtheria-like illness and requires similar treatment.
- *C. jeikeium* colonizes pts with cancer or severe immunodeficiency and can cause severe sepsis, endocarditis, device-related infections, pneumonia, and soft tissue infections. Treatment consists of removal of the source of infection and administration of vancomycin.
- *C. urealyticum* is a cause of nosocomial UTI and sepsis. Vancomycin is an effective therapeutic agent.
- *Rhodococcus* causes tuberculosis-like infections with granulomatous pathology in immunocompromised hosts, often occurring in conjunction with HIV infection. Vancomycin, macrolides, clindamycin, rifampin, and TMP-SMX have been used to treat these infections.
- *Arcanobacterium haemolyticum* can cause pharyngitis and chronic skin ulcers, often in association with a scarlatiniform rash similar to that caused by GAS. The organism is susceptible to β-lactam agents, macrolides, fluoroquinolones, clindamycin, vancomycin, and doxycycline. Penicillin failures have occurred.

For a more detailed discussion, see Wessels MR: Streptococcal and Enterococcal Infections, Chap. 130, p. 881; and Bishai WR, Murphy JR: Diphtheria and Other Infections Caused by Corynebacteria and Related Species, Chap. 131, p. 890, in HPIM-17.

95 Meningococcal and Listerial Infections

MENINGOCOCCAL INFECTIONS

Etiology and Epidemiology *Neisseria meningitidis* (the meningococcus) causes two life-threatening diseases: meningitis and fulminant meningococcemia. Meningococci are gram-negative aerobic diplococci with a polysaccharide capsule. Five serogroups—A, B, C, Y, and W-135—account for >90% of the 300,000–500,000 cases of meningococcal disease that occur worldwide each year. Serogroup A causes recurrent epidemics in sub-Saharan Africa. In the United States, serogroup B causes most sporadic disease, serogroup C causes most outbreaks, and serogroup Y is becoming more prevalent, particularly among older pts and pts with underlying chronic disease. Rates of meningococcal disease are highest among infants and children; a second peak in teenagers is due to residence in barracks, dormitories, or other crowded situations. Meningococci are transmitted via respiratory secretions. Colonization of the nasopharynx or pharynx can persist asymptomatically for months. In nonepidemic situations, 10% of the population is colonized. Household contact with a meningococcal disease pt or a meningococcal carrier, household or institutional crowding, exposure to tobacco smoke, and a recent viral upper respiratory infection are risk factors for colonization and invasive disease.

Pathogenesis Meningococci colonize the upper respiratory tract, are internalized by nonciliated mucosal cells, enter the submucosa, and reach the bloodstream. If bacterial multiplication is slow, the bacteria may seed local sites such as the meninges. If multiplication is rapid, meningococcemia develops. Morbidity and mortality from meningococcemia have been directly correlated with the amount of circulating endotoxin, which can be 10- to 1000-fold higher than levels seen in other gram-negative bacteremias. Deficiencies in antithrombin and proteins C and S can occur during meningococcal disease, and there is a strong negative correlation between protein C activity and mortality risk. Antibodies to serogroup-specific capsular polysaccharide constitute the major host defense. Protective antibodies are induced by colonization with nonpathogenic bacteria possessing cross-reactive antigens. Deficiency of late complement components C5–C9 can result in recurrent infections.

Clinical Features

- Respiratory tract disease that is clinically apparent is most common among adults. Serogroup Y causes pneumonia, particularly often in military populations.
- Meningococcemia without meningitis occurs in ~10–30% of pts with meningococcal disease. Clinical manifestations include the following.

  1. Fever, chills, nausea, vomiting, myalgias, prostration
  2. Rash: erythematous macules, primarily on the trunk and extremities, that become petechial and—in severe cases—purpuric and may coalesce into hemorrhagic bullae that necrose and ulcerate
  3. Fulminant disease is associated with hemorrhagic skin lesions and disseminated intravascular coagulation (DIC) and is perhaps the most rapidly fatal form of septic shock in humans. Waterhouse-Friderichsen syndrome

consists of DIC-induced microthrombosis, hemorrhage, tissue injury, and adrenal insufficiency.
4. Long-term morbidity includes loss of skin, limbs, or digits from ischemic necrosis and infarction.
5. Chronic meningococcemia is a rare syndrome of episodic fever, rash, and arthralgias lasting for weeks to months. If treated with steroids, this condition may become fulminant or evolve into meningitis.

- Meningitis pts usually present after >24 h of illness with headache, nausea and vomiting, neck stiffness, lethargy, and confusion. Petechial or purpuric skin lesions help distinguish this form of bacterial meningitis from other types. Cerebrospinal fluid (CSF) examination reveals an increased protein concentration, a low glucose level, and neutrophilic leukocytosis. Sequelae include mental retardation, deafness, and hemiparesis.
- Arthritis occurs in ~10% of pts with meningococcal disease.

Diagnosis Definitive diagnosis relies on isolation of the organism from normally sterile body fluids. Gram's staining of CSF yields positive results in ~85% of pts with meningococcal meningitis; if results are positive in the absence of CSF leukocytosis, the prognosis is poor. Polymerase chain reaction tests on buffy coat or CSF are more sensitive than Gram's staining or latex agglutination tests for meningococcal polysaccharides and are unaffected by prior antibiotic therapy.

Rx Meningococcal Infections

See Table 95-1. Glucocorticoid therapy (10 mg IV 15 min before the first antibiotic dose and then q6h for 4 days) is controversial, but many experts recommend it. Pts with fulminant meningococcemia need aggressive supportive therapy that can include vigorous fluid resuscitation, elective ventilation, pressor agents, fresh-frozen plasma (in pts with abnormal clotting parameters), and supplemental glucocorticoid treatment (hydrocortisone, 1 mg/kg every 6 h) for impaired adrenal reserve. Activated protein C (24 µg/kg per hour in a continuous infusion for 96 h) is recommended for pts with severe sepsis of any cause and an APACHE II score of >25; pts with meningococcemia may be one group most likely to benefit from this treatment. If the platelet count is <50,000/µL or if there is active bleeding, activated protein C should not be given.

Prognosis Shock, purpuric or ecchymotic rash, low or normal blood leukocyte count, an age of ≥60 years, coma, absence of meningitis, thrombocytopenia, and low erythrocyte sedimentation rate are all associated with increased mortality risk. Receipt of antibiotics prior to hospital admission has been associated with a better outcome in some studies.

Prevention
- Vaccines: A meningococcal conjugate vaccine active against serogroups A, C, Y, and W-135 but not against serogroup B was licensed in 2005 for use in the United States. The conjugate vaccine has increased immunogenicity and probably confers longer-duration protection than the previously available polysaccharide vaccine. The conjugate vaccine is also expected to reduce asymptomatic carriage of *N. meningitidis* and to produce herd immunity. In light of these considerations, the meningococcal conjugate vaccine is now recommended for routine vaccination of all persons 11–18 years old

TABLE 95-1	ANTIBIOTIC TREATMENT, CHEMOPROPHYLAXIS, AND VACCINATIONS FOR INVASIVE MENINGOCOCCAL DISEASE

Antibiotic Treatment[a]

1. Ceftriaxone 2 g IV q12h (100 mg/kg per day) or cefotaxime 2 g IV q4h
2. For penicillin-sensitive *N. meningitidis*: Penicillin G 18–24 million units per day in divided doses q4h (250,000 units/kg per day)
3. Chloramphenicol 75–100 mg/kg per day in divided doses q6h
4. Meropenem 1.0 g (children, 40 mg) IV q8h
5. In an outbreak setting in developing countries: Long-acting chloramphenicol in oil suspension (Tifomycin), single dose
   Adults: 3.0 g (6 mL)
   Children 1–15 years old: 100 mg/kg
   Children <1 year old: 50 mg/kg

Chemoprophylaxis[b]

Rifampin (oral)
   Adults: 600 mg bid for 2 days
   Children ≥1 month old: 10 mg/kg bid for 2 days
   Children <1 month old: 5 mg/kg bid for 2 days
Ciprofloxacin (oral)
   Adults: 500 mg, 1 dose
Ofloxacin (oral)
   Adults: 400 mg, 1 dose
Ceftriaxone (IM)
   Adults: 250 mg, 1 dose
   Children <15 years old: 125 mg, 1 dose
Azithromycin (oral)
   500 mg, 1 dose

Vaccination[c]

A, C, Y, W-135 vaccine (Memomune, Aventis Pasteur) or A, C vaccine
   Single 0.5-mL subcutaneous injection
New C; A, C; and A, C, Y, W-135 meningococcal conjugate vaccines[d]

[a]Patients with meningococcal meningitis should receive antimicrobial therapy for at least 5 days.
[b]Use is recommended for close contacts of cases or if ceftriaxone is not used for primary treatment.
[c]At present, use is generally limited to the control of epidemics and to individuals with increased risk of meningococcal disease. Vaccine efficacy wanes after 3–5 years, and vaccine is not effective in recipients <2 years of age.
[d]These vaccines appear to provide immunity in young children, a prolonged immune response, and herd immunity (decreased transmission and colonization); see "Prevention" section of text.

and of persons 2–55 years old who are at increased risk for meningococcal disease.
- Antimicrobial chemoprophylaxis: See Table 95-1 for prophylaxis options. Household and other close contacts (e.g., day-care center contacts, persons exposed to a pt's oral secretions) have a >400-fold higher risk of meningococcal disease than the population as a whole.
- Respiratory isolation of hospitalized pts during the first 24 h of treatment is required.

LISTERIAL INFECTIONS

Etiology and Epidemiology   *Listeria monocytogenes* is a foodborne pathogen that can cause serious infections, particularly in pregnant women and immuno-compromised individuals. The organism is a nonsporulating, gram-positive rod that demonstrates motility when cultured at low temperatures. Listeriosis can follow the ingestion of contaminated food. *Listeria* can be found in processed and unprocessed foods such as soft cheeses, delicatessen meats, hot dogs, milk, and cold salads.

Clinical Features   *Listeria* causes several clinical syndromes, of which meningitis and septicemia are most common.

- Gastroenteritis: Gastroenteritis can develop within 48 h after the ingestion of contaminated foods containing a large inoculum of bacteria. Listeriosis should be considered in outbreaks of gastroenteritis when cultures for other likely pathogens are negative.
- Bacteremia: Pts present with fever, chills, myalgias, and arthralgias. Neurologic findings or meningeal signs may suggest the diagnosis. Endocarditis is uncommon and is associated with fatality rates of 35–50%.
- Meningitis: *Listeria* causes ~5–10% of cases of community-acquired meningitis in adults. In the United States, case-fatality rates are 15–26%. Listerial meningitis differs from meningitis of other bacterial etiologies in that its presentation is often subacute and the CSF profile usually reveals <1000 white blood cells/μL with a less marked polymorphonuclear leukocyte predominance. Low glucose levels and a positive Gram's stain are seen in ~30–40% of cases.
- Meningoencephalitis and central nervous system (CNS) infection: *Listeria* can directly invade the brain parenchyma and cause cerebritis or focal abscess. Brainstem invasion can cause severe rhombencephalitis. Pts have fever and headache followed by asymmetric cranial nerve defects, cerebellar signs, and hemiparetic/hemisensory defects.
- Infection in pregnant women and neonates: Listeriosis is a serious infection in pregnancy. Pts are usually bacteremic and present with a nonspecific febrile illness that includes myalgias/arthralgias, backache, and headache. CNS involvement is rare. Infection develops in 70–90% of fetuses from infected women; almost 50% of infected fetuses die. This risk can be reduced with prepartum treatment. Infected women usually do well after delivery. Overwhelming listerial fetal infection—granulomatosis infantiseptica—is characterized by miliary microabscesses and granulomas, most often in the skin, liver, and spleen.

Diagnosis   Timely diagnosis requires that the illness be considered in groups at risk: pregnant women, elderly pts, neonates, immunocompromised pts (e.g., transplant recipients, cancer pts, pts being treated with tumor necrosis factor antagonists or glucocorticoids), and pts with chronic underlying medical conditions (e.g., alcoholism, diabetes). Listeriosis is diagnosed when the organism is cultured from a usually sterile site, such as blood, CSF, or amniotic fluid. Listeriae may be confused with "diphtheroids" or pneumococci in gram-stained CSF or may be gram-variable and confused with *Haemophilus* spp.

℞   Listerial Infections

- Ampicillin is the drug of choice for the treatment of listerial infections; penicillin is also highly active. Adults should receive ampicillin at a dosage of 2 g IV every 4 h. Most experts recommend gentamicin (1.0–1.7 mg/kg every 8 h) for synergy. For penicillin-allergic pts, trimethoprim-sulfamethoxazole (15–20 mg of TMP/kg IV daily in divided doses every 6–8 h) should be given. These doses cover CNS infection and bacteremia. Cephalosporins are not effective. Neonates should receive ampicillin and gentamicin, dosed by weight.

- The duration of therapy depends on the syndrome: 2 weeks for bacteremia, 3 weeks for meningitis, 6–8 weeks for brain abscess/encephalitis, and 4–6 weeks for endocarditis. Early-onset neonatal disease can be severe and requires >2 weeks of treatment.

Prognosis With prompt therapy, 50–70% of pts recover fully unless they have brain abscess or rhombencephalitis. Of live-born treated neonates in one series, 60% recovered fully, 24% died, and 13% were left with sequelae or complications.

Prevention Pregnant women and other persons at risk for listeriosis should avoid soft cheeses and should avoid or thoroughly reheat ready-to-eat and delicatessen foods.

For a more detailed discussion, see Wetzler LM: Meningococcal Infections, Chap. 136, p. 908; and Hohmann EL, Portnoy DA: Infections Caused by *Listeria monocytogenes*, Chap. 132, p. 895, in HPIM-17.

96 Infections Caused by *Haemophilus*, *Bordetella*, *Moraxella*, and HACEK Group Organisms

HAEMOPHILUS INFLUENZAE

Etiology and Epidemiology *H. influenzae* is a small, gram-negative, pleomorphic coccobacillus. Strains with a polysaccharide capsule are serotyped *a* through *f*. *H. influenzae* type b (Hib) is most important clinically, causing systemic invasive disease, primarily in infants and children <6 years of age. Use of Hib conjugate vaccine has dramatically decreased rates of Hib colonization and invasive disease. Nontypable strains of *H. influenzae* (NTHi), which are unencapsulated, cause disease by locally invading mucosal surfaces. NTHi strains colonize the upper respiratory tract of up to 75% of healthy adults. *H. influenzae* is spread by airborne droplets or through direct contact with secretions or fomites.

Clinical Features
- Hib

  1. Meningitis is associated with high morbidity; 6% of pts have sensorineural hearing loss; one-fourth have some significant sequelae; mortality is ~5%.

2. Epiglottitis, which occurs in older children and occasionally in adults, involves cellulitis of the epiglottis and supraglottic tissues that begins with a sore throat and progresses rapidly to dysphagia, drooling, and airway obstruction.
3. Miscellaneous: cellulitis, pneumonia, osteomyelitis

- NTHi

   1. Community-acquired pneumonia in adults—especially those with chronic obstructive pulmonary disease (COPD) or AIDS—and exacerbations of COPD
   2. Miscellaneous: childhood otitis media, puerperal sepsis, neonatal bacteremia, sinusitis, and—less commonly—invasive infections (e.g., osteomyelitis, endocarditis)

Diagnosis Gram's staining and culture of clinical samples

℞ *H. influenzae* **Infections**

- Hib meningitis in adults: ceftriaxone (2 g every 12 h for 1–2 weeks)
- Hib meningitis in children: ceftriaxone (75–100 mg/kg per day, split into two doses given every 12 h) plus dexamethasone (0.6 mg/kg per day in four divided doses for 2 days at initiation of antibiotic treatment to prevent hearing loss)
- Epiglottitis: ceftriaxone (50 mg/kg daily for 1–2 weeks)
- NTHi: About 20–35% of clinical isolates produce β-lactamase. Many agents are useful: amoxicillin/ clavulanate, extended-spectrum cephalosporins, newer macrolides (azithromycin or clarithromycin), and fluoroquinolones (in nonpregnant adults).
- Ampicillin-resistant strains of *H. influenzae* in which resistance is due to altered penicillin-binding proteins rather than to β-lactamase production are increasing in prevalence in Europe and Japan.

Prevention Hib vaccine is recommended for all children; the immunization series should be started at ~2 months of age. Secondary attack rates are high among household contacts of pts with Hib disease. All children and adults (except pregnant women) in households with a case of Hib disease and at least one incompletely immunized contact <4 years of age should receive prophylaxis with oral rifampin.

PERTUSSIS

Etiology *Bordetella pertussis* causes pertussis, an acute respiratory tract infection. *B. pertussis* is a fastidious gram-negative aerobic bacillus that attaches to ciliated epithelial cells of the nasopharynx, multiplies locally, and produces a wide array of toxins and biologically active products.

Epidemiology Pertussis is highly communicable. In households, attack rates are 80% among unimmunized contacts and 20% among immunized contacts. Pertussis remains an important cause of infant morbidity and death in developing countries. In the United States, the incidence has increased slowly since 1976, particularly among adolescents and adults. Persistent cough of >2 weeks' duration in an adult may be due to *B. pertussis* in 12–30% of cases. Severe morbidity and mortality are restricted to infants <6 months of age.

Clinical Features   After an incubation period of 7–10 days, a prolonged coughing illness begins. Symptoms are usually more severe in infants and young children.

- The *catarrhal* phase is similar to the common cold and lasts 1–2 weeks.
- The *paroxysmal* phase follows and lasts 2–4 weeks. It is characterized by cough that at times occurs in spasmodic fits of 5–10 coughs each. Episodes are worse at night. Vomiting or a "whoop" may follow a coughing fit. Apnea and cyanosis can occur during spasms. Pts become increasingly fatigued.
- *Convalescent* phase: Symptoms resolve over 1–3 months.

Diagnosis
- Cultures of nasopharyngeal secretions remain positive in untreated cases for a mean of 3 weeks after illness onset. Secretions must be inoculated immediately onto selective media. Results become positive by day 5.
- Compared with culture, polymerase chain reaction of nasopharyngeal specimens provides increased sensitivity and longer duration of a positive result in both treated and untreated pts. Results can be available within hours.
- Although serology can be useful in pts with symptoms lasting >4 weeks, diagnostic criteria are not agreed upon, and antibody tests are not widely available.

Rx Pertussis

- Macrolides: erythromycin (1–2 g/d for 1–2 weeks); clarithromycin (250 mg bid for 1 week); azithromycin (500-mg load on day 1, then 250 mg/d for 4 days)
- Trimethoprim-sulfamethoxazole (TMP-SMX) in macrolide-intolerant pts
- Respiratory isolation for hospitalized pts until antibiotics have been given for 5 days

Prevention
- Chemoprophylaxis with macrolides for household contacts of pts, especially if there are household members at high risk of severe disease (e.g., children <1 year of age)
- Immunization: In the United States, acellular vaccines are safe for older children and adults.

MORAXELLA CATARRHALIS

Etiology   *M. catarrhalis* is a gram-negative coccus that resembles *Neisseria*. It can retain crystal violet on Gram's staining and be confused with *Staphylococcus aureus*. Part of the normal flora of the upper airways, *M. catarrhalis* colonizes up to 50% of healthy children and up to 3–7% of healthy adults. Infection rates peak in late winter/early spring.

Clinical Features
- Otitis media and sinusitis: *M. catarrhalis* is the third most common cause of otitis media in children and is a prominent isolate from cases of acute and chronic sinusitis.
- Purulent tracheobronchitis and pneumonia: Most pts are >50 years of age and have COPD (often with lung cancer as well).
- Symptoms are mild to moderate; invasive disease (e.g., empyema) is rare.

Diagnosis   Gram's staining and cultures of sputum

℞ *M. catarrhalis* Infections

Moraxellae are susceptible to β-lactam/β-lactamase inhibitor combinations, second- and third-generation cephalosporins, doxycycline, newer macrolides, TMP-SMX, and fluoroquinolones. Respiratory infections should be treated with a 5-day course and sinusitis for longer durations.

THE HACEK GROUP

Etiology   The HACEK group consists of fastidious, slow-growing, gram-negative bacteria whose growth requires carbon dioxide. Normal residents of the oral cavity, HACEK bacteria can cause both local oral infections and severe systemic disease, particularly endocarditis. Several *Haemophilus* species, *Actinobacillus actinomycetemcomitans*, *Cardiobacterium hominis*, *Eikenella corrodens*, and *Kingella kingae* make up this group.

Clinical Features

- HACEK endocarditis: Up to 3% of cases of infective endocarditis are caused by HACEK organisms; most of these cases are due to *A. actinomycetemcomitans*, *Haemophilus* species, or *C. hominis*. Pts often have underlying valvular disease. Embolization is common, even in subacute presentations. Major emboli are found in 28–71% of pts and vegetations—often very large—in 85%. Cultures can take 30 days to become positive, although most cultures that ultimately yield HACEK bacteria become positive in the first week, especially with newer detection systems such as BACTEC.
- *Haemophilus* species: *H. aphrophilus*, *H. parainfluenzae*, and *H. paraphrophilus* cause more than half of all cases of HACEK endocarditis. Pts usually present within the first 2 months of illness, and 19–50% of pts develop congestive heart failure.
- *A. actinomycetemcomitans*: This organism is isolated from soft tissue infections in association with *Actinomyces israelii*. It is associated with severe destructive periodontal disease, which also is frequently evident in pts with endocarditis.
- *C. hominis*: Unlike other HACEK bacteria, *C. hominis* most often affects the aortic valve. Long-standing infection usually precedes diagnosis.
- *E. corrodens*: Usually a component of mixed infections, *E. corrodens* is common in human bite wounds, head and neck soft-tissue infections, endocarditis, and infections in IV drug users.
- *K. kingae*: *K. kingae* is the third most common cause of septic arthritis in children <2 years old and a common cause of osteomyelitis in the same age group. *K. kingae* bacteremia is seen in association with stomatitis (e.g., due to herpes simplex virus infection). Unlike other *K. kingae* infections, endocarditis due to this organism occurs in older children and adults. Inoculation of clinical specimens (e.g., synovial fluid) into aerobic blood culture bottles enhances recovery of this organism.

℞ HACEK Group Infections

See Table 96-1 for antibiotic regimens used to treat endocarditis and other serious infections caused by HACEK organisms. Native-valve endocarditis should be treated for 4 weeks and prosthetic-valve endocarditis for 6 weeks. Unlike prosthetic-valve endocarditis caused by other gram-negative organisms, that due to HACEK bacteria can often be cured with antibiotics alone (i.e., without surgery).

TABLE 96-1 TREATMENT OF ENDOCARDITIS AND OTHER SERIOUS INFECTIONS CAUSED BY HACEK GROUP ORGANISMS[a]

Organism	Initial Therapy	Alternative Agents	Comments
Haemophilus species, *Actinobacillus actinomycetemcomitans*	Ceftriaxone (2 g/d)	Ampicillin/sulbactam (3 g of ampicillin q6h) or fluoroquinolones[b]	Ampicillin ± an aminoglycoside can be used if the organism does not produce β-lactamase.[c]
Cardiobacterium hominis	Penicillin (16–18 mU/d in 6 divided doses) or ampicillin (2 g q4h)	Ceftriaxone (2 g/d) or ampicillin/sulbactam (3 g of ampicillin q6h)	An aminoglycoside (gentamicin, 3 mg/kg per day in 3 divided doses) may be added, but its value has not been proven. The organism is usually pan-sensitive, but high-level penicillin resistance has been reported.
Eikenella corrodens	Ampicillin (2 g q4h)	Ceftriaxone (2 g/d) or fluoroquinolones[b]	The organism is typically resistant to clindamycin, metronidazole, and aminoglycosides.
Kingella kingae	Ceftriaxone (2 g/d) or ampicillin/sulbactam (3 g of ampicillin q6h)	Fluoroquinolones[b]	The prevalence of β-lactamase-producing strains is increasing. Efficacy for invasive infections is best demonstrated for first-line treatments.

[a]Susceptibility testing should be performed in all cases to guide therapy.
[b]Fluoroquinolones are not recommended for treatment of children <17 years of age.
[c]European guidelines for endocarditis recommend the addition of gentamicin (3 mg/kg per day in 3 divided doses for 2–4 weeks).

For a more detailed discussion, see Musher DM: *Moraxella* Infections, Chap. 138, p. 921; Murphy TF: *Haemophilus* Infections, Chap. 139, p. 923; Barlam TF, Kasper DL: Infections Due to the HACEK Group and Miscellaneous Gram-Negative Bacteria, Chap. 140, p. 926; and Halperin SA: Pertussis and Other *Bordetella* Infections, Chap. 142, p. 933, in HPIM-17.

97 Diseases Caused by Gram-Negative Enteric Bacteria, *Pseudomonas*, and *Legionella*

INFECTIONS CAUSED BY GRAM-NEGATIVE ENTERIC BACTERIA

GENERAL CONSIDERATIONS

Gram-negative bacilli (GNB) are normal components of the human colonic flora and can colonize mucosal and skin surfaces of pts in long-term-care and hospital settings. Virtually every organ or body cavity can be infected with GNB. *Escherichia coli* and, to a lesser degree, *Klebsiella* and *Proteus* account for most infections. Isolation of GNB from any sterile site almost always implies infection. Isolation from nonsterile sites requires clinical correlation. Early appropriate antimicrobial therapy improves outcomes. Multidrug resistance in GNB [e.g., due to extended-spectrum β-lactamases (ESBLs) and AmpC β-lactamases] is increasing worldwide. Combination empirical antimicrobial therapy may be appropriate pending susceptibility results.

EXTRAINTESTINAL INFECTIONS CAUSED BY PATHOGENIC *E. COLI*

Most *E. coli* isolates from symptomatic infections outside the GI tract are distinct from commensal strains and from pathogenic strains that cause intestinal infections.

Clinical Features
- Urinary tract infection (UTI): *E. coli* is the most prevalent pathogen in all genitourinary syndromes and causes 85–95% of acute uncomplicated UTIs.
- Abdominal and pelvic infection: the second most common site of infection with extraintestinal pathogenic strains of *E. coli* (ExPEC). Syndromes include peritonitis, intraabdominal abscesses, and cholangitis.
- Pneumonia: In pts with underlying illnesses and antibiotic exposure, rates of colonization with and pneumonia due to GNB increase. ExPEC is a common cause of pneumonia in long-term-care residents and hospitalized pts. *E. coli* can cause multifocal nodular infiltrates with tissue necrosis. Mortality rates are high.
- Meningitis: occurs mostly in neonates; caused by strains with the K1 capsular serotype
- Cellulitis/musculoskeletal infection: *E. coli* often contributes to infection of decubitus ulcers and to diabetic lower-extremity ulcers. When close to the

perineum, cellulitis and burn-site or surgical-site infections can be due to *E. coli*. Osteomyelitis, particularly vertebral, is more common than is generally appreciated; *E. coli* accounts for up to 10% of cases in some series.

- Bacteremia: can arise from primary infection at any site, but originates most commonly from the urinary tract and next most commonly from the bowel and biliary tract. Endovascular infections are rare but have been described.

Diagnosis   ExPEC grows readily on standard media. Most strains ferment lactose and are indole-positive.

 Extraintestinal Infections Caused by *E. coli*

Rates of resistance to ampicillin, first-generation cephalosporins, trimethoprim-sulfamethoxazole (TMP-SMX), and fluoroquinolones are increasing. ESBLs are increasingly common in *E. coli*. Currently, cephalosporins (particularly second-, third-, and fourth-generation agents), monobactams, piperacillin-tazobactam, carbapenems, and aminoglycosides retain good activity.

INTESTINAL INFECTIONS CAUSED BY *E. COLI*

At least five "pathotypes" of *E. coli* cause intestinal infections exclusively. (For further discussion, see Chap. 89.)

1. Shiga toxin–producing *E. coli* (STEC)/enterohemorrhagic *E. coli* (EHEC): In contrast to other pathotypes, STEC/EHEC causes infection more frequently in developed countries. *E. coli* O157:H7 belongs to this pathotype. STEC/EHEC is associated with ingestion of contaminated food and water or person-to-person transmission. Ground beef is a common food source.
2. Pathotypes most common in developing countries
   a. Enterotoxigenic *E. coli* (ETEC): the most common agent of traveler's diarrhea
   b. Enteropathogenic *E. coli* (EPEC): an important cause of diarrhea among infants
   c. Enteroinvasive *E. coli* (EIEC): causes inflammatory colitis similar to that caused by *Shigella*
   d. Enteroaggregative and diffusely adherent *E. coli* (EAEC): causes prolonged watery diarrhea

Diagnosis   Specific diagnosis is usually unnecessary except when STEC/EHEC is involved. Bloody diarrhea can be screened for *E. coli* strains that do not ferment sorbitol, and strains can then be typed for *E. coli* O157:H7. However, testing for Shiga toxins or toxin genes is more sensitive, specific, and rapid.

 Intestinal Infections Caused by *E. coli*

Supportive care, replacement of water and electrolytes, and avoidance of antibiotics in STEC/EHEC infection (since antibiotic use may increase the risk of hemolytic-uremic syndrome) are indicated.

KLEBSIELLA INFECTIONS

Etiology   *K. pneumoniae* colonizes the colon in 5–35% of healthy individuals and causes most *Klebsiella* infections. *K. oxytoca* causes infections in long-term-care and hospital settings. *K. rhinoscleromatis* and *K. ozaenae* infect pts in tropical climates.

Clinical Features
- Pneumonia: occurs primarily in pts with underlying disease (e.g., alcoholism, diabetes, chronic obstructive pulmonary disease). Long-term-care facility residents and hospitalized pts have higher rates of oropharyngeal colonization and more frequent *K. pneumoniae* pulmonary infections. The presentation is similar to that of pneumonia caused by other enteric GNB, with purulent sputum production and pulmonary infiltrates on chest x-ray (CXR). Infection can progress to pulmonary necrosis, pleural effusion, and empyema.
- UTI: *K. pneumoniae* causes 1–2% of cases of uncomplicated cystitis and 5–17% of cases of complicated UTI.
- Abdominal infections: spectrum similar to that of *E. coli*, but less frequent occurrence
- Cellulitis and soft tissue infections: most often involve devitalized tissues in compromised hosts. *K. pneumoniae* causes some surgical-site infections.
- Miscellaneous: Bacteremia can arise from a primary infection at any site.
- Other infections: include endophthalmitis, nosocomial sinusitis, osteomyelitis

Diagnosis Klebsiellae usually ferment lactose, although the subspecies *rhinoscleromatis* and *ozaenae* are nonfermenters and are indole-negative.

℞ *Klebsiella* Infections

Klebsiellae are resistant to ampicillin and ticarcillin. Their resistance to third-generation cephalosporins is increasing, as is the frequency of ESBL-containing isolates. Fluoroquinolone resistance is increasing, especially among ESBL-containing strains. Empirical treatment of serious or health care–associated *Klebsiella* infection with amikacin and carbapenems is prudent. Rates of resistance to tigecycline are low, but clinical experience with this drug is limited.

PROTEUS INFECTIONS

Etiology *P. mirabilis* is part of the colonic flora in up to half of healthy people and causes 90% of *Proteus* infections. *P. vulgaris* and *P. penneri* are isolated primarily from pts in hospitals and long-term-care facilities.

Clinical Features *Proteus* causes 1–2% of uncomplicated UTIs, 5% of hospital-acquired UTIs, and 10–15% of complicated UTIs, especially those associated with urinary catheters. Pts with long-term catheterization have *Proteus* infection prevalence rates of 20–45%. *Proteus* produces high levels of urease, alkalinizes urine, and causes formation of struvite calculi. Removal of the stones or the urinary catheter is usually required for cure of infection. Infections rarely occur in other sites.

Diagnosis *Proteus* strains are typically lactose-negative and exhibit swarming motility on agar plates. *P. mirabilis* is indole-negative, whereas most other *Proteus* strains are indole-positive.

℞ *Proteus* Infections

P. mirabilis is susceptible to most agents. Resistance to ampicillin, first-generation cephalosporins, and quinolones is increasing. *P. vulgaris* and *P. penneri* are more resistant. Imipenem, fourth-generation cephalosporins, aminoglycosides, and TMP-SMX exhibit excellent activity.

OTHER GRAM-NEGATIVE ENTERIC PATHOGENS

Enterobacter (e.g., *E. cloacae, E. aerogenes*), *Acinetobacter* (e.g., *A. baumannii*), *Serratia* (e.g., *S. marcescens*), and *Citrobacter* (e.g., *C. freundii, C. koseri*) usually cause nosocomial infections. These organisms are associated with moist environmental foci. Risk factors include immunosuppression, comorbid disease, prior antibiotic use, and intensive care unit (ICU) stays. Infections caused by *Morganella* (e.g., *M. morganii*) and *Providencia* (e.g., *P. stuartii, P. rettgeri*) resemble *Proteus* infections in terms of epidemiology, pathogenicity, and clinical manifestations but occur almost exclusively in persons in long-term-care facilities and, to a lesser degree, in hospitalized pts.

Clinical Features

- Pneumonia, particularly ventilator-associated
- UTI, especially catheter-related. *Morganella* and *Providencia* are particularly strongly associated with long-term catheterization (>30 days).
- Intravascular device–related infection, surgical-site infection, and abdominal infection
- Biliary disease is associated with *Enterobacter*.
- *Acinetobacter* has caused soft tissue and bone infections among soldiers with battlefield injuries.

℞ Other Gram-Negative Enteric Pathogens

Significant antibiotic resistance makes therapy challenging. Imipenem and aminoglycosides (amikacin > gentamicin) are most reliably active, and fourth-generation cephalosporins often display excellent activity. *Enterobacter* is commonly resistant to third-generation cephalosporins and monobactams. *Acinetobacter* may be susceptible to β-lactam/β-lactamase inhibitor agents, but these agents do not have enhanced activity against *Enterobacter* or *Citrobacter*. Susceptibility testing is essential. Some isolates may retain susceptibility only to colistin and polymyxin B.

AEROMONAS INFECTIONS

A. hydrophila is the most common *Aeromonas* species causing infection. *Aeromonas* organisms proliferate in potable and fresh water and are a putative cause of gastroenteritis. *Aeromonas* causes bacteremia and sepsis in infants and compromised hosts, especially those with cancer, hepatobiliary disease, trauma, or burns. The organisms can produce skin lesions similar to the ecthyma gangrenosum lesions seen with *P. aeruginosa*. *Aeromonas* causes nosocomial infections related to catheters, surgical incisions, and use of leeches.

℞ Aeromonas Infections

Aeromonas is usually susceptible to fluoroquinolones (e.g., ciprofloxacin at a dose of 500 mg PO q12h or 400 mg IV q12h), TMP-SMX (10 mg of TMP/kg per day in 3 or 4 divided doses), third-generation cephalosporins, and aminoglycosides.

INFECTIONS DUE TO *PSEUDOMONAS AERUGINOSA* AND RELATED ORGANISMS

PSEUDOMONAS AERUGINOSA

Epidemiology   *P. aeruginosa* is found in most moist environments. The many factors that predispose to *P. aeruginosa* infection include disruption of cutaneous or mucosal barriers (e.g., due to burns or trauma), immunosuppression (e.g., due to neutropenia, AIDS, or diabetes), and disruption of the normal bacterial flora (e.g., due to broad-spectrum antibiotic therapy).

Laboratory Features   *P. aeruginosa* is a motile gram-negative rod that commonly produces green or bluish pigment. *P. aeruginosa* differs from enteric GNB in that it has a positive reaction in the oxidase test and does not ferment lactose.

Clinical Features

- Bacteremia
  1. *P. aeruginosa* is no longer a major cause of life-threatening bacteremia in neutropenic pts or those with burn injury. *P. aeruginosa* bacteremia is currently most common among pts in the ICU.
  2. Pathognomonic skin lesions, called *ecthyma gangrenosum*, develop in a small minority of pts with *P. aeruginosa* bacteremia, beginning as painful reddish maculopapular lesions that become black and necrotic.
- Respiratory tract infections: the most common of all infections caused by *P. aeruginosa*
  1. Acute pneumonia: presents with fever, chills, and cough and can have a fulminant course with cyanosis, tachypnea, and systemic toxicity. CXR shows bilateral pneumonia, often with nodular densities and/or cavitation. This presentation is now uncommon. Community-acquired necrotizing pneumonia can follow inhalation of hot-tub water contaminated with *P. aeruginosa*.
  2. Ventilator-associated pneumonia (VAP): *P. aeruginosa* is considered a major cause of VAP, although colonization may be difficult to distinguish from true infection. Clinically, most pts have a slowly progressive infiltrate, although progression is rapid in some cases. Infiltrates may become necrotic. Bronchoalveolar lavage or protected-brush sampling of distal airways should be done to substantiate *P. aeruginosa* pneumonia.
- Chronic respiratory infections in pts with underlying or predisposing conditions (e.g., cystic fibrosis or bronchiectasis)
- Endocarditis: occurs mostly in IV drug users and pts with prosthetic valves
- Bone and joint infections
  1. Sternoclavicular joint infection: a complication of injection drug use
  2. Vertebral osteomyelitis: associated with UTIs in the elderly and with injection drug use
  3. Osteomyelitis of the foot: follows plantar puncture wounds, typically through sneakers. This infection is most common among children.
- Central nervous system infections: rare, almost always secondary to surgical procedures or head trauma
- Eye infections: keratitis, corneal ulcer, and endophthalmitis can occur, usually resulting from trauma or surface injury by contact lenses. These infections are rapidly progressing entities that demand immediate therapeutic intervention.

- Ear infections
  1. External otitis ("swimmer's ear")
  2. Malignant external otitis: occurs mostly in elderly diabetic pts. Decreased hearing and severe ear pain are the usual presenting symptoms. If the infection is diagnosed late in the course, pts may present with cranial-nerve palsies or cavernous venous sinus thrombosis. Infection involves ear cartilage and sometimes mastoid and petrous ridge bone. Treatment is the same as for osteomyelitis.
- UTIs: complicated or nosocomial
- Skin and soft tissue infections: folliculitis and other papular or vesicular lesions linked to whirlpools, spas, and swimming pools
- Infections in febrile neutropenic pts: *P. aeruginosa* is always targeted in empirical treatment of these pts. The most common clinical syndromes are bacteremia, pneumonia, and soft tissue infections, mainly manifesting as ecthyma gangrenosum.
- Infections in AIDS pts: *P. aeruginosa* infections are more common among AIDS pts. Pneumonia is associated with a high frequency of cavitary disease. Since the advent of antiretroviral therapy, *P. aeruginosa* infection has declined in incidence among these pts but still occurs, presenting particularly often as sinusitis.

℞ *P. aeruginosa* Infections

See Table 97-1 for antibiotic options and schedules. Severe or life-threatening infections are generally treated with two antibiotics to which the infecting strain is sensitive, although evidence that this course is more efficacious than monotherapy has been lacking since the introduction of more active β-lactam agents.

BACTERIA RELATED TO *PSEUDOMONAS* SPECIES

Stenotrophomonas maltophilia and Burkholderia cepacia *S. maltophilia* is a nosocomial pathogen; most cases of infection occur in the setting of prior broad-spectrum antimicrobial therapy that has eradicated the normal flora in immunocompromised pts. *S. maltophilia* causes pneumonia, especially VAP. Bacteremic *S. maltophilia* pneumonia can lead to septic shock in ICU pts. Central venous line infection (most often in cancer pts) and ecthyma gangrenosum in neutropenic pts have been described.

B. cepacia is recognized as an antibiotic-resistant nosocomial pathogen in ICU pts. This organism can colonize airways during broad-spectrum antimicrobial treatment and is a cause of VAP, catheter-associated infection, and wound infection. *B. cepacia* can cause a rapidly fatal syndrome of respiratory distress and septicemia in cystic fibrosis pts.

℞ *S. maltophilia* and *B. cepacia* Infections

Intrinsic resistance to many antibiotics limits treatment. TMP-SMX (15–20 mg of TMP/kg per day) is the preferred agent. In addition, *S. maltophilia* is often susceptible to ticarcillin/clavulanate and levofloxacin, while *B. cepacia* is often susceptible to meropenem and doxycycline.

Miscellaneous Organisms Melioidosis is endemic to Southeast Asia and is caused by *Burkholderia pseudomallei*. Glanders is associated with close con-

TABLE 97-1 ANTIBIOTIC TREATMENT OF INFECTIONS DUE TO *PSEUDOMONAS AERUGINOSA* AND RELATED ORGANISMS

Infection	Antibiotics and Dosages	Other Considerations
Bacteremia		
Nonneutropenic host	*Monotherapy:* Ceftazidime (2 g q8h IV) or cefepime (2 g q12h IV) *Combination therapy:* Piperacillin/tazobactam (3.375 g q4h IV) or imipenem (500 mg q6h IV) or meropenem (1 g q8h IV) *plus* Amikacin (7.5 mg/kg q12h or 15 mg/kg q24h IV)	Add an aminoglycoside for patients in shock and in regions or hospitals where rates of resistance to the primary β-lactam agents are high. Tobramycin may be used instead of amikacin (susceptibility permitting).
Neutropenic host	Cefepime (2 g q8h IV) or all other agents in above dosages	
Endocarditis	Antibiotic regimens as for bacteremia for 6–8 weeks	Resistance during therapy is common. Surgery is required for relapse.
Pneumonia	Drugs and dosages as for bacteremia, except that the available carbapenems should not be the primary drugs because of high rates of resistance during therapy	IDSA guidelines recommend the addition of an aminoglycoside or ciprofloxacin. The duration of therapy is 10–14 days.
Bone infection, malignant otitis externa	Cefepime or ceftazidime at the same dosages as for bacteremia; aminoglycosides not a necessary component of therapy; ciprofloxacin (500–750 mg q12h PO) may be used	Duration of therapy varies with the drug used (e.g., 6 weeks for a β-lactam agent; at least 3 months for oral therapy except in puncture-wound osteomyelitis, for which the duration should be 2–4 weeks).
Central nervous system infection	Ceftazidime or cefepime (2 g q8h IV) or meropenem (1 g q8h IV)	Abscesses or other closed-space infections may require drainage. The duration of therapy is ≥2 weeks.
Eye infection		
Keratitis/ulcer	Topical therapy with tobramycin/ciprofloxacin/levofloxacin eyedrops	Use maximal strengths available or compounded by pharmacy.
Endophthalmitis	Ceftazidime or cefepime as for central nervous system infection *plus* Topical therapy	

(continued)

TABLE 97-1 ANTIBIOTIC TREATMENT OF INFECTIONS DUE TO *PSEUDOMONAS AERUGINOSA* AND RELATED ORGANISMS (CONTINUED)

Infection	Antibiotics and Dosages	Other Considerations
Urinary tract infection	Ciprofloxacin (500 mg q12h PO) or levofloxacin (750 mg q24h) or any aminoglycoside (total daily dose given once daily)	Relapse may occur if an obstruction or a foreign body is present.
Multidrug-resistant *P. aeruginosa* infection	Colistin (100 mg q12h IV) for the shortest possible period to obtain a clinical response	Doses used have varied. Dosage adjustment is required in renal failure. Inhaled colistin may be added for pneumonia (100 mg q12h).
Stenotrophomonas maltophilia infection	TMP-SMX (1600/320 mg q12h IV for 14 days) Ticarcillin/clavulanate (3.1 g q4h IV for 14 days)	Resistance to all agents is increasing. Levofloxacin may be an alternative, but there is little published clinical experience with this agent.
Burkholderia cepacia infection	Meropenem (1 g q8h IV for 14 days) TMP-SMX (1600/320 mg q12h IV for 14 days)	Resistance to both agents is increasing. Do not use them in combination because of possible antagonism.
Melioidosis, glanders	Ceftazidime (2 g q6h for 2 weeks) or meropenem (1 g q8h for 2 weeks) or imipenem (500 mg q6h for 2 weeks) *followed by* TMP-SMX (1600/320 mg q12h PO for 3 months)	See "Further Readings" in HPIM-17, Chap. 145, for more details on therapy and alternative agents.

Note: IDSA, Infectious Diseases Society of America; TMP-SMX, trimethoprim-sulfamethoxazole.

tact with horses or other equines and is caused by *Burkholderia mallei*. These diseases present as acute or chronic pulmonary or extrapulmonary suppurative illnesses or as acute septicemia.

LEGIONELLA INFECTIONS

Microbiology   Legionellaceae are intracellular aerobic gram-negative bacilli that grow on buffered charcoal yeast extract (BCYE) agar. *L. pneumophila* causes 80–90% of cases of human *Legionella* disease; serogroups 1, 4, and 6 are most common. Eighteen other species, including *L. micdadei*, have been linked to human infections.

Epidemiology   *Legionella* is found in fresh water and human-constructed water sources. Outbreaks have been traced to potable-water supplies and occasionally cooling towers. The organisms are transmitted to individuals primarily via aspiration but can also be transmitted by aerosolization and direct instillation into the lung during respiratory tract manipulations. *Legionella* is the fourth most common cause of community-acquired pneumonia, accounting for 2–9% of cases. It causes 10–50% of cases of nosocomial pneumonia if the hospital's water system is colonized with the organism. Pts who have chronic lung disease, who smoke, and/or who are elderly or immunosuppressed are at particularly high risk for disease. Cell-mediated immunity is the primary mechanism of host defense.

Clinical Features
* Pontiac fever: a flulike illness with a 24- to 48-h incubation period. Pneumonia does not develop, but malaise, fatigue, myalgias, and fever are common. The disease is self-limited, and recovery takes place in a few days.
* Legionnaires' disease: more severe than other atypical pneumonias and more likely to result in ICU admission
  1. After an incubation period (usually 2–10 days), nonspecific symptoms (e.g., malaise, fatigue, headache, fever) develop and are followed by a cough that is usually mild and nonproductive.
  2. Chest pain (pleuritic or nonpleuritic) can be prominent, and dyspnea is common. Sputum is usually scant and may be blood-streaked.
  3. GI manifestations (pain, nausea, vomiting, diarrhea) may be pronounced.
  4. Diarrhea, confusion, high fevers, hyponatremia, increased values in liver function tests, hematuria, hypophosphatemia, and elevated creatine phosphokinase levels are documented more frequently than in other pneumonias.
  5. The heart is the most common extrapulmonary site of disease (myocarditis, pericarditis, and occasionally prosthetic valve endocarditis).
  6. CXR reveals pulmonary infiltrates, multilobar involvement in many instances, and pleural effusion in up to 63% of cases. In compromised hosts, nodular infiltrates, abscesses, and cavities can be seen.

Diagnosis
* Sputum or bronchoalveolar samples are subjected to direct fluorescent antibody (DFA) staining and culture. DFA testing is rapid and specific but less sensitive than culture.
* Cultures on BCYE media require 3–5 days to become positive.
* Diagnosis by antibody testing can take 12 weeks.
* Urinary antigen testing is rapid, inexpensive, easy to perform, second only to culture in terms of sensitivity, and highly specific. It is useful only for *L. pneumophila* serogroup 1, which causes 80% of disease cases. Urinary anti-

gen is detectable 3 days after disease onset and generally disappears over 2 months, although positivity can be prolonged if the pt is receiving glucocorticoid therapy.

R_x *Legionella* Infections

- Newer macrolides (e.g., azithromycin at 500 mg/d or clarithromycin at 500 mg bid, IV or PO) or fluoroquinolones (e.g., levofloxacin at 750 mg IV or 500 mg PO daily or moxifloxacin at 400 mg PO daily) are most effective. Rifampin (100–600 mg bid) combined with either class of drug is recommended in severe cases.
- Tetracyclines (doxycycline at 100 mg bid, IV or PO) or TMP-SMX (160/ 800 mg IV q8h or PO bid) are alternatives.
- Immunocompetent hosts can receive 10–14 days of therapy, but immunocompromised hosts should receive a 3-week course of treatment. A 5- to 10-day course of azithromycin is adequate because of this drug's long half-life.

Prognosis   Mortality approaches 80% among compromised hosts who do not receive timely therapy. Among immunocompetent hosts, mortality can approach 31% without treatment but ranges from 0 to 11% if pts receive appropriate therapy. Fatigue, weakness, and neurologic symptoms can persist for >1 year.

For a more detailed discussion, see Barlam TF, Kasper DL: Infections Due to the HACEK Group and Miscellaneous Gram-Negative Bacteria, Chap. 140, p. 926; Sabria M, Yu VL: *Legionella* Infection, Chap. 141, p. 929; Russo TA, Johnson JR: Diseases Caused by Gram-Negative Enteric Bacilli, Chap. 143, p. 937; and Ramphal R: Infections Due to *Pseudomonas* Species and Related Organisms, Chap. 145, p. 949, in HPIM-17.

98   Infections Caused by Miscellaneous Gram-Negative Bacilli

BRUCELLOSIS

Etiology   Brucellae are facultative intracellular parasites in a genus that includes four major species: *B. melitensis* (acquired by humans most commonly from sheep, goats, and camels), *B. suis* (from swine), *B. abortus* (from cattle or buffalo), and *B. canis* (from dogs). Brucellosis is transmitted via ingestion, inhalation, or mucosal or percutaneous exposure; the disease in humans is usually associated with exposure to infected animals or their products in either occupational settings (e.g., slaughterhouse work, farming,) or domestic settings (e.g., consumption of contaminated foods, especially dairy products).

Clinical Features   An incubation period of 1 week to several months is followed by the development of undulating fever; sweats; increasing apathy, fa-

TABLE 98-1	RADIOLOGY OF THE SPINE: DIFFERENTIATION OF BRUCELLOSIS FROM TUBERCULOSIS	
	Brucellosis	Tuberculosis
Site	Lumbar and others	Dorsolumbar
Vertebrae	Multiple or contiguous	Contiguous
Diskitis	Late	Early
Body	Intact until late	Morphology lost early
Canal compression	Rare	Common
Epiphysitis	Anterosuperior (Pom's sign)	General: upper and lower disk regions, central, subperiosteal
Osteophyte	Anterolateral (parrot beak)	Unusual
Deformity	Wedging uncommon	Anterior wedge, gibbus
Recovery	Sclerosis, whole body	Variable
Paravertebral abscess	Small, well-localized	Common and discrete loss, transverse process
Psoas abscess	Rare	More likely

tigue, and anorexia; and nonspecific symptoms such as headache, myalgias, and chills. Brucellosis often presents with one of three patterns: a febrile illness similar to but less severe than typhoid fever; fever and acute monarthritis, typically of the hip or knee, in a young child (septic arthritis); or long-lasting fever and low back or hip pain in an older man (vertebral osteomyelitis). *Brucella* infection can cause lymphadenopathy, hepatosplenomegaly, epididymoorchitis, neurologic involvement, and focal abscess.

Diagnosis Laboratory personnel must be alerted to the potential diagnosis to ensure that they take precautions to prevent occupational exposure. The organism is successfully cultured in 50–70% of cases, but culture identification usually takes up to 6 weeks. Cultures using the BACTEC systems can be deemed negative at 3 weeks. Agglutination assays for IgM are positive early in infection. Single titers of ≥1:160 and 1:320–1:640 are diagnostic in nonendemic and endemic areas, respectively. Brucellosis must be distinguished from tuberculosis; if this distinction is not possible, the regimen should be tailored to avoid inadvertent monotherapy for tuberculosis (see below). Brucellosis tends to cause less bone and joint destruction than tuberculosis (Table 98-1).

Rx Brucellosis

- Streptomycin at a dosage of 750 mg to 1 g daily (or gentamicin at 5–6 mg/kg daily) for 14–21 days plus doxycycline at a dosage of 100 mg bid for 6 weeks is recommended. Complex disease (e.g., significant neurologic disease or endocarditis) requires at least 3–6 months of treatment with multiple agents.
- Alternative: rifampin (600–900 mg/d) plus doxycycline (100 mg bid) for 6 weeks. Trimethoprim-sulfamethoxazole (TMP-SMX) can be given instead of doxycycline—e.g., to children or pregnant women.
- Relapse occurs in ~30% of cases, usually because of poor compliance. Pts should be monitored for at least 2 years.

TULAREMIA

Epidemiology Human infections caused by *Francisella tularensis* occur via interaction with biting or blood-sucking insects (especially ticks and tabanid flies), wild or domestic animals (e.g., wild rabbits, squirrels), or the environment. The organism can persist for months in mud, water, and decaying animal carcasses. More than half of U.S. cases occur in Arkansas, Oklahoma, and Missouri. The organism gains entry into the skin or mucous membranes through bites or inapparent abrasions or is acquired via inhalation or ingestion. *F. tularensis* is a potential agent of bioterrorism (see Chap. 32).

Clinical Features The incubation period is 2–10 days long. Tularemia often starts with an acute onset of fever, chills, headache, and myalgias. One of several syndromes can develop:

1. *Ulceroglandular/glandular tularemia* (75–85% of cases)
   a. The hallmark is an indurated, erythematous, nonhealing ulcer lasting 1–3 weeks (ulceroglandular form) that begins as a pruritic papule, ulcerates, has sharply demarcated edges and a yellow exudate, and develops a black base. A primary skin lesion may not be apparent in 5–10% of cases (glandular form).
   b. Lymphadenopathy is related to the location of the tick bite; inguinal/femoral nodes are most often affected in adults because of the frequency of bites on the legs. Lymph nodes can become fluctuant and drain spontaneously.
2. *Oculoglandular tularemia*: Infection of the conjunctiva, usually by contact with contaminated fingers, results in purulent conjunctivitis with regional adenopathy and debilitating pain. Painful preauricular lymphadenopathy is unique to tularemia.
3. *Oropharyngeal and GI tularemia*: Acquired via ingestion, infection can present with pharyngitis and cervical adenopathy, intestinal ulcerations, mesenteric adenopathy, diarrhea, nausea, vomiting, and abdominal pain.
4. *Pulmonary tularemia*: Infection is acquired via inhalation or hematogenous spread. Pts present with a nonproductive cough, dyspnea, pleuritic chest pain, bilateral patchy or lobar infiltrates, cavities, and occasional pleural effusions and empyema on chest x-ray.
5. *Typhoidal tularemia*: Consists of fever and signs of sepsis without focal findings

Diagnosis

- Polychromatic staining of clinical specimens (Gram's staining of little help)
- Serology via microagglutination or tube agglutination test. A single titer of ≥1:160 or a fourfold increase in titer after 2–3 weeks is considered positive.
- Culture is difficult and poses a significant risk to laboratory personnel. Polymerase chain reaction (PCR) methods have been used to detect *F. tularensis* DNA in clinical specimens.

Rx Tularemia

- Gentamicin is considered the drug of choice for both adults (5 mg/kg daily in 2 divided doses) and children (2.5 mg/kg tid or 5 mg/kg bid) with tularemia. Streptomycin (1 g q12h) is also effective, but tobramycin is not. Defervescence usually occurs within 2 days, but healing of skin lesions and lymph nodes may take 1–2 weeks. Late lymph-node suppuration can occur, with sterile necrotic tissue.

- Rapidly responding mild to moderate disease can be treated for 5–7 days; otherwise, treatment is given for 7–10 days.
- Alternatives include tetracyclines or chloramphenicol (relapse rates of up to 20%).
- Fluoroquinolones have shown promise, but clinical trials are pending.

PLAGUE

Epidemiology   *Yersinia pestis* causes plague, one of the most virulent and lethal of all bacterial diseases. Most often seen in Asia, Africa, and the Americas, plague occurs in the United States, primarily in New Mexico, Arizona, Colorado, and California. Wild rodents and rats are the usual hosts; ground squirrels, prairie dogs, and chipmunks are the main epizootic hosts in the United States. Fleabites or direct contact with infected tissues or airborne droplets can cause human infections. *Y. pestis* is a potential agent of bioterrorism (see Chap. 32).

Clinical Features   There are three major presentations.
1. *Bubonic plague*: the most common form, caused by the bite of an infected flea
   a. After an incubation period of 2–6 days, the pt develops chills, fever, myalgias and arthralgias, headache, weakness, and signs of toxemia.
   b. Within 24 h, adenopathy proximal to the inoculation site occurs. An enlarging node or bubo becomes painful and tender. Edema and erythema—but not cellulitis or lymphangitis—develop in the surrounding tissue.
   c. The primary inoculation site may have a papule, pustule, ulcer, or eschar.
   d. Disease progresses to lethargy, convulsions, shock, organ failure, and death.
2. *Septicemic plague*
   a. Overwhelming infection (no bubo) with disease progression to multiorgan failure, disseminated intravascular coagulation, hypotension, and death
   b. GI symptoms (diarrhea, nausea and vomiting, abdominal pain) are common.
3. *Pneumonic plague*: the most life-threatening form
   a. After an incubation period of 3–5 days, there is a sudden onset of chills, fever, headache, myalgias, weakness, and dizziness.
   b. Pulmonary signs include tachypnea, dyspnea, cough, sputum production, chest pain, hemoptysis, and circulatory collapse. Auscultatory findings are minimal. Sputum is watery, frothy, and blood-tinged or frankly bloody.
   c. Bronchopneumonia progresses rapidly to involve multiple lobes and both lungs, with liquefaction necrosis and cavitation of consolidated areas.
   d. Secondary pneumonic plague is a diffuse interstitial process and may be less infectious because sputum is tenacious and scant.

Diagnosis   A high index of clinical suspicion and a thorough clinical and epidemiologic examination are required for timely diagnosis and treatment. Smear and culture of specimens of blood, lymph node aspirates, pulmonary aspirates, and other sites should be prepared as appropriate. Smears should be examined immediately with Wayson or Giemsa stain (*Y. pestis* has a bipolar appearance resembling closed safety pins) and with Gram's stain and should be submitted for direct fluorescent antibody testing, enzyme linked immunosorbent assay, or PCR. Acute-phase—and, if possible, convalescent-phase—serum samples should undergo serologic testing. Either a single titer of >1:128 or seroconversion (as documented by a fourfold or greater rise in titer) is considered diagnostic. Confirm with the F1 antigen hemagglutination-inhibition test, which is positive in most cases by 1–2 weeks.

Rx Plague

- Without treatment, >50% of pts with bubonic plague and nearly all pts with septicemic or pneumonic plague die.
- Streptomycin or gentamicin is the drug of choice.
- Doxycycline and chloramphenicol are alternative agents.
- National bioterrorism-response protocols recommend administration of gentamicin, ciprofloxacin, and doxycycline in the event of a *Y. pestis* attack.
- Persons who are exposed to pts with pneumonic plague or who have traveled to an area where a plague outbreak is in progress should receive short-term (5-day) prophylaxis with doxycycline (adult dose, 100–200 mg q12–24h), ciprofloxacin (1 g q12h), or TMP-SMX (320 mg of TMP q12h).
- Pts hospitalized with pneumonic plague should remain on respiratory droplet precautions until treatment has been given for at least 48 h.

BARTONELLA INFECTIONS

Bartonella species are gram-negative bacteria that cause an array of infectious disease syndromes. Therapy for these syndromes is summarized in Table 98-2.

TABLE 98-2 TREATMENT OF ADULTS WITH DISEASE CAUSED BY *BARTONELLA* SPECIES[a]

Disease	Treatment
Cat-scratch disease	
Lymphadenopathy	Consider azithromycin (500 mg PO on day 1, then 250 mg PO qd for 4 days)
Retinitis	Doxycycline (100 mg PO bid for 4–6 weeks) *plus* Rifampin (300 mg PO bid for 4–6 weeks)
Bacillary angiomatosis	Erythromycin (500 mg PO qid for 3 months) *or* Doxycycline (100 mg PO bid for 3 months)
Bacillary peliosis	Erythromycin (500 mg PO qid for 4 months) *or* Doxycycline (100 mg PO bid for 4 months)
Bartonella endocarditis	
Suspected	Gentamicin (3 mg/kg qd IV for 14 days) *plus* Ceftriaxone (2 g IV qd for 6 weeks) *with or without* Doxycycline (100 mg PO bid for 6 weeks)
Confirmed	Gentamicin (3 mg/kg qd IV for 14 days) *plus* Doxycycline (100 mg PO bid for 6 weeks)
Trench fever	Doxycycline (200 mg PO qd for 4 weeks) *plus* Gentamicin (3 mg/kg qd IV for 14 days)
Bartonellosis	
Oroya fever	Chloramphenicol (500 mg PO or IV qid for 14 days) *plus* a β-lactam agent *or* Ciprofloxacin (500 mg bid for 10 days)
Verruga peruana	Rifampin (10 mg/kg qd PO for 14 days) *or* Streptomycin (15–20 mg/kg qd IM for 10 days)

[a]Based on recommendations from JM Rolain et al: Antimicrob Agents Chemother 48:1921, 2004; with permission.

CAT-SCRATCH DISEASE

This infection is associated with exposure to cats (especially kittens) with asymptomatic *B. henselae* bacteremia. Infection is transmitted by scratch, bite, or lick; ~40% of cases involve adults.

Clinical Features   Appearance of a localized lesion (papule, vesicle, or nodule) is followed 2–3 weeks later by lymphadenopathy. Unilateral solitary or regional adenopathy develops in >90% of pts. Nodes are tender, firm, and mobile; ~10% suppurate. Systemic symptoms include fever, malaise, headache, myalgias, and anorexia. Lymphadenopathy in untreated pts usually resolves within 3 months. Disseminated disease may occur and most often involves the nervous system (encephalitis, neuroretinitis), visceral organs (granulomatous hepatitis, splenitis), or bone.

Diagnosis

- Serologic testing for antibody to *B. henselae*
- Lymph node biopsy or aspiration. PCR analysis of a tissue sample is preferred; cultures are rarely positive.

BACILLARY ANGIOMATOSIS AND PELIOSIS HEPATIS

Clinical Features   These diseases, caused by *B. henselae* and *B. quintana*, occur most often in HIV-infected pts with CD4+ T cell counts of <100/μL. Pts with bacillary angiomatosis present with painless skin lesions, but subcutaneous masses or nodules, ulcerated plaques, and verrucous growths also occur. Lesions may be single or multiple and vary from tan to red to deep purple. They may invade underlying bone. Dissemination may occur, affecting the oropharynx, lungs, heart, intestines, lymph nodes, muscle, or brain. Pts with peliosis hepatis present with nonspecific systemic symptoms, with or without cutaneous involvement.

Diagnosis

- Radiographic studies of osseous bacillary angiomatosis demonstrate lytic bone lesions, while imaging of pts with peliosis hepatis reveals hypodense regions in the liver.
- Histopathologic findings (sites of angiogenesis and inflammation) and a positive Warthin-Starry stain

TRENCH FEVER

Caused by *B. quintana*, trench fever can occur as any of four patterns: a solitary episode of fever; a febrile illness of <1 week's duration; quintan fever (febrile episodes of ~5 days interspersed with asymptomatic intervals of ~5 days); and a persistent, febrile, debilitating illness lasting >1 month, with fever, headache, weight loss, and leg pain. The diagnosis is made by blood culture or serologic studies.

CULTURE-NEGATIVE ENDOCARDITIS

Bartonella species are an important cause of culture-negative endocarditis. Blood cultures are positive in ~25% of cases; yield is enhanced by extended incubation (4–6 weeks). Serologic tests or PCR testing for *Bartonella* in cardiac valve tissue can establish the diagnosis in pts with negative blood cultures.

OROYA FEVER AND VERRUGA PERUANA

These infections, caused by *B. bacilliformis*, are transmitted by a sandfly vector found in river valleys of the Andes Mountains. Pts present with fever; profound anemia follows. Without treatment, mortality is high. During convalescence, cutaneous lesions—verrugas—can develop; these lesions are typically reddish-purple pruritic papules or nodules similar to the skin lesions of bacillary angiomatosis. The diagnosis is based on detection of intraerythrocytic organisms in a Wright-Giemsa-stained thin blood smear and/or blood culture. Biopsy of verrugas reveals formation of new blood vessels and endothelial hyperplasia.

> For a more detailed discussion, see Corbel MJ, Beeching NJ: Brucellosis, Chap. 150, p. 973; Jacobs RF, Schutze GE: Tularemia, Chap. 151, p. 976; Dennis DT, Campbell GL: Plague and Other *Yersinia* Infections, Chap. 152, p. 980; and Spach DH, Darby E: *Bartonella* Infections, Including Cat-Scratch Disease, Chap. 153, p. 987, in HPIM-17.

99 Anaerobic Infections

DEFINITIONS

- *Anaerobic bacteria:* require reduced oxygen tension for growth; do not grow on the surface of solid media in 10% CO_2 in air
- *Microaerophilic bacteria:* grow in an atmosphere of 10% CO_2 in air or under anaerobic or aerobic conditions, but grow best if only a small amount of atmospheric oxygen is present
- *Facultative bacteria:* grow in the presence or absence of air

TETANUS

Etiology, Epidemiology, and Pathogenesis   Tetanus is a neurologic disorder characterized by increased muscle tone and spasms caused by tetanospasmin, a toxin produced by *Clostridium tetani*. *C. tetani* is a drumstick-shaped, spore-forming, anaerobic gram-positive rod that is ubiquitous in soil. In the United States, disease occurs in inadequately immunized persons, primarily nonwhites and the elderly; in developing countries, neonatal tetanus is most common. After contaminating wounds (typically puncture wounds), spores germinate if there is low oxidation-reduction potential (e.g., due to devitalized tissue or foreign bodies) and produce toxin. The toxin blocks release of inhibitory neurotransmitters (glycine and γ-aminobutyric acid) in presynaptic terminals, and rigidity results from an increased resting firing rate of the α-motor neurons.

Clinical Features

- *Generalized tetanus*: A median of 7 days after injury (range, 3–14 days), pts develop trismus—increased tone of the masseter muscles (lockjaw)—as well as sustained facial muscle contraction (risus sardonicus), dysphagia, neck stiffness or pain, back muscle contraction (opisthotonos), and rigidity of the abdominal wall and proximal limb muscles. Mentation is clear. Pts are often afebrile. Paroxysmal generalized spasms, either entirely spontaneous or provokcd by even the slightest stimulation, may result in cyanosis and ventilatory compromise. Autonomic dysfunction can cause labile hypertension, tachycardia, arrhythmias, and sudden cardiac arrest.

- *Local tetanus:* Only muscles near the wound are affected.
- *Neonatal tetanus:* Occurs in children of unimmunized mothers, often after contamination of the umbilical cord stump, and is usually fatal if not treated.

Diagnosis   The diagnosis is made primarily on clinical grounds. Muscle enzyme levels can be elevated.

℞ Tetanus

- Monitor and give supportive care in a quiet intensive care unit room.
- Give penicillin (10–12 mU/d IV for 10 days) or metronidazole (500 mg q6h or 1 g q12h) to eliminate vegetative cells and a source of further toxin. Clindamycin and erythromycin are alternatives.
- Give one dose of human tetanus immune globulin (TIG, 3000–6000 units IM) to neutralize unbound toxin; divide the dose because of the large volume.
- Control muscle spasms with benzodiazepines such as diazepam. Therapeutic paralysis with neuromuscular blocking agents may be necessary. However, prolonged paralysis may follow discontinuation of these agents.
- Immunize recovering pts. Natural disease does not induce immunity.

Prevention

- Primary vaccination: Adults should receive two doses 4–8 weeks apart and a third dose 6–12 months later. Every 10 years, pts >7 years of age should receive a booster dose of adsorbed tetanus and diphtheria toxoid (Td) or tetanus/diphtheria/attenuated pertussis vaccine (Tdap). A single dose of Tdap should be given to adults 19–64 years of age who have not previously received Tdap.
- Wound management: Administer Td or Tdap if the pt's immune status is unknown, immunization was incomplete, or >10 years have elapsed since the last booster. In contaminated or severe wounds, administer Td if >5 years have elapsed since the last vaccination. Consider TIG (250 units IM) for all but clean or minor wounds if the pt's immune status is unknown or immunization was incomplete. Vaccine and antibody should be given at separate sites.

Prognosis   The mortality rate is <10% with optimal management. Recovery is usually complete but extends over 4–6 weeks. Prolonged ventilator support may be needed. Increased muscle tone and minor spasms may last for months.

BOTULISM

Etiology, Epidemiology, and Pathogenesis   Botulism is a paralytic disease caused by neurotoxins elaborated by *Clostridium botulinum*, an anaerobic spore-forming bacterium. The neurotoxin inhibits the release of the neurotransmitter acetylcholine. *C. botulinum* is found in soil and marine environments worldwide. *C. botulinum* toxin types A, B, E, and rarely F cause human disease. Most U.S. food-borne cases are associated with home-canned food, especially vegetables, fruits, and condiments. Type E is associated with fish products. Disease occurs when (1) spores contaminate food; (2) the food is subsequently preserved in a manner that kills other bacteria but not the spores and provides anaerobic conditions at a pH and temperature permissive for germination and toxin production; and (3) the food is ingested before being heated to a temperature adequate for toxin destruction. Toxin is heat-labile (inactivated when heated for 10 min at 100°C), and spores are heat-resistant (inactivated at 116°–121°C or with steam sterilizers or pressure cookers).

Clinical Features

- *Food-borne botulism* occurs 18–36 h after ingestion of food contaminated with toxin and ranges in severity from mild to fatal (within 24 h). The characteristic presentation is symmetric descending paralysis with early cranial nerve involvement (diplopia, dysarthria, dysphonia, ptosis, and/or dysphagia) that can progress to paralysis, respiratory failure, and death. Sensory findings are absent. Nausea, abdominal pain, and vomiting may occur. Fever is uncommon. Pts are usually alert and oriented but may be drowsy or agitated.
- *Wound botulism* occurs when spores contaminate a wound and germinate—e.g., in wounds of black-tar heroin users. Wound botulism has a longer incubation period (~10 days) than food-borne botulism and causes no GI symptoms. Otherwise, the two diseases are similar.
- In *intestinal botulism*, spores germinate in the intestine and produce toxin, which is absorbed and causes illness. This form in infants has been associated with contaminated honey; thus honey should not be fed to children <12 months of age.
- *Bioterrorism-related botulism* is the potential result of the intentional dispersal (as an aerosol or as a contaminant in ingested material) of the most potent bacterial toxin known.

Diagnosis The clinical symptoms should suggest the diagnosis. The definitive test is the demonstration of the toxin in serum with a mouse bioassay, but this test may yield a negative result, particularly in wound and infant intestinal botulism. Demonstration of the organism or the toxin in clinical samples strongly suggests the diagnosis.

℞ Botulism

- Supportive care with intubation and mechanical ventilation as needed
- Routine administration of bivalent equine antitoxin to types A and B; use of an investigational monovalent antitoxin if exposure to type E toxin (i.e., through seafood ingestion) is suspected.
- Infants should receive human botulism immune globulin, which can be obtained from the California Department of Health Services (510-231-7600 or *www.infantbotulism.org*).
- Wound botulism: exploration, debridement, penicillin treatment (to eradicate the organism from the site), and administration of equine antitoxin
- For antitoxin and management advice, contact state health departments or the Centers for Disease Control and Prevention (emergency number: 770-488-7100).

Prognosis The mortality rate has been reduced to ~7.5%. Type A disease tends to be the most severe. Respiratory support may be required for months. Residual weakness and autonomic dysfunction may persist for as long as a year.

OTHER CLOSTRIDIAL INFECTIONS

Etiology and Pathogenesis Clostridia are gram-positive, spore-forming obligate anaerobes. In humans, they reside in the GI and female genital tracts. *Clos-*

tridium perfringens is the most common clostridial species isolated from tissue infections and bacteremias; next in frequency are *C. novyi* and *C. septicum*. Tissue necrosis and low oxidation-reduction potential are factors that allow rapid growth and toxin production and are essential for the development of severe disease. *C. perfringens* produces multiple virulence factors and toxins, including α toxin, which causes hemolysis, destroys platelets and polymorphonuclear leukocytes, causes widespread capillary damage, and is probably important in the initiation of muscle infections that can progress to gas gangrene.

Clinical Features

I. Intestinal disorders: food poisoning and antibiotic-associated colitis (see Chap. 89)

II. Suppurative deep-tissue infections: severe local inflammation without systemic signs (e.g., intraabdominal infection, empyema, pelvic abscess). Clostridia can be identified in association with other bacteria or as the sole isolate. These organisms are isolated from two-thirds of pts with intraabdominal infections resulting from intestinal perforation. *C. perfringens* is isolated from 20% of diseased gallbladders at surgery and from at least 50% of pts with emphysematous cholecystitis.

III. Skin and soft tissue infections

A. Localized infection without systemic signs (also called *anaerobic cellulitis*): An indolent infection that may spread to contiguous areas, it causes little pain or edema and does not involve the muscles. Gas production may be more noticeable than in more severe infections because of the lack of edema. If not treated appropriately, infection may progress to severe systemic toxic illness.

B. The onset of spreading cellulitis and fasciitis with systemic toxicity is abrupt, with rapid spread through fascial planes. On examination, SC crepitus with little localized pain is evident. The infection can be rapidly fatal (within 48 h) despite aggressive treatment. It is associated with malignancy, especially of the sigmoid or cecum. This infection differs from necrotizing fasciitis by its rapid mortality, rapid tissue invasion, and massive hemolysis.

C. Gas gangrene (clostridial myonecrosis) is characterized by rapid and extensive necrosis of muscle accompanied by gas formation and systemic toxicity. It is typically associated with traumatic wounds that are deep, necrotic, and without communication to the surface. *C. perfringens* causes 80% of cases. *C. septicum* can cause spontaneous nontraumatic clostridial myonecrosis, often in the setting of leukemia or solid tumors (especially of the GI tract and in particular the colon).

1. Incubation period: <3 days and often <24 h

2. Sudden onset of pain that is localized to the infected area and increases steadily. Infection progresses with swelling; edema; cool, tense, white skin; and profuse serous discharge with a sweetish, mousy odor. Gram's stain reveals few white cells and many gram-positive rods. Pts have a heightened sense of awareness.

IV. Bacteremia and clostridial sepsis: Transient clostridial bacteremia can arise from a focus in the GI or biliary tract or the uterus and resolves quickly without treatment. Clostridial sepsis is an uncommon but usually fatal clostridial infection, primarily of the uterus, colon, or biliary tract. The majority of cases follow septic abortion within 1–3 days. Pts are hyperalert and have fever, chills, malaise, headache, severe myalgias, abdominal pain, nausea, vomiting, oliguria, hypotension, hemolysis with jaundice (less common with *C. septicum*), and hemoglobinuria. Death occurs within 12 h.

Diagnosis Isolation of clostridia from clinical sites does not alone indicate severe disease. Clinical findings and presentation must be taken into account.

℞ **Other Clostridial Infections**

- Surgical intervention and debridement are the mainstays of treatment.
- Antibiotics: Penicillin (3–4 million units q4h) in conjunction with clindamycin (600 mg q6h) is indicated for severe clostridial disease. Clostridial wound contamination alone does not require antibiotics, and localized skin and soft tissue infections without systemic signs can be treated by debridement alone. Because suppurative infections are often mixed, they require broader-spectrum treatment. Use of hyperbaric oxygen for gas gangrene may be beneficial but is controversial and should not delay surgical treatment.

MIXED ANAEROBIC INFECTIONS

Etiology and Pathogenesis Nonsporulating anaerobic bacteria are components of the normal flora of mucosal surfaces of the mouth, lower GI tract, skin, and female genital tract. Infection results when reduced tissue redox potentials occur—e.g., from tissue ischemia, trauma, surgery, perforated viscus, shock, or aspiration. Infections often involve multiple species of anaerobes combined with microaerophilic and facultative bacteria. Most anaerobes associated with human infections are relatively aerotolerant and can survive for as long as 72 h in the presence of oxygen. Anaerobic bacteria produce exoproteins that enhance virulence; e.g., *Bacteroides fragilis* has a polysaccharide capsule that promotes abscess formation. Major anaerobic gram-positive cocci include *Peptostreptococcus* spp. Major anaerobic gram-positive rods include spore-forming clostridia and non-spore-forming *Propionibacterium acnes* (a rare cause of foreign-body infections). Major anaerobic gram-negative bacilli include the *B. fragilis* group (normal bowel flora), *Fusobacterium* spp. (oral cavity and GI tract), *Prevotella* spp. (oral cavity and female genital tract), and *Porphyromonas* spp. (oral flora).

Clinical Features
Anaerobic Infections of the Mouth, Head, and Neck
- Gingivitis and periodontal disease: can progress to involve bone, sinuses, and adjacent soft tissue
- Necrotizing ulcerative gingivitis (trench mouth, Vincent's angina): The pt has a sudden onset of bleeding tender gums, foul breath, and ulceration with gray exudates; widespread destruction of bone and soft tissue can develop (acute necrotizing ulcerative mucositis; cancrum oris, noma) after a debilitating illness, in malnourished children, or in leukemic pts. Lesions heal but leave disfiguring defects.
- Acute necrotizing infections of the pharynx: associated with ulcerative gingivitis. Pts have sore throat, foul breath, fever, a choking sensation, and tonsillar pillars that are swollen, red, ulcerated, and covered with a gray membrane. Lymphadenopathy and leukocytosis are common. Aspiration, lung abscesses, or soft tissue infection can result.
- Peripharyngeal space infections: Peritonsillar abscess (quinsy) is a complication of acute tonsillitis caused by a mixed flora including anaerobes and group A streptococci. Ludwig's angina is an infection arising from the second and third molars and associated with submandibular soft tissue infection, swelling, pain, trismus, and displacement of the tongue. Swelling can cause respiratory obstruction.

- Sinusitis and otitis: Anaerobes are important, especially in chronic infections.
- Lemierre syndrome: acute oropharyngeal *F. necrophorum* infection causing septic thrombophlebitis of the internal jugular vein and metastatic infections
- Other complications of anaerobic mouth, head, and neck infections: osteomyelitis, brain abscess, subdural empyema, mediastinitis or pleuropulmonary infection, hematogenous dissemination

Central Nervous System Infections Up to 85% of brain abscesses yield anaerobic bacteria, usually *Peptostreptococcus*, *Fusobacterium*, *Bacteroides*, and *Prevotella* spp.

Pleuropulmonary Infections

- Aspiration pneumonia: Mendelson's syndrome is characterized by aspiration of the stomach contents, with consequent destruction of the alveolar lining and rapid transudation of fluid into the alveolar space. This condition initially represents a chemical injury and not an infection, and antibiotics should be withheld unless bacterial infection supervenes.
- Bacterial aspiration pneumonia: due to depressed gag reflex, impaired swallowing, or altered mental status. Illness develops over days with low-grade fevers, malaise, and sputum production. Sputum contains a mixed flora, and cultures are usually unreliable because of contamination by oral flora components.
- Necrotizing pneumonitis: numerous small abscesses throughout the lung. The clinical course can be either indolent or fulminant.
- Anaerobic lung abscess: usually a subacute infection, often from a dental source. Pts have constitutional symptoms and foul-smelling sputum.
- Empyema: usually follows long-standing anaerobic pulmonary infection. Pts have symptoms resembling other anaerobic pulmonary infections but may report pleuritic chest pain and marked chest-wall tenderness.

Intraabdominal Infections See Chap. 88.

Pelvic Infections (Chap. 90) Most infections of the female genital tract and pelvis are mixed infections that include anaerobes and coliforms. Pure anaerobic infections occur more often at pelvic sites than at other intraabdominal sites. Pts may have foul-smelling drainage or pus from the uterus, generalized uterine or local pelvic tenderness, and fever. Suppurative thrombophlebitis of the pelvic veins may complicate the picture and lead to septic pulmonary emboli. Anaerobes are also thought to contribute to bacterial vaginosis.

Skin and Soft Tissue Infections (Chap. 91)

- Trauma, ischemia, or surgery may create a suitable environment for skin or soft tissue infections caused by anaerobic bacteria, usually as part of a mixed etiology. There is a higher frequency of fever, foul-smelling drainage, gas in the tissues, and visible foot ulcer in cases involving anaerobic bacteria.
- Meleney's gangrene (synergistic gangrene), a rare infection of the superficial fascia, is characterized by exquisite pain, redness, swelling, and induration with erythema around a central zone of necrosis, usually at the site of a surgical wound or an ulcer on an extremity.
- Necrotizing fasciitis is a rapidly destructive disease that is usually due to group A *Streptococcus* but can be a mixed anaerobic-aerobic infection. *Fournier's gangrene* involves the scrotum, perineum, and anterior abdominal wall.

Bone and Joint Infections Anaerobic bone and joint infections usually occur adjacent to soft tissue infections.

TABLE 99-1	DOSES AND SCHEDULES FOR TREATMENT OF SERIOUS INFECTIONS DUE TO COMMONLY ENCOUNTERED ANAEROBIC GRAM-NEGATIVE RODS	
First-Line Therapy	**Dose**	**Schedule**[a]
Metronidazole[b]	500 mg	q6h
Ticarcillin/clavulanic acid	3.1 g	q4h
Piperacillin/tazobactam	3.375 g	q6h
Imipenem	0.5 g	q6h
Meropenem	1.0 g	q8h

[a]See disease-specific chapters in HPIM-17 for recommendations on duration of therapy.
[b]Should generally be used in conjunction with drugs active against aerobic or facultative organisms.
Note: All drugs are given by the IV route.

Bacteremia *B. fragilis* is the most common cause of significant anaerobic bacteremia. The clinical course can resemble septic shock, and pts can become extremely ill.

Diagnosis When infections develop in close proximity to mucosal surfaces normally harboring anaerobic flora, the involvement of anaerobes should be considered. The three critical steps in successfully culturing anaerobic bacteria from clinical samples are (1) proper specimen collection, with avoidance of contamination by normal flora; (2) rapid specimen transport to the microbiology laboratory in anaerobic transport media; and (3) proper specimen handling.

℞ Mixed Anaerobic Infections

Appropriate treatment requires antibiotic administration (Table 99-1), surgical resection or debridement of devitalized tissues, and drainage.

1. Infections above the diaphragm: Metronidazole treatment gives unpredictable results in infections caused by peptostreptococci, and penicillin resistance is increasing because of β-lactamase production. Either clindamycin or a penicillin/metronidazole combination is an option.
2. Infections below the diaphragm: must be treated with agents active against *Bacteroides* spp., such as metronidazole, β-lactam/β-lactamase inhibitor combinations, or carbapenems. Aerobic gram-negative flora should also be treated, with coverage for enterococci when indicated.

For a more detailed discussion, see Abrutyn E: Tetanus, Chap. 133, p. 898; Abrutyn E: Botulism, Chap. 134, p. 901; Kasper DL, Madoff LC: Gas Gangrene and Other Clostridial Infections, Chap. 135, p. 903; and Kasper DL, Cohen-Poradosu R: Infections Due to Mixed Anaerobic Organisms, Chap. 157, p. 999, in HPIM-17.

100 Nocardiosis and Actinomycosis

NOCARDIOSIS

Nocardiae are saprophytic aerobic actinomycetes common in soil. Several species are associated with human disease. *N. asteroides* is the species most commonly associated with invasive disease. *N. brasiliensis* is most often associated with localized skin lesions.

Epidemiology In the United States, ~1100 cases of nocardial infection occur annually, of which 85% are pulmonary or systemic. The risk of disease is greater than usual among persons with deficient cell-mediated immunity—e.g., that associated with lymphoma, transplantation, glucocorticoid therapy, or AIDS.

Pathology and Pathogenesis Pneumonia and disseminated disease follow inhalation of bacterial mycelia. Nocardiosis causes abscesses with neutrophilic infiltration and necrosis. Organisms survive within phagocytes.

Clinical Features

- Pulmonary disease is usually subacute, presenting over days to weeks. Extrapulmonary disease is documented in >50% of cases, and some pulmonary involvement is evident in 80% of pts with extrapulmonary disease. A prominent cough productive of small amounts of thick purulent sputum, fever, anorexia, weight loss, and malaise are common; dyspnea, hemoptysis, and pleuritic chest pain are less common. Chest x-ray (CXR) typically shows single or multiple nodular infiltrates of varying sizes that tend to cavitate. Empyema is noted in one-third of cases. Infection may spread to adjacent tissues, such as pericardium or mediastinum.
- Extrapulmonary disease typically manifests as subacute abscesses in brain, skin, kidneys, bone, and/or muscle. Some abscesses form fistulae and discharge small amounts of pus, but not those in the lungs or brain. Brain abscesses are usually supratentorial, are often multiloculated, can be single or multiple, and tend to burrow into ventricles or extend into the subarachnoid space.
- Disease after transcutaneous inoculation
  1. Cellulitis: Subacute cellulitis may present 1–3 weeks after a break in the skin (often contaminated with soil). The firm, tender, erythematous, warm, and nonfluctuant lesions may involve underlying structures.
  2. Lymphocutaneous syndrome: A pyodermatous lesion develops at the inoculation site, with central ulceration and purulent discharge. This lesion is often drained by SC nodules along lymphatics. This form resembles sporotrichosis.
  3. Actinomycetoma: A nodular swelling forms at the site of local trauma, typically on the feet or hands. Fistulae form and discharge serous or purulent drainage that can contain granules consisting of masses of mycelia. Lesions, which spread slowly along fascial planes to involve adjacent skin and SC tissue and bone, can cause extensive deformity.
- Eye infections: Keratitis usually follows eye trauma. Endophthalmitis can occur after eye surgery or during disseminated disease.

Diagnosis

- Sputum or pus should be examined for branching, beaded, gram-positive filaments. Nocardiae usually give positive results with modified acid-fast stains. Sputum smears are often negative, and bronchoscopy may be needed to obtain adequate specimens.
- Cultures take 2–4 weeks to yield the organism. The laboratory should be alerted if nocardiosis is being considered. Sputum cultures positive for nocardiae should be assumed to reflect disease in immunocompromised hosts but may represent colonization in immunocompetent pts. Brain imaging should be considered in pts with pulmonary or disseminated disease.

Rx Nocardiosis

Table 100-1 lists the drugs, dosages, and durations used for treatment of nocardiosis.

- Sulfonamides are the drugs of choice. For serious disease, serum sulfonamide levels should be monitored and maintained at 100–150 μg/mL. Once disease is controlled, the trimethoprim-sulfamethoxazole dose may be decreased by 50%.
- Susceptibility testing can guide alternative treatments.
- Therapy for nocardiosis should continue while pts remain immunosuppressed.
- Brain abscesses that are large or unresponsive to antibiotics should be aspirated.
- Relapse is common. Pts should be followed for at least 6 months after therapy is complete. Mortality rates are high among pts with nocardiosis of the brain.

TABLE 100-1 TREATMENT FOR NOCARDIOSIS

Disease	Duration	Drugs (Daily Dose)[a]
Pulmonary or systemic		Systemic therapy
Intact host defenses	6–12 mo	Oral
Deficient host defenses	12 mo[b]	1. Trimethoprim (10–20 mg/kg) and sulfamethoxazole (50–100 mg/kg)
CNS disease	12 mo[c]	2. Minocycline (200–400 mg)
Cellulitis, lymphocutaneous syndrome	2 mo	3. Linezolid (1200 mg) Parenteral
Osteomyelitis, arthritis, laryngitis, sinusitis	4 mo	1. Amikacin (10–15 mg/kg)
Actinomycetoma	6–12 mo after clinical cure	2. Cefotaxime (6 g), ceftizoxime (6 g), ceftriaxone (1–2 g), or imipenem (2 g)
Keratitis	Topical: Until apparent cure Systemic: Until 2–4 mo after apparent cure	1. Sulfonamide drops 2. Amikacin drops Drugs for systemic therapy as listed above

[a]For each category, choices are numbered in order of preference.
[b]In some patients with AIDS or chronic granulomatous disease, therapy for pulmonary or systemic disease must be continued indefinitely.
[c]If all apparent CNS disease has been excised, the duration of therapy may be reduced to 6 months.
Note: CNS, central nervous system.

ACTINOMYCOSIS

Actinomycosis is caused by anaerobic or microaerophilic bacteria primarily of the genus *Actinomyces* (e.g., *A. israelii*). This diagnosis should be considered when a chronic progressive process with mass-like features crosses tissue boundaries, a sinus tract develops, and/or the pt has evidence of a refractory or relapsing infection despite short courses of antibiotics. Most infections are polymicrobial, but the role of other species in the pathogenesis of the disease is unclear.

Epidemiology   Actinomycosis is associated with poor dental hygiene, use of intrauterine contraceptive devices (IUCDs), and immunosuppression. Its incidence is decreasing, probably as a result of better dental hygiene and earlier initiation of antibiotic treatment.

Pathogenesis   The agents of actinomycosis are members of the normal oral flora and are commonly cultured from the GI and female genital tracts. Disease occurs only after disruption of the mucosal barrier. Local infection spreads contiguously in a slow, progressive manner, ignoring tissue planes. In vivo growth produces clumps called *grains* or *sulfur granules*. Central necrosis of lesions with neutrophils and sulfur granules is virtually diagnostic of the disease. The fibrotic walls of the mass are often described as "wooden."

Clinical Features

- Oral-cervicofacial disease: Infection starts as a soft tissue swelling, abscess, or mass, often at the angle of the jaw with contiguous extension to the brain, cervical spine, or thorax. Pain, fever, and leukocytosis are variable.
- Thoracic disease: The pulmonary parenchyma and/or pleural space is usually involved. Chest pain, fever, and weight loss occur. CXR shows a mass lesion or pneumonia. Cavitary disease or hilar adenopathy may occur, and >50% of pts have pleural thickening, effusion, or empyema. Lesions cross fissures or pleura and may involve the mediastinum, contiguous bone, or the chest wall.
- Abdominal disease: The diagnosis is challenging and may not be made until months after the initial event (e.g., diverticulitis, bowel surgery). The disease usually presents as an abscess, mass, or lesion fixed to underlying tissue and is often mistaken for cancer. Sinus tracts to the abdominal wall, perianal region, or other organs may develop and mimic inflammatory bowel disease. Involvement of the urogenital tract can present as pyelonephritis or perinephric abscess.
- Pelvic disease: Pelvic actinomycosis is often associated with IUCDs. The presentation is indolent and may follow removal of the device. Pts have fever, weight loss, abdominal pain, and abnormal vaginal bleeding. Endometritis progresses to pelvic masses or tuboovarian abscess. When there are no symptoms and actinomycosis-causing organisms are isolated, it is not clear whether an IUCD should be removed, but the pt should be carefully observed over time.
- Miscellaneous sites: Actinomycosis can involve musculoskeletal tissue, soft tissue, or the central nervous system and can disseminate hematogenously, most commonly to the lungs and liver.

Diagnosis   Aspirations, biopsies, or surgical excision may be required to obtain material for diagnosis. Microscopic identification of sulfur granules in pus or tissues establishes the diagnosis. Occasionally, sulfur granules are grossly identified from draining sinus tracts or pus. Cultures usually require 5–7 days but may take 2–4 weeks to become positive; even a single antibiotic dose can affect the yield of cultures.

℞ Actinomycosis

Like nocardiosis, actinomycosis requires prolonged treatment. IV therapy for 2–6 weeks (usually with penicillin) followed by oral therapy for 6–12 months (e.g., with penicillin or ampicillin) is suggested for serious infection and bulky disease. Less extensive disease, particularly that involving the oral-cervicofacial region, may be cured with a shorter course. If treatment is extended beyond the point of resolution of measurable disease (as quantified by CT or MRI), relapse is minimized. Suitable alternative agents include the tetracyclines (e.g., minocycline, 200 mg/d given IV or PO q12h) or clindamycin (2.7 g/d given IV q8h or 1.2–1.8 g/d given PO q6–8h).

For a more detailed discussion, see Filice GA: Nocardiosis, Chap. 155, p. 992; and Russo TA: Actinomycosis, Chap. 156, p. 996, in HPIM-17.

101 Tuberculosis and Other Mycobacterial Infections

TUBERCULOSIS

Tuberculosis (TB) is caused by organisms of the *Mycobacterium tuberculosis* complex. This complex includes *M. tuberculosis* (MTB), the most frequent and important agent of human mycobacterial disease, and *M. bovis*, which is acquired via ingestion of unpasteurized milk. MTB is a thin aerobic bacterium that is neutral on Gram's staining but that, once stained, is acid-fast—i.e., it cannot be decolorized by acid alcohol because of the cell wall's high content of mycolic acids and other lipids.

Epidemiology

- It is estimated that >8.8 million new cases of TB occurred worldwide in 2005, mostly in developing countries. In 2005, 1.6 million deaths due to TB are estimated to have occurred. In the United States, TB tends to be a disease of elderly persons, HIV-infected young adults, immigrants, and the poor. Rates increased during the late 1980s as a result of disease in these populations and the emergence of multidrug-resistant (MDR) TB but have since decreased as a result of strong TB control programs. TB rates are stable or falling globally as well.
- Disease from a pt with pulmonary TB is spread by droplet nuclei that are aerosolized by coughing, sneezing, or speaking. Droplets may be suspended in air for several hours. Transmission is determined by the intimacy and duration of contact with a pt with TB, the degree of infectiousness of the pt, and the shared environment. Pts with cavitary or laryngeal disease are most infectious, with as many as 10^5–10^7 acid-fast bacilli (AFB)/mL of sputum.
- Risk factors for development of active disease after MTB infection include recent acquisition (within the preceding year), comorbidity (e.g., HIV dis-

ease, diabetes, silicosis, immunosuppression, gastrectomy), malnutrition, and presence of fibrotic lesions.

Pathogenesis AFB that reach alveoli are ingested by macrophages. If the bacilli are not contained, they multiply, lyse the macrophages, and spread to regional lymph nodes, from which dissemination throughout the body may occur. About 2–4 weeks after infection, delayed-type hypersensitivity (DTH) destroys nonactivated macrophages that contain multiplying bacilli, and a macrophage-activating response activates cells capable of killing AFB. DTH is the basis for tuberculin skin testing (TST). A granuloma forms at the site of the primary lesion and at sites of dissemination. The lesions can then either heal by fibrosis or undergo further evolution. Despite "healing," viable bacilli can remain dormant within macrophages or in necrotic material for years. Cell-mediated immunity confers partial protection against TB. Cytokines secreted by alveolar macrophages contribute to disease manifestations, granuloma formation, and mycobacterial killing.

Clinical Features **Pulmonary TB** TB is limited to the lungs in >80% of cases in HIV-negative pts.

1. *Primary* disease: The initial infection is frequently located in the middle and lower lobes. The primary lesion usually heals spontaneously, and a calcified nodule (Ghon lesion) remains. Hilar and paratracheal lymphadenopathy are common. In immunosuppressed pts and children, primary disease may progress rapidly to clinical disease, with cavitation, pleural effusions, and hematogenous dissemination.
2. *Postprimary* (adult-type, reactivation, or secondary) disease: usually localized to the apical and posterior segments of the upper lobes and the superior segments of the lower lobes
   a. Early symptoms of fever, night sweats, weight loss, anorexia, malaise, and weakness are nonspecific and insidious.
   b. Cough and purulent sputum production, often with blood streaking, occur. Occasionally, massive hemoptysis follows erosion of a vessel located in the wall of a cavity.
   c. Disease can be limited, or extensive cavitation may develop. Extensive disease may cause dyspnea and respiratory distress.

Extrapulmonary TB Any site in the body can be involved. Up to two-thirds of HIV-infected pts with TB have extrapulmonary disease.

1. *Lymphadenitis* occurs in >40% of extrapulmonary TB cases, especially among HIV-infected pts. Painless swelling of cervical and supraclavicular nodes (*scrofula*) is typical. Early on, nodes are discrete but can be inflamed with a fistulous tract. Fine-needle aspiration or surgical biopsy of the node is required for diagnosis. AFB smears are positive in ~50% of cases and cultures in 70–80%.
2. *Pleural involvement* is common in primary TB, resulting from penetration of bacilli into the pleural space or contiguous spread of parenchymal inflammation.
   a. DTH in response to these bacilli can result in effusion. Fluid is straw-colored and exudative, with protein levels >50% of those in serum, normal to low glucose levels, a usual pH of ~7.3 (occasionally <7.2), and pleocytosis (500–6000 cells/μL). Mononuclear cells are most common, although neutrophils may be present early in disease, and mesothelial cells are rare or absent. The pleural concentration of adenosine deami-

nase (ADA), if low, virtually excludes TB. Pleural biopsy is often required for diagnosis, with up to 80% of biopsy cultures positive.

b. Empyema is uncommon and results from rupture of a cavity with many bacilli into the pleural space.

3. In *genitourinary* disease, local symptoms predominate (e.g., frequency and dysuria). Calcifications and ureteral strictures can be seen. In >90% of cases, urinalysis shows pyuria and hematuria with negative bacterial cultures; in 90% of cases, culture of three morning urine specimens is diagnostic. Genital TB is more common among women than among men. Fallopian tube and uterine disease can cause infertility.

4. *Skeletal* disease: The spine, hips, and knees are the most common sites. Spinal TB (Pott's disease) often involves two or more adjacent vertebral bodies; in adults, lower thoracic/upper lumbar vertebrae are usually affected. Disease spreads to adjacent vertebral bodies, later affecting the intervertebral disk and causing collapse of vertebral bodies in advanced disease (kyphosis, gibbus). Paravertebral cold abscesses may form.

5. *Meningitis* occurs most often in young children and HIV-seropositive pts. Disease typically evolves over 1–2 weeks.

a. Cranial nerve involvement (particularly of ocular nerves) is common. Disease progresses to coma, hydrocephalus, and intracranial hypertension.

b. Cerebrospinal fluid (CSF) has a high lymphocyte count, an elevated protein level, and a low glucose concentration. Cultures are positive in 80% of cases. Polymerase chain reaction is ~80% sensitive but gives a false-positive result 10% of the time.

c. Neurologic sequelae are seen in ~25% of treated pts; adjunctive glucocorticoids enhance survival among pts >14 years of age but do not reduce the frequency of neurologic sequelae.

6. *Gastrointestinal* disease affects the terminal ileum and cecum, causing abdominal pain and diarrhea, and can present with a clinical picture similar to that of Crohn's disease. A palpable mass and bowel obstruction may occur. TB peritonitis presents with fever, abdominal pain, and ascites that is exudative with a high protein content and lymphocytic leukocytosis. Peritoneal biopsy is usually required for diagnosis.

7. *Pericarditis* is characterized by an acute or subacute onset of fever, dull retrosternal pain, and sometimes a friction rub. Effusion is common. Chronic constrictive pericarditis is a potentially fatal complication, even in treated pts. Adjunctive glucocorticoids may help manage acute disease but do not seem to reduce constriction.

8. *Miliary* disease arises from hematogenous spread of MTB throughout the body. Lesions are small (1- to 2-mm) granulomas, and symptoms are nonspecific. Hepatomegaly, splenomegaly, lymphadenopathy, and choroidal tubercles of the eye may occur.

HIV-Associated TB The manifestations of TB vary with the stage of HIV infection. When cell-mediated immunity is only partly compromised, pulmonary TB presents as typical upper-lobe cavitary disease. In late HIV infection, a primary TB–like pattern may be evident, with diffuse interstitial or miliary infiltrates, little or no cavitation, and intrathoracic lymphadenopathy. Extrapulmonary disease occurs frequently; common forms include lymphadenitis, meningitis, pleuritis, pericarditis, mycobacteremia, and disseminated disease.

Diagnosis

- Maintain a high index of suspicion, perform appropriate radiographic studies, and obtain appropriate clinical specimens.

- Examine diagnostic specimens for AFB with auramine-rhodamine stain and fluorescence microscopy.
- Isolate and identify MTB on culture; liquid media and speciation by molecular methods have decreased the time required for diagnostic confirmation to 2–3 weeks.
- Nucleic acid amplification is useful for rapid confirmation of TB in AFB-positive specimens.
- The results of drug susceptibility testing are most rapid if liquid medium is used.
- TST is of limited value in active disease because of low sensitivity and specificity but is the most widely used screening test for latent TB infection. Interferon γ (IFN-γ) release assays (IGRAs) measure the release of IFN-γ by T cells after stimulation with TB-specific antigens. IGRAs are as sensitive as TST in active disease and are more specific; however, further studies must assess their performance in this setting.

R_x Tuberculosis

DRUGS
First-Line Agents
- *Rifampin*: the most important and potent antituberculous agent. The standard dosage in adults is 600 mg/d. The drug distributes well throughout body tissues, including inflamed meninges. It turns body fluids (e.g., urine, saliva, tears) red-orange and is excreted through bile and the enterohepatic circulation. Rifampin is usually well tolerated but may cause GI upset. The drug can cause hepatitis when given in combination with isoniazid or pyrazinamide. Rash, anemia, and thrombocytopenia are less common side effects. Of note, rifampin is a potent inducer of hepatic microsomal enzymes and decreases the half-life of many other drugs.
- *Isoniazid (INH)*: the best agent available after rifampin. The usual adult dosage is 300 mg/d or 900 mg 2 or 3 times per week. INH is distributed well throughout the body and infected tissues, including CSF and caseous granulomas. The most important toxicities are hepatotoxicity and peripheral neuropathy. INH-associated hepatitis is idiosyncratic and increases with age, alcohol use, pregnancy or the postpartum period, active hepatitis B infection, and concomitant use of rifampin. Because peripheral neuropathy can result from interference with pyridoxine metabolism, pyridoxine (25–50 mg/d) should be given to pts with other risk factors for neuropathy, such as diabetes, alcohol abuse, or malnutrition.
- *Ethambutol*: the least potent first-line agent, ethambutol is usually given at a dosage of 15–20 mg/kg daily. It is distributed throughout the body but reaches only low levels in CSF. At higher doses, retrobulbar optic neuritis can occur, causing central scotoma and impairing both visual acuity and the ability to see green.
- *Pyrazinamide*: the usual dosage is 15–30 mg/kg daily (maximum, 2 g/d). The drug distributes well throughout the body, including the CSF. At current doses, hepatotoxicity is no greater than with INH or rifampin. Hyperuricemia and—in rare instances—gout can occur.

Other Effective Agents
- *Streptomycin*: the usual adult dose is 0.5–1.0 g IM daily or 5 times per week. Streptomycin causes ototoxicity, affecting both hearing and vestibular function, but is less nephrotoxic than other aminoglycosides.
- *Rifabutin*: may be as effective as rifampin, eliciting fewer drug interactions, and is active against some rifampin-resistant TB strains. Tissue le-

vels are 5–10 times higher than plasma levels. Most adverse effects are dose-related.

- *Rifapentine*: similar to rifampin but can be given once or twice weekly. This drug is not approved by the U.S. Food and Drug Administration for the treatment of HIV-infected pts because rifampin monoresistance has been documented in pts taking INH and once-weekly rifapentine.

Second-Line Agents

- *Fluoroquinolones* (e.g., levofloxacin, ciprofloxacin, and moxifloxacin) have solid, broad antimycobacterial activity. Other agents are used uncommonly but may be needed in disease caused by resistant strains of MTB.

REGIMENS

See Table 101-1.

- Nonadherence to the regimen is the most important impediment to cure. Directly observed treatment (especially during the initial 2 months) and fixed-drug-combination products should be used if possible.
- Bacteriologic evaluation is the preferred method of monitoring response to treatment. Virtually all pts should have negative sputum cultures by the end of 2–3 months of treatment. If the culture remains positive, treatment failure and drug resistance should be suspected.
- Drug resistance may be either primary (i.e., infection caused by a strain resistant prior to therapy) or acquired (i.e., resistance arising during treatment because of an inadequate regimen or the pt's noncompliance). MDR TB is defined as that caused by strains resistant to isoniazid and rifampin.
- Close monitoring for drug toxicity should take place during treatment and should include baseline liver function tests (LFTs) and monthly questioning about possible hepatitis symptoms. High-risk pts (e.g., older pts, pts who use alcohol daily) should have LFT values monitored during treatment.
- HIV-associated TB: Three considerations are important for HIV-infected pts receiving TB treatment.
  1. Immune reconstitution inflammatory syndrome (IRIS) may occur when antiretroviral therapy (ART) is initiated. Symptoms and signs of TB are exacerbated as immune function improves.
  2. ART agents and rifamycin may interact.
  3. Rifampin monoresistance may develop with widely spaced intermittent treatment.

Prevention

- Vaccination: An attenuated strain of *M. bovis*, bacille Calmette-Guérin (BCG), protects infants and young children from serious forms of TB. Its efficacy is unclear in other situations.
- Treatment of latent infection: Candidates for chemoprophylaxis are usually identified by TST. Positive skin tests are determined by reaction size and risk group (Table 101-2), and, if the test is positive, drug treatment is considered (Table 101-3). INH should not be given to persons with active liver disease.

LEPROSY

Etiology and Epidemiology Leprosy, a nonfatal chronic infectious disease caused by *M. leprae*, is a disease of the developing world; its global prevalence is difficult to assess and is variously estimated at 0.6–8 million. Africa has the

TABLE 101-1 RECOMMENDED ANTITUBERCULOSIS TREATMENT REGIMENS

	Initial Phase		Continuation Phase	
Indication	Duration, Months	Drugs	Duration, Months	Drugs
New smear- or culture-positive cases	2	HRZE[a,b]	4	HR[a,c,d]
New culture-negative cases	2	HRZE[a]	2	HR[a]
Pregnancy	2	HRE[e]	7	HR
Failure and relapse[f]	—	—	—	—
Resistance (or intolerance) to H	Throughout (6)	RZE[g]		
Resistance to H + R	Throughout (12–18)	ZEQ + S (or another injectable agent[h])		
Resistance to all first-line drugs	Throughout (24)	1 injectable agent[h] + 3 of these 4: ethionamide, cycloserine, Q, PAS		
Standardized re-treatment (susceptibility testing unavailable)	3	HRZES[i]	5	HRE
Drug intolerance to R	Throughout (12)[j]	HZE		
Drug intolerance to Z	2	HRE	7	HR

[a]All drugs can be given daily or intermittently (three times weekly throughout or twice weekly after 2–8 weeks of daily therapy during the initial phase).

[b]Streptomycin can be used in place of ethambutol but is no longer considered to be a first-line drug by ATS/IDSA/CDC.

[c]The continuation phase should be extended to 7 months for pts with cavitary pulmonary tuberculosis who remain sputum culture–positive after the initial phase of treatment.

[d]HIV-negative pts with noncavitary pulmonary tuberculosis who have negative sputum AFB smears after the initial phase of treatment can be given once-weekly rifapentine/isoniazid in the continuation phase.

[e]The 6-month regimen with pyrazinamide can probably be used safely during pregnancy and is recommended by the WHO and the International Union Against Tuberculosis and Lung Disease. If pyrazinamide is not included in the initial treatment regimen, the minimum duration of therapy is 9 months.

[f]Regimen is tailored according to the results of drug susceptibility tests.

[g]A fluoroquinolone may strengthen the regimen for pts with extensive disease.

[h]Amikacin, kanamycin, or capreomycin. All these agents should be discontinued after 2–6 months, depending on tolerance and response.

[i]Streptomycin should be discontinued after 2 months. This regimen is less effective for pts in whom treatment has failed, who have an increased probability of rifampin-resistant disease. In such cases, the re-treatment regimen might include second-line drugs chosen in light of the likely pattern of drug resistance.

[j]Streptomycin for the initial 2 months or a fluoroquinolone might strengthen the regimen for pts with extensive disease.

Note: H, isoniazid; R, rifampin; Z, pyrazinamide; E, ethambutol; S, streptomycin; Q, a quinolone antibiotic; PAS, para-aminosalicylic acid.

highest prevalence, and Asia has the most cases. More than 80% of the world's cases occur in a few countries: India, China, Myanmar, Indonesia, Nepal, Brazil, Nigeria, and Madagascar. Leprosy is associated with poverty and rural residence. The route of transmission is uncertain but may be via nasal droplets, contact with infected soil, or insect vectors.

TABLE 101-2 TUBERCULIN REACTION SIZE AND TREATMENT OF LATENT TB INFECTION

Risk Group	Tuberculin Reaction Size, mm
HIV-infected persons or persons receiving immuno-suppressive therapy	≥5
Close contacts of TB pts	≥5[a]
Persons with fibrotic lesions on chest radiography	≥5
Recently infected persons (≤2 years)	≥10
Persons with high-risk medical conditions[b]	≥10
Low-risk persons[c]	≥15

[a]Tuberculin-negative contacts, especially children, should receive prophylaxis for 2–3 months after contact ends and should then undergo repeat TST. Those whose results remain negative should discontinue prophylaxis. HIV-infected contacts should receive a full course of treatment regardless of TST results.
[b]Including diabetes mellitus, some hematologic and reticuloendothelial diseases, injection drug use (with HIV seronegativity), end-stage renal disease, and clinical situations associated with rapid weight loss.
[c]Except for employment purposes where longitudinal TST screening is anticipated, TST is not indicated for these low-risk persons. A decision to treat should be based on individual risk/benefit considerations.

Clinical, Histologic, and Immunologic Spectrum The spectrum of clinical and histologic manifestations of leprosy is attributable to variability in the immune response to *M. leprae*. The spectrum from polar tuberculoid leprosy (TL) to polar lepromatous leprosy (LL) is associated with an evolution from localized to more generalized disease manifestations and an increasing bacterial load. Prognosis, complications, and intensity of antimicrobial therapy depend on where a pt presents on the clinical spectrum. The incubation period ranges from 2 to 40 years but is usually 5–7 years.

Tuberculoid Leprosy
- Disease is confined to the skin and peripheral nerves. AFB are few or absent.
- One or several hypopigmented macules or plaques with sharp margins that are hypesthetic and have lost sweat glands and hair follicles are present.
- There is asymmetric enlargement of one or several peripheral nerves—most often the ulnar, posterior auricular, peroneal, and posterior tibial nerves—associated with hypesthesia and myopathy.

Lepromatous Leprosy
- Symmetrically distributed skin nodules, raised plaques, and diffuse dermal infiltration that can cause leonine facies, loss of eyebrows and lashes, pendulous earlobes, and dry scaling
- Numerous bacilli in skin, nerves, and all organs except lungs and central nervous system
- Nerve enlargement and damage are usually symmetric; symmetric nerve-trunk enlargement and acral distal peripheral neuropathy are seen.

Complications
- Reactional states: inflammatory conditions at the site of lesions. Erythema nodosum leprosum (ENL) occurs in pts near the LL end of the disease spectrum as they tend toward TL after treatment.

TABLE 101-3   REVISED DRUG REGIMENS FOR TREATMENT OF LATENT TB INFECTION (LTBI) IN ADULTS

Drug	Interval and Duration	Comments[a]	Rating[b] (Evidence[c]) HIV-Negative	Rating[b] (Evidence[c]) HIV-Infected
Isoniazid	Daily for 9 months[d,e]	In HIV-infected persons, isoniazid may be administered concurrently with nucleoside reverse transcriptase inhibitors, protease inhibitors, or nonnucleoside reverse transcriptase inhibitors (NNRTIs).	A (II)	A (II)
	Twice weekly for 9 months[d,e]	Directly observed therapy (DOT) must be used with twice-weekly dosing.	B (II)	B (II)
	Daily for 6 months[e]	Regimen is not indicated for HIV-infected persons, those with fibrotic lesions on chest radiographs, or children.	B (I)	C (I)
	Twice weekly for 6 months[e]	DOT must be used with twice-weekly dosing.	B (II)	C (I)
Rifampin[f]	Daily for 4 months	Regimen is used for contacts of pts with isoniazid-resistant, rifampin-susceptible TB. In HIV-infected pts, most protease inhibitors and delavirdine should not be administered concurrently with rifampin. Rifabutin, with appropriate dose adjustments, can be used with protease inhibitors (saquinavir should be augmented with ritonavir) and NNRTIs (except delavirdine). Consult web-based updates for the latest specific recommendations.	B (II)	B (III)

(continued)

TABLE 101-3	REVISED DRUG REGIMENS FOR TREATMENT OF LATENT TB INFECTION (LTBI) IN ADULTS (CONTINUED)			
			Rating[b] (Evidence[c])	
Drug	Interval and Duration	Comments[a]	HIV-Negative	HIV-Infected
Rifampin plus pyrazin-amide (RZ)	Daily for 2 months	Regimen generally should not be offered for treatment of LTBI in either HIV-infected or HIV-negative pts.	D (II)	D (II)
	Twice weekly for 2–3 months		D (III)	D (III)

[a]Interactions with HIV-related drugs are updated frequently and are available at *www.aidsinfo.nih.gov/guidelines.*

[b]Strength of the recommendation: A. Both strong evidence of efficacy and substantial clinical benefit support recommendation for use. Should always be offered. B. Moderate evidence for efficacy or strong evidence for efficacy but only limited clinical benefit supports recommendation for use. Should generally be offered. C. Evidence for efficacy is insufficient to support a recommendation for or against use, or evidence for efficacy might not outweigh adverse consequences (e.g., drug toxicity, drug interactions) or cost of the treatment or alternative approaches. Optional. D. Moderate evidence for lack of efficacy or for adverse outcome supports a recommendation against use. Should generally not be offered. E. Good evidence for lack of efficacy or for adverse outcome supports a recommendation against use. Should never be offered.

[c]Quality of evidence supporting the recommendation: I. Evidence from at least one properly randomized controlled trial. II. Evidence from at least one well-designed clinical trial without randomization, from cohort or case-controlled analytic studies (preferably from more than one center), from multiple time-series studies, or from dramatic results in uncontrolled experiments. III. Evidence from opinions of respected authorities based on clinical experience, descriptive studies, or reports of expert committees.

[d]Recommended regimen for persons <18 years old.

[e]Recommended regimen for pregnant women.

[f]The substitution of rifapentine for rifampin is not recommended because rifapentine's safety and effectiveness have not been established for pts with LTBI.

Source: Adapted from CDC: Targeted tuberculin testing and treatment of latent tuberculosis infection. MMWR 49(RR-6), 2000.

- Extremities: Neuropathy results in insensitivity and affects fine touch, pain, and heat receptors. Ulcerations, trauma, secondary infections, and (at times) a profound osteolytic process can take place.
- Nose: chronic nasal congestion, epistaxis, destruction of cartilage with saddle-nose deformity or anosmia
- Eye: trauma, secondary infection, corneal ulcerations, opacities, uveitis, cataracts, glaucoma, blindness
- Testes: orchitis, aspermia, impotence, infertility

Diagnosis In TL, the advancing edge of a skin lesion should be biopsied. In LL, biopsy of even normal-appearing skin often yields positive results.

 Leprosy

DRUGS
- Rifampin (600 mg daily or monthly) is the only agent bactericidal against *M. leprae*.

- Dapsone (50–100 mg/d). Hemolysis and methemoglobinemia are common adverse effects. G6PD deficiency must be ruled out before therapy to avoid hemolytic anemia. GI intolerance, headache, pruritus, peripheral neuropathies, and rash can occur.
- Clofazimine (50–100 mg/d, 100 mg 3 times per week, or 300 mg monthly). A phenazine iminoquinone dye, clofazimine is weakly active against *M. leprae*. Adverse effects include skin discoloration and GI intolerance.

REGIMENS
- Paucibacillary disease in adults (<6 skin lesions)
  1. Dapsone (100 mg/d) and rifampin (600 mg monthly, supervised) for 6 months or dapsone (100 mg/d) for 5 years
  2. With a single lesion: a single dose of rifampin (600 mg), ofloxacin (400 mg), and minocycline (100 mg)
- Multibacillary disease in adults (≥6 skin lesions)
  1. Dapsone (100 mg/d) plus clofazimine (50 mg/d) unsupervised as well as rifampin (600 mg monthly) plus clofazimine (300 mg monthly) supervised for 1–2 years
  2. Relapse can occur years later; prolonged follow-up is needed.
  3. Some experts prefer rifampin (600 mg/d for 3 years) and dapsone (100 mg/d) for life.
- Reactional states
  1. Mild reactions: glucocorticoids (40–60 mg/d for at least 3 months)
  2. If ENL is present and persists despite two courses of steroids, thalidomide (100–300 mg nightly) should be given. Because of thalidomide's teratogenicity, its use is strictly regulated.

INFECTIONS WITH NONTUBERCULOUS MYCOBACTERIA (NTM)

Mycobacteria other than MTB and *M. leprae* are distributed widely throughout the environment in water, biofilms, and soil as well as in numerous animal species. Isolation of NTM from a clinical specimen may reflect colonization and requires an assessment of the organism's significance.

Microbiology   *M. abscessus*, *M. fortuitum*, and *M. chelonae* grow rapidly (within 7 days). Other NTM species, such as *M. avium* and *M. intracellulare* (the *M. avium* complex, or MAC), *M. kansasii*, *M. ulcerans*, and *M. marinum*, more typically grow within 2–3 weeks, although newer broth culture systems can isolate these organisms more quickly.

Clinical Features
MAC
1. Pulmonary disease: Compared with MTB, MAC organisms more commonly cause lung disease in pts born in the United States.
   a. Pts present with chronic cough, dyspnea, and fatigue but no fever. Two patterns are seen: (1) primary pulmonary disease presenting as nodules or bronchiectasis and (2) secondary disease (sometimes cavitary) in pts with underlying lung disease [e.g., chronic obstructive pulmonary disease (COPD), prior TB, cystic fibrosis]. MAC can also cause hypersensitivity pneumonitis after a pt's repeated exposure to indoor hot tubs containing MAC-contaminated water.
   b. CT of the chest should be performed to document the extent of disease at baseline.
   c. Most pts with secondary MAC pulmonary disease should be treated. Pts with primary MAC pulmonary disease may not need treatment if there

is no disease progression and the pts' age or underlying disease is likely to be the critical determinant of survival over the next few years. Agents include clarithromycin (250–500 mg bid) or azithromycin (250 mg daily or three times a week) plus ethambutol (15 mg/kg daily). Some authorities include rifampin or rifabutin. Streptomycin or amikacin can be included in the first 2 months for severe disease, and a fluoroquinolone can be considered if one of the first-line agents cannot be tolerated. A macrolide-containing regimen should be given for ≥12 months after sputum cultures become negative.

2. Disseminated disease occurs primarily in immunocompromised pts, including those with advanced HIV disease who are not receiving ART.

   a. Pts present with fever, weakness, wasting, and adenopathy. Laboratory studies reveal anemia, hypoalbuminemia, increased alkaline phosphatase levels, and blood cultures positive for MAC.

   b. Blood cultures yield positive results within 2–3 weeks. AFB staining of bone marrow, intestine, and/or liver can provide the diagnosis.

   c. Pts in whom ART is initiated may experience IRIS 1–12 weeks later and develop localized or generalized culture-positive lymphadenitis.

   d. Treatment should consist of a macrolide—clarithromycin (500 mg bid) or azithromycin (500 mg/d)—plus ethambutol (15 mg/kg daily) and ART. Rifabutin may be included as well. Therapy can be stopped after 12 months if CD4+ T cell counts have been >100/μL for at least 6 months.

   e. Chemoprophylaxis with azithromycin (1200 mg weekly) or clarithromycin (500 mg bid) is indicated to prevent MAC disease in pts with CD4+ T cell counts of <50/μL or when another AIDS-defining illness occurs. Prophylaxis should be continued until the CD4+ T cell count has been >100/μL for at least 3 months.

M. kansasii *M. kansasii* is the second most common cause of lung disease due to NTM in the United States. The average age of onset is 60 years, and most pts have COPD, lung cancer, silicosis, or prior TB. Clinical features resemble those of pulmonary TB. A sputum culture positive for *M. kansasii* is usually clinically significant, especially in HIV-positive pts. Treatment with rifampin (600 mg/d), isoniazid (300 mg/d), and ethambutol (15 mg/kg daily) should be administered for at least 12 months after the last positive culture. Disseminated disease can occur in pts with advanced AIDS and resembles disseminated MAC infection but has more prominent pulmonary findings. Treatment is the same as for pulmonary disease. Pts should be given an ART regimen compatible with a rifamycin.

M. abscessus, M. chelonae, and M. fortuitum Disseminated cutaneous disease is the most common clinical manifestation of infection with the rapidly growing NTM species. Lesions are cellulitic or nodular, erythematous, indurated, and tender. They may ulcerate and exude purulent drainage and may spread proximally along lymphatics. These organisms may infect surgical or traumatic wounds, contaminated injection sites, or sites of body piercing. Pulmonary infections, usually due to *M. abscessus*, are the next most common manifestation and occur in pts with an underlying lung disease such as cystic fibrosis. Susceptibility testing should be performed, although all three species are usually susceptible to clarithromycin (500 mg bid) and amikacin (10–15 mg/kg daily). Cefoxitin (3 g q6h) or imipenem (500 mg q6–12h) is effective for most *M. abscessus* and *M. fortuitum* infections. Experts recommend up to 6 months of treatment for bacteremic or disseminated cutaneous disease and 12 months of treatment after sputum cultures are negative for pulmonary disease. Localized cutaneous lesions may respond to a single agent, such as clarithromycin, administered for 2 weeks.

M. marinum *M. marinum* is widely distributed in water and causes chronic cutaneous infections when open wounds are exposed to a colonized water source, usually via fish tanks, shellfish, or marine settings. *M. marinum* grows best at 30°C, a temperature lower than that at which other mycobacteria thrive. After a median incubation period of 21 days, a granulomatous or ulcerating skin lesion develops, with subsequent proximal spread along lymphatics; extension to deeper structures may occur in pts receiving immunosuppressive therapy, resulting in tenosynovitis or osteomyelitis. Administration of clarithromycin and ethambutol for 1–2 months after lesion resolution (usually a 3- to 4-month course) is recommended.

M. ulcerans *M. ulcerans* causes a cutaneous infection (Buruli ulcer) in endemic regions (e.g., in Central and West Africa and Central and South America). The initial lesion is a painless nodule that progresses to a deep ulcer with sloughing of skin and SC tissue. Osteomyelitis may occur, and deforming scarring and contractures may result from extensive necrosis. Antimycobacterial treatment has not yet been shown to be helpful; surgical treatment is important.

For a more detailed discussion, see Raviglione MC, O'Brien RJ: Tuberculosis, Chap. 158, p. 1006; Gelber RH: Leprosy (Hansen's Disease), Chap. 159, p. 1021; von Reyn CF: Nontuberculous Mycobacteria, Chap. 160, p. 1027; and Wallace RJ Jr., Griffith DE: Antimycobacterial Agents, Chap. 161, p. 1032, in HPIM-17.

102 Lyme Disease and Other Nonsyphilitic Spirochetal Infections

LYME BORRELIOSIS

Etiology and Epidemiology Lyme disease, caused by the spirochete *Borrelia burgdorferi*, is the most common vector-borne illness in the United States. *B. burgdorferi sensu stricto* causes disease in North America; *B. garinii* and *B. afzelii* are more common in Europe. *Ixodes* ticks transmit the disease: *I. scapularis*, which also transmits babesiosis and anaplasmosis, is found in the northeastern and midwestern United States; *I. pacificus* is found in the western United States. The white-footed mouse is the preferred host for larval and nymphal ticks. Adult ticks prefer the white-tailed deer as host. The tick must feed for 24 h to transmit the disease.

Clinical Features **Early Infection, Stage 1: Localized Infection** After an incubation period of 3–32 days, erythema migrans (EM) develops at the site of the tick bite in 80% of pts. The classic presentation is a red macule that expands slowly to form an annular lesion with a bright red outer border and central clearing; central erythema, induration, necrosis, or vesicular changes or many red rings within an outer ring are also possible.

Early Infection, Stage 2: Disseminated Infection

- Hematogenous spread occurs within days to weeks after infection. Secondary annular lesions may develop.
- Pts develop headache, mild neck stiffness, fever, chills, migratory musculoskeletal pain, arthralgias, malaise, and fatigue. These symptoms subside within a few weeks, even in untreated pts.
- Meningeal irritation: CSF is initially normal; however, weeks to months later, ~15% of pts progress to frank neurologic abnormalities (meningitis; encephalitis; cranial neuritis, including bilateral facial palsy; motor or sensory radiculoneuropathy; mononeuritis multiplex; ataxia; and myelitis).
- Cardiac involvement occurs in ~8% of pts. Atrioventricular (AV) block of fluctuating degree is most common, but acute myopericarditis is possible.

Late Infection, Stage 3: Persistent Infection

- Lyme arthritis develops in ~60% of untreated pts in the United States. It usually consists of intermittent attacks of oligoarticular arthritis in large joints (especially the knees) lasting weeks to months. Joint fluid cell counts range from 500 to 110,000/μL. Recurrent attacks decrease yearly, but a few pts have chronic arthritis with bony and cartilage erosion. Arthritis can persist despite eradication of spirochetes.
- Chronic neurologic involvement is less common. Encephalopathy affecting memory, mood, or sleep can be accompanied by axonal polyneuropathy manifested as either distal paresthesia or spinal radicular pain. In Europe, severe encephalomyelitis is seen with *B. garinii* infection.
- Acrodermatitis chronica atrophicans, a late skin manifestation, is seen in Europe and Asia and is associated with *B. afzelii* infection.

Diagnosis

- Culture of the organism in Barbour-Stoenner-Kelly medium is largely a research tool. Cultures are positive only early in illness, with the organism isolated primarily from EM skin lesions.
- Polymerase chain reaction (PCR) is most useful for joint fluid, is less sensitive for cerebrospinal fluid (CSF), and has little utility for plasma or urine testing.
- Serology can be problematic because tests do not clearly distinguish between active and inactive infection. Serologic testing should be undertaken when the pt has at least an intermediate pretest likelihood of having Lyme disease.
- Two-step testing: enzyme-linked immunosorbent assay (ELISA) screening with Western blot testing in cases with positive or equivocal results. IgM and IgG testing should be done in the first month of illness, after which IgG testing alone is adequate.

℞ Lyme Borreliosis

Except for neurologic and cardiac disease, most treatment can be oral.

1. Doxycycline (100 mg bid) is the agent of choice for men and nonpregnant women and is also effective against anaplasmosis.
2. Amoxicillin (500 mg tid), cefuroxime (500 mg bid), erythromycin (250 mg qid), and newer macrolides are alternative agents, preferred in that order.
3. More than 90% of pts have good outcomes with a 14-day course of treatment for localized infection or a 21-day course for disseminated infection.
4. Neuroborreliosis: IV treatment with ceftriaxone (2 g/d for 14–28 days) should be given. Cefotaxime or penicillin is an alternative.

5. Pts with high-degree AV block should receive a 28-day course that commences with IV ceftriaxone (or alternative IV drugs) until the high-degree AV block has resolved; oral agents can then be used to complete treatment.
6. Lyme arthritis: 30–60 days of PO antibiotic. For pts who do not respond to oral agents, re-treatment with IV ceftriaxone for 28 days is appropriate. If joint inflammation persists after therapy but PCR testing for *B. burgdorferi* DNA in joint fluid gives negative results, anti-inflammatory agents or synovectomy may be successful.
7. Chronic Lyme disease: Persistent musculoskeletal and neurocognitive symptoms with fatigue occur in a small percentage of pts after antibiotic treatment. Further antibiotic courses are not helpful; treatment consists of symptom-based supportive care.

Prophylaxis If an attached, engorged *I. scapularis* nymph is found or if follow-up will be difficult, a single 200-mg dose of doxycycline, given within 72 h of the tick bite, effectively prevents the disease. This measure is not routinely recommended.

Prognosis Early treatment results in an excellent prognosis. Although convalescence is longer the later antibiotics are given, the overall prognosis remains excellent, with minimal or no residual deficits. Reinfection can occur. No vaccine is commercially available.

ENDEMIC TREPONEMATOSES

Etiology and Epidemiology The endemic treponematoses—yaws, endemic syphilis, and pinta—are nonvenereal chronic childhood diseases caused by organisms closely related to the agent of syphilis, *Treponema pallidum*. Early skin lesions are infectious; disease is transmitted by direct contact.

Clinical Features Disease is manifest by primary skin lesions that become disseminated with time. After a latency phase, destructive gummas in skin, bone, and joints occur as late manifestations. Pinta causes dyschromic macules but not destructive lesions.

Diagnosis Diagnosis is based on clinical presentation and dark-field microscopy of scrapings from lesions. Serologic tests for syphilis are also used to diagnose endemic treponematoses.

℞ Endemic Treponematoses

Benzathine penicillin (1.2 million units for adults, 600,000 units for children <10 years of age) is the treatment of choice. Doxycycline is probably an effective alternative.

LEPTOSPIROSIS

Etiology and Epidemiology Leptospires are spirochetal organisms that cause an important zoonosis with a broad spectrum of clinical manifestations. Rodents, particularly rats, are the most important disease reservoir, but many mammalian species can harbor the organisms. Transmission can occur during contact with urine, blood, or tissue from infected animals or during exposure to contaminated environments. Organisms are found in urine and can survive in water for many months. The disease is particularly common in developing tropical nations. Approximately 40–120 cases are reported each year in the United States, but these numbers are likely to represent significant underestimates. Risk factors in the United States include recreational water activities, occupational activities that result in exposure to animals or animal waste (e.g., sewage work), and residence in urban settings with expanding rat populations.

Pathogenesis Entry of the organisms via skin abrasions or intact mucous membranes is followed by leptospiremia and widespread dissemination. Organisms can be isolated from blood and CSF for the first 4–10 days of illness. Leptospires damage blood vessel walls and cause vasculitis, leakage, and extravasation, including hemorrhages. Vasculitis is responsible for most manifestations.

Clinical Features

- Incubation period, 1–2 weeks (range, 2–20 days)
- Anicteric leptospirosis, a biphasic illness, is the milder form and is found in 90% of symptomatic cases.
  1. Flulike illness: fever, severe headache, nausea, vomiting. Myalgias, especially of the calves, back, and abdomen, are a dominant feature.
  2. Conjunctival suffusion and fever are the most common physical findings; rash develops occasionally. Symptoms subside within 1 week and recur after 1–3 days in conjunction with antibody development.
  3. Symptoms are generally milder in phase 2, but up to 15% of pts can develop clinically evident aseptic meningitis. A higher percentage of pts have asymptomatic CSF pleocytosis. Iritis, chorioretinitis, and uveitis can occur. Symptoms usually subside in days but can persist for weeks to months.
- Icteric leptospirosis (Weil's syndrome) is severe, with a mortality rate of 5–15%.
  1. After 4–9 days of mild illness, more severe symptoms develop; however, illness is not truly biphasic.
  2. Pts have jaundice, hepatosplenomegaly, and abdominal tenderness.
  3. Renal failure with acute tubular necrosis may develop.
  4. Cough, dyspnea, chest pain, and hemoptysis can occur.
  5. Hemorrhagic manifestations commonly include epistaxis, petechiae, purpura, and ecchymoses.
  6. Rhabdomyolysis, hemolysis, myocarditis, pericarditis, congestive heart failure, shock, adult respiratory distress syndrome, pancreatitis, and multiorgan failure have all been described.
- Laboratory findings
  1. Azotemia, abnormal urinary sediment, proteinuria
  2. Elevated erythrocyte sedimentation rate, marked leukocytosis, thrombocytopenia
  3. Elevated bilirubin and alkaline phosphatase levels, mild aminotransferase increases
  4. Prolonged prothrombin time, elevated creatine phosphokinase level
  5. Patchy alveolar pattern due to hemorrhage on chest x-ray

Diagnosis

- Serology: Microscopic agglutination test (MAT) done at Centers for Disease Control and Prevention; ELISA available at reference laboratories
- The organism can be cultured from blood or CSF in the first 10 days of illness or from urine after the first week. Cultures most often become positive within 2–4 weeks (range, 1 week to 4 months).
- Differential: dengue, malaria, viral hepatitis, hantavirus disease, rickettsial disease

℞ Leptospirosis

Treatment should be started as early as possible but should be given even if delayed. IV agents, including penicillin G (1.5 million units qid), ampicillin (1 g qid), ceftriaxone (1 g once daily), and erythromycin (500 mg qid), are all effective. Milder cases can be treated with oral doxycycline (100 mg bid) or amoxicillin (500 mg qid).

RELAPSING FEVER

Etiology *Borrelia recurrentis* causes louse-borne relapsing fever (LBRF). LBRF is transmitted from person to person by the body louse. Tick-borne relapsing fever (TBRF), a zoonosis usually transmitted from rodents to humans via the bite of various *Ornithodoros* ticks, is caused by multiple *Borrelia* species. DNA rearrangement within *vmp* genes on linear plasmids results in variation in expression of surface antigens, allowing evasion of host immune responses.

Epidemiology Rates of LBRF have decreased markedly with improvements in the standard of living. TBRF still occurs worldwide and often goes unrecognized or underreported. About 35 cases per year are reported in the United States, mostly in forested mountainous areas of far western states and among persons sleeping in rustic mountain cabins and vacation homes. Ticks feed painlessly and quickly (20–45 min).

Clinical Features Symptoms are similar in the two types of relapsing fever.
1. Mean incubation period, 7 days; range, 2–18 days
2. Sudden onset of high fever, headache, shaking chills, sweats, dizziness, nausea, vomiting, myalgias, arthralgias (sometimes severe); no arthritis
3. Tachycardia, tachypnea, dehydration, scleral icterus, and petechiae can occur. Conjunctivae are often injected, and photophobia is common.
4. Epistaxis, blood-tinged sputum, and gastrointestinal or central nervous system hemorrhage can occur.
5. Symptoms increase for 2–7 days, then end in a crisis with two phases.
   a. *Chill phase*: rigors, rising temperature, hypermetabolism
   b. *Flush phase*: falling temperature, diaphoresis, decreased effective circulating blood volume
6. Spirochetemia and symptoms recur after days to weeks. LBRF is associated with 1 or 2 relapses, TBRF with up to 10. Each episode is less severe and is followed by a longer afebrile interval than the last.

Diagnosis Spirochetes can be demonstrated in blood, bone marrow aspirates, or CSF by dark-field microscopy or in thick or thin smears of peripheral blood or buffy-coat preparations treated with Wright, Giemsa, or acridine orange stain. Organisms are most numerous during high fevers before the crisis.

℞ Relapsing Fever

One dose of doxycycline (100 mg), erythromycin (500 mg), or chloramphenicol (500 mg) is effective for LBRF. A 7-day course is recommended for TBRF. A Jarisch-Herxheimer-like reaction within 1–4 h of the first dose occurs in >50% of TBRF cases but is more severe in LBRF cases or when high numbers of spirochetes are circulating at treatment outset. The reaction can last up to 8 h; pts should be closely monitored.

Prognosis Untreated LBRF has a high case-fatality rate, but the mortality rate is <5% with therapy. TBRF is generally a milder disease.

> For a more detailed discussion, see Lukehart SA: Endemic Trepone-
> matoses, Chap. 163, p. 1046; Speelman P, Hartskeerl R: Leptospiro-
> sis, Chap. 164, p. 1048; Dennis DT: Relapsing Fever, Chap. 165, p.
> 1052; and Steere AC: Lyme Borreliosis, Chap. 166, p. 1055, in
> HPIM-17. For a discussion of syphilis, see Chap. 90 in this manual.

103 Rickettsial Diseases

Rickettsiae are obligate intracellular gram-negative coccobacilli and short bacilli usually transmitted by tick, mite, flea, or louse vectors. Except in the case
of louse-borne typhus, humans are incidental hosts.

TICK- AND MITE-BORNE SPOTTED FEVERS

ROCKY MOUNTAIN SPOTTED FEVER (RMSF)

Epidemiology Caused by *R. rickettsii*, RMSF is the most severe rickettsial
disease. In the United States, the prevalence is highest in the south-central and
southeastern states. Most cases occur between May and September. RMSF is
transmitted by different ticks in different geographic areas; e.g., the American
dog tick (*Dermacentor variabilis*) transmits RMSF in the eastern two-thirds of
the United States and in California.

Pathogenesis Rickettsiae are inoculated by the tick after ≥6 h of feeding,
spread lymphohematogenously, and infect numerous foci of contiguous infected endothelial cells. Increased vascular permeability, with edema, hypovolemia, and ischemia, causes tissue and organ injury.

Clinical Features The incubation period is ~1 week (range, 2–14 days). Symptoms in the first 3 days of illness are nonspecific and include fever, headache,
malaise, myalgias, nausea, vomiting, and anorexia. By day 3, half of pts have a
rash. Macules typically appear on the wrists and ankles, subsequently spreading
to the rest of the extremities and the trunk. Lesions initially blanch; however, because of vascular damage, central hemorrhage later develops and the lesions become petechial. Such petechiae eventually develop in 41–59% of pts, appearing
on or after day 6 of illness in ~74% of all cases that include a rash. The palms
and soles become involved after day 5 in 43% of pts but do not become involved
at all in 18–64%. Pts develop hypovolemia, prerenal azotemia, hypotension,
noncardiogenic pulmonary edema, and cardiac involvement with dysrhythmias.
Pulmonary disease is an important factor in fatal cases and develops in 17% of
cases overall. Central nervous system (CNS) involvement is the other important
determinant of outcome. Encephalitis can progress to stupor or delirium, ataxia,
coma, seizures, cranial nerve palsy, hearing loss, severe vertigo, nystagmus, dys-

arthria, aphasia, and other CNS signs. Meningoencephalitis can develop, with cerebrospinal fluid notable for pleocytosis, mononuclear cell predominance, and increased protein and normal glucose levels. Renal and hepatic injury can occur, and bleeding is a rare but potentially life-threatening consequence of severe vascular damage. Other laboratory findings may include increased plasma levels of acute-phase reactants such as C-reactive protein, hyponatremia, and elevated levels of creatine kinase.

Prognosis Without treatment, the pt usually dies in 8–15 days; a rare fulminant presentation can result in death within 5 days. The mortality rate was 20–25% in the preantibiotic era and remains at 3–5% despite the availability of effective antibiotics, mostly because of delayed diagnosis.

Diagnosis Within the first 3 days, diagnosis is difficult, since only 3% of pts have the classic triad of fever, rash, and known history of tick exposure. When the rash appears, the diagnosis should be considered. Immunohistologic examination of a cutaneous biopsy sample from a rash lesion is the only diagnostic test of use during acute illness. Serology, most commonly the indirect immunofluorescence assay (IFA), is usually positive 7–10 days after disease onset, and a diagnostic titer of ≥1:64 is usually documented.

℞ Rocky Mountain Spotted Fever

Doxycycline (100 mg bid PO or IV) is the treatment of choice for both children and adults but not for pregnant women and pts allergic to this drug, who should receive chloramphenicol. Treatment is given until the pt is afebrile and has been improving for 2 or 3 days.

OTHER TICK-BORNE SPOTTED FEVERS

R. conorii causes disease in southern Europe, Africa, and Asia. The name for *R. conorii* infection varies by region (e.g., Mediterranean spotted fever, Kenya tick typhus). Disease is characterized by high fever, rash, and—in most locales—an inoculation eschar (tache noire) at the site of the tick bite. A severe form of disease with ~50% mortality occurs in pts with diabetes, alcoholism, or heart failure. African tick-bite fever, caused by *R. africae*, occurs in sub-Saharan Africa and the Caribbean and is the rickettsiosis most frequently imported into Europe and North America. Tick-borne spotted fever is diagnosed on clinical grounds. Doxycycline (100 mg bid for 1–5 days), ciprofloxacin (750 mg bid for 5 days), or chloramphenicol (500 mg qid for 7–10 days) is effective for treatment.

RICKETTSIALPOX

Epidemiology Rickettsialpox is caused by *R. akari* and is maintained by mice and their mites. Recognized principally in New York City, rickettsialpox has been reported in other urban and rural locations in the United States as well as in Ukraine, Croatia, and Turkey. This infection is more common than was previously thought.

Clinical Features A papule forms at the site of the mite bite and develops a central vesicle that becomes a painless black-crusted eschar surrounded by an erythematous halo. Lymph nodes draining the region of the eschar enlarge. After an incubation period of 10–17 days, malaise, chills, fever, headache, and myalgia mark disease onset. A macular rash appears on day 2–6 of illness and evolves sequentially into papules, vesicles, and crusts that heal without scarring. Some pts have nausea, vomiting, abdominal pain, cough, conjunctivitis, or photophobia. Disease resolves within 6–10 days and is not fatal.

 Rickettsialpox

Doxycycline is the drug of choice for treatment.

FLEA- AND LOUSE-BORNE TYPHUS GROUP RICKETTSIOSES

ENDEMIC MURINE TYPHUS (FLEA-BORNE)

Epidemiology　Caused by *R. typhi*, endemic murine typhus has a rat reservoir and is transmitted by fleas. Humans become infected when rickettsia-laden flea feces are scratched into pruritic bite lesions; less often, the flea bite itself transmits the organisms. In the United States, endemic typhus occurs mainly in southern Texas and southern California; globally, it occurs in warm (often coastal) areas throughout the tropics and subtropics. Flea bites are not often recalled by pts, but exposure to animals such as cats, opossums, raccoons, skunks, and rats is reported by ~40%.

Clinical Features　The incubation period averages 11 days (range, 8–16 days). Prodromal symptoms 1–3 days before the abrupt onset of chills and fever include headache, myalgia, arthralgia, nausea, and malaise. Nausea and vomiting are common early in illness. The duration of untreated disease averages 12 days (range, 9–18 days). Rash is apparent at presentation (usually ~4 days after symptom onset) in 13% of pts; 2 days later, half of the remaining pts develop a maculopapular rash that involves the trunk more than the extremities, is seldom petechial, and rarely involves the face, palms, or soles. Pulmonary disease is common, causing a hacking, nonproductive cough. Almost one-fourth of pts who undergo chest x-ray (CXR) have pulmonary densities due to interstitial pneumonia, pulmonary edema, and pleural effusions. Abdominal pain, confusion, stupor, seizures, ataxia, coma, and jaundice occur less commonly. Laboratory abnormalities include anemia, leukocytosis, thrombocytopenia, hyponatremia, hypoalbuminemia, increased hepatic aminotransferase levels, and prerenal azotemia. Disease can be severe enough for admission to an intensive care unit, and complications include respiratory failure requiring intubation and mechanical ventilation, hematemesis, cerebral hemorrhage, and hemolysis. The disease is more severe in older pts, those with underlying disease, and those treated with a sulfonamide drug.

Diagnosis　The diagnosis can be based on cultivation, polymerase chain reaction (PCR), cross-adsorption serologic studies of acute- and convalescent-phase sera, or immunohistology.

 Endemic Murine Typhus (Flea-Borne)

Doxycycline (100 mg bid for 7–15 days) is effective.

EPIDEMIC TYPHUS (LOUSE-BORNE)

Epidemiology　Epidemic typhus is caused by *R. prowazekii* and is transmitted by the human body louse. The louse lives in clothing under poor hygienic conditions, particularly in colder climates and classically at times of war or natural disaster. Eastern flying-squirrel lice and fleas maintain *R. prowazekii* in a zoonotic cycle. Lice feed on pts with epidemic typhus and then defecate the organism into the bite at their next meal. The pt autoinoculates the organism while scratching. Because lice abandon pts with high fevers, they effectively spread disease. *Brill-Zinsser disease* is a recrudescent and mild form of epidemic typhus whose occurrence years after acute illness suggests that *R. prowazekii* remains dormant in the host, reactivating when immunity wanes.

Clinical Features   After an incubation period of ~1 week (range, 7–14 days), there is an abrupt onset of high fevers, prostration, severe headache, cough, and severe myalgias. Rash appears on the upper trunk around the fifth day of illness and spreads to involve all body-surface areas except the face, palms, and soles. Photophobia with conjunctival injection and eye pain is also common. Confusion and coma, skin necrosis, and gangrene of the digits are noted in severe cases. Untreated, the disease is fatal in 7–40% of cases. Pts develop renal failure, multiorgan involvement, and prominent neurologic manifestations.

Diagnosis   The diagnosis can be based on serology or immunohistochemistry or on detection of the organism in a louse found on a pt. Cross-adsorption IFA can distinguish *R. prowazekii* from *R. typhi*.

 Epidemic Typhus (Louse-Borne)

Doxycycline (a 200-mg dose once or 100 mg bid until 2–3 days after the pt has defervesced).

SCRUB TYPHUS

Orientia tsutsugamushi, the agent of scrub typhus, is a member of the family Rickettsiaceae that is transmitted by larval mites or chiggers in environments of heavy scrub vegetation. Disease occurs during the wet season. It is endemic in Asia, northern Australia, and the Pacific islands. Clinical manifestations range from mild to fatal disease. Pts have an eschar at the site of chigger feeding, regional lymphadenopathy, and maculopapular rash. Severe cases include encephalitis and interstitial pneumonia. Scrub typhus can be diagnosed by serologic assays (IFA, indirect immunoperoxidase and enzyme immunoassays). A 7- to 15-day course of doxycycline (100 mg bid) or chloramphenicol (500 mg qid) is effective.

EHRLICHIOSES AND ANAPLASMOSIS

Ehrlichiae are obligately intracellular organisms transmitted by ticks. Two distinct *Ehrlichia* species and one *Anaplasma* species cause human infections.

HUMAN MONOCYTOTROPIC EHRLICHIOSIS (HME)

HME is caused by *Ehrlichia chaffeensis*. Most cases of HME occur in southeastern, south-central, and mid-Atlantic states. Most pts are male; the median age of pts is 53 years. After a median incubation period of 8 days, pts develop fever, headache, myalgia, and malaise. Nausea, vomiting, diarrhea, cough, rash, and confusion may be noted. Disease can be severe: up to 62% of pts are hospitalized. Complications include a toxic shock–like syndrome, respiratory distress, meningoencephalitis, fulminant infection, and hemorrhage. Leukopenia, thrombocytopenia, and elevated serum aminotransferase levels are common. The diagnosis is usually based on clinical presentation, but PCR testing before initiation of antibiotic therapy or retrospective serodiagnosis to detect increased antibody titers can be performed. Bone marrow examination reveals hypercellular marrow, and noncaseating granulomas may be evident. Morulae are rarely seen in peripheral blood. Treatment with doxycycline (100 mg bid) or tetracycline (250–500 mg q6h) is effective and should be continued for 3–5 days after defervescence.

EHRLICHIOSIS EWINGII

Ehrlichiosis ewingii resembles HME but is less severe. Most cases are diagnosed in immunocompromised pts. Treatment is the same as for HME.

HUMAN GRANULOCYTOTROPIC ANAPLASMOSIS (HGA)

HGA is caused by *Anaplasma phagocytophilum*. Most cases of human anaplasmosis occur in northeastern and upper midwestern states. After an incubation period of 4–8 days, pts develop fever, myalgia, headache, and malaise. A minority of pts develop nausea, vomiting, diarrhea, cough, or confusion. Severe complications—respiratory insufficiency, a toxic shock–like syndrome, and opportunistic infections—occur most often in the elderly. Although the mortality rate is low, nearly 7% of pts require intensive care. On laboratory examination, pts are found to have leukopenia, thrombocytopenia, and elevated serum aminotransferase levels. HGA is not associated with vasculitis or granulomas. Anaplasmosis should be considered in pts with atypical severe presentations of Lyme disease. Co-infection with either *Borrelia burgdorferi* (the agent of Lyme disease) or *Babesia microti* should be considered in all cases because these three agents share the *Ixodes scapularis* vector and have the same geographic distribution. Peripheral blood films may reveal morulae in neutrophils in 20–75% of infections. PCR testing before antibiotic therapy or retrospective serologic testing for rises in antibody can confirm the diagnosis. Treatment with doxycycline (100 mg bid) is effective, and most pts defervesce within 24–48 h. Pregnant women may be treated with rifampin.

PREVENTION

These diseases are prevented by avoidance of ticks in endemic areas, use of protective clothing and tick repellents, careful tick searches after exposures, and prompt removal of attached ticks.

Q FEVER

Etiology *Coxiella burnetii* causes Q fever. The organism can exist as a highly infectious phase I form within humans or as an avirulent phase II form. *C. burnetii* can form spores that allow its prolonged survival in harsh environments.

Epidemiology Q fever is a zoonosis that occurs worldwide. The primary sources of human infection are infected cattle, sheep, and goats, but cats, rabbits, pigeons, and dogs can transmit the disease as well. *C. burnetii* localizes to the uterus and mammary glands of infected female mammals. It is reactivated in pregnancy and is found at high concentrations in the placenta. At parturition, the organism is dispersed as an aerosol, and infection usually follows inhalation. Abattoir workers, veterinarians, and others persons who have contact with infected animals are at risk. Exposure to newborn animals or infected products of conception poses the highest risk. *C. burnetii* is shed in the milk for weeks to months after parturition. Ingestion of contaminated milk is believed to be an important route of transmission in some areas, although the evidence on this point is contradictory.

Clinical Features

- Acute Q fever: The incubation period lasts 3–30 days. Clinical presentations include flulike syndromes, prolonged fever, pneumonia, hepatitis, pericarditis, myocarditis, meningoencephalitis, and infection during pregnancy. Symptoms are often nonspecific (e.g., fever, fatigue, headache, chills, sweats, nausea, vomiting, diarrhea, cough, and occasionally rash). Multiple rounded opacities on CXR are common and are highly suggestive of Q fever pneumonia. The white blood cell count is usually normal, but thrombocytopenia occurs. During recovery, reactive thrombocytosis can develop. Pts with acute Q fever and lesions of native or prosthetic heart valves should be monitored serologically for 2 years. If phase I IgG titers are >1:800, further evaluation is indicated. Some authorities treat pts with acute Q fever and valvulopathy for 1 year with doxycycline and hydroxychloroquine to prevent chronic Q fever.
- Chronic Q fever: This uncommon entity almost always implies endocarditis, occurring in pts with prior valvular heart disease, immunosuppression, or chronic renal failure. Fever is absent or low grade; nonspecific symptoms may be present for a year before diagnosis. Vegetations are seen in only 12% of cases and manifest as nodules on the valve. Hepatomegaly and/or splenomegaly in combination with a positive rheumatoid factor, high erythrocyte sedimentation rate, high C-reactive protein level, and/or increased γ-globulin concentration suggests the diagnosis. Although *C. burnetii* can be isolated by a shell-vial technique, most laboratories are not permitted to attempt isolation because of its highly contagious nature. PCR testing of tissue or biopsy specimens can be used, but serology is the most common diagnostic tool; IFA is the method of choice. In chronic Q fever, titers of antibody to phase I antigen are much higher than those to phase II; the reverse is true in acute infection. Acute infection can be diagnosed by a fourfold rise in antibody titer. Chronic infection is associated with an IgG titer of ≥1:800 to phase I antigen.

Rx Q Fever

Acute Q fever is treated with doxycycline (100 mg bid for 14 days). Quinolones are also efficacious. If Q fever is diagnosed during pregnancy, trimethoprim-sulfamethoxazole should be administered up to term. The currently recommended treatment for chronic Q fever is doxycycline (100 mg bid) and hydroxychloroquine (200 mg tid; plasma concentrations maintained at 0.8–1.2 μg/mL) for 18 months. In vitro, hydroxychloroquine renders doxycycline bactericidal against *C. burnetii*. The minimal inhibitory concentration (MIC) of doxycycline for the pt's isolate should be determined and serum levels monitored. Pts should be advised about photosensitivity and retinal toxicity risks with treatment. Pts who cannot receive this regimen should be treated with at least two agents active against *C. burnetii*. The combination of rifampin (300 mg once daily) plus doxycycline (100 mg bid) or ciprofloxacin (750 mg bid) has been used with success. Treatment should be given for at least 3 years and discontinued only if phase I IgA and IgG antibody titers are ≤1:50 and ≤1:200, respectively.

For a more detailed discussion, see Walker DH et al: Rickettsial Diseases, Chap. 167, p. 1059, in HPIM-17.

104 MYCOPLASMA INFECTIONS

Mycoplasmas are the smallest free-living organisms. Lacking a cell wall and bounded only by a plasma membrane, they colonize mucosal surfaces of the respiratory and urogenital tracts.

M. PNEUMONIAE

Epidemiology *M. pneumoniae* causes upper and lower respiratory tract disease, with the highest attack rates among persons 5–20 years old. Infection is acquired by inhalation of aerosols. Children <5 years old usually have only upper respiratory tract disease; children >5 years old and adults usually have bronchitis and pneumonia. Infection can be severe in pts with sickle cell disease as a result of functional asplenia.

Clinical Features The incubation period is longer than those for other respiratory infections, typically lasting for 2–3 weeks. Pts often have antecedent upper respiratory tract symptoms and then develop fever, sore throat, and prominent headache and cough. Myalgias, arthralgias, and GI symptoms are uncommon. Sputum production is lacking or minimal. If present, sputum is usually white but may be blood-tinged. Pharyngeal injection is common. Bullous myringitis (blisters on the tympanic membrane) is an uncommon but unique manifestation. Physical findings are minimal, and pleural effusion is documented in <20% of pts. Extrapulmonary manifestations suggest *M. pneumoniae* infection because, although unusual in the latter illness, they are even rarer in other respiratory illnesses. These manifestations include erythema multiforme, digital necrosis (due to high titers of cold agglutinins) in pts with sickle cell disease, myocarditis, pericarditis, encephalitis, cerebellar ataxia, Guillain-Barré syndrome, transverse myelitis, peripheral neuropathy, hemolytic anemia, coagulopathies, and arthritis (in pts with hypogammaglobulinemia).

Diagnosis Chest x-ray may show reticulonodular or interstitial infiltrates, primarily in the lower lobes. Most infections are not definitively diagnosed. Gram's staining gives negative results because mycoplasmas lack a cell wall; culture is possible but very difficult; and serologic tests are not positive early enough to help guide clinical decisions (although they may be helpful retrospectively when acute- and convalescent-phase sera are available). Cold agglutinins are nonspecific but develop within the first 7–10 days in >50% of pts with *M. pneumoniae* pneumonia. A titer of ≥1:32 suggests the diagnosis. Antigen detection tests have been developed but are not yet widely available.

℞ *M. pneumoniae* Infections

Upper respiratory infections due to *M. pneumoniae* do not require antibiotic treatment. Pneumonia is usually self-limited, but effective antibiotics shorten the duration of illness and reduce coughing and therefore may also reduce transmission. If the diagnosis is known, doxycycline (100 mg bid), macrolides (e.g., clarithromycin, 500 mg bid; or azithromycin, 500 mg/d), or fluoroquinolones (e.g., levofloxacin, 750 mg/d) are effective and should be administered for 14–21 days. For empirical treatment of community-acquired pneumonia, a fluoroquinolone alone or a macrolide plus ceftriaxone (1 g/d) is recommended for better coverage of *Streptococcus pneumoniae* and *Haemophilus influenzae*.

GENITAL MYCOPLASMAS
See Chap. 90.

 For a more detailed discussion, see McCormack WM: Infections Due to Mycoplasmas, Chap. 168, p. 1068, in HPIM-17.

105 Chlamydial Infections

Three chlamydial species infect humans: *Chlamydia trachomatis*, *Chlamydophila psittaci*, and *Chlamydophila pneumoniae* (formerly the TWAR agent). Chlamydiae are obligate intracellular bacteria, possess both DNA and RNA, and have a cell wall and ribosomes similar to those of gram-negative bacteria. These organisms have a complex reproductive cycle and exist in two forms. The *elementary body* (the infective form) is adapted for extracellular survival, while the *reticulate body* is adapted for intracellular survival and multiplication. After replication, reticulate bodies condense into elementary bodies that are released to infect other cells or people. *C. trachomatis*, *C. psittaci*, and *C. pneumoniae* share group-specific antigens; the microimmunofluorescence test can differentiate among the three species.

C. TRACHOMATIS INFECTIONS

GENITAL INFECTIONS, INCLUDING LYMPHOGRANULOMA VENEREUM
See Chap. 90.

TRACHOMA AND ADULT INCLUSION CONJUNCTIVITIS (AIC)

Definitions and Etiology   Trachoma is a chronic conjunctivitis caused by *C. trachomatis* serovars A, B, Ba, and C. AIC is an acute eye infection in adults exposed to infected genital secretions and in their newborns; this infection is caused by sexually transmitted *C. trachomatis* strains, usually serovars D through K.

Epidemiology   Trachoma causes ~20 million cases of blindness worldwide, primarily in northern and sub-Saharan Africa, the Middle East, and parts of Asia. Transmission occurs from eye to eye via hands, flies, towels, and other fomites, particularly among young children in rural communities with limited water supplies.

Clinical Features   Both trachoma and AIC present initially as conjunctivitis, with small lymphoid follicles in the conjunctiva. Trachoma usually starts insidiously before 2 years of age. Reinfection and persistent infection are common. With progression, there is inflammatory leukocytic infiltration and superficial vascularization (pannus formation) of the cornea. Scarring eventually distorts the eyelids, turning lashes inward and abrading the eyeball. Eventually, the corneal epithelium ulcerates, with subsequent scarring and blindness. Destruction of goblet cells, lacrimal ducts, and glands causes dry-eye syndrome, with resultant corneal opacity and secondary bacterial corneal ulcers. AIC is an acute unilateral follicular conjunctivitis with preauricular lymphadenopathy. Corneal inflammation is evidenced by discrete opacities, punctate epithelial erosions, and superficial corneal vascularization.

Diagnosis Clinical diagnosis is based on the presence of two of the following signs: lymphoid follicles on the upper tarsal conjunctiva, typical conjunctival scarring, vascular pannus, or limbal follicles. Intracytoplasmic chlamydial inclusions are found in 10–60% of Giemsa-stained conjunctival smears. Chlamydial polymerase chain reaction or ligase chain reaction is more sensitive and often gives positive results when smears or cultures are negative.

℞ Treatment and Prevention

- AIC responds to azithromycin (a single 1-g dose) or doxycycline (100 mg bid for 7 days); treatment of sexual partners is needed to prevent ocular reinfection and chlamydial genital disease.
- The World Health Organization's Global Campaign to Eliminate Trachoma promotes surgery for deformed eyelids; periodic mass treatment with azithromycin; face washing; and environmental improvements.

C. PSITTACI INFECTIONS

Epidemiology and Pathogenesis Psittacosis is primarily an infection of birds and mammals. Most avian species can harbor *C. psittaci*, but psittacine birds (e.g., parrots, parakeets) are most often infected. Psittacosis is an occupational disease in pet-shop owners, poultry workers, and other individuals with regular avian contact. Present in nasal secretions, excreta, tissues, and feathers of infected birds, *C. psittaci* is transmitted to humans mainly by the respiratory route, gains access to the upper respiratory tract, spreads hematogenously, and localizes in the pulmonary alveoli and reticuloendothelial cells of the spleen and liver. The pathognomonic histologic finding is the presence of macrophages with typical cytoplasmic inclusion bodies in alveoli filled with fluid, erythrocytes, and lymphocytes.

Clinical Features After an incubation period of 7–14 days or longer, disease onset may be gradual or may be abrupt with shaking chills and fever to 40.6°C (105°F). Headache is prominent, and many pts have a dry, hacking, nonproductive cough. Small amounts of mucoid or bloody sputum may be produced as disease progresses. An increased respiratory rate and dyspnea with cyanosis can develop with extensive pulmonary involvement. Pts also report myalgias, spasm and stiffness of back and neck muscles, lethargy, depression, agitation, insomnia, and disorientation. Occasionally, pts are comatose at presentation. GI symptoms can occur. Physical findings are less prominent than symptoms and x-ray findings would suggest. Splenomegaly is evident in 10–70% of pts.

Diagnosis This diagnosis should be considered in a pt with pneumonia and splenomegaly and is confirmed by serologic studies. A rise in the titer of complement-fixing antibody between acute- and convalescent-phase serum samples suggests the diagnosis.

 C. psittaci Infections

Tetracycline (2 4 g/d in four divided doses) or doxycycline (100 mg bid) is consistently effective, resulting in defervescence and symptom alleviation within 24–48 h. Treatment is continued for 7–14 days after defervescence to avoid relapse. Erythromycin is an alternative agent; azithromycin and some fluoroquinolones are active in vitro and are likely to be effective.

C. PNEUMONIAE INFECTIONS

Epidemiology   Infections are most common among young adults but can occur throughout life, and reinfection is common. Seroprevalence exceeds 40% in the many adult populations tested throughout the world. Epidemics occur in close residential quarters such as military barracks. There is an epidemiologic association between serologic evidence of *C. pneumoniae* infection and atherosclerotic disease. *C. pneumoniae* has been identified in atherosclerotic plaques by electron microscopy, DNA hybridization, immunocytochemistry, and culture. It is hypothesized that the organism's presence accelerates atherosclerosis, especially in the setting of high cholesterol levels.

Clinical Features   Manifestations of *C. pneumoniae* infection include pharyngitis, sinusitis, bronchitis, and pneumonitis. Primary infection is more severe than reinfection. Pneumonia due to *C. pneumoniae* resembles that due to *Mycoplasma pneumoniae*: pts have antecedent upper respiratory tract symptoms, fever, dry cough, minimal findings on auscultation, small segmental infiltrates on chest x-ray, and no leukocytosis. Elderly pts can have severe disease.

Diagnosis   Diagnosis is difficult. Serology does not reliably distinguish *C. pneumoniae* from *C. trachomatis* or *C. psittaci*.

 C. pneumoniae Infections

Erythromycin or tetracycline (2 g/d for 10–14 days) is recommended. Other macrolides (e.g., azithromycin) or quinolones (e.g., levofloxacin) are alternative agents.

For a more detailed discussion, see Stamm WE: Chlamydial Infections, Chap. 169, p. 1070, in HPIM-17.

106 Herpesvirus Infections

HERPES SIMPLEX VIRUSES

Etiology and Pathogenesis   The herpes simplex viruses HSV-1 and HSV-2 are linear, double-stranded DNA viruses. There is ~50% sequence homology between HSV-1 and HSV-2. Exposure to HSV at mucosal surfaces or abraded skin sites permits viral entry and replication in cells of the epidermis and dermis. HSV enters sensory or autonomic neuronal cells and is transported to nerve cell bodies in ganglia, where it can cause latency. The virus is maintained in a repressed state compatible with the survival and normal activities of the cell. Reactivation occurs when normal viral gene expression resumes, with reappearance of the virus on mucosal surfaces. Both antibody-mediated and cell-mediated immunity (including type-specific immunity) are clinically important.

Epidemiology   HSV-1 is acquired more frequently and at an earlier age than HSV-2. More than 90% of adults have antibodies to HSV-1 by the fifth decade of life. Antibodies to HSV-2 usually are not detected until adolescence and correlate with sexual activity. In the United States, 15–20% of the population has antibody to HSV-2. Infection with HSV-2 is an independent risk factor for the acquisition and transmission of infection with HIV-1, which can be shed from genital herpes lesions. HSV is transmitted by contact with active lesions or with virus shed from mucocutaneous surfaces by asymptomatic persons. During the first years after primary infection with HSV-1 or HSV-2, viral shedding from mucosal sites of immunocompetent and immunocompromised adults can occur on 30–50% and up to 80% of days, respectively. Pts with long-term infection can shed HSV on as many as 20–30% of days. The large reservoir of unidentified carriers and the frequent asymptomatic reactivation of HSV-2 have fostered the continued spread of HSV throughout the world.

Clinical Spectrum   The incubation period for primary infection is 1–26 days (median, 6–8 days). Reactivation depends on anatomic site and virus type as well as the pt's age and immune status. Overall, genital HSV-2 is twice as likely to reactivate as genital HSV-1 and recurs 8–10 times more often. In contrast, oral-labial HSV-1 recurs more frequently than oral-labial HSV-2.

Oral-Facial Infections

- Primary HSV-1 infection: seen most often in children and young adults. Pts commonly have gingivostomatitis, pharyngitis, and up to 2 weeks of fever, malaise, myalgia, inability to eat, and cervical adenopathy with lesions on the palate, gingiva, tongue, lip, face, posterior pharynx, and/or tonsillar pillars. Exudative pharyngitis may occur.
- Reactivation: Viral excretion in the saliva, intraoral mucosal ulcerations, or ulcers on the vermilion border of the lip or external facial skin can occur with reactivation of latent virus in the trigeminal ganglia. Pts undergoing trigeminal nerve root decompression or dental extraction can develop oral-labial herpes a median of 3 days after the procedure.
- Infection in compromised hosts: Compromised hosts (e.g., AIDS pts, pts undergoing induction chemotherapy or in the early phases of transplanta-

tion) can have a severe infection that extends into the mucosa and skin, causing friability, necrosis, bleeding, pain, and inability to eat or drink.

- Eczema herpeticum: Severe oral-facial HSV infection, with extensive skin lesions and occasional visceral dissemination, may develop in pts with atopic eczema.
- Erythema multiforme: HSV infection is the precipitating event in ~75% of cases.
- Bell's palsy: A flaccid paralysis of the mandibular portion of the facial nerve, Bell's palsy has been linked to HSV and varicella-zoster virus (VZV). Antiviral therapy and a short course of glucocorticoids may be helpful.

Genital Infections

- Primary infection (see Chap. 90): Pts with prior HSV-1 infection have milder cases. About 15% of cases are associated with other clinical syndromes, such as aseptic meningitis, cervicitis, and urethritis.
- Reactivation: Reactivation infections are often subclinical or can cause genital lesions or urethritis with dysuria. Even without a history of rectal intercourse, perianal lesions can occur as a result of latency established in the sacral dermatome from prior genital tract infection. Proctitis can cause anorectal pain, discharge, tenesmus, and constipation. Ulcerative lesions can be seen in the distal 10 cm of the rectal mucosa.

Whitlow   In HSV infection of the finger, pts experience an abrupt onset of edema, erythema, pain, and vesicular or pustular lesions of the fingertips that are often confused with the lesions of pyogenic bacterial infection. Fever and lymphadenitis are common.

Herpes Gladiatorum   HSV infection caused by trauma to the skin during wrestling can occur anywhere on the body but commonly affects the thorax, ears, face, and hands.

Eye Infections   HSV is the most frequent cause of corneal blindness in the United States.

- Keratitis: acute onset of pain, blurred vision, chemosis, conjunctivitis, and dendritic lesions of the cornea. Topical glucocorticoids may exacerbate disease. Recurrences are common.
- Chorioretinitis: usually seen with disseminated HSV infection
- Acute necrotizing retinitis: a rare, serious manifestation of HSV or VZV infection

Central and Peripheral Nervous System Infections

- Encephalitis: In the United States, HSV causes 10–20% of all cases of sporadic viral encephalitis, and 95% of these cases are due to HSV-1. The estimated incidence is 2.3 cases per 1 million persons per year. Encephalitis can occur during primary infection or in pts already seropositive for HSV-1. Pts present with an acute onset of fever and focal neurologic symptoms and signs, especially in the temporal lobe. Neurologic sequelae are common, especially in pts >50 years of age. Antiviral treatment should be started empirically until the diagnosis is confirmed or an alternative diagnosis is made. IV treatment is recommended until cerebrospinal fluid (CSF) levels of viral DNA are reduced or undetectable.
- Aseptic meningitis: HSV DNA is found in CSF from 3–15% of pts with aseptic meningitis, usually in association with primary genital HSV infection. This acute, self-limited disease without sequelae is manifested by head-

ache, fever, and photophobia. Pts have symptoms for 2–7 days. Lymphocytic pleocytosis in the CSF is documented. HSV is the most common cause of recurrent lymphocytic meningitis (Mollaret's meningitis).

- Autonomic dysfunction caused by either HSV or VZV most commonly affects the sacral region. Numbness, tingling of the buttocks or perineal areas, urinary retention, constipation, and impotence can occur. Symptoms take days to weeks to resolve. Hypesthesia and/or weakness of the lower extremities may develop and persist for months. Rarely, transverse myelitis or Guillain-Barré syndrome follows HSV infection.

Visceral Infections
- Viremia can cause multiorgan involvement.
- Esophagitis: Pts present with odynophagia, dysphagia, substernal pain, and weight loss. Ulcers are most common in the distal esophagus. Cytologic examination and culture of secretions obtained by endoscopy are indicated to distinguish this entity from esophagitis of other etiologies (e.g., *Candida* esophagitis).
- Pneumonitis: Rarely, focal necrotizing pneumonitis due to extension of herpetic tracheobronchitis into the lung parenchyma occurs in severely immunocompromised pts. Hematogenous dissemination from other sites can cause bilateral interstitial pneumonitis. Mortality rates exceed 80% in compromised pts.

Neonatal Infections The frequency of neonatal visceral and/or central nervous system (CNS) infection is highest among pts <6 weeks of age. The mortality rate is 65% without therapy but drops to 25% with IV acyclovir treatment. Fewer than 10% of neonates with CNS disease develop normally. Infection is usually acquired perinatally from contact with infected genital secretions during delivery. More than two-thirds of cases are due to HSV-2. The risk is 10 times higher for infants born to a mother who has recently acquired HSV.

Diagnosis
- Tzanck preparation: This method entails Wright's, Giemsa's, or Papanicolaou's staining of scrapings from the base of lesions to detect giant cells or intranuclear inclusions, which are typical of both HSV and VZV infection. Few clinicians are skilled in the technique, the sensitivity of staining is low, and these cytologic methods do not differentiate between HSV and VZV infections.
- Culture: Positive results are seen within 48–96 h after inoculation. Spin-amplified culture with HSV antigen staining can yield a diagnosis in <24 h.
- Polymerase chain reaction (PCR) detection of HSV DNA: This method is the most sensitive for detection of HSV. Its sensitivity is higher in vesicular rather than ulcerative mucosal lesions, in primary rather than recurrent disease, and in compromised rather than immunocompetent hosts. PCR examination of CSF for viral DNA is the most sensitive noninvasive method for early diagnosis of HSV encephalitis. Examination of tissue obtained by brain biopsy for HSV antigen, DNA, or replication is also highly sensitive and has a low complication rate.
- Serologic assays can identify and distinguish between carriers of HSV-1 and HSV-2.

Rx Infections with Herpes Simplex Viruses

Table 106-1 details antiviral chemotherapy for HSV infection. Acyclovir and other drugs of its class serve as substrates for the HSV enzyme thymidine kinase. These drugs are phosphorylated to the monophosphate form in herpes-

TABLE 106-1 ANTIVIRAL CHEMOTHERAPY FOR HSV INFECTION

I. Mucocutaneous HSV infections

A. *Infections in immunosuppressed pts*

1. *Acute symptomatic first or recurrent episodes:* IV acyclovir (5 mg/kg q8h) or oral acyclovir (400 mg qid), famciclovir (500 mg bid or tid), or vala-cyclovir (500 mg bid) is effective. Treatment duration may vary from 7 to 14 days.

2. *Suppression of reactivation disease (genital or oral-labial):* IV acyclovir (5 mg/kg q8h) or oral valacyclovir (500 mg bid) or acyclovir (400–800 mg 3–5 times per day) prevents recurrences during the 30-day period imme-diately after transplantation. Longer-term HSV suppression is often used for pts with continued immunosuppression. In bone marrow and renal transplant recipients, oral valacyclovir (2 g/d) is also effective in reduc-ing cytomegalovirus infection. Oral valacyclovir at a dose of 4 g/d has been associated with thrombotic thrombocytopenic purpura after ex-tended use in HIV-positive pts. In HIV-infected pts, oral acyclovir (400–800 mg bid), valacyclovir (500 mg bid), or famciclovir (500 mg bid) is effective in reducing clinical and subclinical reactivations of HSV-1 and HSV-2.

B. *Infections in immunocompetent pts*

1. *Genital herpes*

   a. *First episode:* Oral acyclovir (200 mg 5 times per day or 400 mg tid), valacyclovir (1 g bid), or famciclovir (250 mg bid) for 7–14 days is ef-fective. IV acyclovir (5 mg/kg q8h for 5 days) is given for severe dis-ease or neurologic complications such as aseptic meningitis.

   b. *Symptomatic recurrent genital herpes:* Short-course (1- to 3-day) regi-mens are preferred because of low cost and convenience. Oral acyclo-vir (800 mg tid for 2 days), valacyclovir (500 mg bid for 3 days), or famciclovir (750 or 1000 mg bid for 1 day, a 1500-mg single dose, or 500 mg stat followed by 250 mg q12h for 3 days) effectively shortens lesion duration. Other options include oral acyclovir (200 mg 5 times per day), valacyclovir (500 mg bid), and famciclovir (125 mg bid) for 5 days.

   c. *Suppression of recurrent genital herpes:* Oral acyclovir (200-mg cap-sules tid or qid, 400 mg bid, or 800 mg qd), famciclovir (250 mg bid), or valacyclovir (500 mg qd) is effective. Pts with >9 episodes per year should take oral valacyclovir at a dosage of 1 g qd or 500 mg bid.

2. *Oral-labial HSV infections*

   a. *First episode:* Oral acyclovir (200 mg) is given 4 or 5 times per day; an oral acyclovir suspension can be used (600 mg/m^2 qid). Oral famciclovir (250 mg bid) or valacyclovir (1 g bid) has been used clinically.

   b. *Recurrent episodes:* If initiated at onset of the prodrome, single-dose or 1-day therapy effectively reduces pain and speeds healing. Regi-mens include oral famciclovir (a 1500-mg single dose or 750 mg bid for 1 day) or valacyclovir (a 2-g single dose or 2 g bid for 1 day). Self-initiated therapy with 6-times-daily topical penciclovir cream effec-tively speeds healing of oral-labial HSV. Topical acyclovir cream has also been shown to speed healing.

   c. *Suppression of reactivation of oral-labial HSV:* If started before expo-sure and continued for the duration of exposure (usually 5–10 days), oral acyclovir (400 mg bid) prevents reactivation of recurrent oral-la-bial HSV infection associated with severe sun exposure.

(continued)

TABLE 106-1 ANTIVIRAL CHEMOTHERAPY FOR HSV INFECTION (*CONTINUED*)

3. *Surgical prophylaxis of oral or genital HSV infection:* Several surgical procedures (e.g., laser skin resurfacing, trigeminal nerve-root decompression, and lumbar disk surgery) have been associated with HSV reactivation. IV acyclovir (5 mg/kg q8h) or oral acyclovir (800 mg bid), valacyclovir (500 mg bid), or famciclovir (250 mg bid) effectively reduces reactivation. Therapy should be initiated 48 h before surgery and continued for 3–7 days.

4. *Herpetic whitlow:* Oral acyclovir (200 mg) is given 5 times daily for 7–10 days.

5. *HSV proctitis:* Oral acyclovir (400 mg 5 times per day) is useful in shortening the course of infection. In immunosuppressed pts or in pts with severe infection, IV acyclovir (5 mg/kg q8h) may be useful.

6. *Herpetic eye infections:* In acute keratitis, topical trifluorothymidine, vidarabine, idoxuridine, acyclovir, penciclovir, and interferon are all beneficial. Debridement may be required. Topical steroids may worsen disease.

II. **CNS HSV infections**

A. *HSV encephalitis:* IV acyclovir (10 mg/kg q8h; 30 mg/kg per day) is given for 10 days or until HSV DNA is no longer detected in CSF.

B. *HSV aseptic meningitis:* No studies of systemic antiviral chemotherapy exist. If therapy is to be given, IV acyclovir (15–30 mg/kg per day) should be used.

C. *Autonomic radiculopathy:* No studies are available. Most authorities recommend a trial of IV acyclovir.

III. **Neonatal HSV infections:** IV acyclovir (60 mg/kg per day, divided into 3 doses) is given. The recommended duration of treatment is 21 days. Monitoring for relapse should be undertaken, and some authorities recommend continued suppression with oral acyclovir suspension for 3–4 months.

IV. **Visceral HSV infections**

A. *HSV esophagitis:* IV acyclovir (15 mg/kg per day). In some pts with milder forms of immunosuppression, oral therapy with valacyclovir or famciclovir is effective.

B. *HSV pneumonitis:* No controlled studies exist. IV acyclovir (15 mg/kg per day) should be considered.

V. **Disseminated HSV infections:** No controlled studies exist. IV acyclovir (5 mg/kg q8h) should be tried. Adjustments for renal insufficiency may be needed. No definite evidence indicates that therapy will decrease the risk of death.

VI. **Erythema multiforme associated with HSV:** Anecdotal observations suggest that oral acyclovir (400 mg bid or tid) or valacyclovir (500 mg bid) will suppress erythema multiforme.

VII. **Infections due to acyclovir-resistant HSV:** IV foscarnet (40 mg/kg q8h) should be given until lesions heal. The optimal duration of therapy and the usefulness of its continuation in suppressing lesions are unclear. Some pts may benefit from cutaneous application of trifluorothymidine or 5% cidofovir gel.

Note: HSV, herpes simplex virus; CSF, cerebrospinal fluid.

virus-infected cells. Cellular enzymes then convert the monophosphate form into the triphosphate form, which incorporates into the viral DNA chain and inhibits viral DNA polymerase. Acyclovir-resistant strains of HSV have been identified but are uncommon. Almost all resistance—more often to HSV-2 than to HSV-1—has been seen in strains from immunocompromised pts. The level of clinical suspicion of resistance should rise if HSV persists despite adequate acyclovir treatment.

- Acyclovir: This agent is available for IV, oral, and topical administration. IV acyclovir can cause transient renal insufficiency due to crystallization of the compound in the renal parenchyma. The drug should be given slowly over 1 h to a well-hydrated pt. CSF levels are 30–50% of plasma levels, so doses are doubled for treatment of CNS infection over those used to treat mucocutaneous disease. Even higher doses are used for neonatal infections.
- Valacyclovir: The L-valyl ester of acyclovir, this agent is converted to acyclovir by intestinal and hepatic hydrolysis after oral administration, with greater bioavailability, higher blood levels, and less frequent administration than acyclovir. Thrombotic thrombocytopenic purpura has been reported in compromised pts who have received high doses (8 g/d) and after extended use in HIV-seropositive pts receiving 4 g daily.
- Famciclovir: This drug offers excellent bioavailability and a twice-daily dosing schedule.

Prevention   The use of barrier forms of contraception, especially condoms, decreases the likelihood of HSV transmission, particularly during asymptomatic viral excretion.

VARICELLA-ZOSTER VIRUS

VZV causes two distinct entities: primary infection (varicella or chickenpox) and reactivation infection (herpes zoster or shingles). Primary infection is transmitted by the respiratory route. The virus replicates and causes viremia, which is reflected by the diffuse and scattered skin lesions in varicella; it then establishes latency in the dorsal root ganglia.

Chickenpox
- VZV causes disease only in humans. Chickenpox is highly contagious, with an attack rate of 90% among susceptible persons. Household attack rates among susceptible siblings are 70–90%. Before vaccine became available, children 5–9 years old accounted for half of all cases. With vaccine use, the annualized incidence of chickenpox has decreased significantly.
- The incubation period ranges from 10 to 21 days, but most pts evince disease within 14–17 days. Pts are infectious for 48 h before onset of rash and remain infectious until all vesicles have crusted.
- Pts present with fever, rash, and malaise. In immunocompetent hosts, the disease is benign and lasts 3–5 days. Skin lesions include maculopapules, vesicles, and scabs in various stages of evolution. Most lesions are small and have an erythematous base of 5–10 mm. Successive crops appear over 2–4 days. Lesions can occur on the mucosa of the pharynx or vagina. Severity varies from person to person, but older pts tend to have more severe disease.
- Compromised hosts (e.g., leukemic pts) have numerous lesions (often with a hemorrhagic base) that take longer to heal. These pts are more likely than immunocompetent pts to have visceral complications that, if not treated, are fatal in 15% of cases.

Complications
- Bacterial superinfection is usually caused by *Streptococcus pyogenes* or *Staphylococcus aureus* (including methicillin-resistant *S. aureus*).

- The CNS is the most common extracutaneous site of VZV disease in children. Acute cerebellar ataxia and meningeal irritation usually appear ~21 days after the onset of rash and run a benign course. CSF contains lymphocytes and has elevated protein levels. Aseptic meningitis, encephalitis, transverse myelitis, Guillain-Barré syndrome, or Reye's syndrome (which mandates the avoidance of aspirin administration to children) can occur. There is no specific therapy other than supportive care.
- The most serious complication of chickenpox, pneumonia develops more frequently among adults (occurring in up to 20% of cases) than among children. The onset comes 3–5 days into illness, with tachypnea, cough, dyspnea, and fever. Cyanosis, pleuritic chest pain, and hemoptysis are common. Chest x-ray shows nodular infiltrates and interstitial pneumonitis.
- Perinatal varicella has a high mortality rate when maternal disease occurs within 5 days before delivery or within 48 h afterward. Congenital varicella causing birth defects is rare.

Herpes Zoster (Shingles) Herpes zoster represents a reactivation of VZV from dorsal root ganglia.

- The incidence is highest among pts ≥60 years of age.
- There is usually a unilateral vesicular eruption within a dermatome, often associated with severe pain. Dermatomes T3 to L3 are most frequently involved. Dermatomal pain may precede lesions by 48–72 h. The usual duration of disease is 7–10 days, but it may take as long as 2–4 weeks for the skin to return to normal.

Complications

- Zoster ophthalmicus: Zoster of the ophthalmic division of the trigeminal nerve is a debilitating condition that can cause blindness if not treated.
- Ramsay Hunt syndrome is characterized by pain and vesicles in the external auditory canal, loss of taste in the anterior two-thirds of the tongue, and ipsilateral facial palsy.
- Postherpetic neuralgia (PHN) is a debilitating complication of shingles. Pain persists for months after resolution of cutaneous disease. At least 50% of pts over age 50 report some degree of PHN.
- Abnormal CSF in the absence of symptoms is not uncommon. Symptomatic meningoencephalitis can occur.
- Compromised pts—particularly those with Hodgkin's disease and non-Hodgkin's lymphoma—are at greatest risk for severe zoster and progressive disease. Cutaneous dissemination occurs in up to 40% of these pts; among those with cutaneous dissemination, the risk of visceral and other complications (pneumonitis, meningoencephalitis, hepatitis) increases by 5–10%. Bone marrow transplant recipients are also at high risk of VZV infection; these pts can have cutaneous or visceral dissemination. Mortality rates are 10%. PHN, scarring, and bacterial superinfection are common in VZV infection developing within 9 months of transplantation. Concomitant graft-versus-host disease increases the chance of dissemination and/or death.

Diagnosis

- Isolation of VZV in tissue culture, detection of VZV DNA by PCR, or direct immunofluorescent staining of cells from the lesion base
- Seroconversion or a fourfold or greater rise in antibody titer between convalescent- and acute-phase serum specimens. The fluorescent antibody to membrane antigen (FAMA) test, immune adherence hemagglutination test, and enzyme-linked immunosorbent assay (ELISA) are the most frequently used techniques.

Rx **Varicella-Zoster Virus Infections**

- Chickenpox
  1. Antiviral therapy: Acyclovir for children <12 years of age (20 mg/kg q6h, if initiated early in disease) and for adolescents and adults (800 mg five times daily for 5–7 days for chickenpox of ≤24 h duration) is recommended. Valacyclovir and famciclovir are probably as efficacious or more so.
  2. Good hygiene, meticulous skin care, and antipruritic drugs are important to relieve symptoms and prevent bacterial superinfection of skin lesions.
- Zoster: Lesions heal more quickly with antiviral treatment: acyclovir, 800 mg five times daily for 7–10 days; famciclovir, 500 mg tid for 7 days (one study also showed twofold faster resolution of PHN with this agent); or valacyclovir, 1 g tid for 5–7 days.
- Compromised hosts: Acyclovir (10–12.5 mg/kg q8h for 7 days) should be given IV, at least at the outset, for chickenpox and herpes zoster to reduce the risk of complications, although this regimen does not speed the healing or relieve the pain of skin lesions. Low-risk immunocompromised pts can be treated with oral valacyclovir or famciclovir.
- Pneumonia: This complication may require ventilatory support in addition to antiviral treatment.
- Zoster ophthalmicus: Antiviral treatment and consultation with an ophthalmologist are required.
- PHN: Gabapentin, amitriptyline, lidocaine patches, and fluphenazine may relieve pain and can be given along with routine analgesic agents. Prednisone (administered at a dosage of 60 mg/d for the first week of zoster, tapered over 21 days, and given with antiviral therapy) can accelerate quality-of-life improvements, including a return to usual activity; this treatment is indicated only for healthy elderly persons with moderate or severe pain at presentation.

Prevention
- Vaccine
    Varicella: Two doses of a live attenuated vaccine are recommended for all children: the first at 12–15 months of age and the second at ~4–6 years of age. VZV-seronegative pts >13 years of age should receive two doses of vaccine at least 1 month apart.
    Zoster: A vaccine with 18 times the viral content of varicella vaccine, given to pts >60 years of age, reduces the incidence of zoster and PHN. Zoster vaccine is recommended for routine use in this age group.
- Varicella-zoster immune globulin (VZIg): given to VZV-susceptible hosts within 96 h of a significant exposure if the risk of complications from varicella is high (e.g., immunocompromised pts, pregnant women, premature infants, neonates whose mother had chickenpox onset within 5 days before or 2 days after delivery). VZIg is no longer manufactured in the United States; a new product is awaiting FDA approval.
- Antiviral treatment: Seven days after intense exposure, prophylaxis can be given to high-risk pts who are ineligible for vaccine or for whom the 96-h window after direct contact has passed. This intervention may lessen illness severity.

HUMAN HERPESVIRUS (HHV) TYPES 6, 7, AND 8

- HHV-6 causes exanthem subitum (roseola infantum), a common childhood febrile illness with rash, and is a major cause of febrile seizures without rash in infancy. Older pts can have an infectious mononucleosis syndrome or encephalitis. Compromised hosts can have disseminated disease and pneumonitis. More than 80% of adults are seropositive for HHV-6. This virus has been implicated in graft dysfunction and increased all-cause mortality in transplant recipients and may contribute to the pathogenesis of multiple sclerosis.

- HHV-7 is commonly present in saliva. Manifestations of childhood HHV-7 infection include fever and seizures. HHV-7 may have an association with pityriasis rosea.

- HHV-8 is associated with Kaposi's sarcoma (KS), body cavity–based lymphoma in AIDS pts, and multicentric Castleman's disease. The virus appears to be sexually spread and may also be transmitted in saliva, by organ transplantation, and through IV drug use. Primary HHV-8 infection in healthy children can present as fever and rash. In immunocompromised hosts, primary infection may present as fever, splenomegaly, pancytopenia, and rapid-onset KS. Neoplastic disorders develop only after immunocompromise.

For a more detailed discussion, see Baden LR, Dolin R: Antiviral Chemotherapy, Excluding Antiretroviral Drugs, Chap. 171, p. 1087; Corey L: Herpes Simplex Viruses, Chap. 172, p. 1095; Whitley RJ: Varicella-Zoster Virus Infections, Chap. 173, p. 1102; and Hirsch MS: Cytomegalovirus and Human Herpesvirus Types 6, 7, and 8, Chap. 175, p. 1109, in HPIM-17.

107   Cytomegalovirus and Epstein-Barr Virus Infections

CYTOMEGALOVIRUS (CMV)

Etiology   CMV is a herpesvirus that renders infected cells 2–4 times the size of surrounding cells. These cytomegalic cells contain an eccentrically placed intranuclear inclusion surrounded by a clear halo, with an "owl's-eye" appearance.

Epidemiology   CMV disease is found worldwide. In the United States, ~1% of newborns are infected. The virus may be spread in breast milk, saliva, feces, and urine. Transmission requires repeated or prolonged contact. In adolescents and adults, sexual transmission is common, and CMV has been identified in semen and cervical secretions. Latent CMV infection persists throughout life unless reactivation is triggered by depressed cell-mediated immunity (e.g., in transplant recipients or HIV-infected pts).

Pathogenesis   Primary CMV infection is associated with a vigorous T lymphocyte response; atypical lymphocytes are predominantly activated CD8+ T cells. Latent infection occurs in multiple cell types and various organs. Chronic antigen stimulation in the presence of immunosuppression (e.g., in the transplantation setting) and certain immunosuppressive agents (e.g., antithymocyte globulin) promote CMV reactivation. CMV disease increases the risk of infection with opportunistic pathogens by depressing T lymphocyte responsiveness.

Clinical Features **Congenital CMV Infection** Cytomegalic inclusion disease occurs in ~5% of infected fetuses in the setting of primary maternal CMV infection in pregnancy. Pts have petechiae, hepatosplenomegaly, and jaundice. Other findings include microcephaly with or without cerebral calcifications, intrauterine growth retardation, prematurity, and chorioretinitis. Laboratory findings include abnormal liver function tests (LFTs), thrombocytopenia, hemolysis, and increased cerebrospinal fluid (CSF) protein levels. The mortality rate is 20–30% among infants with severe disease; survivors have intellectual or hearing difficulties.

Perinatal CMV Infection Perinatal infection with CMV is acquired by breast-feeding or contact with infected maternal secretions. Most pts are asymptomatic, but interstitial pneumonitis and other opportunistic infections can occur, particularly in premature infants.

CMV Mononucleosis This heterophile antibody–negative illness is the most common CMV syndrome in immunocompetent hosts. The incubation period ranges from 20 to 60 days. Symptoms last 2–6 weeks and include fevers, profound fatigue and malaise, myalgias, headache, and splenomegaly; pharyngitis and cervical lymphadenopathy are rare. Laboratory findings include relative lymphocytosis with >10% atypical lymphocytes. Increased serum levels of aminotransferases and alkaline phosphatase as well as immunologic abnormalities (e.g., the presence of cryoglobulins or cold agglutinins) can be evident. Recovery is complete, but postviral asthenia can persist for months. CMV excretion in urine, genital secretions, and/or saliva can continue for months or years.

CMV Infection in the Immunocompromised Host CMV is the most common and important viral pathogen complicating organ transplantation; CMV infection is a risk factor for graft loss and death. The risk of infection is greatest 1–4 months after transplantation, but retinitis can occur later. Primary CMV infection is more likely than reactivation to cause severe disease with high viral loads. Seropositive recipients can develop reinfection with a new, donor-derived strain of CMV. Reactivation infection is common but less important clinically. The transplanted organ is at particular risk; e.g., CMV pneumonitis tends to follow lung transplantation. Around 15–20% of bone marrow transplant recipients develop CMV pneumonia 5–13 weeks after transplantation, with a case-fatality rate of 84–88%. The risk of severe disease may be reduced by antiviral prophylaxis or preemptive therapy.

CMV is an important pathogen in pts with HIV infection whose CD4+ cell counts have fallen below 50–100/μL. In this setting, CMV produces retinitis, colitis, and disseminated disease.

Immunocompromised pts with CMV infection develop fever, malaise, anorexia, fatigue, night sweats, and arthralgias or myalgias. Tachypnea, hypoxia, and unproductive cough precede respiratory involvement. Involvement of the GI tract may be localized or extensive, with ulcers that can bleed or perforate developing in any part of the tract. Hepatitis is common. Central nervous system (CNS) disease, most often affecting HIV-infected pts, takes one of two forms: encephalitis with dementia or ventriculoencephalitis with cranial nerve deficits, disorientation, and lethargy. Subacute progressive polyradiculopathy has also been described. CMV retinitis can result in blindness. Lesions begin as small white areas of granular retinal necrosis, with later development of hemorrhages, vessel sheathing, and retinal edema. Fatal infection is associated with persistent viremia and multiorgan involvement. Extensive adrenal necrosis is often seen at autopsy.

Diagnosis

- Viral culture: A shell-vial assay gives more rapid results from tissue culture; samples are centrifuged, and monoclonal antibodies are used to detect immediate-early CMV antigen.
- Detection of CMV antigens (pp65) in peripheral-blood leukocytes or of CMV DNA in blood, CSF, or tissues [e.g., with polymerase chain reaction (PCR) assays]: Positive results may be obtained days sooner than with culture methods, allowing earlier interventions.
- Antibodies may not be detectable for up to 4 weeks in primary infection, and titers may remain elevated for years. IgM may be useful in diagnosing acute infection.

℞ Cytomegalovirus Infections

- When possible, seronegative donors should be used for seronegative transplant recipients.
- CMV immune or hyperimmune globulin may reduce the risk of CMV disease in seronegative renal transplant recipients and prevent congenital CMV infection in infants of women with primary CMV infection during pregnancy.
- Ganciclovir (or valganciclovir, the oral prodrug of ganciclovir) produces response rates of 70–90% among HIV-infected pts with CMV retinitis or colitis. Induction therapy with ganciclovir (5 mg/kg bid IV) or valganciclovir (900 mg bid PO) is given for 14–21 days. In bone marrow transplant recipients, CMV pneumonia should be treated with both ganciclovir and CMV immune globulin; clinical response rates are 50–70% with combination therapy. Neutropenia is an adverse reaction to ganciclovir treatment that may require administration of colony-stimulating factors. Maintenance therapy (ganciclovir, 5 mg/kg qd IV; or valganciclovir, 900 mg qd PO) is needed for prolonged periods except in AIDS pts receiving antiretroviral treatment who have a sustained (>6-month) increase in CD4+ T cell counts to levels of >100–150/μL. Prophylactic or suppressive ganciclovir or valganciclovir can be given to high-risk transplant recipients (those who are seropositive before transplantation or culture positive afterward).
- Ganciclovir can be administered via a slow-release pellet sutured into the eye, but this intervention does not provide treatment for the contralateral eye or for systemic disease.
- Foscarnet is active against CMV infection but is reserved for cases of ganciclovir failure or intolerance because of its toxicities, which include renal dysfunction, hypomagnesemia, hypokalemia, hypocalcemia, and paresthesia. This drug must be given via an infusion pump, and its administration must be closely monitored. An induction regimen of 60 mg/kg q8h or 90 mg/kg q12h for 2 weeks is followed by maintenance regimens of 90–120 mg/kg daily.
- Cidofovir has a long intracellular half-life. Induction regimens of 5 mg/kg per week for 2 weeks are followed by maintenance regimens of 3–5 mg/kg every 2 weeks. Cidofovir causes severe nephrotoxicity by proximal tubular cell injury. The use of saline hydration and probenecid reduces this adverse effect.

EPSTEIN-BARR VIRUS (EBV)

Epidemiology EBV is a herpesvirus that infects >90% of persons by adulthood. Infectious mononucleosis (IM) is a disease of young adults and is more common in areas with higher standards of hygiene; infection occurs at a younger age in poorer areas. EBV is spread by contact with oral secretions (e.g., by transfer of saliva during kissing) and is shed in oropharyngeal secretions by >90% of asymptomatic seropositive individuals.

Pathogenesis   EBV infects the epithelium of the oropharynx and salivary glands as well as B cells in tonsillar crypts. The virus spreads through the bloodstream. Reactive T cells proliferate, and there is polyclonal activation of B cells. Memory B cells are the reservoir for EBV. Cellular immunity is more important than humoral immunity in controlling infection. If T cell immunity is compromised, EBV-infected B cells may proliferate—a step toward neoplastic transformation.

Clinical Features

I. Infants and young children: asymptomatic or mild pharyngitis

II. Adolescents and adults: IM, with an incubation period of ~4–6 weeks

    A. A prodrome of fatigue, malaise, and myalgia may last for 1–2 weeks before fever onset.

    B. Illness lasts for 2–4 weeks and is characterized by fever, sore throat, lymphadenopathy (especially of the posterior cervical nodes), malaise, and headache. Signs include pharyngitis or exudative tonsillitis that can resemble streptococcal infection, splenomegaly (usually in the second or third week), hepatomegaly, rash, and periorbital edema. Ampicillin treatment can cause a rash that does not represent a true penicillin allergy. Erythema nodosum or erythema multiforme can occur.

    C. Malaise and difficulty with concentration can persist for months.

    D. Laboratory findings: Lymphocytosis occurs in the second or third week, with >10% atypical lymphocytes (enlarged cells with abundant cytoplasm and vacuoles). Most atypical lymphocytes are CD8+ T cells. Neutropenia, thrombocytopenia, and abnormal LFTs are common.

    E. Complications

        1. CNS: In the first 2 weeks of IM, meningitis or encephalitis can present as headache, meningismus, cerebellar ataxia, acute hemiplegia, or psychosis. The CSF contains lymphocytes. Most cases resolve without sequelae.

        2. Autoimmune hemolytic anemia (Coombs-positive, with cold agglutinins directed against the i RBC antigen) can last for 1–2 months. Severe disease (red cell aplasia, severe granulocytopenia or pancytopenia, or hemophagocytic syndrome) can occur.

        3. Splenic rupture is more common among males than among females and may manifest as abdominal pain, referred shoulder pain, or hemodynamic compromise.

        4. Upper airway obstruction due to hypertrophy of lymphoid tissue may occur.

        5. Hepatitis, myocarditis, pericarditis, pneumonia, interstitial nephritis, and vasculitis are rare complications.

III. EBV-associated lymphoproliferative disease occurs in immunodeficient pts (e.g., pts infected with HIV, transplant recipients, pts receiving immunosuppressive therapy). Proliferating EBV-infected B cells infiltrate lymph nodes and multiple organs; there is B cell hyperplasia or lymphoma. Pts have fever and lymphadenopathy or GI symptoms.

IV. Oral hairy leukoplakia consists of white corrugated lesions on the tongue in HIV-infected pts.

V. EBV-associated malignancies include Burkitt's lymphoma, anaplastic nasopharyngeal carcinoma, Hodgkin's disease (especially the mixed-cellularity

TABLE 107-1 SEROLOGIC FEATURES OF EBV-ASSOCIATED DISEASES

		Result in Indicated Test				
		Anti-VCA		Anti-EA		Anti-EBNA
Condition	Heterophile	IgM	IgG	EA-D	EA-R	
Acute infectious mononucleosis	+	+	++	+	−	−
Convalescence	±	−	+	−	±	+
Past infection	−	−	+	−	−	+
Reactivation with immunodeficiency	−	−	++	+	+	±
Burkitt's lymphoma	−	−	+++	±	++	+
Nasopharyngeal carcinoma	−	−	+++	++	±	+

Note: VCA, viral capsid antigen; EA, early antigen; EA-D antibody, antibody to early antigen in diffuse pattern in nucleus and cytoplasm of infected cells; EA-R antibody, antibody to early antigen restricted to the cytoplasm; EBNA, Epstein-Barr nuclear antigen.
Source: Adapted from M. Okano et al: Clin Microbiol Rev 1:300, 1988.

type), and CNS lymphoma (especially HIV-related). The risk of Hodgkin's disease is significantly increased in young adults after EBV-seropositive IM.

Diagnosis

- Heterophile test (Table 107-1): The heterophile titer is defined as the highest serum dilution that agglutinates sheep, horse, or cow erythrocytes after adsorption with guinea pig kidney. A titer of ≥40-fold is diagnostic of acute EBV infection. Heterophile titers are positive in 40% of pts during the first week and in 80–90% of pts by the third week. The test remains positive for 3 months—or as long as a year—after the onset of acute infection. The monospot test for heterophile antibodies is ~75% sensitive and ~90% specific compared with EBV-specific serologies.
- EBV-specific antibody testing (Table 107-1): Specific antibody testing can be useful in heterophile-negative pts (a group that includes many young children) and pts with atypical disease. Antibodies to viral capsid antigen occur in >90% of cases. IgM titers are elevated only during the first 2–3 months of disease and are most useful in diagnosing acute infection. Documented seroconversion to Epstein-Barr nuclear antigen (EBNA) is also useful. EBNA antibodies are not detected until 3–6 weeks after symptom onset and then persist for life. Other antibodies may be elevated but are less useful diagnostically.
- Other studies: Detection of EBV DNA by PCR is useful in demonstrating the association with various malignancies (e.g., positive EBV DNA of the CSF in HIV-associated CNS lymphoma) and in monitoring EBV DNA levels in the blood of pts with lymphoproliferative disease. High EBV DNA levels in plasma correlate with lower survival rates in anaplastic nasopharyngeal carcinoma.

℞ Epstein-Barr Virus Infections

IM is treated with supportive measures. Excessive physical activity should be avoided in the first month of illness to reduce the possibility of splenic rupture. Splenectomy is required if rupture occurs. Administration of glucocorticoids may be indicated for some complications of IM; e.g., these agents may be given to prevent airway obstruction or for autoimmune hemolytic anemia. Antiviral therapy (e.g., with acyclovir) is generally not effective. Treatment of posttransplantation EBV lymphoproliferative syndrome is generally directed toward reduction of immunosuppression, although other treatments—e.g., with interferon α or antibody to CD20 (rituximab)—and donor lymphocyte infusions have been used with varying success.

For a more detailed discussion, see Baden LR, Dolin R: Antiviral Chemotherapy, Excluding Antiretroviral Drugs, Chap. 171, p. 1087; Cohen JI: Epstein-Barr Virus Infections, Including Infectious Mononucleosis, Chap. 174, p. 1106; and Hirsch MS: Cytomegalovirus and Human Herpesvirus Types 6, 7, and 8, Chap. 175, p. 1109, in HPIM-17.

108 Influenza and Other Viral Respiratory Diseases

INFLUENZA

Etiology   Influenza A, B, and C viruses are RNA viruses and members of the Orthomyxoviridae family. Influenza A viruses are subtyped by surface hemagglutinin (H) and neuraminidase (N) antigens. Influenza A and B viruses are major human pathogens and are morphologically similar. Virus attaches to cell receptors via the hemagglutinin. Neuraminidase degrades the receptor and plays a role in the release of virus from infected cells after replication has occurred. Antibodies to the H antigen are the major determinants of immunity, while antibodies to the N antigen limit viral spread and contribute to reduction of the infection.

Epidemiology   Influenza outbreaks occur each year but vary in extent and severity. Until 30 years ago, there were influenza A epidemics or pandemics every 10–15 years due in part to the propensity of the H and N antigens to undergo periodic antigenic variation. Major changes (which are restricted to influenza A viruses) are called *antigenic shifts* and are associated with pandemics. Minor variations are called *antigenic drifts*. The segmented genome of influenza A and B viruses allows reassortment. Prior pandemic strains of influenza A virus have been linked to genetic reassortment between human and avian strains, with adaptation of an avian virus to efficient infection of humans. The avian influenza strain A/H5N1, first detected in 1997, has not resulted in a pandemic because efficient person-to-person transmission has not been observed; infection is linked to direct contact with infected poultry. Thus far, influenza A/H5N1 has caused 261 cases of infection in 10 countries in Asia and the Middle East.

Generally, influenza A epidemics begin abruptly, peak over 2–3 weeks, last 2–3 months, and then subside rapidly. They take place almost exclusively during the winter months in temperate climates but occur year-round in the tropics. The morbidity and mortality associated with influenza outbreaks continue to be substantial, particularly among persons with comorbid disease. Chronic cardiac and pulmonary disease and old age are prominent risk factors for severe illness. Influenza B viruses have a more restricted host range and do not undergo antigenic shifts, although they do exhibit antigenic drift. Outbreaks are less extensive and less severe than those of influenza A, occurring most commonly in schools and military camps. Influenza C causes subclinical infection.

Pathogenesis Influenza is acquired from respiratory secretions of acutely ill individuals through aerosols generated by coughs and sneezes and possibly by hand-to-hand contact or other personal or fomite contact. Virus then infects the ciliated columnar epithelial cells and spreads quickly to infect other respiratory cells. Cells undergo degenerative changes, become necrotic, and desquamate. Extrapulmonary sites of infection are rare, but cytokine induction causes systemic symptoms. Host defenses include production of humoral antibody, local IgA antibody, cell-mediated immune responses, and interferon. Viral shedding usually stops 2–5 days after disease onset.

Clinical Features

- Systemic symptoms: abrupt onset of headache, fever, chills, myalgia, malaise
- Respiratory tract symptoms: cough and sore throat that can become more prominent as systemic symptoms subside
- Physical findings are minimal in uncomplicated disease.
- Pts with uncomplicated influenza improve over 2–5 days and have largely recovered at 1 week, although cough can persist for 1–2 weeks. Postinfluenzal asthenia may persist for weeks.

Complications Complications are more common among pts >64 years old, pregnant women, and pts with chronic disorders (e.g., cardiac or pulmonary disease, diabetes, renal diseases, hemoglobinopathies, or immunosuppression).

- Pneumonia: the most significant complication of influenza. Pts can have tachypnea, cyanosis, diffuse rales, and signs of consolidation.
  1. Primary viral: least common but most severe. Acute influenza progresses relentlessly, with persistent fever, dyspnea, cyanosis, and hemoptysis. Chest x-ray (CXR) may show diffuse infiltrates. Acute respiratory distress syndrome (ARDS) can result. Cultures of respiratory secretions yield high viral titers. Primary pneumonia is especially common among pts with cardiac disease, particularly mitral stenosis.
  2. Secondary bacterial: usually due to *Streptococcus pneumoniae*, *Staphylococcus aureus*, or *Haemophilus influenzae*. Pts improve over 2–3 days of illness and then have a recurrence of fever and clinical signs of bacterial pneumonia (e.g., cough, sputum production, and consolidation on CXR).
  3. Pts can have features of both primary and secondary pneumonia.
- Extrapulmonary complications
  1. Reye's syndrome: associated with influenza B more often than with influenza A; also associated with varicella-zoster virus infection and with aspirin use. Aspirin should not be given to children with acute viral respiratory infections.
  2. Miscellaneous: Myositis, rhabdomyolysis, and myoglobinuria are rare despite the prevalence of severe myalgia. Myocarditis and pericarditis, encephalitis, transverse myelitis, and Guillain-Barré syndrome have been reported.
- Avian influenza (A/H5N1): Infected pts have high rates of pneumonia and extrapulmonary manifestations such as diarrhea and CNS involvement. Deaths are associated with multisystem dysfunction, including cardiac and renal failure. Mortality rates have approached 60%.

Laboratory Findings Tissue culture of virus from throat swabs, nasopharyngeal washes, or sputum usually gives a positive result within 48–72 h. Rapid tests for viral nucleoprotein or neuraminidase are highly sensitive, with a specificity of 60–90%. Serology requires the availability of acute- and convalescent-phase sera and is useful only retrospectively.

Rx **Influenza**

- Symptom-based therapy (e.g., acetaminophen, rest, hydration)
- Antiviral agents (Table 108-1)
  1. Antiviral treatment has been tested in healthy adults with uncomplicated influenza but not in pts with severe disease.
  2. The neuraminidase inhibitors oseltamivir and zanamivir decrease the duration of signs and symptoms by 1–1.5 days if therapy is begun with-

TABLE 108-1 ANTIVIRAL MEDICATIONS FOR TREATMENT AND PROPHYLAXIS OF INFLUENZA

Antiviral Drug	Age Group (years)		
	Children (≤12)	13–64	≥65
Oseltamivir			
Treatment, influenza A and B	Age 1–12, dose varies by weight[a]	75 mg PO bid	75 mg PO bid
Prophylaxis, influenza A and B	Age 1–12, dose varies by weight[b]	75 mg PO qd	75 mg PO qd
Zanamivir			
Treatment, influenza A and B	Age 7–12, 10 mg bid by inhalation	10 mg bid by inhalation	10 mg bid by inhalation
Prophylaxis, influenza A and B	Age 5–12, 10 mg qd by inhalation	10 mg qd by inhalation	10 mg qd by inhalation
Amantadine[c]			
Treatment, influenza A	Age 1–9, 5 mg/kg in 2 divided doses, up to 150 mg/d	Age ≥10, 100 mg PO bid	≤100 mg/d
Prophylaxis, influenza A	Age 1–9, 5 mg/kg in 2 divided doses, up to 150 mg/d	Age ≥10, 100 mg PO bid	≤100 mg/d
Rimantadine[c]			
Treatment, influenza A	Not approved	100 mg PO bid	100–200 mg/d
Prophylaxis, influenza A	Age 1–9, 5 mg/kg in 2 divided doses, up to 150 mg/d	Age ≥10, 100 mg PO bid	100–200 mg/d

[a]<15 kg: 30 mg bid; >15–23 kg: 45 mg bid; >23–40 kg: 60 mg bid; >40 kg: 75 mg bid.
[b]<15 kg: 30 mg qd; >15–23 kg: 45 mg qd; >23–40 kg: 60 mg qd; >40 kg: 75 mg qd.
[c]Amantadine and rimantadine are not currently recommended (2006–2007) because of widespread resistance in influenza A/H3N2 viruses. Their use may be reconsidered if viral susceptibility is reestablished.

in 2 days of illness onset. Zanamivir may exacerbate bronchospasm in asthmatic pts, while oseltamivir has been associated with nausea and vomiting (reactions whose incidence is reduced if the drug is given with food) and with neuropsychiatric side effects in children. Antiviral resistance to neuraminidase inhibitors is infrequent but can occur.

3. Amantadine and rimantadine are not recommended at present because of widespread resistance among influenza A/H3N2 viruses. Amantadine causes mild CNS side effects (e.g., jitteriness, anxiety, insomnia, difficulty concentrating) in ~5–10% of pts. Rimantadine has fewer CNS side effects.

Prophylaxis

- Vaccination: Influenza vaccine is derived from the influenza A and B viruses that have circulated during the previous influenza season. If the currently circulating virus is similar to the vaccine strain, 50–80% protection is expected. Influenza vaccination is recommended for any individual >6 months of age who is at increased risk for complications (Table 108-2). The commercially available vaccines are inactivated and may be given to immunocompromised pts. A live attenuated influenza vaccine given by intranasal spray has been approved and can be used for healthy children and adults up to 49 years of age.
- Chemoprophylaxis: Efficacy rates in preventing illness are 84–89% for oseltamivir or zanamivir. Amantadine and rimantadine are not recommended

---

TABLE 108-2   PERSONS FOR WHOM ANNUAL INFLUENZA VACCINATION IS RECOMMENDED

Children 6–59 months old

Women who will be pregnant during the influenza season

Persons ≥50 years old

Children and adolescents (6 months to 18 years old) who are receiving long-term aspirin therapy and therefore may be at risk for developing Reye's syndrome after influenza

Adults and children who have chronic disorders of the pulmonary or cardiovascular systems, including asthma[a]

Adults and children who have required regular medical follow-up or hospitalization during the preceding year because of chronic metabolic diseases (including diabetes mellitus), renal dysfunction, hemoglobinopathies, or immunodeficiency (including immunodeficiency caused by medications or by HIV)

Adults and children who have any condition (e.g., cognitive dysfunction, spinal cord injuries, seizure disorders, or other neuromuscular disorders) that can compromise respiratory function or the handling of respiratory secretions or can increase the risk of aspiration

Residents of nursing homes and other chronic-care facilities that house persons of any age who have chronic medical conditions

Persons who live with or care for persons at high risk for influenza-related complications, including healthy household contacts of and caregivers for children from birth through 59 months of age

Health care workers

---

[a]Hypertension itself is not considered a chronic disorder for which influenza vaccination is recommended.
Source: Centers for Disease Control and Prevention: Prevention and control of influenza: Recommendations of the Advisory Committee on Immunization Practices (ACIP). MMWR 55(RR-11):1, 2006.

at this time. Prophylaxis is useful for high-risk individuals who have not received vaccine and are exposed to influenza; it can be administered simultaneously with inactivated—but not with live—vaccine.

OTHER COMMON VIRAL RESPIRATORY INFECTIONS

(See also Chap. 62)

RHINOVIRUSES

Rhinoviruses are RNA viruses of the Picornaviridae family.

- Major cause of the "common cold" (up to 50% of cases)
- Spread by direct contact with infected secretions, usually respiratory droplets
- Short incubation period (1–2 days). Pts develop rhinorrhea, sneezing, nasal congestion, and sore throat. Fever and systemic symptoms are unusual.
- Severe disease is rare but is described in bone marrow transplant recipients.
- Diagnosis is not usually attempted. PCR and tissue culture methods are available.

CORONAVIRUSES

General Information   Coronaviruses are RNA viruses that account for 10–35% of common colds and cause typical presentations. A coronavirus was identified as the cause of severe acute respiratory syndrome (SARS).

The SARS Outbreak   Epidemiology   SARS began in China in 2002. Although >8000 cases were ultimately identified in 28 countries of Asia, Europe, and North America, ~90% of all cases occurred in China and Hong Kong. Case-fatality rates were ~9.5% overall. Transmission appeared to take place by both large and small aerosols and perhaps also by the fecal-oral route. The last reported cases occurred in 2004.

Pathogenesis   SARS virus probably enters and infects cells of the respiratory tract but also causes viremia and is found in the urine and in the stool. Viral titers in the respiratory tract peak ~10 days after the onset of illness. Pulmonary pathology consists of hyaline membrane formation, pneumocyte desquamation in alveolar spaces, and an interstitial infiltrate.

Clinical Features   The incubation period lasts 2–7 days. A systemic illness with fever, malaise, headache, and myalgias is followed in 1–2 days by nonproductive cough, dyspnea, diarrhea, and abnormal CXR. Respiratory function deteriorates in the second week of illness and can progress to ARDS and multiorgan dysfunction. A worse prognosis is associated with an age of >50 years and with comorbidities such as cardiovascular disease, diabetes, and hepatitis. Pregnant women have particularly severe disease.

Diagnosis   Lymphopenia affecting mostly CD4+ T cells, thrombocytopenia, and increased serum levels of aminotransferases, creatine kinase, and lactate dehydrogenase (LDH) are described. Diagnosis is based on clinical, epidemiologic, and laboratory features. Virus can be isolated from respiratory tract secretions. A rapid diagnosis can be made by reverse-transcriptase polymerase chain reaction (PCR) of respiratory tract samples and plasma early in illness and of urine and stool later in the course. Serum antibodies are detectable by enzyme-linked immunosorbent assay (ELISA) or immunofluorescence and develop within 28 days of illness onset.

SARS

Aggressive supportive care is most important. No specific therapy has established efficacy.

Prevention SARS caused a worldwide public health response; case definitions were established, travel advisories issued, and quarantines imposed in certain locales. Transmission to health care workers was frequent; strict infection control measures were found to be essential.

HUMAN RESPIRATORY SYNCYTIAL VIRUS

Human respiratory syncytial virus (HRSV) is so named because its replication in vitro leads to fusion of neighboring cells into large multinucleated syncytia. HRSV is an RNA virus and a member of the Paramyxoviridae family. It is a major respiratory pathogen among young children and the foremost cause of lower respiratory disease among infants. Rates of illness peak at 2–3 months of age, when attack rates among susceptible individuals approach 100%. HRSV accounts for 20–25% of hospital admissions of infants and young children for pneumonia and for up to 75% of cases of bronchiolitis in this age group. The virus is transmitted efficiently via contact with contaminated fingers or fomites and by spread of coarse aerosols. The incubation period is 4–6 days. Viral shedding can last for >2 weeks in children and compromised hosts. HRSV is an important nosocomial pathogen.

Clinical Features
- Infants: Around 20–40% of infections result in lower tract disease, including pneumonia, bronchiolitis, and tracheobronchitis. Mild disease begins with rhinorrhea, low-grade fever, cough, and wheezing, and recovery comes within 1–2 weeks. Severe disease is marked by tachypnea and dyspnea; hypoxia, cyanosis, and apnea can ensue. Examination reveals wheezing, rhonchi, and rales. CXR may reveal hyperexpansion, peribronchial thickening, and variable infiltrates. Mortality rates can be high, especially among infants with prematurity, bronchopulmonary dysplasia, congenital heart disease, nephrotic syndrome, or immunosuppression.
- Milder disease results from reinfection among older children and adults.
- The common cold is the most common presentation in adults, but HRSV can cause lower respiratory tract disease with fever, including severe pneumonia in elderly pts. HRSV pneumonia can be a significant cause of morbidity and death among transplant recipients, with case-fatality rates of 20–80%.

Diagnosis Immunofluorescence, ELISA, and other techniques can identify HRSV isolates in tissue culture. Rapid viral diagnosis is available by immunofluorescence or ELISA of nasopharyngeal washes, aspirates, or swabs. Serologic testing is also available.

R͟x͟ Human Respiratory Syncytial Virus

For upper tract disease, treatment is symptom-based. For severe lower tract disease, aerosolized ribavirin is beneficial to infants, but its efficacy in older children and adults (including immunocompromised pts) has not been established. Health care workers exposed to the drug have experienced minor toxicity, including eye and respiratory tract irritation. Ribavirin is mutagenic, teratogenic, and embryotoxic; its use is contraindicated in pregnancy, and its aerosolized administration is a risk to pregnant health care workers. IV immunoglobulin (IVIg), immunoglobulin with high titers of antibody to HRSV (RSVIg), and monoclonal IgG antibody to HRSV (palivizumab) are available but have not been shown to be beneficial.

Prevention Monthly RSVIg or palivizumab is approved for prophylaxis in children <2 years of age who have bronchopulmonary dysplasia or cyanotic heart disease or who were born prematurely.

METAPNEUMOVIRUS

Metapneumovirus is an RNA virus of the Paramyxoviridae family. This newly described respiratory pathogen causes disease in a wide variety of age groups, with clinical manifestations similar to those caused by HRSV. Diagnosis is made by PCR or tissue culture of nasal aspirates or respiratory secretions. Treatment is primarily supportive and symptom-based.

PARAINFLUENZA VIRUS

This RNA virus of the Paramyxoviridae family ranks second only to HRSV as a cause of lower respiratory tract disease among young children and is the most common cause of croup (laryngotracheobronchitis). Infections are milder among older children and adults, but severe, prolonged, and fatal infection is reported among pts with severe immunosuppression, including transplant recipients. Tissue culture, rapid testing, or PCR of respiratory tract secretions or nasopharyngeal washings can detect the virus. Glucocorticoids are beneficial in severe cases. Ribavirin has been used on occasion, and anecdotal reports indicate some efficacy.

ADENOVIRUSES

Adenoviruses are DNA viruses that cause ~10% of acute respiratory infections among children but <2% of respiratory illnesses among civilian adults. Some serotypes are associated with outbreaks among military recruits. Transmission can take place via inhalation of aerosolized virus, through inoculation of the conjunctival sacs, and probably via the fecal-oral route.

- In children, adenovirus causes acute upper and lower respiratory tract infections; upper tract infections are more common. The virus causes outbreaks of pharyngoconjunctival fever (often at summer camps), an illness characterized by bilateral conjunctivitis, granular conjunctivae, rhinitis, sore throat, and cervical adenopathy.
- In adults, adenovirus causes sore throat, fever, cough, coryza, and regional adenopathy.
- Other manifestations include diarrheal illness, hemorrhagic cystitis, and epidemic keratoconjunctivitis.
- Immunocompromised pts, especially transplant recipients, can develop disseminated disease, pneumonia, hepatitis, nephritis, colitis, encephalitis, and hemorrhagic cystitis. Adenovirus may involve the transplanted organ.
- Definitive diagnosis can be made by isolation in tissue culture; by rapid testing (with immunofluorescence or ELISA) of nasopharyngeal aspirates, conjunctival or respiratory secretions, urine, or stool; or by PCR testing.
- Treatment is supportive. Ribavirin and cidofovir exhibit in vitro activity against adenovirus.

For a more detailed discussion, see Baden LR, Dolin R: Antiviral Chemotherapy, Excluding Antiretroviral Drugs, Chap. 171, p. 1087; Dolin R: Common Viral Respiratory Infections and Severe Acute Respiratory Syndrome (SARS), Chap. 179, p. 1120; and Dolin R: Influenza, Chap. 180, p. 1127, in HPIM-17.

109 Rubeola, Rubella, Mumps, and Parvovirus Infections

MEASLES (RUBEOLA)

Definition and Etiology   Measles is a highly contagious, acute, exanthematous respiratory disease with a characteristic clinical picture and a pathognomonic enanthem (Koplik's spots). Measles is caused by an RNA virus of the genus *Morbillivirus* and the family Paramyxoviridae.

Epidemiology   Routine administration of the measles vaccine has markedly decreased the number of cases in the United States. Most of the 37 U.S. cases reported in 2004 were attributable to international importation of the virus. The disease is spread by respiratory secretions through exposure to aerosols and through direct contact with larger droplets. Pts are contagious from 1–2 days before symptom onset until 4 days after the rash appears; infectivity peaks during the prodromal phase.

Clinical Features

- Symptoms and rash occur a mean of 10 and 14 days, respectively, after infection.
- Prodrome: 2–4 days of malaise, cough, coryza, conjunctivitis, nasal discharge, and fever. Fever starts to resolve by day 4 or 5 after rash onset.
- Koplik's spots: 1- to 2-mm blue-white spots on a bright red background; typically occur on the buccal mucosa, alongside the second molars, 1–2 days before rash
- An erythematous, nonpruritic, maculopapular rash begins at the hairline and behind the ears, spreads down the trunk and limbs to include the palms and soles, can become confluent, and begins to fade by day 4. Rash is often more severe in adults.
- Lymphadenopathy, diarrhea and vomiting, and splenomegaly are common.
- Pts with defects in cell-mediated immunity are at risk for severe, protracted, and fatal disease and may have no rash.
- Complications
    Respiratory tract: otitis media in children, croup in infants. Adults and immunocompromised children can develop primary viral giant cell pneumonia.
    CNS disease
        Acute encephalitis: headache, drowsiness, coma, seizures; 10% mortality; retardation, epilepsy, and other sequelae in survivors
        Risk of progressive fatal encephalitis 1–6 months after illness in immunocompromised pts

Subacute sclerosing panencephalitis: protracted, chronic, rare form of encephalitis with progressive dementia over several months; more common among children who contract measles at <2 years of age; rare in the United States because of widespread vaccination

GI tract: hepatitis, colitis, adenitis, appendicitis

Myocarditis, glomerulonephritis, thrombocytopenic purpura

- Atypical measles occurs in pts who contract measles after receiving inactivated vaccine (in use before 1967). Pts have a peripheral rash that moves centrally, high fevers, edema of the extremities, interstitial pulmonary infiltrates, hepatitis, and occasionally pleural effusions. Full recovery is typical, but convalescence may be prolonged. Inactivated vaccine has not been available for >35 years; atypical measles has virtually disappeared.

Diagnosis Lymphopenia and neutropenia are common. Immunofluorescent staining of respiratory secretions for measles antigen or examination of secretions for multinucleated giant cells can help establish the diagnosis. Virus can be isolated from respiratory secretions or urine. Polymerase chain reaction (PCR) is available as well. IgM antibody appears 1–2 days before rash.

℞ Measles

- Supportive care; antibiotics for bacterial superinfections (e.g., otitis or pneumonia)
- Vitamin A for young children hospitalized with measles and for pediatric measles pts with immunodeficiency, vitamin A deficiency, impaired intestinal absorption, malnutrition, or immigration from areas with high measles mortality rates
- Ribavirin may be considered for use in immunocompromised pts.

Prevention Live attenuated vaccine containing measles, mumps, and rubella (MMR) antigens is given routinely at 12–15 months; a second dose is given to school-age children at 4–12 years of age. MMR vaccine is being supplanted by MMRV vaccine, which also covers varicella. Older individuals without prior documented illness or vaccination should be immunized. Asymptomatic HIV-infected children should receive MMR vaccine, but pts with severe immunosuppression, others with impaired cell-mediated immunity, pregnant women, and persons with anaphylaxis to egg protein or neomycin should not receive the vaccine.

Postexposure prophylaxis with immunoglobulin should be considered in susceptible children or adults exposed to measles; a dose of 0.25 mL/kg is given to healthy pts and a dose of 0.5 mL/kg to immunocompromised hosts, with a maximal dose of 15 mL.

RUBELLA (GERMAN MEASLES)

Etiology and Epidemiology Rubella is a contagious infectious disease caused by an RNA togavirus of the genus *Rubivirus*. Virus is shed in respiratory secretions during the prodromal phase, and shedding continues for a week after symptom onset. Transmission occurs via droplets or direct contact with nasopharyngeal secretions. Infants with congenital disease can shed virus from the respiratory tract and urine for 2 years. Rubella vaccine, introduced in 1969, has eliminated most disease. In 2001–2004, an average of 14 cases of postnatally acquired rubella were reported annually in the United States; 4 confirmed cases of congenital rubella syndrome were reported to the Centers for Disease

Control and Prevention during this 4-year period. Young immigrants from Latin America and the Caribbean, where childhood vaccination against the disease is not routine, are at increased risk.

Clinical Features

- Incubation period: average, 18 days; range, 12–23 days
- Usually a mild or subclinical illness; may be more severe in adults
- A prodrome of malaise, fever, and anorexia is followed by posterior auricular, cervical, and suboccipital lymphadenopathy; fever; mild coryza; and conjunctivitis.
- Rash follows, beginning on the face, spreading down the body, and lasting 3–5 days.
- Women are more prone to arthritis of the fingers, wrists, and/or knees; this condition can take weeks to resolve.
- Congenital rubella is the most serious manifestation of rubella infection and can include cataracts, heart disease, deafness, and other deficits. Maternal infection results in fetal infection in ~50% of cases in the first trimester and in about one-third of cases in the second trimester. Fetal disease is more severe the earlier infection occurs.

Diagnosis

- Enzyme-linked immunosorbent assay (ELISA) testing for IgG and IgM antibodies
- Congenital rubella can be diagnosed by isolation of the virus, a positive PCR assay, detection of IgM antibodies in a single serum sample, and/or documentation of either the persistence of antibodies beyond 1 year of age or a rising antibody titer at any time during infancy in an unvaccinated child.
- Biopsy tissue samples or blood or CSF samples can be analyzed for rubella antigen with monoclonal antibodies or for rubella RNA via in situ hybridization or PCR.

Prevention See MMR recommendations under "Measles (Rubeola)," above. Pregnancy should be avoided for at least 3 months after vaccination. However, the occurrence of vaccine-related congenital rubella has not been proven in women inadvertently vaccinated during pregnancy.

MUMPS

Definition and Etiology Mumps is an acute systemic communicable viral infection whose most distinctive feature is swelling of one or both parotid glands. It is caused by the mumps virus, an RNA paramyxovirus with only one antigenic type.

Epidemiology The introduction of mumps vaccine in 1967 resulted in a marked decline in new mumps cases in the United States. Currently, there are ~231–277 cases annually, a >99% reduction from prevaccine levels. Pts may shed virus before clinical disease onset or during subclinical infection (which occurs in one-third of pts). The virus is transmitted by droplet nuclei, saliva, and fomites. Transmission occurs 1–2 days before parotitis onset and can continue for up to 5 days afterward. Viral replication in the upper respiratory tract leads to viremia, which is followed by infection of glandular tissues and/or the central nervous system.

Clinical Features

- The incubation period is generally 14–18 days (range, 7–23 days).
- A prodrome of fever, malaise, myalgia, and anorexia is followed 1–7 days later by tender parotitis that is bilateral in two-thirds of pts. Pts have trouble

eating, swallowing, or talking. Swelling slowly resolves within a week. Submaxillary and sublingual glands are involved less often.

- After parotitis, orchitis is the most common manifestation among postpubertal males, occurring in about one-fifth of cases. The testes are painful, tender, and enlarged, and atrophy can develop in half of affected men. Orchitis is bilateral in <15% of cases, and sterility is rare. In women, oophoritis can occur but does not lead to sterility.
- Aseptic meningitis: Cerebrospinal fluid (CSF) pleocytosis can occur in half of mumps cases, but clinical meningitis is evident in only 5–25%. CSF glucose levels may be very low, and polymorphonuclear leukocytes may predominate in the first 24 h, leading to a consideration of bacterial meningitis. Disease is self-limited; cranial nerve palsies occasionally lead to permanent sequelae, particularly deafness.
- Pancreatitis, myocarditis, and other unusual manifestations can occur. High serum amylase levels due to parotitis make pancreatitis difficult to diagnose. First-trimester maternal infection can cause spontaneous abortions but not congenital malformations.

Diagnosis   Mumps virus is easily isolated and can be rapidly identified in shell-vial cultures by immunofluorescence. Virus can be recovered from saliva, throat, urine (in which it is shed for up to 2 weeks), and CSF. PCR is also available. ELISA is useful for serologic diagnosis.

Prevention   See MMR recommendations under "Measles (Rubeola)," above.

PARVOVIRUS INFECTION

Etiology   Parvovirus B19, a DNA virus of the family Parvoviridae, is the only member shown definitively to be a human pathogen.

Pathogenesis   B19 replicates in erythroid progenitors. Infection leads to high-titer viremia and arrest of erythropoiesis. When an IgM and IgG antibody response is mounted, normal erythropoiesis resumes. Pts with increased erythropoiesis (especially with hemolytic anemia) can develop a transient crisis with severe anemia, while pts who do not mount an adequate antibody response can develop chronic anemia. At 2–3 weeks after infection, an immune-mediated phase of illness, with rash and/or arthritis, occurs in the healthy host in the presence of rising antibody titers.

Epidemiology   B19 is endemic worldwide and is transmitted via the respiratory route. By the age of 15 years, ≥50% of children have antibody; >90% of elderly pts are antibody-positive.

Clinical Features

- Erythema infectiosum (fifth disease) is a mild viral illness with a facial "slapped-cheek" rash (more common in children) and low-grade fever. A lacy, reticular rash develops primarily on the arms and legs.
- Polyarthropathy syndrome: occurs in ~50% of adults and in women more often than in men. The arthritis is typically symmetric and affects the small joints of the hands and occasionally the ankles, knees, and wrists. Most cases resolve in 3 weeks, but some persist for months.
- Transient aplastic crisis (TAC): Pts with chronic hemolytic conditions (e.g., hemoglobinopathies, autoimmune hemolytic anemia) can develop aplastic crisis with B19 infection that can be life-threatening. Pts display symptoms associated with severe anemia.

- Pure red cell aplasia/chronic anemia: Pts have persistent anemia, high levels of B19 DNA in serum, and absent or low-level B19 IgG. HIV-infected pts, transplant recipients, and pts with other immunodeficiencies are at risk.
- Hydrops fetalis: B19 infection during pregnancy can lead to hydrops fetalis and/or fetal loss. The risk of transplacental fetal infection is ~30%, and the risk of fetal loss (which occurs predominantly early in the second trimester) is ~9%. The risk of congenital infection is <1%.

Diagnosis Diagnosis relies on measurement of B19-specific IgM and IgG antibodies. Detection of B19 DNA via quantitative PCR should be used to diagnose TAC or chronic anemia. In acute infection, the viremia load can exceed >10^{12} B19 DNA genome equivalents (ge)/mL of serum; pts with TAC or chronic anemia generally have >10^5 B19 DNA ge/mL. Bone marrow examination demonstrates characteristic giant pronormoblasts and the absence of erythroid precursors.

 Parvovirus Infection

Aplastic crisis should be treated with transfusions as needed; in pts receiving chemotherapy, this treatment should be temporarily discontinued if possible. Commercial IV immunoglobulin should be given to immunodeficient anemic pts to control and possibly cure B19 infection.

Prevention Pts with chronic B19 infection or TAC should be considered infectious. Hospitalized pts with chronic B19 infection or TAC pose a risk of nosocomial transmission and should be placed on contact and respiratory isolation precautions.

 For a more detailed discussion, see Brown KE: Parvovirus Infections, Chap. 177, p. 1114; Gershon A: Measles (Rubeola), Chap. 185, p. 1214; Rubella (German Measles), Chap. 186, p. 1217; and Mumps, Chap. 187, p. 1220, in HPIM-17.

110 Enteroviral Infections

ETIOLOGY

Enteroviruses are so named because of their ability to multiply in the GI tract, but they do not typically cause gastroenteritis. This group of viruses includes 3 serotypes of poliovirus, 23 serotypes of coxsackievirus A, 6 serotypes of coxsackievirus B, 29 serotypes of echovirus, and enteroviruses 68–71. Enteroviruses 73–102 have recently been identified in humans, but the clinical features of these viruses have not yet been defined. In the United States, echovirus causes most enteroviral infections.

PATHOGENESIS AND IMMUNITY

Of the enteroviruses, poliovirus is best characterized. After ingestion, poliovirus infects GI tract mucosal epithelial cells, spreads to regional lymph nodes, causes viremia, and replicates in the reticuloendothelial system; in some cases, a second round of viremia occurs. Virus gains access to the central nervous system (CNS) either via the bloodstream or via direct spread from neural pathways. Virus is present in blood for 3–5 days. It is shed from the oropharynx for up to 3 weeks and from the GI tract for up to 12 weeks after infection. Immunocompromised pts can shed virus for up to 20 years. Infection is controlled by humoral and secretory immunity in the GI tract.

EPIDEMIOLOGY

Enteroviruses cause disease worldwide, especially in areas with crowded conditions and poor hygiene. Infants and young children are most often infected and are the most frequent shedders. Transmission takes place mainly by the fecal-oral route, but airborne transmission and placental transmission have been described. Pts are most infectious shortly before or after the onset of symptoms. The incubation period ranges from 2 to 14 days but usually is <1 week in duration.

CLINICAL FEATURES

Poliovirus

- Most infections are asymptomatic. Mild illness resolves in 3 days and is manifest by fever, malaise, sore throat, myalgias, and headache.
- Aseptic meningitis (nonparalytic) occurs in ~1% of pts. Examination of cerebrospinal fluid (CSF) reveals normal glucose and protein concentrations and lymphocytic pleocytosis [with polymorphonuclear leukocytes (PMNs) sometimes predominating early].
- Paralytic disease is least common. Risk factors include older age, pregnancy, and trauma or strenuous exercise at the onset of CNS symptoms. Aseptic meningitis is followed ≥1 day later by severe back, neck, and muscle pain as well as a gradual development of motor weakness. This weakness is usually asymmetric and proximal and is most common in the legs; the arms and the abdominal, thoracic, and bulbar muscles are other frequently involved sites. Paralysis occurs only during the febrile phase. Physical examination reveals weakness, fasciculations, decreased muscle tone, and reduced or absent reflexes in affected areas; hyperreflexia may precede the loss of reflexes. Bulbar paralysis is associated with dysphagia, difficulty handling secretions, or dysphonia. Respiratory insufficiency due to aspiration or neurologic involvement may develop. Severe medullary infection may lead to circulatory collapse. Most pts recover some function, but around two-thirds have residual neurologic sequelae.
- Live poliovirus vaccine–associated disease: The risk is estimated to be 1 case per 2.5 million doses and is ~2000 times higher among immunodeficient persons.
- Postpolio syndrome: new weakness 20–40 years after poliomyelitis. Onset is insidious, progression is slow, and plateau periods can last 1–10 years.

Coxsackievirus, Echovirus, and Other Enteroviruses   In the United States, 5–10 million cases of symptomatic enteroviral disease other than poliomyelitis occur each year.

- *Nonspecific febrile illness* (summer grippe) occurs during the summer and early fall. Pts experience an acute onset of fever, malaise, and headache;

upper respiratory symptoms; nausea; and vomiting. Disease resolves within a week.

- *Generalized disease of the newborn* occurs from the first week of life to 3 months of age. The illness resembles bacterial sepsis and has a high associated mortality rate. Myocarditis, hypotension, hepatitis, disseminated intravascular coagulation, meningitis, and pneumonia are complications.
- *Aseptic meningitis and encephalitis*: Enteroviruses cause 90% of aseptic meningitis cases among children and young adults. Pts have an acute onset of fever, chills, headache, photophobia, nausea, and vomiting, with meningismus on examination. Diarrhea, rashes, myalgias, pleurodynia, myocarditis, and herpangina may occur. CSF examination reveals pleocytosis, with PMNs sometimes predominating early but a shift to lymphocyte predominance within 24 h. Total cell counts usually do not exceed 1000/μL. CSF glucose and protein levels are typically normal. Symptoms resolve within a week, but CSF abnormalities persist longer. Encephalitis is much less common and is usually mild, with an excellent prognosis in healthy hosts. However, pts with γ globulin defects can develop chronic meningitis or encephalitis. Pts receiving γ globulin replacement may develop neurologic disease due to echovirus.
- *Pleurodynia (Bornholm disease)*: Pts have an acute onset of fever associated with spasms of pleuritic chest pain (more common among adults) or upper abdominal pain (more common among children). Fever subsides when pain resolves. A pleural rub may be present. Coxsackievirus B is the most common cause. Disease lasts for several days and can be treated with nonsteroidal anti-inflammatory drugs and heat application to the affected muscles.
- *Myocarditis and pericarditis*: Enteroviruses (e.g., coxsackievirus B) cause up to one-third of cases of acute myocarditis. Disease is more common among males and occurs most often in newborns (who have the most severe disease), adolescents, and young adults. Pts have upper respiratory symptoms followed by fever, chest pain, dyspnea, arrhythmias, and occasionally congestive heart failure. A pericardial friction rub, ST-segment and T-wave abnormalities on electrocardiogram, and elevated serum levels of myocardial enzymes can be present. Up to 10% of pts develop chronic dilated cardiomyopathy. Constrictive pericarditis may occur.
- *Exanthems*: Enteroviral infection is a leading cause of exanthems among children in the summer and fall. Echoviruses 9 and 16 are common causes.
- *Hand-foot-and-mouth disease*: Pts present with fever, anorexia, and malaise, followed by sore throat and vesicles on the buccal mucosa, tongue, and dorsum or palms of the hands and occasionally on the palate, uvula, tonsillar pillars, or feet. Lesions can become bullous and ulcerate. The disease is highly infectious, with attack rates of almost 100% among young children. Symptoms resolve within a week. Coxsackievirus A16 and enterovirus 71 are the most common etiologic agents. A Taiwan epidemic of enterovirus 71 infection was associated with CNS disease, myocarditis, and pulmonary hemorrhage. Deaths occurred primarily among children ≤5 years old.
- *Herpangina*: associated with coxsackievirus A infection. Pts have fever, sore throat, and dysphagia and develop grayish-white papulovesicular lesions that ulcerate and are concentrated in the posterior portion of the mouth. Lesions can persist for weeks. In contrast to herpes simplex stomatitis, enteroviral herpangina is not associated with gingivitis.
- *Acute hemorrhagic conjunctivitis*: associated with enterovirus 70 and coxsackievirus A24. Pts experience an acute onset of severe eye pain, blurred vision, photophobia, watery eye discharge, fever, and headache. Edema, chemosis, and subconjunctival hemorrhage are evident. Symptoms resolve within 10 days.

DIAGNOSIS

Enterovirus can be isolated from throat or rectal swabs, stool, and/or normally sterile body fluids. Stool and throat cultures may reflect colonization, but throat cultures are more likely to be associated with disease because virus is shed for shorter periods from the throat. Positive results for normally sterile body fluids, such as CSF and serum, reflect disease. Serotyping is not clinically useful. Polymerase chain reaction (PCR) detects >92% of the serotypes that infect humans. PCR of the CSF is sensitive and specific and is more rapid than culture; however, the result of PCR is less likely to be positive if pts present ≥3 days after meningitis onset. In those cases, PCR of fecal specimens, although less specific, should be considered. PCR of the serum is also useful in disseminated disease. Tests are more likely to be positive early in disease.

 Enteroviral Infections

Most enteroviral illness resolves spontaneously, but immunoglobulin may be helpful in pts with γ globulin defects and chronic infection and in neonates with severe disease. Glucocorticoids are contraindicated.

PREVENTION

Hand hygiene, use of gowns and gloves, and enteric precautions (for 7 days after disease onset) prevent nosocomial transmission of enteroviruses during epidemics. The availability of poliovirus vaccines and the implementation of polio eradication programs have largely eliminated disease due to wild-type poliovirus; of 1959 cases in 2006, ~90% were from Nigeria and India. Outbreaks and sporadic disease due to vaccine-derived poliovirus occur. Both oral poliovirus vaccine (OPV) and inactivated poliovirus vaccine (IPV) induce IgG and IgA antibodies that persist for at least 5 years. OPV causes less viral shedding, reduces the risk of community transmission of wild-type virus, costs less, and is easier to administer than IPV. Most developing countries, particularly those with persistent wild-type poliomyelitis, use OPV. Developed countries without wild-type disease but with cases of vaccine-associated polio have adopted all-IPV childhood vaccination programs. Doses are given at 2, 4, and 6–18 months and at 4–6 years of age. Unvaccinated adults in the United States do not need routine poliovirus vaccination but should receive three doses of IPV (the second dose 1–2 months after the first and the final dose 6–12 months later) if they are traveling to polio-endemic areas or might be exposed to wild-type poliovirus in their communities or workplaces. Adults at increased risk of exposure who have received their primary vaccination series should receive a single dose of IPV.

For a more detailed discussion, see Cohen JI: Enteroviruses and Reoviruses, Chap. 184, p. 1208, in HPIM-17.

111 Insect- and Animal-Borne Viral Infections

RABIES

Rabies is a zoonosis generally transmitted to humans by the bite of a rabid animal and caused by rabies virus: a rodlike, enveloped, single-stranded RNA virus in the family Rhabdoviridae of the genus *Lyssavirus*. Each animal reservoir harbors distinct rabies virus variants.

Epidemiology   Worldwide, canine rabies causes ~55,000 human deaths each year, most in Asia and Africa. In North America, bats, raccoons, skunks, and foxes carry endemic rabies. Bats cause the most human cases in the United States; rabies can be transmitted by minor or unrecognized bat bites.

Pathogenesis   The incubation period varies from 2 weeks to >1 year (mean, 1–3 months). During most of this period, rabies virus is present at or close to the site of the bite. Virus replicates at the inoculation site and spreads to peripheral nerves and then to the central nervous system (CNS), dispersing rapidly throughout the gray matter. Establishment of CNS infection is followed by centrifugal spread along peripheral nerves to other tissues, including salivary glands—hence the excretion of virus in the saliva of rabid animals. The most characteristic pathologic CNS finding is the *Negri body*—an eosinophilic cytoplasmic inclusion that is found within neurons and is composed of rabies virus particles in an amorphous matrix.

Clinical Features   Rabies has the highest case-fatality rate of any infectious disease. Clinical rabies can be divided into three phases.

- *Prodrome* (1–7 days): Pts have fever, headache, malaise, nausea, vomiting, and anxiety or agitation. Paresthesia and/or fasciculations at or near the site of viral inoculation are found in 50–80% of cases and are suggestive of rabies.
- *Acute neurologic phase*: presents as the encephalitic (furious) form in 80% of cases and as the paralytic form in 20%

   Encephalitic form (1–7 days): Pts develop fever, confusion, hallucinations, combativeness, muscle spasms, hyperactivity, and seizures. Autonomic dysfunction is common and includes hypersalivation, excessive perspiration, pupillary dilation, gooseflesh, and/or priapism. Prominent early brainstem dysfunction distinguishes rabies from other viral encephalitides. Hydrophobia and aerophobia occur as a consequence of involuntary, painful contraction of the diaphragm and the accessory respiratory, laryngeal, and pharyngeal muscles in response to swallowing liquid or air. Hypersalivation and pharyngeal dysfunction produce characteristic foaming at the mouth.

   Paralytic form (2–10 days): For unknown reasons, muscle weakness predominates but cardinal features of rabies encephalitis are lacking.
- *Coma and death* (1–14 days): Even with aggressive supportive measures, recovery is rare.

Diagnosis

- Examination of cerebrospinal fluid (CSF) can show a mild pleocytosis and a slightly increased protein level.

- Rabies virus–specific antibodies may be detected in serum and CSF a few days after symptom onset, but pts may die without detectable antibodies. Rabies virus–specific antibodies in the CSF suggest rabies regardless of immunization status.
- Reverse-transcription polymerase chain reaction (RT-PCR) can detect virus in fresh saliva, CSF, and tissue. RT-PCR can also distinguish among rabies virus variants and may indicate the likely source of infection.
- Direct fluorescent antibody (DFA) testing: DFA testing is sensitive and specific and can be applied to brain tissue or skin biopsies from the nape of the neck (where virus is found in cutaneous nerves at the base of hair follicles).
- Differential diagnosis: Other viral encephalitides [e.g., those due to herpes simplex virus (HSV) type 1, varicella-zoster virus, and enteroviruses as well as arboviruses] should be considered.

Rx Rabies

Treatment is palliative and supportive. There is no established treatment for rabies.

Prevention
- Rabies is almost uniformly fatal but is nearly always preventable with appropriate postexposure prophylaxis during the incubation period.
- The wound should be thoroughly scrubbed with soap and flushed with water; these measures can reduce the risk of rabies by 90%.
- Postexposure prophylaxis (PEP; Fig. 111-1)
  Passive immunization with rabies immune globulin (RIG): RIG should be given to previously unvaccinated persons as soon as possible but no later than 7 days after the first vaccine dose (see below). If possible, the full dose of RIG (20 IU/kg) should be infused at the bite site; any residual RIG should be given IM at a distant site.
  Inactivated rabies vaccine should be given as soon as possible (1 mL IM in the deltoid region) and repeated on days 3, 7, 14, and 28.
- Preexposure prophylaxis is occasionally given to persons at high risk. A primary vaccine schedule is given on days 0, 7, and 21 or 28. Serum neutralizing antibody titers can be monitored to determine the need for booster doses of vaccine.

INFECTIONS CAUSED BY ARTHROPOD- AND RODENT-BORNE VIRUSES

More than 500 distinct RNA viruses are maintained in arthropods or chronically infected rodents. Arthropod-borne viruses infect their vector after a blood meal from a viremic vertebrate; the viruses penetrate the gut and spread throughout the vector; when in the salivary glands, they can be transmitted to another vertebrate during a blood meal. The rodent-borne viruses cause chronic infections transmitted between rodents. Humans become infected by inhalation of aerosols containing the viruses and through close contact with rodents and their excreta. These infections are most common in the tropics but also occur in temperate and frigid climates.

Clinical Features Infection usually causes one of four major clinical syndromes: fever and myalgia, encephalitis, arthritis and rash, or hemorrhagic fever (HF).

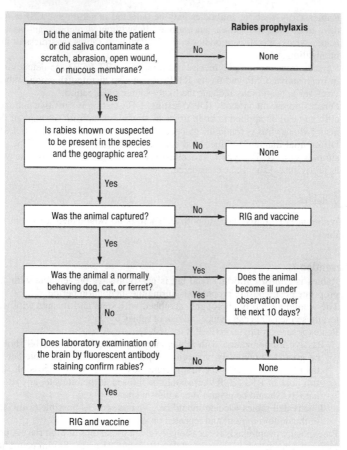

FIGURE 111-1 Algorithm for rabies postexposure prophylaxis. RIG, rabies immune globulin. *[From L Corey, in Harrison's Principles of Internal Medicine, 15th ed. E Braunwald et al (eds): New York, McGraw-Hill, 2001, adapted with permission.]*

Fever and Myalgia   This is the most common syndrome associated with these viruses. Typically, pts have an acute onset of fever, severe myalgia, and headache. Complete recovery is usual. Important examples include the following.

- *Lymphocytic choriomeningitis* (LCM): This infection is transmitted from the common house mouse and pet hamsters via aerosols of excreta and secreta. Unlike other viral infections that cause fever and myalgia, LCM has a gradual onset. Other manifestations include transient alopecia, arthritis, cough, maculopapular rash, and orchitis. About one-fourth of infected pts have a biphasic illness. After a 3- to 6-day febrile phase, there is a remission followed by recurrent fever, headache, nausea, vomiting, and meningeal signs lasting ~1 week. Pregnant women can have mild infection yet pass on the virus to the fetus, who can develop hydrocephalus and chorioretinitis. The diagnosis should be considered in adult pts who have aseptic meningitis in the autumn months and who have had a febrile prodrome. CSF examination reveals mononuclear cell counts that can exceed 1000/µL and low glucose levels. Marked leukopenia and thrombocytopenia are common. Recovery of LCM virus from blood or CSF is most likely in the initial phase of illness. Diagnosis can be made by IgM-capture enzyme-linked immunosorbent assay (ELISA) of serum or CSF or by RT-PCR of CSF (if this test is available).

• *Dengue fever:* The vector of all four distinct dengue viruses (serotypes 1–4) is *Aedes aegypti*, which is also a vector for yellow fever. A second infection with a different dengue serotype can lead to dengue hemorrhagic fever (DHF; see "Hemorrhagic Fever," below). Year-round transmission occurs between latitudes 25°N and 25°S. After an incubation period of 2–7 days, pts experience the sudden onset of fever, headache, retroorbital pain, back pain, severe myalgia (break-bone fever), adenopathy, palatal vesicles, and scleral injection. The illness usually lasts 1 week, and a maculopapular rash often appears near the time of defervescence. Epistaxis, petechiae, and GI bleeding may occur. Leukopenia, thrombocytopenia, and increased serum aminotransferase levels may be documented. IgM ELISA, antigen-detection ELISA, or RT-PCR during the acute phase permits the diagnosis. Virus is easily isolated from blood during the acute phase.

Encephalitis Depending on the causative virus, there is much variability in the ratio of clinical to subclinical disease, mortality, and residua (Table 111-1). The pt usually presents with a prodrome of nonspecific symptoms followed quickly by headache, meningeal signs, photophobia, and vomiting. Complications include deepening lethargy and ultimately coma, tremors, cranial nerve palsies, and focal neurologic signs and seizures. Acute encephalitis usually lasts from a few days to 2–3 weeks, but recovery may be slow. Treatable causes of encephalitis (e.g., HSV) should be ruled out quickly. Many viruses cause arboviral encephalitis. Some important examples follow.

• *Japanese encephalitis:* This infection is present throughout Asia and is occasionally found in the western Pacific islands. An effective vaccine (given on days 0, 7, and 30) is available and is indicated for summer travelers to rural Asia, where the risk can be as high as 2.1 cases per 10,000 per week. Expatriates have an especially high risk of severe and often fatal disease. There is a 0.1–1% chance of a vaccine reaction (which may be severe but is rarely fatal) beginning 1–9 days after vaccination. Spinal and motor neuron disease can be documented in addition to the encephalitis.

• *West Nile encephalitis:* Usually a mild or asymptomatic disease, West Nile virus infection can cause aseptic meningitis or encephalitis. Introduced into New York City in 1999, it has now spread throughout the United States. Encephalitis, serious sequelae, and death are more common among elderly pts, diabetic pts, and pts with previous CNS disease. Unusual clinical features include chorioretinitis and flaccid paralysis.

• *Eastern equine encephalitis:* This disease is found primarily within endemic swampy foci along the eastern coast of the United States, with inland foci as distant as Michigan. It is most common in the summer and early fall. One of the most severe arboviral conditions, eastern equine encephalitis is characterized by rapid onset, rapid progression, high mortality risk, and frequent residua. Necrotic lesions and polymorphonuclear leukocyte (PMN) infiltrates are found in the brain at autopsy. PMN-predominant pleocytosis of the CSF within the first 3 days of disease is common, as is leukocytosis with a left shift in peripheral blood.

Arthritis and Rash Arboviruses are common causes of true arthritis accompanied by a febrile illness and maculopapular rash. Examples include the following:

TABLE 111-1	PROMINENT FEATURES OF ARBOVIRAL ENCEPHALITIS		
Virus	Natural Cycle	Incubation Period, Days	Annual No. of Cases
La Crosse	*Aedes triseriatus*—chipmunk (transovarial component in mosquito also important)	~3–7	70 (U.S.)
St. Louis	*Culex tarsalis, C. pipiens, C. quinquefasciatus*—birds	4–21	85, with hundreds to thousands in epidemic years (U.S.)
Japanese	*Culex tritaeniorhynchus*—birds	5–15	>25,000
West Nile	*Culex* mosquitoes—birds	3–6	?
Central European	*Ixodes ricinus*—rodents, insectivores	7–14	Thousands
Russian spring-summer	*I. persulcatus*—rodents, insectivores	7–14	Hundreds
Powassan	*I. cookei*—wild mammals	~10	~1 (U.S.)
Eastern equine	*Culiseta melanura*—birds	~5–10	5 (U.S.)
Western equine	*Culex tarsalis*—birds	~5–10	~20 (U.S.)
Venezuelan equine (epidemic)	Unknown (multiple mosquito species and horses in epidemics)	1–5	?

- *Sindbis virus*: found in northern Europe and the independent states of the former Soviet Union
- *Chikungunya virus*: of African origin. In a massive epidemic in 2004 in the Indian Ocean region, the disease appeared to be spread solely by travelers.
- *Ross River virus*: a cause of epidemic polyarthritis in Australia since the start of the twentieth century

Hemorrhagic Fever   The viral HF syndrome is a constellation of findings based on vascular instability and decreased vascular integrity. Pts develop local hemorrhage, hypotension, and—in severe cases—shock. All HF syndromes begin with the abrupt onset of fever and myalgia and can progress to severe prostration, headache, dizziness, photophobia, abdominal and/or chest pain, anorexia, and GI disturbances. On initial physical examination, there is conjunctival suffusion, muscle or abdominal tenderness to palpation, hypotension, petechiae, and periorbital edema. Laboratory examination usually reveals elevated serum aminotrans-

Case-to-Infection Ratio	Age of Cases	Case-Fatality Rate, %	Residua
<1:1000	<15 years	<0.5	Recurrent seizures in ~10%; severe deficits in rare cases; decreased school performance and behavioral change suspected in small proportion
<1:200	Milder cases in the young; more severe cases in adults >40 years old, particularly the elderly	7	Common in the elderly
1:200–300	All ages; children in highly endemic areas	20–50	Common (approximately half of cases); may be severe
Very low	Mainly the elderly	5–10	Uncommon
1:12	All ages; milder in children	1–5	20%
—	All ages; milder in children	20	Approximately half of cases; often severe; limb-girdle paralysis
—	All ages; some predilection for children	~10	Common (approximately half of cases)
1:40 adult 1:17 child	All ages; predilection for children	50–75	Common
1:1000 adult 1:50 child 1:1 infant	All ages; predilection for children <2 years old (increased mortality in elderly)	3–7	Common only among infants <1 year old
1:250 adult 1:25 child (approximate)	All ages; predilection for children	~10	—

ferase levels, proteinuria, and hemoconcentration. Shock, multifocal bleeding, and CNS involvement (encephalopathy, coma, convulsions) are poor prognostic signs. Early recognition is important; appropriate supportive measures and, in some cases, virus-specific therapy can be instituted.

• *Lassa fever*: Endemic and epidemic in West Africa, Lassa fever virus is spread to humans by aerosols from chronically infected rodents. Transmission by close person-to-person contact can occur. A gradual onset gives way to more severe constitutional symptoms and prostration. Bleeding is evident in 15–30% of cases. CNS dysfunction is marked by confusion, tremors of the upper extremity and tongue, and cerebellar signs; effusions, including pericarditis in men, are common. Pregnant women have higher mortality rates, and the fetal death rate is 92% in the last trimester. Pts who are pregnant should consider termination of the pregnancy. Pts with high-level viremia or a serum aspartate aminotransferase level of >150 IU/mL are at an elevated risk of death, and the administration of ribavirin, which appears to reduce this risk, should be considered. Ribavirin is given by slow IV infusion; an initial dose of 32 mg/kg is followed by 16 mg/kg every 6 h for 4 days and then by 8 mg/kg every 8 h for 6 days.

- *South American HF syndromes* (Argentine, Bolivian, Venezuelan, Brazilian): These syndromes resemble Lassa fever; however, thrombocytopenia and bleeding are common, whereas CNS dysfunction is not. Passive antibody treatment for Argentine HF is effective, and an effective vaccine exists. Ribavirin is likely to be effective in all South American HF syndromes.
- *Rift Valley fever*: Although Rift Valley virus typically causes fever and myalgia, HF can occur with prominent liver involvement, renal failure, and disseminated intravascular coagulation (DIC). Retinal vasculitis can occur in ~10% of infections, and pts' vision can be permanently impaired. There is no proven therapy for Rift Valley fever.
- *Crimean-Congo HF*: This disease is similar to other HF syndromes but causes extensive liver damage and jaundice. Ribavirin should be given in severe cases.
- *HF with renal syndrome*

  This entity is most often caused in Europe by Puumala virus (rodent reservoir, the bank vole) and in Asia by Hantaan virus (rodent reservoir, the striped field mouse). More than 100,000 cases of severe disease occur annually in endemic areas of Asia. Severe classic Hantaan disease has four stages.

  Febrile stage: abrupt onset of fever, headache, myalgia, thirst
  Hypotensive stage: falling blood pressure; relative bradycardia; laboratory findings including leukocytosis with a left shift, atypical lymphocytosis, proteinuria, vascular leakage causing hemoconcentration, and renal tubular necrosis
  Oliguric stage: continuing hemorrhage; oliguria persisting for 3–10 days before renal function returns
  Polyuric stage: As renal function returns, there is a danger of dehydration and electrolyte abnormalities.

  The diagnosis can be made by IgM-capture ELISA, which should yield a positive result within 48 h of admission. RT-PCR of a blood clot gives a positive result early in the clinical course.
  Treatment: Expectant management of shock and renal failure is crucial. Ribavirin may reduce mortality and morbidity in severe cases if treatment is begun within the first 4 days of illness.
- *Hantavirus pulmonary syndrome* (HPS): The disease is linked to rodent exposure and particularly affects rural residents in dwellings permeable to rodent entry. Sin Nombre virus infects the deer mouse and is the most important virus causing HPS in the United States.

  Clinical findings include the following:
  Prodrome (3–4 days; range, 1–11 days): fever, myalgia, dizziness, vertigo, malaise, nausea, vomiting, abdominal pain
  Cardiopulmonary phase: tachycardia, hypotension, tachypnea, early signs of pulmonary edema
  Final phase: rapid decompensation with hypoxemia, respiratory failure, low cardiac output, myocardial depression, increased pulmonary vascular permeability, shock
  Laboratory findings include thrombocytopenia (an important early clue), atypical lymphocytes, and a left shift, often with leukocytosis; hemoconcentration; hypoalbuminemia; and proteinuria. IgM testing of acute-phase serum can yield positive results, even during the prodromal stage.

RT-PCR of blood clots or tissue usually gives a positive result in the first 7–9 days of illness.

Treatment: Intensive respiratory management and other supportive measures are crucial in the first few hours after presentation. Shock should be managed with pressor agents and modest amounts of fluid.

Prognosis: Most pts who survive for 48 h recover without residua. Mortality rates are ~30–40% despite optimal management.

- *Yellow fever*: Yellow fever is a former cause of major epidemics. Hundreds of cases in South America and thousands of cases in Africa still occur. Yellow fever causes a typical HF syndrome with prominent hepatic necrosis. Pts are viremic for 3–4 days and can have jaundice, hemorrhage, black vomit, anuria, and terminal delirium. Vaccination of visitors to endemic areas and control of the mosquito vector *A. aegypti* prevent disease.

- *Dengue hemorrhagic fever* (DHF)/*dengue shock syndrome* (DSS): Previous infection with a heterologous dengue virus serotype may elicit nonprotective antibodies and enhanced disease if pts are reinfected. The risk decreases considerably after age 12; DHF/DSS is more common among females than among males, more severe among Caucasians than among blacks, and more common among well-nourished than among malnourished persons. DHF is marked by bleeding tendencies. DSS is more serious because of vascular permeability leading to shock. In mild cases, lethargy, thrombocytopenia, and hemoconcentration occur 2–5 days after typical dengue fever, usually at the time of defervescence. In severe cases, frank shock occurs with cyanosis, hepatomegaly, ascites and pleural effusions, and GI bleeding. Shock lasts for 1–2 days and usually responds to supportive measures. With good care, the overall mortality rate is as low as 1%. Control of *A. aegypti*, the mosquito vector, is the key to control of the disease.

EBOLA AND MARBURG VIRUS INFECTIONS

Etiology Marburg and Ebola viruses are two distinct single-stranded RNA viruses of the family Filoviridae. Almost all Filoviridae are African viruses that cause severe disease with high mortality rates. Both Marburg virus and Ebola virus are biosafety level 4 pathogens because of the high mortality rate from infection and the aerosol infectivity of the agents.

Epidemiology The first human cases of Marburg virus infection occurred in laboratory workers exposed to infected African green monkeys from Uganda. In 2004–2005, a massive Marburg virus epidemic occurred in Angola, with a case-fatality rate of 90%. Ebola virus has been associated with epidemics of severe HF. The first two epidemics were due to different subtypes: Zaire, with 90% mortality, and Sudan, with 50% mortality. Interhuman spread was noted. However, epidemiologic studies have failed to yield evidence for an important role (like that documented in Ebola disease in monkeys) of airborne particles in human Ebola disease. The reservoir is unknown, but speculation currently centers on bats.

Pathogenesis Both viruses replicate well in virtually all cell types, and viral replication is associated with cellular necrosis. Acute infection is associated with high levels of circulating virus and viral antigen until antibody development, evidence of which is usually lacking in fatal cases. Virions are abundant in fibroblasts, interstitium, and SC tissues and may escape through breaks in the skin or through sweat glands—a potential scenario that may be correlated with the risk of transmission through close pt contact or by touching of deceased pts. High levels of circulating proinflammatory cytokines contribute to disease severity.

Clinical Features After a 7- to 10-day incubation period, pts experience an abrupt onset of fever, headache, severe myalgia, nausea, vomiting, diarrhea, prostration, and depressed mentation. A maculopapular rash may appear at day 5–7 and be followed by desquamation. Bleeding can occur from any mucosal site and into the skin. The fever may break after 10–12 days, and the pt may eventually recover. Recrudescence and secondary bacterial infection may occur.

Laboratory Findings Leukopenia is common early on and is followed by neutrophilia. Thrombocytopenia, DIC, and increases in serum aminotransferase and amylase levels can develop. Proteinuria and renal failure are proportional to shock.

Diagnosis High concentrations of virus in blood can be documented by antigen detection ELISA, virus isolation, or RT-PCR. Antibodies can be detected in recovering pts.

℞ Ebola and Marburg Virus Infections

Supportive measures may not be as useful as had been hoped, but studies in rhesus monkeys suggest that treatment with an inhibitor of factor VIIa/tissue factor or with activated protein C may improve survival rates.

For a more detailed discussion, see Jackson AC, Johannsen EC: Rabies and Other Rhabdovirus Infections, Chap. 188, p. 1222; Peters CJ: Infections Caused by Arthropod- and Rodent-Borne Viruses, Chap. 189, p. 1226; and Peters CJ: Ebola and Marburg Viruses, Chap. 190, p. 1240, in HPIM-17.

112 HIV Infection and AIDS

DEFINITION

AIDS was originally defined empirically by the Centers for Disease Control and Prevention (CDC) as "the presence of a reliably diagnosed disease that is at least moderately indicative of an underlying defect in cell-mediated immunity." Following the recognition of the causative virus, HIV, and the development of sensitive and specific tests for HIV infection, the definition of AIDS has undergone substantial revision. The current surveillance definition categorizes HIV-infected persons on the basis of clinical conditions associated with HIV infection and CD4+T lymphocyte counts (Tables 182-1 and 182-2, p. 1138, in HPIM-17). From a practical standpoint, the clinician should view HIV disease as a spectrum of disorders ranging from primary infection, with or without the acute HIV syndrome, to the asymptomatic infected state to advanced disease.

ETIOLOGY

AIDS is caused by infection with the human retroviruses HIV-1 or -2. HIV-1 is the most common cause worldwide; HIV-2 has about 40% sequence homology with HIV-1, is more closely related to simian immunodeficiency viruses, and has been identified predominantly in western Africa. HIV-2 infection has also been reported in Europe, South America, Canada, the United States, and elsewhere. These viruses are passed through sexual contact; through transfusion of contaminated blood or blood products, through sharing of contaminated needles and syringes among injection drug abusers; intrapartum or perinatally from mother to infant; or via breast milk. There is no evidence that the virus can be passed through casual or family contact or by insects such as mosquitoes. There is a definite, though small, occupational risk of infection for health care workers and laboratory personnel who work with HIV-infected specimens. The risk of transmission of HIV from an infected health care worker to his or her pts through invasive procedures is extremely low.

EPIDEMIOLOGY

Through 2006, an estimated 982,498 cumulative cases of AIDS had been diagnosed in the United States; ~56% of those have died. However, the death rate from AIDS has decreased substantially in the past 10 years primarily due to the increased use of potent antiretroviral drugs. At the end of 2003, an estimated 1.0–1.2 million HIV-infected persons were living in the United States. Major risk groups continue to be men who have had sex with men and men and women injection drug users (IDUs). However, the number of cases that are transmitted heterosexually, particularly to women, is increasing rapidly (see Figs. 182-8, p. 1143; 182-14 through 182-16, pp. 1148 and 1149, in HPIM-17). As the majority of IDU-associated cases are among inner-city minority populations, the burden of HIV infection and AIDS falls increasingly and disproportionately on minorities, especially in the cities of the northeast and southeast United States. Cases of AIDS are still being found among individuals who have received contaminated blood products in the past, although the risk of acquiring new infection through this route is extremely small in the United States. HIV infection/AIDS is a global pandemic, especially in developing countries. The current estimate of the number of cases of HIV infection worldwide is ~33.2 million, two-thirds of whom are in sub-Saharan Africa; ~50% of cases are in women (Figs. 182-7, p. 1142; 182-9, p. 1143; 182-11 through 182-13, pp. 1147 and 1148, in HPIM-17).

PATHOPHYSIOLOGY AND IMMUNOPATHOGENESIS

The hallmark of HIV disease is a profound immunodeficiency resulting from a progressive quantitative and qualitative deficiency of the subset of T lymphocytes referred to as helper or inducer T cells. This subset of T cells is defined phenotypically by the expression on the cell surface of the CD4 molecule, which serves as the primary cellular receptor for HIV. A co-receptor must be present with CD4 for efficient entry of HIV-1 into target cells. The two major co-receptors for HIV-1 are the chemokine receptors CCR5 and CXCR4. Although the CD4+ T lymphocyte and CD4+ monocyte lineage are the principal cellular targets of HIV, virtually any cell that expresses CD4 along with one of the co-receptors can potentially be infected by HIV; however, viral replication is not efficient in these other cell types.

Primary Infection Following initial transmission, the virus infects CD4+ cells, probably T lymphocytes, monocytes, or bone marrow–derived dendritic cells. Both during this initial stage and later in infection, the lymphoid system is a major site for the establishment and propagation of HIV infection. The gut-associated lymphoid tissue (GALT) plays a major role in the establishment of infection and in the early depletion of memory CD4+ T cells.

Essentially all pts undergo a viremic stage during primary infection; in some pts this is associated with the "acute retroviral syndrome," a mononucleosis-like illness (see below). This phase is important in disseminating virus to lymphoid and other organs throughout the body, and it is ultimately contained partially by the development of an HIV-specific immune response.

Establishment of Chronic and Persistent Infection Despite the robust immune response that is mounted following primary infection, the virus is not cleared from the body. Instead, a chronic infection develops that persists for a median time of 10 years before the untreated patient becomes clinically ill. During this period of clinical latency, the number of CD4+ T cells gradually declines but few, if any, clinical signs and symptoms may be evident; however, active viral replication can almost always be detected by measurable plasma viremia and the demonstration of virus replication in lymphoid tissue. The level of steady-state viremia (referred to as the *viral set point*) at ~6 months to 1 year postinfection has important prognostic implications for the progression of HIV disease; individuals with a low viral set point at 6 months to 1 year after infection progress to AIDS more slowly than those whose set point is very high at this time (see Fig. 182-20, p. 1152, in HPIM-17).

Advanced HIV Disease In untreated pts or in pts in whom therapy has not controlled viral replication (see below), after some period of time (often years), CD4+ T cell counts will fall below a critical level (~200/μL) and pts become highly susceptible to opportunistic disease. The presence of a CD4+ T cell count of <200/μL or an AIDS-defining opportunistic disease establishes a diagnosis of AIDS. Control of plasma viremia by effective antiretroviral therapy, particularly maintaining the plasma viral load at <50 copies of RNA per ml, even in individuals with low CD4+ T cell counts, has increased survival in these pts, including those whose CD4+ T cell counts may not increase significantly as a result of therapy.

IMMUNE ABNORMALITIES IN HIV DISEASE

A broad range of immune abnormalities has been documented in HIV-infected pts resulting in varying degrees of immunodeficiency. These include both quantitative and qualitative defects in lymphocyte, monocyte/macrophage, and natural killer (NK) cell function. Autoimmune phenomena have also been observed in HIV-infected individuals.

IMMUNE RESPONSE TO HIV INFECTION

Both humoral and cellular immune responses to HIV develop soon after primary infection (see summary in Table 182-5, p. 1163, and Fig. 182-24, p. 1163, in HPIM-17). Humoral responses include antibodies with HIV binding and neutralizing activity, as well as antibodies participating in antibody-dependent cellular cytotoxicity (ADCC). Cellular immune responses include the generation of HIV-specific CD4+ and CD8+ T lymphocytes, as well as NK cells and mononuclear cells mediating ADCC. CD8+ T lymphocytes may also suppress HIV replication in a noncytolytic, non-MHC restricted manner. This effect is mediated by soluble factors such as the CC-chemokines RANTES, MIP-1α, and MIP-1β. For the most part, the natural immune response to HIV is not adequate. Broadly reacting neutralizing antibodies against HIV are not easily generated in infected individuals, and eradication of the virus from infected individuals by naturally occurring immune responses has not been reported.

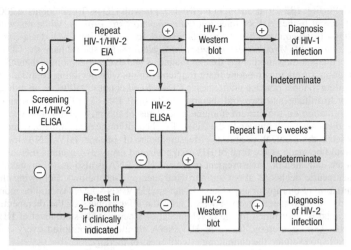

FIGURE 112-1 Algorithm for the use of serologic tests in the diagnosis of HIV-1 or HIV-2 infection. *Stable indeterminate Western blot 4–6 weeks later makes HIV infection unlikely. However, it should be repeated twice at 3-month intervals to rule out HIV infection. Alternatively, one may test for HIV-1 p24 antigen on HIV RNA.

DIAGNOSIS OF HIV INFECTION

Laboratory diagnosis of HIV infection depends on the demonstration of anti-HIV antibodies and/or the detection of HIV or one of its components.

The standard screening test for HIV infection is the detection of anti-HIV antibodies using an enzyme immunoassay (EIA). This test is highly sensitive (>99.5%) and is quite specific. Most commercial EIA kits are able to detect antibodies to both HIV-1 and -2. Western blot is the most commonly used confirmatory test and detects antibodies to HIV antigens of specific molecular weights. Antibodies to HIV begin to appear within 2 weeks of infection, and the period of time between initial infection and the development of detectable antibodies is rarely >3 months. The HIV p24 antigen can be measured using an EIA-type capture assay. Plasma p24 antigen levels rise during the first few weeks following infection, prior to the appearance of anti-HIV antibodies. A guideline for the use of these serologic tests in the diagnosis of HIV infection is depicted in Fig. 112-1.

HIV can be cultured directly from tissue, peripheral blood cells, or plasma, but this is most commonly done in a research setting. HIV genetic material can be detected using reverse transcriptase PCR (RT-PCR), branched DNA (bDNA), or nucleic acid sequence–based assay (NASBA). These tests are useful in pts with a positive or indeterminate EIA and an indeterminate Western blot, as may be seen early in infection, or in pts in whom serologic testing may be unreliable (such as those with hypogammaglobulinemia).

LABORATORY MONITORING OF PATIENTS WITH HIV INFECTION

Measurement of the CD4+ T cell count and level of plasma HIV RNA are important parts of the routine evaluation and monitoring of HIV-infected individuals. The CD4+ T cell count is a generally accepted indicator of the immunologic competence of the pt with HIV infection, and there is a close relationship between the CD4+ T cell count and the clinical manifestations of

AIDS (Fig. 182-29, p. 1168, in HPIM-17). Pts with CD4+ T cell counts < 200/ μL are at higher risk of infection with *Pneumocystis jiroveci*, while pts with CD4+ T cell counts < 50/μL are at higher risk for developing CMV disease and infection with *Mycobacterium avium intracellulare*. Pts should have the CD4+ T cell count measured at the time of diagnosis and every 3–6 months thereafter (measurements may be done more frequently in pts with declining counts). According to most practice guidelines, a CD4+ T cell count < 350/μL is an indication to initiate antiretroviral therapy. While the CD4+ T cell count provides information on the current immunologic status of the pt, the HIV RNA level predicts what will happen to the CD4+ T cell count in the near future and hence reflects the clinical prognosis. Measurements of plasma HIV RNA levels should be made at the time of HIV diagnosis and every 3–4 months thereafter in the untreated pt. Measurement of plasma HIV RNA is also useful in making therapeutic decisions about antiretroviral therapy (see below). Following the initiation of therapy or any change in therapy, HIV RNA levels should be monitored approximately every 4 weeks until the effectiveness of the therapeutic regimen is determined by the development of a new steady-state level of HIV RNA. During therapy, levels of HIV RNA should be monitored every 3–4 months to evaluate the continuing effectiveness of therapy.

The sensitivity of an individual's HIV virus(es) to different antiretroviral agents can be tested by either genotypic or phenotypic assays. In the hands of experts, the use of resistance testing to select a new antiretroviral regimen in patients failing their current regimen leads to a ~0.5-log greater decline in viral load compared to the efficacy of regimens selected solely on the basis of drug history. HIV resistance testing may also be of value in selecting an initial treatment regimen in geographic areas with a high prevalence of baseline resistance.

CLINICAL MANIFESTATIONS OF HIV INFECTION

A complete discussion is beyond the scope of this chapter. The major clinical features of the various stages of HIV infection are summarized below (see also Chap. 182, HPIM-17).

Acute HIV (Retroviral) Syndrome   Approximately 50–70% of infected individuals experience an acute syndrome following primary infection. The acute syndrome follows infection by 3–6 weeks. It can have multiple clinical features (Table 112-1), lasts 1–2 weeks, and resolves spontaneously as an immune response to HIV develops and the viral load diminishes from its peak levels. Most pts will then enter a phase of clinical latency, although an occasional pt will experience rapidly progressive immunologic and clinical deterioration.

TABLE 112-1   CLINICAL FINDINGS IN THE ACUTE HIV SYNDROME

General	Neurologic
Fever	Meningitis
Pharyngitis	Encephalitis
Lymphadenopathy	Peripheral neuropathy
Headache/retroorbital pain	Myelopathy
Arthralgias/myalgias	Dermatologic
Lethargy/malaise	Erythematous maculopapular rash
Anorexia/weight loss	Mucocutaneous ulceration
Nausea/vomiting/diarrhea	

Source: From B Tindall, DA Cooper: AIDS 5:1, 1991.

Asymptomatic Infection   The length of time between HIV infection and development of disease varies greatly, but the median is estimated to be 10 years in untreated individuals. HIV disease with active viral replication usually progresses during this asymptomatic period, and CD4+ T cell counts fall. The rate of disease progression is directly correlated with plasma HIV RNA levels. Pts with high levels of HIV RNA progress to symptomatic disease faster than do those with low levels of HIV RNA.

Symptomatic Disease   Symptoms of HIV disease can develop at any time during the course of HIV infection. In general, the spectrum of illness changes as the CD4+ T cell count declines. The more severe and life-threatening complications of HIV infection occur in patients with a CD4+ T cell count < 200/μl. Overall, the clinical spectrum of HIV disease is constantly changing as pts live longer and new and better approaches to treatment and prophylaxis of opportunistic infections are developed. In addition, a variety of neurologic, cardiovascular, and hepatic problems are increasingly seen in pts with HIV infection and may be a direct consequence of HIV infection. The key element to treating symptomatic complications of HIV disease, whether primary or secondary, is achieving good control of HIV replication through the use of combination antiretroviral therapy and instituting primary and secondary prophylaxis as indicated. Major clinical syndromes seen in the symptomatic stage of HIV infection are summarized below.

- *Persistent generalized lymphadenopathy*: Palpable adenopathy at two or more extrainguinal sites that persists for >3 months without explanation other than HIV infection. Many pts will go on to disease progression.
- *Constitutional symptoms*: Fever persisting for >1 month, involuntary weight loss of >10% of baseline, diarrhea for >1 month in absence of explainable cause.
- *Neurologic disease*: Most common is HIV encephalopathy (AIDS dementia complex); other neurologic complications include opportunistic infections, primary CNS lymphoma, CNS Kaposi's sarcoma, aseptic meningitis, myelopathy, peripheral neuropathy and myopathy.
- *Secondary infectious diseases*: P. jiroveci pneumonia is most common opportunistic infection, occurring in ~80% of untreated individuals during the course of their illness. Other common pathogens include CMV (chorioretinitis, colitis, pneumonitis, adrenalitis), *Candida albicans* (oral thrush, esophagitis), *M. avium intracellulare* (localized or disseminated infection), *M. tuberculosis, Cryptococcus neoformans* (meningitis, disseminated disease), *Toxoplasma gondii* (encephalitis, intracerebral mass lesion), herpes simplex virus (severe mucocutaneous lesions, esophagitis), diarrhea due to *Cryptosporidium* spp. or *Isospora belli*, bacterial pathogens (especially in pediatric cases).
- *Secondary neoplasms*: Kaposi's sarcoma (cutaneous and visceral, more fulminant course than in non-HIV-infected pts), lymphoid neoplasms (especially B cell lymphomas of brain, marrow, GI tract).
- *Other diseases*: A variety of organ-specific syndromes can be seen in HIV-infected pts, either as primary manifestations of the HIV infection or as complications of treatment.

Rx   **HIV Infection**   (See Chap. 182, HPIM-17)

General principles of pt management include counseling, psychosocial support, and screening for infections and other conditions and require comprehensive knowledge of the disease processes associated with HIV infection.

ANTIRETROVIRAL THERAPY (See Table 112-2)
The cornerstone of medical management of HIV infection is highly active combination antiretroviral therapy, or HAART. Suppression of HIV replication is an important component in prolonging life as well as in improving the quality of life of pts with HIV infection. However, several important questions related to the treatment of HIV disease lack definitive answers. Among them are questions of when antiretroviral therapy should be started, what is the best HAART regimen, when should a given regimen be changed, and what drugs in a regimen should be changed when a change is made. The drugs that are currently licensed for the treatment of HIV infection are listed in Table 112-2. These drugs fall into four main categories: those that inhibit the viral reverse transcriptase enzyme, those that inhibit the viral protease enzyme, those that inhibit viral entry, and those that inhibit the viral integrase. There are numerous drug-drug interactions that must be taken into consideration when using these medications. One of the main problems that has been encountered with the widespread use of HAART regimens has been a syndrome of hyperlipidemia and fat redistribution often referred to as *lipodystrophy syndrome* (Chap. 182, HPIM-17).

Nucleoside Analogues
These agents act by causing premature DNA-chain termination during the reverse transcription of viral RNA to proviral DNA and should be used in combination with other antiretroviral agents. The most common usage is together with another nucleoside analogue and a nonnucleoside reverse transcriptase inhibitor or a protease inhibitor (see below).

Nonnucleoside Reverse Transcriptase Inhibitors
These agents interfere with the function of HIV-1 reverse transcriptase by binding to regions outside the active site and causing conformational changes in the enzyme that render it inactive. These agents are very potent; however, when they are used as monotherapy, they induce rapid emergence of drug-resistant mutants. Four members of this class, *nevirapine, delavirdine, efavirenz,* and *etravirine* are currently available for clinical use. These drugs are licensed for use in combination with other antiretrovirals.

Protease Inhibitors
These drugs are potent and selective inhibitors of the HIV-1 protease enzyme and are active in the nanomolar range. Unfortunately, as in the case of the nonnucleoside reverse transcriptase inhibitors, this potency is accompanied by the rapid emergence of resistant isolates when these drugs are used as monotherapy. Thus, the protease inhibitors should be used only in combination with other antiretroviral drugs.

HIV Entry Inhibitors
These agents act by interfering with the binding of HIV to its receptor or co-receptor or by interfering with the process of fusion. A variety of small molecules that bind to HIV-1 co-receptors are currently in clinical trials. The first drugs in this class to be licensed are the fusion inhibitor *enfuvirtide* and the entry inhibitor *maraviroc.*

HIV Integrase Inhibitors
These drugs interfere with the integration of proviral DNA into the host cell genome. The first agent in this class, *raltegravir,* was approved in 2007 for use in treatment-experienced patients.

TABLE 112-2 ANTIRETROVIRAL DRUGS USED IN THE TREATMENT OF HIV INFECTION

Drug	Status	Indication	Dose in Combination	Supporting Data	Toxicity
Reverse Transcriptase Inhibitors					
Zidovudine (AZT, azidothymidine, Retrovir, 3'azido-3'-deoxythymidine)	Licensed	Treatment of HIV infection in combination with other antiretroviral agents Prevention of maternal-fetal HIV transmission	200 mg q8h or 300 mg bid	19 vs 1 death in original placebo-controlled trial in 281 patients with AIDS or ARC. Decreased progression to AIDS in patients with CD4+ T cell counts <500/μL, $n = 2051$. In pregnant women with CD4+ T cell count ≥200/μL, AZT PO beginning at weeks 14–34 of gestation plus IV drug during labor and delivery plus PO AZT to infant for 6 wk decreased transmission of HIV by 67.5% (from 25.5% to 8.3%), $n = 363$	Anemia, granulocytopenia, myopathy, lactic acidosis, hepatomegaly with steatosis, headache, nausea
Didanosine (Videx, Videx EC, ddI, dideoxyinosine, 2',3'-dideoxyinosine)	Licensed	For treatment of HIV infection in combination with other antiretroviral agents	Buffered: Requires 2 tablets to achieve adequate buffering of stomach acid; should be administered on an empty stomach ≥60 kg: 200 mg bid <60 kg: 125 mg bid Enteric coated: ≥60 kg: 400 mg qd < 60 kg: 250 mg qd	Clinically superior to AZT as monotherapy in 913 patients with prior AZT therapy. Clinically superior to AZT and comparable to AZT + ddI and AZT + ddC in 1067 AZT-naive patients with CD4+ T cell counts of 200–500/μL.	Pancreatitis, peripheral neuropathy, abnormalities on liver function tests, lactic acidosis, hepatomegaly with steatosis

(continued)

TABLE 112-2 ANTIRETROVIRAL DRUGS USED IN THE TREATMENT OF HIV INFECTION (CONTINUED)

Drug	Status	Indication	Dose in Combination	Supporting Data	Toxicity
Zalcitabine (ddC, HIVID, 2'3'-dideoxycytidine)	Licensed Discontinued in 2006	In combination with other antiretroviral agents for the treatment of HIV infection	0.75 mg tid	Clinically inferior to AZT monotherapy as initial treatment. Clinically as good as ddI in advanced patients intolerant to AZT. In combination with AZT, was clinically superior to AZT alone in patients with AIDS or CD4+ T cell count <350/μL.	Peripheral neuropathy, pancreatitis, lactic acidosis, hepatomegaly with steatosis, oral ulcers
Stavudine (d4T, Zerit, 2'3'-didehydro-3'-dideoxythymidine)	Licensed	Treatment of HIV-infected patients in combination with other antiretroviral agents	≥60 kg: 40 mg bid <60 kg: 30 mg bid	Superior to AZT with respect to changes in CD4+ T cell counts in 359 patients who had received ≥24 wk of AZT. Following 12 wk of randomization, the CD4+ T cell count had decreased by a mean of 22/μL in stavudine-treated patients, while in AZT-treated controls it had increased by a mean of 22/μL.	Peripheral neuropathy, pancreatitis, lactic acidosis, hepatomegaly with steatosis, ascending neuromuscular weakness, lipodystrophy
Lamivudine (Epivir, 2'3'-dideoxy-3'-thiacytidine, 3TC)	Licensed	In combination with other antiretroviral agents for the treatment of HIV infection	150 mg bid 300 mg qd	Superior to AZT alone with respect to changes in CD4 counts in 495 patients who were zidovudine-naive and 477 patients who were zidovudine-experienced. Overall CD4+ T cell counts for the zidovudine group were at baseline by 24 wk, while in the group treated with zidovudine plus lamivudine, they were 10–50 cells/μL above baseline. 54% decrease in progression to AIDS/death compared to AZT alone.	Hepatotoxicity

Drug	Status	Indication	Dose	Comments	Adverse effects
Emtricitabine (FTC, Emtriva)	Licensed	In combination with other antiretroviral agents for the treatment of HIV infection	200 mg qd	Comparable to d4T in combination with ddI and efavirenz in 571 treatment-naive patients. Similar to 3TC in combination with AZT or d4T + NNRTI or PI in 440 patients doing well for at least 12 weeks on a 3TC regimen.	Hepatotoxicity
Abacavir (Ziagen)	Licensed	For treatment of HIV infection in combination with other antiretroviral agents	300 mg bid	Abacavir + AZT + 3TC equivalent to indinavir + AZT + 3TC with regard to viral load suppression (~60% in each group with <400 HIV RNA copies/mL plasma) and CD4 cell increase (~100/μL in each group) at 24 weeks	Hypersensitivity reaction (can be fatal); fever, rash, nausea, vomiting, malaise or fatigue, and loss of appetite
Tenofovir (Viread)	Licensed	For use in combination with other antiretroviral agents when treatment is indicated	300 mg qd	Reduction of ~0.6 log in HIV-1 RNA levels when added to background regimen in treatment-experienced patients	Potential for renal toxicity
Delavirdine (Rescriptor)	Licensed	For use in combination with appropriate antiretrovirals when treatment is warranted	400 mg tid	Delavirdine + AZT superior to AZT alone with regard to viral load suppression at 52 weeks	Skin rash, abnormalities in liver function tests
Nevirapine (Viramune)	Licensed	In combination with other antiretroviral agents for treatment of progressive HIV infection	200 mg/d × 14 days then 200 mg bid	Increases in CD4+ T cell count, decrease in HIV RNA when used in combination with nucleosides	Skin rash, hepatotoxicity

(continued)

TABLE 112-2 ANTIRETROVIRAL DRUGS USED IN THE TREATMENT OF HIV INFECTION (CONTINUED)

Drug	Status	Indication	Dose in Combination	Supporting Data	Toxicity
Efavirenz (Sustiva)	Licensed	For treatment of HIV infection in combination with other antiretroviral agents	600 mg qhs	Efavirenz + AZT + 3TC comparable to indinavir + AZT + 3TC with regard to viral load suppression (a higher percentage of the efavirenz group achieved viral load <50 copies/mL; however, the discontinuation rate in the indinavir group was unexpectedly high, accounting for most treatment "failures"); CD4 cell increase (~140/μL in each group) at 24 weeks.	Rash, dysphoria, elevated liver function tests, drowsiness, abnormal dreams, depression
Etravirine	Licensed	In combination with other antiretroviral agents in treatment-experienced adult pts who have evidence of viral replication and HIV-1 strains resistant to an NNRTI inhibitor and other antiretroviral agents	200 mg bid (or twice daily)	At 24 weeks in treatment-experienced pts with 1 or more NNRTI mutation and 3 or more PI mutations at screening, 74% of pts randomized to etravirine + background had HIV levels <400 copies/mL compared to 51.5% of pts randomized to background regimen + placebo. All subjects received darunavir/ritonavir as part of their background regimen. CD4+ T cell counts increased by 81 cells/mL in the etravirine arm and 64 cells/mL in the placebo arm.	Skin rash

Protease Inhibitors

Saquinavir mesylate (Invirase—hard gel capsule)	Licensed	In combination with other antiretroviral agents when therapy is warranted	1000 mg + 100 mg ritonavir bid	Increases in CD4+ T cell counts, reduction in HIV RNA most pronounced in combination therapy with ddC. 50% reduction in first AIDS-defining event or death in combination with ddC compared to either agent alone.	Diarrhea, nausea, headaches, hyperglycemia, fat redistribution, lipid abnormalities
(Fortovase—soft gel capsule)	Licensed Discontinued 2006	For use in combination with other antiretroviral agents when treatment is warranted	1200 mg tid	Reduction in the mortality rate and AIDS-defining events for patients who received hard-gel formulation in combination with ddC	Diarrhea, nausea, abdominal pain, headaches, hyperglycemia, fat redistribution, lipid abnormalities
Ritonavir (Norvir)	Licensed	In combination with other antiretroviral agents for treatment of HIV infection when treatment is warranted	600 mg bid	Reduction in the cumulative incidence of clinical progression or death from 34 to 17% in patients with CD4+ T cell count <100/µL treated for a median of 6 months	Nausea, abdominal pain, hyperglycemia, fat redistribution, lipid abnormalities, may alter levels of many other drugs, including saquinavir

(continued)

TABLE 112-2 ANTIRETROVIRAL DRUGS USED IN THE TREATMENT OF HIV INFECTION (CONTINUED)

Drug	Status	Indication	Dose in Combination	Supporting Data	Toxicity
Indinavir sulfate (Crixivan)	Licensed	For treatment of HIV infection in combination with other antiretroviral agents when antiretroviral treatment is warranted	800 mg q8h or 800 mg + 100 mg ritonavir bid or 1000 mg q8h when used with efavirenz or nevirapine	Increase in CD4+ T cell count by 100/μL and 2-log decrease in HIV RNA levels when given in combination with zidovudine and lamivudine. Decrease of 50% in risk of progression to AIDS or death when given with zidovudine and lamivudine compared with zidovudine and lamivudine alone.	Nephrolithiasis, indirect hyperbilirubinemia, hyperglycemia, fat redistribution, lipid abnormalities
Nelfinavir mesylate (Viracept)	Licensed	For treatment of HIV infection in combination with other antiretroviral agents when antiretroviral therapy is warranted	750 mg tid or 1250 mg bid	2.0-log decline in HIV RNA when given in combination with stavudine	Diarrhea, loose stools, hyperglycemia, fat redistribution, lipid abnormalities. May contain traces of the potential carcinogen/teratogen ethyl methane sulfonate

Drug	Status	Indication	Dosage	Comments	Adverse effects
Amprenavir (Agenerase)	Licensed	In combination with other antiretroviral agents for treatment of HIV infection	1200 mg bid or 600 mg + 100 mg ritonavir bid or 1200 mg + 200 mg ritonavir qd	In treatment-naïve patients, amprenavir + AZT + 3TC superior to AZT + 3TC with regard to viral load suppression (53% vs 11% with <400 HIV RNA copies/mL plasma at 24 weeks). CD4+ T cell responses similar between treatment groups. In treatment-experienced patients, amprenavir + NRTIs similar to indinavir + NRTIs with regard to viral load suppression (43% vs 53% with <400 HIV RNA copies/mL plasma at 24 weeks). CD4+ T cell responses superior in the indinavir + NRTIs group.	Nausea, vomiting, diarrhea, rash, oral paresthesias, elevated liver function tests, hyperglycemia, fat redistribution, lipid abnormalities
Fosamprenavir (Lexiva)	Licensed		1400 mg bid or 700 mg + 100 mg ritonavir bid		
Lopinavir/ritonavir (Kaletra)	Licensed	For treatment of HIV infection in combination with other antiretroviral agents	400 mg/100 mg bid	In treatment-naïve patients, lopinavir/ritonavir + d4T + 3TC superior to nelfinavir + d4T + 3TC with regard to viral load suppression (79% vs 64% with <400 HIV RNA copies/µL at 40 weeks). CD4+ T cell increases similar in both groups.	Diarrhea, hyperglycemia, fat redistribution, lipid abnormalities
Atazanavir (Reyataz)	Licensed	For treatment of HIV infection in combination with other antiretroviral agents	400 mg qd or 300 mg qd + ritonavir 100 mg qd when given with efavirenz	Comparable to efavirenz when given in combination with AZT + 3TC in a study of 810 treatment-naïve patients. Comparable to nelfinavir when given in combination with d4T + 3TC in a study of 467 treatment-naïve patients.	Hyperbilirubinemia, PR prolongation, nausea, vomiting, hyperglycemia, fat maldistribution

(continued)

TABLE 112-2 ANTIRETROVIRAL DRUGS USED IN THE TREATMENT OF HIV INFECTION (CONTINUED)

Drug	Status	Indication	Dose in Combination	Supporting Data	Toxicity
Tipranavir (Aptivus)	Licensed	In combination with 200 mg ritonavir for combination therapy in treatment-experienced adults	500 mg + 200 mg ritonavir twice daily	At 24 weeks, patients with prior extensive exposure to ARVs showed a –0.8 log change in HIV RNA levels and a 34 cell increase in CD4+ T cells compound to –0.25 log and 4 cells in the control arm. Inferior to lopinavir/ritonavir in a randomized, controlled trial in naive patients.	Diarrhea, nausea, fatigue, headache, skin rash, hepatotoxicity, intracranial hemorrhage
Darunavir (Prezista)	Licensed	In combination with 100 mg ritonavir for combination therapy in treatment-experienced adults	600 mg + 100 mg ritonavir twice daily with food	At 24 weeks, patients with prior extensive exposure to antiretrovirals treated with a new combination including darunavir showed a –1.89 log change in HIV RNA levels and a 92 cell increase in CD4+ T cells compared to –0.48 log and 17 cells in the control arm.	Diarrhea, nausea, headache
Entry Inhibitors					
Enfuvirtide (Fuzeon)	Licensed	In combination with other agents in treatment-experienced patients with evidence of HIV-1 replication despite ongoing antiretroviral therapy	90 mg SC bid	In treatment of experienced patients, superior to placebo when added to new optimized background (37% vs 16% with <400 HIV RNA copies/mL at 24 weeks; +71 vs +35 CD4+ T cells at 24 weeks)	Local injection reactions, hypersensitivity reactions, increased rate of bacterial pneumonia

Maraviroc (Selzentry)	Licensed	In combination with other antiretroviral agents in treatment experienced adults infected with only CCR5-tropic HIV-1 that is resistant to multiple antiretroviral agents	150–600 mg bid depending upon concomitant medications (see text)	At 24 weeks, among 635 patients with CCR5-tropic virus and HIV-1 RNA >5000 copies/mL despite at least 6 months of prior therapy with at least one agent from 3 of the 4 antiretroviral drug classes, 61% of patients randomized to maraviroc achieved HIV RNA levels <400 copies/mL compared to 28% of patients randomized to placebo	Hepatotoxicity, nasopharyngitis, fever, cough, rash, abdominal pain, dizziness, fever, musculoskeletal symptoms
Integrase Inhibitor					
Raltegravir (Isentress)	Licensed	In combination with other antiretroviral agents in treatment experienced patients with evidence of ongoing HIV-1 replication	400 mg bid	At 24 weeks, among 436 patients with three-class drug resistance, 76% of patients randomized to receive raltegravir achieved HIV RNA levels <400 copies/mL compared to 41% of patients randomized to receive placebo	Nausea, rash

Note: ARC, AIDS-related complex; NRTIs, nonnucleoside reverse transcriptase inhibitors.

615

CHOICE OF ANTIRETROVIRAL TREATMENT STRATEGY

The large number of available antiretroviral agents coupled with relatively few clinical end-point studies make the subject of antiretroviral therapy one of the more controversial in the management of HIV-infected pts.

The principles of therapy for HIV infection have been articulated by a panel sponsored by the U.S. Department of Health and Human Services (Table 112-3). Treatment decisions must take into account the fact that one is dealing with a chronic infection and that complete eradication of HIV infection is probably not possible with currently available HAART regimens. Thus, immediate treatment of HIV infection upon diagnosis may not be prudent, and therapeutic decisions must take into account the balance between risks and benefits. At present a reasonable course of action is to initiate antiretroviral therapy in anyone with the acute HIV syndrome; pts with symptomatic disease; pts with evidence of renal disease; pts with asymptomatic infection and CD4+ counts < 350/μL; and pts with hepatitis B infection when hepatitis B treatment is indicated, to avoid development of resistant strains of HIV. In addition, one may wish to administer a 4-week course of therapy to uninfected individuals immediately following a high-risk exposure to HIV (see below).

When the decision to initiate therapy is made, the physician must decide which drugs to use in the initial regimen. The two options for initial therapy most commonly in use today are: two nucleoside analogues (one of which is usually lamivudine or emtricitabine) combined with a protease inhibitor; or

---

TABLE 112-3 PRINCIPLES OF THERAPY OF HIV INFECTION

1. Ongoing HIV replication leads to immune system damage and progression to AIDS.
2. Plasma HIV RNA levels indicate the magnitude of HIV replication and the rate of CD4+ T cell destruction. CD4+ T cell counts indicate the current level of competence of the immune system.
3. Rates of disease progression differ among individuals, and treatment decisions should be individualized based upon plasma HIV RNA levels and CD4+ T cell counts.
4. Maximal suppression of viral replication is a goal of therapy; the greater the suppression the less likely the appearance of drug-resistant quasispecies.
5. The most effective therapeutic strategies involve the simultaneous initiation of combinations of effective anti-HIV drugs with which the patient has not been previously treated and that are not cross-resistant with antiretroviral agents that the patient has already received.
6. The antiretroviral drugs used in combination regimens should be used according to optimum schedules and dosages.
7. The number of available drugs is limited. Any decisions on antiretroviral therapy have a long-term impact on future options for the patient.
8. Women should receive optimal antiretroviral therapy regardless of pregnancy status.
9. The same principles apply to children and adults. The treatment of HIV-infected children involves unique pharmacologic, virologic, and immunologic considerations.
10. Compliance is an important part of ensuring maximal effect from a given regimen. The simpler the regimen, the easier it is for the patient to be compliant.

Source: Modified from *Principles of Therapy of HIV Infection*, USPHS, and the Henry J. Kaiser Family Foundation.

TABLE 112-4	INDICATIONS FOR CHANGING ANTIRETROVIRAL THERAPY IN PATIENTS WITH HIV INFECTION[a]

Less than a 1-log drop in plasma HIV RNA by 4 weeks following the initiation of therapy

A reproducible significant increase (defined as 3-fold or greater) from the nadir of plasma HIV RNA level not attributable to intercurrent infection, vaccination, or test methodology

Persistently declining CD4+ T cell numbers

Clinical deterioration

Side effects

---

[a]Generally speaking, a change should involve the initiation of at least 2 drugs felt to be effective in the given patient. The exception to this is when change is being made to manage toxicity, in which case a single substitution is reasonable.
Source: *Guidelines for the Use of Antiretroviral Agents in HIV-Infected Adults and Adolescents.* USPHS.

two nucleoside analogues and a nonnucleoside reverse transcriptase inhibitor. There are no clear data at present on which to base distinctions between these two approaches. Following the initiation of therapy, one should expect a 1-log (tenfold) reduction in plasma HIV RNA within 1–2 months; eventually a decline in plasma HIV RNA to <50 copies/mL; and a rise in CD4+ T cell count of 100–150/μL. Failure to achieve and maintain an HIV RNA level <50 copies/mL is an indication to consider a change in therapy. Other reasons for changing therapy are listed in Table 112-4. When changing therapy because of treatment failure, it is important to attempt to provide a regimen with at least two new drugs. In the pt in whom a change is made for reasons of drug toxicity, a simple replacement of one drug is reasonable.

Treatment of Secondary Infections and Neoplasms
Specific for each infection and neoplasm (see Chap. 182, in HPIM-17).

Prophylaxis Against Secondary Infections   (Table 182-8, pp. 1170, 1171, in HPIM-17)
Primary prophylaxis is clearly indicated for *P. jiroveci* pneumonia (especially when CD4+ T cell counts fall to <200 cells/μL), for *M. avium* complex infections in pts with CD4+ T cell counts <50 cells/μL, and for *M. tuberculosis* infections in pts with a positive PPD or anergy if at high risk of TB. Vaccination with the influenza and pneumococcal polysaccharide vaccines is generally recommended for all pts with CD4+ T cell counts >200/μL (see Table 182-8, pp. 1170, 1171, in HPIM-17). Secondary prophylaxis, when available, is indicated for virtually every infection experienced by HIV-infected pts.

HIV AND THE HEALTH CARE WORKER

There is a small but definite risk to health care workers of acquiring HIV infection via needle stick exposures, large mucosal surface exposures, or exposure of open wounds to HIV-infected secretions or blood products. The risk of HIV transmission after a skin puncture by an object contaminated with blood from a person with documented HIV infection is ~0.3%, compared to 20–30% risk for hepatitis B infection from a similar incident. Postexposure prophylaxis appears to be effective in decreasing the likelihood of acquisition of infection through accidental exposure in the health care setting. In this regard, a U.S. Public Health Service working group has recommended that chemoprophylaxis be given as soon as possible after occupational exposure. While the precise regimen remains a subject of debate, the U.S. Public Health Service guidelines recommend (1) a combination of two nucleoside analogue reverse transcriptase inhibitors given for 4 weeks for routine exposures, or (2) a combination of two nucleoside analogue reverse transcriptase inhibitors plus a third drug given for 4 weeks for high-risk or otherwise complicated exposures. Most clinicians administer the latter regimen in all cases in which a decision to treat is made. Regardless of which regimen is used, treatment should be initiated as soon as possible after exposure.

Prevention of exposure is the best strategy and includes following universal precautions and proper handling of needles and other potentially contaminated objects.

Transmission of TB is another potential risk for all health care workers, including those dealing with HIV-infected pts. All workers should know their PPD status, which should be checked yearly.

VACCINES

Development of a safe and effective HIV vaccine is the object of active investigation at present. The first series of clinical trials of candidate vaccines in humans have not proven the candidates to be effective in preventing acquisition of infection or in lowering the viral set point after acquisition of infection.

PREVENTION

Education, counseling, and behavior modification remain the cornerstones of HIV prevention efforts. While abstinence is an absolute way to prevent sexual transmission, other strategies include "safe sex" practices such as use of condoms. Avoidance of shared needle use by IDUs is critical. If possible, breastfeeding should be avoided by HIV-positive women, as the virus can be transmitted to infants via this route. In societies where withholding of breastfeeding is not feasible, treatment of the mother, if possible, greatly decreases the chances of transmission.

For a more detailed discussion, see Fauci AS, Lane HC: Human Immunodeficiency Virus (HIV) Disease: AIDS and Related Disorders, Chap. 182, p. 1137, in HPIM-17.

113 Fungal Infections

GENERAL CONSIDERATIONS

Yeasts (e.g., *Candida*, *Cryptococcus*) appear microscopically as round, budding forms; *molds* (e.g., *Aspergillus*, *Rhizopus*) appear as filamentous forms called hyphae; and *dimorphic fungi* (e.g., *Histoplasma*) are spherical in tissue but appear as molds in culture. *Endemic* fungi pathogenic for humans are saprophytic in nature and infect hosts preferentially by inhalation. *Opportunistic* fungi invade the host from normal sites of colonization (e.g., mucous membranes or the GI tract). Definitive diagnosis of any fungal infection requires histopathologic identification of the fungus invading tissue and evidence of an accompanying inflammatory response.

ANTIFUNGAL AGENTS

Amphotericin B (AmB)
- The broadest-spectrum antifungal agent
- Significant toxicities include nephrotoxicity and fever, chills, and nausea during treatment.
- Lipid formulations are used to circumvent nephrotoxicity and infusion reactions; whether there is truly a clinically significant difference remains controversial. Lipid formulations are expensive.

Imidazoles and Triazoles Azoles cause little or no nephrotoxicity. Unlike AmB, which is considered fungicidal, azoles are fungistatic.

Fluconazole
- Useful for coccidioidal and cryptococcal meningitis and for candidal infections, including candidemia
- Not effective against aspergillosis or mucormycosis
- Effective as fungal prophylaxis in bone marrow and high-risk liver transplant recipients
- Has oral and IV formulations and a long half-life
- Penetrates into most body fluids, including ocular fluids and cerebrospinal fluid (CSF)
- Toxicity is minimal but includes hepatotoxicity (at high doses), alopecia, muscle weakness, dry mouth, and metallic taste.

Voriconazole
- Available in oral and IV preparations
- First-line agent against *Aspergillus*
- Active against *Scedosporium* and *Fusarium*
- Has broader spectrum than fluconazole against *Candida* species
- Multiple drug interactions
- Common side effects include hepatotoxicity, skin rashes (including photosensitivity), and visual disturbances.
- Metabolized completely by the liver; dose adjustments required in pts with hepatic dysfunction
- Because of renal excretion of cyclodextrin after receipt of the IV formulation, oral treatment is indicated for pts with severe renal insufficiency.

Itraconazole
- Useful for blastomycosis, histoplasmosis, cutaneous candidiasis, coccidioidomycosis, sporotrichosis, onychomycosis, tinea versicolor, tinea capitis, and indolent aspergillosis
- Absorption is variable after administration in capsule form; blood levels should be monitored during treatment for disseminated mycosis.
- Minimal CSF penetration
- Cyclodextrin is used in both the oral solution and the IV formulation.

Posaconazole
- Approved for prophylaxis of aspergillosis and candidiasis in high-risk immunocompromised pts

- Effective against fluconazole-resistant *Candida* isolates
- May be useful as salvage therapy for aspergillosis

Echinocandins

- Caspofungin, anidulafungin, and micafungin are approved echinocandin agents that are available for IV administration only.
- Among the safest antifungal agents
- Broad-spectrum fungicidal activity against *Candida* species; also efficacious as salvage therapy for aspergillosis
- Cyclosporine increases caspofungin levels, but no dose adjustment is needed with anidulafungin or micafungin.

Flucytosine Used in combination with AmB (e.g., for cryptococcal meningitis); has excellent CSF penetration. Adverse effects include bone marrow suppression.

Griseofulvin and Terbinafine Griseofulvin is used primarily for ringworm infection. Terbinafine is used for onychomycosis and ringworm and is as effective as itraconazole.

Topical Agents Many drug classes are used for topical treatment of common fungal skin infections: azoles (e.g., clotrimazole, miconazole), polyene agents (e.g., nystatin), and other classes (e.g., ciclopirox olamine, terbinafine).

CANDIDIASIS

Etiology *Candida* is a small, thin-walled ovoid yeast that reproduces by budding and occurs in three forms in tissue: blastospores, pseudohyphae, and hyphae. *Candida* is ubiquitous in nature and inhabits the GI tract, the female genital tract, and the skin. *C. albicans* is common, but non-*albicans* species (e.g., *C. glabrata*, *C. krusei*, *C. parapsilosis*, *C. tropicalis*) now cause ~50% of all cases of candidemia and disseminated candidiasis.

Pathogenesis

- *Candida* probably enters the bloodstream from mucosal surfaces after multiplying to large numbers as a result of bacterial suppression by antibacterial drugs.
- Other risk factors for hematogenous dissemination include indwelling intravascular or urinary catheters and hyperalimentation fluids.
- Neonates of low birth weight, neutropenic pts, pts taking high-dose glucocorticoids, and pts with other impairments of host defenses are also susceptible to hematogenous seeding.

Clinical Features

1. *Oral thrush*: white, adherent, painless, discrete or confluent patches in the mouth, tongue, or esophagus. *Vulvovaginal thrush*: pruritus, pain, vaginal discharge
2. *Cutaneous candidiasis*: includes paronychia, balanitis, and intertrigo, manifesting as redness, pain, pustules
3. *Chronic mucocutaneous candidiasis*: infection of hair, nails, skin, and mucous membranes that persists despite therapy and is associated with a specific immunologic dysfunction
4. *Esophageal candidiasis*: substernal pain or sense of blockage on swallowing
5. *Urinary tract candidiasis*: Candidal colonization secondary to indwelling catheters is common; if the urinary tract is obstructed, *Candida* causes cystitis and upper tract disease.

6. *Candidemia*: often originating from the GI tract or from skin via an intra-vascular catheter

   a. The brain, chorioretina, heart, and kidneys are most commonly infected. Except in neutropenic pts, the liver and spleen are less often infected. Ocular involvement may require partial vitrectomy to prevent permanent blindness.

   b. Skin involvement manifests as macronodular lesions.

   c. Chorioretinal or skin involvement predicts a high probability of abscess formation in deep organs from generalized hematogenous seeding. Nearly any organ can become infected.

Diagnosis

- Demonstration of pseudohyphae on wet mount with culture confirmation
- Recovery of *Candida* from sputum, urine, or peritoneal catheters may reflect colonization rather than deep infection. The most challenging aspect of diagnosis is determining which pts have hematogenously disseminated disease.

℞ Candidiasis

- *Cutaneous*: topical azoles or nystatin
- *Vulvovaginal*: vaginal azole suppositories or fluconazole (150 mg PO once)
- *Thrush*: clotrimazole troches or nystatin
- *Esophageal*: fluconazole (100–200 mg/d) or itraconazole (200 mg/d). Caspofungin, micafungin, and AmB are alternatives.
- *Deeply invasive candidiasis*
  1. Foreign materials (e.g., catheters) should be removed or replaced, when possible.
  2. AmB (including lipid formulations), echinocandins, and fluconazole or voriconazole are used; no agent is clearly superior to the others.
  3. Nonneutropenic, hemodynamically stable pts: Unless azole resistance is considered likely, fluconazole is the agent of choice.
  4. Neutropenic or hemodynamically unstable pts: Initial treatment should consist of broader-spectrum agents such as AmB or echinocandins. Once the pt's condition has stabilized and the infecting strain has been isolated and identified, treatment can be adjusted.
  5. *Candida* endocarditis should be treated with valve removal and long-term antifungal administration.
  6. *Candida* endophthalmitis requires ophthalmologic consultation.

Prevention

- Allogeneic stem-cell and high-risk liver transplant recipients typically receive prophylaxis with fluconazole (400 mg/d).
- Prophylaxis in acute leukemic and other neutropenic pts is controversial. Prophylaxis may be useful in high-risk postoperative pts but should not be given routinely to pts in general surgical or medical intensive care units.
- HIV-infected pts generally should not receive chronic prophylaxis against mucocutaneous disease unless they have frequent recurrences.

ASPERGILLOSIS

Etiology *Aspergillus* is a mold with septate branching hyphae. It has a worldwide distribution and typically grows in decomposing plant materials. *A. fumigatus* is the most common cause of invasive aspergillosis.

Pathogenesis

- Inhalation is common; only intense exposures cause disease in healthy, immunocompetent individuals.
- The primary risk factors for invasive aspergillosis are profound neutropenia and glucocorticoid use. Risk increases with longer duration of these conditions. Pts with chronic pulmonary aspergillosis have a wide spectrum of underlying pulmonary diseases (e.g., tuberculosis, sarcoidosis).

Clinical Features

1. *Invasive pulmonary aspergillosis*: The frequency of invasive disease and the pace of progression increase with greater degrees of immunocompromise. Acute and subacute forms have courses of ≤1 month and 1–3 months, respectively. Of invasive aspergillosis cases, >80% involve the lungs. Pts can be asymptomatic or can present with fever, cough, chest discomfort, hemoptysis, and shortness of breath. Early diagnosis requires a high index of suspicion, screening for circulating antigen, and urgent CT of the chest.
2. *Invasive sinusitis*: The sinuses are involved in 5–10% of cases of invasive aspergillosis, especially in leukemic pts and hematopoietic stem-cell transplant recipients. Pts have fever, nasal or facial discomfort, and nasal discharge. CT or MRI of the sinuses is essential.
3. *Disseminated aspergillosis*: occurs in the most immunocompromised pts. *Aspergillus* disseminates from lung to brain, skin, thyroid, bone, and other organs. Pts develop skin lesions and deteriorate clinically over 1–3 days, developing fever and signs of mild sepsis with multiple abnormalities in laboratory tests. Blood cultures are usually negative.
4. *Cerebral aspergillosis*: Single or multiple lesions, hemorrhagic infarction, and cerebral abscess are common. The presentation can be acute or subacute, with mood changes, focal signs, seizures, and a decline in mental status. MRI is the most useful investigation.
5. *Chronic pulmonary aspergillosis* is characterized by one or more cavities expanding over months to years, with pulmonary symptoms, fatigue, and weight loss. Pericavitary infiltrates and multiple cavities are typical. Without treatment, pulmonary fibrosis can develop.
6. *Aspergilloma*: fungal ball in residual chest cavities. Life-threatening hemoptysis may occur.
7. *Chronic sinusitis*: three presentations
   a. Fungal ball without invasion in a diseased, chronically infected sinus
   b. Chronic invasive, slowly progressive disease
   c. Chronic granulomatous inflammation
8. *Allergic bronchopulmonary aspergillosis* (ABPA)
   a. Seen in asthmatics and cystic fibrosis pts
   b. Intermittent wheezing, infiltrates due to bronchial plugging, eosinophilia, sputum

Diagnosis

- Histologic examination of affected tissue reveals either infarction, with invasion of blood vessels by fungal hyphae, or acute necrosis.
- Culture is important in confirming the diagnosis but may be falsely positive (e.g., in pts with airway colonization) or falsely negative.
- Galactomannan antigen testing of serum from high-risk pts is best done prospectively, as positive results precede clinical disease; false-positive results can occur.

- Definitive diagnosis requires a positive culture of an ordinarily sterile site or positive results of histologic testing and culture of a sample taken from the affected organ.
- Data suggestive of the diagnosis include a halo sign on high-resolution thoracic CT scan (a localized ground-glass appearance representing hemorrhagic infarction surrounding a nodule).
- IgE antibody to *Aspergillus* antigens is seen in ABPA.

℞ Aspergillosis

- See Table 113-1 for recommended treatments and doses.
- Invasive aspergillosis: Duration of treatment varies from ~3 months to years, depending on the host and the response.
- Chronic and allergic forms of aspergillosis: Voriconazole or posaconazole can be substituted for itraconazole in instances of treatment failure, adverse events, or emergence of resistance. Itraconazole blood levels should be monitored. Chronic cavitary pulmonary aspergillosis probably requires treatment for life.
- Surgical treatment is important for some forms of aspergillosis (e.g., maxillary sinus fungal ball; single aspergilloma; invasive disease of bone, heart valve, brain, or sinuses).

Outcome   Invasive aspergillosis is curable if immune reconstitution occurs. Poor outcomes are seen in pts with cerebral aspergillosis, endocarditis, bilateral extensive invasive pulmonary disease, late-stage AIDS, relapsed uncontrolled leukemia, or allogeneic hematopoietic stem cell transplants. The overall mortality rate is ~50% with treatment, but the disease is uniformly fatal without therapy.

CRYPTOCOCCOSIS

Etiology   *Cryptococcus* is a yeast-like fungus. *C. neoformans* and *C. gattii* are pathogenic for humans and can cause cryptococcosis.

Epidemiology   *C. neoformans* is found in soil contaminated with pigeon droppings, whereas *C. gattii* is associated with eucalyptus trees. *C. neoformans* infection is strongly associated with advanced HIV disease, treatment with glucocorticoids or immunosuppressive drugs, transplantation, and hematologic malignancy. *C. gattii* infection is not associated with specific immune deficits.

Pathogenesis   Most cases are acquired via inhalation, with consequent pulmonary infection. Spread to the brain can occur. *C. neoformans* has a polysaccharide capsule that is antiphagocytic and interferes with local immune responses.

Clinical Features

1. *Meningoencephalitis*: most common presentation
   a. Early: headache, fever, lethargy, cranial nerve paresis, visual deficits, meningismus
   b. Symptoms can be of several weeks' duration.
2. *Pulmonary manifestations*
   a. Usually asymptomatic but can present as cough, increased sputum production, and chest pain
   b. Often runs an indolent course; often is associated with prior disease (e.g., malignancy, diabetes, tuberculosis)
   c. Cryptococcomas: usually seen in immunocompetent pts; associated with *C. gattii* infections

TABLE 113-1 TREATMENT OF ASPERGILLOSIS

Indication	Primary Treatment	Evidence Level[a]	Secondary Treatment	Precautions	Comments
Invasive[a]	Voriconazole	AI	Amphotericin B, caspofungin, posaconazole, micafungin	Drug interactions (especially with rifampin), renal failure (IV only)	As primary therapy, voriconazole carries 20% more responses than amphotericin B. If azole prophylaxis fails, it is unclear whether a class change is required for therapy.
Prophylaxis	Itraconazole solution, posaconazole	AI	Micafungin, aerosolized amphotericin B	Diarrhea and vomiting with itraconazole, vincristine interaction	Some centers monitor plasma levels of itraconazole.
ABPA	Itraconazole	AI	Voriconazole	Some glucocorticoid interactions, including with inhaled formulations	Long-term therapy is helpful in most patients. Others can discontinue treatment. No evidence indicates whether or not therapy modifies progression to bronchiectasis/fibrosis.
Single aspergilloma	Surgery	BII	Itraconazole, voriconazole, intracavity amphotericin B	Multicavity disease: poor outcome of surgery; medical therapy preferable	Single large cavities with an aspergilloma are best resected.

| Chronic pulmonary[b] | Itraconazole | BII | Poor absorption of capsules with proton pump inhibitors or H_2 blockers | Voriconazole, IV amphotericin B | Resistance may emerge during treatment, especially if plasma drug levels are subtherapeutic. |

Note: The oral dose is usually 200 mg bid for voriconazole and itraconazole and 400 mg bid for posaconazole. The IV dose of voriconazole is 6 mg/kg twice at 12-h intervals (loading doses) followed by 4 mg/kg q12h. Plasma monitoring is helpful in optimizing the dosage. Caspofungin is given as a single loading dose of 70 mg, followed by 50 mg/d; some authorities use 70 mg/d for patients weighing >80 kg, and lower doses are required with hepatic dysfunction. Micafungin is given as 50 mg/d for prophylaxis and as at least 150 mg/d for treatment; this drug is not yet approved by the U.S. Food and Drug Administration (FDA) for this indication. Amphotericin B deoxycholate is given at a daily dose of 1 mg/kg if tolerated. Several strategies are available for minimizing renal dysfunction. Lipid-associated amphotericin B is given at 3 mg/kg (AmBisome) or 5 mg/kg (Abelcet). Different regimens are available for aerosolized amphotericin B, but none is FDA approved. Other considerations that may alter dose selection or route include age; concomitant medications; renal, hepatic, or intestinal dysfunction; and drug tolerability.

[a]Evidence levels are those used in treatment guidelines (Stevens DA et al: Practice guidelines for diseases caused by *Aspergillus*. Clin Infect Dis 30:696, 2000).

[b]An infectious disease consultation is appropriate for these patients.

3. *Skin lesions*
   a. Associated with disseminated cryptococcosis
   b. Lesions can be papules, plaques, purpura, vesicles, tumor-like lesions, or rashes.

Diagnosis

- Diagnosis requires the demonstration of *C. neoformans* in normally sterile tissue. Positive cultures of CSF and blood are diagnostic.
- India ink smear of CSF is a useful rapid diagnostic technique. Pts have high protein levels in CSF, with mononuclear cell pleocytosis.
- Cryptococcal antigen testing of CSF, serum

℞ Cryptococcosis

1. Pulmonary cryptococcosis in an immunocompetent pt: fluconazole (200–400 mg/d for 3–6 months)
2. Extrapulmonary cryptococcosis may initially require AmB (0.5–1.0 mg/kg daily for 4–6 weeks).
3. Central nervous system (CNS) cryptococcal disease in HIV-seronegative pts: induction phase with AmB (0.5–1.0 mg/kg daily) followed by prolonged consolidation therapy with fluconazole (400 mg/d)
4. Meningoencephalitis in immunocompetent pts: AmB (0.5–1.0 mg/kg) plus flucytosine (100 mg/kg) daily for 6–10 weeks or the same drugs at the same dosages for 2 weeks followed by fluconazole (400 mg/d) for 10 weeks
5. HIV-infected pts with CNS involvement: AmB (0.7–1.0 mg/kg daily) plus flucytosine for at least 2 weeks followed by fluconazole (400 mg/d) for 10 weeks and then by lifelong maintenance therapy with fluconazole (200 mg/d). If antiretroviral therapy results in immunologic improvement, it may be possible to stop fluconazole.
6. Prognosis depends on the underlying disease process.

MUCORMYCOSIS

Etiology   Mucormycosis is caused by fungi from the order Mucorales, primarily those of the genera *Rhizopus* and *Rhizomucor*. Mucorales appear as broad, usually nonseptate hyphae with branches at right angles; organisms are described as ribbon-like.

Epidemiology   Mucorales are ubiquitous in the environment, and spores of these fungi are likely to be inhaled daily. Pts at high risk include those with diabetes, immunocompromise (e.g., after organ transplantation), or iron overload syndromes (e.g., in pts on hemodialysis) and associated use of deferoxamine therapy; in those pts, spores germinate, hyphae develop, and the fungi invade blood vessels and surrounding tissues in the lungs. Dissemination can occur.

Clinical Features

1. *Rhinocerebral mucormycosis*
   a. Pts may present with typical symptoms of sinusitis: low-grade fever, dull sinus pain, nasal congestion, and thin bloody nasal discharge.
   b. The disease may progress to hypesthesia or numbness of the face overlying the infection, headache, bloody nasal discharge, and altered mental status.
   c. Hyperemic areas of the palate can progress to a black eschar.

    d. Orbit involvement causes double vision, blindness, reduction of ocular motion, proptosis, and ptosis.

    e. Cavernous sinus thrombosis is an ominous sign.

2. *Pulmonary mucormycosis*: Neutropenia is a common predisposing factor.

    a. Progressive, severe, tissue-destructive pneumonia with high fever and toxicity

    b. Rapidly developing cavitation

    c. Hematogenous spread beyond the lungs to the brain and other organs

3. *GI and cutaneous infections* have been reported.

Diagnosis   Biopsy of sites of infection for histology and culture is critical for an accurate diagnosis; as much tissue as possible should be submitted for examination.

 Mucormycosis

Three factors are key to successful outcomes: reversal of underlying predisposing condition, if possible; aggressive surgical debridement; and aggressive antifungal treatment.

- AmB dosing is often limited by nephrotoxicity. Use of liposomal AmB (15–20 mg/kg per day of Ambisome or 15 mg/kg per day of Abelcet) maximizes the drug's delivery to tissues as well as the speed of its delivery, with nephrotoxicity occurring in <50% of pts. Posaconazole may also prove to be efficacious.
- Although the optimal duration is unknown, treatment should continue for at least 3 months after (1) clinical abnormalities resolve or stabilize, leaving no clinical evidence of disease at the involved site(s); and (2) scans, x-rays, and laboratory studies yield normal or stable results.
- Follow-up should continue for at least 1 year to confirm that infection does not recur.

HISTOPLASMOSIS

Etiology   *Histoplasma capsulatum,* a dimorphic fungus, causes histoplasmosis. Mycelia are infectious and have microconidial and macroconidial forms.

Epidemiology   Histoplasmosis is the most prevalent endemic mycosis in North America and is also found in Central and South America, Africa, and Asia. In the United States, histoplasmosis is endemic in the Ohio and Mississippi river valleys. The fungus is found in soil, particularly that enriched by droppings of certain birds and bats.

Pathogenesis and Pathology   Microconidia are inhaled, reach the alveoli, and are transformed into yeasts with occasional narrow budding. A granulomatous reaction results, but, in pts with impaired cellular immunity, infection may disseminate.

Clinical Features

1. *Acute pulmonary histoplasmosis*

    a. Asymptomatic or mild respiratory disease with cough, fever, hilar adenopathy, pneumonitis

    b. Occasionally associated with arthralgia or arthritis, erythema nodosum, or pericarditis

2. *Progressive disseminated histoplasmosis (PDH)*

    a. Typically seen in immunocompromised pts (e.g., pts with HIV infection, those at the extremes of age, and those using immunosuppressive agents)

b. The clinical spectrum ranges from a rapidly fatal course with diffuse interstitial or reticulonodular lung infiltrates, shock, and multiorgan failure to a subacute course with focal organ involvement, hepatosplenomegaly, fever, and weight loss. Meningitis, oral mucosal ulcerations, GI ulcerations, and adrenal insufficiency can occur.

3. *Chronic cavitary histoplasmosis*
   a. Most often affects smokers with structural lung disease (e.g., emphysema)
   b. Cough, weight loss, night sweats, apical infiltrates, cavitation, pleural thickening similar to that in tuberculosis

4. *Fibrosing mediastinitis associated with histoplasmosis* (rare): progressive fibrosis around hilar and mediastinal nodes resulting in superior vena cava syndrome, obstruction of pulmonary vessels, and recurrent airway obstruction

5. *African histoplasmosis*: distinct clinical presentation with frequent skin and bone involvement

Diagnosis

- Fungal culture: may take 1 month to become positive. In 75% of cases, pts with PDH and chronic cavitary disease have positive cultures of bronchoalveolar lavage fluid, bone marrow aspirate, and/or blood.
- Fungal stains of cytopathology or biopsy materials
- *Histoplasma* antigen assay of blood or urine is useful in diagnosing PDH or acute disease and in monitoring the response to treatment.
- Serologic tests can diagnose self-limited acute pulmonary and chronic cavitary histoplasmosis.

℞ Histoplasmosis

See Table 113-2 for treatment recommendations. Fibrosing mediastinitis does not respond to antifungal treatment.

COCCIDIOIDOMYCOSIS

Etiology Coccidioidomycosis is caused by the two species of the dimorphic soil-dwelling fungus *Coccidioides*: *C. immitis* and *C. posadasii*.

Epidemiology Coccidioidomycosis is highly endemic in California, Arizona, and other areas of the southwestern United States; northern Mexico and localized regions in Central and South America also account for cases of infection. Direct exposure to soil harboring *Coccidioides* increases risk, but infection can occur without overt soil exposure and may be related to other climatic factors (e.g., periods of dryness after rainy seasons). The frequency of cases has recently increased dramatically in south-central Arizona, perhaps because of the influx of older, susceptible persons into the area.

Pathogenesis and Pathology Infection, which results from inhalation of airborne arthroconidia, incites necrotizing granulomas in host tissue.

Clinical Features

1. *Primary pulmonary infection*: symptomatic in 40% of cases
   a. Fever, cough, chest pain; also erythema nodosum, erythema multiforme, other hypersensitivity reactions, night sweats, arthralgias
   b. Chest x-ray: infiltrate, hilar and mediastinal adenopathy, pleural effusion in ~10%

TABLE 113-2 RECOMMENDATIONS FOR THE TREATMENT OF HISTOPLASMOSIS

Type of Histoplasmosis	Treatment Recommendations	Comments
Acute pulmonary, moderate to severe illness with diffuse infiltrates and/or hypoxemia	Lipid amphotericin B (3–5 mg/kg per day) ± glucocorticoids for 1–2 weeks; then itraconazole (200 mg twice daily) for 12 weeks. Monitor renal and hepatic function.	Patients with mild cases usually recover without therapy, but itraconazole should be considered if the patient's condition has not improved after 1 month.
Chronic/cavitary pulmonary	Itraconazole (200 mg once or twice daily) for at least 12 months. Monitor hepatic function.	Continue treatment until radiographic findings show no further improvement. Monitor for relapse after treatment is stopped.
Progressive disseminated	Lipid amphotericin B (3–5 mg/kg per day) for 1–2 weeks; then itraconazole (200 mg twice daily) for at least 12 months. Monitor renal and hepatic function.	Liposomal amphotericin B is preferred, but the amphotericin B lipid complex may be used because of cost. Chronic maintenance therapy may be necessary if the degree of immunosuppression cannot be reduced.
Central nervous system	Liposomal amphotericin B (5 mg/kg per day) for 4–6 weeks; then itraconazole (200 mg 2 or 3 times daily) for at least 12 months. Monitor renal and hepatic function.	A longer course of lipid amphotericin B is recommended because of the high risk of relapse. Itraconazole should be continued until cerebrospinal fluid or CT abnormalities clear.

   c. Occasionally presents as diffuse reticulonodular pulmonary process with dyspnea and fever

   d. Mild peripheral-blood eosinophilia

2. *Cavitary pulmonary disease*: chronic thin-walled cavities. Symptomatic pts have cough, hemoptysis, and pleuritic chest pain.

3. *Disseminated infection*

   a. More likely in pts with cell-mediated immunosuppression (e.g., Hodgkin's disease, HIV infection), pregnant women, and certain racial and ethnic groups

   b. Common sites for dissemination include bone, skin, joint, soft tissue, and meninges

   c. Meningitis: fatal if untreated. Pts have persistent headache, lethargy, and confusion. Examination of CSF reveals lymphocytic pleocytosis, elevated protein levels, profound hypoglycorrhachia, and occasional eosinophilia.

Diagnosis

- Serology: Tube-precipitin (TP) and complement-fixation (CF) assays, immunodiffusion, and enzyme immunoassay (EIA) to detect IgM and IgG antibodies. TP antibody does not gauge disease progression and is not found in CSF. Rising CF titers in serum are associated with clinical progression, and CF antibody in CSF indicates meningitis. EIA frequently yields false-positive results.
- Examine tissue by smear and culture. Alert the laboratory of the possible diagnosis to avoid exposure.

R_x Coccidioidomycosis

- *Focal primary pneumonia*: no therapy except in pts with underlying cellular immunodeficiency or prolonged symptoms
- *Diffuse pulmonary disease*: AmB (0.7–1.0 mg/kg daily or three times a week IV) followed by itraconazole or fluconazole (minimum oral dose of 400 mg/d) after clinical improvement occurs
- *Pulmonary cavities*: Most do not require treatment.
- *Chronic pulmonary disease and disseminated infection*: prolonged triazole therapy (i.e., for ≥1 year)
- *Meningitis*: lifelong therapy with a triazole. Fluconazole is the drug of choice (≥400 mg/d). If triazole therapy fails, intrathecal AmB may be used.

BLASTOMYCOSIS

Blastomyces dermatitidis is a dimorphic fungus that is found in the southeastern and south-central states bordering the Mississippi and Ohio river basins, in areas of the United States and Canada bordering the Great Lakes and the St. Lawrence River, and in Africa. Infection is caused by inhalation of *Blastomyces* from moist soil rich in organic debris. Acute pulmonary infection can present as an abrupt onset of fever, chills, pleuritic chest pain, and arthralgias. However, most pts have chronic indolent pneumonia with fever, weight loss, productive cough, and hemoptysis. Skin disease is common and can present as verrucous or ulcerative lesions. Osteomyelitis is seen in up to one-fourth of infections.

Diagnosis

Smears of clinical samples or cultures of sputum, pus, or tissue are required for diagnosis. Antigen detection in urine and serum may assist in diagnosing infection and in monitoring pts during therapy.

Blastomycosis

Every pt should be treated because of the high risk of dissemination. AmB should be given for rapidly progressive infections or severe illness; when the pt's condition stabilizes (usually after 2 weeks of AmB therapy in non-CNS disease), the regimen can be switched to itraconazole (200-400 mg/d for 6–12 months). CNS disease is treated initially with AmB; after a total dose of ≥2 g, a switch can be made to fluconazole (800 mg/d for 6–12 months). More indolent infections can be treated with itraconazole (200–400 mg/d for 6–12 months). Among compliant immunocompetent pts, clinical and mycologic response rates are 90–95%.

MALASSEZIA INFECTION

Malassezia species are components of the normal skin flora and can cause tinea (pityriasis) versicolor, the most common superficial skin infection. *M. furfur* causes catheter-related fungemia in premature neonates and immunocompromised adults receiving IV lipids by central venous catheter.

SPOROTRICHOSIS

Sporothrix schenckii is a dimorphic fungus found in soil, plants, and moss and on animals. Infection, which results from inoculation of the organism into the skin, is seen especially often in florists, gardeners, and nursery workers.

Clinical Features
- *Plaque disease*: Sporotrichosis is limited to the site of inoculation. The lesion enlarges; it may ulcerate and become verrucous.
- *Lymphocutaneous disease*: 80% of cases. Secondary lesions ascend along lymphatics draining the area, producing small painless nodules that erupt, drain, and ulcerate.
- *Osteoarticular disease*: granulomatous tenosynovitis and bursitis, especially in alcoholic pts
- *Pulmonary sporotrichosis and disseminated disease*: can occur in compromised hosts

Diagnosis   Culture or skin biopsy

 Sporotrichosis

Cutaneous sporotrichosis is treated with itraconazole (100–200 mg/d). For extracutaneous disease, itraconazole (200 mg bid) can be given, but AmB is more effective for life-threatening pulmonary disease or disseminated infection.

PARACOCCIDIOIDOMYCOSIS

Paracoccidioidomycosis (South American blastomycosis) is caused by *Paracoccidioides brasiliensis*, a dimorphic fungus acquired by inhalation from environmental sources. Pulmonary infection follows inhalation of conidia and may disseminate to skin, lymph nodes, and adrenal glands. Diagnosis relies on culture of the organism. Itraconazole is effective, but AmB may be required for seriously ill pts.

PENICILLIOSIS

Penicillium marneffei is a leading cause of opportunistic infection in pts with immunocompromise (e.g., due to AIDS) in Southeast Asia and is acquired by spore inhalation. Clinical manifestations are similar to those of disseminated histoplasmosis, with fever, weight loss, generalized lymphadenopathy, and hepatomegaly. Diffuse papular lesions are common in pts with AIDS. AmB is the treatment of choice for severely ill pts; less severe disease may be treated with itraconazole. Primary therapy is usually given for 2 months; suppressive therapy with itraconazole may be indicated for pts with HIV infection or AIDS.

FUSARIOSIS

Fusarium species cause necrotic skin lesions in immunocompetent pts at sites of trauma; these fungi cause disseminated disease in immunocompromised pts, especially those who are severely neutropenic. The clinical presentation is generally nonspecific, with fever and skin lesions that become necrotic and resemble ecthyma gangrenosum. Blood cultures are positive in 50% of cases; in contrast, blood cultures are rarely positive in aspergillosis or zygomycosis. *Fusarium* species are often resistant to antifungal agents; high-dose AmB or voriconazole (6 mg/kg q12h for the first 24 h; then 4 mg/kg q12h) has been successful in some pts.

PSEUDALLESCHERIASIS AND SCEDOSPORIOSIS

Pseudallescheria boydii, Scedosporium apiospermum, and *S. prolificans* are molds that cause severe pneumonia, invasive sinusitis, and hematogenous dissemination (including brain abscess) in immunocompromised hosts. Most disseminated infections are fatal. AmB is not effective, but some infections have been cured with voriconazole at the doses used to treat fusariosis. Surgical drainage or debridement may be helpful.

DERMATOPHYTOSIS

See Chap. 64.

For a more detailed discussion, see Edwards JE Jr: Diagnosis and Treatment of Fungal Infections, Chap. 191, p. 1242; Hage CA, Wheat LJ: Histoplasmosis, Chap. 192, p. 1244; Ampel NM: Coccidioidomycosis, Chap. 193, p. 1247; Chapman SW, Sullivan DC: Blastomycosis, Chap. 194, p. 1249; Casadevall A: Cryptococcosis, Chap. 195, p. 1251; Edwards JE Jr: Candidiasis, Chap. 196, p. 1254; Denning DW: Aspergillosis, Chap. 197, p. 1256; Sugar AM: Mucormycosis, Chap. 198, p. 1261; and Chapman SW, Sullivan DC: Miscellaneous Mycoses and Algal Infections, Chap. 199, p. 1263, in HPIM-17.

114   *Pneumocystis* Infections

Pneumocystis, an opportunistic fungal pulmonary pathogen, is an important cause of pneumonia in immunocompromised hosts. *P. jirovecii* infects humans, whereas *P. carinii*—the original species described—infects rats. In contrast to most fungi, *Pneumocystis* lacks ergosterol and is not susceptible to antifungal drugs that inhibit ergosterol synthesis. Developmental stages include the small trophic form, the cyst, and the intermediate precyst stage.

EPIDEMIOLOGY

Pneumocystis is found worldwide. Most healthy children have been exposed to the organism by 3–4 years of age. Both airborne transmission and person-to-person transmission have been demonstrated.

PATHOGENESIS

Defects in cellular and humoral immunity predispose to *Pneumocystis* pneumonia. HIV-infected pts are at particular risk, and the risk rises dramatically when CD4+ T cell counts fall below 200/μL. Other persons at risk include those receiving immunosuppressive therapy (particularly glucocorticoids) for cancer and organ transplantation; those taking biologic agents (e.g., infliximab and etanercept for rheumatoid arthritis and inflammatory bowel disease); malnourished premature infants; and children with primary immunodeficiency disorders. The organisms are inhaled and attach tightly to type I cells in alveoli, although they remain extracellular. On histology, alveoli are seen to be filled with foamy, vacuolated exudates. Severe disease may cause interstitial edema, fibrosis, and hyaline membrane formation.

CLINICAL AND LABORATORY FEATURES

Pts develop dyspnea, fever, and nonproductive cough. Pts without HIV infection often become symptomatic after their glucocorticoid dose has been tapered, and symptoms last 1–2 weeks. HIV-infected pts are usually ill for several weeks or longer with more subtle manifestations. On physical examination, pts are found to have tachypnea, tachycardia, and cyanosis, but findings on pulmonary examination are often unremarkable. Reduced arterial oxygen pressure, increased alveolar-arterial oxygen gradient, and respiratory alkalosis are evident. Gallium scans can be positive, with nonspecific uptake in the lungs. Serum lactate dehydrogenase levels can be elevated, but this finding is nonspecific. Chest x-ray classically reveals bilateral diffuse infiltrates beginning in the perihilar regions. Other findings (e.g., nodular densities, cavitary lesions) have been described. Pneumothorax may occur. Rare cases of disseminated infection have been described, mainly in HIV pts taking aerosolized pentamidine. Lymph nodes, spleen, liver, and bone marrow are most often involved.

DIAGNOSIS

Histopathologic staining makes the definitive diagnosis. Methenamine silver and other cell wall stains selectively stain the wall of *Pneumocystis* cysts. Wright-Giemsa stains the nuclei of all developmental stages. Immunofluorescence with monoclonal antibodies increases diagnostic sensitivity. DNA amplification by polymerase chain reaction is most sensitive but may not distinguish colonization from infection. Proper specimens are key. HIV-infected pts have a higher organism burden, and their *Pneumocystis* infections can often be diagnosed by means of sputum induction. However, fiberoptic bronchoscopy with bronchoalveolar lavage (BAL) remains the mainstay of diagnosis. Transbronchial biopsy and open lung biopsy are used only when BAL results are negative.

COURSE AND PROGNOSIS

Therapy is most effective if started early, before there is extensive alveolar damage. The mortality rate is 15–20% at 1 month and 50–55% at 1 year among HIV-infected pts. The risk of early death remains high among people who need mechanical ventilation (60%) and among non-HIV-infected pts (40%).

R̲x̲ *Pneumocystis* Infections

Pts are classified as having disease that is mild (a $Pa_{O_2} >70$ mmHg or a $PA_{O_2} - Pa_{O_2}$ gradient <35 mmHg on room air) or moderate to severe (a $Pa_{O_2} \leq 70$ mmHg or a $PA_{O_2} - Pa_{O_2}$ gradient ≥ 35 mmHg). Trimethoprim-sulfamethoxazole (TMP-SMX) is the drug of choice for all pts. For doses and adverse effects of TMP-SMX and alternative regimens, see Table 114-1. For mild to moderate

TABLE 114-1 TREATMENT OF PNEUMOCYSTOSIS

Drug(s), Dose, Route	Adverse Effects
First Choice[a]	
TMP-SMX (5 mg/kg TMP, 25 mg/kg SMX[b]) q6–8h PO or IV	Fever, rash, cytopenias, hepatitis, hyperkalemia, GI disturbances
Other Agents[a]	
TMP, 5 mg/kg q6–8h, plus dapsone, 100 mg qd PO	Hemolysis (G6PD deficiency), methemoglobinemia, fever, rash, GI disturbances
Atovaquone, 750 mg bid PO	Rash, fever, GI and hepatic disturbances
Clindamycin, 300–450 mg q6h PO or 600 mg q6–8h IV, plus primaquine, 15–30 mg qd PO	Hemolysis (G6PD deficiency), methemoglobinemia, rash, colitis, neutropenia
Pentamidine, 3–4 mg/kg qd IV	Hypotension, azotemia, cardiac arrhythmias, pancreatitis, dysglycemias, hypocalcemia, neutropenia, hepatitis
Trimetrexate, 45 mg/m² qd IV, plus leucovorin,[c] 20 mg/kg q6h PO or IV	Cytopenias, peripheral neuropathy, hepatic disturbances
Adjunctive Agent	
Prednisone, 40 mg bid × 5 d, 40 mg qd × 5 d, 20 mg qd × 11 d; PO or IV	Immunosuppression, peptic ulcer, hyperglycemia, mood changes, hypertension

[a]Therapy is administered for 14 days to non-HIV-infected pts and for 21 days to HIV-infected pts.
[b]Equivalent of 2 double-strength (DS) tablets. (One DS tablet contains 160 mg of TMP and 800 mg of SMX.)
[c]Leucovorin prevents bone marrow toxicity from trimetrexate.

TABLE 114-2	PROPHYLAXIS OF PNEUMOCYSTOSIS[a]
Drug(s), Dose, Route	**Comments**
First Choice	
TMP-SMX, 1 DS tablet or 1 SS tablet qd PO[b]	TMP-SMX can be safely reintroduced in some pts who have experienced mild to moderate side effects.
Other Agents	
Dapsone, 50 mg bid or 100 mg qd PO	—
Dapsone, 50 mg qd PO, plus pyrimethamine, 50 mg weekly PO, plus leucovorin, 25 mg weekly PO	Leucovorin prevents bone marrow toxicity from pyrimethamine.
Dapsone, 200 mg weekly PO, plus pyrimethamine, 75 mg weekly PO, plus leucovorin, 25 mg weekly PO	Leucovorin prevents bone marrow toxicity from pyrimethamine.
Pentamidine, 300 mg monthly via Respirgard II nebulizer	Adverse reactions include cough and bronchospasm.
Atovaquone, 1500 mg qd PO	—
TMP-SMX, 1 DS tablet 3 times weekly PO	TMP-SMX can be safely reintroduced in some pts who have experienced mild to moderate side effects.

[a]For list of adverse effects, see Table 114-1.
[b]One DS tablet contains 160 mg of TMP and 800 mg of SMX.
Note: DS, double-strength; SS, single-strength.

cases, alternatives include TMP plus dapsone or clindamycin plus primaquine. Atovaquone is less effective than TMP-SMX but is better tolerated. Alternative treatments for moderate to severe infection include parenteral pentamidine, IV clindamycin plus primaquine, or trimetrexate. Clindamycin plus primaquine may be more efficacious than pentamidine. Adjunctive administration of tapering doses of glucocorticoids to HIV-infected pts with moderate to severe disease reduces the risk of respiratory function deterioration shortly after initiation of treatment. The use of glucocorticoids in other pts remains to be evaluated.

PREVENTION

Primary prophylaxis is indicated for HIV-infected pts with CD4+ T cell counts <200/μL or a history of oropharyngeal candidiasis. Guidelines for other compromised hosts are less clear. Secondary prophylaxis is indicated for all pts who have recovered from pneumocystosis. In HIV infection, once CD4+ counts have risen to >200/μL and have remained above that cutoff for ≥3 months, prophylaxis may be stopped. For prophylaxis regimens, see Table 114-2. TMP-SMX is the drug of choice for both primary and secondary prophylaxis and also protects against toxoplasmosis and some bacterial infections.

For a more detailed discussion, see Smulian AG, Walzer PD: *Pneumocystis* Infection, Chap. 200, p. 1267, in HPIM-17.

115 Protozoal Infections

MALARIA

Epidemiology   Malaria is the most important parasitic disease in humans, causing 1–3 million deaths each year.

Etiology   Four major species of *Plasmodium* cause nearly all human disease: *P. falciparum*, *P. vivax*, *P. ovale*, and *P. malariae*. *P. falciparum*, the cause of most cases of severe disease and most deaths, predominates in Africa, New Guinea, and Haiti. *P. vivax* is more common in Central America. *P. falciparum* and *P. vivax* are equally prevalent in South America, the Indian subcontinent, eastern Asia, and Oceania. *P. malariae* is less common but is found in most areas (especially throughout sub-Saharan Africa).

Pathogenesis

- Female anopheline mosquitoes inoculate *sporozoites* into humans during a blood meal. Sporozoites are carried to the liver, reproduce asexually, and produce *merozoites* that enter the bloodstream, invade red blood cells (RBCs), and become *trophozoites*. After progressively consuming and degrading intracellular proteins (principally hemoglobin), trophozoites become *schizonts*. When RBCs rupture, the cycle repeats with invasion of new RBCs.
- In *P. vivax* or *P. ovale* infection, dormant forms called *hypnozoites* remain in liver cells and may cause disease 3 weeks to >1 year later.
- Some parasites develop into long-lived sexual forms called *gametocytes*.
- RBCs infected with *P. falciparum* may exhibit *cytoadherence* (attachment to venular and capillary endothelium), *rosetting* (adherence to uninfected RBCs), and *agglutination* (adherence to other infected RBCs). The result is sequestration of *P. falciparum* in vital organs, with consequent underestimation (through parasitemia determinations) of parasite numbers in the body. Sequestration is central to the pathogenesis of falciparum malaria but is not evident in the other three "benign" forms.
- In nonimmune individuals, infection triggers nonspecific host defense mechanisms such as splenic filtration. With repeated exposure to malaria, a specific immune response develops and limits the degree of parasitemia. Over time, pts are rendered immune to disease but remain susceptible to infection. Genetic disorders more common in endemic areas protect against death from malaria (e.g., sickle cell disease, ovalocytosis, thalassemia, and G6PD deficiency).

Clinical Features

- Fever and nonspecific symptoms (headache, fatigue, muscle aches) occur at the onset of disease. Nausea, vomiting, and orthostasis are also common.
- Febrile paroxysms at regular intervals can occur and suggest infection with *P. vivax* or *P. ovale*.
- Splenomegaly may develop along with mild anemia, hepatomegaly, and jaundice.
- Severe falciparum malaria causes multiorgan dysfunction.
  1. Cerebral malaria: coma, obtundation, delirium, diffuse symmetric encephalopathy without focal neurologic signs. Seizures are common in children.

2. Poor prognostic signs: hypoglycemia, especially in children and pregnant women (may be exacerbated by quinine or quinidine treatment); acidosis; noncardiogenic pulmonary edema; renal failure; severe anemia and coagulation abnormalities; severe jaundice and liver dysfunction

- Malaria in pregnancy: Pregnant women have unusually severe illness. Premature labor, stillbirths, delivery of low-birth-weight infants, and fetal distress are common.
- Malaria in children: Most persons who die of malaria are children. Convulsions, coma, hypoglycemia, acidosis, and severe anemia occur at high rates.
- Transfusion malaria: has a shorter incubation period than naturally acquired disease
- Tropical splenomegaly: abnormal response to repeated infections. Pts have massive splenomegaly and, to a lesser degree, hepatomegaly. Pts have a dragging sensation in the abdomen.

Diagnosis

- Demonstration of asexual forms of the parasite on peripheral blood smears is required for diagnosis. Giemsa is the preferred stain, but other stains (e.g., Wright's) can be used. Both thick and thin smears should be examined. Thick smears concentrate parasites by 40- to 100-fold compared with thin smears and increase diagnostic sensitivity. If the level of clinical suspicion is high and smears are initially negative, they should be repeated q12–24h for 2 days.
- Rapid antibody-based diagnostic stick or card tests are available for *P. falciparum*.
- The parasitemia level should be calculated from a thin smear and is expressed as the number of parasitized erythrocytes per 1000 RBCs.
- Other laboratory studies: anemia, elevated erythrocyte sedimentation rate, reduced platelet count (to $10^5/\mu L$)

Rx Malaria

See Table 115-1 for treatment options.

- Artemisinin-based combinations are recommended as first-line treatments for falciparum malaria. These agents are not available in the United States for treatment of uncomplicated *P. falciparum* disease, however.
- Severe falciparum malaria: Treatment with parenteral water-soluble artemisinin derivatives reduces mortality rates by 35% from rates obtained with quinine. IV artesunate is available for emergency use in the United States through the Centers for Disease Control and Prevention (CDC) drug service; contact the CDC Malaria Hotline at 770-488-7788 or the CDC Emergency Operations Center at 770-488-7100.
- If falciparum malaria is treated with quinidine, pts should undergo cardiac monitoring; increased QT intervals (>0.6 s) and QRS widening by >25% are indications for slowing the infusion rate.
- Pts with severe falciparum malaria require intensive nursing care and monitoring. Ancillary drugs, including glucocorticoids or heparin, should not be given. Exchange transfusions can be considered for severely ill pts, although indications for their use are not yet agreed upon. Unconscious pts should have blood glucose levels measured q4–6h. Pts with glucose levels of <2.2 mmol/L (<40 mg/dL) and pts treated with IV quinine or quinidine should receive IV dextrose.
- Parasite counts and hematocrits should be measured q6–12h.

TABLE 115-1 **REGIMENS FOR THE TREATMENT OF MALARIA**

Type of Disease or Treatment	Regimen(s)
Uncomplicated Malaria	
Known chloroquine-sensitive strains of *Plasmodium vivax, P. malariae, P. ovale, P. falciparum*[a]	Chloroquine (10 mg of base/kg stat followed by 5 mg/kg at 12, 24, and 36 h or by 10 mg/kg at 24 h and 5 mg/kg at 48 h) *or* Amodiaquine (10–12 mg of base/kg qd for 3 days)
Radical treatment for *P. vivax* or *P. ovale* infection	In addition to chloroquine or amodiaquine as detailed above, primaquine (0.25 mg of base/kg qd; 0.375–0.5 mg of base/kg qd in Southeast Asia and Oceania) should be given for 14 days to prevent relapse. In mild G6PD deficiency, 0.75 mg of base/kg should be given once weekly for 6 weeks. Primaquine should not be given in severe G6PD deficiency.
Sensitive *P. falciparum* malaria[b]	Artesunate[c] (4 mg/kg qd for 3 days) plus sulfadoxine (25 mg/kg)/pyrimethamine (1.25 mg/kg) as a single dose *or* Artesunate[c] (4 mg/kg qd for 3 days) plus amodiaquine (10 mg of base/kg qd for 3 days)[d]
Multidrug-resistant *P. falciparum* malaria	Either artemether-lumefantrine[c] (1.5/9 mg/kg bid for 3 days with food) or artesunate[c] (4 mg/kg qd for 3 days) *plus* Mefloquine (25 mg of base/kg—either 8 mg/kg qd for 3 days or 15 mg/kg on day 2 and then 10 mg/kg on day 3)[d]
Second-line treatment/treatment of imported malaria	Either artesunate[c] (2 mg/kg qd for 7 days) or quinine (10 mg of salt/kg tid for 7 days) *plus 1 of the following 3:* 1. Tetracycline[e] (4 mg/kg qid for 7 days) 2. Doxycycline[e] (3 mg/kg qd for 7 days) 3. Clindamycin (10 mg/kg bid for 7 days) *or* Atovaquone-proguanil (20/8 mg/kg qd for 3 days with food)

(continued)

TABLE 115-1	REGIMENS FOR THE TREATMENT OF MALARIA (CONTINUED)
Type of Disease or Treatment	**Regimen(s)**
Severe Falciparum Malaria[f]	
	Artesunate[c] (2.4 mg/kg stat IV followed by 2.4 mg/kg at 12 and 24 h and then daily if necessary)[g]
	or
	Artemether[c] (3.2 mg/kg stat IM followed by 1.6 mg/kg qd)
	or
	Quinine dihydrochloride (20 mg of salt/kg[h] infused over 4 h, followed by 10 mg of salt/kg infused over 2–8 h q8h[i])
	or
	Quinidine (10 mg of base/kg[h] infused over 1–2 h, followed by 1.2 mg of base/kg per hour[i] with electrocardiographic monitoring)

[a]Very few areas now have chloroquine-sensitive malaria (Fig. 203-2).

[b]In areas where the partner drug to artesunate is known to be effective.

[c]Artemisinin derivatives are not registered in the United States and some other temperate countries.

[d]Fixed-dose coformulated combinations are available.

[e]Tetracycline and doxycycline should not be given to pregnant women or to children <8 years of age.

[f]Oral treatment should be substituted as soon as the patient recovers sufficiently to take fluids by mouth.

[g]Artesunate is the drug of choice when available. The data from large studies in Southeast Asia showed a 35% reduction in mortality rate from that with quinine. Severe malaria in children in high-transmission settings has different characteristics; thus trials are ongoing in Africa comparing artesunate with quinine to determine whether there is a survival benefit in African children.

[h]A loading dose should not be given if therapeutic doses of quinine or quinidine have definitely been adminstered in the previous 24 h. Some authorities recommend a lower dose of quinidine.

[i]Infusions can be given in 0.9% saline and 5% or 10% dextrose in water. Infusion rates for quinine and quinidine should be carefully controlled.

Note: G6PD, glucose-6-phosphate dehydrogenase.

- Pts should be monitored for vomiting for 1 h after oral malaria treatment, and the dose should be repeated if vomiting occurs.
- Primaquine eradicates persistent liver stages and prevents relapse in *P. vivax* or *P. ovale* infection. G6PD deficiency must be ruled out before treatment.

Prevention   **Personal Protection Measures**   Measures that can protect persons against infection include avoidance of mosquito exposure at peak feeding times (dusk and dawn) and use of insect repellents containing DEET (10–35%) or (if DEET is unacceptable) picaridin (7%), suitable clothing, and insecticide-impregnated bed nets.

Chemoprophylaxis   See Table 115-2 for prophylaxis options.
- Mefloquine is the only drug advised for pregnant women traveling to areas with drug-resistant malaria and is generally considered safe in the second and third trimesters.
- The CDC offers 24-h travel and malaria information at 877-FYI-TRIP.

TABLE 115-2 DRUGS USED IN THE PROPHYLAXIS OF MALARIA

Drug	Usage	Adult Dose	Pediatric Dose	Comments
Atovaquone/proguanil (Malarone)	Prophylaxis in areas with chloroquine- or mefloquine-resistant *Plasmodium falciparum*	1 adult tablet PO[a]	5–8 kg: 1/2 pediatric tablet[b] daily ≥8–10 kg: 3/4 pediatric tablet daily ≥10–20 kg: 1 pediatric tablet daily ≥20–30 kg: 2 pediatric tablets daily ≥30–40 kg: 3 pediatric tablets daily ≥40 kg: 1 adult tablet daily	Begin 1–2 days before travel to malarious areas. Take daily at the same time each day while in the malarious area and for 7 days after leaving such areas. Atovaquone-proguanil is contraindicated in persons with severe renal impairment (creatinine clearance rate <30 mL/min). It is not recommended for children weighing <5 kg, pregnant women, or women breast-feeding infants weighing <5 kg. Atovaquone/proguanil should be taken with food or a milky drink.
Chloroquine phosphate (Aralen and generic)	Prophylaxis only in areas with chloroquine-sensitive *P. falciparum*[c]	300 mg of base (500 mg of salt) PO once weekly	5 mg of base/kg (8.3 mg of salt/kg) PO once weekly, up to a maximum adult dose of 300 mg of base	Begin 1–2 weeks before travel to malarious areas. Take weekly on the same day of the week while in the malarious areas and for 4 weeks after leaving such areas. Chloroquine phosphate may exacerbate psoriasis.
Doxycycline (many brand names and generic)	Prophylaxis in areas with chloroquine- or mefloquine-resistant *P. falciparum*[c]	100 mg PO qd	≥8 years of age: 2 mg/kg, up to adult dose	Begin 1–2 days before travel to malarious areas. Take daily at the same time each day while in the malarious areas and for 4 weeks after leaving such areas. Doxycycline is contraindicated in children <8 years of age and in pregnant women.
Hydroxychloroquine sulfate (Plaquenil)	An alternative to chloroquine for primary prophylaxis only in areas with chloroquine-sensitive *P. falciparum*[c]	310 mg of base (400 mg of salt) PO once weekly	5 mg of base/kg (6.5 mg of salt/kg) PO once weekly, up to maximum adult dose of 310 mg of base	Begin 1–2 weeks before travel to malarious areas. Take weekly on the same day of the week while in the malarious areas and for 4 weeks after leaving such areas. Hydroxychloroquine may exacerbate psoriasis.

Drug	Indication	Adult dose	Pediatric dose	Comments
Mefloquine (Lariam and generic)	Prophylaxis in areas with chloroquine-resistant *P. falciparum*	228 mg of base (250 mg of salt) PO once weekly	≤9 kg: 4.6 mg of base/kg (5 mg of salt/kg) PO once weekly 10–19 kg: 1/4 tablet once weekly 20–30 kg: 1/2 tablet once weekly 31–45 kg: 3/4 tablet once weekly ≥46 kg: 1 tablet once weekly	Begin 1–2 weeks before travel to malarious areas. Take weekly on the same day of the week while in the malarious areas and for 4 weeks after leaving such areas. Mefloquine is contraindicated in persons allergic to this drug or related compounds (e.g., quinine and quinidine) and in persons with active or recent depression, generalized anxiety disorder, psychosis, schizophrenia, other major psychiatric disorders, or seizures. Use with caution in persons with psychiatric disturbances or a history of depression. Mefloquine is not recommended for persons with cardiac conduction abnormalities.
Primaquine	An option for prophylaxis in special circumstances	30 mg of base (52.6 mg of salt) PO qd	0.5 mg of base/kg (0.8 mg of salt/kg) PO qd, up to adult dose; should be taken with food	Begin 1–2 days before travel to malarious areas. Take daily at the same time each day while in the malarious areas and for 7 days after leaving such areas. Primaquine is contraindicated in persons with G6PD1 deficiency. It is also contraindicated during pregnancy and in lactation unless the infant being breast-fed has a documented normal G6PD level. Use in consultation with malaria experts.
Primaquine	Used for presumptive antirelapse therapy (terminal prophylaxis) to decrease risk of relapses of *P. vivax* and *P. ovale*	30 mg of base (52.6 mg of salt) PO qd for 14 days after departure from the malarious area	0.5 mg of base/kg (0.8 mg of salt/kg), up to adult dose, PO qd for 14 days after departure from the malarious area	This therapy is indicated for persons who have had prolonged exposure to *P. vivax* and/or *P. ovale*. It is contraindicated in persons with G6PD1 deficiency as well as during pregnancy and in lactation unless the infant being breast-fed has a documented normal G6PD level.

[a]An adult tablet contains 250 mg of atovaquone and 100 mg of proguanil hydrochloride.
[b]A pediatric tablet contains 62.5 mg of atovaquone and 25 mg of proguanil hydrochloride.
[c]Very few areas now have chloroquine-sensitive malaria (Fig. 203-2 in HPIM-17).
Source: CDC: *http://wwwn.cdc.gov/travel/contentMalariaDrugsHC.aspx.*

BABESIOSIS

Etiology   Babesiosis is caused by intraerythrocytic protozoa of the genus *Babesia*. *B. microti* is the most common species in the United States. *B. divergens* causes disease in Europe.

Epidemiology   In the United States, infections occur most frequently along the northeastern coast. Hard-bodied ticks (*Ixodes scapularis* in the United States and *I. ricinus* in Europe) transmit the parasite.

Clinical Features

- The incubation period is usually 1–6 weeks. There is a gradual onset of fevers, fatigue, myalgias, arthralgias, and—less often—dyspnea, headache, anorexia, and nausea. Pts have mild hepatosplenomegaly, anemia, thrombocytopenia, and elevated liver enzymes. Parasitemia levels may range from 1 to 10% in immunocompetent pts and up to 85% in asplenic pts.
- Complications include respiratory failure, disseminated intravascular coagulation, congestive heart failure, and renal failure. Immunocompromised pts (e.g., HIV-infected pts, asplenic pts), pts with concurrent Lyme disease, and pts >50 years of age have more severe disease.
- *B. divergens* causes severe—often fatal—disease in asplenic pts. This illness is characterized by high fevers, hemolytic anemia, jaundice, and renal failure.

Diagnosis   Giemsa-stained thin smears identify intraerythrocytic *Babesia* parasites, which appear annular, oval, or piriform. Ring forms resembling *P. falciparum* but without pigment are most common. Tetrads ("Maltese crosses")—formed by four budding merozoites—are pathognomonic for *B. microti* and other small *Babesia* species. An indirect immunofluorescence antibody test for *B. microti* is available from the CDC. Persistent low-grade infection is best diagnosed by polymerase chain reaction (PCR) testing of blood.

Rx **Babesiosis**

- Mild disease: atovaquone (750 mg q12h PO) plus azithromycin (500–1000 mg/d PO on day 1 followed by 250 mg/d PO for immunocompetent pts or 600–1000 mg/d PO for immunocompromised pts) for 7–10 days
- Severe infections: clindamycin (300–600 mg q6h IV or 600 mg q8h PO) plus quinine (650 mg q6–8h PO). Also consider exchange transfusion.
- *B. divergens* infection: immediate exchange transfusion; clindamycin (600 mg q6–8h IV) and quinine (650 mg q8h PO)

LEISHMANIASIS

Etiology   *Leishmania* spp. are obligate intracellular protozoa endemic in the tropics, subtropics, and southern Europe. Organisms of the *L. donovani* complex usually cause visceral leishmaniasis; *L. tropica*, *L. major*, and *L. aethiopica* cause Old World cutaneous leishmaniasis; and the *L. mexicana* complex causes New World or American cutaneous leishmaniasis. Leishmaniasis is typically a vector-borne zoonosis caused by the bite of female phlebotomine sandflies. The parasite's flagellated promastigote is introduced into the mammalian host and transforms into the nonflagellated amastigote within macrophages.

Epidemiology, Prevention, and Control

- Around 90% of visceral leishmaniasis cases occur in southern Asia, the Indian subcontinent, eastern Africa, and the Americas (with particularly high rates in northeastern Brazil). More than 90% of cutaneous cases occur in Afghanistan, the Middle East, Brazil, and Peru.
- Prevention and control measures must be tailored to the specific setting. Personal protective measures include minimizing nocturnal outdoor activities (when sandflies are active) and using protective clothing and insect repellent.

Clinical Features
Visceral Leishmaniasis

- The incubation period can range from weeks to months or even years. Disease manifestations can be acute, subacute, or chronic.
- Kala-azar: The classic picture is of cachectic, febrile pts with massive splenomegaly, hepatomegaly, and life-threatening disease.
- Abnormal laboratory findings include pancytopenia, hypergammaglobulinemia, and hypoalbuminemia.
- The diagnosis should be considered in HIV-infected pts with visceral disease who have been in endemic areas.

Cutaneous Leishmaniasis

- After an incubation period of weeks to months, papular lesions progress to plaques (which can be smooth, scaly, or nodular and can develop central ulceration) and then to atrophic scars. Both active and healed lesions can cause significant morbidity. *L. aethiopica* and *L. mexicana* cause chronic, disseminated, nonulcerative skin lesions. Leishmaniasis recidivans, caused by *L. tropica*, manifests as a chronic solitary cheek lesion that expands slowly with central healing.
- Regional adenopathy, multiple primary and satellite lesions, and bacterial superinfection can occur.

Mucosal Leishmaniasis This disfiguring sequela of New World cutaneous leishmaniasis results from dissemination of parasites from the skin to the naso-oro-pharyngeal mucosa. Persistent nasal symptoms, such as epistaxis with erythema and edema of the mucosa, are followed by progressive ulcerative destruction.

Diagnosis

- Visceral leishmaniasis: Identification of amastigotes on slides that have been stained (e.g., with Giemsa) or by culture of tissue aspirates or biopsy samples of spleen, liver, bone marrow, or lymph nodes yields the diagnosis. Spleen aspiration poses a high risk of hemorrhage. Seropositivity can be diagnostic in an appropriate setting; the sensitivity of serology is lower in HIV-infected pts.
- Cutaneous and mucosal leishmaniasis: Diagnosis is made by examination of aspirates and biopsy specimens of skin lesions and lymph nodes. Serology is not useful.

R_x Leishmaniasis

- Visceral leishmaniasis: The pentavalent antimonial (Sb^v) compounds sodium stibogluconate and meglumine antimonate (20 mg/kg per day IV or IM for 28 days) are the first-line therapeutic agents. Amphotericin B (AmB; either deoxycholate or a lipid formulation) is recommended (total dose, 15–20 mg/kg) in areas with Sb^v resistance (e.g., northeastern India). The oral agent miltefosine (2.5 mg/kg daily for 28 days) is effective but must be used carefully to prevent the emergence of resistance. Sb^v treatment is associated with significant but reversible toxicity (body aches, malaise, elevated liver function test values, chemical pancreatitis) whose incidence increases as treatment continues.

- Cutaneous leishmaniasis: The decision to treat cutaneous leishmaniasis should be based on therapeutic goals (e.g., accelerating healing, decreasing morbidity), parasite factors (e.g., tissue tropisms and drug sensitivities), and the extent to which the lesions are of concern (e.g., location on the face). Administration of Sb^v (20 mg/kg daily for 20 days) constitutes the most effective treatment; conventional AmB is likely to be highly effective. The efficacy of oral agents is dependent on species and strain. Local therapies may be considered for cases without demonstrable local dissemination.
- Mucosal leishmaniasis: Sb^v or conventional AmB is effective. Oral miltefosine shows promise. Glucocorticoid therapy is indicated if respiratory compromise develops after the start of therapy.

TRYPANOSOMIASIS

CHAGAS' DISEASE

Etiology and Pathology   *Trypanosoma cruzi* causes Chagas' disease (also known as American trypanosomiasis) and is transmitted among mammalian hosts by hematophagous reduviid bugs. One week after parasitic invasion, an indurated inflammatory lesion appears at the portal of entry, and organisms disseminate through the lymphatics and the bloodstream, often parasitizing muscles particularly heavily.

Epidemiology   Chagas' disease is the most important parasitic disease in Latin America. *T. cruzi* is found mostly among the poor in rural Mexico and Central and South America. An estimated 12 million persons are infected, with 25,000 deaths annually.

Clinical Features

- *Acute disease*: An indurated area of erythema and swelling (the *chagoma*) with local lymphadenopathy may appear. *Romaña's sign*—unilateral painless edema of the palpebrae and periocular tissues—occurs when the conjunctiva is the portal of entry.
  1. Malaise, fever, anorexia, rash, lymphadenopathy, and hepatosplenomegaly develop.
  2. After symptoms resolve spontaneously, pts enter an asymptomatic phase.
- *Chronic disease*: becomes apparent years to decades after initial infection
  1. Heart: rhythm disturbances, dilated cardiomyopathy, thromboembolism. Right bundle branch block and other conduction abnormalities may occur.
  2. Megaesophagus: dysphagia, odynophagia, chest pain, and aspiration. Weight loss, cachexia, or pulmonary infection can cause death.
  3. Megacolon: abdominal pain, chronic constipation. Advanced megacolon can cause obstruction, volvulus, septicemia, and death.

Diagnosis   Microscopic examination of fresh anticoagulated blood or the buffy coat may reveal motile organisms. Giemsa-stained thin and thick blood smears can also be used. If attempts to visualize the organism fail, PCR or hemoculture can be performed. Chronic Chagas' disease is diagnosed by detection of specific antibodies. The assays vary in specificity and sensitivity; false-positive results pose a particular problem. A positive result should be confirmed by at least two assays. The U.S. Food and Drug Administration has approved a test to screen blood and organ donors for *T. cruzi*.

R̲x̲ Chagas' Disease

Acute Chagas' disease is treated with nifurtimox, which reduces symptom duration, parasitemia level, and mortality rate but cures only ~70% of pts. Treatment should be initiated as early as possible in acute disease. Adults should receive 8–10 mg/kg daily in four divided oral doses for 90–120 days. Higher doses are given to children and adolescents. Adverse drug effects include abdominal pain, anorexia, nausea, vomiting, weight loss, and neurologic reactions such as restlessness, disorientation, insomnia, paresthesia, and seizures. In Latin America, the drug of choice is benznidazole (5 mg/kg per day for 60 days). Benznidazole is associated with peripheral neuropathy, rash, and granulocytopenia. Treatment of chronic Chagas' disease is controversial. The current consensus of Latin American authorities is that pts up to 18 years of age should receive treatment.

SLEEPING SICKNESS

Etiology and Epidemiology   Sleeping sickness (human African trypanosomiasis) is caused by parasites of the *T. brucei* complex and is transmitted via tsetse flies. *T. b. rhodesiense* causes the East African form and *T. b. gambiense* the West African form. During stage I of infection, the parasites disseminate through the lymphatics and the bloodstream. Central nervous system (CNS) invasion occurs during stage II. West African infection occurs primarily in rural populations and rarely develops in tourists. East African disease has reservoirs in antelope and cattle; tourists can be infected when visiting areas where infected game and vectors are present.

Clinical Features   A painful chancre sometimes appears at the site of inoculation. Stage I is marked by bouts of high fever alternating with afebrile periods and by lymphadenopathy with discrete, rubbery, nontender nodes. *Winterbottom's sign*—the enlargement of nodes of the posterior cervical triangle—is a classic sign. Pruritus and maculopapular rashes are common. Malaise, headache, arthralgias, hepatosplenomegaly, and other nonspecific manifestations can develop. In stage II, pts develop progressive indifference and daytime somnolence, a state that sometimes alternates with restlessness and insomnia. Extrapyramidal signs may include choreiform movements, tremors, and fasciculations; ataxia is common. Progressive neurologic impairment may end in coma and death. East African disease is a more acute illness that, without treatment, generally leads to death in weeks or months.

Diagnosis   Examination of fluid from the chancre, thin or thick blood smears, lymph node aspirates, bone marrow biopsy specimens, or cerebrospinal fluid (CSF) samples can reveal the parasite. CSF should be examined whenever the diagnosis is being considered. Increased opening pressure, increased protein level, and increased mononuclear cell counts are common. Parasites can be visualized in the sediment of centrifuged CSF.

R̲x̲ Sleeping Sickness

Treatment is toxic and must be closely supervised.
- Stage I disease
    East African: suramin (a test dose of 100–200 mg followed by 20 mg/kg IV on days 1, 5, 12, 18, and 26). Fever, photophobia, pruritus, arthralgias, skin eruptions, and renal damage can occur. Severe reactions (shock, seizures) can be fatal.

West African: pentamidine (4 mg/kg daily IM or IV for 10 days). Serious adverse reactions include nephrotoxicity, abnormal liver function, neutropenia, hypoglycemia, and sterile abscesses. Suramin is the alternative treatment.

- Stage II disease

East African: melarsoprol (2–3.6 mg/kg daily in 3 divided doses for 3 days; 1 week later, 3.6 mg/kg per day in 3 divided doses for 3 days; 1 week later, the latter course repeated). To reduce melarsoprol-induced encephalopathy, administer prednisolone (1 mg/kg up to 40 mg daily, starting 1–2 days before the first dose of melarsoprol and continuing through the last dose).

West African: Eflornithine (400 mg/kg per day in 4 divided doses for 2 weeks) is the first-line agent, with melarsoprol as an alternative.

TOXOPLASMOSIS

Etiology and Epidemiology Toxoplasmosis is caused by the intracellular parasite *Toxoplasma gondii*. In the United States and most European countries, seroconversion rates increase with age and exposure. Cats and their prey are the definitive hosts. Transmission occurs when humans ingest oocysts from contaminated soil or tissue cysts from undercooked meat. Acute infection with *T. gondii* during pregnancy results in transmission to the fetus in about one-third of cases. Congenital infection can occur if the mother is infected <6 months before conception and becomes increasingly likely throughout pregnancy, with a 65% likelihood if the mother is infected in the third trimester.

Pathogenesis Both humoral and cellular immunity are important, but infection commonly persists. Such lifelong infection usually remains subclinical. Compromised hosts do not control infection; progressive focal destruction and organ failure occur.

Clinical Features

- Disease in immunocompetent hosts is usually asymptomatic and self-limited and does not require therapy; 80–90% of cases go unrecognized. Cervical lymphadenopathy is the most common finding; nodes are nontender and discrete. Generalized lymphadenopathy can occur. Fever, headache, malaise, and fatigue are documented in 20–40% of pts with lymphadenopathy.
- Immunocompromised pts, including those with AIDS and those receiving immunosuppressive treatment for lymphoproliferative disorders, are at greatest risk. Most clinical disease is due to reactivated latent infection.
  1. CNS: principal site of involvement. Findings include encephalopathy, meningoencephalitis, and mass lesions. Pts may exhibit changes in mental status, fever, seizures, headaches, and aphasia. The brainstem, basal ganglia, pituitary gland, and corticomedullary junction are most often involved.
  2. Pneumonia: Dyspnea, fever, and nonproductive cough can progress to respiratory failure. *Toxoplasma* pneumonia is often confused with *Pneumocystis* pneumonia.
  3. Miscellaneous sites: GI tract, pancreas, eyes, heart, liver
- Congenital infection affects 400–4000 infants each year in the United States. Severe disease, manifesting as hydrocephalus, microcephaly, mental retardation, and chorioretinitis, is more common the earlier the infection is contracted.

- Ocular infection: *T. gondii* is estimated to cause ~35% of all cases of chorioretinitis in the United States and Europe. Most cases are associated with congenital infection. Blurred vision, scotoma, photophobia, and eye pain are manifestations of infection; macular involvement can occur with loss of central vision. On examination, yellow-white cotton-like patches with indistinct margins of hyperemia are seen. Older lesions appear as white plaques with distinct borders and black spots.

Diagnosis
- Acute toxoplasmosis can be diagnosed by the demonstration of tachyzoites in tissue or by documentation of the simultaneous presence of serum IgM and IgG antibodies to *T. gondii*.
- In AIDS pts, the infection is diagnosed presumptively on the basis of clinical presentation and a positive test for IgG antibody to *T. gondii*. In these pts, CT or MRI of the brain shows lesions that are often multiple and contrast enhancing. A single lesion may prove to be a CNS lymphoma rather than toxoplasmosis.
- Congenital toxoplasmosis is diagnosed by PCR of the amniotic fluid (to detect the B1 gene of the parasite) and by the persistence of IgG antibody or a positive IgM titer after the first week of life; IgG antibody determinations should be repeated every 2 months.
- Ocular toxoplasmosis is diagnosed by the detection of typical lesions on ophthalmologic examination and the demonstration of a positive IgG titer.

℞ Toxoplasmosis

- Congenital infection: daily pyrimethamine (0.5–1 mg/kg) and sulfadiazine (100 mg/kg) for 1 year. If infection is diagnosed and treated early, up to 70% of children can have normal findings at follow-up evaluations.
- Ocular disease: pyrimethamine and sulfadiazine or clindamycin for 1 month
- Immunocompromised pts: pyrimethamine (200-mg PO loading dose followed by 50–75 mg/d) plus sulfadiazine (4–6 g/d PO, divided into 4 doses) plus leucovorin (10–15 mg/d). Pyrimethamine (75 mg/d) plus clindamycin (450 mg tid) is an alternative. Glucocorticoids are often used to treat intracerebral edema. After 4–6 weeks (or after radiographic improvement), the pt may be switched to chronic suppressive therapy (secondary prophylaxis) with pyrimethamine (25–50 mg/d) plus sulfadiazine (2–4 g/d), pyrimethamine (75 mg/d) plus clindamycin (450 mg tid), or pyrimethamine alone (50–75 mg/d).

Chemoprophylaxis The risk of disease is very high among AIDS pts who are seropositive for *T. gondii* and have a CD4+ T lymphocyte count of <100/μL. Trimethoprim-sulfamethoxazole (one double-strength tablet daily) should be given to these pts as prophylaxis against both *Pneumocystis* pneumonia and toxoplasmosis. Primary or secondary prophylaxis can be stopped if, after institution of antiretroviral treatment, the CD4+ T lymphocyte count increases to >200/μL and remains above that cutoff for 3 months.

Personal Protection Measures *Toxoplasma* infection can be prevented by avoiding undercooked meats and oocyst-contaminated materials (e.g., cats' litter boxes).

For a more detailed discussion, see Reed SL, Davis CE: Laboratory Diagnosis of Parasitic Infections, Chap. e16; and Moore TA: Pharmacology of Agents Used to Treat Parasitic Infections, Chap. e17, in *Harrison's Online*; and Moore TA: Agents Used to Treat Parasitic Infections, Chap. 201, p. 1270; White NJ, Breman JG: Malaria, Chap. 203, p. 1280; Gelfand JA, Vannier E: Babesiosis, Chap. 204, p. 1294; Herwaldt BL: Leishmaniasis, Chap. 205, p. 1296; Kirchhoff LV: Trypanosomiasis, Chap. 206, p. 1300; and Kasper LH: *Toxoplasma* Infections, Chap. 207, p. 1305, in HPIM-17.

116 Helminthic Infections and Ectoparasite Infestations

HELMINTHS

NEMATODES

The nematodes, or roundworms, that are of medical significance can be broadly classified as either tissue or intestinal parasites.

Tissue Nematode Infections

Trichinellosis *Etiology* *T. spiralis* and seven other *Trichinella* species cause human infection.

Life Cycle and Epidemiology Infection results when humans ingest meat (usually pork) that contains cysts with *Trichinella* larvae. During the first week of infection, the larvae invade the small-bowel mucosa; during the second and third weeks, they mature into adult worms, which release new larvae that migrate to striated muscle via the circulation and encyst.

Clinical Features Light infections (<10 larvae per gram of muscle) are asymptomatic. A burden of >50 larvae per gram can cause fatal disease.

- Week 1: diarrhea, abdominal pain, constipation, nausea, and/or vomiting
- Week 2: hypersensitivity reactions with fever and hypereosinophilia; periorbital and facial edema; hemorrhages in conjunctivae, retina, and nail beds; maculopapular rash; headache; cough; dyspnea; dysphagia. Deaths are usually due to myocarditis with arrhythmias or congestive heart failure and are less often caused by pneumonitis or encephalitis.
- Weeks 2–3: myositis, myalgias, muscle edema, weakness (especially in extraocular muscles, biceps, neck, lower back, and diaphragm). Symptoms peak at 3 weeks; convalescence is prolonged.

Diagnosis
- Eosinophilia in >90% of pts, peaking at a level of >50% at 2–4 weeks
- Elevated IgE and muscle enzyme levels; increase in specific antibody titers by week 3
- A definitive diagnosis is made by the detection of larvae on biopsy of at least 1 g of muscle tissue. Yields are highest near tendon insertions.

R̽ Trichinellosis

Drugs are ineffective against muscle larvae, but mebendazole (200–400 mg tid for 3 days; then 400 mg tid for 8–14 days) and albendazole (400 mg bid for 8–14 days) may be active against enteric-stage parasites. Glucocorticoids (1 mg/kg daily for 5 days) may reduce severe myositis and myocarditis.

Prevention   Cooking pork until it is no longer pink or freezing it at 15°C for 3 weeks kills larvae and prevents infection.

Visceral and Ocular Larva Migrans   *Etiology*   Most cases of larva migrans are caused by *Toxocara canis*.

Life Cycle and Epidemiology   Infection results when humans—most often preschool children—ingest soil contaminated by puppy feces that contain infective *T. canis* eggs. Larvae penetrate the intestinal mucosa and disseminate hematogenously to a wide variety of organs [e.g., liver, lungs, central nervous system (CNS)], provoking intense eosinophilic granulomatous responses.

Clinical Features   Heavy infections may cause fever, malaise, anorexia, weight loss, cough, wheezing, rashes, and hepatosplenomegaly. Ocular disease usually develops in older children or young adults and includes endophthalmitis, uveitis, chorioretinitis, and/or an eosinophilic mass that mimics retinoblastoma.

Diagnosis   No eggs are found in the stool because larvae do not develop into adult worms. Blood eosinophilia up to 90%, leukocytosis, and hypergammaglobulinemia may be evident. Toxocaral antibodies can be detected by enzyme-linked immunosorbent assay (ELISA).

R̽ Visceral and Ocular Larva Migrans

Glucocorticoids can reduce inflammatory complications. Ocular infections can be treated with albendazole (800 mg bid for adults and 400 mg bid for children) for 5–20 days in conjunction with glucocorticoids.

Cutaneous Larva Migrans   This disease is caused by larvae of animal hookworms, usually the dog and cat hookworm *Ancylostoma braziliense*. Larvae in contaminated soil penetrate human skin; erythematous lesions form along the tracks of their migration and advance several centimeters each day. Pruritus is intense. Vesicles or bullae may form. Ivermectin (a single dose of 200 µg/kg) or albendazole (200 mg bid for 3 days) can relieve the symptoms of this self-limited infestation.

Intestinal Nematode Infections   Intestinal nematodes infect >1 billion persons worldwide in regions with poor sanitation, particularly in developing countries in the tropics or subtropics. These parasites contribute to malnutrition and diminished work capacity.

Ascariasis   *Etiology*   Ascariasis is caused by *Ascaris lumbricoides*, the largest intestinal nematode, which reaches lengths up to 40 cm. The parasite is transmitted via fecally contaminated soil.

Life Cycle   Swallowed eggs hatch in the intestine, invade the mucosa, migrate to the lungs, break into the alveoli, ascend the bronchial tree, are swallowed, reach the small intestine, mature, and produce up to 240,000 eggs per day that pass in the feces.

Clinical Features   Most infections have a low worm burden and are asymptomatic. During lung migration of the parasite, pts may develop a cough and substernal discomfort, occasionally with dyspnea or blood-tinged sputum, fever, and eosinophilia. Eosinophilic pneumonitis (Löffler's syndrome) may be evident. Heavy infections occasionally cause pain, small-bowel obstruction, perforation, volvulus, biliary obstruction and colic, or pancreatitis.

Laboratory Findings   *Ascaris* eggs (65 by 45 μm) can be found in fecal samples. Adult worms can pass in the stool or through the mouth or nose. During the transpulmonary migratory phase, larvae can be found in sputum or gastric aspirates.

 Ascariasis

A single dose of albendazole (400 mg), mebendazole (500 mg), or ivermectin (150–200 μg/kg) is effective. Pyrantel pamoate (a single dose of 11 mg/kg, up to 1 g) is safe in pregnancy.

Hookworm   *Etiology*   Two hookworm species, *Ancylostoma duodenale* and *Necator americanus*, cause human infections.

Life Cycle   Infectious larvae penetrate the skin, reach the lungs via the bloodstream, invade the alveoli, ascend the airways, are swallowed, reach the small intestine, mature into adult worms, attach to the mucosa, and suck blood and interstitial fluid.

Clinical Features   Most infections are asymptomatic. Chronic infection causes iron deficiency and—in marginally nourished persons—progressive anemia and hypoproteinemia, weakness, shortness of breath, and skin depigmentation.

Laboratory Findings   Hookworm eggs (40 by 60 μm) can be found in the feces. Stool concentration may be needed for the diagnosis of light infections.

 Hookworm

Albendazole (400 mg once), mebendazole (500 mg once), or pyrantel pamoate (11 mg/kg daily for 3 days) is effective. Nutritional support, iron replacement, and deworming are undertaken as needed.

Strongyloidiasis   *Etiology and Epidemiology*   Unlike other helminths, *Strongyloides stercoralis* can replicate in the human host, permitting ongoing cycles of autoinfection from endogenously produced larvae. Autoinfection is most common among immunocompromised hosts, including those receiving glucocorticoids. Hyperinfection and widespread larval dissemination can occur in these pts. However, severe disease due to *Strongyloides* is unusual in HIV-infected pts.

Life Cycle   Infection results when filariform larvae in fecally contaminated soil penetrate the skin or mucous membranes. Larvae travel through the bloodstream to the lungs, break through alveolar spaces, ascend the bronchial tree, are swallowed, reach the small intestine, mature into adult worms, and penetrate the mucosa of the proximal small bowel; eggs hatch in the intestinal mucosa. Rhabditiform larvae can pass with the feces into the soil or can develop into filariform larvae that penetrate the colonic wall or perianal skin and enter the circulation to establish ongoing autoinfection.

Clinical Features Uncomplicated disease is associated with mild cutaneous and/or abdominal manifestations such as urticaria, larva currens (a pathognomonic serpiginous, pruritic, erythematous eruption along the course of larval migration that may advance up to 10 cm/h), abdominal pain, nausea, diarrhea, bleeding, and weight loss. Colitis, enteritis, or malabsorption can develop. Disseminated disease involves extraintestinal tissues, including the CNS, peritoneum, liver, and kidney. Bacteremia can develop when enteric flora components enter the bloodstream through disrupted mucosal barriers. Gram-negative sepsis, pneumonia, or meningitis can complicate the disease.

Diagnosis Eosinophilia is common, with levels that fluctuate over time. Eggs are rarely found in feces because they hatch in the colon. A single stool examination detects rhabditiform larvae (~250 μm long) in about one-third of uncomplicated infections. Duodenojejunal contents can be sampled if stool examinations are negative. Antibodies can be detected by ELISA. In disseminated infection, filariform larvae can be found in stool or at sites of larval migration.

 Strongyloidiasis

Ivermectin (200 μg/kg daily for 2 days) is more effective than albendazole (400 mg daily for 3 days). Disseminated disease should be treated with ivermectin for ≥5–7 days.

Enterobiasis *Etiology* Enterobiasis (pinworm) is caused by *Enterobius vermicularis*.

Life Cycle Adult worms in the bowel lumen migrate nocturnally out into the perianal region, releasing immature eggs that become infective within hours. Autoinfection results from perianal scratching and transport of infective eggs to the mouth. Person-to-person spread occurs. Pinworm is common among schoolchildren and their household contacts and among institutionalized populations.

Clinical Features Perianal pruritus is the cardinal symptom and is often worst at night.

Diagnosis Eggs in the perianal region are detected by application of cellulose acetate tape in the morning. Eggs measure 55 by 25 μm and are flattened on one side.

 Enterobiasis

One dose of mebendazole (100 mg), albendazole (400 mg), or pyrantel pamoate (11 mg/kg; maximum, 1 g) is given, with the same treatment repeated after 2 weeks. Household members should also be treated.

Filarial and Related Infections Filarial worms are nematodes that dwell in the SC tissue and lymphatics. More than 170 million people are infected worldwide. Infection is established only with repeated and prolonged exposures to infective larvae. Disease tends to be more intense and acute in newly exposed individuals than in natives of endemic areas.

Life Cycle Insects transmit infective larvae to humans. Adult worms reside in lymphatics or SC tissues; their offspring are microfilariae (200–250 μm long, 5–7 μm wide) that either circulate in the blood or migrate through the skin.

Subperiodic forms are those that are present in peripheral blood at all times and peak in the afternoon. *Nocturnally periodic* forms are scarce in peripheral blood by day and increase by night. Adult worms live for years; microfilariae live for 3–36 months. A rickettsia-like endosymbiont, *Wolbachia*, is found in all stages of the four major filarial species that cause human disease and may prove to be a target for future antifilarial chemotherapy.

Lymphatic Filariasis *Etiology* *Wuchereria bancrofti*, *Brugia malayi*, or *B. timori* can reside in lymphatic channels or lymph nodes. *W. bancrofti* is most common and usually is nocturnally periodic.

Pathology Adult worms cause inflammatory damage to the lymphatics.

Clinical Features Asymptomatic microfilaremia, hydrocele, acute adenolymphangitis (ADL), and chronic lymphatic disease are the main clinical presentations. ADL is associated with high fever, lymphatic inflammation, and transient local edema. *W. bancrofti* particularly affects genital lymphatics. ADL may progress to lymphatic obstruction and elephantiasis with brawny edema, thickening of the SC tissues, and hyperkeratosis. Superinfection is a problem.

Diagnosis Detection of the parasite is difficult, but microfilariae can be found in peripheral blood, hydrocele fluid, and occasionally other body fluids. Timing of blood collection is critical. Two assays are available to detect *W. bancrofti* circulating antigens, and a polymerase chain reaction (PCR) has been developed to detect DNA of both *W. bancrofti* and *B. malayi* in the blood. High-frequency ultrasound of the scrotum or the female breast can identify motile adult worms. Pts have eosinophilia and elevated IgE levels. The presence of antifilarial antibody supports the diagnosis, but cross-reactivity with other helminthic infections makes interpretation difficult.

℞ **Lymphatic Filariasis**

Diethylcarbamazine (DEC) given at 6 mg/kg daily for 12 days is the standard regimen, but one dose may be equally efficacious. An alternative is albendazole (400 mg bid for 21 days), but this drug may be less effective than DEC. An 8-week course of daily doxycycline, which targets *Wolbachia* endosymbionts, has significant macrofilaricidal activity and sustained microfilaricidal activity, as does a 7-day course of daily DEC/albendazole.

Prevention
- Mosquito control or personal protective equipment can minimize bites.
- Mass annual distribution of albendazole with DEC or ivermectin for community-based control reduces microfilaremia and interrupts transmission.

Onchocerciasis *Etiology* Onchocerciasis ("river blindness") is caused by *Onchocerca volvulus*, is the second leading cause of infectious blindness worldwide, and is transmitted by the bite of an infected blackfly. The blackfly vector breeds along free-flowing rivers and streams and restricts its flight to an area within several kilometers of these breeding sites.

Life Cycle Larvae develop into adult worms that are found in SC nodules (*onchocercomata*). After months or years, microfilariae migrate out of the nodules and concentrate in the dermis. Onchocerciasis affects primarily the skin, eyes, and lymph nodes. Microfilariae cause inflammation and fibrosis. Neovascularization and corneal scarring cause corneal opacities and blindness.

Clinical Features
- Skin: Pruritus and rash are the most common manifestations.
- Onchocercomata: palpable and/or visible, firm and nontender
- Ocular tissue: Conjunctivitis with photophobia is an early finding. Sclerosing keratitis, anterior uveitis, iridocyclitis, and secondary glaucoma due to anterior uveal tract deformity are complications.
- Lymphadenopathy: especially in the inguinal and femoral areas

Diagnosis   A definitive diagnosis is based on the finding of an adult worm in an excised nodule or of microfilariae in a skin snip. Eosinophilia and elevated serum IgE levels are common. Specific antibody assays and PCR to detect onchocercal DNA are available in some laboratories.

 Onchocerciasis

Nodules on the head should be excised to avoid ocular infection. Ivermectin in a single dose of 150 μg/kg, given yearly or semiannually, is the mainstay of treatment. In regions where *O. volvulus* is co-endemic with *Loa loa*, ivermectin is contraindicated because of the risk of severe posttreatment encephalopathy. Doxycycline therapy for 6 weeks may render adult female worms sterile for long periods and also targets the *Wolbachia* endosymbiont.

TREMATODES

The trematodes, or flatworms, may be classified according to the tissues invaded by the adult flukes. The life cycle involves a definitive mammalian host in which adult worms produce eggs and an intermediate host (e.g., snails) in which larval forms multiply. Worms do not multiply within the definitive host. Human infection results from either direct penetration of intact skin or ingestion.

Schistosomiasis   *Etiology*   Schistosomes are blood flukes that infect 200–300 million persons in South America, the Caribbean, Africa, the Middle East, and Southeast Asia. Five species cause human schistosomiasis: the intestinal species *Schistosoma mansoni*, *S. japonicum*, *S. mekongi*, and *S. intercalatum* and the urinary species *S. haematobium*. Infection is initiated by penetration of intact skin by infective cercariae—the form of the parasite released from snails in freshwater bodies. As they mature into schistosomes, the parasites reach the portal vein; they mate and then migrate to the venules of the bladder and ureters (*S. haematobium*) or the mesentery (*S. mansoni*, *S. japonicum*, *S. mekongi*, *S. intercalatum*) and deposit eggs. Some mature ova are extruded into the intestinal or urinary lumina, from which they may be voided and ultimately may reach water and perpetuate the life cycle. The persistence of other ova in tissues leads to a granulomatous host response and fibrosis. Factors governing disease manifestations include the intensity and duration of infection, the site of egg deposition, and the genetic characteristics of the host.

Pathogenesis   In the liver, granulomata cause presinusoidal portal blockage, hemodynamic changes (including portal hypertension), and periportal fibrosis. Similar processes occur in the bladder.

Clinical Features   Clinical manifestations vary by species, intensity of infection, and host factors.
- Cercarial invasion ("swimmers' itch"): An itchy maculopapular rash develops 2–3 days after parasitic invasion. This condition is most frequently

caused by *S. mansoni* or *S. japonicum* but is most severe if due to avian schistosomes, which invade human skin but then die in SC tissue.

- Acute schistosomiasis (Katayama fever): A serum sickness–like illness with fever, generalized lymphadenopathy, hepatosplenomegaly, and peripheral blood eosinophilia may develop during worm maturation and at the start of oviposition. Parasite-specific antibodies may be detected before eggs are seen in excreta.
- Chronic schistosomiasis causes manifestations that depend primarily on the schistosome species.
  1. Intestinal species cause colicky abdominal pain, bloody diarrhea, anemia, hepatosplenomegaly, and portal hypertension. Esophageal varices with bleeding, ascites, hypoalbuminemia, and coagulation defects are late complications.
  2. Urinary species cause dysuria, frequency, hematuria, obstruction with hydroureter and hydronephrosis, fibrosis of bladder granulomas, and late development of squamous cell carcinoma of the bladder.
  3. Granulomata and fibrosis at other sites (e.g., in the lungs and the CNS) may occur.

Diagnosis Diagnosis is based on clinical presentation, blood eosinophilia, and a positive serologic assay for schistosomal antibodies. Examination of stool or urine can yield positive results. Infection may also be diagnosed by examination of tissue samples (e.g., rectal biopsies).

Rx Schistosomiasis

Severe acute schistosomiasis requires hospitalization and supportive measures along with a consideration of glucocorticoid treatments. After the acute critical phase has resolved, praziquantel results in parasitologic cure in ~85% of cases. The recommended doses are 20 mg/kg bid for 1 day for *S. mansoni*, *S. intercalatum*, and *S. haematobium* infections and 20 mg/kg tid for 1 day for *S. japonicum* and *S. mekongi* infections. Late established manifestations, such as fibrosis, do not improve with treatment.

Prevention Travelers should avoid contact with all freshwater bodies.

Liver (Biliary) Flukes Stool ova and parasite (O & P) examination diagnoses infection with liver flukes.

- Clonorchiasis and opisthorchiasis occur in Southeast Asia. Infection is acquired by ingestion of contaminated raw freshwater fish. Chronic infection causes cholangitis, cholangiohepatitis, and biliary obstruction and is associated with cholangiocarcinoma. Therapy for acute infection consists of praziquantel administration (25 mg/kg tid for 1 day).
- Fascioliasis is endemic in sheep-raising countries. Infection is acquired by ingestion of contaminated aquatic plants (e.g., watercress). Acute disease causes fever, right upper quadrant (RUQ) pain, hepatomegaly, and eosinophilia. Chronic infection is associated with bile duct obstruction and biliary cirrhosis. For treatment, triclabendazole is given as a single dose of 10 mg/kg.

Lung Flukes Infection with *Paragonimus* spp. is acquired by ingestion of contaminated crayfish and freshwater crabs. Acute infection causes lung hemorrhage, necrosis with cyst formation, and parenchymal eosinophilic infiltrates. A productive cough, with brownish or bloody sputum, in association with peripheral blood eosinophilia is the usual presentation in pts with heavy infection. In chronic cases, bronchitis or bronchiectasis may predominate. CNS disease can also occur and can result in seizures. The diagnosis is made by O & P examination of sputum or stool. Praziquantel (25 mg/kg tid for 2 days) is the therapeutic agent of choice.

CESTODES

The cestodes, or tapeworms, can be classified into two groups, according to whether humans are the definitive or the intermediate hosts. The tapeworm attaches to intestinal mucosa via sucking cups or hooks located on the scolex. Proglottids (segments) form behind the scolex and constitute the bulk of the tapeworm. Eggs of the various *Taenia* species are identical; thus diagnosis to the species level relies on differences in the morphology of the scolex or proglottids.

Taeniasis Saginata   *Etiology and Pathogenesis*   Humans are the definitive host for *Taenia saginata*, the beef tapeworm, which inhabits the upper jejunum. Eggs are excreted in feces and ingested by cattle or other herbivores; larvae encyst (cysticerci) in the striated muscles of these animals. When humans ingest raw or undercooked beef, the cysticerci mature into adult worms.

Clinical Features   Pts may experience perianal discomfort, mild abdominal pain, nausea, change in appetite, weakness, and weight loss.

Diagnosis   The diagnosis is made by detection of eggs or proglottids in the stool. Eggs may be found in the perianal area. Eosinophilia may develop, and IgE levels may be elevated.

 Taeniasis Saginata

Praziquantel is given in a single dose of 10 mg/kg.

Taeniasis Solium and Cysticercosis   *Etiology and Pathogenesis*   Humans are the definitive host and pigs the usual intermediate host for *T. solium*, the pork tapeworm. The disease, which is due to ingestion of pork infected with cysticerci, is similar to taeniasis saginata. If humans ingest *T. solium* eggs (e.g., as a result of close contact with a tapeworm carrier or via autoinfection), they develop cysticercosis. Larvae penetrate the intestinal wall and are carried to many tissues, where cysticerci develop.

Clinical Features

- Intestinal infections: Epigastric discomfort, nausea, a sensation of hunger, weight loss, and diarrhea can occur, but most infections are asymptomatic.
- Cysticercosis: Cysticerci can be found anywhere in the body but most often are detected in the brain, skeletal muscle, SC tissue, or eye. Neurologic manifestations are most common and include seizures due to inflammation surrounding cysticerci in the brain, hydrocephalus (from obstruction of cerebrospinal fluid flow by cysticerci and accompanying inflammation or by arachnoiditis), headache, nausea, vomiting, changes in vision, dizziness, ataxia, and confusion.

Diagnosis   Intestinal infection is diagnosed by detection of eggs or proglottids in stool. A consensus conference has delineated criteria for the diagnosis of cysticercosis (Table 116-1). Findings on neuroimaging include cystic lesions with or without enhancement, one or more nodular calcifications, or focal enhancing lesions.

TABLE 116-1 **DIAGNOSTIC CRITERIA FOR HUMAN CYSTICERCOSIS**[a]

1. Absolute criteria
   a. Demonstration of cysticerci by histologic or microscopic examination of biopsy material
   b. Visualization of the parasite in the eye by funduscopy
   c. Neuroradiologic demonstration of cystic lesions containing a characteristic scolex
2. Major criteria
   a. Neuroradiologic lesions suggestive of neurocysticercosis
   b. Demonstration of antibodies to cysticerci in serum by enzyme-linked immunoelectrotransfer blot
   c. Resolution of intracranial cystic lesions spontaneously or after therapy with albendazole or praziquantel alone
3. Minor criteria
   a. Lesions compatible with neurocysticercosis detected by neuroimaging studies
   b. Clinical manifestations suggestive of neurocysticercosis
   c. Demonstration of antibodies to cysticerci or cysticercal antigen in CSF by ELISA
   d. Evidence of cysticercosis outside the CNS (e.g., cigar-shaped soft tissue calcifications)
4. Epidemiologic criteria
   a. Residence in a cysticercosis-endemic area
   b. Frequent travel to a cysticercosis-endemic area
   c. Household contact with an individual infected with *Taenia solium*

[a]Diagnosis is confirmed by either one absolute criterion or a combination of two major criteria, one minor criterion, and one epidemiologic criterion. A probable diagnosis is supported by the fulfillment of (1) one major criterion plus two minor criteria; (2) one major criterion plus one minor criterion and one epidemiologic criterion; or (3) three minor criteria plus one epidemiologic criterion.
Note: CSF, cerebrospinal fluid; ELISA, enzyme-linked immunosorbent assay; CNS, central nervous system.
Source: Modified from Del Brutto et al.

℞ Taeniasis Solium and Cysticercosis

Intestinal infections respond to a single dose of praziquantel (10 mg/kg). Neurocysticercosis can be treated with albendazole (15 mg/kg per day for 8–28 days) or praziquantel (50–60 mg/kg daily in 3 divided doses for 15–30 days). Pts should be carefully monitored, given the potential for an inflammatory response to treatment, and high-dose glucocorticoids should be used during treatment. Since glucocorticoids induce praziquantel metabolism, cimetidine should be given with praziquantel to inhibit this effect. Supportive measures include antiepileptic administration and treatment of hydrocephalus as indicated.

Echinococcosis   *Etiology and Pathogenesis*   Echinococcosis is an infection of humans that is caused by *Echinococcus* larvae. The adult worm of *E. granulosus* lives in the jejunum of dogs and releases eggs that humans may ingest. Disease is prevalent in areas where livestock is raised in association with dogs. After ingestion, embryos escape from the eggs, penetrate the intestinal mucosa, enter the portal circulation, and are carried to many organs but particularly the liver and lungs. Larvae develop into fluid-filled unilocular hydatid cysts within which daughter cysts develop, as do germinating cystic structures. Cysts expand over years. *E. multilocularis*, found in arctic or subarctic regions, is similar, but rodents are the intermediate hosts. The parasite is multilocular, and vesicles progressively invade host tissue by peripheral extension of processes from the germinal layer.

Clinical Features Expanding cysts exert the effects of space-occupying lesions, causing symptoms in the affected organ. Pts with hepatic disease most commonly present with abdominal pain or a palpable mass in the RUQ. Compression of a bile duct may cause biliary obstruction or may mimic cholelithiasis. Rupture or leakage from a hydatid cyst may cause fever, pruritus, urticaria, eosinophilia, or anaphylaxis. Pulmonary cysts may rupture into the bronchial tree or the peritoneal cavity and cause cough, chest pain, or hemoptysis. Rupture of cysts may result in multifocal dissemination. *E. multilocularis* disease may present as a hepatic tumor, with destruction of the liver and extension into vital structures.

Diagnosis Radiographic imaging is important in evaluating echinococcal cysts. Daughter cysts within a larger cyst are pathognomonic of *E. granulosus*. Eggshell or mural calcification on CT is also indicative of *E. granulosus* infections. Serology may be useful but can be negative in up to half of pts with lung cysts. Serology is usually positive in pts with hepatic disease. Aspiration of cysts usually is not attempted because leakage of cyst fluid can cause dissemination or anaphylactic reactions.

℞ Echinococcosis

Ultrasound staging is recommended for *E. granulosus* infection. Therapy is based on considerations of the size, location, and manifestations of cysts and the overall health of the pt. For some uncomplicated lesions, percutaneous aspiration, infusion of scolicidal agents, and reaspiration are recommended. Albendazole (15 mg/kg daily in 2 divided doses for 4 days before the procedure and for at least 4 weeks afterward) is given for prophylaxis of secondary peritoneal echinococcosis due to inadvertent spillage of fluid during this treatment. Surgery is the treatment of choice for complicated *E. granulosus* cysts. Albendazole should also be given prophylactically, as just described. Praziquantel (50 mg/kg daily for 2 weeks) may hasten the death of protoscolices. Medical therapy alone with albendazole for 12 weeks to 6 months results in cure in ~30% of cases and in clinical improvement in another 50%. *E. multilocularis* infection is treated surgically, and albendazole is given for at least 2 years after presumptively curative surgery. If surgery is not curative, albendazole should be continued indefinitely.

Diphyllobothriasis *Diphyllobothrium latum*, the longest tapeworm (up to 25 cm), attaches to the ileal and occasionally the jejunal mucosa. Humans are infected by eating raw fish. Symptoms are rare and usually mild, but infection can cause vitamin B_{12} deficiency because the tapeworm absorbs large amounts of vitamin B_{12} and interferes with ileal B_{12} absorption. Up to 2% of infected pts, especially the elderly, have megaloblastic anemia resembling pernicious anemia and can suffer neurologic sequelae due to B_{12} deficiency. The diagnosis is made by detection of eggs in the stool. Praziquantel (5–10 mg/kg once) is highly effective.

ECTOPARASITES

Ectoparasites are arthropods or helminths that infest the skin of other animals, from which they derive sustenance. These organisms can incidentally inflict direct injury, elicit hypersensitivity, or inoculate toxins or pathogens.

Scabies *Etiology* Scabies is caused by the human itch mite *Sarcoptes scabiei.*

Life Cycle and Epidemiology Gravid female mites burrow beneath the stratum corneum, deposit eggs that mature in 2 weeks, and emerge as adults to reinvade the same or another host. Scabies transmission is facilitated by intimate contact with an infested person and by crowding, uncleanliness, or contact with multiple sexual partners. The itching and rash are due to a sensitization reaction against excreta of the mite. Immunity and associated scratching limit most infestations to <15 mites per person. Norwegian or crusted scabies—hyperinfestation with thousands of mites—is associated with glucocorticoid use and immunodeficiency diseases.

Clinical Features Itching is worst at night and after a hot shower. Burrows appear as dark wavy lines that end in a pearly bleb containing the female mite. Most lesions are between the fingers or on the volar wrists, elbows, and penis. Bacterial superinfection can occur.

Diagnosis Scrapings from unroofed burrows reveal the mite, its eggs, or fecal pellets.

 Scabies

Permethrin cream (5%) should be applied thinly behind the ears and from the neck down after bathing and removed 8 h later with soap and water. A dose of ivermectin (200 µg/kg) is also effective but is not yet approved by the U.S. Food and Drug Administration for scabies treatment. For crusted scabies, first a keratolytic agent (e.g., 6% salicylic acid) and then scabicides are applied to the scalp, face, and ears in addition to the rest of the body. Two doses of ivermectin, separated by an interval of 1–2 weeks, may be required in pts with crusted scabies. Itching and hypersensitivity may persist for weeks or months in scabies and should be managed with symptom-based treatment. Bedding and clothing should be washed in hot water and dried in a heated dryer, and close contacts should be treated to prevent reinfestations.

Pediculiasis *Etiology and Epidemiology* Nymphs and adults of human lice— *Pediculus capitis* (the head louse), *P. humanus* (the body louse), and *Pthirus pubis* (the pubic louse)—feed at least once a day and ingest human blood exclusively. The saliva of these lice produces an irritating rash in sensitized persons. Eggs are cemented firmly to hair or clothing, and empty eggs (nits) remain affixed for months after hatching. Lice are generally transmitted from person to person. Head lice are transmitted among schoolchildren and body lice among persons who do not change their clothes often; pubic lice are usually transmitted sexually. The body louse is a vector for the transmission of diseases such as louse-borne typhus, relapsing fever, and trench fever.

Diagnosis The diagnosis can be suspected if nits are detected, but confirmatory measures should include the demonstration of a live louse.

 Pediculiasis

If live lice are found, treatment with 1% permethrin (two 10-min applications 10 days apart) is usually adequate. If this course fails, treatment for ≤12 h with 0.5% malathion may be indicated. Ivermectin may be useful in cases resistant to permethrin and malathion. Eyelid infestations should be treated with petrolatum applied for 3–4 days. The hair should be combed with a fine-toothed comb to remove nits. Pediculicides applied from head to foot may be needed in hirsute pts to remove body lice. Clothes and bedding should be deloused by placement in a hot dryer for 30 minutes or by heat pressing.

Myiasis In this infestation, maggots invade living or necrotic tissue or body cavities and produce clinical syndromes that vary with the species of fly. In wound and body-cavity myiasis, flies are attracted to blood and pus, and newly hatched larvae enter wounds or diseased skin. Treatment consists of maggot removal and tissue debridement.

Leech Infestations Medicinal leeches can reduce venous congestion in surgical flaps or replanted body parts. *Aeromonas hydrophila* colonizes the gullets of commercially available leeches.

For a more detailed discussion, see Reed SL, Davis CE: Laboratory Diagnosis of Parasitic Infections, Chap. e16; and Moore TA: Pharmacology of Agents Used to Treat Parasitic Infections, Chap. e17, in *Harrison's Online*; and Moore TA: Agents Used to Treat Parasitic Infections, Chap. 201, p. 1270; Weller PF: *Trichinella* and Other Tissue Nematodes, Chap. 209, p. 1316; Weller PF, Nutman TB: Intestinal Nematodes, Chap. 210, p. 1319; Nutman TB, Weller PF: Filarial and Related Infections, Chap. 211, p. 1324; Mahmoud AAF: Schistosomiasis and Other Trematode Infections, Chap. 212, p. 1330; White AC Jr, Weller PF: Cestodes, Chap. 213, p. 1336; and Pollack RJ, Maguire JH: Ectoparasite Infestations and Arthropod Bites and Stings, Chap. 392, p. 2748, in HPIM-17.

117 Physical Examination of the Heart

General examination of a pt with suspected heart disease should include vital signs (respiratory rate, pulse, blood pressure), skin color (e.g., cyanosis, pallor), clubbing, edema, evidence of decreased perfusion (cool and sweaty skin), and hypertensive changes in optic fundi. Examine abdomen for evidence of hepatomegaly, ascites, or abdominal aortic aneurysm. An ankle-brachial index (systolic bp at ankle divided by arm systolic bp) <0.9 indicates lower extremity arterial obstructive disease. Important findings on cardiovascular examination include:

CAROTID ARTERY PULSE (Fig. 117-1)

- *Pulsus parvus*: Weak upstroke due to decreased stroke volume (hypovolemia, LV failure, aortic or mitral stenosis).
- *Pulsus tardus*: Delayed upstroke (aortic stenosis).
- *Bounding (hyperkinetic) pulse*: Hyperkinetic circulation, aortic regurgitation, patent ductus arteriosus, marked vasodilatation.
- *Pulsus bisferiens*: Double systolic pulsation in aortic regurgitation, hypertrophic cardiomyopathy.
- *Pulsus alternans*: Regular alteration in pulse pressure amplitude (severe LV dysfunction).
- *Pulsus paradoxus*: Exaggerated inspiratory fall (>10 mmHg) in systolic bp (pericardial tamponade, severe obstructive lung disease).

JUGULAR VENOUS PULSATION (JVP)

Jugular venous distention develops in right-sided heart failure, constrictive pericarditis, pericardial tamponade, obstruction of superior vena cava. JVP normally

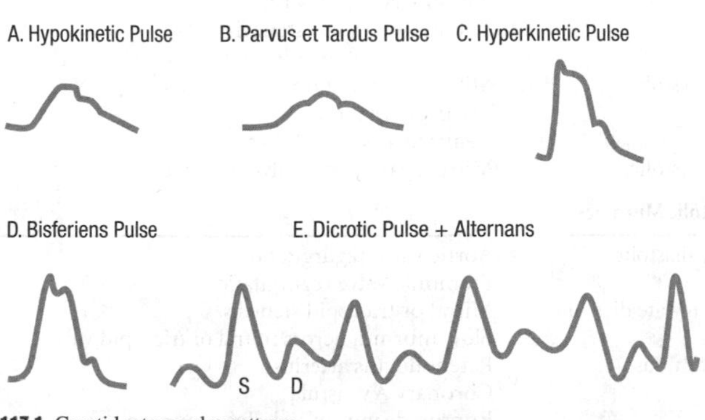

A. Hypokinetic Pulse   B. Parvus et Tardus Pulse   C. Hyperkinetic Pulse

D. Bisferiens Pulse   E. Dicrotic Pulse + Alternans

FIGURE 117-1 Carotid artery pulse patterns.

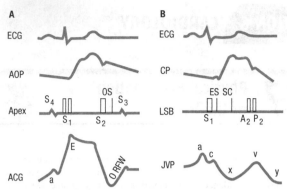

FIGURE 117-2 *A.* Schematic representation of electrocardiogram, aortic pressure pulse (AOP), phonocardiogram recorded at the apex, and apex cardiogram (ACG). On the phonocardiogram, S_1, S_2, S_3, and S_4 represent the first through fourth heart sounds; OS represents the opening snap of the mitral valve, which occurs coincident with the O point of the apex cardiogram. S_3 occurs coincident with the termination of the rapid-filling wave (RFW) of the ACG, while S_4 occurs coincident with the *a* wave of the ACG. *B.* Simultaneous recording of electrocardiogram, indirect carotid pulse (CP), phonocardiogram along the left sternal border (LSB), and indirect jugular venous pulse (JVP). ES, ejection sound; SC, systolic click.

falls with inspiration but may rise (Kussmaul's sign) in constrictive pericarditis. Abnormalities in examination include:

- *Large "a" wave*: Tricuspid stenosis (TS), pulmonic stenosis, AV dissociation (right atrium contracts against closed tricuspid valve).
- *Large "v" wave*: Tricuspid regurgitation, atrial septal defect.
- *Steep "y" descent*: Constrictive pericarditis.
- *Slow "y" descent*: Tricuspid stenosis.

TABLE 117-1   HEART MURMURS

Systolic Murmurs	
Ejection-type	Aortic outflow tract
	Aortic valve stenosis
	Hypertrophic obstructive cardiomyopathy
	Aortic flow murmur
	Pulmonary outflow tract
	Pulmonic valve stenosis
	Pulmonic flow murmur
Holosystolic	Mitral regurgitation
	Tricuspid regurgitation
	Ventricular septal defect
Late-systolic	Mitral or tricuspid valve prolapse
Diastolic Murmurs	
Early diastolic	Aortic valve regurgitation
	Pulmonic valve regurgitation
Mid-to-late diastolic	Mitral or tricuspid stenosis
	Flow murmur across mitral or tricuspid valves
Continuous	Patent ductus arteriosus
	Coronary AV fistula
	Ruptured sinus of Valsalva aneurysm

PRECORDIAL PALPATION

Cardiac apical impulse is normally localized in the fifth intercostal space, mid-clavicular line (Fig. 117-2). Abnormalities include:

- *Forceful apical thrust*: Left ventricular hypertrophy.
- *Lateral and downward displacement of apex impulse*: Left ventricular dilatation.
- *Prominent presystolic impulse*: Hypertension, aortic stenosis, hypertrophic cardiomyopathy.
- *Double systolic apical impulse*: Hypertrophic cardiomyopathy.
- *Sustained "lift" at lower left sternal border*: Right ventricular hypertrophy.
- *Dyskinetic (outward bulge) impulse*: Ventricular aneurysm, large dyskinetic area post MI, cardiomyopathy.

AUSCULTATION

HEART SOUNDS (Fig. 117-2)

S_1 *Loud*: Mitral stenosis, short PR interval, hyperkinetic heart, thin chest wall. *Soft*: Long PR interval, heart failure, mitral regurgitation, thick chest wall, pulmonary emphysema.

TABLE 117-2	**EFFECTS OF PHYSIOLOGIC AND PHARMACOLOGIC INTERVENTIONS ON THE INTENSITY OF HEART MURMURS AND SOUNDS**
Respiration	Systolic murmurs due to TR or pulmonic blood flow through a normal or stenotic valve and diastolic murmurs of TS or PR generally increase with inspiration, as do right-sided S_3 and S_4. Left-sided murmurs and sounds usually are louder during expiration, as is the PES.
Valsalva maneuver	Most murmurs decrease in length and intensity. Two exceptions are the systolic murmur of HCM, which usually becomes much louder, and that of MVP, which becomes longer and often louder. Following release of the Valsalva maneuver, right-sided murmurs tend to return to control intensity earlier than left-sided murmurs.
After VPB or AF	Murmurs originating at normal or stenotic semilunar valves increase in the cardiac cycle following a VPB or in the cycle after a long cycle length in AF. By contrast, systolic murmurs due to AV valve regurgitation either do not change, diminish (papillary muscle dysfunction), or become shorter (MVP).
Positional changes	With *standing*, most murmurs diminish, two exceptions being the murmur of HCM, which becomes louder, and that of MVP, which lengthens and often is intensified. With *squatting*, most murmurs become louder, but those of HCM and MVP usually soften and may disappear. Passive leg raising usually produces the same results.
Exercise	Murmurs due to blood flow across normal or obstructed valves (e.g., PS, MS) become louder with both isotonic and submaximal isometric (handgrip) exercise. Murmurs of MR, VSD, and AR also increase with handgrip exercise. However, the murmur of HCM often decreases with near maximum handgrip exercise. Left-sided S_4 and S_3 are often accentuated by exercise, particularly when due to ischemic heart disease.

Note: TR, tricuspid regurgitation; TS, tricuspid stenosis; PR, pulmonic regurgitation; HCM, hypertrophic cardiomyopathy; MVP, mitral valve prolapse; PS, pulmonic stenosis; MS, mitral stenosis; MR, mitral regurgitation; PES, pulmonic ejection sound; VSD, ventricular septal defect; AR, aortic regurgitation; VPB, ventricular premature beat; AF, atrial fibrillation.

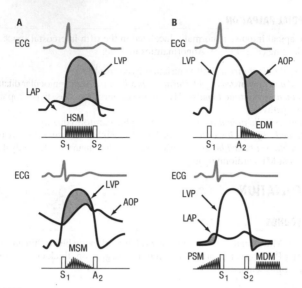

FIGURE 117-3 *A.* Schematic representation of ECG, aortic pressure (AOP), left ventricular pressure (LVP), and left atrial pressure (LAP). The gray areas indicated a transvalvular pressure difference during systole. HSM, holosystolic murmur; MSM, midsystolic murmur. *B.* Graphic representation of ECG, aortic pressure (AOP), left ventricular pressure (LVP), and left atrial pressure (LAP) with gray areas indicating transvalvular diastolic pressure difference. EDM, early diastolic murmur; PSM, presystolic murmur; MDM, middiastolic murmur.

S_2 Normally A_2 precedes P_2 and splitting increases with inspiration; abnormalities include:

- *Widened* splitting: Right bundle branch block, pulmonic stenosis, mitral regurgitation.
- *Fixed* splitting (no respiratory change in splitting): Atrial septal defect.
- *Narrow* splitting: Pulmonary hypertension.
- *Paradoxical* splitting (splitting narrows with inspiration): Aortic stenosis, left bundle branch block, CHF.
- *Loud* A_2: Systemic hypertension.
- *Soft* A_2: Aortic stenosis (AS).
- *Loud* P_2: Pulmonary arterial hypertension.
- *Soft* P_2: Pulmonic stenosis (PS).

S_3 Low-pitched, heard best with bell of stethoscope at apex, following S_2; normal in children; after age 30–35, indicates LV failure or volume overload.

S_4 Low-pitched, heard best with bell at apex, preceding S_1; reflects atrial contraction into a noncompliant ventricle; found in AS, hypertension, hypertrophic cardiomyopathy, and coronary artery disease (CAD).

Opening Snap (OS)   High-pitched; follows S_2 (by 0.06–0.12 s), heard at lower left sternal border and apex in mitral stenosis (MS); the more severe the MS, the shorter the S_2–OS interval.

Ejection Clicks   High-pitched sounds following S_1; observed in dilatation of aortic root or pulmonary artery, congenital AS (loudest at apex) or PS (upper left sternal border); the latter decreases with inspiration.

Midsystolic Clicks   At lower left sternal border and apex, often followed by late systolic murmur in mitral valve prolapse.

HEART MURMURS   (Tables 117-1 and 117-2, Fig. 117-3)

Systolic Murmurs   May be "crescendo-decrescendo" ejection type, pansystolic, or late systolic; right-sided murmurs (e.g., tricuspid regurgitation) typically increase with inspiration.

Diastolic Murmurs

- *Early diastolic murmurs*: Begin immediately after S_2, are high-pitched, and are usually caused by aortic or pulmonary regurgitation.
- *Mid-to-late diastolic murmurs*: Low-pitched, heard best with bell of stethoscope; observed in MS or TS; less commonly due to atrial myxoma.
- *Continuous murmurs*: Present in systole and diastole (envelops S_2); found in patent ductus arteriosus and sometimes in coarctation of aorta; less common causes are systemic or coronary AV fistula, aortopulmonary septal defect, ruptured aneurysm of sinus of Valsalva.

For a more detailed discussion, see O'Rourke RA, Braunwald E: Physical Examination of the Cardiovascular System, Chap. 220, p. 1382, in HPIM-17.

118 Electrocardiography

STANDARD APPROACH TO THE ECG

Normally, standardization is 1.0 mV per 10 mm, and paper speed is 25 mm/s (each horizontal small box = 0.04 s).

Heart Rate   Beats/min = 300 divided by the number of *large* boxes (each 5 mm apart) between consecutive QRS complexes. For faster heart rates, divide 1500 by number of *small* boxes (1 mm apart) between each QRS.

Rhythm   *Sinus rhythm* is present if every P wave is followed by a QRS, PR interval ≥ 0.12 s, every QRS is preceded by a P wave, and the P wave is upright in leads I, II, and III. Arrhythmias are discussed in Chaps. 129 and 130.

Mean Axis   If QRS is primarily positive in limb leads I and II, then axis is *normal*. Otherwise, find limb lead in which QRS is most isoelectric (R = S). The mean axis is perpendicular to that lead (Fig. 118-1). If the QRS complex is *positive* in that perpendicular lead, then mean axis is in the direction of that lead; if *negative*, then mean axis points directly away from that lead.

   Left-axis deviation (more negative than –30°) occurs in diffuse left ventricular disease, inferior MI; also in left anterior hemiblock (small R, deep S in leads II, III, and aVF).

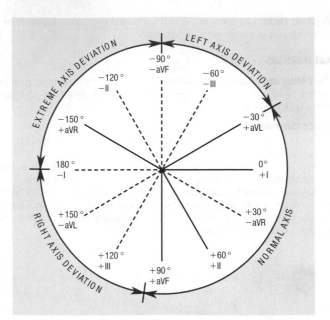

FIGURE 118-1 Electrocardiographic lead systems: The hexaxial frontal plane reference system to estimate electrical axis. Determine leads in which QRS deflections are maximum and minimum. For example, a maximum positive QRS in I which is isoelectric in aVF is oriented to 0°. Normal axis ranges from −30° to +90°. An axis > +90° is right-axis deviation and < 30° is left-axis deviation.

Right-axis deviation (>90°) occurs in right ventricular hypertrophy (R > S in V_1) and left posterior hemiblock (small Q and tall R in leads II, III, and aVF). Mild right-axis deviation is seen in thin, healthy individuals (up to 110°).

Intervals (Normal Values in Parentheses)
PR (0.12–0.20 s)
- *Short:* (1) preexcitation syndrome (look for slurred QRS upstroke due to "delta" wave), (2) nodal rhythm (inverted P in aVF).
- *Long:* first-degree AV block (Chap. 129).

QRS (0.06–0.10 s)   *Widened:* (1) ventricular premature beats, (2) bundle branch blocks: *right* (RsR′ in V_1, deep S in V_6) and *left* [RR′ in V_6 (Fig. 118-2)], (3) toxic levels of certain drugs (e.g., quinidine), (4) severe hypokalemia.

QT (<50% of RR interval; corrected QT ≤ 0.44 s)   *Prolonged:* congenital, hypokalemia, hypocalcemia, drugs (e.g., quinidine, procainamide, tricyclics).

Hypertrophy
- *Right atrium:* P wave ≥ 2.5 mm in lead II.
- *Left atrium:* P biphasic (positive, then negative) in V_1, with terminal negative force wider than 0.04 s.
- *Right ventricle:* R > S in V_1 and R in V_1 > 5 mm; deep S in V_6; right-axis deviation.
- *Left ventricle:* S in V_1 plus R in V_5 or V_6 ≥ 35 mm or R in aVL > 11 mm.

Infarction (Figs. 118-3 and 118-4)   *Q-wave MI:* Pathologic Q waves (≥0.04 s and ≥25% of total QRS height) in leads shown in Table 118-1; acute *non-Q-*

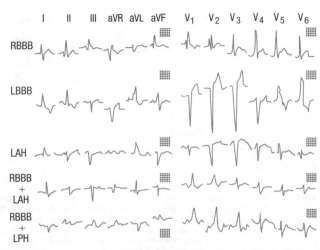

I   II   III   aVR   aVL   aVF   V₁   V₂   V₃   V₄   V₅   V₆

RBBB

LBBB

LAH

RBBB + LAH

RBBB + LPH

FIGURE 118-2 Intraventricular conduction abnormalities. Illustrated are right bundle branch block (RBBB); left bundle branch block (LBBB); left anterior hemiblock (LAH); right bundle branch block with left anterior hemiblock (RBBB + LAH); and right bundle branch block with left posterior hemiblock (RBBB + LPH). (*Reproduced from RJ Myerburg: HPIM-12.*)

wave MI shows ST-T changes in these leads without Q wave development. A number of conditions (other than acute MI) can cause Q waves (Table 118-2).

ST-T Waves

- *ST elevation*: Acute MI, coronary spasm, pericarditis (concave upward) (see Fig. 123-1 and Table 123-2), LV aneurysm, Brugada pattern (RBBB with ST elevation in V_1–V_2).
- *ST depression*: Digitalis effect, strain (due to ventricular hypertrophy), ischemia, or nontransmural MI.

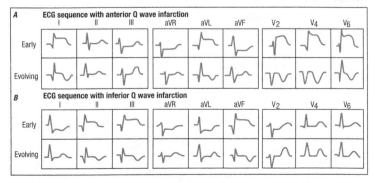

FIGURE 118-3 Sequence of depolarization and repolarization changes with (*A*) acute anterior and (*B*) acute inferior wall Q-wave infarctions. With anterior infarcts, ST elevation in leads I, aVL, and the precordial leads may be accompanied by reciprocal ST depressions in leads II, III, and aVF. Conversely, acute inferior (or posterior) infarcts may be associated with reciprocal ST depressions in leads V_1 to V_3. (*After AL Goldberger: Clinical Electrocardiography: A Simplified Approach, 7th ed. St. Louis, Mosby/Elsevier, 2006.*)

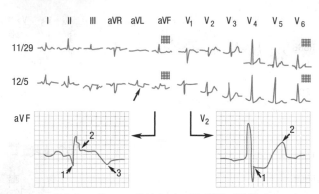

FIGURE 118-4 Acute inferior wall myocardial infarction. The ECG of 11/29 shows minor nonspecific ST-segment and T-wave changes. On 12/5 an acute myocardial infarction occurred. There are pathologic Q waves (1), ST-segment elevation (2), and terminal T-wave inversion (3) in leads II, III, and aVF indicating the location of the infarct on the inferior wall. Reciprocal changes in aVL (small arrow). Increasing R-wave voltage with ST depression and increased voltage of the T wave in V_2 are characteristic of true posterior wall extension of the inferior infarction. (*Reproduced from RJ Myerburg: HPIM-12.*)

TABLE 118-1	LEADS WITH ABNORMAL Q WAVES IN MI
Leads with Abnormal Q Waves	**Site of Infarction**
V_1–V_2	Anteroseptal
V_3–V_4	Apical
I, aVL, V_5–V_6	Anterolateral
II, III, aVF	Inferior
V_1–V_2 (tall R, *not* deep Q)	True posterior

TABLE 118-2	DIFFERENTIAL DIAGNOSIS OF Q WAVES (WITH SELECTED EXAMPLES)

Physiologic or positional factors
1. Normal variant "septal" Q waves
2. Normal variant Q waves in V_1 to V_2, aVL, III, and aVF
3. Left pneumothorax or dextrocardia
Myocardial injury or infiltration
1. Acute processes: myocardial ischemia or infarction, myocarditis, hyperkalemia
2. Chronic processes: myocardial infarction, idiopathic cardiomyopathy, myocarditis, amyloid, tumor, sarcoid, scleroderma
Ventricular hypertrophy/enlargement
1. Left ventricular (poor R-wave progression)[a]
2. Right ventricular (reversed R-wave progression)
3. Hypertrophic cardiomyopathy
Conduction abnormalities
1. Left bundle branch block
2. Wolff-Parkinson-White patterns

[a]Small or absent R waves in the right to midprecordial leads.
Source: After AL Goldberger: *Myocardial Infarction: Electrocardiographic Differential Diagnosis*, 4th ed. St. Louis, Mosby-Year Book, 1991.

- *Tall peaked T*: Hyperkalemia; acute MI ("hyperacute T").
- *Inverted T*: Non-Q-wave MI, ventricular "strain" pattern, drug effect (e.g., digitalis), hypokalemia, hypocalcemia, increased intracranial pressure (e.g., subarachnoid bleed).

For a more detailed discussion, see Goldberger AL: Electrocardiography, Chap. 221, p. 1398 in HPIM-17.

119 Noninvasive Examination of the Heart

ECHOCARDIOGRAPHY (Table 119-1 and Fig. 119-1)

Visualizes heart in real time with ultrasound; Doppler recordings noninvasively assess hemodynamics and abnormal flow patterns. Imaging may be compromised in patients with chronic obstructive lung disease, thick chest wall, or narrow intercostal spaces.

Chamber Size and Ventricular Performance Size of atria and ventricles can be accurately measured. Global and regional systolic wall motion abnormalities of both ventricles can be assessed; ventricular hypertrophy/infiltration may be visualized; evidence of pulmonary hypertension may be obtained. RV systolic pressure (RVSP) is calculated from maximum velocity of tricuspid regurgitation (TR):

$$RVSP = 4 \times (TR \text{ velocity})^2 + RA \text{ pressure}$$

(RA pressure is same as JVP estimated by physical exam). In absence of RV outflow obstruction, RVSP = pulmonary artery systolic pressure.

LV diastolic function is assessed by transmitral Doppler (see Fig. 222-5, page 1399 in HPIM-17) and Doppler tissue imaging, which measures velocity of myocardial relaxation.

TABLE 119-1   CLINICAL USES OF ECHOCARDIOGRAPHY

2-D echo	Transesophageal echocardiography
Cardiac chambers: size, hypertrophy, wall motion abnormalities	Superior to 2-D echo to identify:
	Infective endocarditis
Valves: morphology and motion	Cardiac source of embolism
Pericardium: effusion, tamponade	Prosthetic valve dysfunction
Aorta: Aneurysm, dissection	Aortic dissection
Assess intracardiac masses	**Stress echocardiography**
Doppler echocardiography	Assess myocardial ischemia and viability
Valvular stenosis and regurgitation	ability
Intracardiac shunts	
Diastolic filling/dysfunction	
Approximate intracardiac pressures	

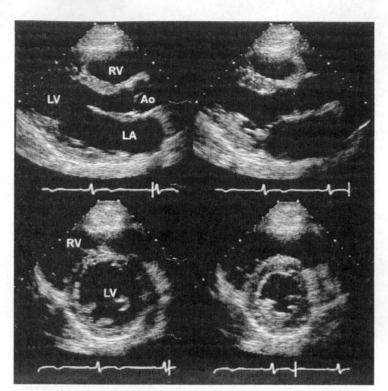

FIGURE 119-1 Two-dimensional echocardiographic still-frame images of a normal heart. *Upper*: Parasternal long axis view during systole and diastole (*left*) and systole (*right*). During systole, there is thickening of the myocardium and reduction in the size of the left ventricle (LV). The valve leaflets are thin and open widely. *Lower*: Parasternal short axis view during diastole (*left*) and systole (*right*) demonstrating a decrease in the left ventricular cavity size during systole as well as an increase in wall thickness. LA, left atrium; RV, right ventricle; Ao, aorta. (*Reproduced from RJ Myerburg in HPIM-12.*)

Valvular Abnormalities   Thickness, mobility, calcification, and regurgitation of each cardiac valve can be assessed. Severity of valvular stenosis is calculated by Doppler [peak gradient = $4 \times$ (peak velocity)^2]. Structural lesions (e.g., flail leaflet, vegetation) resulting in regurgitation may be identified and Doppler (Fig. 119-2) estimates severity of regurgitation.

Pericardial Disease   Echo is noninvasive modality of choice to rapidly identify pericardial effusion and assess its hemodynamic significance; in tamponade there is diastolic RA and RV collapse, dilatation of IVC, exaggerated respiratory alterations in transvalvular Doppler velocities. Actual thickness of pericardium (e.g., in suspected constrictive pericarditis) is better measured by CT or MRI.

Intracardiac Masses   May visualize atrial or ventricular thrombus, intracardiac tumors, and valvular vegetations. Yield of identifying cardiac source of embolism is *low* in absence of cardiac history or physical findings. Transesophageal echocardiography (TEE) is more sensitive than standard transthoracic study for masses < 1 cm in diameter.

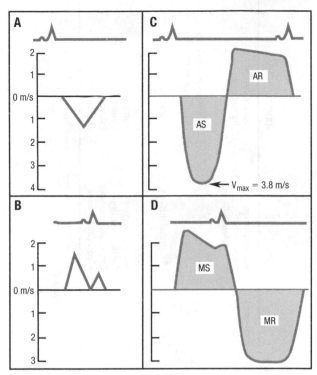

FIGURE 119-2 Schematic presentation of normal Doppler flow across the aortic (*A*) and mitral valves (*B*). Abnormal continuous wave Doppler profiles: *C.* Aortic stenosis (AS) [peak transaortic gradient = $4 \times V_{max}^2 = 4 \times (3.8)^2 = 58$ mmHg] and regurgitation (AR). *D.* Mitral stenosis (MS) and regurgitation (MR).

Aortic Disease   Aneurysm and dissection of the aorta may be evaluated and complications (aortic regurgitation, tamponade) assessed (Chap. 132) by standard transthoracic echo. TEE is more sensitive and specific for aortic dissection.

Congenital Heart Disease   (See Chap. 120)

Echo, Doppler, and contrast echo (rapid IV injection of agitated saline) are useful in identifying congenital lesions and shunts.

Stress Echocardiography   Echo performed prior to, and after, treadmill or bicycle exercise identifies regions of prior MI and inducible myocardial ischemia ($\downarrow$ regional contraction with exercise) Dobutamine pharmacologic stress echo can be substituted for patients who cannot exercise.

NUCLEAR CARDIOLOGY

Uses nuclear isotopes to assess LV perfusion and contractile function.

Ventricular Function Assessment   Blood pool imaging is obtained by injecting intravenous ^{99m}Tc-labeled albumin or RBCs to quantify LV ejection fraction. Contractile function can also be assessed during gated single photon emission CT (SPECT) myocardial perfusion exercise test imaging (see below).

TABLE 119-2 SELECTION OF IMAGING TESTS

	Echo	Nuclear	CT[a]	MRI[b]
LV Size/function	Initial modality of choice Low cost, portable Provides ancillary structural and hemo- dynamic information	Available from gated SPECT stress imaging	Best resolution Highest cost	Best resolution Highest cost
Valve disease	Initial modality of choice Valve motion Doppler hemodynamics			Visualize valve motion Delineate abnormal flow
Pericardial disease	Pericardial effusion Doppler hemodynamics		Pericardial thickening	Pericardial thickening
Aortic disease	TEE rapid diagnosis[c] Acute dissection		Image entire aorta Acute aneurysm Aortic dissection	Image entire aorta Aortic aneurysm Chronic dissection
Cardiac masses	TTE—large intracardiac masses TEE—smaller intracardiac masses[c]		Extracardiac masses Myocardial masses	Extracardiac masses Myocardial masses

Note: Echo, echocardiography; SPECT, single-photon emission CT; TEE, transesophageal echocardiography; TTE, transthoracic echocardiogram.

[a]Contrast required.
[b]Relative contraindication: pacemakers, metallic objects, claustrophobic.
[c]When not seen on TTE.

Nuclear Myocardial Perfusion Assessment SPECT imaging using ^{201}Tl or ^{99m}Tc-labeled compounds (sestamibi or tetrofosmin), obtained at peak exercise and at rest, depicts zones of prior infarction as fixed defects and regions of inducible myocardial ischemia as reversible defects. Nuclear imaging is more sensitive, but less specific, than stress echocardiography for detection of ischemia.

For patients who can't exercise, pharmacologic perfusion imaging with adenosine, dipyridamole, or dobutamine is used instead (see Chap. 128). For patients with LBBB, perfusion imaging with adenosine or dipyridamole is preferred to avoid artifactual septal defects that are common with exercise imaging.

Pharmacologic positron emission tomography scanning is especially useful in imaging obese patients and to assess myocardial viability.

MAGNETIC RESONANCE IMAGING (MRI)

Delineates cardiac structures with high resolution without ionizing radiation. Excellent technique to characterize intracardiac masses, the pericardium, great vessels, and anatomic relationships in congenital heart disease. MRI with delayed gadolinium enhancement (avoid in patients with renal insufficiency) differentiates ischemic from nonischemic cardiomyopathy and is useful in assessing myocardial viability.

COMPUTED TOMOGRAPHY (CT)

Provides high-resolution images of cardiac structures and detects coronary calcification in atherosclerosis with high sensitivity (but low specificity). CT angiography delineates abnormalities of the great vessels, including aortic aneurysms and dissection, and pulmonary embolism. Multislice spiral CT is evolving technology that provides high-resolution images of coronary anatomy; it is currently most useful for evaluating suspected coronary anatomic anomalies and to "rule out" high-grade coronary stenoses in patients with chest pain and intermediate pretest probability of coronary artery disease.

Table 119-2 summarizes key diagnostic features of the noninvasive imaging modalities.

For a more detailed discussion, see Nishimura RA, Gibbons RJ, Glockner JF, Tajik AJ: Noninvasive Cardiac Imaging: Echocardiography, Nuclear Cardiology, and MRI/CT Imaging, Chap. 222, p. 1397 in HPIM-17.

120 Congenital Heart Disease in the Adult

ACYANOTIC CONGENITAL HEART LESIONS WITH LEFT-TO-RIGHT SHUNT

ATRIAL SEPTAL DEFECT (ASD)

Most common is *ostium secundum* ASD, located at mid interatrial septum. *Sinus venosus* type ASD involves the high atrial septum and may be associated with anomalous pulmonary venous drainage to the right heart. *Ostium primum* ASDs (e.g., typical of Down's syndrome) appear at lower atrial septum, adjacent to atrioventricular (AV) valves.

History   Usually asymptomatic until third or fourth decades when exertional dyspnea, fatigue, and palpitations may occur. Onset of symptoms may be associated with development of pulmonary hypertension (see below).

Physical Examination   Prominent right ventricular (RV) impulse, wide fixed splitting of S_2, systolic murmur from flow across pulmonic valve, diastolic flow rumble across tricuspid valve, prominent jugular venous v wave.

ECG   Incomplete RBBB (rSR' in right precordial leads) common. Left axis deviation frequently present with ostium primum defect.

CXR   Increased pulmonary vascular markings, prominence of right atrium (RA), RV, and main pulmonary artery (LA enlargement *not* usually present).

Echocardiogram   RA, RV, and pulmonary artery enlargement; Doppler shows abnormal turbulent transatrial flow. Echo contrast (agitated saline injection into peripheral systemic vein) may visualize transatrial shunt. Transesophageal echo usually diagnostic if transthoracic echo is ambiguous.

℞ Atrial Septal Defect

In the absence of contraindications an ASD with pulmonary-to-systemic flow ratio (PF:SF) > 2.0:1.0 should be repaired surgically or by percutaneous transcatheter closure. Surgery is contraindicated with significant pulmonary hypertension and PF:SF < 1.2:1.0. Medical management includes antiarrhythmic therapy for associated atrial fibrillation or supraventricular tachycardia (Chap. 130) and standard therapy for symptoms of heart failure (Chap. 131).

VENTRICULAR SEPTAL DEFECT (VSD)

Congenital VSDs may close spontaneously during childhood. Symptoms relate to size of the defect and pulmonary vascular resistance.

History   CHF may develop in infancy. Adults may be asymptomatic or develop fatigue and reduced exercise tolerance.

Physical Examination Systolic thrill and holosystolic murmur at lower left sternal border, loud P_2, S_3; diastolic flow murmur across mitral valve.

ECG Normal with small defects. Large shunts result in LA and LV enlargement.

CXR Enlargement of main pulmonary artery, LA, and LV, with increased pulmonary vascular markings.

Echocardiogram LA and LV enlargement; defect may be directly visualized. Color Doppler demonstrates flow across the defect.

Rx Ventricular Septal Defect

Fatigue and mild dyspnea are treated with diuretics and afterload reduction (Chap. 131). Surgical closure is indicated if PF:SF > 1.5:1 in absence of very high pulmonary vascular resistance.

PATENT DUCTUS ARTERIOSUS (PDA)

Abnormal communication between the descending aorta and pulmonary artery; associated with birth at high altitudes and maternal rubella.

History Asymptomatic or fatigue and dyspnea on exertion.

Physical Examination Hyperactive LV impulse; loud continuous "machinery" murmur at upper left sternal border. If pulmonary hypertension develops, diastolic component of the murmur may disappear.

ECG LV hypertrophy is common; RV hypertrophy if pulmonary hypertension develops.

CXR Increased pulmonary vascular markings: enlarged main pulmonary artery, LV, ascending aorta; occasionally, calcification of ductus.

Echocardiography Hyperdynamic, enlarged LV; the PDA can often be visualized on two-dimensional echo; Doppler demonstrates abnormal flow through it.

Rx Patent Ductus Arteriosus

In absence of pulmonary hypertension, PDA should be surgically ligated or divided to prevent infective endocarditis, LV dysfunction, and pulmonary hypertension. Transcatheter closure is possible in selected pts.

PROGRESSION TO PULMONARY HYPERTENSION (PHT)

Pts with large, uncorrected left-to-right shunts (e.g., ASD, VSD, or PDA) may develop progressive, irreversible PHT with reverse shunting of desaturated blood into the arterial circulation (right-to-left direction), resulting in *Eisenmenger syndrome*. Fatigue, lightheadedness, and chest pain due to RV ischemia are common, accompanied by cyanosis, clubbing of digits, loud P_2, murmur of pulmonary valve regurgitation, and signs of RV failure. ECG and echocardiogram show RV hypertrophy. Therapeutic options are limited and include pulmonary artery vasodilators and consideration of single lung transplant with repair of cardiac defect, or heart-lung transplantation.

ACYANOTIC CONGENITAL HEART LESIONS WITHOUT A SHUNT

PULMONIC STENOSIS (PS)

A transpulmonary valve gradient < 50 mmHg rarely causes symptoms, and progression tends not to occur. Higher gradients result in dyspnea, fatigue, lightheadedness, chest pain (RV ischemia).

Physical Examination   Jugular venous distention with prominent a wave, RV parasternal impulse, wide splitting of S_2 with soft P_2, ejection click followed by "diamond-shaped" systolic murmur at upper left sternal border, right-sided S_4.

ECG   Normal in mild PS; RA and RV enlargement in advanced PS.

CXR   Often shows poststenotic dilatation of the pulmonary artery and RV enlargement.

Echocardiography   RV hypertrophy and systolic "doming" of the pulmonic valve. Doppler accurately measures transvalvular gradient.

 Pulmonic Stenosis

Moderate or severe stenosis (gradient > 50 mmHg) requires surgical (or balloon) valvuloplasty.

CONGENITALLY BICUSPID AORTIC VALVE

One of the most common congenital heart malformations; rarely results in childhood aortic stenosis (AS), but is a cause of AS and/or regurgitation later in life. May go undetected in early life or suspected by the presence of a systolic ejection click; often identified during echocardiography that was obtained for another reason. See Chap. 121 for typical history, physical findings, and treatment of subsequent clinical aortic valve disease.

COARCTATION OF THE AORTA

Aortic constriction just distal to the origin of the left subclavian artery is a surgically correctable form of hypertension (Chap. 124). Usually asymptomatic, but it may cause headache, fatigue, or claudication of lower extremities. Often accompanied by bicuspid aortic valve.

Physical Examination   Hypertension in upper extremities; delayed femoral pulses with decreased pressure in lower extremities. Pulsatile collateral arteries can be palpated in the intercostal spaces. Systolic (and sometimes also diastolic) murmur is best heard over the mid-upper back at left interscapular space.

ECG   LV hypertrophy.

CXR   Notching of the ribs due to collateral arteries; "figure 3" appearance of distal aortic arch.

Echocardiography   Can delineate site and length of coarctation, and Doppler determines the pressure gradient across it. MR or CT angiography also visualizes the site of coarctation and can identify associated collateral vessel formation.

R_x Coarction of the Aorta

Surgical correction (or percutaneous transcatheter stent dilation in selected patients), although hypertension may persist. Recoarctation after surgical repair may be amenable to percutaneous balloon dilatation.

COMPLEX CONGENITAL HEART LESIONS

Such lesions are often accompanied by cyanosis. Examples include:

TETRALOGY OF FALLOT

The four main components are: (1) malaligned VSD, (2) obstruction to RV outflow, (3) aorta that overrides the VSD, (4) RV hypertrophy (RVH). Degree of RV outflow obstruction largely determines clinical presentation; when severe, the large right-to-left shunt causes cyanosis and systemic hypoxemia. *ECG* shows RVH. *CXR* demonstrates "boot-shaped" heart with prominent RV. *Echocardiography* delineates VSD, overriding aorta, and RVH and quantitates degree of RV outflow obstruction.

COMPLETE TRANSPOSITION OF THE GREAT ARTERIES

Accounts for 10% of patients with cyanotic congenital heart disease. Aorta and pulmonary artery arise abnormally from the right and left ventricles respectively, creating two separate parallel circulations; a communication must exist between the two sides (ASD, PDA, or VSD) to sustain life. Development of RV dysfunction and heart failure are common by the third decade. *Echocardiography* reveals the aberrant anatomy.

EBSTEIN ANOMALY

Abnormal downward placement of tricuspid valve within the RV; tricuspid regurgitation, hypoplasia of RV, and a right-to-left shunt are common. *Echocardiography* shows apical displacement of tricuspid septal leaflet, abnormal RV size, and quantitates degree of tricuspid regurgitation.

ENDOCARDITIS PROPHYLAXIS IN CONGENITAL HEART DISEASE

American Heart Association 2007 Guidelines recommend antibiotic prophylaxis is only in specific patients with congential heart disease, i.e., those who are to undergo a dental procedure associated with bacteremia who have:

1. Unrepaired cyanotic congenital heart disease (e.g., tetralogy of Fallot)
2. Repaired congenital heart disease with residual defects adjacent to site of a prosthetic patch or transcatheter device
3. A history of complete repair of congenital defects with prosthetic material or a transcatheter device within the previous 6 months.

For a more detailed discussion, see Child JS: Congenital Heart Disease in the Adult, Chap. 229, p. 1458, in HPIM-17.

121 Valvular Heart Disease

MITRAL STENOSIS (MS)

Etiology   Most commonly rheumatic, although history of acute rheumatic fever is now uncommon; congenital MS is an uncommon cause, observed primarily in infants.

History   Symptoms most commonly begin in the fourth decade, but MS often causes severe disability at earlier ages in developing nations. Principal symptoms are dyspnea and pulmonary edema precipitated by exertion, excitement, fever, anemia, paroxysmal tachycardia, pregnancy, sexual intercourse, etc.

Physical Examination   Right ventricular lift; palpable S_1; opening snap (OS) follows A_2 by 0.06–0.12 s; OS–A_2 interval inversely proportional to severity of obstruction. Diastolic rumbling murmur with presystolic accentuation in sinus rhythm. Duration of murmur correlates with severity of obstruction.

Complications   Hemoptysis, pulmonary embolism, pulmonary infection, systemic embolization; endocarditis is *uncommon* in pure MS.

Laboratory   ECG   Typically shows atrial fibrillation (AF) or left atrial (LA) enlargement when sinus rhythm is present. Right-axis deviation and RV hypertrophy in the presence of pulmonary hypertension.

CXR   Shows LA and RV enlargement and Kerley B lines.

Echocardiogram   Most useful noninvasive test; shows inadequate separation, calcification and thickening of valve leaflets and subvalvular apparatus, and LA enlargement. Doppler flow recordings provide estimation of transvalvular gradient, mitral valve area, and degree of pulmonary hypertension (Chap. 119).

> **℞   Mitral Stenosis**   See Fig. 121-1.
>
> Pts should receive prophylaxis for recurrent rheumatic fever (penicillin V 250–500 mg PO bid or benzathine penicillin G 1–2 M units IM monthly.) In the presence of dyspnea, sodium restriction and oral diuretic therapy; beta blockers; digitalis, or rate-limiting calcium channel antagonists (i.e., verapamil or diltiazem) to slow ventricular rate in AF. Warfarin (with target INR 2.0–3.0) for pts with AF and/or history of systemic and pulmonic emboli. For AF of recent onset, consider reversion (chemical or electrical) to sinus rhythm, ideally after ≥3 weeks of anticoagulation. Mitral valvotomy in the presence of symptoms and mitral orifice ≤ ~1.5 cm². In uncomplicated MS, percutaneous balloon valvuloplasty is the procedure of choice; if not feasible, then open surgical valvotomy (Fig. 121-1).

MITRAL REGURGITATION (MR)

Etiology   Rheumatic heart disease in ~33% of patients with chronic MR. Other causes: mitral valve prolapse, ischemic heart disease with papillary muscle dysfunction, LV dilatation of any cause, mitral annular calcification, hypertrophic cardiomyopathy, infective endocarditis, congenital.

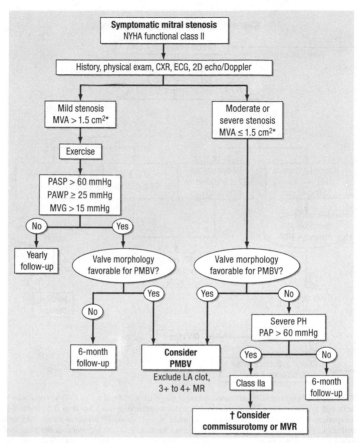

FIGURE 121-1 Management of mitral stenosis (MS). [†]There is controversy as to whether patients with severe MS (MVA <1.0 cm²) and severe pulmonary hypertension (PH) (PASP >60 mmHg) should undergo percutaneous mitral balloon valvotomy (PMBV) or mitral valve replacement (MVR) to prevent right ventricular failure. CXR, chest x-ray; ECG, electrocardiogram; echo, echocardiography; LA, left atrial; MR, mitral regurgitation; MVA, mitral valve area; MVG, mean mitral valve pressure gradient; NYHA, New York Heart Association; PASP, pulmonary artery systolic pressure; PAWP, pulmonary artery wedge pressure; 2D, 2-dimensional. (*Modified from RO Bonow et al: Circulation 114:450, 2006; with permission.*)

Clinical Manifestations   Fatigue, weakness, and exertional dyspnea. Physical examination: sharp upstroke of arterial pulse, LV lift, S_1 diminished: wide splitting of S_2; S_3; loud holosystolic murmur and often a brief early-mid-diastolic murmur.

Echocardiogram   Enlarged LA, hyperdynamic LV; Doppler echocardiogram helpful in diagnosing and assessing severity of MR and degree of pulmonary hypertension.

℞ Mitral Regurgitation   See Fig. 121-2.

For severe/decompensated MR, treat as for heart failure (Chap. 131), including diuretics, ACE inhibitors, beta blockers, and digoxin. Intravenous vasodilators

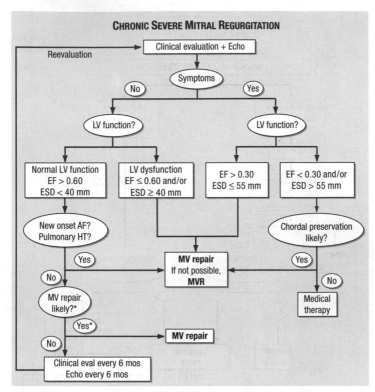

FIGURE 121-2 Management of advanced mitral regurgitation. *Mitral valve (MV) repair may be performed in asymptomatic patients with normal left ventricular (LV) function if performed by an experienced surgical team and if the likelihood of successful MV repair is >90%. AF, atrial fibrillation; Echo, echocardiography; EF, ejection fraction; ESD, end-systolic dimension; eval, evaluation; HT, hypertension; MVR, mitral valve replacement. (*Modified from RO Bonow et al: Circulation 114:450, 2006; with permission.*)

(e.g., IV nitroprusside) are beneficial for acute, severe MR. Anticoagulation is indicated in the presence of atrial fibrillation. Surgical treatment, either valve repair or replacement, is indicated if patient has symptoms or evidence of progressive LV dysfunction [LV ejection fraction (LVEF) < 60% or end-systolic LV diameter by echo >40 mm]. Operation should be carried out *before* development of severe chronic heart failure.

MITRAL VALVE PROLAPSE (MVP)

Etiology Most commonly idiopathic; may accompany rheumatic fever, ischemic heart disease, atrial septal defect, the Marfan syndrome.

Pathology Redundant mitral valve tissue with myxedematous degeneration and elongated chordae tendineae.

Clinical Manifestations More common in females. Most pts are asymptomatic and remain so. Most common symptoms are atypical chest pain and a variety of supraventricular and ventricular arrhythmias. Most important complication is severe MR resulting in LV failure. Rarely, systemic emboli from platelet-fibrin deposits on valve. Sudden death is a *very rare* complication.

Physical Examination   Mid or late systolic click(s) followed by late systolic murmur at the apex; exaggeration by Valsalva maneuver, reduced by squatting and isometric exercise (Chap. 117).

Echocardiogram   Shows posterior displacement of one or both mitral leaflets late in systole.

℞ Mitral Valve Prolapse

Asymptomatic pts should be reassured. Beta blockers may lessen chest discomfort and palpitations. Prophylaxis for infective endocarditis is indicated only if prior history of endocarditis. Valve repair or replacement for pts with severe mitral regurgitation; aspirin or anticoagulants for pts with history of TIA or embolization.

AORTIC STENOSIS (AS)

Etiology   Most common cause in adults is age-related degenerative calcific AS and is usually mild. Other causes are congenital (bicuspid valves) or rheumatic (almost always associated with rheumatic mitral valve disease).

Symptoms   Dyspnea, angina, and syncope are cardinal symptoms; they occur late, after years of obstruction.

Physical Examination   Weak and delayed arterial pulses with carotid thrill. Double apical impulse; A_2 soft or absent; S_4 common. Diamond-shaped systolic murmur $\geq$ grade 3/6, often with systolic thrill. Murmur is typically loudest at 2nd right intercostal space, with radiation to carotids.

Laboratory   ECG and CXR   Often show LV hypertrophy, but not useful for predicting gradient.

Echocardiogram   Shows thickening of LV wall, calcification and thickening of aortic valve cusps with reduced systolic opening. Dilatation and reduced contraction of LV indicate poor prognosis. Doppler useful for estimating gradient and calculating valve area.

℞ Aortic Stenosis   See Fig. 121-3.

Avoid strenuous activity in severe AS, even in asymptomatic phase. Treat heart failure in standard fashion (Chap. 131), but use vasodilators with caution in patients with advanced disease. Valve replacement is indicated in adults with symptoms resulting from AS and hemodynamic evidence of severe obstruction. Operation should be carried out *before* frank failure has developed.

AORTIC REGURGITATION (AR)

Etiology   Rheumatic etiology is common, especially if rheumatic mitral disease present; may also be due to infective endocarditis, syphilis, aortic dissec-

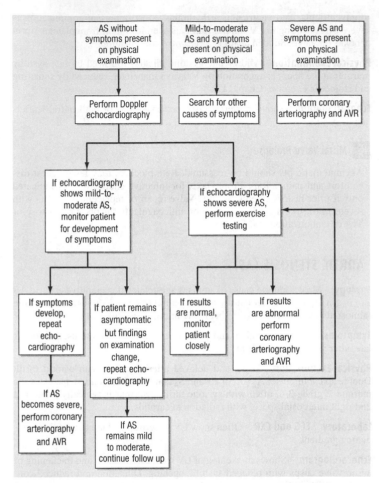

FIGURE 121-3 Algorithm for the management of aortic stenosis (AS). AVR, aortic valve replacement. (*From BA Carabello: N Engl J Med 346:677, 2002.*)

tion, or aortic dilatation due to cystic medial necrosis; three-fourths of pts are males.

Clinical Manifestations   Exertional dyspnea and awareness of heartbeat, angina pectoris, and signs of LV failure. Wide pulse pressure, waterhammer pulse, capillary pulsations (Quincke's sign), A_2 soft or absent, S_3 common. Blowing, decrescendo diastolic murmur along left sternal border (along right sternal border with aortic dilatation). May be accompanied by systolic murmur of augmented blood flow.

Laboratory   ECG and CXR   LV enlargement.

Echocardiogram   LA enlargement, LV enlargement, high-frequency diastolic fluttering of mitral valve. Failure of coaptation of aortic valve leaflets may be present. Doppler studies useful in detection and quantification of AR.

Rx Aortic Regurgitation

Standard therapy for LV failure (Chap. 131). Vasodilators (long-acting nifedipine or ACE inhibitors) are recommended as antihypertensive agents. Surgical valve replacement should be carried out in pts with severe AR when symptoms develop or in asymptomatic pts with LV dysfunction (LVEF < 50%, LV end-systolic volume > 55 mL/m^2, end-systolic diameter > 55 mm or LV diastolic dimension > 75 mm) by echocardiography.

TRICUSPID STENOSIS (TS)

Etiology   Usually rheumatic; most common in females; almost invariably associated with MS.

Clinical Manifestations   Hepatomegaly, ascites, edema, jaundice, jugular venous distention with slow y descent (Chap. 117). Diastolic rumbling murmur along left sternal border increased by inspiration with loud presystolic component. Right atrial and superior vena caval enlargement on chest x-ray. Doppler echocardiography demonstrates thickened valve and impaired separation of leaflets and provides estimate of transvalvular gradient.

Rx Tricuspid Stenosis

In severe TS, surgical relief is indicated, with valvular repair or replacement.

TRICUSPID REGURGITATION (TR)

Etiology   Usually functional and secondary to marked RV dilatation of any cause and often associated with pulmonary hypertension.

Clinical Manifestations   Severe RV failure, with edema, hepatomegaly, and prominent v waves in jugular venous pulse with rapid y descent (Chap. 117). Systolic murmur along lower left sternal edge is increased by inspiration. Doppler echocardiography confirms diagnosis and estimates severity.

Rx Tricuspid Regurgitation

Intensive diuretic therapy when right-sided heart failure signs are present. In severe cases (in absence of severe pulmonary hypertension), surgical treatment consists of tricuspid annuloplasty or valve replacement.

For a more detailed discussion, see O'Gara P, Braunwald E: Valvular Heart Disease, Chap. 230, p. 1465, in HPIM-17.

122 Cardiomyopathies and Myocarditis

Table 122-1 summarizes distinguishing features of the cardiomyopathies.

DILATED CARDIOMYOPATHY (CMP)

Symmetrically dilated left ventricle (LV), with poor systolic contractile function; right ventricle (RV) commonly involved.

TABLE 122-1	**LABORATORY EVALUATION OF THE CARDIOMYOPATHIES**		
	Dilated	**Restrictive**	**Hypertrophic**
Chest roentgenogram	Moderate to marked cardiac silhouette enlargement Pulmonary venous hypertension	Mild cardiac silhouette enlargement	Mild to moderate cardiac silhouette enlargement
Electrocardiogram	ST-segment and T-wave abnormalities	Low voltage, conduction defects	ST-segment and T-wave abnormalities Left ventricular hypertrophy Abnormal Q waves
Echocardiogram	Left ventricular dilatation and dysfunction	Increased left ventricular wall thickness Normal or mildly reduced systolic function	Asymmetric septal hypertrophy (ASH) Systolic anterior motion (SAM) of the mitral valve
Radionuclide studies	Left ventricular dilatation and dysfunction (RVG)	Normal or mildly reduced systolic function (RVG)	Vigorous systolic function (RVG) Perfusion defect (^{201}Tl or technetium sestamibi)
Cardiac catheterization	Left ventricular dilatation and dysfunction Elevated left- and often right-sided filling pressures Diminished cardiac output	Normal or mildly reduced systolic function Elevated left- and right-sided filling pressures	Vigorous systolic function Dynamic left ventricular outflow obstruction Elevated left- and right-sided filling pressures

Note: RVG, radionuclide ventriculogram; ^{201}Tl, thallium 201.
Source: J Wynne, E Braunwald, Table 231-3 in HPIM-17.

Etiology Up to $1/3$ of patients have a familial form, including those cases due to mutations in genes encoding sarcomeric proteins. Other causes include previous myocarditis, toxins [ethanol, certain antineoplastic agents (doxorubicin, truastuzumab, imatinib mesylate)], connective tissue disorders, muscular dystrophies, "peripartum." Severe coronary disease/infarctions or chronic aortic/mitral regurgitation may behave similarly.

Symptoms Congestive heart failure (Chap. 131); tachyarrhythmias and peripheral emboli from LV mural thrombus occur.

Physical Examination Jugular venous distention (JVD), rales, diffuse and dyskinetic LV apex, S_3, hepatomegaly, peripheral edema; murmurs of mitral and tricuspid regurgitation are common.

Laboratory ECG Left bundle branch block and ST-T-wave abnormalities common.

CXR Cardiomegaly, pulmonary vascular redistribution, pulmonary effusions common.

Echocardiogram, CT, and Cardiac MRI LV and RV enlargement with globally impaired contraction. *Regional* wall motion abnormalities suggest coronary artery disease rather than primary cardiomyopathy.

Brain Natriuretic Peptide (BNP) Level elevated in heart failure/cardiomyopathy but not in patients with dyspnea due to lung disease.

℞ Dilated Cardiomyopathy

Standard therapy of CHF (Chap. 131); vasodilator therapy with ACE inhibitor (preferred), angiotensin receptor blocker or hydralazine-nitrate combination shown to improve longevity. Add beta blocker in most pts (Chap. 131). Add spironolactone for patients with advanced heart failure. Chronic anticoagulation with warfarin, recommended for very low ejection fraction (<25%), if no contraindications. Antiarrhythmic drugs (Chap. 130), e.g., amiodarone, indicated only for symptomatic or sustained arrhythmias as they may cause proarrhythmic side effects; implanted internal defibrillator is often a better alternative. Consider biventricular pacing for persistently symptomatic patients with widened (≥130 ms) QRS complex and ejection fraction <35%. Possible trial of immunosuppressive drugs, if active myocarditis present on RV biopsy (controversial as long-term efficacy has not been demonstrated). In selected pts, consider cardiac transplantation.

RESTRICTIVE CARDIOMYOPATHY

Increased myocardial "stiffness" impairs ventricular relaxation; diastolic ventricular pressures are elevated. Etiologies include infiltrative disease (amyloid, sarcoid, hemochromatosis, eosinophilic disorders), endomyocardial fibrosis, Fabry's disease, and prior mediastinal irradiation.

Symptoms Are of CHF, although right-sided heart failure often predominates, with peripheral edema and ascites.

Physical Examination Signs of right-sided heart failure: JVD, hepatomegaly, peripheral edema, murmur of tricuspid regurgitation. Left-sided signs may also be present.

Laboratory ECG Low limb lead voltage, sinus tachycardia, ST-T-wave abnormalities.

CXR Mild LV enlargement.

Echocardiogram, CT, Cardiac MRI Bilateral atrial enlargement; increased ventricular thickness ("speckled pattern") in infiltrative disease, especially amyloidosis. Systolic function is usually normal but may be mildly reduced.

Cardiac Catheterization Increased LV and RV diastolic pressures with "dip and plateau" pattern; RV biopsy useful in detecting infiltrative disease (rectal or fat pad biopsy useful in diagnosis of amyloidosis).

Note: Must distinguish restrictive cardiomyopathy from constrictive pericarditis, which is surgically correctable. Thickening of pericardium in pericarditis usually apparent in CT or MRI.

℞ Restrictive Cardiomyopathy

Salt restriction and diuretics ameliorate pulmonary and systemic congestion; digitalis is not indicated unless systolic function is impaired or atrial arrhythmias are present. *Note:* Increased sensitivity to digitalis in amyloidosis. Anticoagulation often indicated, particularly in pts with eosinophilic endomyocarditis. For specific therapy of hemochromatosis and sarcoidosis, see Chaps. 351 and 322, respectively, in HPIM-17.

HYPERTROPHIC CARDIOMYOPATHY

Marked LV hypertrophy; often asymmetric, without underlying cause. Systolic function is usually normal; increased LV stiffness results in elevated diastolic filling pressures. Typically results from mutations in sarcomeric proteins (autosomal dominant transmission).

Symptoms Secondary to elevated diastolic pressure, dynamic LV outflow obstruction (if present), and arrhythmias; dyspnea on exertion, angina, and presyncope; sudden death may occur.

Physical Examination Brisk carotid upstroke with pulsus bisferiens; S_4, harsh systolic murmur along left sternal border, blowing murmur of mitral regurgitation at apex; murmur changes with Valsalva and other maneuvers (Chap. 117).

Laboratory ECG LV hypertrophy with prominent "septal" Q waves in leads I, aVL, V_{5-6}. Periods of atrial fibrillation or ventricular tachycardia are often detected by Holter monitor.

Echocardiogram LV hypertrophy, often with asymmetric septal hypertrophy (ASH) and ≥1.3 × thickness of LV posterior wall; LV contractile function excellent with small end-systolic volume. If LV outflow tract obstruction is present, systolic anterior motion (SAM) of mitral valve and midsystolic partial closure of aortic valve are present. Doppler shows early systolic accelerated blood flow through LV outflow tract.

℞ Hypertrophic Cardiomyopathy

Strenuous exercise should be avoided. Beta blockers, verapamil, diltiazem, or disopyramide used individually to reduce symptoms. Digoxin, other inotropes, diuretics, and vasodilators are generally *contraindicated*. Endocarditis antibiotic prophylaxis (Chap. 87) is necessary only in patients with a prior history of endocarditis. Antiarrhythmic agents, especially amiodarone, may suppress atrial and ventricular arrhythmias. In selected pts, LV outflow gradient can be reduced by controlled septal infarction by ethanol injection into the septal artery. Consider implantable automatic defibrillator for pts with high-risk profile, e.g., history of syncope or aborted cardiac arrest, ventricular tachycardia, marked LVH (>3 cm), family history of sudden death. Surgical myectomy may be useful in pts refractory to medical therapy.

MYOCARDITIS

Inflammation of the myocardium most commonly due to acute viral infection; may progress to chronic dilated cardiomyopathy. Myocarditis may develop in pts with HIV infection or Lyme disease. Chagas disease is a common cause of myocarditis in endemic areas, typically Central and South America.

History   Fever, fatigue, palpitations; if LV dysfunction develops, then symptoms of CHF are present. Viral myocarditis may be preceded by URI.

Physical Examination   Fever, tachycardia, soft S_1; S_3 common.

Laboratory   CK-MB isoenzyme and cardiac troponins may be elevated in absence of MI. Convalescent antiviral antibody titers may rise.

ECG   Transient ST-T-wave abnormalities.

CXR   Cardiomegaly

Echocardiogram, Cardiac MRI   Depressed LV function; pericardial effusion present if accompanying pericarditis present. MRI demonstrates contrast enhancement.

℞ Myocarditis

Rest; treat as CHF (Chap. 131); immunosuppressive therapy (steroids and azathioprine) may be considered if RV biopsy shows active inflammation, but long-term efficacy has not been demonstrated. In fulminant cases, cardiac transplantation may be indicated.

For a more detailed discussion, see Wynne J, Braunwald E: Cardiomyopathy and Myocarditis, Chap. 231, p. 1481, in HPIM-17.

123 Pericardial Disease

ACUTE PERICARDITIS

Causes   See Table 123-1

History   Chest pain, which may be intense, mimicking acute MI, but characteristically sharp, pleuritic, and positional (relieved by leaning forward); fever and palpitations are common.

Physical Examination   Rapid or irregular pulse, coarse pericardial friction rub, which may vary in intensity and is loudest with pt sitting forward.

Laboratory ECG   (See Table 123-2 and Fig. 123-1)   Diffuse ST elevation (concave upward) usually present in all leads except aVR and V_1; PR-segment depression may be present; *days* later (unlike acute MI), ST returns to baseline and T-wave inversion develops. Atrial premature beats and atrial fibrillation may appear. Differentiate from ECG of early repolarization variant (ERV) (ST-T ratio <0.25 in ERV, but >0.25 in pericarditis).

CXR   Increased size of cardiac silhouette if large (>250 mL) pericardial effusion is present, with "water bottle" configuration.

Echocardiogram   Most readily available test for detection of pericardial effusion, which commonly accompanies acute pericarditis.

℞ Acute Pericarditis

Aspirin 650–975 mg qid or other NSAIDs (e.g., ibuprofen 400–800 mg qid or indomethacin 25–75 mg qid); addition of colchicine 0.6 mg bid may be useful. For *severe, refractory* pain, prednisone 40–80 mg/d is used and tapered over several weeks or months. Intractable, prolonged pain or frequently recurrent episodes may require pericardiectomy. Anticoagulants are relatively contraindicated in acute pericarditis because of risk of pericardial hemorrhage.

TABLE 123-1   MOST COMMON CAUSES OF PERICARDITIS

"Idiopathic"
Infections (particularly viral)
Acute myocardial infarction
Metastatic neoplasm
Mediastinal radiation therapy
Chronic renal failure
Connective tissue disease (e.g., rheumatoid arthritis, SLE)
Drug reaction (e.g., procainamide, hydralazine)
"Autoimmune" following heart surgery or myocardial infarction (several weeks/
   months later)

TABLE 123-2	**ECG IN ACUTE PERICARDITIS VS. ACUTE (Q-WAVE) MI**		
ST-Segment Elevation	ECG Lead Involvement	Evolution of ST and T Waves	PR-Segment Depression
Pericarditis			
Concave upward	All leads involved except aVR and V_1	ST remains elevated for several days; after ST returns to baseline, T waves invert	Yes, in majority
Acute ST Elevation MI			
Convex upward	ST elevation over infarcted region only; reciprocal ST depression in opposite leads	T waves invert within hours, while ST still elevated; followed by Q wave development	No

CARDIAC TAMPONADE

Life-threatening condition resulting from accumulation of pericardial fluid under pressure; impaired filling of cardiac chambers and decreased cardiac output.

Etiology Previous pericarditis (most commonly metastatic tumor, uremia, viral or idiopathic pericarditis), cardiac trauma, or myocardial perforation during catheter or pacemaker placement.

History Hypotension may develop suddenly; subacute symptoms include dyspnea, weakness, confusion.

Physical Examination Tachycardia, hypotension, pulsus paradoxus (inspiratory fall in systolic blood pressure >10 mmHg), jugular venous distention with preserved x descent, but loss of y descent; heart sounds distant. If tamponade develops subacutely, peripheral edema, hepatomegaly, and ascites are frequently present.

Laboratory **ECG** Low limb lead voltage; large effusions may cause electrical alternans (alternating size of QRS complex due to swinging of heart).

CXR Enlarged cardiac silhouette if large (>250 mL) effusion present.

Echocardiogram Swinging motion of heart within large effusion; prominent respiratory alteration of RV dimension with RA and RV collapse during diastole. Doppler shows marked respiratory variation of transvalvular flow velocities.

Cardiac Catheterization Confirms diagnosis; shows equalization of diastolic pressures in all four chambers; pericardial = RA pressure.

 Cardiac Tamponade

Immediate pericardiocentesis and IV volume expansion.

CONSTRICTIVE PERICARDITIS

Rigid pericardium leads to impaired cardiac filling, elevation of systemic and pulmonary venous pressures, and decreased cardiac output. Results from healing and

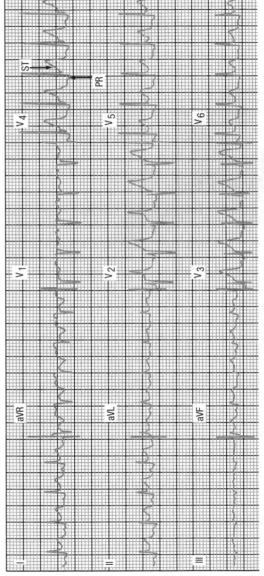

FIGURE 123-1 Electrocardiogram in acute pericarditis. Note diffuse ST-segment elevation and PR-segment depression.

scar formation in some pts with previous pericarditis. Viral, tuberculosis (mostly in developing nations), previous cardiac surgery, collagen vascular disorders, uremia, neoplastic and radiation-associated pericarditis are potential causes.

History Gradual onset of dyspnea, fatigue, pedal edema, abdominal swelling; symptoms of LV failure uncommon.

Physical Examination Tachycardia, jugular venous distention (prominent y descent), which increases further on inspiration (Kussmaul's sign); hepatomegaly, ascites, peripheral edema are common; sharp diastolic sound, "pericardial knock" following S_2 sometimes present.

Laboratory **ECG** Low limb lead voltage; atrial arrhythmias are common.

CXR Rim of pericardial calcification is most common in tuberculous pericarditis.

Echocardiogram Thickened pericardium, normal ventricular contraction; abrupt halt in ventricular filling in early diastole. Dilatation of IVC is common. Dramatic effects of respiration are typical: During inspiration the ventricular septum shifts to the left with prominent reduction of blood flow velocity across mitral valve; pattern reverses during expiration (Fig 123-2).

CT or MRI More precise than echocardiogram in demonstrating thickened pericardium.

Cardiac Catheterization Equalization of diastolic pressures in all chambers; ventricular pressure tracings show "dip and plateau" appearance. Differentiate from restrictive cardiomyopathy (Table 123-3).

℞ Constrictive Pericarditis

Surgical stripping of the pericardium. Progressive improvement ensues over several months.

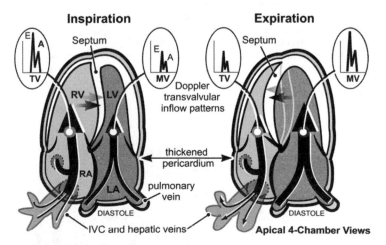

FIGURE 123-2 Constrictive pericarditis Doppler schema of respirophasic changes in mitral and tricuspid inflow. Reciprocal patterns of ventricular filling are assessed on pulsed Doppler examination of mitral (MV) and tricuspid (TV) inflow. (*Courtesy of Bernard E. Bulwer, MD; with permission.*)

	Constrictive Pericarditis	Restrictive Cardiomyopathy
TABLE 123-3	**FEATURES THAT DIFFERENTIATE CONSTRICTIVE PERICARDITIS FROM RESTRICTIVE CARDIOMYOPATHY**	
Physical Exam		
Kussmaul's sign	Present	Absent
Pericardial knock	May be present	Absent
Chest X-ray		
Pericardial calcification	May be present	Absent
Echocardiography		
Thickened pericardium	Present	Absent
Thickened myocardium	Absent	Present
Exaggerated variation in trans-valvular velocities	Present	Absent
CT or MRI		
Thickened pericardium	Present	Absent
Cardiac Catheterization		
Equalized RV and LV diastolic pressures	Yes	Often LV > RV
Elevated PA systolic pressure	Uncommon	Usual
Effect of inspiration on systolic pressures	Discordant: LV↓, RV↑	Concordant: LV↓, RV↓
Endomyocardial biopsy	Normal	Usually abnormal (e.g., amyloid)

Note: LV, left ventricle; PA, pulmonary artery; RV, right ventricle.

APPROACH TO THE PATIENT WITH ASYMPTOMATIC PERICARDIAL EFFUSION OF UNKNOWN CAUSE

If careful history and physical exam do not suggest etiology, the following may lead to diagnosis:

- Skin test and cultures for tuberculosis (Chap. 101)
- Serum albumin and urine protein measurement (nephrotic syndrome)
- Serum creatinine and BUN (renal failure)
- Thyroid function tests (myxedema)
- ANA (SLE and other collagen-vascular disease)
- Search for a primary tumor (especially lung and breast)

For a more detailed discussion, see Braunwald E: Pericardial Disease, Chap. 232, p. 1488, in HPIM-17.

124   Hypertension

Definition   Chronic elevation in bp >140/90; etiology unknown in 80–95% of pts ("essential hypertension"). Always consider a secondary correctable form of hypertension, especially in pts under age 30 or those who become hypertensive after 55. Isolated systolic hypertension (systolic ≥ 140, diastolic < 90) most common in elderly pts, due to reduced vascular compliance.

SECONDARY HYPERTENSION

Renal Artery Stenosis (Renovascular Hypertension)   Due either to atherosclerosis (older men) or fibromuscular dysplasia (young women). Presents with recent onset of hypertension, refractory to usual antihypertensive therapy. Abdominal bruit is present in 50% of cases; often audible; mild hypokalemia due to activation of the renin-angiotensin-aldosterone system may be present.

Renal Parenchymal Disease   Elevated serum creatinine and/or abnormal urinalysis, containing protein, cells, or casts.

Coarctation of Aorta   Presents in children or young adults; constriction is usually present in aorta at origin of left subclavian artery. Exam shows diminished, delayed femoral pulsations; late systolic murmur loudest over the midback. CXR shows indentation of the aorta at the level of the coarctation and rib notching (due to development of collateral arterial flow).

Pheochromocytoma   A catecholamine-secreting tumor, typically of the adrenal medulla or extraadrenal paraganglion tissue, that presents as paroxysmal or sustained hypertension in young to middle-aged pts. Sudden episodes of headache, palpitations, and profuse diaphoresis are common. Associated findings include chronic weight loss, orthostatic *hypotension*, and impaired glucose tolerance. Pheochromocytomas may be localized to the bladder wall and may present with micturition-associated symptoms of catecholamine excess. Diagnosis is suggested by elevated plasma metanephrine level or urinary catecholamine metabolites in a 24-h urine collection (see below); the tumor is then localized by CT scan or MRI.

Hyperaldosteronism   Usually due to aldosterone-secreting adenoma or bilateral adrenal hyperplasia. Should be suspected when hypokalemia is present in a hypertensive pt off diuretics (Chap. 180).

Other Causes   Oral contraceptive usage, obstructive sleep apnea (Chap. 144), Cushing's and adrenogenital syndromes (Chap. 180), thyroid disease (Chap. 179), hyperparathyroidism (Chap. 179), and acromegaly (Chap. 177). In patients with systolic hypertension and wide pulse pressure, consider thyrotoxicosis, aortic regurgitation (Chap. 121), and systemic AV fistula.

APPROACH TO THE PATIENT

HISTORY   Most pts are asymptomatic. Severe hypertension may lead to headache, dizziness, or blurred vision.

Clues to Specific Forms of Secondary Hypertension

Use of medications (e.g., birth control pills, glucocorticoids, decongestants, erythropoietin, NSAIDs, cyclosporine); paroxysms of headache, sweating, or tachycardia (pheochromocytoma); history of renal disease or abdominal traumas (renal hypertension); daytime somnolence and snoring (sleep apnea).

PHYSICAL EXAMINATION

Measure bp with appropriate-sized cuff (large cuff for large arm). Measure bp in both arms as well as a leg (to evaluate for coarctation). Signs of hypertension include retinal arteriolar changes (narrowing/nicking); left ventricular lift, loud A_2, S_4. Clues to secondary forms of hypertension include cushingoid appearance, thyromegaly, abdominal bruit (renal artery stenosis), delayed femoral pulses (coarctation of aorta).

LABORATORY WORKUP
Screening Tests for Secondary Hypertension

Should be carried out on all pts with documented hypertension: (1) serum creatinine, BUN, and urinalysis (renal parenchymal disease); (2) serum K measured off diuretics (hypokalemia prompts workup for hyperaldosteronism or renal artery stenosis); (3) CXR (rib notching or indentation of distal aortic arch in coarctation of the aorta); (4) ECG (LV hypertrophy suggests chronicity of hypertension); (5) other useful screening blood tests include CBC, glucose, lipid levels, calcium, uric acid; (6) thyroid-stimulating hormone if thyroid disease suspected.

Further Workup

Indicated for specific diagnoses if screening tests are abnormal or bp is refractory to antihypertensive therapy: (1) *renal artery stenosis*: magnetic resonance angiography, captopril renogram, renal duplex ultrasound, digital subtraction angiography, renal arteriography, and measurement of renal vein renin; (2) *Cushing's syndrome*: dexamethasone suppression test (Chap. 180); (3) *pheochromocytoma*: 24-h urine collection for catecholamines, metanephrines, and vanillylmandelic acid and/or measurement of plasma metanephrine; (4) *primary hyperaldosteronism*: depressed plasma renin activity and hypersecretion of aldosterone, both of which fail to change with volume expansion; (5) *renal parenchymal disease* (Chaps. 147,150,151).

℞ Hypertension

Helpful lifestyle modifications include weight reduction (to attain BMI < 25 kg/m^2); sodium restriction; diet rich in fruits, vegetables, and low-fat dairy products; regular exercise; and moderation of alcohol consumption.

DRUG THERAPY OF ESSENTIAL HYPERTENSION (See Table 124-1 and Fig. 124-1) Goal is to control hypertension with minimal side effects. A combination of medications with complementary actions is often required. First-line agents include diuretics, beta blockers, ACE inhibitors, angiotensin receptor antagonists, and calcium antagonists. On-treatment blood pressure goal is <135–140 systolic, <80–85 diastolic (<130/80 in patients with diabetes or chronic kidney disease).

Diuretics

Should be cornerstone of most antihypertensive regimes. Thiazides preferred over loop diuretics because of longer duration of action; however, the latter are more potent when serum creatinine > 2.5 mg/dL. Major side effects include hypokalemia, hyperglycemia, and hyperuricemia, which can be mini-

TABLE 124-1	ORAL DRUGS COMMONLY USED IN TREATMENT OF HYPERTENSION		

Drug Class	Examples	Usual Total Daily Dose (Dosing Frequency/Day)	Potential Adverse Effects
Diuretics			
Thiazides	Hydrochloro-thiazide	6.25–50 mg (1–2)	Hypokalemia, hyperuricemia, hyperglycemia, ↑cholesterol, ↑triglycerides
Thiazide-like	Chlorthali-done	25–50 mg (1)	
Loop diuretics	Furosemide	40–80 mg (2–3)	Hypokalemia, hyperuricemia
K⁺-retaining	Spironolactone	25–100 mg (1–2)	Hyperkalemia, gynecomastia
	Eplerenone	50–100 mg (1–2)	Hyperkalemia
	Amiloride	5–10 mg (1–2)	
	Triamterene	50–100 mg (1–2)	
Beta blockers			
β_1-selective	Atenolol	25–100 mg (1–2)	Bronchospasm, bradycardia, heart block, fatigue, sexual dysfunction, ↑triglycerides, ↓HDL
	Metoprolol	25–100 mg (1–2)	
Nonselective	Propranolol	40–160 mg (2)	
	Propranolol LA	60–180 mg (1)	
Combined alpha/ beta	Labetolol	200–800 mg (2)	Bronchospasm, bradycardia, heart block
	Carvedilol	12.5–50 mg (2)	
ACE inhibitors	Captopril	25–200 mg (2)	Cough, hyperkalemia, azotemia, angioedema
	Lisinopril	10–40 mg (1)	
	Ramipril	2.5–20 mg (1–2)	
Angiotensin II receptor blockers	Losartan	25–100 mg (1–2)	Hyperkalemia, azotemia
	Valsartan	80–320 mg (1)	
	Candesartan	2–32 mg (1–2)	
Calcium channel antagonists			
Dihydropyri-dines	Nifedipine long-acting	30–60 mg (1)	Edema, constipation
Nondihydro-pyridines	Verapamil long-acting	120–360 mg (1–2)	Edema, constipation, bradycardia, heart block
	Diltiazem long-acting	180–420 mg (1)	

mized by using low dosage (e.g., hydrochlorothiazide 6.25–50 mg qd). Diuretics are particularly effective in elderly and black pts. Prevention of hypokalemia is especially important in pts on digitalis glycosides.

Beta Blockers

Particularly useful in young pts with "hyperkinetic" circulation. Begin with low dosage (e.g., metoprolol succinate 25–50 mg daily). Relative contraindications: bronchospasm, CHF, AV block, bradycardia, and "brittle" insulin-dependent diabetes.

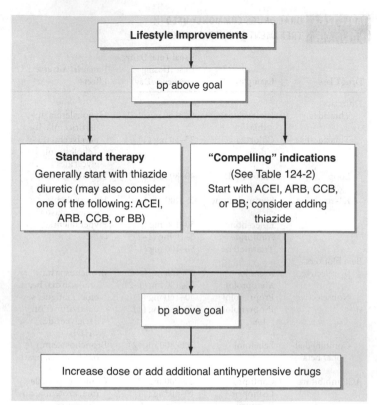

FIGURE 124-1 Initiation of therapy in patients with hypertension. ACEI, angiotensin-converting enzyme inhibitor; ARB, angiotensin receptor blocker; CCB, calcium channel blocker; BB, beta blocker.

ACE Inhibitors and Angiotensin II Receptor Blockers

ACE inhibitors are well tolerated with low frequency of side effects. May be used as monotherapy or in combination with a diuretic, calcium antagonist, or beta blocker. Side effects are uncommon and include angioedema, hyperkalemia and azotemia (particularly in pts with elevated baseline serum creatinine). A nonproductive cough may develop in the course of therapy in up to 15% of patients, requiring an alternative regimen. Note that renal function may deteriorate rapidly as a result of ACE inhibition in pts with bilateral renal artery stenosis.

Potassium supplements and potassium-sparing diuretics should be used cautiously with ACE inhibitors to prevent hyperkalemia. If pt is intravascularly volume depleted, hold diuretics for 2–3 days prior to initiation of ACE inhibitor, which should then be administered at very low dosage (e.g., captopril, 6.25 mg bid).

For pts who do not tolerate an ACE inhibitor because of cough, substitute an angiotensin receptor antagonist.

Calcium Antagonists

Direct arteriolar vasodilators; all have negative inotropic effects (particularly verapamil) and should be used cautiously if LV dysfunction is present. Vera-

TABLE 124-2 GUIDELINES FOR SELECTING INITIAL DRUG TREATMENT OF HYPERTENSION

Class of Drug	Compelling Indications	Possible Indications	Compelling Contraindications	Possible Contraindications
Diuretics	Heart failure Elderly patients Systolic hypertension	Diabetes	Gout	Dyslipidemia
β-Blockers	Angina After myocardial infarct Tachyarrhythmias	Heart failure Pregnancy	Asthma and COPD Heart block[a]	Dyslipidemia Athletes and physically active patients Peripheral vascular disease
ACE inhibitors	Heart failure Left ventricular dysfunction After myocardial infarct Diabetic nephropathy	Chronic renal parenchymal disease	Pregnancy Hyperkalemia Bilateral renal artery stenosis	
Angiotensin receptor blockers	ACE inhibitor cough Heart failure Diabetic nephropathy	Chronic renal parenchymal disease	Pregnancy Bilateral renal artery stenosis Hyperkalemia	
Calcium channel blocker	Angina Elderly patients Systolic hypertension	Peripheral vascular disease	Heart block[b]	Congestive heart failure[c]

[a]Grade 2 or 3 atrioventricular block.
[b]Grade 2 or 3 atrioventricular block with verapamil or diltiazem.
[c]Verapamil or diltiazem.

Note: COPD, chronic obstructive pulmonary disease; ACE, angiotensin-converting enzyme; ARB, angiotensin receptor blocker.
Source: Adapted with permission from 1999 WHO.

TABLE 124-3	USUAL INTRAVENOUS DOSES OF ANTIHYPERTENSIVE AGENTS USED IN HYPERTENSIVE EMERGENCIES[a]
Antihypertensive Agent	**Intravenous Dose**
Nitroprusside	Initial 0.3 (mg/kg)/min; usual 2–4 (mg/kg)/min; maximum 10 (mg/kg)/min for 10 min
Nicardipine	Initial 5 mg/h; titrate by 2.5 mg/h at 5–15 min intervals; max 15 mg/h
Labetalol	2 mg/min up to 300 mg *or* 20 mg over 2 min, then 40–80 mg at 10-min intervals up to 300 mg total
Enalaprilat	Usual 0.625–1.25 mg over 5 min every 6–8 h; maximum 5 mg/dose
Esmolol	Initial 80–500 mg/kg over 1 min, then 50–300 (mg/kg)/min
Phentolamine	5–15 mg bolus
Nitroglycerin	Initial 5 mg/min, then titrate by 5 mg/min at 3–5 min intervals; if no response is seen at 20 mg/min, incremental increases of 10–20 mg/min may be used
Hydralazine	10–50 mg at 30-min intervals

[a]Constant blood pressure monitoring is required. Start with the lowest dose. Subsequent doses and intervals of administration should be adjusted according to the blood pressure response and duration of action of the specific agent.

pamil, and to a lesser extent diltiazem, can result in bradycardia and AV block, so combination with beta blockers is generally avoided. Use sustained-release formulations, as short-acting dihydropyridine calcium channel blockers may increase incidence of coronary events. Common side effects include peripheral edema and constipation.

If bp proves refractory to drug therapy, workup for secondary forms of hypertension, especially renal artery stenosis and pheochromocytoma.

Table 124-2 lists compelling indications for specific initial drug treatment.

SPECIAL CIRCUMSTANCES
Pregnancy
Most commonly used antihypertensives include methyldopa (250–1000 mg PO bid-tid), labetalol (100–200 mg bid), and hydralazine (10–150 mg PO bid-tid). Calcium channel blockers (e.g., nifedipine, long-acting, 30–60 mg daily) also appear to be safe in pregnancy. Beta blockers need to be used cautiously–fetal hypoglycemia and low birth weights have been reported. ACE inhibitors and angiotensin receptor antagonists are contraindicated in pregnancy.

Renal Disease
Standard thiazide diuretics may not be effective. Consider metolazone, furosemide, or bumetanide, alone or in combination.

Diabetes
Goal bp < 130/80. Consider ACE inhibitors and angiotensin receptor blockers as first-line therapy to control bp and slow renal deterioration.

Malignant Hypertension
Defined as an abrupt increase in bp in patient with chronic hypertension or sudden onset of severe hypertension, and is a medical emergency. Immediate therapy is mandatory if there is evidence of cardiac decompensation (CHF, angina), encephalopathy (headache, seizures, visual disturbances), or deterio-

rating renal function. Drugs to treat hypertensive crisis are listed in Table 124-3. Replace with PO antihypertensive as pt becomes asymptomatic and diastolic bp improves.

For a more detailed discussion, see Kotchen TA: Hypertensive Vascular Disease, Chap. 241, p. 1549, in HPIM-17.

125 Metabolic Syndrome

The *metabolic syndrome* (*insulin resistance syndrome*, *syndrome X*) is an important risk factor for cardiovascular disease and type 2 diabetes; it consists of a constellation of metabolic abnormalities that includes insulin resistance, hypertension, dyslipidemia, central obesity, and endothelial dysfunction.

ETIOLOGY

Overweight/obesity, sedentary lifestyle, increasing age, and lipodystrophy are all risk factors for the metabolic syndrome. The exact cause is not known and may be multifactorial. Insulin resistance is central to the development of the metabolic syndrome. Increased intracellular fatty acid metabolites contribute to insulin resistance by impairing insulin-signaling pathways and accumulating as triglycerides in skeletal and cardiac muscle, while stimulating hepatic glucose and triglyceride production. Excess adipose tissue leads to increased production of proinflammatory cytokines.

CLINICAL FEATURES

There are no specific symptoms of the metabolic syndrome. The major features include central obesity, hypertriglyceridemia, low HDL cholesterol, hyperglycemia, and hypertension (Table 125-1). Associated conditions include cardiovascular disease, type 2 diabetes, nonalcoholic fatty liver disease, hyperuricemia, polycystic ovary syndrome, and obstructive sleep apnea.

DIAGNOSIS

The diagnosis of the metabolic syndrome relies on satisfying the criteria listed in Table 125-1. Screening for associated conditions should be considered.

Rx Metabolic Syndrome

Obesity is the driving force behind the metabolic syndrome. Thus, weight reduction is the primary approach to this disorder. In general, recommendations for weight loss include a combination of caloric restriction, increased physical activity, and behavior modification. Weight loss drugs or bariatric surgery are adjuncts that may be considered for obesity management (Chap. 181). Hypertension (Chap. 124), impaired fasting glucose or diabetes (Chap. 182), and lipid

TABLE 125-1	NCEP:ATPIII 2001 AND IDF CRITERIA FOR THE METABOLIC SYNDROME

NCEP:ATPIII 2001

Three or more of the following:
Central obesity: Waist circumference >102 cm (M), >88 cm (F)
Hypertriglyceridemia: Triglycerides ≥150 mg/dL or specific medication
Low HDL cholesterol: <40 mg/dL and <50 mg/dL, respectively, or specific medication
Hypertension: Blood pressure ≥130 mm systolic or ≥85 mm diastolic or specific medication
Fasting plasma glucose ≥100 mg/dL or specific medication or previously diagnosed type 2 diabetes

Abbreviations: NCEP:ATPIII, National Cholesterol Education Program, Adult Treatment Panel III; HDL, high-density lipoprotein; IDF, International Diabetes Foundation.

abnormalities (Chap. 187) should be managed according to current guidelines. The antihypertensive regimen should include an angiotensin-converting enzyme (ACE) inhibitor or angiotensin receptor blocker when possible.

For a more detailed discussion, see Eckel RH: The Metabolic Syndrome, Chap. 236, p. 1509, in HPIM-17.

126 ST-Segment Elevation Myocardial Infarction (STEMI)

Early recognition and immediate treatment of acute MI are essential; diagnosis is based on characteristic history, ECG, and serum cardiac markers.

Symptoms Chest pain similar to angina (Chap. 33) but more intense and persistent; not fully relieved by rest or nitroglycerin, often accompanied by nausea, sweating, apprehension. However, ~25% of MIs are clinically silent.

Physical Examination Pallor, diaphoresis, tachycardia, S_4, dyskinetic cardiac impulse may be present. If CHF exists, rales and S_3 are present. Jugular venous distention is common in right ventricular infarction.

ECG ST elevation, followed by T-wave inversion, then Q-wave development over several hours (see Figs. 118-3 and 118-4).

Non-ST Elevation MI, or NSTEMI ST depression followed by persistent ST-T-wave changes *without* Q-wave development. Comparison with old ECG helpful (see Chap. 127).

Cardiac Biomarkers Cardiac-specific troponins T and I are highly specific for myocardial injury and are the preferred biochemical markers for diagnosis of acute MI. They remain elevated for 7–10 days. Creatine phosphokinase (CK) level rises within 4–8 h, peaks at 24 h, returns to normal by 48–72 h. CK-MB isoenzyme is more specific for MI but may also be elevated with myocarditis or after electrical cardioversion. Total CK (but not CK-MB) rises (two- to three-fold) after IM injection, vigorous exercise, or other skeletal muscle trauma. A ratio of CK-MB mass:CK activity ≥ 2.5 suggests acute MI. CK-MB peaks earlier (about 8 h) following acute reperfusion therapy (see below). Serum cardiac markers should be measured at presentation, 6–9 h later, then at 12–24 h.

Noninvasive Imaging Techniques   Useful when diagnosis of MI is not clear. *Echocardiography* detects infarct-associated regional wall motion abnormalities (but cannot distinguish acute MI from a previous myocardial scar). Echo is also useful in detecting RV infarction, LV aneurysm, and LV thrombus. *Myocardial perfusion imaging* (thallium 201 or technetium 99m-sestamibi) is sensitive for regions of decreased perfusion but is not specific for acute MI. *MRI with delayed gadolinium enhancement* accurately indicates regions of infarction but is technically difficult to obtain in acutely ill patients.

Rx STEMI

Initial Therapy
Initial goals are to: (1) quickly identify if patient is candidate for reperfusion therapy, (2) relieve pain, and (3) prevent/treat arrhythmias and mechanical complications.

- Aspirin should be administered immediately (162–325 mg chewed at presentation, then 162–325 mg PO qd), unless pt is aspirin-intolerant.
- Perform targeted history, exam, and ECG to identify STEMI (>1 mm ST elevation in two contiguous limb leads, ≥ 2mm ST elevation in two contiguous precordial leads, or new LBBB) and appropriateness of reperfusion therapy [percutaneous coronary intervention (PCI) or intravenous fibrinolytic agent], which reduces infarct size, LV dysfunction, and mortality.
- Primary PCI is generally more effective than fibrinolysis and is preferred at experienced centers capable of performing procedure rapidly (Fig. 126-1), especially when diagnosis is in doubt, cardiogenic shock is present, bleeding risk is increased, or if symptoms have been present for >3 h.
- Proceed with IV fibrinolysis if PCI is not available or if logistics would delay PCI >1 h longer than fibrinolysis could be initiated (Fig. 126-1). Door-to-needle time should be <30 min for maximum benefit. Ensure absence of contraindications (Fig. 126-2) before administering fibrinolytic agent. Those treated within 1–3 h benefit most; can still be useful up to 12 h if chest pain is persistent or ST remains elevated in leads that have not developed new Q waves. Complications include bleeding, reperfusion arrhythmias, and, in case of streptokinase (SK), allergic reactions. Enoxaparin or heparin [60 U/kg (maximum 4000 U), then 12 (U/kg)/h (maximum 1000 U/h)] should be initiated with fibrinolytic agents (Fig. 126-2); maintain activated partial thromboplastin time (aPTT) at 1.5–2.0 × control (~50–70 s).
- If chest pain or ST elevation persists >90 min after fibrinolysis, consider referral for rescue PCI. Later coronary angiography after fibrinolysis generally reserved for pts with recurrent angina or positive stress test.

The initial management of NSTEMI (non-Q MI) is different (Chap. 127). In particular, fibrinolytic therapy should not be administered.

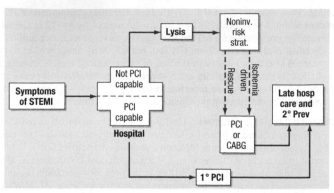

FIGURE 126-1 Reperfusion choices in STEMI. If hospital is capable, percutaneous coronary intervention (PCI) is undertaken. Otherwise, patient is considered for fibrinolytic therapy (Fig. 126-2). Patients who receive fibrinolytic therapy undergo noninvasive risk stratification (Noninv. risk strat). Those with continued chest pain or failure to resolve ST-segment elevation by 90 min after fibrinolysis should be considered for rescue PCI. Later in hospitalization, spontaneous recurrent ischemia or provoked ischemia on noninvasive testing should lead to coronary angiography and consideration of PCI or coronary artery bypass graft (CABG) surgery. (*Adapted from PW Armstrong, D Collen, EM Antman. Circulation 107:2533, 2003.*)

Additional Standard Treatment

(Whether or not reperfusion therapy is undertaken):

- *Hospitalize in CCU* with continuous ECG monitoring.
- *IV line* for emergency arrhythmia treatment.
- *Pain control*: (1) Morphine sulfate 2–4 mg IV q5–10min until pain is relieved or side effects develop [nausea, vomiting, respiratory depression (treat with naloxone 0.4–1.2 mg IV), hypotension (if bradycardic, treat with atropine 0.5 mg IV; otherwise use careful volume infusion)]; (2) nitroglycerin 0.3 mg SL if systolic bp > 100 mmHg; for refractory pain: IV nitroglycerin (begin at 10 μg/min, titrate upward to maximum of 200 μg/min, monitoring bp closely); do not administer nitrates within 24 h of sildenafil or within 48 h of tadalafil (used for erectile dysfunction); (3) β-adrenergic antagonists (see below).
- *Oxygen*: 2–4 L/min by nasal cannula (if needed to maintain O_2 saturation > 90%).
- Mild *sedation* (e.g., diazepam 5 mg, oxazepam 15–30 mg or lorazepam 0.5–2 mg PO three to four times daily).
- *Soft diet* and stool softeners (e.g., docusate sodium 100–200 mg/d).
- β-*Adrenergic blockers* (Chap. 124) reduce myocardial O_2 consumption, limit infarct size, and reduce mortality. Especially useful in pts with hypertension, tachycardia, or persistent ischemic pain; contraindications include active CHF, systolic bp < 95 mmHg, heart rate < 50 beats/min, AV block, or history of bronchospasm. Consider IV (e.g., metoprolol 5 mg q5–10min to total dose of 15 mg), if patient is hypertensive. Otherwise, begin PO regimen (e.g., metoprolol 25–100 mg two times daily).
- *Anticoagulation/antiplatelet agents:* Pts who receive fibrinolytic therapy are begun on heparin and aspirin as indicated above. In absence of fibrinolytic therapy, administer aspirin, 160–325 mg qd, and low-dose heparin (5000 U SC q12h) or enoxaparin (40 mg SC daily) for DVT prevention. Full-dose IV heparin (PTT 2 × control) or low-molecular-weight heparin (e.g., enoxaparin 1 mg/kg SC q12h) followed by oral anticoagulants is rec-

SELECTION CRITERIA

1. Acute chest discomfort characteristic of myocardial infarction
2. ECG criteria for ST-elevation MI (a, b, or c):
   a. ST elevation ≥ 0.1 mV (1 mm) in at least 2 leads of either:
      Inferior group: II, III, aVF
      Lateral gorup: I, aVL, V_5, V_6
   b. ST elevation ≥ 0.2 mV (1 mm) in at least 2 contiguous anterior leads (V_1–V_4)
   c. New LBBB
3. Primary PCI not available, or delay to PCI would be >1 h longer than initiation of fibrinolysis

↓

ASSESS FOR CONTRAINDICATIONS

- Prior intracranial bleeding
- Intracranial malignancy or vascular malformation
- Ischemic stroke or head trauma in previous 3 months
- Aortic dissection
- Active bleeding (with exception of menses)
- Internal bleeding in previous 4 weeks
- Severe hypertension (systolic >180 or diastolic >110)
- Prolonged (>10 min) CPR chest compressions
- INR ≥ 2.0 on warfarin, or known bleeding diathesis
- Pregnancy

↓

FIBRINOLYTIC DRUG	INTRAVENOUS DOSAGE
Streptokinase	1.5 million U over 60 min
Alteplase*	15-mg bolus, then 0.75 mg/kg (up to 50 mg) over 30 min, then 0.5 mg/kg (up to 35 mg) over 60 min
Reteplase*	10 U over 2 min; repeat same dose 30 min later
Tenecteplase*	Single bolus over 5 s, based on weight: <60 kg: 30 mg 60–69 kg: 35 mg 70–79 kg: 40 mg 80–89 kg: 45 mg ≥90 kg: 50 mg

*If alteplase, reteplase, or tenecteplase used, also administer IV heparin 60-U/kg bolus (maximum 4000 U) followed by 12 (U/kg)/h (maximum 1000 U/h), then adjusted to maintain aPTT at 1.5–2 x control (~50–70 s) for 48 h

↓

SUBSEQUENT CORONARY ANGIOGRAPHY RESERVED FOR

- Failure of reperfusion (persistent chest pain or ST elevation after 90 min)
- Spontaneous recurrent ischemia during hospitalization
- Positive exercise test prior to or soon after discharge

FIGURE 126-2 Algorithm for fibrinolytic therapy of acute STEMI.

ommended for pts with severe CHF, presence of ventricular thrombus by echocardiogram, or large dyskinetic region in anterior MI. Oral anticoagulants are continued for 3–6 months, then replaced by aspirin.

- *ACE inhibitors* reduce mortality in pts following acute MI and should be prescribed within 24 h of hospitalization for pts with STEMI—e.g., captopril (6.25 mg PO test dose) advanced to 50 mg PO tid. ACE inhibitors should be continued indefinitely after discharge in pts with CHF or those with asymptomatic LV dysfunction [ejection fraction (EF) ≤ 40%]; if ACE inhibitor intolerant, use angiotensin receptor blocker (ARB; e.g., valsartan or candesartan).

- *Serum magnesium* level should be measured and repleted if necessary to reduce risk of arrhythmias.

COMPLICATIONS

(For arrhythmias, see also Chaps. 129 and 130)

Ventricular Arrhythmias   Isolated ventricular premature beats (VPBs) occur frequently. Precipitating factors should be corrected [hypoxemia, acidosis, hypokalemia (maintain serum K^+ ~4.5 mmol/L), hypercalcemia, hypomagnesemia, CHF, arrhythmogenic drugs]. Routine beta-blocker administration (see above) diminishes ventricular ectopy. Other in-hospital antiarrhythmic therapy should be reserved for pts with sustained ventricular arrhythmias.

Ventricular Tachycardia   If hemodynamically unstable, perform immediate electrical countershock (unsynchronized discharge of 200–300 J or 50% less if using biphasic device). If hemodynamically tolerated, use IV amiodarone (bolus of 150 mg over 10 min; infusion of 1.0 mg/min for 6 h, then 0.5 mg/min).

Ventricular Fibrillation (VF)   VF requires immediate defibrillation (200–400 J). If unsuccessful, initiate cardiopulmonary resuscitation (CPR) and standard resuscitative measures (Chap. 11). Ventricular arrhythmias that appear several days or weeks following MI often reflect pump failure and may warrant invasive electrophysiologic study and use of an implantable cardioverter defibrillator (ICD).

Accelerated Idioventricular Rhythm   Wide QRS complex, regular rhythm, rate 60–100 beats/min, is common and usually benign; if it causes hypotension, treat with atropine 0.6 mg IV.

Supraventricular Arrhythmias   *Sinus tachycardia* may result from CHF, hypoxemia, pain, fever, pericarditis, hypovolemia, administered drugs. If no cause is identified, may treat with beta blocker. Other *supraventricular arrhythmias* (paroxysmal supraventricular tachycardia, atrial flutter, and fibrillation) are often secondary to CHF, in which case digoxin (Chap. 131) is treatment of choice. In absence of CHF, may use beta blocker, verapamil, or diltiazem (Chap. 130). If hemodynamically unstable, proceed with electrical cardioversion.

Bradyarrhythmias and AV Block   (See Chap. 129)   In *inferior MI*, usually represent heightened vagal tone or discrete AV nodal ischemia. If hemodynamically compromised (CHF, hypotension, emergence of ventricular arrhythmias), treat with atropine 0.5 mg IV q5min (up to 2 mg). If no response, use temporary external or transvenous pacemaker. Isoproterenol should be avoided. In *anterior MI*, AV conduction defects usually reflect extensive tissue necrosis. Consider temporary external or transvenous pacemaker for (1) complete heart block, (2) Mobitz type II block (Chap. 129), (3) new bifascicular block (LBBB, RBBB

+ left anterior hemiblock, RBBB + left posterior hemiblock), (4) any bradyarrhythmia associated with hypotension or CHF.

Congestive Heart Failure   CHF may result from systolic "pump" dysfunction,
increased LV diastolic "stiffness," and/or acute mechanical complications.

Symptoms   Dyspnea, orthopnea, tachycardia.

Examination   Jugular venous distention, S_3 and S_4 gallop, pulmonary rales;
systolic murmur if acute mitral regurgitation or ventricular septal defect (VSD)
has developed.

℞ Congestive Heart Failure   (See Chaps. 14 and 131)

Initial therapy includes diuretics (begin with furosemide 10–20 mg IV), inhaled O_2, and vasodilators, particularly nitrates [PO, topical, or IV (Chap. 131)
unless pt is hypotensive (systolic bp < 100 mmHg)]; digitalis is usually of little
benefit in acute MI unless supraventricular arrhythmias are present. Diuretic,
vasodilator, and inotropic therapy (Table 126-1) may be guided by invasive
hemodynamic monitoring (Swan-Ganz pulmonary artery catheter, arterial
line), particularly in pts with accompanying hypotension (Table 126-2; Fig.
126-3). In acute MI, optimal pulmonary capillary wedge pressure (PCW) is
15–20 mmHg; in the absence of hypotension, PCW > 20 mmHg is treated with
diuretic plus vasodilator therapy [IV nitroglycerin (begin at 10 µg/min) or nitroprusside (begin at 0.5 µg/kg per min)] and titrated to optimize bp, PCW, and
systemic vascular resistance (SVR).

$$SVR = \frac{(\text{mean arterial pressure} - \text{mean RA pressure}) \times 80}{\text{cardiac output}}$$

**TABLE 126-1   INTRAVENOUS VASODILATORS AND INOTROPIC
DRUGS USED IN ACUTE MI**

Drug	Usual Dosage Range	Comment
Nitroglycerin	5–100 µg/min	May improve coronary blood flow to ischemic myocardium
Nitroprusside	0.5–10 (µg/kg)/min	More potent vasodilator, but improves coronary blood flow less than nitroglycerin
		With therapy >24 h or in renal failure, watch for thiocyanate toxicity (blurred vision, tinnitus, delirium)
Dobutamine	2–20 (µg/kg)/min	Results in ↑ cardiac output, ↓ PCW, but does not raise bp
Dopamine	2–20 (µg/kg)/min	More appropriate than dobutamine if hypotensive
		Hemodynamic effect depends on dose: (µg/kg)/min <5:↑ renal blood flow 2.5–10:positive inotrope >10:vasoconstriction
Milrinone	50-µg/kg over 10 min, then 0.375–0.75 (µg/kg)/min	Ventricular arrhythmias may result

	Cardiac Index,	PCW,	Systolic bp,	
TABLE 126-2	**HEMODYNAMIC COMPLICATIONS IN ACUTE MI**			
Condition	(L/min)/m²	mmHg	mmHg	Treatment
Uncomplicated	>2.5	≤18	>100	—
Hypovolemia	<2.5	<15	<100	Successive boluses of normal saline
				In setting of inferior wall MI, consider RV infarction (esp. if RA pressure >10)
Volume overload	>2.5	>20	>100	Diuretic (e.g., furosemide 10–20 mg IV)
				Nitroglycerin, topical paste or IV (Table 126-1)
LV failure	<2.5	>20	>100	Diuretic (e.g., furosemide 10–20 mg IV)
				IV nitroglycerin (or if hypertensive, use IV nitroprusside)
Severe LV failure	<2.5	>20	<100	If bp ≥90: IV dobutamine ± IV nitroglycerin or sodium nitroprusside
				If bp <90: IV dopamine
				If accompanied by pulmonary edema: attempt diuresis with IV furosemide; may be limited by hypotension
				If new systolic murmur present, consider acute VSD or mitral regurgitation
Cardiogenic shock	<2.2	>20	<90 with oliguria and confusion	IV dopamine
				Intraaortic balloon pump
				Reperfusion by PCI or CABG may be life-saving

Note: PCW, pulmonary artery wedge pressure; RV, right ventricle; LV, left ventricle; PCI, percutaneous coronary intervention; VSD, ventricular septal defect; CABG, coronary artery bypass graft.

Normal SVR = 900 – 1350 dyn•s/cm⁵. If PCW > 20 mmHg and pt is hypotensive (Table 126-2 and Fig. 126-3), evaluate for VSD or acute mitral regurgitation, add dobutamine [begin at 1–2 (μg/kg)/min], titrate upward to maximum of 10 (μg/kg)/min; beware of drug-induced tachycardia or ventricular ectopy.

After stabilization on parenteral vasodilator therapy, oral therapy follows with an ACE inhibitor, an ARB, or the combination of nitrates plus hydrala-

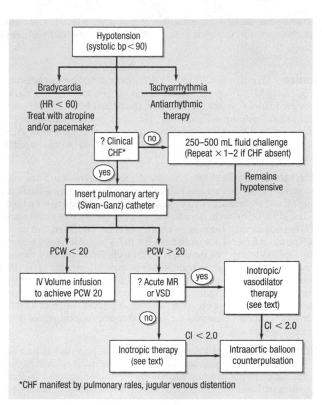

FIGURE 126-3 Approach to hypotension in pts with acute myocardial infarction; PCW, pulmonary capillary wedge pressure.

zine (Chap. 131). Consider addition of long-term aldosterone antagonist (spironolactone 25–50 mg daily, or eplerenone 25 mg daily) to ACE inhibitor if LV ejection fraction (LVEF) ≤ 40% or symptomatic heart failure or diabetes are present—do not use if renal insufficiency or hyperkalemia are present.

Cardiogenic Shock   (See Chap. 12)   Severe LV failure with hypotension (bp < 90 mmHg) *and* elevated PCW (>20 mmHg), accompanied by oliguria (<20 mL/h), peripheral vasoconstriction, dulled sensorium, and metabolic acidosis.

℞ Cardiogenic Shock

Swan-Ganz catheter and intraarterial bp monitoring are essential; aim for mean PCW of 18–20 mmHg with adjustment of volume (diuretics or infusion) as needed. Vasopressors [e.g. dopamine (Table 126-1)] and/or intraaortic balloon counterpulsation may be necessary to maintain systolic bp > 90 mmHg and reduce PCW. Administer high concentration of O_2 by mask; if pulmonary edema coexists, consider bilateral positive airway pressure (Bi-PAP) or intubation and mechanical ventilation. Acute mechanical complications (see below) should be sought and promptly treated.

If cardiogenic shock develops within 36 h of acute STEMI, reperfusion by PCI or coronary artery bypass grafting (CABG) may markedly improve LV function.

Hypotension May also result from *RV MI*, which should be suspected in inferior or posterior MI, if jugular venous distention and elevation of right-heart pressures predominate (rales are typically absent and PCW may be normal); right-sided ECG leads typically show ST elevation, and echocardiography may confirm diagnosis. *Treatment* consists of volume infusion, gauged by PCW and arterial pressure. Noncardiac causes of hypotension should be considered: hypovolemia, acute arrhythmia, or sepsis.

Acute Mechanical Complications Ventricular septal rupture and acute mitral regurgitation due to papillary muscle ischemia/infarct develop during the first week following MI and are characterized by sudden onset of CHF and new systolic murmur. Echocardiography with Doppler can confirm presence of these complications. PCW tracings may show large *v* waves in either condition, but an oxygen "step-up" as the catheter is advanced from RA to RV suggests septal rupture.

Acute medical therapy of these conditions includes vasodilator therapy (IV nitroprusside: begin at 10 μg/min and titrate to maintain systolic bp $\approx$ 100 mmHg); intraaortic balloon pump may be required to maintain cardiac output. Surgical correction is the definitive therapy. Acute ventricular free-wall rupture presents with sudden loss of bp, pulse, and consciousness, while ECG shows an intact rhythm (pulseless electrical activity); emergent surgical repair is crucial, and mortality is high.

Pericarditis Characterized by *pleuritic, positional* pain and pericardial rub (Chap. 123); atrial arrhythmias are common; must be distinguished from recurrent angina. Often responds to aspirin, 650 mg PO qid. Anticoagulants should be avoided when pericarditis is suspected to avoid development of tamponade.

Ventricular Aneurysm Localized "bulge" of LV chamber due to infarcted myocardium. *True aneurysms* consist of scar tissue and do not rupture. However, complications include CHF, ventricular arrhythmias, and thrombus formation. Typically, ECG shows persistent ST-segment elevation, >2 weeks after initial infarct; aneurysm is confirmed by echocardiography and by left ventriculography. The presence of thrombus within the aneurysm, or a large aneurysmal segment due to anterior MI, warrants oral anticoagulation with warfarin for 3–6 months.

Pseudoaneurysm is a form of cardiac rupture contained by a local area of pericardium and organized thrombus; direct communication with the LV cavity is present; surgical repair usually necessary to prevent rupture.

Recurrent Angina Usually associated with transient ST-T wave changes; signals high incidence of reinfarction; when it occurs in early post-MI period, proceed directly to coronary arteriography, to identify those who would benefit from percutaneous coronary intervention or coronary artery bypass surgery.

SECONDARY PREVENTION

For pts who have not already undergone coronary angiography and PCI, submaximal exercise testing should be performed prior to or soon after discharge. A positive test in certain subgroups (angina at a low workload, a large region of provocable ischemia, or provocable ischemia with a reduced LVEF) suggests need for cardiac catheterization to evaluate myocardium at risk of recurrent infarction.

Beta blockers (e.g., timolol, 10 mg bid; metoprolol, 25–100 mg bid) should be prescribed routinely for at least 2 years following acute MI (Table 124-1), unless contraindications present (asthma, CHF, bradycardia, "brittle" diabetes). Aspirin (80–325 mg/d) is administered to reduce incidence of subsequent infarction, unless contraindicated (e.g., active peptic ulcer, allergy). In aspirin-intolerant pts, use clopidogrel (75 mg/d) instead. If the LVEF ≤ 40%, an ACE inhibitor (e.g., captopril 6.25 mg PO tid, advanced to target dose of 50 mg PO tid) or ARB (if ACE inhibitor is not tolerated) should be used indefinitely. Consider addition of aldosterone antagonist (see "Congestive Heart Failure" section above).

Modification of cardiac risk factors must be encouraged: discontinue smoking; control hypertension, diabetes, and serum lipids (typically atorvastatin 80 mg daily in immediate post-MI period—see Chap. 187); and pursue graduated exercise.

For a more detailed discussion, see Antman EM, Braunwald E: ST-Segment Elevation Myocardial Infarction, Chap. 239, p. 1532, in HPIM-17.

127 Unstable Angina and Non-ST-Elevation Myocardial Infarction

Unstable angina (UA) and non-ST-elevation MI (NSTEMI) are acute coronary syndromes with similar mechanisms, clinical presentations, and treatment strategies.

Clinical Presentation UA includes (1) new onset of severe angina, (2) angina at rest or with minimal activity, and (3) recent increase in frequency and intensity of chronic angina. NSTEMI is diagnosed when symptoms of UA are accompanied by evidence of myocardial necrosis (e.g., elevated cardiac biomarkers). Some patients with NSTEMI present with symptoms identical to STEMI—the two are differentiated by ECG (see Chap. 126).

Physical Examination May be normal or include diaphoresis, pale cool skin, tachycardia, S_4, basilar rales; if large region of ischemia, may demonstrate S_3, hypotension.

Electrocardiogram Most commonly ST depression and/or T-wave inversion; unlike STEMI, there is no Q-wave development.

Cardiac Biomarkers CK-MB and/or cardiac-specific troponins (more specific and sensitive markers of myocardial necrosis) are elevated in NSTEMI. Small troponin elevations may also occur in pts with CHF, myocarditis, or pulmonary embolism.

℞ Unstable Angina and Non-ST-Elevation Myocardial Infarction

First step is appropriate triage based on likelihood of coronary artery disease (CAD) and acute coronary syndrome (Fig. 127-1) as well as identification of

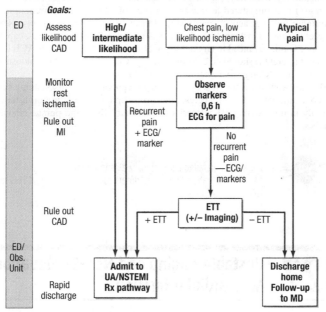

**Critical Pathway for ED Evaluation of Chest Pain/
"Rule Out MI"**

FIGURE 127-1 Diagnostic evaluation of patients presenting with suspected UA/NSTEMI. The first step is to assess the likelihood of coronary artery disease (CAD). Patients at high or intermediate likelihood are admitted to the hospital. Those with clearly atypical chest pain are discharged home. Patients with a *low* likelihood of ischemia enter the pathway and are observed in a monitored bed in the emergency department (ED) or observation unit over a period of 6 h and 12-lead electrocardiograms are performed if the patient has recurrent chest discomfort. A panel of cardiac markers (e.g., troponin and CK-MB) are drawn at baseline and 6 h later. If the patient develops recurrent pain, has ST-segment or T-wave changes, or had positive cardiac markers, he/she is admitted to the hospital and treated for UA/NSTEMI. If the patient has negative markers and no recurrence of pain, he/she is sent for stress testing, with imaging reserved for patients with abnormal baseline ECGs (e.g., left bundle branch block or left ventricular hypertrophy). If positive, the patient is admitted; if negative, the patient is discharged home with follow-up to his/her physician. (ETT, exercise tolerance test; OBS, observation unit.) [*Adapted from CP Cannon, in E Braunwald et al (eds): Heart Disease: A Textbook of Cardiovascular Medicine, 6th ed. Philadelphia, Saunders, 2001.*]

higher-risk pts (Fig. 127-2). Patients with low likelihood of active ischemia are initially monitored by serial ECGs, serum cardiac biomarkers, and for recurrent chest discomfort; if these are negative, stress testing (or CT angiography if probability of CAD is low) can be used for further therapeutic planning.

Therapy of UA/NSTEMI is directed: (1) against the inciting intracoronary thrombus, and (2) toward restoration of balance between myocardial oxygen supply and demand. Patients with the highest risk scores (Fig. 127-2) benefit the most from aggressive interventions.

ANTITHROMBOTIC THERAPIES
- Aspirin (162–325 mg, then 75–325 mg/d)
- Clopidogrel (300 mg PO load, then 75 mg/d) unless excessive risk of bleeding or immediate coronary artery bypass grafting (CABG) likely

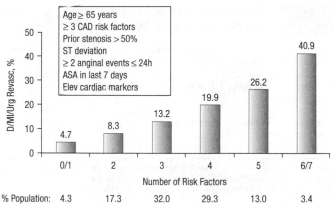

FIGURE 127-2 The TIMI Risk Score for UA/NSTEMI. The quantity of listed attributes correlates with risk of death, MI, or need for urgent revascularization over 14 days. (*Modified from E Antman et al: JAMA 284:835, 2000.*)

- Unfractionated heparin [60 U/kg then 12 (U/kg)/h (maximum 1000 U/h)] to achieve aPTT 1.5–2.5 × control, *or* low-molecular-weight heparin (e.g., enoxaparin 1 mg/kg SC q12h)
- Add intravenous GP IIb/IIIa antagonist for high-risk pts for whom invasive management is planned [e.g., tirofiban, 0.4 (μg/kg)/min × 30 min, then 0.1 (μg/kg)/min for 48–96 h; or eptifibatide, 180-μg/kg bolus, then 2.0 (μg/kg)/min for 72–96 h].
- Do not administer fibrinolytic therapy to pts with UA/NSTEMI.

ANTI-ISCHEMIC THERAPIES
- Nitroglycerin 0.3–0.6 mg sublingually or by buccal spray. If chest discomfort persists after three doses given 5 min apart, consider IV nitroglycerin (5–10 μg/min, then increase by 10 μg/min every 3–5 min until symptoms relieved or systolic bp < 100 mmHg). Do not use nitrates in pts with recent use of phosphodiesterase-5 inhibitors for erectile dysfunction (e.g., not within 24 h of sildenafil or within 48 h of tadalafil).
- Beta blockers (e.g., metoprolol 5 mg IV q5–10min to total dose of 15 mg, then 25–50 mg PO q6h) targeted to a heart rate of 50–60 beats/min. In pts with contraindications to beta blockers (e.g., bronchospasm), consider long-acting verapamil or diltiazem (Table 124-1).

ADDITIONAL RECOMMENDATIONS
- Admit to unit with continuous ECG monitoring, initially with bed rest.
- Consider morphine sulfate 2–5 mg IV q5–30min for refractory chest discomfort (Chap. 126).
- Add HMG-CoA reductase inhibitor (initially at high dose, e.g., atorvastatin 80 mg daily) and consider ACE inhibitor (Chap. 126).

INVASIVE VS. CONSERVATIVE STRATEGY
In highest risk pts (Table 127-1), an early invasive strategy (coronary arteriography within ~48 h followed by percutaneous intervention or CABG) improves outcomes. In lower-risk pts, angiography can be deferred but should be pursued if myocardial ischemia recurs spontaneously (angina or ST deviations at rest or with minimal activity) or is provoked by stress testing.

TABLE 127-1	**CLASS I RECOMMENDATIONS FOR USE OF AN EARLY INVASIVE STRATEGY**

Recurrent angina/ischemia at rest or minimal exertion despite anti-ischemic therapy
Elevated cardiac TnI or TnT
New ST-segment depression
Recurrent ischemia with CHF or worsening mitral regurgitation
Positive stress test
LVEF < 0.40
Hemodynamic instability or hypotension
Sustained ventricular tachycardia
PCI within previous 6 months, or prior CABG

Note: TnI, troponin I; TnT, troponin T; LVEF, left ventricular ejection fraction; PCI, percutaneous coronary intervention; CABG, coronary artery bypass grafting.
Source: Modified from E Braunwald et al: Circulation 106:1893, 2002.

LONG-TERM MANAGEMENT

* Stress importance of smoking cessation, achieving optimal weight, diet low in saturated and trans-fats, regular exercise; these principles can be reinforced by encouraging patient to enter cardiac rehabilitation program.
* Continue aspirin, clopidogrel (for at least 9–12 months), beta-blocker, statin, and ACE inhibitor (especially if hypertensive or diabetic or LV ejection fraction is reduced).

For a more detailed discussion, see Cannon CP, Braunwald E: Unstable Angina and Non-ST-Elevation Myocardial Infarction, Chap. 238, p. 1527, in HPIM-17.

128 Chronic Stable Angina

ANGINA

Angina pectoris, the most common clinical manifestation of coronary artery disease (CAD), results from an imbalance between myocardial O_2 supply and demand, most often due to atherosclerotic coronary artery obstruction. Other major conditions that upset this balance and result in angina include aortic valve disease (Chap. 121), hypertrophic cardiomyopathy (Chap. 122), and coronary artery spasm (see below).

Symptoms   Angina is typically associated with exertion or emotional upset; relieved quickly by rest or nitroglycerin (Chap. 33). Major risk factors are cigarette smoking, hypertension, hypercholesterolemia (↑LDL fraction; ↓HDL), diabetes, obesity, and family history of CAD before age 55.

Physical Examination   Often normal; arterial bruits or retinal vascular abnormalities suggest generalized atherosclerosis; S_4 is common. During acute anginal episode, other signs may appear: loud S_3 or S_4, diaphoresis, rales, and a transient murmur of mitral regurgitation due to papillary muscle ischemia.

Laboratory ECG May be normal between anginal episodes or show old infarction (Chap. 118). During angina, ST- and T-wave abnormalities typically appear (ST-segment depression reflects subendocardial ischemia; ST-segment elevation may reflect acute infarction or transient coronary artery spasm). Ventricular arrhythmias frequently accompany acute ischemia.

Stress Testing Enhances diagnosis of CAD (Fig. 128-1). Exercise is performed on treadmill or bicycle until target heart rate is achieved or pt becomes symptomatic (chest pain, light-headedness, hypotension, marked dyspnea, ventricular tachycardia) or develops diagnostic ST-segment changes. Useful information includes duration of exercise achieved; peak heart rate and bp; depth, morphology, and persistence of ST-segment depression; and whether at and at which level of exercise pain, hypotension, or ventricular arrhythmias develop. Exercise testing with radionuclide or echocardiographic imaging increases sensitivity and specificity and is particularly useful if baseline ECG abnormalities prevent interpretation of test. *Note:* Exercise testing should not be performed in pts with acute MI, unstable angina, or severe aortic stenosis. If the pt is unable to exercise, pharmacologic stress with intravenous dipyridamole (or adenosine) or dobutamine can be performed in conjunction

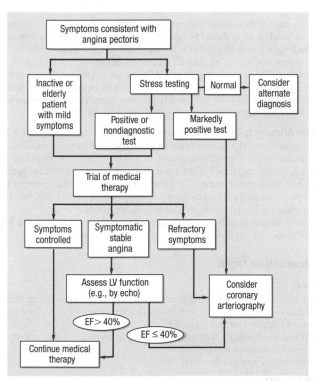

FIGURE 128-1 Role of exercise testing in management of CAD; EF, left ventricular ejection fraction. [*Modified from LS Lilly, in Textbook of Primary Care Medicine, 3d ed., J Nobel (ed.) St. Louis, Mosby, 2001, p. 552.*]

TABLE 128-1 STRESS TESTING RECOMMENDATIONS	
Subgroup	Recommended Study
Patient able to exercise	
If baseline ST-T on ECG is normal	Standard exercise test (treadmill, bicycle, or arm ergometry)
If baseline ST-T impairs test interpretation (e.g., LVH with strain, digoxin)	Standard exercise test (above) combined with *either*
	Perfusion scintigraphy (thallium 201, ^{99m}Tc-sestamibi or rubidium-82 PET) *or*
	Echocardiography
Patient *not* able to exercise (regardless of baseline ST-T abnormality)	Pharmacologic stress test (IV dobutamine, dipyridamole, or adenosine combined with *either*
	Perfusion scintigraphy (thallium 201, ^{99m}Tc-sestamibi or rubidium-82 PET) *or*
	Echocardiography
LBBB on baseline ECG	Adenosine (or dipyridamole) ^{99m}Tc-sestamibi
Alternative choice (if baseline ST-T normal)	Ambulatory ECG monitor

with radionuclide or echocardiographic imaging. (Table 128-1). Patients with LBBB on baseline ECG should be referred for adenosine or dipyridamole radionuclide imaging, which is most specific for diagnosis of CAD in this setting.

The prognostic utility of coronary calcium detection (by electron-beam or multidetector CT) in the diagnosis of CAD has not yet been fully characterized.

Some pts do not experience chest pain during ischemic episodes with exertion ("silent ischemia") but are identifed by transient ST-T-wave abnormalities during stress testing or ambulatory ECG monitoring (see below).

Coronary Arteriography   The definitive test for assessing severity of CAD; major indications are (1) angina refractory to medical therapy, (2) markedly positive exercise test (≥2-mm ST-segment depression, onset of ischemia at low workload, or ventricular tachycardia or hypotension with exercise) suggestive of left main or three-vessel disease, (3) recurrent angina or positive exercise test after MI, (4) to assess for coronary artery spasm, and (5) to evaluate pts with perplexing chest pain in whom noninvasive tests are not diagnostic.

The role of new *noninvasive* coronary imaging techniques (CT and MR angiography) has not yet been defined.

℞ Chronic Stable Angina

GENERAL
- Identify and treat risk factors: mandatory cessation of smoking; treatment of diabetes, hypertension, and lipid disorders (Chap. 187); advocate a diet low in saturated fat and trans-fats.
- Correct exacerbating factors contributing to angina: morbid obesity, CHF, anemia, hyperthyroidism.
- Reassurance and pt education.

DRUG THERAPY
Sublingual nitroglycerin (TNG 0.3–0.6 mg); may be repeated at 5-min intervals; warn pts of possible headache or light-headedness; teach prophylactic

TABLE 128-2 EXAMPLES OF COMMONLY USED NITRATES

	Usual Dose	Recommended Dosing Frequency
Short-Acting Agents		
Sublingual TNG	0.3–0.6 mg	As needed
Aerosol TNG	0.4 mg (1 inhalation)	As needed
Sublingual ISDN	2.5–10 mg	As needed
Long-Acting Agents		
ISDN		
Oral	5–30 mg	tid
Sustained-action	40 mg	bid (once in A.M., then 7 h later)
TNG ointment (2%)	0.5–2	qid (with one 7- to 10-h nitrate-free interval)
TNG skin patches	0.1–0.6 mg/h	Apply in morning, remove at bedtime
ISMO		
Oral	20–40 mg	bid (once in A.M., then 7 h later)
Sustained-action	30–240 mg	Daily

Note: TNG, nitroglycerin; ISDN, isosorbide dinitrate; ISMO, isosorbide mononitrate.

use of TNG prior to activity that regularly evokes angina. If chest pain persists for >10 min despite 2–3 TNG, pt should report promptly to nearest medical facility for evaluation of possible unstable angina or acute MI.

LONG-TERM ANGINA SUPPRESSION
Three classes of drugs are used, frequently in combination:

Long-Acting Nitrates
May be administered by many routes (Table 128-2); start at the lowest dose and frequency to limit tolerance and side effects of headache, light-headedness, tachycardia.

Beta Blockers (See Table 128-1)
All have antianginal properties; β_1-selective agents are less likely to exacerbate airway or peripheral vascular disease. Dosage should be titrated to resting heart rate of 50–60 beats/min. *Contraindications* to beta blockers include CHF, AV block, bronchospasm, "brittle" diabetes. Side effects include fatigue, bronchospasm, depressed LV function, impotence, depression, and masking of hypoglycemia in diabetics.

Calcium Antagonists (See Table 124-1)
Useful for stable and unstable angina, as well coronary vasospasm. Combination with other antianginal agents is beneficial, but verapamil should be administered very cautiously, or not at all, to pts on beta blockers or disopyramide (additive effects on LV dysfunction). Use sustained-release, not short-acting, calcium antagonists; the latter increase coronary mortality.

Ranolazine
For patients who continue to experience stable angina despite the above standard medications, consider addition of ranolazine (500–1000 mg PO bid), which reduces anginal frequency and improves exercise capacity without af-

fecting blood pressure or heart rate. Ranolazine is contraindicated in hepatic impairment, prolongation of the QT_c interval, or in combination with drugs that inhibit its metabolism (e.g., ketoconazole, macrolide antibiotics, HIV protease inhibitors, diltiazem and verapamil).

Aspirin

80–325 mg/d reduces the incidence of MI in chronic stable angina, following MI, and in asymptomatic men. It is recommended in pts with CAD in the absence of contraindications (GI bleeding or allergy). Consider clopidogrel (75 mg/d) for aspirin-intolerant individuals.

The addition of an ACE inhibitor is recommended in patients with CAD and LV ejection fraction < 40%, hypertension, diabetes, or chronic kidney disease.

MECHANICAL REVASCULARIZATION

Percutaneous Coronary Intervention (PCI)

Includes percutaneous transluminal angioplasty (PTCA) and/or stenting. Performed on anatomically suitable stenoses of native vessels and bypass grafts; more effective than medical therapy for relief of angina. Has not been shown to reduce risk of MI or death in chronic stable angina; should not be performed on asymptomatic or only mildly symptomatic individuals. With PCI initial relief of angina occurs in 95% of pts; however, with PTCA alone stenosis recurs in 30–45% within 6 months (more commonly in pts with initial unstable angina, incomplete dilation, diabetes, or stenoses containing thrombi). If restenosis occurs, PTCA can be repeated with success and risks like original procedure. Potential complications include dissection or thrombosis of the vessel and uncontrolled ischemia or CHF. Complications are most likely to occur in pts with CHF, long eccentric stenoses, calcified plaque, female gender, and dilation of an artery that perfuses a large segment of myocardium with inadequate collaterals. Placement of a bare metal intracoronary stent in suitable pts reduces the restenosis rate to ~30% at 6 months. Restenosis is nearly abolished when drug-eluting stents are used, but late stent thrombosis can rarely occur. The latter is prevented by prolonged antiplatelet therapy (aspirin indefinitely and clopidogrel for a minimum of 12 months).

Coronary Artery Bypass Surgery (CABG)

For angina refractory to medical therapy or when the latter is not tolerated (and when lesions are not amenable to PCI) or if severe CAD is present (e.g., left main, three-vessel disease with impaired LV function). CABG is currently preferred over PCI in diabetics with CAD in ≥2 vessels because of better survival.

The relative advantages of PCI and CABG are summarized in Table 128-3.

PRINZMETAL'S VARIANT ANGINA (CORONARY VASOSPASM)

Intermittent focal spasm of coronary artery; often associated with atherosclerotic lesion near site of spasm. Chest discomfort is similar to angina but more severe and occurs typically at rest, with transient ST-segment elevation. Acute infarction or malignant arrhythmias may develop during spasm-induced ischemia. Evaluation includes observation of ECG (or ambulatory Holter monitor) for transient ST elevation; diagnosis confirmed at coronary angiography using provocative (e.g., IV acetylcholine) testing. Primary treatment consists of long-acting nitrates and calcium antagonists. Prognosis is better in pts with anatomically normal coronary arteries than in those with fixed coronary stenoses.

TABLE 128-3	**COMPARISON OF REVASCULARIZATION PROCEDURES IN MULTIVESSEL DISEASE**	
Procedure	Advantages	Disadvantages
Percutaneous coronary revascularization (angioplasty and/or stenting)	Less invasive Shorter hospital stay Lower initial cost Easily repeated Effective in relieving symptoms	Restenosis Possible incomplete revascularization Unknown outcomes in pts with severe left ventricular dysfunction Limited to specific anatomic subsets ? Less beneficial outcome in diabetics with 2- to 3-vessel coronary disease
Coronary artery bypass grafting	Effective in relieving symptoms Improved survival in certain subsets, including diabetics Ability to achieve complete revascularization	Cost Risk of a repeat procedure due to late graft closure Morbidity and mortality of major surgery

Source: Modified from DP Faxon, in GA Beller (ed), *Chronic Ischemic Heart Disease*, in E Braunwald (series ed), *Atlas of Heart Disease*, Philadelphia, Current Medicine, 1994.

For a more detailed discussion, see Antman EM, Selwyn AP, Braunwald E, Loscalzo J: Ischemic Heart Disease, Chap. 237, p. 1514, in HPIM-17.

129 Bradyarrhythmias

Bradyarrhythmias arise from: (1) failure of impulse initiation (sinoatrial node dysfunction) or (2) impaired electrical conduction (e.g., AV conduction blocks).

SINOATRIAL (SA) NODE DYSFUNCTION

Etiologies are either *intrinsic* [degenerative, ischemic, inflammatory, infiltrative (e.g., senile amyloid), or rare mutations in sodium channel or pacemaker current genes] or *extrinsic* [e.g., drugs (beta blockers, Ca^{++} channel blockers, digoxin), autonomic dysfunction, hypothyroidism].

Symptoms are due to *bradycardia* (fatigue, weakness, lightheadedness, syncope) and/or episodes of associated *tachycardia* (e.g., rapid palpitations, angina) in patients with sick sinus syndrome (SSS).

Diagnosis Examine ECG for evidence of sinus bradycardia (sinus rhythm at <60 beats/min) or failure of rate to increase with exercise, sinus pauses, or exit block. In patients with SSS, periods of tachycardia (i.e., atrial fibrillation/flutter) occur. Prolonged ECG monitoring (24-h Holter or 30-day loop event monitor) aids in identifying these abnormalities. Invasive electrophysiologic testing is rarely necessary to establish diagnosis.

℞ Sinoatrial Node Dysfunction

Remove or treat extrinsic causes such as contributing drugs or hypothyroidism. Otherwise, symptoms of bradycardia respond to permanent pacemaker placement. In SSS, treat associated atrial fibrillation or flutter as indicated in Chap. 130.

AV BLOCK

Impaired conduction from atria to ventricles may be structural and permanent, or reversible (e.g., autonomic, metabolic, drug-related)—see Table 129-1.

TABLE 129-1 ETIOLOGIES OF ATRIOVENTRICULAR BLOCK

Autonomic

Carotid sinus hypersensitivity	Vasovagal

Metabolic/endocrine

Hyperkalemia	Hypothyroidism
Hypermagnesemia	Adrenal insufficiency

Drug-related

Beta blockers	Adenosine
Calcium channel blockers	Antiarrhythmics (class I & III)
Digitalis	Lithium

Infectious

Endocarditis	Tuberculosis
Lyme disease	Diphtheria
Chagas disease	Toxoplasmosis
Syphilis	

Heritable/congenital

Congenital heart disease	Kearns-Sayre syndrome, OMIM #530000
Maternal SLE	Myotonic dystrophy

Inflammatory

SLE	MCTD
Rheumatoid arthritis	Scleroderma

Infiltrative

Amyloidosis	Hemochromatosis
Sarcoidosis	

Neoplastic/traumatic

Lymphoma	Radiation
Mesothelioma	Catheter ablation
Melanoma	

Degenerative

Lev disease	Lenègre disease

Coronary artery disease

Acute MI

Note: SLE, systemic lupus erythematosus; OMIM, Online Mendelian Inheritance in Man (database); MCTD, mixed connective tissue disease; MI, myocardial infarction.

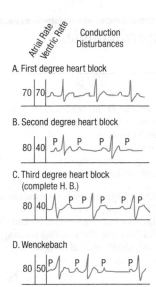

Conduction
Disturbances

A. First degree heart block

70 | 70

B. Second degree heart block

80 | 40

C. Third degree heart block
(complete H. B.)

80 | 40

D. Wenckebach

80 | 50

FIGURE 129-1 Tachyarrhythmias. (*Modified from BE Sobel, E Braunwald: HPIM-9, p. 1052.*)

First Degree (See Fig. 129-1A) Prolonged, constant PR interval (>0.20 s). May be normal or secondary to increased vagal tone or drugs (e.g., beta-blocker, diltiazem, verapamil, digoxin); treatment not usually required.

Second Degree (See Fig. 129-1B)
Mobitz I (Wenckebach) Narrow QRS, progressive increase in PR interval until a ventricular beat is dropped, then sequence is repeated (Fig. 129-1D). Seen with drug intoxication (digitalis, beta blockers), increased vagal tone, inferior MI. Usually transient, no therapy required; if symptomatic, use atropine (0.6 mg IV, repeated × 3–4) or temporary pacemaker.

Mobitz II Fixed PR interval with occasional dropped beats, in 2:1, 3:1, or 4:1 pattern; the QRS complex is usually wide. Seen with MI or degenerative conduction system disease; more serious than Mobitz I—may progress suddenly to complete AV block; permanent pacemaker is indicated.

Third Degree (Complete AV Block) (See Fig. 129-1C) Complete failure of conduction from atria to ventricles; atria and ventricles depolarize independently. May occur with MI, digitalis toxicity, or degenerative conduction system disease. Permanent pacemaker is usually indicated, except when reversible (e.g., drug-related or appears only transiently in MI without associated bundle branch block).

For a more detailed discussion, see Tomaselli GF: The Bradyarrhythmias, Chap. 225, p. 1416, in HPIM-17.

130 Tachyarrhythmias

Tachyarrhythmias may appear in the presence or absence of structural heart disease; they are more serious in the former. Conditions that provoke arrhythmias include (1) myocardial ischemia, (2) CHF, (3) hypoxemia, (4) hypercapnia, (5) hypotension, (6) electrolyte disturbances (e.g., hypokalemia and/or hypomagnesemia), (7) drug toxicity (digoxin, pharmacologic agents that prolong QT interval), (8) caffeine, (9) ethanol.

Diagnosis Examine ECG for evidence of ischemic changes (Chap. 118), prolonged or shortened QT interval, characteristics of Wolff-Parkinson-White (WPW) syndrome (see below), or ST elevation in leads V_1–V_3 typical of Brugada syndrome. See Fig. 130-1 and Table 130-1 for diagnosis of tachyarrhythmias; always identify atrial activity and relationship between P waves and QRS complexes. To aid the diagnosis:

- Obtain long rhythm strip of lead II, aVF, or V_1. Double the ECG voltage and increase paper speed to 50 mm/s to help identify P waves.
- Place accessory ECG leads (e.g., right-sided chest leads) to help identify P waves. Record ECG during carotid sinus massage (Table 130-1). Note: Do not massage both carotids simultaneously.
- For intermittent symptoms, consider 24-h Holter monitor (if symptoms occur daily), a patient-activated event monitor, or, if symptoms are very infrequent but severely symptomatic, an implanted loop monitor. A standard exercise test may help provoke arrhythmias for diagnostic purposes.

Tachyarrhythmias with wide QRS complex beats may represent ventricular tachycardia or supraventricular tachycardia with aberrant conduction. Factors favoring ventricular tachycardia include (1) AV dissociation, (2) QRS > 0.14 s, (3) rightward and superior QRS axis, (4) no response to carotid sinus massage, (5) morphology of QRS unlike typical RBBB or LBBB, and similar to that of previous ventricular premature beats (Table 130-2).

Rx **Tachyarrhythmias** (Tables 130-1 and 130-3)

Precipitating causes (listed above) should be corrected. If pt is hemodynamically compromised (angina, hypotension, CHF), proceed to immediate cardioversion.

Do not cardiovert sinus tachycardia; exercise caution if digitalis toxicity is suspected. Initiate drugs as indicated in the tables; follow drug levels and ECG intervals (esp. QRS and QT). Reduce dosage for pts with hepatic or renal dysfunction as indicated in Table 130-3. Drug efficacy is confirmed by ECG (or Holter) monitoring, stress testing, and, in special circumstances, invasive electrophysiologic study.

Antiarrhythmic agents all have potential toxic side effects, including provocation of ventricular arrhythmias, esp. in pts with LV dysfunction or history of sustained ventricular arrhythmias. Drug-induced QT prolongation and associated torsades de pointes ventricular tachycardia (Table 130-1) is most common with group IA and III agents; the drug should be discontinued if the

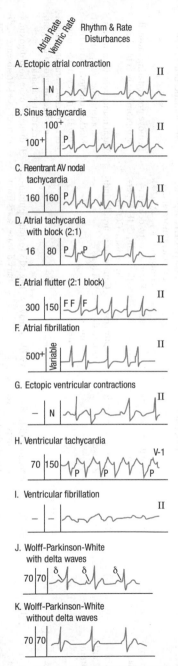

FIGURE 130-1 Tachyarrhythmias. (*Modified from BE Sobel, E Braunwald: HPIM-9, p. 1052.*)

TABLE 130-1 CLINICAL AND ELECTROCARDIOGRAPHIC FEATURES OF COMMON ARRHYTHMIAS

Rhythm	Example (See Fig. 130-1)	Atrial Rate	Features	Carotid Sinus Massage	Precipitating Conditions	Initial Treatment
Narrow QRS Complex						
Atrial premature beats	A	—	P wave abnormal; QRS width normal	—	Can be normal; or due to anxiety, CHF, hypoxia, caffeine, abnormal electrolytes ($\downarrow$K+, $\downarrow$Mg2+)	Remove precipitating cause; if symptomatic: beta blocker
Sinus tachycardia	B	100–160	Normal P wave contour	Rate gradually slows	Fever, anxiety, dehydration, pain, CHF, hyperthyroidism, COPD	Remove precipitating cause; if symptomatic: beta blocker
AV nodal tachycardia (reentrant)	C	120–250	Absent or retrograde P wave	Abruptly converts to sinus rhythm (or no effect)	Can occur in healthy individuals	Vagal maneuvers; if unsuccessful: adenosine, verapamil, beta blocker, cardioversion (100–200 J). To prevent recurrence: beta blocker, verapamil, diltiazem, digoxin, group IC agent, or catheter ablation
Atrial tachycardia	D	130–200	P contour different from sinus P wave; AV block may occur; automatic form shows "warm-up" in rate in first several beats	AV block may $\uparrow$	Digitalis toxicity; pulmonary disease; scars from cardiac surgery	If digitalis toxic: hold digoxin, correct [K+]. In absence of digoxin toxicity: slow rate with beta blocker, verapamil, or diltiazem; can attempt conversion with IV procainamide or amiodarone

		Rate	ECG	Effect	Associated Conditions	Treatment
Atrial flutter	E	250–350	"Sawtooth" flutter waves; 2:1, 4:1 block	↑AV block: ventricular rate ↓	Mitral valve disease, hypertension, pulmonary embolism, pericarditis, postcardiac surgery; hyperthyroidism; obstructive lung disease, EtOH, idiopathic	1. Slow the ventricular rate: beta blocker, verapamil, diltiazem, or digoxin 2. Convert to NSR (after anticoagulation if chronic) electrically (50–100 J for atrial flutter, 100–200 J for atrial fibrillation) or chemically with IV ibutilide or oral group IC, III, or IA[a] agent. Atrial flutter may respond to rapid atrial pacing, and radio frequency ablation highly effective to prevent recurrences
Atrial fibrillation	F	>350	No discrete P; irregularly spaced QRS	↓Ventricular rate		
Multifocal atrial tachycardia		100–150	More than 3 different P wave shapes with varying PR intervals	No effect	Severe respiratory insufficiency	Treat underlying lung disease; verapamil may be used to slow ventricular rate; group IC agents or amiodarone may ↓ episodes

(continued)

TABLE 130-1 CLINICAL AND ELECTROCARDIOGRAPHIC FEATURES OF COMMON ARRHYTHMIAS (CONTINUED)

Rhythm	Example (See Fig. 130-1)	Atrial Rate	Features	Carotid Sinus Massage	Precipitating Conditions	Initial Treatment
Wide QRS Complex						
Ventricular premature beats	G		Fully compensatory pause between normal beats	No effect	CAD, MI, CHF, hypoxia, hypokalemia, digitalis toxicity, prolonged QT interval (congenital or drugs: quinidine and other antiarrhythmics, tricyclics, phenothiazines)	May not require therapy; if needed, use beta blocker
Ventricular tachycardia	H		QRS rate 100–250; slightly irregular rate	No effect		If unstable: electrical conversion/defibrillation (> 200 J); otherwise: Acute (IV): amiodarone, lidocaine, procainamide; chronic management: usually ICD. Patients without structural heart disease (focal outflow tract VT) may respond to beta blockers or verapamil.
Accelerated idioventricular rhythm (AIVR)			Gradual onset and offset; QRS rate 40–120		Acute MI, cocaine, myocarditis	Usually none; for symptoms, use atropine or atrial pacing
Ventricular fibrillation	I		Erratic electrical activity only	No effect		Immediate defibrillation

| Torsades de pointes | Ventricular tachycardia with sinusoidal oscillations of QRS height | No effect | Prolonged QT interval (congenital or drugs: quinidine and other antiarrhythmics, tricyclics, phenothiazines) | IV magnesium (1–2 g bolus); overdrive pacing; isoproterenol (unless CAD present); lidocaine. Drugs that prolong QT interval are contraindicated. |
| Supraventricular tachycardias with aberrant ventricular conduction | P wave typical of the supraventricular rhythm; wide QRS complex due to conduction through partially refractory pathways | | Etiologies of the respective supraventricular rhythms listed above; atrial fibrillation with rapid, wide QRS may be due to preexcitation (WPW) | Same as treatment of respective supraventricular rhythm; if ventricular rate rapid (>200), treat as WPW (see text). |

[a]Antiarrhythmic drug groups listed in Table 130-3.

Note: CAD, coronary artery disease; COPD, chronic obstructive pulmonary disease; EtOH, ethyl alcohol; ICD, implantable cardioverter defibrillator; NSR, normal sinus rhythm; WPW, Wolff-Parkinson-White.

TABLE 130-2	**WIDE COMPLEX TACHYCARDIA**

ECG Criteria That Favor Ventricular Tachycardia

1. AV dissociation
2. QRS width: >0.14 s with RBBB configuration
   >0.16 s with LBBB configuration
3. QRS axis: Left axis deviation with RBBB morphology
   Extreme left axis deviation (northwest axis) with LBBB morphology
4. Concordance of QRS in precordial leads
5. Morphologic patterns of the QRS complex
   RBBB: Mono-or biphasic complex in V_1
   RS (*only with left axis deviation*) or QS inV_6

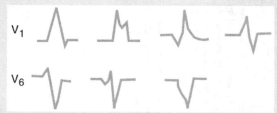

   LBBB: Broad R wave in V_1 or V_2 ≥0.04 s
   Onset of QRS to nadir of S wave in V_1 or V2 of ≥0.07 s
   Notched downslope of S wave in V_1 or V_2
   Q wave in V_6

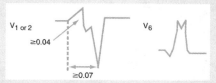

Note: AV, atrioventricular; BBB, bundle branch block.

QTc interval (QT divided by square root of RR interval) increases by >25%. Antiarrhythmic drugs should be avoided in pts with asymptomatic ventricular arrhythmias after MI, since mortality risk increases.

CHRONIC ATRIAL FIBRILLATION

Evaluate potential underlying cause (e.g., thyrotoxicosis, mitral stenosis, excessive ethanol consumption, pulmonary embolism). Pts with risk factors for stroke (e.g., rheumatic mitral valve disease, history of cerebrovascular accident or transient ischemic attack, hypertension, diabetes, CHF, age >75) should receive warfarin anticoagulation (INR 2.0–3.0). Substitute aspirin, 325 mg/d, for pts without these risk factors or if contraindication to warfarin exists.

Control ventricular rate (60–80 beats/min at rest, <100 beats/min with mild exercise) with beta blocker, calcium channel blocker (verapamil, diltiazem), or digoxin.

Consider cardioversion (100–200 J) after ≥3 weeks therapeutic anticoagulation, or acutely if no evidence of left atrial thrombus by transesophageal echo, especially if symptomatic despite rate control. Initiation of group IC, III, or IA agent (usually initiate with inpatient monitoring) prior to electrical cardioversion facilitates maintenance of sinus rhythm after successful procedure. Type IC (Table 130-3) drugs are preferred in pts without structural heart

TABLE 130-3 ANTIARRHYTHMIC DRUGS

Drug	Loading Dose	Maintenance Dose	Side Effects	Excretion
Group IA				
Quinidine sulfate		PO: 200–400 mg q6h	Diarrhea, tinnitus, QT prolongation, hypotension, anemia, thrombocytopenia	Hepatic
Quinidine gluconate		PO: 324–628 mg q8h		Hepatic
Procainamide	IV: 15 mg/kg over 60 min	IV: 1–4 mg/min	Nausea, lupus-like syndrome, agranulocytosis, QT prolongation	Renal and hepatic
		PO: 500–1000 mg q4h		
Sustained-release:		PO: 1000–2500 mg q12h		
Disopyramide		PO: 100–300 mg q6–8h	Myocardial depression, AV block, QT prolongation anticholinergic effects	Renal and hepatic
Sustained-release:		PO: 200–400 mg q12h		
Group IB				
Lidocaine	IV: 1 mg/kg bolus followed by 0.5 mg/kg bolus q8–10 min to total 3 mg/kg	IV: 1–4 mg/min	Confusion, seizures, respiratory arrest	Hepatic
Mexiletine		PO: 150–300 mg q8–12h	Nausea, tremor, gait disturbance	Hepatic
Group IC				
Flecainide		PO: 50–200 mg q12h	Nausea, exacerbation of ventricular arrhythmia, prolongation of PR and QRS intervals	Hepatic and renal
Propafenone		PO: 150–300 mg q8h		Hepatic
Group II				
Metroprolol	IV: 5–10 mg q5min × 3	PO: 25–100 mg q6h	CHF, bradycardia, AV block, bronchospasm	Hepatic
Esmolol	IV: 500 µg/kg over 1 min	IV: 50 (µg/kg)/min		

727

TABLE 130-3 ANTIARRHYTHMIC DRUGS (CONTINUED)

Drug	Loading Dose	Maintenance Dose	Side Effects	Excretion
Group III				
Amiodarone	PO: 800–1600 mg qd × 1–2 weeks, then 400–600 mg/d × 3 weeks	PO: 100–400 mg qd	Thyroid abnormalities, pulmonary fibrosis, hepatitis, corneal microdeposits, bluish skin, QT prolongation	—
	IV: 150 mg over 10 min	IV: 1 mg/min × 6 h, then 0.5 mg/min		
Ibutilide	IV (≥60 kg): 1 mg over 10 min, can repeat after 10 min	—	Torsades de pointes, hypotension, nausea	Hepatic
Dofetilide		PO: 125–500 µg bid	Torsades de pointes, headache, dizziness	Renal
Sotalol		PO: 80–160 mg q12h	Fatigue, bradycardia, exacerbation of ventricular arrhythmia	Renal
Group IV				
Verapamil	IV: 2.5–10 mg over 3–5 min	IV: 2.5–10 mg/h	AV block, CHF, hypotension, constipation	Hepatic
		PO: 80–120 mg q6–8 h		
Diltiazem	IV: 0.25 mg/kg over 3–5 min; can repeat with 0.35 mg/kg after 15 min	IV: 5–15 mg/h	—	Hepatic
		PO: 30–60 mg q6h		
Other				
Digoxin	IV, PO: 0.75–1.5 mg over 24 h	IV, PO: 0.125–0.25 mg qd	Nausea, AV block, ventricular and supraventricular arrhythmias	Renal
Adenosine	IV: 6-mg rapid bolus; if no effect then 12-mg bolus	—	Transient hypotension or atrial standstill	—

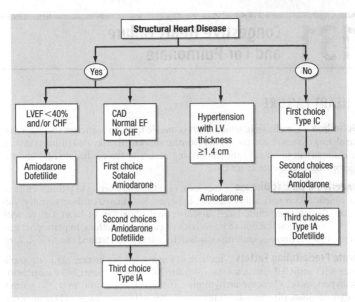

FIGURE 130-2 Recommendations for the selection of antiarrhythmic medications to prevent the recurrence of atrial fibrillation. See Table 130-3 for definition of type IA and IC drugs. An atrioventricular nodal blocking agent (i.e., beta blocker, calcium channel blocker, or digoxin) should be added to all type IC and IA agents as well as to dofetilide. LVEF, left ventricular ejection fraction; CHF, congestive heart failure; CAD, coronary artery disease; EF, ejection fraction.

disease, and type III drugs are recommended in presence of left ventricular dysfunction or coronary artery disease (Fig. 130-2). Anticoagulation should be continued for a minimum of 3 weeks after successful cardioversion.

Catheter-based ablation can be considered for recurrent symptomatic atrial fibrillation (AF) refractory to pharmacologic measures.

PREEXCITATION SYNDROME (WPW)

Conduction occurs through an accessory pathway between atria and ventricles. Baseline ECG typically shows a short PR interval and slurred upstroke of the QRS ("delta" wave) (Fig. 130-1J). Associated tachyarrhythmias are of two types:

- Narrow QRS complex tachycardia (antegrade conduction through AV node). Treat cautiously with IV adenosine or beta blocker, verapamil, or diltiazem (Table 130-2).
- Wide QRS complex tachycardia (antegrade conduction through accessory pathway); may also be associated with AF with a very rapid (>250/min) ventricular rate, which can degenerate into VF. If hemodynamically compromised, immediate cardioversion is indicated; otherwise, treat with IV procainamide or ibutilide (Table 130-3), *not* digoxin, beta blocker, or verapamil.

Consider catheter ablation of accessory pathway for long-term prevention.

For a more detailed discussion, see Marchlinski F: The Tachyarrhythmias, Chap. 226, p. 1425, in HPIM-17.

131 Congestive Heart Failure and Cor Pulmonale

HEART FAILURE

Definition   Condition in which heart is unable to pump sufficient blood for metabolizing tissues or can do so only from an abnormally elevated filling pressure. It is important to identify the underlying nature of the cardiac disease and the factors that precipitate acute CHF.

Underlying Cardiac Disease   Includes: (1) states that depress systolic ventricular function (coronary artery disease, hypertension, dilated cardiomyopathy, valvular disease, congenital heart disease); and (2) states of heart failure with preserved ejection fraction (e.g., restrictive cardiomyopathies, hypertrophic cardiomyopathy, fibrosis, endomyocardial disorders), also termed *diastolic failure*.

Acute Precipitating Factors   Include (1) increased Na intake, (2) noncompliance with anti-CHF medications, (3) acute MI (may be silent), (4) exacerbation of hypertension, (5) acute arrhythmias, (6) infections and/or fever, (7) pulmonary embolism, (8) anemia, (9) thyrotoxicosis, (10) pregnancy, (11) acute myocarditis or infective endocarditis, and (12) certain drugs (e.g., nonsteroidal antiinflammatory agents, verapamil).

Symptoms   Due to inadequate perfusion of peripheral tissues (fatigue, dyspnea) and elevated intracardiac filling pressures (orthopnea, paroxysmal nocturnal dyspnea, peripheral edema).

Physical Examination   Jugular venous distention, S_3, pulmonary congestion (rales, dullness over pleural effusion, peripheral edema, hepatomegaly, and ascites). Sinus tachycardia is common.

In patients with diastolic dysfunction, an S_4 is often present.

Laboratory   *CXR* can reveal cardiomegaly, pulmonary vascular redistribution, Kerley B lines, pleural effusions. Left ventricular contraction and diastolic dysfunction can be assessed by *echocardiography* with Doppler recordings. In addition, echo can identify underlying valvular, pericardial, or congenital heart disease, as well as regional wall motion abnormalities typical of coronary artery disease. Measurement of brain natriuretic peptide (BNP) differentiates cardiac from pulmonary causes of dyspnea (>100 pg/mL in heart failure).

Conditions That Mimic CHF   Pulmonary Disease   Chronic bronchitis, emphysema, and asthma (Chaps. 136 and 138); look for sputum production and abnormalities on CXR and pulmonary function tests.

Other Causes of Peripheral Edema   Liver disease, varicose veins, and cyclic edema, none of which results in jugular venous distention. Edema due to renal dysfunction is often accompanied by elevated serum creatinine and abnormal urinalysis (Chap. 49).

 Heart Failure   (See Fig. 131-1)

Aimed at symptomatic relief, removal of precipitating factors, control of underlying cardiac disease, and prevention of adverse cardiac remodeling. Over-

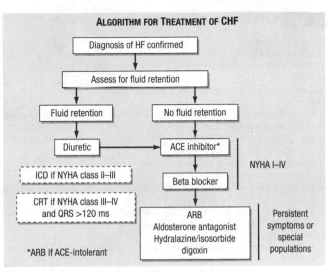

ALGORITHM FOR TREATMENT OF CHF

FIGURE 131-1 Treatment algorithm for chronic heart failure with reduced ejection fraction.

view of treatment shown in Table 131-1; notably, ACE inhibitors and beta blockers are cornerstones of therapy in patients with impaired ejection fraction (EF). Once symptoms develop:

- *Decrease cardiac workload*: Reduce physical activity; include periods of bed rest. Prevent deep venous thrombosis of immobile pts with heparin, 5000 U SC bid, or enoxaparin, 40 mg SC qd.
- *Control excess fluid retention*: (1) *Dietary sodium restriction* (eliminate salty foods, e.g., potato chips, canned soups, bacon, salt added at table); more stringent requirements (<2 g NaCl/d) in advanced CHF. If dilutional hyponatremia present, restrict fluid intake (<1000 mL/d). (2) *Diuretics* (see Chap. 49): *Loop diuretics* [e.g., furosemide (see Table 131-2)] are most potent and unlike thiazides remain effective when GFR < 25 mL/min. Combine loop diuretic with thiazide or metolazone for augmented effect. Potassium-sparing diuretics are useful adjunct to reduce potassium loss; should be used cautiously when combined with ACE inhibitor or angiotensin receptor blocker (ARB) to avoid hyperkalemia.

During diuresis, obtain daily weights, aiming for loss of 1–1.5 kg/d.

- *ACE inhibitors* (Table 131-2): Recommended as standard initial CHF therapy. ACE inhibitors are mixed (arterial and venous) dilators and are particularly effective and well tolerated. They have been shown to prolong life in pts with symptomatic CHF. ACE inhibitors have also been shown to delay the onset of CHF in pts with asymptomatic LV dysfunction and to lower mortality when begun soon after acute MI. ACE inhibitors may result in significant hypotension in pts who are volume depleted, so start at lowest dosage (e.g., captopril 6.25 mg PO tid). ARBs (Table 131-2) may be substituted if pt is intolerant of ACE inhibitor (because of cough or angioedema). Consider hydralazine plus an oral nitrate instead in pts who develop hyperkalemia or renal insufficiency on ACE inhibitor.

TABLE 131-1	**THERAPY FOR HEART FAILURE**

1. General measures
    a. Restrict salt intake
    b. Avoid antiarrhythmics for asymptomatic arrhythmias
    c. Avoid NSAIDs
    d. Immunize against influenza and pneumococcal pneumonia
2. Diuretics
    a. Use in volume-overloaded pts to achieve normal JVP and relief of edema
    b. Weigh daily to adjust dose
    c. For diuretic resistance, administer IV or use 2 diuretics in combination
    (e.g., furosemide plus metolazone)
    d. Low-dose dopamine to enhance renal flow
3. ACE inhibitors
    a. For all patients with LV systolic heart failure or asymptomatic LV dysfunction
    b. Contraindications: Serum $K^+ > 5.5$, advanced renal failure (e.g., creatinine > 3 mg/dL), bilateral renal artery stenosis, pregnancy
4. Beta blockers
    a. For patients with class II–III heart failure, combined with ACE inhibitor and diuretics
    b. Contraindications: Bronchospasm, symptomatic bradycardia or advanced heart block, unstable heart failure or class IV symptoms
5. Digitalis
    a. For persistently symptomatic pts with systolic heart failure (especially if atrial fibrillation present) added to ACE inhibitor, diuretics, beta blocker
6. Other measures
    a. Consider angiotensin receptor blocker or combination of hydralazine and oral nitrate if not tolerant of ACE inhibitor
    b. Consider spironolactone in class III–IV heart failure
    c. Consider ventricular resynchronization in pts with class III or IV heart failure and QRS > 120 ms
    d. Consider implantable cardioverter-defibrillator in pts with class III heart failure and ejection fraction <30%

Source: Modified from E Braunwald: HPIM-15, p. 1318.

- *Beta blockers* (Table 131-2) administered in gradually augmented dosage improve symptoms and prolong survival in pts with moderate (NYHA class II–III) heart failure and reduced EF. After pt stabilized on ACE inhibitor and diuretic, begin at low dosage and increase gradually [e.g., carvedilol 3.125 mg bid, double q2weeks as tolerated to maximum of 25 mg bid (for weight < 85 kg) or 50 mg bid (weight > 85 kg)].
- Aldosterone antagonists, e.g., *spironolactone*, 25 mg/d, added to standard therapy in patients with advanced heart failure have been shown to reduce mortality. Its diuretic properties may also be beneficial, and it should be considered in patients with class III/IV heart failure symptoms.
- *Digoxin* is useful in heart failure due to (1) marked systolic dysfunction (LV dilatation, low EF, S_3) and (2) heart failure associated with atrial fibrillation (AF) and rapid ventricular rate. Unlike ACE inhibitors and beta blockers, digoxin does not prolong survival in heart failure pts but reduces hospitalizations. Not indicated in CHF due to pericardial disease, restrictive cardiomyopathy, or mitral stenosis (unless AF is present). Digoxin is contraindicated in hypertrophic cardiomyopathy and in pts with AV conduction blocks.

TABLE 131-2	DRUGS FOR THE TREATMENT OF CHRONIC HEART FAILURE (EF <40%)	
	Initiating Dose	**Maximal Dose**
Diuretics		
Furosemide	20–40 mg qd or bid	400 mg/d[a]
Torsemide	10–20 mg qd bid	200 mg/d[a]
Bumetanide	0.5–1.0 mg qd or bid	10 mg/d[a]
Hydrochlorthiazide	25 mg qd	100 mg/d[a]
Metolazone	2.5–5.0 mg qd or bid	20 mg/d[a]
Angiotensin-Converting Enzyme Inhibitors		
Captopril	6.25 mg tid	50 mg tid
Enalapril	2.5 mg bid	10 mg bid
Lisinopril	2.5–5.0 mg qd	20–35 mg qd
Ramipril	1.25–2.5 mg bid	2.5–5 mg bid
Trandolapril	0.5 mg qd	4 mg qd
Angiotensin Receptor Blockers		
Valsartan	40 mg bid	160 mg bid
Candesartan	4 mg qd	32 mg qd
Irbesartan	75 mg qd	300 mg qd[b]
Losartan	12.5 mg qd	50 mg qd
β Receptor Blockers		
Carvedilol	3.125 mg bid	25–50 mg bid
Bisoprolol	1.25 mg qd	10 mg qd
Metoprolol succinate CR	12.5–25 mg qd	Target dose 200 mg qd
Additional Therapies		
Spironolactone	12.5–25 mg qd	25–50 mg qd
Eplerenone	25 mg qd	50 mg qd
Combination of hydralazine/ isosorbide dinitrate	10–25 mg/10 mg tid	75 mg/40 mg tid
Fixed dose of hydralazine/iso- sorbide dinitrate	37.5 mg/20 mg (one tablet) tid	75 mg/40 mg (two tablets) tid
Digoxin	0.125 mg qd	≤0.375 mg/d[b]

[a]Dose must be titrated to reduce the patient's congestive symptoms.
[b]Target dose not established.

Digoxin loading dose is administered over 24 h (0.5 mg PO/IV, followed by 0.25 mg q6h to achieve total of 1.0–1.5 mg). Subsequent dose (0.125–0.25 mg qd) depends on age, weight, and renal function and is guided by measurement of serum digoxin level (maintain level < 1.0 ng/mL).

Digitalis toxicity may be precipitated by hypokalemia, hypoxemia, hypercalcemia, hypomagnesemia, hypothyroidism, or myocardial ischemia. Early signs of toxicity include anorexia, nausea, and lethargy. *Cardiac toxicity* includes ventricular extrasystoles and ventricular tachycardia and fibrillation; atrial tachycardia with block; sinus arrest and sinoatrial block; all degrees of AV block. *Chronic* digitalis intoxication may cause cachexia, gynecomastia, "yellow" vision, or confusion. At first sign of digitalis toxicity, discontinue the drug; maintain serum K concentration between 4.0 and 5.0 mmol/L.

Bradyarrhythmias and AV block may respond to atropine (0.6 mg IV); otherwise, a temporary pacemaker may be required. Digitalis-induced ventricular arrhythmias are usually treated with lidocaine (Chap. 130). Antidigoxin antibodies are available for massive overdose.

- The combination of the oral vasodilators hydralazine and isosorbide dinitrate may be of benefit for chronic administration in pts intolerant of ACE inhibitors and ARBs and is also recommended as part of standard therapy in African Americans with class II–IV heart failure.

- In sicker, hospitalized patients, IV vasodilator therapy (Table 131-2) is monitored by placement of a pulmonary artery catheter and indwelling arterial line. Nitroprusside is a potent mixed vasodilator for pts with markedly elevated systemic vascular resistance. It is metabolized to thiocyanate, then excreted via the kidneys. To avoid thiocyanate toxicity (seizures, altered mental status, nausea), follow thiocyanate levels in pts with renal dysfunction or if administered for >2 days.

IV *nesiritide* (Table 131-3), a purified preparation of BNP, is a vasodilator that reduces pulmonary capillary wedge pressure and dyspnea in patients with acutely decompensated CHF. It should be used only in patients with refractory heart failure.

- *IV inotropic agents* (see Table 131-3) are administered to hospitalized pts for refractory symptoms or acute exacerbation of CHF to augment cardiac output. They are contraindicated in hypertrophic cardiomyopathy. *Dobutamine* augments cardiac output without significant peripheral vasoconstriction or tachycardia. *Dopamine* at low dosage [1–5 $(\mu g/kg)/min$] facilitates diuresis; at higher dosage [5–10 $(\mu g/kg)/min$] positive inotropic effects predominate; peripheral vasoconstriction is greatest at dosage >10 $(\mu g/kg)/min$. *Milrinone* [0.375 $(\mu g/kg)/min$ after 50-$\mu g/kg$ loading dose] is a non-

TABLE 131-3 DRUGS FOR TREATMENT OF ACUTE HEART FAILURE

	Initiating Dose	Maximal Dose
Vasodilators		
Nitroglycerin	20 µg/min	40–400 µg/min
Nitroprusside	10 µg/min	30–350 µg/min
Nesiritide	Bolus 2 µg/kg	0.01–0.03 µg/kg per min[a]
Inotropes		
Dobutamine	1–2 µg/kg per min	2–10 µg/kg per min[b]
Milrinone	Bolus 50 µg/kg	0.1–0.75 µg/kg per min[b]
Dopamine	1–2 µg/kg per min	2–4 µg/kg per min[b]
Levosimendan	Bolus 12 µg/kg	0.1–0.2 µg/kg per min[c]
Vasoconstrictors		
Dopamine for hypotension	5 µg/kg per min	5–20 µg/kg per min
Epinephrine	0.5 µg/kg per min	50 µg/kg per min
Phenylephrine	0.3 µg/kg per min	3 µg/kg per min
Vasopressin	0.05 units/min	0.1–0.4 units/min

[a]Usually <4 µg/kg/min.
[b]Inotropes will also have vasodilatory properties.
[c]Approved outside of the United States for the management of acute heart failure.

sympathetic positive inotrope and vasodilator. The above vasodilators and inotropic agents may be used together for additive effect.

Consider implantable cardioverter defibrillator prophylactically for class II–III heart failure and LVEF < 30–35%. Patients with an LVEF <35%, refractory CHF, and QRS > 120 ms may be candidates for biventricular pacing (cardiac resynchronization therapy). Pts with severe disease and <6 months expected survival, who meet stringent criteria, may be candidates for a ventricular assist device or cardiac transplantation.

- Patients with predominantly diastolic heart failure are treated with salt restriction and diuretics. Beta blockers and ACE inhibitors may be of benefit in blunting neurohormonal activation.

COR PULMONALE

RV enlargement resulting from *primary* lung disease; leads to RV hypertrophy and eventually to RV failure. Etiologies include:

- *Pulmonary parenchymal or airway disease.* Chronic obstructive lung disease (COPD), interstitial lung diseases, bronchiectasis, cystic fibrosis (Chaps. 138 and 141).
- *Pulmonary vascular disease.* Recurrent pulmonary emboli, primary pulmonary hypertension (PHT) (Chap. 134), vasculitis, sickle cell anemia.
- *Inadequate mechanical ventilation.* Kyphoscoliosis, neuromuscular disorders, marked obesity, sleep apnea.

Symptoms Depend on underlying disorder but include dyspnea, cough, fatigue, and sputum production (in parenchymal diseases).

Physical Examination Tachypnea, cyanosis, clubbing are common. RV impulse along left sternal border, loud P_2, right-sided S_4. If RV failure develops, elevated jugular venous pressure, hepatomegaly with ascites, pedal edema. Murmur of tricuspid regurgitation (Chap. 117) may appear.

Laboratory **ECG** RV hypertrophy and RA enlargement (Chap. 118); tachyarrhythmias are common.

Radiologic Studies CXR shows RV and pulmonary artery enlargement; if PHT present, tapering of the pulmonary artery branches. Chest CT identifies emphysema, interstitial lung disease, and acute pulmonary embolism; V̇/Q̇ scan more reliable for diagnosis of chronic thromboemboli. Pulmonary function tests and ABGs characterize intrinsic pulmonary disease.

Echocardiogram RV hypertrophy; LV function typically normal. RV systolic pressure can be estimated from Doppler measurement of tricuspid regurgitant flow. If imaging is difficult because of air in distended lungs, RV volume and wall thickness can be evaluated by MRI.

Rx Cor Pulmonale

Aimed at underlying pulmonary disease and may include bronchodilators, antibiotics, and oxygen administration. If RV failure is present, treat as CHF, instituting low-sodium diet and diuretics; digoxin must be administered cautiously (toxicity increased due to hypoxemia, hypercapnia, acidosis). Loop diuretics must also be used with care to prevent significant metabolic alkalosis that blunts respiratory drive. Supraventricular tachyarrhythmias are common and treated with digoxin or verapamil (should typically avoid beta blockers). Chronic anticoagulation with warfarin is indicated when pulmonary hypertension is accompanied by RV failure. See Chap. 140 for treatment of pulmonary embolism, and Chap. 134 for management of pulmonary hypertension.

For a more detailed discussion, see Mann DL: Heart Failure and Cor Pulmonale, Chap. 227, p. 1443, in HPIM-17.

132 Diseases of the Aorta

AORTIC ANEURYSM

Abnormal dilatation of the abdominal or thoracic aorta; in ascending aorta most commonly secondary to cystic medial necrosis; aneurysms of descending thoracic and abdominal aorta are primarily atherosclerotic. Rare causes of aneurysms are infections (syphilitic, tuberculous, mycotic) and vasculitides (e.g., Takayasu's arteritis, giant cell arteritis).

History May be clinically silent, but thoracic aortic aneurysms can result in deep, diffuse chest pain, dysphagia, hoarseness, hemoptysis, dry cough; abdominal aneurysms may result in abdominal pain or thromboemboli to the lower extremities.

Physical Examination Abdominal aneurysms are often palpable, most commonly in periumbilical area. Pts with ascending thoracic aneurysms may show features of the Marfan syndrome (HPIM-17, Chap. 357).

Laboratory Suspect thoracic aneurysm by abnormal *CXR* (enlarged aortic silhouette) and confirm by *echocardiography, contrast CT,* or *MRI.* Confirm abdominal aneurysm by *abdominal plain film* (rim of calcification), *ultrasound, CT, MRI,* or *contrast aortography.* If clinically suspected, obtain serologic test for syphilis, especially if ascending thoracic aneurysm shows thin shell of calcification.

℞ Aortic Aneurysm

Control of hypertension (Chap. 124) is essential. Surgical resection of thoracic aortic aneurysms >5.5–6 cm in diameter (abdominal aortic aneurysms >5.5 cm), for persistent pain despite bp control, or for evidence of rapid expansion. In pts with the Marfan syndrome, thoracic aortic aneurysms >5 cm usually warrant repair.

AORTIC DISSECTION (Fig. 132-1)

Potentially life-threatening condition in which disruption or aortic intima allows dissection of blood into vessel wall; may involve ascending aorta (type II), descend-

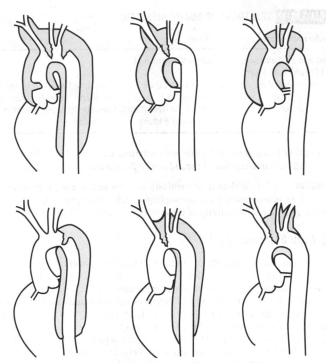

FIGURE 132-1 Classification of aortic dissections. Stanford classification: Top panels illustrate type A dissections that involve the ascending aorta independent of site of tear and distal extension; type B dissections (bottom panels) involve transverse and/or descending aorta without involvement of the ascending aorta. DeBakey classification: Type I dissection involves ascending to descending aorta (top left); type II dissection is limited to ascending or transverse aorta, without descending aorta (top center + top right); type III dissection involves descending aorta only (bottom left). *[From DC Miller, in RM Doroghazi, EE Slater (eds.), Aortic Dissection. New York, McGraw-Hill, 1983, with permission.]*

ing aorta (type III), or both (type I). Alternative classification: Type A—dissection involves ascending aorta; type B—limited to descending aorta. Involvement of the ascending aorta is most lethal form. Variant acute aortic syndromes include intramural hematoma without an intimal flap, and penetrating atherosclerotic ulcer.

Etiology Ascending aortic dissection associated with hypertension, cystic medial necrosis, the Marfan and Ehlers-Danlos syndromes; descending dissections commonly associated with atherosclerosis or hypertension. Incidence is increased in pts with coarctation of aorta, bicuspid aortic valve, and rarely in third trimester of pregnancy in otherwise normal women.

Symptoms Sudden onset of severe anterior or posterior chest pain, with "ripping" quality; maximal pain may travel if dissection propagates. Additional symptoms relate to obstruction of aortic branches (stroke, MI), dyspnea (acute aortic regurgitation), or symptoms of low cardiac output due to cardiac tamponade (dissection into pericardial sac).

Physical Examination Sinus tachycardia common; if cardiac tamponade develops, hypotension, pulsus paradoxus, and pericardial rub appear. Asymmetry

TABLE 132-1 TREATMENT OF AORTIC DISSECTION	
Preferred Regimen	Dose
Sodium nitroprusside *plus* a beta blocker:	20–400 µg/min IV
Propranolol *or*	0.5 mg IV; then 1 mg q5min, to total of 0.15 mg/kg
Esmolol or	500 µg/kg IV over 1 min; then 50–200 (µg/kg)/min
Labetalol	20 mg IV over 2 min, then 40–80 mg q10–15min to max of 300 mg

of carotid or brachial pulses, aortic regurgitation, and neurologic abnormalities associated with interruption of carotid artery flow are common findings.

Laboratory   *CXR:* Widening of mediastinum; dissection can be confirmed by *CT, MRI,* or *ultrasound* (esp. transesophageal echocardiography). Aortography is rarely required, as sensitivity of these noninvasive techniques is >90%.

Rx | Aortic Dissection

Reduce cardiac contractility and treat hypertension to maintain systolic bp between 100 and 120 mmHg using IV agents (Table 132-1), e.g., sodium nitroprusside accompanied by a beta blocker (aiming for heart rate of 60 beats per min), followed by oral therapy. If beta blocker contraindicated, consider IV verapamil or diltiazem (see Table 130-3). Direct vasodilators (hydralazine, diazoxide) are contraindicated because they may increase shear stress. Ascending aortic dissection (type A) requires surgical repair emergently or, if pt can be stabilized with medications, semielectively. Descending aortic dissections are stabilized medically (maintain systolic bp between 110 and 120 mmHg) with oral antihypertensive agents (esp. beta blockers); immediate surgical repair is not necessary unless continued pain or extension of dissection is observed (by serial MRI or CT performed every 6–12 months).

OTHER ABNORMALITIES OF THE AORTA

Atherosclerotic Occlusive Disease of Abdominal Aorta   Particularly common in presence of diabetes mellitus or cigarette smoking. Symptoms include intermittent claudication of the buttocks and thighs and impotence (Leriche syndrome); femoral and other distal pulses are absent. Diagnosis is established by noninvasive leg pressure measurements and Doppler velocity analysis, and confirmed by MRI, CT, or aortography. Catheter-based endovascular treatment or aortic-femoral bypass surgery is required for symptomatic treatment.

Takayasu's ("Pulseless") Disease   Arteritis of aorta and major branches in young women. Anorexia, weight loss, fever, and night sweats occur. Localized symptoms relate to occlusion of aortic branches (cerebral ischemia, claudication, and loss of pulses in arms). ESR is increased; diagnosis confirmed by aortography. Glucocorticoid and immunosuppressive therapy may be beneficial, but mortality is high.

For a more detailed discussion, see Creager MA, Loscalzo J: Diseases of the Aorta, Chap. 242, p. 1563, in HPIM-17.

133 Peripheral Vascular Disease

Occlusive or inflammatory disease that develops within the peripheral arteries, veins, or lymphatics.

ARTERIOSCLEROSIS OF PERIPHERAL ARTERIES

History *Intermittent claudication* is muscular cramping with exercise; quickly relieved by rest. Pain in buttocks and thighs suggests aortoiliac disease; calf muscle pain implies femoral or popliteal artery disease. More advanced arteriosclerotic obstruction results in pain at rest; painful ulcers of the feet (painless in diabetics) may result.

Physical Examination Decreased peripheral pulses (ankle:brachial index <1.0), blanching of affected limb with elevation, dependent rubor (redness). Ischemic ulcers or gangrene of toes may be present.

Laboratory Doppler ultrasound of peripheral pulses before and during exercise localizes stenoses; magnetic resonance angiography or contrast arteriography performed only if reconstructive surgery or angioplasty is considered.

℞ Arteriosclerosis

Most pts can be managed medically with daily exercise program, careful foot care (especially in diabetics), treatment of hypercholesterolemia, and local debridement of ulcerations. Abstinence from cigarettes is mandatory. Some, but not all, pts note symptomatic improvement with drug therapy (pentoxifylline or cilostazol). Pts with severe claudication, rest pain, or gangrene are candidates for arterial reconstructive surgery; percutaneous transluminal angioplasty or stent placement can be performed in selected pts.

OTHER CONDITIONS THAT IMPAIR PERIPHERAL ARTERIAL FLOW

Arterial Embolism This is due to thrombus or vegetation within the heart or aorta or paradoxically from a venous thrombus through a right-to-left intracardiac shunt.

History Sudden pain or numbness in an extremity in the absence of previous history of claudication.

Physical Examination Absent pulse, pallor, and decreased temperature of limb distal to the occlusion. Lesion is identified by angiography.

℞ Arterial Embolism

Intravenous heparin is administered to prevent propagation of clot. For acute severe ischemia, immediate endovascular or surgical embolectomy is indicated. Thrombolytic therapy (e.g., tissue plasminogen activator or urokinase) may be effective for thrombus within atherosclerotic vessel or arterial bypass graft.

Atheroembolism A subset of acute arterial occlusion due to embolization of fibrin, platelets, and cholesterol debris from more proximal atheromas or aneurysm; typically occurs after intraarterial instrumentation. Depending on location, may lead to stroke, renal insufficiency, or pain and tenderness in embolized tissue. Atheroembolism to lower extremities results in blue toe syndrome, which can progress to necrosis and gangrene. Treatment is supportive; for recurrent episodes, surgical intervention in the proximal atherosclerotic vessel or aneurysm may be required.

Vasospastic Disorders This manifests by Raynaud's phenomenon in which cold exposure results in triphasic color response: blanching of the fingers, followed by cyanosis, then redness. Usually a benign disorder. However, suspect an underlying disease (Table 133-1) if tissue necrosis occurs, if disease is unilateral, or if it develops after age 50.

℞ Vasospastic Disorders

Keep extremities warm; calcium channel blockers (e.g., nifedipine XL 30–90 mg PO qd) or α-adrenergic antagonists (e.g., prazocin 1–5 mg tid) may be effective.

Thromboangiitis Obliterans (Buerger's Disease) Occurs in young men who are heavy smokers and involves both upper and lower extremities; nonatheromatous inflammatory reaction develops in veins and small arteries leading to superficial thrombophlebitis and arterial obstruction with ulceration or gangrene of digits. Abstinence from tobacco is essential.

VENOUS DISEASE

Superficial Thrombophlebitis A benign disorder characterized by erythema, tenderness, and edema along involved vein. Conservative therapy includes local heat, elevation, and anti-inflammatory drugs such as aspirin. More serious conditions such as cellulitis or lymphangitis may mimic this, but these are associated with fever, chills, lymphadenopathy, and red superficial streaks along inflamed lymphatic channels.

TABLE 133-1 CLASSIFICATION OF RAYNAUD'S PHENOMENON

Primary or idiopathic Raynaud's phenomenon: Raynaud's disease
Secondary Raynaud's phenomenon
    Collagen vascular diseases: scleroderma, systemic lupus erythematosus, rheumatoid arthritis, dermatomyositis, polymyositis
    Arterial occlusive diseases: atherosclerosis of the extremities, thromboangiitis obliterans, acute arterial occlusion, thoracic outlet syndrome
    Pulmonary hypertension
    Neurologic disorders: intervertebral disk disease, syringomyelia, spinal cord tumors, stroke, poliomyelitis, carpal tunnel syndrome
    Blood dyscrasias: cold agglutinins, cryoglobulinemia, cryofibrinogenemia, myeloproliferative disorders, Waldenström's macroglobulinemia
    Trauma: vibration injury, hammer hand syndrome, electric shock, cold injury, typing, piano playing
    Drugs: ergot derivatives, methysergide, β-adrenergic receptor blockers, bleomycin, vinblastine, cisplatin

TABLE 133-2	**CONDITIONS ASSOCIATED WITH AN INCREASED RISK FOR DEVELOPMENT OF VENOUS THROMBOSIS**

Surgery: Orthopedic, thoracic, abdominal, and genitourinary procedures
Neoplasms: Pancreas, lung, ovary, testes, urinary tract, breast, stomach
Trauma: Fractures of spine, pelvis, femur, tibia
Immobilization: Acute MI, CHF, stroke, postoperative convalescence
Pregnancy: Estrogen use (for replacement or contraception)
Hypercoagulable states: Resistance to activated protein C; prothrombin 20210A
   mutation; deficiencies of antithrombin III, protein C, or protein S; antiphos-
   pholipid antibodies; myeloproliferative disease; dysfibrinogenemia; DIC
Venulitis: Thromboangiitis obliterans, Behçet's disease, homocysteinuria
Previous deep vein thrombosis

Deep Venous Thrombosis (DVT)   This is a more serious condition that may lead to pulmonary embolism (Chap. 140). Particularly common in pts on prolonged bed rest, those with chronic debilitating disease, and those with malignancies (Table 133-2).

History   Pain or tenderness in calf or thigh, usually unilateral; may be asymptomatic, with pulmonary embolism as primary presentation.

Physical Examination   Often normal; local swelling or tenderness to deep palpation may be present over affected vein.

Laboratory   D-Dimer testing is sensitive but not specific for diagnosis. Most helpful noninvasive testing is ultrasound imaging of the deep veins with Doppler interrogation. These noninvasive studies are most sensitive for proximal (upper leg) DVT, less sensitive for calf DVT. Invasive venography is used when diagnosis is not clear. MRI may be useful for diagnosis of proximal DVT and DVT within the pelvic veins or in the superior or inferior vena cavae.

℞ Venous Disease

Systemic anticoagulation with heparin [5000- to 10,000-U bolus, followed by continuous IV infusion to maintain a PTT at 2 × normal (or using a nomogram: 80 U/kg bolus followed by initial infusion of 18 U/kg/hour)] or low-molecular-weight heparin (e.g., enoxaparin 1 mg/kg SC bid), followed by warfarin PO (overlap with heparin for at least 4–5 days and continue for at least 3 months if proximal deep veins involved). Adjust warfarin dose to maintain prothrombin time at INR 2.0–3.0.
   DVT can be prevented by early ambulation following surgery or with low-dose unfractionated heparin during prolonged bed rest (5000 U SC bid-tid) or low-molecular-weight heparin (e.g., enoxaparin 40 mg SC daily), supplemented by pneumatic compression boots. Following knee or hip surgery, warfarin (INR 2.0–3.0) is an effective regimen. Low-molecular-weight heparins are also effective in preventing DVT after general or orthopedic surgery.

Chronic Venous Insufficiency   This results from prior DVT or venous valvular incompetence and manifests as chronic dull ache in leg that worsens with prolonged standing, edema, and superficial varicosities. May lead to erythema, hyperpigmentation, and recurrent cellulitis; ulcers may appear at medial and lateral malleoli. Treatment includes graduated compression stockings and leg elevation.

LYMPHEDEMA

Chronic, painless edema, usually of the lower extremities; may be primary (inherited) or secondary to lymphatic damage or obstruction (e.g., recurrent lymphangitis, tumor, filariasis).

Physical Examination Marked pitting edema in early stages; limb becomes indurated with *non*pitting edema chronically. Differentiate from chronic *venous* insufficiency, which displays hyperpigmentation, stasis dermatitis, and superficial venous varicosities.

Laboratory Abdominal and pelvic ultrasound or CT or MRI to identify obstructing lesions. Lymphangiography or lymphoscintigraphy (rarely done) to confirm diagnosis. If *unilateral* edema, differentiate from DVT by noninvasive venous studies (above).

℞ Lymphedema

(1) Meticulous foot hygiene to prevent infection, (2) leg elevation, (3) compression stockings and /or pneumatic compression boots. Diuretics should be *avoided* to prevent intravascular volume depletion.

For a more detailed discussion, see Creager MA, Loscalzo J: Vascular diseases of the extremities, Chap. 243, in HPIM-17.

134 Pulmonary Hypertension

Definition Elevation of pulmonary artery (PA) pressure due to pulmonary vascular or parenchymal disease, increased left heart filling pressure, or a combination. Table 134-1 lists most common etiologies. Pulmonary hypertension is most common cause of cor pulmonale (Chap. 131).

Symptoms Exertional dyspnea, fatigue, angina (due to RV ischemia), syncope, peripheral edema.

Physical Examination Jugular venous distention, RV lift, increased P_2, right-sided S_4. Tricuspid regurgitation appears in advanced stages.

Laboratory *CXR* shows enlarged central PA. *ECG* may demonstrate RV hypertrophy and RA enlargement. *Echocardiogram* shows RV and RA enlargement; RV systolic pressure can be estimated from Doppler recording of tricuspid

TABLE 134-1	CAUSES OF PULMONARY HYPERTENSION

Pulmonary Arterial Hypertension
  Primary pulmonary hypertension
  Collagen vascular diseases (e.g., CREST, scleroderma, SLE, RA)
  Congenital systemic to pulmonary shunts (e.g., ventricular septal defect,
    patent ductus arteriosus, atrial septal defect)
  Portal hypertension
  HIV infection
  Anorexigen use (e.g., fenfluramines)
Pulmonary Venous Hypertension
  LV diastolic dysfunction (e.g., LV hypertrophy, coronary artery disease)
  Mitral stenosis or regurgitation
Lung Disease and Hypoxemia
  Chronic obstructive pulmonary disease
  Interstitial lung disease
  Sleep apnea
  Chronic hypoventilation
Pulmonary Thromboembolic Disease
  Acute pulmonary embolism (Chap. 140)
  Chronic pulmonary embolism

Note: CREST, calcinosis, Raynaud's phenomenon, esophageal involvement, sclerodactyly, and telangiectasia (syndrome).

regurgitation (Chap. 118). *Pulmonary function tests* identify underlying obstructive or restrictive lung disease; impaired CO diffusion capacity is common. *V/Q nuclear scan* or contrast-enhanced *high-resolution chest CT* can identify thromboembolic pulmonary vascular disease. *ANA titer* is elevated in collagen vascular diseases. *HIV testing* should be performed in individuals at risk. *Cardiac catheterization* accurately measures PA pressures, cardiac output, identifies underlying congenital vascular shunts; during procedure, response to short-acting vasodilators can be assessed.

Figure 134-1 summarizes workup of patient with unexplained pulmonary hypertension.

PRIMARY PULMONARY HYPERTENSION

Uncommon (2 cases/million), very serious form of pulmonary hypertension. Most pts present in 4th and 5th decades, female >> male predominance; up to 20% of cases are familial. Major symptom is dyspnea, often with insidious onset. Mean survival < 3 years in absence of therapy.

Physical Examination   Prominent *a* wave in jugular venous pulse, right ventricular heave, narrowly split S_2 with accentuated P_2. Terminal course is characterized by signs of right-sided heart failure. CXR: RV and central pulmonary arterial prominence. Pulmonary arteries taper sharply. PFT: usually normal or mild restrictive defect. ECG: RV enlargement, right axis deviation, and RV hypertrophy. Echocardiogram: RA and RV enlargement and tricuspid regurgitation.

Differential Diagnosis   Other disorders of heart, lungs, and pulmonary vasculature must be excluded. Lung function studies will identify chronic pulmonary disease causing pulmonary hypertension and cor pulmonale. Interstitial diseases (PFTs, CT scan) and hypoxic pulmonary hypertension (ABGs, Sa_{O_2}) should be excluded. Perfusion lung scan should be performed to exclude chronic pulmo-

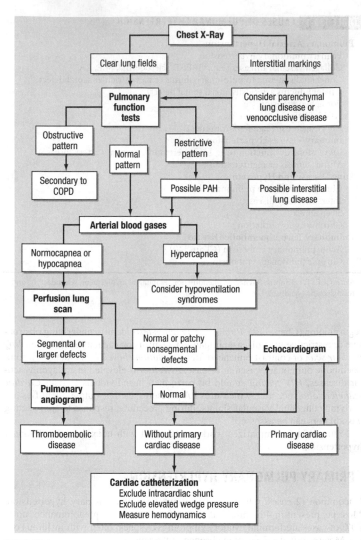

FIGURE 134-1 An algorithm for the workup of a patient with unexplained pulmonary hypertension. Note: COPD, chronic obstructive pulmonary disease; PAH, pulmonary arterial hypertension. (*Adapted with permission from S Rich: HPIM-17.*)

nary embolism (PE). Spiral CT scan, pulmonary arteriogram, and even open-lung biopsy may be required to distinguish PE from idiopathic pulmonary arterial hypertension. Rarely, pulmonary hypertension is due to parasitic disease (schistosomiasis, filariasis). Cardiac disorders to be excluded include pulmonary artery and pulmonic valve stenosis. Pulmonary artery and ventricular and atrial shunts with pulmonary vascular disease (Eisenmenger reaction) should be sought. Silent mitral stenosis should be excluded by echocardiography.

℞ Primary Pulmonary Hypertension

Limit physical activities, use diuretics for peripheral edema, O_2 supplemenation if PO_2 reduced, and chronic warfarin anticoagulation (target INR = 2.0–3.0).

If short-acting vasodilators are beneficial during acute testing in catheter laboratory, pt may benefit from high-dose *calcium channel blocker* (e.g., nifedipine, up to 240 mg/d), but must monitor for hypotension or worsening of right heart failure.

For patients with advanced refractory symptoms, options to improve symptoms and functional class include prostaglandins [*epoprostenol* (which has been shown to increase survival) via continuous central IV access, or *treprostinil* via continuous subcutaneous infusion pump] and the orally active endothelin receptor antagonist *bosentan*.

For selected patients with persistent right heart failure, lung transplantation can be considered.

For a more detailed discussion, see Rich S: Pulmonary Hypertension, Chap. 244, p. 1576, in HPIM-17.

Primary pulmonary hypertension

135 Respiratory Function and Pulmonary Diagnostic Procedures

RESPIRATORY FUNCTION

The respiratory system includes not only the lungs but also the chest wall, pulmonary circulation, and central nervous system. Three major types of respiratory system disturbances will be reviewed: ventilatory function, pulmonary circulation, and gas exchange.

Disturbances in Ventilatory Function   Ventilation involves the delivery of gas to the alveoli. Pulmonary function tests are used to assess ventilatory function. The classification of lung volumes, which are measured with pulmonary function testing, is shown in Fig. 135-1. Spirometry involves forced exhalation from total lung capacity (TLC) to residual volume (RV); key measurements from a spirogram are the forced expiratory volume in 1 s (FEV_1) and the forced vital capacity (FVC). Expiratory flow rates may be plotted against lung volumes to yield a flow-volume curve. Other lung volumes, including TLC and RV, are measured under static conditions using either helium dilution or body plethysmography. Lung volumes and flow rates are typically compared with population-based normal values that adjust for the age, height, sex, and race of the pt.

There are two major patterns of abnormal ventilatory function detected by pulmonary function testing: restrictive and obstructive (Tables 135-1 and 135-2). The presence of obstruction is determined by a reduced ratio of FEV_1/FVC, and

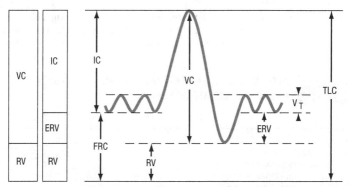

FIGURE 135-1 Lung volumes, shown by block diagrams (*left*) and by a spirographic tracing (*right*). TLC, total lung capacity; VC, vital capacity; RV, residual volume; IC, inspiratory capacity; ERV, expiratory reserve volume; FRC, functional residual capacity; V_T, tidal volume. (*From SE Weinberger: Principles of Pulmonary Medicine, 4th ed. Philadelphia, Saunders, 2004; with permission.*)

TABLE 135-1	COMMON RESPIRATORY DISEASES BY DIAGNOSTIC CATEGORIES

Obstructive

Asthma	Bronchiectasis
Chronic obstructive pulmonary	Cystic fibrosis
disease	Bronchiolitis

Restrictive—Parenchymal

Sarcoidosis	Pneumoconiosis
Idiopathic pulmonary fibrosis	Drug- or radiation-induced interstitial
	lung disease

Restrictive—Extraparenchymal

Neuromuscular	Chest wall
Diaphragmatic weakness/paralysis	Kyphoscoliosis
Myasthenia gravis	Obesity
Guillain-Barré syndrome	Ankylosing spondylitis
Muscular dystrophies	
Cervical spine injury	

the severity of airflow obstruction is determined by the level of reduction of FEV_1. With airflow obstruction, TLC may be normal or increased, and RV is typically elevated. With severe airflow obstruction, the FVC is often reduced.

The presence of a restrictive pattern is determined by a reduction in lung volumes, especially TLC. When pulmonary parenchymal processes cause restriction, RV is also decreased, but the FEV_1/FVC is normal. With extraparenchymal etiologies of restrictive ventilatory defects, such as neuromuscular weakness or chest wall abnormalities, the impact on RV and FEV_1/FVC is more variable.

Disturbances in Pulmonary Circulation The pulmonary vasculature normally handles the right ventricular output (~5 L/min) at a low pressure. Normal mean pulmonary artery pressure (PAP) is 15 mmHg. When cardiac output increases, pulmonary vascular resistance (PVR) normally falls, leading to only small increases in mean PAP.

Assessment of the pulmonary vasculature requires measuring pulmonary vascular pressures and cardiac output to derive PVR. PVR rises with hypoxemia (due to vasoconstriction), intraluminal thrombi (due to diminished cross-

TABLE 135-2	ALTERATIONS IN VENTILATORY FUNCTION IN DIFFERENT PULMONARY DISEASE CATEGORIES

	TLC	RV	VC	FEV_1/FVC
Obstructive	N to ↑	↑	↓	↓
Restrictive				
Pulmonary parenchymal	↓	↓	↓	N to ↑
Extraparenchymal— neuromuscular weakness	↓	Variable	↓	Variable
Extraparenchymal—chest wall deformity	↓	Variable	↓	N

Note: N, normal; for other abbreviations, see text.

sectional area from obstruction), or destruction of small pulmonary vessels (due to scarring or loss of the alveolar walls).

All diseases of the respiratory system causing hypoxemia are capable of causing pulmonary hypertension. However, pts with prolonged hypoxemia related to chronic obstructive pulmonary disease, interstitial lung disease, chest wall disease, and obesity-hypoventilation–sleep apnea are particularly likely to develop pulmonary hypertension. When pulmonary vessels are directly affected, as with recurrent pulmonary emboli, the decrease in cross-sectional area of the pulmonary vasculature is the primary mechanism for increased PVR, rather than hypoxemia.

Disturbances in Gas Exchange   The primary functions of the respiratory system are to remove CO_2 from blood entering the pulmonary circulation and to provide O_2 to blood leaving the pulmonary circulation. Normal tidal volume is approximately 500 mL and normal respiratory rate is approximately 15 breaths/min, leading to a total minute ventilation of approximately 7.5 L/min. Because of anatomic dead space, alveolar ventilation is approximately 5 L/min. Gas exchange depends on alveolar ventilation rather than total minute ventilation.

Partial pressure of CO_2 in arterial blood (Pa_{CO_2}) is directly proportional to the amount of CO_2 produced each minute ($\dot{V}_{CO_2}$) and inversely proportional to alveolar ventilation ($\dot{V}A$).

$$Pa_{CO_2} = 0.863 \times \dot{V}_{CO_2} / \dot{V}A$$

Adequate movement of gas between alveoli and pulmonary capillaries by diffusion is required for normal gas exchange. Diffusion can be tested by measuring the diffusing capacity of the lung for a low concentration of carbon monoxide (DLCO). DLCO measurement is typically corrected for the pt's hemoglobin level. Diffusion abnormalities rarely result in arterial hypoxemia at rest but can cause hypoxemia with exercise. Gas exchange is critically dependent on proper matching of ventilation and perfusion.

Assessment of gas exchange is commonly performed with arterial blood gases, which provide measurements of the partial pressures of O_2 and CO_2. The actual content of O_2 in blood is determined by both P_{O_2} and hemoglobin concentration. The alveolar-arterial O_2 difference [(A – a) gradient] can provide useful information when assessing abnormalities in gas exchange. The normal (A – a) gradient is <15 mmHg under age 30 but increases with aging. In order to calculate the (A – a) gradient, the alveolar P_{O_2} (PA_{O_2}) must be calculated:

$$PA_{O_2} = FI_{O_2} \times (PB - P_{H_2O}) - Pa_{CO_2}/R$$

where FI_{O_2} = fractional concentration of inspired O_2 (0.21 while breathing room air), PB = barometric pressure (760 mmHg at sea level), P_{H_2O} = water vapor pressure (47 mmHg when air is saturated at 37°C), and R = respiratory quotient (the ratio of CO_2 production to O_2 consumption, usually assumed to be 0.8). The (A – a) gradient is calculated by subtracting the measured Pa_{O_2} from the calculated PA_{O_2}.

Adequacy of CO_2 removal is reflected in the partial pressure of CO_2 measured in an arterial blood gas. Pulse oximetry is a valuable, widely used, and noninvasive tool to assess O_2 saturation, but it provides no information about Pa_{CO_2}. Other limitations of pulse oximetry include relative insensitivity to oxygenation changes when Pa_{O_2} is >60 mmHg, problems with obtaining an adequate signal when cutaneous perfusion is decreased, and inability to distinguish oxyhemoglobin from other forms of hemoglobin, such as carboxyhemoglobin and methemoglobin.

Mechanisms of Abnormal Respiratory Function The four basic mechanisms of hypoxemia are (1) decrease in inspired P_{O_2}, (2) hypoventilation, (3) shunt, and (4) ventilation/perfusion mismatch. Decrease in inspired P_{O_2} (e.g., at high altitude) and hypoventilation (characterized by an increased Pa_{CO_2}) both lower arterial oxygenation by reducing alveolar oxygenation; thus, the $(A - a)$ gradient is normal. Shunting (e.g., intracardiac shunt) causes hypoxemia by bypassing the alveolar capillaries. Shunting is characterized by an elevated $(A - a)$ gradient and is relatively refractory to oxygenation improvement with supplemental O_2. Ventilation/perfusion mismatch is the most common cause of hypoxemia; it is associated with an elevated $(A - a)$ gradient, but supplemental O_2 corrects the hypoxemia by raising the O_2 content of blood from regions with low ventilation/perfusion ratios. An algorithm for approaching the hypoxemic pt is shown in **Fig. 135-2**.

Hypercapnia is caused by inadequate alveolar ventilation. Potential contributing factors include (1) increased CO_2 production, (2) decreased ventilatory drive, (3) malfunction of the respiratory pump or increased airway resistance, and (4) inefficiency of gas exchange (increased dead space or ventilation/perfusion mismatch).

Although diffusion abnormalities rarely cause hypoxemia at rest, assessment of DLCO can be used to determine the functional integrity of the alveolar-capillary membrane. Diseases that solely affect the airways typically do not reduce the DLCO. DLCO is reduced in interstitial lung disease, emphysema, and pulmonary vascular disease. DLCO can be elevated in alveolar hemorrhage and congestive heart failure.

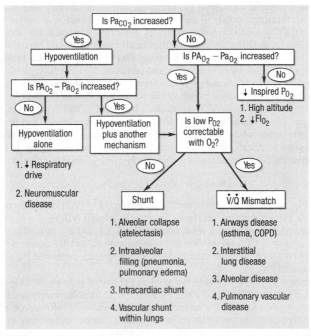

FIGURE 135-2 Flow diagram outlining the diagnostic approach to the pt with hypoxemia (Pa_{O_2} <80 mmHg). $PA_{O_2} - Pa_{O_2}$ is usually <15 mmHg for subjects ≤30 years old and increases ~3 mmHg per decade after age 30. COPD, chronic obstructive pulmonary disease. (*From SE Weinberger: Principles of Pulmonary Medicine, 4th ed. Philadelphia, Saunders, 2004; with permission.*)

DIAGNOSTIC PROCEDURES

Noninvasive Procedures **Radiographic Studies** The chest x-ray (CXR), generally including both posteroanterior and lateral views, is often the first diagnostic study in pts presenting with respiratory symptoms. With some exceptions (e.g., pneumothorax), the CXR pattern is usually not sufficiently specific to *establish* a diagnosis; instead, the CXR serves to *detect* disease, assess magnitude, and guide further diagnostic investigation. CXRs can detect a localized opacification that is classified as a nodule (<3 cm in diameter), a mass(≥3 cm in diameter), or an infiltrate. With diffuse lung disease, CXR can detect an alveolar, interstitial, or nodular pattern. CXR can also detect pleural effusion and pneumothorax, as well as abnormalities in the hila and mediastinum.

Chest CT is widely used to clarify radiographic abnormalities detected by CXR. Advantages of chest CT compared with CXR include (1) ability to distinguish superimposed structures due to cross-sectional imaging; (2) superior assessment of tissue density, permitting accurate assessment of the size and density of pulmonary nodules and improved identification of abnormalities adjacent to the chest wall, such as pleural disease; (3) with the use of IV contrast, ability to distinguish vascular from nonvascular structures; (4) with CT angiography, ability to detect pulmonary emboli; and (5) due to superior visible detail, improved recognition of parenchymal and airway diseases, including emphysema, bronchiectasis, and interstitial lung disease.

A variety of other imaging techniques are used less commonly to assess respiratory disease. MRI is generally less useful than CT but is preferred in the evaluation of intrathoracic cardiovascular pathology and to distinguish vascular and nonvascular structures without IV contrast. Ultrasound is not useful for assessing the pulmonary parenchyma, but it can detect pleural abnormalities and guide thoracentesis of a pleural effusion. Pulmonary angiography can assess the pulmonary arterial system for venous thromboembolism but has largely been replaced by CT angiography.

Nuclear Medicine Imaging Ventilation-perfusion lung scans can be used to assess for pulmonary thromboembolism but have also largely been replaced by CT angiography. Positron emission tomography (PET) scanning assesses the uptake and metabolism of a radiolabeled glucose analogue. Because malignant lesions have increased metabolic activity, PET scanning is useful to assess pulmonary nodules for potential malignancy and to stage lung cancer.

Sputum Exam Sputum can be obtained by spontaneous expectoration or induced by inhalation of an irritating aerosol like hypertonic saline. Sputum is distinguished from saliva by the presence of bronchial epithelial cells and alveolar macrophages as opposed to squamous epithelial cells. Sputum exam should include gross inspection for blood, color, and odor, as well as Gram's stain and routine bacterial culture. Bacterial culture of expectorated sputum may be misleading due to contamination with oropharyngeal flora. Sputum samples can also be assessed for a variety of other pathogens, including mycobacteria, fungi, and viruses. Sputum samples induced by hypertonic saline can be stained for the presence of *Pneumocystis jiroveci*.

Pulmonary Function Tests As discussed previously in this chapter, pulmonary function tests (PFTs) may indicate abnormalities of airway function, alterations of lung volume, and disturbances of gas exchange. PFTs may also provide objective measures of therapeutic response, e.g., to bronchodilators.

Invasive Procedures **Bronchoscopy** Bronchoscopy is a procedure that provides direct visualization of the tracheobronchial tree. The fiberoptic bronchoscope is used in most cases, but rigid bronchoscopy is valuable in specific circumstances, including massive hemorrhage and foreign body removal. Flexible fiberoptic bronchoscopy allows visualization of the airways; identification of endobronchial abnormalities, including tumors and sites of bleeding; and collection of diagnostic specimens by washing, brushing, biopsy, or lavage. Washing involves instilling sterile saline through the bronchoscope channel onto the surface of a lesion; part of the saline is suctioned back through the bronchoscope and processed for cytology and microorganisms. Bronchial brushings can be obtained from the surface of an endobronchial lesion or from a more distal mass or infiltrate (potentially with fluoroscopic guidance) for cytologic and microbiologic studies. Biopsy forceps can be used to obtain biopsies of endobronchial lesions or passed into peribronchial alveolar tissue (often with fluoroscopic guidance) to obtain transbronchial biopsies of more distal lung tissue. Transbronchial biopsy is particularly useful in diagnosing diffuse infectious processes, lymphangitic spread of cancer, and granulomatous diseases. Complications of transbronchial biopsy include hemorrhage and pneumothorax.

Bronchoalveolar lavage (BAL) is an adjunct to fiberoptic bronchoscopy, permitting collection of cells and liquid from distal air spaces. After wedging the bronchoscope in a subsegmental airway, saline is instilled and then suctioned back through the bronchoscope for analyses, which can include cytology, microbiology, and cell counts. BAL is especially useful in the diagnosis of *P. jiroveci* pneumonia and some other infections.

Video-Assisted Thoracic Surgery Video-assisted thoracic surgery (VATS), also known as thoracoscopy, is widely used for the diagnosis of pleural lesions as well as peripheral parenchymal infiltrates and nodules. VATS involves passing a rigid scope with a camera through a trocar and into the pleural space; instruments can be inserted and manipulated through separate intercostal incisions. VATS has largely replaced "open biopsy," which requires a thoracotomy.

Percutaneous Needle Aspiration of the Lung A needle can be inserted through the chest wall and into a pulmonary lesion to aspirate material for cytologic and microbiologic studies. Percutaneous needle aspiration is usually performed under CT guidance. Owing to the small size of the sample obtained, sampling error is a limitation of the procedure.

Thoracentesis and Pleural Biopsy Thoracentesis should be performed as an early step in the evaluation of a pleural effusion of uncertain etiology. Analysis of pleural fluid can determine the etiology of the effusion (Chap. 143). Large-volume thoracentesis can be therapeutic by palliating dyspnea. Closed pleural biopsy can also be done when a pleural effusion is present but has largely been replaced by VATS.

Mediastinoscopy Tissue biopsy is often required to assess mediastinal masses or lymph nodes. Mediastinoscopy is performed from a suprasternal approach, and a rigid mediastinoscope is inserted—from which biopsies can be obtained. Lymph nodes in the left paratracheal or aortopulmonary locations typically require a parasternal mediastinotomy to provide access for biopsy.

For a more detailed discussion, see Lipson DA, Weinberger SE: Approach to the Patient with Disease of the Respiratory System, Chap. 245, p. 1583, in HPIM-17; Weinberger SE, Rosen IM: Disturbances of Respiratory Function, Chap. 246, p. 1586, in HPIM-17; and Manaker S, Weinberger SE: Diagnostic Procedures in Respiratory Disease, Chap. 247, p. 1593, in HPIM-17.

136 Asthma

Definition and Epidemiology   Asthma is a syndrome characterized by airflow obstruction that varies both spontaneously and with specific treatment. Chronic airway inflammation causes airway hyperresponsiveness to a variety of triggers, leading to airflow obstruction and respiratory symptoms including dyspnea and wheezing. Although asthmatics typically have periods of normal lung function with intermittent airflow obstruction, a subset of pts develop chronic airflow obstruction.

The prevalence of asthma has increased markedly over the past 30 years. In developed countries, approximately 10% of adults and 15% of children have asthma. Most asthmatics are atopic, and they often have allergic rhinitis and/or eczema. The majority of asthmatics have childhood-onset disease. A minority of asthmatic pts do not have atopy (negative skin prick tests to common allergens and normal serum total IgE levels). These individuals, occasionally referred to as *intrinsic asthmatics*, often have adult-onset disease. Occupational asthma can result from a variety of chemicals, including toluene diisocyanate and trimellitic anhydride, and also can have an adult onset.

Asthmatics can develop increased airflow obstruction and respiratory symptoms in response to a variety of different triggers. Inhaled allergens can be potent asthma triggers for individuals with specific sensitivity to those agents. Viral URIs commonly trigger asthma exacerbations. β-adrenergic blocking medications can markedly worsen asthma symptoms and should typically be avoided in asthmatics. Exercise often triggers increased asthma symptoms, which usually begin after exercise has ended. Other triggers of increased asthma symptoms include air pollution, occupational exposures, and stress.

Clinical Evaluation of the Patient   History   Common respiratory symptoms in asthma include wheezing, dyspnea, and cough. These symptoms often vary widely within a particular individual, and they can change spontaneously or with age, season of the year, and treatment. Symptoms may be worse at night, and nocturnal awakenings are an indicator of inadequate asthma control. The severity of their asthmatic symptoms, as well as their need for systemic steroid treatment, hospitalization, and intensive care treatment, are important to ascertain. Types of asthmatic triggers for the particular pt, and their recent exposure to them, should be determined.

Physical Exam   It is important to assess for signs of respiratory distress, including tachypnea, use of accessory respiratory muscles, and cyanosis. On lung exam, there may be wheezing and rhonchi throughout the chest, typically more prominent in expiration than inspiration. Localized wheezing may indicate an endobronchial lesion. Evidence of allergic nasal, sinus, or skin disease should be assessed. When asthma is adequately controlled, the physical exam may be normal.

Pulmonary Function Tests   Spirometry often shows airflow obstruction, with a reduction in the FEV_1 and FEV_1/FVC ratio. However, spirometry may be normal, especially if asthma symptoms are adequately treated. Bronchodilator reversibility is demonstrated by an increase in FEV_1 by ≥ 200 mL and $\geq 12\%$ from baseline FEV_1 15–20 min after a short-acting β agonist (often albuterol MDI two puffs or 180 μg). Many but not all asthmatics will demonstrate significant bronchodilator reversibility; optimal pharmacologic treatment may reduce bronchodilator reversibility. The peak expiratory flow rate (PEF) can be used by the pt to track asthma control objectively at home. Measurement of lung volumes is not typically performed, but increases in total lung capacity and residual volume may be observed. The diffusing capacity for carbon monoxide is usually normal.

Other Laboratory Tests Blood tests are usually not helpful. CBC may demonstrate eosinophilia. Specific IgE measurements for inhaled allergens (RAST) or allergy skin testing may assist in determining allergic triggers. Total serum IgE is markedly elevated in allergic bronchopulmonary aspergillosis (ABPA).

Radiographic Findings Chest x-ray is usually normal. In acute exacerbations, pneumothorax may be identified. In ABPA, eosinophilic pulmonary infiltrates may be observed. Chest CT scan is not typically performed in routine asthma but may show central bronchiectasis in ABPA.

Differential Diagnosis The differential diagnosis of asthma includes other disorders that can cause wheezing and dyspnea. Upper airway obstruction by tumor or laryngeal edema can mimic asthma, but stridor in the large airways is typically noted on physical examination. Localized wheezing in the chest may indicate an endobronchial tumor or foreign body. CHF can cause wheezing but is typically accompanied by bibasilar crackles. Eosinophilic pneumonias and Churg-Strauss syndrome may present with wheezing. Vocal cord dysfunction can mimic severe asthma and may require direct laryngoscopy to assess. When asthma involves chronic airflow obstruction, distinguishing it from chronic obstructive pulmonary disease (COPD) can be very difficult.

 Chronic Asthma

If a specific inciting agent for asthmatic symptoms can be identified and eliminated, that is an optimal part of treatment. In most cases, pharmacologic therapy is required. The two major classes of drugs are bronchodilators, which provide rapid symptomatic relief by relaxing airway smooth muscle, and controllers, which limit the airway inflammatory process.

Bronchodilators

The most widely used class of bronchodilators is β_2-adrenergic agonists, which relax airway smooth muscle by activating β_2-adrenergic receptors. Two types of inhaled β_2 agonists are widely used in asthma treatment: short-acting (SABA) and long-acting (LABA). SABAs, which include albuterol, have rapid onset of action and last for up to 6 h. SABAs are effective rescue medications, but excessive use indicates inadequate asthma control. SABAs can prevent exercise-induced asthma if administered before exercise. LABAs, which include salmeterol and formoterol, have a slower onset of action but last for >12 h. Combinations of LABAs with inhaled corticosteroids reduce asthma exacerbations and provide an excellent long-term treatment option for asthma severity of moderate persistent degree or greater.

Common side effects of β_2-adrenergic agonists include muscle tremors and palpitations. These side effects are more prominent with oral formulations, which should not generally be used. There have been ongoing concerns about mortality risks associated with β_2-adrenergic agonists, which have not been completely resolved. LABAs taken without concomitant inhaled steroid treatment may increase this risk.

Other available bronchodilator medications include anticholinergics and theophylline. Anticholinergics, which are available in short-acting and long-acting inhaled formulations, are commonly used in COPD. They appear to be considerably less effective than β_2-adrenergic agonists in asthma, and they are considered only if other asthma medications do not provide adequate asthma control. Theophylline may have both bronchodilator and anti-inflammatory effects; it is not widely used due to the potential toxicities associated with high plasma levels.

Controller Therapies

Inhaled corticosteroids (ICS) are the most effective controller treatments for asthma. ICS are usually given twice daily; a variety of ICS medications are available, including fluticasone, triamcinolone, budesonide, flunisolide, and beclomethasone. Although they do not provide immediate symptom relief, respiratory symptoms and lung function often begin to improve within several days of initiating treatment. ICS reduce exercise-induced symptoms, nocturnal symptoms, and acute exacerbations.

ICS side effects include hoarseness and oral candidiasis; these effects may be minimized by use of a spacer device and by rinsing out the mouth after taking ICS.

Other available controller therapies for asthma include systemic corticosteroids. Although quite helpful in the management of acute asthma exacerbations, oral or IV steroid use should be avoided if at all possible in the chronic management of asthma due to multiple potential side effects. Antileukotrienes, such as montelukast and zafirlukast, may be quite beneficial in some pts. Cromolyn sodium and nedocromil sodium are not widely used due to their brief durations of action and typically modest effects. Omalizumab is an antibody that neutralizes IgE; with SC injection it appears to reduce acute asthma exacerbation frequency in severe asthmatics. However, it is expensive and considered only for highly selected pts with elevated total serum IgE levels and refractory asthma symptoms.

Overall Treatment Approach

In addition to limiting exposure to their environmental triggers for asthma, pts should receive stepwise therapy appropriate for their disease severity (Figure 136-1). Asthmatics with mild intermittent symptoms are typically managed adequately with SABAs taken on an as-needed basis. Use of SABAs more than three times a week suggests that controller therapy, typically with an ICS twice per day, is required. If symptoms are not adequately controlled with ICS, LABAs can be added. If symptoms are still not adequately controlled, higher doses of ICS and/or alternative controller therapies should be considered.

ASTHMA EXACERBATIONS

Clinical Features Asthma exacerbations are periods of acute worsening of asthma symptoms that may be life-threatening. Exacerbations are commonly triggered by viral URIs, but other triggers also can be involved. Symptoms often include increased dyspnea, wheezing, and chest tightness. Physical examination can reveal pulsus paradoxus as well as tachypnea, tachycardia, and lung hyperinflation. Pulmonary function testing reveals a reduction in FEV_1 and PEF. Hypoxemia can result; P_{CO_2} is usually reduced due to hyperventilation. Normal or rising P_{CO_2} can signal impending respiratory failure.

Rx Asthma Exacerbations

The mainstays of asthma exacerbation treatment are high doses of SABAs and systemic corticosteroids. SABAs may be administered by nebulizer or

FIGURE 136-1 Step-wise approach to asthma therapy according to the severity of asthma and ability to control symptoms. ICS, inhaled corticosteroid; LABA, long-acting β₂-agonists; OCS, oral corticosteroid.

metered-dose inhaler with a spacer; very frequent dosing (q1h or more) may be required initially. IV corticosteroids, such as methylprednisolone (e.g., 80 mg IV q8h) may be used, although oral corticosteroids also may be used. Supplemental oxygen should be provided to maintain adequate oxygen saturation (>90%). If respiratory failure occurs, mechanical ventilation should be instituted, with care to minimize airway pressures and auto-PEEP. Because bacterial infections rarely trigger asthma exacerbations, antibiotics are not routinely administered.

In an effort to treat asthma exacerbations before they become severe, asthma pts should receive written action plans with instructions for self-initiation of treatment based on respiratory symptoms and reductions in PEF.

For a more detailed discussion, see Barnes PJ: Asthma, Chap. 248, p. 1596 in HPIM-17.

137 Environmental Lung Diseases

The susceptibility to develop many pulmonary diseases is influenced by environmental factors. This chapter will focus on occupational and toxic chemical exposures. However, a variety of non-occupational indoor exposures such as environmental tobacco smoke exposure (lung cancer), radon gas (lung cancer), and biomass cooking (COPD) also should be considered. Particle size is an important determinant of the impact of environmental exposures on the respiratory system. Particles >10 μm in diameter typically are captured by the upper airway. Particles 2.5–10 μm in diameter will likely deposit in the upper tracheobronchial tree, while smaller particles will reach the alveoli.

APPROACH TO THE PATIENT WITH ENVIRONMENTAL LUNG DISEASES

Because there are many types of occupational lung disease (pneumoconiosis) that can mimic diseases not known to relate to environmental factors, obtaining a careful occupational history is essential. In addition to the types of occupation performed by the pt, the specific environmental exposures, use of protective respiratory devices, and ventilation of the work environment can provide key information. Assessing the temporal development of symptoms relative to the pt's work schedule also can be very useful.

The chest x-ray is very valuable in the assessment of environmental lung disease, but it may over- or underestimate the functional impact of pneumoconioses. Pulmonary function tests should be used to assess the severity of impairment, but they typically do not suggest a specific diagnosis. Changes in spirometry before and after a work shift can provide strong evidence for bronchoconstriction in suspected occupational asthma. Some radiologic patterns are distinctive for certain occupational lung diseases; chest x-rays are widely used, and chest CT scans can provide more detailed evaluation.

OCCUPATIONAL EXPOSURES AND PULMONARY DISEASE

Inorganic Dusts   Asbestos-Related Diseases   In addition to exposures to asbestos that may occur during the production of asbestos products (from mining to manufacturing), common occupational asbestos exposures occur in shipbuilding and other construction trades (e.g., pipefitting, boilermaking) and in the manufacture of safety garments and friction materials (e.g., brake and clutch linings). Along with worker exposure in these areas, bystander exposure (e.g., spouses) can be responsible for some asbestos-related lung diseases.

A range of respiratory diseases has been associated with asbestos exposure. Pleural plaques indicate that asbestos exposure has occurred, but they are typically not symptomatic. Interstitial lung disease, often referred to as *asbestosis*, is pathologically and radiologically similar to idiopathic pulmonary fibrosis; it is typically accompanied by a restrictive ventilatory defect on pulmonary function testing. Asbestosis can develop after 10 years of exposure, and no specific therapy is available.

Benign pleural effusions can also occur from asbestos exposure. Lung cancer is clearly associated with asbestos exposure but does not typically present for at least 15 years after initial exposure. The lung cancer risk increases multiplicatively with cigarette smoking. In addition, mesotheliomas (both pleural and peritoneal) are strongly associated with asbestos exposure, but they are not related to smoking. Relatively brief asbestos exposures may lead to mesotheliomas, which typically do not develop for decades after the initial exposure. Biopsy of pleural tissue, typically by thoracoscopic surgery, is required for diagnosing mesothelioma.

Silicosis   Silicosis results from exposure to free silica (crystalline quartz), which occurs in mining, stone cutting, abrasive industries (e.g., stone, clay, glass, and cement manufacturing), foundry work, and quarrying. Heavy exposures over relatively brief time periods (as little as 10 months) can cause acute silicosis—which is pathologically similar to pulmonary alveolar proteinosis and associated with a characteristic chest CT pattern known as "crazy paving." Acute silicosis can be severe and progressive; whole lung lavage may be of some therapeutic benefit.

Longer-term exposures can result in simple silicosis, with small rounded opacities in the upper lobes of the lungs. Calcification of hilar lymph nodes can give a characteristic "eggshell" appearance. Progressive nodular fibrosis can result in masses >1 cm in diameter in complicated silicosis. When such masses become very large, the term *progressive massive fibrosis* is used to describe the condition. Due to impaired cell-mediated immunity, silicosis pts are at increased risk of tuberculosis, atypical mycobacterial infections, and fungal infections. Silica may also be a lung carcinogen.

Coal Worker's Pneumoconiosis   Occupational exposure to coal dust predisposes to coal worker's pneumoconiosis (CWP), which is less common among coal workers in the western United States due to a lower risk from the bituminous coal found in that region. Simple CWP is defined radiologically by small nodular opacities and is not typically symptomatic. The development of larger nodules (>1 cm in diameter), usually in the upper lobes, characterizes complicated CWP. Complicated CWP is often symptomatic and is associated with reduced pulmonary function and increased mortality.

Berylliosis   Beryllium exposure may occur in the manufacturing of alloys, ceramics, and electronic devices. Although acute beryllium exposure can rarely produce acute pneumonitis, a chronic granulomatous disease very similar to sarcoidosis is much more common. Radiologically, chronic beryllium disease, like sarcoidosis, is characterized by pulmonary nodules along septal lines. As in sarcoidosis, either a restrictive or obstructive ventilatory pattern on pulmonary function testing can be seen. Bronchoscopy with transbronchial biopsy is typically required to diagnose chronic beryllium disease. The most effective way to distinguish chronic beryllium disease from sarcoidosis is to perform a beryllium lymphocyte proliferation test using blood or bronchoalveolar lavage lymphocytes. Removal from further beryllium exposure is required, and corticosteroids may be beneficial.

Organic Dusts   Cotton Dust (Byssinosis)   Dust exposures occur in the production of yarns for cotton, linen, and rope-making. Flax, hemp, and jute produce a similar syndrome. At the early stages of byssinosis, chest tightness occurs near the end of the first day of the work week. In progressive cases, symptoms are present throughout the work week. After at least 10 years of exposure, chronic airflow obstruction can develop. In symptomatic individuals, limiting further exposure is essential.

Grain Dust   Farmers and grain elevator operators are at risk for grain dust–related lung disease, which is similar to COPD. Symptoms include cough, wheezing, and dyspnea. Pulmonary function tests show airflow obstruction.

Farmer's Lung   Exposure to moldy hay containing thermophilic actinomycetes can lead to the development of hypersensitivity pneumonitis. Within 8 h after exposure, the acute presentation of farmer's lung includes fever, cough, and dyspnea. With repeated exposures, chronic and patchy interstitial lung disease can develop.

Toxic Chemicals   Many toxic chemicals can affect the lung in the form of vapors and gases.

Smoke inhalation can be lethal to firefighters and fire victims through a variety of mechanisms. Carbon monoxide poisoning can cause life-threatening hypoxemia. Combustion of plastics and polyurethanes can release toxic agents including cyanide.

Occupational asthma can result from exposure to diisocyanates in polyurethanes and acid anhydrides in epoxides.

PRINCIPLES OF MANAGEMENT

Treatment of environmental lung diseases typically involves limiting or avoiding exposures to the toxic substance. Chronic interstitial lung diseases (e.g., asbestosis, CWP) are not responsive to glucocorticoids, but acute organic dust exposures may respond to corticosteroids. Therapy of occupational asthma (e.g., diisocyanates) follows usual asthma guidelines (Chap. 136) and therapy of occupational COPD (e.g., byssinosis) follows usual COPD guidelines (Chap 138).

> For a more detailed discussion, see Speizer FE and Balmes JR: Environmental Lung Disease, Chap. 250, p. 1611, in HPIM-17.

138 Chronic Obstructive Pulmonary Disease

DEFINITION AND EPIDEMIOLOGY

Chronic obstructive pulmonary disease (COPD) is a disease state characterized by chronic airflow obstruction; thus, pulmonary function testing is central to its diagnosis. The presence of airflow obstruction is determined by a reduced ratio of the forced expiratory volume in 1 s (FEV_1) to the forced vital capacity (FVC). Among individuals with a reduced FEV_1/FVC, the severity of airflow obstruction is determined by the level of reduction in FEV_1 (Table 138-1): ≥80% is stage I, 50–80% is stage II, 30–50% is stage III, and <30% is stage IV. Cigarette smoking is the major environmental risk factor for COPD. The risk of COPD increases with cigarette smoking intensity, which is typically quantified as pack-years. (One pack of cigarettes smoked per day for 1 year equals 1 pack-year.) Individuals with airway hyperresponsiveness and certain occupational exposures (e.g., coal mining, gold mining, and cotton textiles) are likely also at increased risk for COPD. In countries in which biomass combustion with poor ventilation is used for cooking, an increased risk of COPD among women has been reported. COPD is a progressive disorder; however, the rate of loss of lung function often slows markedly if smoking cessation occurs. In normal individuals, FEV_1 reaches a lifetime peak at around age 25 years, enters a plateau phase, and subsequently declines gradually and progressively. Subjects can develop COPD by having reduced maximally attained lung function, shortened plateau phase, or accelerated decline in lung function.

Symptoms often occur only when COPD is advanced; thus, early detection requires spirometric testing. The Pa_{O_2} typically remains near normal until the FEV_1 falls to <50% of the predicted value. Hypercarbia and pulmonary hypertension are most common after FEV_1 has fallen to <25% of predicted. COPD pts with similar FEV_1 values can vary markedly in their respiratory symptoms and functional impairment. COPD often includes periods of increased respiratory symptoms, such as dyspnea, cough, and phlegm production, which are known as exacerbations. Exacerbations are often triggered by bacterial and/or viral respiratory infections. These exacerbations become more common as COPD severity

TABLE 138-1   GOLD CRITERIA FOR COPD SEVERITY

GOLD Stage	Severity	Symptoms	Spirometry
I	Mild	With or without chronic cough or sputum production	$FEV_1/FVC < 0.7$ and $FEV_1 \geq 80\%$ predicted
II	Moderate	With or without chronic cough or sputum production	$FEV_1/FVC < 0.7$ and $50\% \leq FEV_1 < 80\%$ predicted
III	Severe	With or without chronic cough or sputum production	$FEV_1/FVC < 0.7$ and $30\% \leq FEV_1 < 50\%$ predicted
IV	Very Severe	With or without chronic cough or sputum production	$FEV_1/FVC < 0.7$ and $FEV_1 < 30\%$ predicted *or* $FEV_1 < 50\%$ predicted with respiratory failure or signs of right heart failure

Note: GOLD, Global Initiative for Chronic Obstructive Pulmonary Disease (COPD).
Source: From RA Pauwels et al. *Am J Respir Crit Care Med* 163:1256, 2001; with permission.

increases, but some individuals are much more susceptible to developing exacerbations than others with similar degrees of airflow obstruction.

CLINICAL MANIFESTATIONS

History   Subjects with COPD usually have smoked ≥ 20 pack-years of cigarettes. Common symptoms include cough and phlegm production; individuals with chronic productive cough for 3 months per year for the preceding 2 years have chronic bronchitis. However, chronic bronchitis without airflow obstruction is not included within COPD. Dyspnea, especially with exertion, is a common and potentially disabling symptom in COPD subjects. Exercise involving upper-body activity is especially difficult for severe COPD pts. Weight loss and cachexia are common in advanced disease. Hypoxemia and hypercarbia may result in fluid retention, morning headaches, sleep disruption, erythrocytosis, and cyanosis.

Exacerbations are more frequent as disease progresses and are most often triggered by respiratory infections, often with a bacterial component. Exacerbations may also be precipitated by left ventricular failure, cardiac arrhythmia, pneumothorax, pneumonia, and pulmonary thromboembolism.

Physical Findings   The physical examination may be normal until COPD is fairly advanced. As disease progresses, signs of hyperinflation may become more prominent. Wheezing is occasionally observed, but it does not predict the severity of obstruction or response to therapy. Persistently localized wheezing raises the possibility of lung cancer.

During COPD exacerbations, signs of respiratory distress may be prominent, including tachycardia, tachypnea, use of accessory muscles of respiration, and cyanosis.

Radiographic Findings   Plain chest x-ray may show hyperinflation, emphysema, and pulmonary hypertension. It is typically performed to exclude other disease processes during routine evaluation, and to exclude pneumonia during exacerbations. Chest CT scanning has much greater sensitivity for detecting emphysema but is typically reserved for the evaluation of advanced disease when surgical options such as lung volume reduction and lung transplantation are being considered.

Pulmonary Function Tests Objective documentation of airflow obstruction is essential for diagnosing COPD. Standardized staging of COPD is based on post-bronchodilator spirometry. In COPD, the FEV_1/FVC ratio is reduced below 0.7. Despite prolonged expiratory efforts, subjects may not be able to achieve a plateau in their FVC. Increases in total lung capacity and residual volume, as well as reduced diffusing capacity for carbon monoxide, are typically seen in emphysema.

Laboratory Tests α_1 antitrypsin ($\alpha_1 AT$) testing, typically by measurement of the protein level in the bloodstream, is recommended to exclude severe $\alpha_1 AT$ deficiency. Augmentation therapy (a weekly IV infusion) is available for individuals with severe $\alpha_1 AT$ deficiency (e.g., PI Z). Pulse oximetry can determine the O_2 saturation. However, arterial blood gases remain useful to assess the severity of CO_2 retention as well as acid-base disorders. During acute exacerbations, arterial blood gases should be considered in pts with mental status changes, significant respiratory distress, very severe COPD, or a history of hypercarbia. Complete blood counts are useful in advanced disease to assess for erythrocytosis, which can occur secondary to hypoxemia, and anemia, which can worsen dyspnea.

 COPD

OUTPATIENT MANAGEMENT
Smoking Cessation
Elimination of tobacco smoking has been convincingly shown to reduce decline in pulmonary function and to prolong survival in pts with COPD. Although lung function does not typically improve substantially after smoking cessation, the rate of decline in FEV_1 often reverts to that of nonsmokers. Pharmacologic treatment to assist with smoking cessation is often beneficial. Use of nicotine replacement therapy (available as a patch, gum, nasal spray, and oral inhaler) can increase rates of smoking cessation; oral bupropion (150 mg bid after starting at 150 mg qd for 3 days) also produces significant benefit and can be combined successfully with nicotine replacement. Varenicline, a partial agonist for nicotinic acetylcholine receptors, also can promote smoking cessation. All adult, nonpregnant smokers without specific contraindications should be offered pharmacologic treatment to assist with smoking cessation.

Nonpharmacologic Treatment
Pulmonary rehabilitation improves functional status and reduces hospitalizations. Annual influenza vaccinations are strongly recommended; in addition, pneumococcal vaccination is recommended.

Bronchodilators
Although inhaled bronchodilator medications do not increase longevity in COPD, they may significantly reduce respiratory symptoms. Short- and long-acting β-adrenergic agonists, short- and long-acting anticholinergics, and theophylline derivatives all may be used. Although oral medications are associated with greater rates of adherence, inhaled medications generally have fewer side effects.

Pts with mild disease can usually be managed with an inhaled short-acting anticholinergic such as ipratropium or a short acting β agonist such as albuterol. Combination therapy and long-acting β agonists and/or anticholinergics should be added in pts with severe disease. The narrow toxic-therapeutic ratio of theophylline compounds limits their use, and either low doses or regular monitoring of serum levels are required.

Corticosteroids

Chronic systemic corticosteroid treatment is not recommended in COPD pts due to the risk of multiple complications, including osteoporosis, weight gain, cataracts, and diabetes mellitus. Although multiple studies have demonstrated that inhaled steroids do not reduce the rate of decline of FEV_1 in COPD, inhaled steroid medications may reduce the frequency of exacerbations in individuals with severe COPD. Combinations of inhaled steroids and long-acting β agonists reduce COPD exacerbations and may reduce mortality—although that has not been conclusively shown.

Oxygen

Long-term supplemental oxygen therapy has been shown to reduce symptoms and improve survival in COPD pts who are chronically hypoxemic. Documentation of the need for O_2 requires a measurement of Pa_{O_2} or oxygen saturation (Sa_{O_2}) after a period of stability. Pts with a Pa_{O_2} ≤55 mmHg or Sa_{O_2} ≤88% should receive O_2 to raise the Sa_{O_2} to ≥90%. O_2 is also indicated for pts with Pa_{O_2} of 56–59 mmHg or Sa_{O_2} ≤89% if associated with signs and symptoms of pulmonary hypertension or cor pulmonale. For individuals who meet these guidelines, continuous O_2 therapy is recommended because the number of hours per day of oxygen use is directly related to the mortality benefit. Supplemental oxygen may also be prescribed for selected COPD pts who desaturate only with exercise or during sleep, although the evidence for benefit is less compelling.

Surgical Options for Severe COPD

Two main types of surgical options are available for end-stage COPD. Lung volume reduction surgery can reduce mortality and improve lung function in selected pts with upper lobe–predominant emphysema and low exercise capacity (after pulmonary rehabilitation). Individuals who meet the criteria for the high-risk group (FEV_1 <20% predicted and either a diffuse distribution of emphysema or lung carbon monoxide diffusing capacity <20% predicted) should not be considered for lung volume reduction surgery. In addition to surgical lung volume reduction, several bronchoscopic lung volume reduction approaches are in clinical trials. Lung transplantation should be considered for COPD pts who have very severe chronic airflow obstruction and disability at a relatively young age despite maximal medical therapy.

MANAGEMENT OF COPD EXACERBATIONS

COPD exacerbations are a major cause of morbidity and mortality. Critical decisions in management include whether hospitalization is required. Although there are not definitive guidelines to determine which COPD pts require hospitalization for an exacerbation, the development of respiratory acidosis, significant hypercarbia, worsening hypoxemia, pneumonia, or social situations without adequate home support for the treatment required should prompt consideration of hospitalization.

Key components of exacerbation treatment include bronchodilators, antibiotics, and short courses of systemic glucocorticoids.

Antibiotics

Because bacterial infections often trigger COPD exacerbations, antibiotic therapy should be strongly considered, especially with increased sputum volume or change in sputum color. Common pathogens include *Streptococcus pneumoniae, Haemophilus influenzae*, and *Moraxella catarrhalis*. Antibiotic choice should depend on the local antibiotic sensitivity patterns, previous sputum culture results for a particular pt, and the severity of disease. Trimethoprim-sulfamethoxazole, doxycycline, and amoxicillin are reasonable choices for subjects with mild to moderate COPD; broader-spectrum antibiotics should be considered for subjects with more severe underlying COPD and/or more severe exacerbations. Outside of the setting of an acute exacerbation, chronic antibiotic therapy is not recommended in COPD.

Bronchodilators

Bronchodilator therapy is essential during COPD exacerbations. Short-acting β-adrenergic agonists by inhalation (e.g., albuterol q1–2h) are used; addition of anticholinergics is likely of benefit (e.g., ipratropium q4–6h). Administration of bronchodilators by nebulizer is often used initially because it is easier to administer to pts in respiratory distress. Conversion to metered-dose inhaler administration can be successfully achieved with appropriate training of the pt and staff.

Glucocorticoids

Systemic steroids hasten resolution of symptoms and reduce relapses and subsequent exacerbations for up to 6 months. Dosing is not well worked out, but 30–40 mg of prednisone daily (or IV equivalent) is standard, with a total course of 10–14 days. Hyperglycemia is the most commonly reported complication and should be monitored.

Oxygen

Hypoxemia often worsens during COPD exacerbations. Supplemental O_2 should be administered to maintain $Sa_{O_2} \geq 90\%$. Delivery systems include nasal prongs at 1–2 L/min or 24% Venturi mask. Very high O_2 delivery can worsen hypercarbia, primarily due to increasing ventilation-perfusion mismatch. However, providing adequate O_2 to obtain saturation of ~90% is the key goal. Therefore, supplemental O_2 delivery should be focused on providing adequate oxygenation without providing unnecessarily high O_2 saturations. Pts may require use of supplemental O_2 after hospital discharge until the exacerbation completely resolves.

Ventilatory Support

The diagnosis of acute respiratory failure is made on the basis of a decrease in Pa_{O_2} by 10–15 mmHg from baseline or an increase in Pa_{O_2} associated with a pH <7.30. Numerous studies suggest that noninvasive mask ventilation [noninvasive positive pressure ventilation (NPPV)] can improve outcomes in acute COPD exacerbations with respiratory failure (Pa_{CO_2} >45 mmHg). Contraindications to NPPV include cardiovascular instability, impaired mental status, inability to cooperate, copious secretions, craniofacial abnormalities or facial trauma, extreme obesity, or significant burns. Progressive hypercarbia, refractory hypoxemia, or alterations in mental status that compromise ability to comply with NPPV therapy may necessitate endotracheal intubation for mechanical ventilation.

For a more detailed discussion, see Reilly JJ Jr., Silverman EK, Shapiro SD: Chronic Obstructive Pulmonary Disease, Chap. 254, p. 1635, in HPIM-17.

139 Pneumonia and Lung Abscess

Pneumonia, an infection of the pulmonary parenchyma, is classified as community-acquired (CAP) or health care–associated (HCAP). The HCAP category is subdivided into hospital-acquired pneumonia (HAP) and ventilator-associated pneumonia (VAP). HCAP is associated with hospitalization for ≥48 h, hospitalization for ≥2 days in the prior 3 months, nursing home or extended-care facility residence, antibiotic therapy in the preceding 3 months, chronic dialysis, home infusion therapy, home wound care, and contact with a family member who has a multidrug-resistant (MDR) infection.

PATHOPHYSIOLOGY

- Microorganisms gain access to the lower respiratory tract via microaspiration from the oropharynx (the most common route), inhalation of contaminated droplets, hematogenous spread, or contiguous extension from an infected pleural or mediastinal space.
- Classic pneumonia (typified by that due to *Streptococcus pneumoniae*) presents as a lobar pattern and evolves through four phases.
  Edema: Proteinaceous exudates are present in the alveoli.
  Red hepatization: Erythrocytes and neutrophils are present in the intraalveolar exudate.
  Gray hepatization: Neutrophils predominate, with abundant fibrin deposition. Bacteria are absent.
  Resolution: Macrophages are the dominant cell type in the alveolar space. Debris and inflammation have cleared.
- In VAP, respiratory bronchiolitis can precede pneumonia. A bronchopneumonia pattern is most common.

COMMUNITY-ACQUIRED PNEUMONIA

Epidemiology and Etiology CAP, which affects ~4 million adults each year in the United States, is more common among pts with severe underlying illness. Many factors (e.g., alcoholism, asthma, age >70 years, immunosuppression, smoking, and HIV infection) influence the types of pathogens that should be considered in identifying the etiologic agent. Relatively few pathogens cause most cases.

- Typical bacterial pathogens: *S. pneumoniae*, *Haemophilus influenzae*, *Staphylococcus aureus* [including community-acquired methicillin-resistant *S. aureus* (CA-MRSA)], gram-negative bacteria such as *Klebsiella pneumoniae* and *Pseudomonas aeruginosa*
- Atypical organisms: *Mycoplasma pneumoniae*, *Chlamydophila pneumoniae*, *Legionella* spp., respiratory viruses (e.g., influenza viruses)
- Anaerobes play a significant role in CAP only when aspiration occurs days to weeks before presentation.

Clinical Features

- Typical symptoms are fever, chills, sweats, cough (either nonproductive or productive of mucoid, purulent, or blood-tinged sputum), pleuritic chest pain, and dyspnea.
- Other common symptoms include nausea, vomiting, diarrhea, fatigue, headache, myalgias, and arthralgias. Elderly pts may present atypically with confusion.
- Physical examination: tachypnea, increased or decreased tactile fremitus, dull to flat percussion reflecting consolidation or pleural fluid, crackles, bronchial breath sounds, pleural friction rub

Diagnosis

- Chest x-ray (CXR) is usually adequate for diagnosis, but CT of the chest may be required in some cases. Some patterns suggest an etiology; e.g., pneumatoceles suggest *S. aureus*.
- Sputum stains and culture: The presence of >25 white blood cells and <10 squamous epithelial cells per high-power field suggests that a sample is appropriate for culture. A single, predominant organism on Gram's stain suggests the etiology. Other stains should be used as indicated (e.g., for *Mycobacterium tuberculosis* or fungi).
- Blood cultures are positive in 5–14% of cases, most commonly yielding *S. pneumoniae*. Blood cultures are optional for most CAP pts but should be performed for high-risk pts (e.g., pts with neutropenia or asplenia).
- Urine antigen tests for *S. pneumoniae* and *Legionella pneumophila* type 1 can be helpful.
- Serology: A fourfold rise in titer of specific IgM antibody can assist in the diagnosis of pneumonia due to some pathogens. The time required to obtain a final result makes serology of limited clinical utility.

Rx Community-Acquired Pneumonia

Site of Care

Two sets of criteria identify pts who will benefit from hospital care. It is not clear which set is superior, and application of each tool should be tempered by a consideration of factors relevant to the individual pt.

- Pneumonia Severity Index (PSI): Points are given for 20 variables, including age, coexisting illness, and abnormal physical and laboratory findings. On this basis, pts are assigned to one of five classes of mortality risk.
- CURB-65: Five variables are included: confusion (C); urea >7 mmol/L (U); respiratory rate ≥30/min (R); blood pressure, systolic ≤90 mmHg or diastolic ≤60 mmHg (B); and age ≥65 years (65). Pts with a score of 0 can be treated at home, pts with a score of 2 should be hospitalized, and pts with a score of ≥3 may require management in the ICU.

Antibiotic Therapy

For recommendations on empirical antibiotic treatment of CAP, see Table 139-1. U.S. guidelines always target *S. pneumoniae* and atypical pathogens. A retrospective review of pts >65 years of age suggests that this approach lowers the mortality rate. A pt initially treated with IV antibiotics can be switched to oral agents when he or she can ingest and absorb drugs, is hemodynamically stable, and is showing clinical improvement. CAP is typically treated for 10–14 days, but a 5-day course of a fluoroquinolone is sufficient for cases of uncomplicated CAP. A longer course is required for pts with bacteremia, metastatic infection, or infection with a particularly virulent pathogen and in most cases of severe CAP.

TABLE 139-1   EMPIRICAL ANTIBIOTIC TREATMENT OF COMMUNITY-ACQUIRED PNEUMONIA

Outpatients
  Previously healthy and no antibiotics in past 3 months
  • A macrolide [clarithromycin (500 mg PO bid) or azithromycin (500 mg PO once, then 250 mg od)] *or*
  • Doxycycline (100 mg PO bid)
  Comorbidities or antibiotics in past 3 months: select an alternative from a different class
  • A respiratory fluoroquinolone [moxifloxacin (400 mg PO od), gemifloxacin (320 mg PO od), levofloxacin (750 mg PO od)] *or*
  • A β-lactam [preferred: high-dose amoxicillin (1 g tid) or amoxicillin/clavulanate (2 g bid); alternatives: ceftriaxone (1–2 g IV od), cefpodoxime (200 mg PO bid), cefuroxime (500 mg PO bid)] *plus* a macrolide[a]
  In regions with a high rate of "high-level" pneumococcal macrolide resistance,[b] consider alternatives listed above for pts with comorbidities.

Inpatients, non-ICU
  • A respiratory fluoroquinolone [moxifloxacin (400 mg PO or IV od), gemifloxacin (320 mg PO od), levofloxacin (750 mg PO or IV od)]
  • A β-lactam[c] [cefotaxime (1–2 g IV q8h), ceftriaxone (1–2 g IV od), ampicillin (1–2 g IV q4–6h), ertapenem (1 g IV od in selected pts)] *plus a* macrolide[d] [oral clarithromycin or azithromycin (as listed above for previously healthy patients) or IV azithromycin (1 g once, then 500 mg od)]

Inpatients, ICU
  • A β-lactam[e] [cefotaxime (1–2 g IV q8h), ceftriaxone (2 g IV od), ampicillin-sulbactam (2 g IV q8h)] *plus*
  • Azithromycin or a fluoroquinolone (as listed above for inpatients, non-ICU)

Special concerns
  If *Pseudomonas* is a consideration
  • An antipneumococcal, antipseudomonal β-lactam [piperacillin/tazobactam (4.5 g IV q6h), cefepime (1–2 g IV q12h), imipenem (500 mg IV q6h), meropenem (1 g IV q8h)] *plus* either ciprofloxacin (400 mg IV q12h) or levofloxacin (750 mg IV od)
  • The above β-lactams *plus* an aminoglycoside [amikacin (15 mg/kg od) or tobramycin (1.7 mg/kg od) and azithromycin]
  • The above β-lactams[f] *plus* an aminoglycoside *plus* an antipneumococcal fluoroquinolone
  If CA-MRSA is a consideration
  • Add linezolid (600 mg IV q12h) or vancomycin (1 g IV q12h)

Note: CA-MRSA, community-acquired methicillin-resistant *Staphylococcus aureus*; ICU, intensive care unit.
[a]Doxycycline (100 mg PO bid) is an alternative to the macrolide.
[b]MICs of >16 μg/mL in 25% of isolates.
[c]A respiratory fluoroquinolone should be used for penicillin-allergic pts.
[d]Doxycycline (100 mg IV q12h) is an alternative to the macrolide.
[e]For penicillin-allergic pts, use a respiratory fluoroquinolone and aztreonam (2 g IV q8h).
[f]For penicillin-allergic pts, substitute aztreonam.

Complications

• Common complications of severe CAP include respiratory failure, shock and multiorgan failure, bleeding diatheses, and exacerbation of comorbid disease.
• Metastatic infection (e.g., brain abscess, endocarditis) may occur and requires immediate attention.

- Lung abscess may occur in association with aspiration or infection caused by single CAP pathogens (e.g., CA-MRSA or *P. aeruginosa*). Drainage should be established and proper antibiotics administered.
- Pleural effusion should be tapped for diagnostic and therapeutic purposes. If the fluid has a pH <7, a glucose level <2.2 mmol/L, and a lactate dehydrogenase content >1000 U or if bacteria are seen or cultured, fluid should be drained; a chest tube is usually required.

Follow-Up
- CXR abnormalities may require 4–12 weeks to clear.
- Pts should receive influenza and pneumococcal vaccines, as appropriate.

HEALTH CARE–ASSOCIATED PNEUMONIA (see also Chap. 85)

VENTILATOR-ASSOCIATED PNEUMONIA

VAP is a common complication in pts on mechanical ventilation, with prevalence estimates of 6–52 cases per 100 pts. Three factors important in the pathogenesis of VAP are colonization of the oropharynx with pathogenic microorganisms, aspiration of these organisms to the lower respiratory tract, and compromise of normal host defense mechanisms. Potential etiologic agents include MDR and non-MDR pathogens; the prominence of the various pathogens depends on the length of hospital stay at the time of infection. Clinical manifestations are similar to those in other forms of pneumonia.

Diagnosis Diagnosis is difficult. Application of clinical criteria consistently results in overdiagnosis of VAP. Use of quantitative cultures to discriminate between colonization and true infection by determining bacterial burden may be helpful; the more distal in the respiratory tree the diagnostic sampling, the more specific the results.

TABLE 139-2 EMPIRICAL ANTIBIOTIC TREATMENT OF HEALTH CARE–ASSOCIATED PNEUMONIA

Patients without Risk Factors for MDR Pathogens

Ceftriaxone (2 g IV q24h) *or*
Moxifloxacin (400 mg IV q24h), ciprofloxacin (400 mg IV q8h), or levofloxacin (750 mg IV q24h) *or*
Ampicillin/sulbactam (3 g IV q6h) *or*
Ertapenem (1 g IV q24h)

Patients with Risk Factors for MDR Pathogens

1. A β-lactam:
Ceftazidime (2 g IV q8h) or cefepime (2 g IV q8–12h) *or*
Piperacillin/tazobactam (4.5 g IV q6h), imipenem (500 mg IV q6h or 1 g IV q8h), or meropenem (1 g IV q8h) *plus*
2. A second agent active against gram-negative bacterial pathogens:
Gentamicin or tobramycin (7 mg/kg IV q24h) or amikacin (20 mg/kg IV q24h) *or*
Ciprofloxacin (400 mg IV q8h) or levofloxacin (750 mg IV q24h) *plus*
3. An agent active against gram-positive bacterial pathogens:
Linezolid (600 mg IV q12h) *or*
Vancomycin (15 mg/kg, up to 1 g IV, q12h)

Note: MDR, multidrug-resistant.

℞ Ventilator-Associated Pneumonia

Higher mortality rates are associated with inappropriate initial empirical treatment. See Table 139-2 for recommended options for empirical therapy for HCAP. Broad-spectrum treatment should be modified when a pathogen is identified. Treatment failure in VAP is not uncommon, especially when MDR pathogens are involved; MRSA and *P. aeruginosa* are associated with high failure rates. VAP complications include prolongation of mechanical ventilation, increased length of stay in the ICU, and necrotizing pneumonia with pulmonary hemorrhage or bronchiectasis. VAP is associated with significant mortality risk. Strategies effective for the prevention of VAP are listed in Table 139-3.

TABLE 139-3	PATHOGENIC MECHANISMS AND CORRESPONDING PREVENTION STRATEGIES FOR VENTILATOR-ASSOCIATED PNEUMONIA
Pathogenic Mechanism	**Prevention Strategy**
Oropharyngeal colonization with pathogenic bacteria	
Elimination of normal flora	Avoidance of prolonged antibiotic courses
Large-volume oropharyngeal aspiration around time of intubation	Short course of prophylactic antibiotics for comatose pts[a]
Gastroesophageal reflux	Postpyloric enteral feeding[b]; avoidance of high gastric residuals, prokinetic agents
Bacterial overgrowth of stomach	Avoidance of gastrointestinal bleeding due to prophylactic agents that raise gastric pH[b]; selective decontamination of digestive tract with nonabsorbable antibiotics[b]
Cross-infection from other colonized patients	Hand washing, especially with alcohol-based hand rub; intensive infection control education[a]; isolation; proper cleaning of reusable equipment
Large-volume aspiration	Endotracheal intubation; avoidance of sedation; decompression of small-bowel obstruction
Microaspiration around endotracheal tube	
Endotracheal intubation	Noninvasive ventilation[a]
Prolonged duration of ventilation	Daily awakening from sedation,[a] weaning protocols[a]
Abnormal swallowing function	Early percutaneous tracheostomy[a]
Secretions pooled above endotracheal tube	Head of bed elevated[a]; continuous aspiration of subglottic secretions with specialized endotracheal tube[a]; avoidance of reintubation; minimization of sedation and pt transport
Altered lower respiratory host defenses	Tight glycemic control[a]; lowering of hemoglobin transfusion threshold; specialized enteral feeding formula

[a]Strategies demonstrated to be effective in at least one randomized controlled trial.
[b]Strategies with negative randomized trials or conflicting results.

HOSPITAL-ACQUIRED PNEUMONIA

Less well studied than VAP, HAP more commonly involves non-MDR pathogens. Anaerobes may also be more commonly involved in non-VAP pts because of the increased risk of macroaspiration in pts who are not intubated.

> For a more detailed discussion, see Mandell LA, Wunderink R:
> Pneumonia, Chap. 251, p. 1619, in HPIM-17.

140 Pulmonary Thromboembolism and Deep-Vein Thrombosis

DEFINITION AND NATURAL HISTORY

Venous thromboembolism includes both deep-vein thrombosis (DVT) and pulmonary thromboembolism (PE). DVT results from blood clot formation within large veins, usually in the legs. PE results from DVTs that have broken off and traveled to the pulmonary arterial circulation. DVT is approximately three times more common than PE. Although DVTs are typically related to thrombus formation in the legs and/or pelvis, indwelling venous catheters have increased the occurrence of upper extremity DVT. In the absence of PE, the major complication of DVT is postphlebitic syndrome, which causes chronic leg swelling and discomfort due to damage to the venous valves of the affected leg. PE is often fatal, usually due to progressive right ventricular failure. Chronic thromboembolic pulmonary hypertension is another long-term complication of PE.

Some genetic risk factors, including factor V Leiden and the prothrombin G20210A mutation, have been identified, but they account for only a minority of venous thromboembolic disease. A variety of other risk factors have been identified, including immobilization during prolonged travel, obesity, smoking, surgery, trauma, oral contraceptives, and postmenopausal hormone replacement. Medical conditions that increase the risk of venous thromboembolism include cancer and antiphospholipid antibody syndrome.

CLINICAL EVALUATION

History DVTs often present with progressive lower calf discomfort. For PE, dyspnea is the most common presenting symptom. Chest pain can indicate pulmonary infarction with pleural irritation. Syncope can occur with massive PE.

Physical Examination Tachypnea and tachycardia are common in PE. Low-grade fever, neck vein distention, and a loud P_2 on cardiac examination can be seen. Hypotension and cyanosis suggest massive PE. Physical examination with DVT may be notable only for mild calf tenderness. However, with massive DVT, marked thigh swelling and inguinal tenderness can be observed.

Laboratory Tests Normal D-dimer level (<500 µg/mL by enzyme-linked immunosorbent assay) essentially rules out PE, although hospitalized pts often have elevated D-dimer levels due to other disease processes. Although hypoxemia and an increased alveolar-arterial O_2 gradient may be observed in PE, arterial blood gases are rarely useful in diagnosing PE. Elevated serum troponin and brain natriuretic peptide levels are associated with increased risk of complications in PE. The electrocardiogram can show an S1Q3T3 sign in PE, but that finding is not frequently observed.

Imaging Studies Venous ultrasonography can detect DVT by demonstrating loss of normal venous compressibility. When combined with Doppler imaging of venous flow, the detection of DVT by ultrasonography is excellent. For pts with nondiagnostic venous ultrasound studies, CT or MRI can be used to assess for DVT. Contrast phlebography is very rarely required.

In PE, a normal chest x-ray (CXR) is common. Although not commonly observed, focal oligemia and peripheral wedge-shaped densities on CXR are well-established findings in PE. Chest CT with IV contrast has become the primary diagnostic imaging test for PE. Ventilation/perfusion lung scanning is primarily used for subjects unable to tolerate IV contrast. Transthoracic echocardiography is valuable to assess for RV hypokinesis with moderate to large PE, but it is not typically useful for diagnosing the presence of a PE. With the advent of contrast chest CT scans for PE diagnosis, pulmonary angiography studies are rarely performed.

Integrated Diagnostic Approach An integrated diagnostic approach that considers the clinical suspicion for DVT and PE is required. For individuals with a low clinical likelihood of DVT or with a low to moderate clinical likelihood of PE, the D-dimer level can be used to determine if further imaging studies are required. An algorithm for imaging studies in both DVT and PE is shown in Fig. 140-1. The differential diagnosis of DVT includes a ruptured Baker's cyst and cellulitis. The differential diagnosis of PE is broad and includes pneumonia, acute myocardial infarction, and aortic dissection.

 Deep-Vein Thrombosis and Pulmonary Thromboembolism

Anticoagulation

Although anticoagulants do not dissolve existing clots in DVT or PE directly, they limit further thrombus formation and allow fibrinolysis to occur. In order to provide effective anticoagulation rapidly, parenteral anticoagulation is used for the initial treatment of venous thromboembolism. Traditionally, unfractionated heparin (UFH) has been used, with a target activated partial thromboplastin time (aPTT) of 2–3 times the upper limit of the normal laboratory value. UFH is typically administered with a bolus of 5000–10,000 U followed by a continuous infusion of approximately 1000 U/h. Frequent dosage adjustments are often required to achieve and maintain a therapeutic aPTT with UFH. Heparin-induced thrombocytopenia can occur with UFH. However, the short-half life of UFH remains a significant advantage.

Alternatives to UFH for acute anticoagulation include low-molecular-weight heparins (LMWHs) such as enoxaparin and tinzaparin. Laboratory monitoring is not required, but doses are adjusted for renal impairment or obesity. Fondaparinux, a pentasaccharide, is another parenteral alternative to UFH that does not require laboratory monitoring but does require dose adjustment for renal insufficiency.

After initiating treatment with a parenteral agent, warfarin is typically used for long-term oral anticoagulation. Warfarin can be initiated soon after a parenteral agent is given; however, 5–7 days are typically required for warfarin to achieve therapeutic anticoagulation. Warfarin is given to achieve a therapeutic international normalized ratio (INR) of the prothrombin time, which is typi-

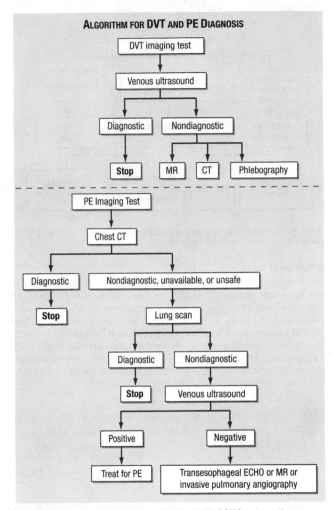

FIGURE 140-1 Imaging tests useful to diagnose DVT and PE. ECHO, echocardiogram.

cally an INR of 2–3. Pts vary widely in their required warfarin doses; dosing often begins at 5 mg/d, with adjustment based on the INR.

The most troublesome adverse event from anticoagulation treatment is hemorrhage. For severe hemorrhage while undergoing treatment with UFH or LMWH, protamine can be given to reverse anticoagulation. Severe bleeding while anticoagulated with warfarin can be treated with fresh frozen plasma or cryoprecipitate; milder hemorrhage or markedly elevated INR values can be treated with vitamin K. Warfarin should be avoided in pregnant pts.

The duration of anticoagulation for an initial DVT or PE is at least 3–6 months. Recurrent DVT or PE typically requires lifelong anticoagulation.

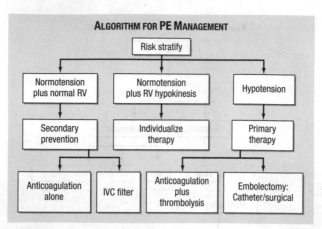

ALGORITHM FOR PE MANAGEMENT

Risk stratify

- Normotension plus normal RV
- Normotension plus RV hypokinesis
- Hypotension

- Secondary prevention
- Individualize therapy
- Primary therapy

- Anticoagulation alone
- IVC filter
- Anticoagulation plus thrombolysis
- Embolectomy: Catheter/surgical

FIGURE 140-2 Acute management of pulmonary thromboembolism: RV, right ventricular; IVC, inferior vena cava.

Other Treatment Modalities

Although anticoagulation is the mainstay of therapy for venous thromboembolism, additional therapeutic modalities also can be employed (Fig. 140-2). Inferior vena cava filters can be used if thrombosis recurs despite adequate anticoagulation. Fibrinolytic therapy (often with tissue plasminogen activator) should be considered for massive PE, although the risk of hemorrhage is significant. Surgical embolectomy also can be considered for massive PE.

If PE pts develop chronic thromboembolic pulmonary hypertension, surgical intervention (pulmonary thromboendarterectomy) can be performed.

For a more detailed discussion, see Goldhaber SZ: Deep Venous Thrombosis and Pulmonary Thromboembolism, Chap. 256, p. 1651, in HPIM-17.

141 Interstitial Lung Disease

Interstitial lung diseases (ILDs) are a group of >200 disease entities characterized by diffuse parenchymal abnormalities. ILDs can be classified into two major groups: (1) diseases associated with predominant inflammation and fibrosis, and (2) diseases with predominantly granulomatous reaction in interstitial or vascular areas (Table 141-1). ILDs are nonmalignant and noninfectious, and they are typically chronic. The differential diagnosis of ILDs often includes infections (e.g., atypical mycobacteria, fungi) and malignancy (e.g., bronchoalveolar cell carcinoma, lymphangitic carcinomatosis). One of the most common

TABLE 141-1	MAJOR CATEGORIES OF ALVEOLAR AND INTERSTITIAL INFLAMMATORY LUNG DISEASE

Lung Response: Alveolitis, Interstitial Inflammation, and Fibrosis

Known Cause

Asbestos	Radiation
Fumes, gases	Aspiration pneumonia
Drugs (antibiotics, amiodarone, gold) and chemotherapy drugs	Residual of adult respiratory distress syndrome

Unknown Cause

Idiopathic interstitial pneumonias	Pulmonary alveolar proteinosis
Idiopathic pulmonary fibrosis (usual interstitial pneumonia)	Lymphocytic infiltrative disorders (lymphocytic interstitial pneumonitis associated with connective tissue disease)
Desquamative interstitial pneumonia	
Respiratory bronchiolitis-associated interstitial lung disease	Eosinophilic pneumonias
Acute interstitial pneumonia (diffuse alveolar damage)	Lymphangioleiomyomatosis
	Amyloidosis
Cryptogenic organizing pneumonia (bronchiolitis obliterans with organizing pneumonia)	Inherited diseases
	Tuberous sclerosis, neurofibromatosis, Niemann-Pick disease, Gaucher's disease, Hermansky-Pudlak syndrome
Nonspecific interstitial pneumonia	
Connective tissue diseases	
Systemic lupus erythematosus, rheumatoid arthritis, ankylosing spondylitis, systemic sclerosis, Sjögren's syndrome, polymyositis-dermatomyositis	GI or liver diseases (Crohn's disease, primary biliary cirrhosis, chronic active hepatitis, ulcerative colitis)
	Graft-versus-host disease (bone marrow transplantation; solid organ transplantation)
Pulmonary hemorrhage syndromes	
Goodpasture's syndrome, idiopathic pulmonary hemosiderosis, isolated pulmonary capillaritis	

Lung Response: Granulomatous

Known Cause

Hypersensitivity pneumonitis (organic dusts)	Inorganic dusts: beryllium, silica

Unknown Cause

Sarcoidosis	Bronchocentric granulomatosis
Langerhans cell granulomatosis (eosinophilic granuloma of the lung)	Lymphomatoid granulomatosis
Granulomatous vasculitides	
Wegener's granulomatosis, allergic granulomatosis of Churg-Strauss	

ILDs associated with a granulomatous reaction, sarcoidosis, is discussed in Chap. 175. Many ILDs are of unknown etiology; however, some ILDs are known to be associated with specific environmental exposures including asbestos, radiation therapy, and organic dusts.

APPROACH TO THE PATIENT WITH INTERSTITIAL LUNG DISEASE

History

Common presenting symptoms for pts with ILDs include dyspnea and nonproductive cough. Symptom onset and duration can assist in the differential diagnosis. Chronic symptoms (over months to years) are typically seen in most ILDs, including idiopathic pulmonary fibrosis (IPF) and pulmonary Langerhans cell histiocytosis (PLCH or eosinophilic granuloma). Subacute symptoms (over weeks to months) can also be observed in most ILDs, especially in sarcoidosis, drug-induced ILDs, and alveolar hemorrhage syndromes. Acute presentations are uncommon for ILDs but are typically observed with acute interstitial pneumonia (AIP), and they can also occur with eosinophilic pneumonia and hypersensitivity pneumonitis. Sudden onset of dyspnea can indicate a pneumothorax, which occurs in PLCH and tuberous sclerosis/lymphangioleiomyomatosis. Episodic presentations also are unusual, but they are more typical for eosinophilic pneumonia, hypersensitivity pneumonitis, and cryptogenic organizing pneumonia [COP, also known as bronchiolitis obliterans with organizing pneumonia (BOOP)].

Age at presentation also can guide the differential diagnosis. IPF pts typically present at age >50, while PLCH, LAM, and connective tissue disease—related ILD often present between the ages of 20–40. LAM occurs exclusively in women, while ILD in rheumatoid arthritis (RA) typically occurs in men. Cigarette smoking is a risk factor for several ILDs including IPF, PLCH, Goodpasture's syndrome, and respiratory bronchiolitis. Occupational exposures can be important risk factors for many types of hypersensitivity pneumonitis as well as pneumoconioses. Medical treatment with radiation and drugs also should be assessed.

Physical Examination

Tachypnea and end-inspiratory crackles are commonly observed in inflammatory ILDs, but they are less frequent in granulomatous ILDs. Clubbing of the digits is observed in some pts with advanced ILD.

Laboratory Studies

Antinuclear antibodies and rheumatoid factor at low titers are observed in some IPF pts without a connective tissue disorder. Specific serum antibodies can confirm exposure to relevant antigens in hypersensitivity pneumonitis, but they do not prove causation.

Chest Imaging

Chest x-ray (CXR) does not typically provide a specific diagnosis but often raises the possibility of ILD by demonstrating a bibasilar reticular pattern. Upper-lung-zone predominance of nodular opacities is noted in several ILDs, including PLCH, sarcoidosis, and silicosis. High-resolution chest CT scans provide improved sensitivity for the early detection of ILDs and may be sufficiently specific to allow a diagnosis to be made in ILDs such as IPF, PLCH, and asbestosis. Honeycombing is indicative of advanced fibrosis.

Tissue and Cellular Examination

In order to provide a specific diagnosis and assess disease activity, lung biopsy is often required. Bronchoscopy with transbronchial biopsies can be diagnostic in some ILDs, including sarcoidosis. In addition, bronchoscopy can assist by excluding chronic infections or lymphangitic carcinomatosis. However, the more extensive tissue samples provided by open lung biopsies, often obtained by video-assisted thoracic surgery, are often required to establish a specific diagnosis. Evidence for diffuse end-stage disease, such as widespread honeycombing, or other major operative risks, are relative contraindications to lung biopsy procedures.

PRINCIPLES OF MANAGEMENT

If a causative agent can be identified (e.g., thermophilic actinomyces in hypersensitivity pneumonitis), cessation of exposure to that agent is imperative. Because the response to treatment among different ILDs is so variable, identification of treatable causes is essential. Glucocorticoids can be highly effective for eosinophilic pneumonias, COP, HP, radiation pneumonitis, and drug-induced ILD. Prednisone at 0.5–1.0 mg/kg qd is commonly given for 4–12 weeks, followed by a gradual tapering dose. On the other hand, glucocorticoids are typically not beneficial in IPF. Smoking cessation is essential, especially for smoking-related ILDs such as PLCH and respiratory bronchiolitis.

Supportive therapeutic measures include providing supplemental O_2 for pts with significant hypoxemia (Pa_{O_2} <55 mmHg at rest). Pulmonary rehabilitation may also be beneficial. For young pts with end-stage ILD, lung transplantation should be considered.

SELECTED INDIVIDUAL ILDS

Idiopathic Pulmonary Fibrosis   IPF, which is also known as usual interstitial pneumonia (UIP), is the most common idiopathic interstitial pneumonia. Cigarette smoking is a risk factor for IPF. Common respiratory symptoms include dyspnea and a nonproductive cough. Physical examination is notable for inspiratory crackles at the lung bases. Clubbing may occur. High-resolution chest CT scans show subpleural reticular opacities predominantly in the lower lung fields, which are associated with honeycombing in advanced disease. Pulmonary function tests reveal a restrictive ventilatory defect with reduced lung carbon monoxide diffusing capacity (DLCO). Surgical lung biopsy is usually required to confirm the diagnosis, although classic presentations may not require a biopsy. IPF can include acute exacerbations characterized by accelerated clinical deterioration over days to weeks. IPF is poorly responsive to available pharmacologic treatment.

ILD Associated with Connective Tissue Disorders   Pulmonary manifestations may precede systemic manifestations of a connective tissue disorder. In addition to direct pulmonary involvement, it is necessary to consider complications of therapy (e.g., opportunistic infections), respiratory muscle weakness, esophageal dysfunction, and associated malignancies as contributors to pulmonary parenchymal abnormalities in pts with connective tissue disorders.

Progressive systemic sclerosis (scleroderma) commonly includes ILD as well as pulmonary vascular disease. Lung involvement tends to be highly resistant to available treatment.

In addition to pulmonary fibrosis (ILD), RA can involve a range of pulmonary complications, including pleural effusions, pulmonary nodules, and pulmonary vasculitis. ILD in RA pts is more common in men.

Systemic lupus erythematosus (SLE) also can involve a range of pulmonary complications, including pleural effusions, pulmonary vascular disease, pulmonary hemorrhage, and BOOP. Chronic, progressive ILD is not commonly observed.

Cryptogenic Organizing Pneumonia   When the BOOP pathologic pattern occurs without another primary pulmonary disorder, the term *cryptogenic organizing pneumonia (COP)* is used. COP may present with a flu-like illness. Recurrent and migratory pulmonary opacities are common. Glucocorticoid therapy is often effective.

Pulmonary Alveolar Proteinosis   Pulmonary alveolar proteinosis (PAP) is a diffuse lung disease that involves the accumulation of lipoproteinaceous material in the distal airspaces, rather than a classic ILD. More common in males, PAP usually presents insidiously, with dyspnea, fatigue, weight loss, and low-grade fever. Whole lung lavage may be of therapeutic benefit.

Pulmonary Infiltrates with Eosinophilia   Several disorders are characterized by pulmonary infiltrates and peripheral blood eosinophilia. Tropical eosinophilia relates to parasitic infection; drug-induced eosinophilic pneumonias are more common in the United States. Loeffler's syndrome typically includes migratory pulmonary infiltrates and minimal clinical symptoms. Acute eosinophilic pneumonia involves pulmonary infiltrates with severe hypoxemia. Chronic eosinophilic pneumonia is often in the differential diagnosis with other ILDs; it includes fever, cough, and weight loss, with a CXR notable for peripheral infiltrates. Eosinophilic pneumonias tend to be rapidly responsive to glucocorticoid therapy.

Alveolar Hemorrhage Syndromes   A variety of diseases can cause diffuse alveolar hemorrhage, including systemic vasculitic syndromes (e.g., Wegener's granulomatosis), connective tissue diseases (e.g., SLE), and Goodpasture's syndrome. Although typically an acute process, recurrent episodes can lead to pulmonary fibrosis. Hemoptysis may not occur initially in one-third of cases. CXR typically shows patchy or diffuse alveolar opacities. The DLCO may be increased. High doses of IV methylprednisolone are typically required, followed by gradual tapering of systemic steroid doses. Plasmapheresis may be effective for Goodpasture's Syndrome.

Pulmonary Langerhans Cell Histiocytosis   PLCH is a smoking-related diffuse lung disease that typically affects men 20–40 years of age. Presenting symptoms often include cough, dyspnea, chest pain, weight loss, and fever. Pneumothorax occurs in 25% of pts. High-resolution chest CT scan reveals upper-zone-predominant nodular opacities and thin-walled cysts. Smoking cessation is the key therapeutic intervention.

Hypersensitivity Pneumonitis   HP is an inflammatory lung disorder caused by repeated inhalation of an organic agent in a susceptible individual. Many organic agents have been implicated. Clinical presentations can be acute, with cough, fever, and dyspnea developing within 6–8 h after exposure; subacute, with cough and dyspnea that can become progressively worse over weeks; and chronic, which can appear similar to IPF. Peripheral blood eosinophilia is not observed. Serum precipitins can be measured as an indicator of an environmental exposure. Although helpful in implicating specific agents, the presence of a specific serum precipitin is not diagnostic since many exposed individuals without HP will have such precipitins; false-negative results can also occur. Diagnosis is made based on symptoms, physical exam, pulmonary function tests, and radiographic studies that are consistent with HP; history of exposure to a recognized antigen; and presence of an antibody to that antigen. In some cases, lung biopsy (transbronchial or open lung) may be required to confirm the diagnosis. Treatment involves avoiding exposure to the causative antigen; systemic corticosteroids may be required in subacute or chronic HP.

> For a more detailed discussion, see King TE Jr: Interstitial Lung Diseases, Chap. 255 (p. 1643); Kline JN and Hunninghake GW: Hypersensitivity Pneumonitis and Pulmonary Infiltrates with Eosinophilia, Chap. 249 (p. 1607); in HPIM-17.

142 Diseases of the Pleura and Mediastinum

PLEURAL EFFUSION

Etiology and Diagnostic Approach   Pleural effusion is defined as excess fluid accumulation in the pleural space. It can result from increased pleural fluid formation in the lung interstitium, parietal pleura, or peritoneal cavity, or from decreased pleural fluid removal by the parietal pleural lymphatics.

The two major classes of pleural effusions are transudates, which are caused by systemic influences on pleural fluid formation or resorption, and exudates, which are caused by local influences on pleural fluid formation and resorption. Common causes of transudative effusions are left ventricular heart failure, cirrhosis, and nephrotic syndrome. Common causes of exudative effusions are pneumonia, malignancy, and pulmonary embolism. A more comprehensive list of the etiologies of transudative and exudative pleural effusions is provided in Table 142-1.

Exudates fulfill at least one of the following three criteria: high pleural fluid/serum protein ratio (>0.5), pleural fluid lactate dehydrogenase (LDH) greater than two-thirds of the laboratory normal upper limit for serum LDH, or pleural/serum LDH ratio >0.6. Transudative effusions typically do not meet any of these criteria. For exudative effusions, pleural fluid should also be tested for pH, glucose, white blood cell count with differential, microbiologic studies, cytology, and amylase. An algorithm for determining the etiology of a pleural effusion is presented in Fig. 142-1.

Despite full evaluation, no cause for the pleural effusion will be found in 25% of pts; many of these effusions are likely due to viral infections. A subset of the most common types of pleural effusions is described in the following sections.

Transudative Pleural Effusions   Transudative pleural effusions related to left ventricular failure are often bilateral; if unilateral, right-sided effusions are more common than left-sided effusions. Thoracentesis is not always required to confirm the transudative nature of the pleural effusions if congestive heart failure is present; however, if the effusions are not comparable in size, if the pt is febrile, or if pleuritic chest pain is present, thoracentesis should be strongly considered.

Parapneumonic Effusion/Empyema   Parapneumonic effusions are exudates that are associated with contiguous bacterial lung infections, including pneumo-

TABLE 142-1 DIFFERENTIAL DIAGNOSES OF PLEURAL EFFUSIONS

Transudative Pleural Effusions

1. Congestive heart failure	5. Peritoneal dialysis
2. Cirrhosis	6. Superior vena cava obstruction
3. Pulmonary embolization	7. Myxedema
4. Nephrotic syndrome	8. Urinothorax

Exudative Pleural Effusions

1. Neoplastic diseases	6. Post–coronary artery bypass surgery
a. Metastatic disease	7. Asbestos exposure
b. Mesothelioma	8. Sarcoidosis
2. Infectious diseases	9. Uremia
a. Bacterial infections	10. Meigs' syndrome
b. Tuberculosis	11. Yellow nail syndrome
c. Fungal infections	12. Drug-induced pleural disease
d. Viral infections	a. Nitrofurantoin
e. Parasitic infections	b. Dantrolene
3. Pulmonary embolization	c. Methysergide
4. Gastrointestinal disease	d. Bromocriptine
a. Esophageal perforation	e. Procarbazine
b. Pancreatic disease	f. Amiodarone
c. Intraabdominal abscesses	13. Trapped lung
d. Diaphragmatic hernia	14. Radiation therapy
e. After abdominal surgery	15. Post–cardiac injury syndrome
f. Endoscopic variceal sclerotherapy	16. Hemothorax
g. After liver transplant	17. Iatrogenic injury
5. Collagen-vascular diseases	18. Ovarian hyperstimulation syndrome
a. Rheumatoid pleuritis	19. Pericardial disease
b. Systemic lupus erythematosus	20. Chylothorax
c. Drug-induced lupus	
d. Immunoblastic lymphadenopathy	
e. Sjögren's syndrome	
f. Wegener's granulomatosis	
g. Churg-Strauss syndrome	

nia and lung abscess. In the setting of pulmonary infections, the presence of free pleural fluid can be demonstrated with a lateral decubitus x-ray, chest CT scan, or ultrasound. If the pleural fluid is grossly purulent, it is referred to as an empyema.

Tube thoracostomy (i.e., chest tube) for management of parapneumonic effusions is likely indicated if any of the following applies (in descending order of importance): (1) gross pus is present, (2) Gram's stain or culture of pleural fluid is positive, (3) pleural fluid glucose is <3.3 mmol/L (<60 mg/dL), (4) pleural pH is <7.20, or (5) there is loculated pleural fluid.

If chest tube drainage does not result in complete removal of pleural fluid, streptokinase (250,000 units) can be instilled through the tube, or thoracoscopy can be performed to lyse adhesions. If these approaches are not effective, surgical decortication may be required.

Malignant Pleural Effusions Metastatic cancer is a common cause of exudative pleural effusions. Tumors that frequently cause malignant effusions include lung cancer, breast cancer, and lymphoma. The pleural fluid glucose level may be markedly reduced. Cytologic examination of the pleural fluid is usually diagnostic. If cytologic examination of thoracentesis fluid is negative, thoracosco-

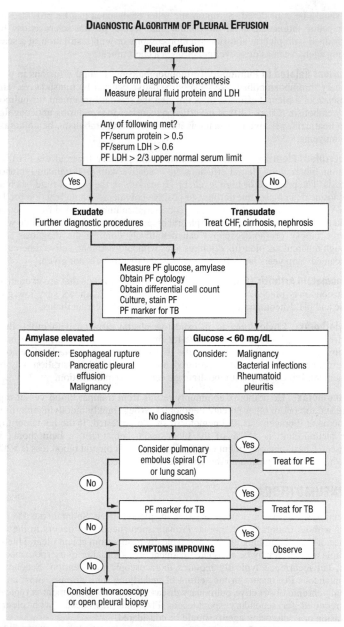

FIGURE 142-1 Approach to the diagnosis of pleural effusions. PF, pleural fluid; PE, pulmonary embolism; CHF, congestive heart failure; TB, tuberculosis; LDH, lactate dehydrogenase; CT, computed tomography.

py should be considered. Symptomatic relief of dyspnea can be provided by therapeutic thoracentesis. If the pleural fluid recurs, pleural sclerosis can be performed with pleural abrasion via thoracoscopy or with instillation of a sclerosing agent, such as doxycycline, through a chest tube.

Effusions Related to Pulmonary Thromboembolism Pleural effusions in pulmonary thromboembolism are usually exudative but can be transudative. The presence of a pleural effusion does not alter the standard treatment for pulmonary embolism (Chap. 140). If the effusion increases in size during anticoagulation treatment, possible explanations include recurrent embolism, hemothorax, or empyema.

Tuberculous Pleuritis Usually associated with primary tuberculosis (Tb) infection, tuberculous pleural effusions are exudative with predominant lymphocytosis. The presence of high levels of Tb markers in the pleural fluid, such as adenosine deaminase, interferon γ, or positive polymerase chain reaction for Tb DNA, can establish the diagnosis. Mycobacterial cultures obtained from pleural fluid (low positive culture rate) or pleural biopsy (high positive culture rate with needle biopsy or thoracoscopy) can definitively confirm the diagnosis. Although tuberculous pleuritis often resolves without treatment, active tuberculosis can develop years later if antimycobacterial treatment is not given.

Rheumatoid Arthritis (RA) RA can cause pleural effusions that are exudative. Effusions may precede articular symptoms. Pleural fluid shows very low glucose and pH. Rheumatoid pleural effusions are usually seen in males.

Chylothorax Chylothorax is an exudative pleural effusion with milky fluid and an elevated triglyceride level (>1.2 mmol/L or >110 mg/dL). The most common etiologies are trauma to the thoracic duct and mediastinal tumors. Chest tube placement is often required, and octreotide administration may be beneficial. Prolonged chest tube drainage can lead to malnutrition.

Hemothorax Hemothorax commonly results from trauma; blood vessel rupture and tumor are other potential etiologies. When frankly bloody pleural fluid is noted at thoracentesis, the hematocrit should be tested. If the hematocrit of the pleural fluid is >50% of the bloodstream hematocrit, a hemothorax is present. Chest tube placement is typically required. If pleural blood loss is >200 mL/h, thoracic surgical intervention should be pursued.

PNEUMOTHORAX

Pneumothorax (Ptx) is defined as gas in the pleural space. Spontaneous Ptx occurs without trauma to the thorax. Primary spontaneous Ptx occurs in the absence of underlying lung disease and typically results from apical pleural blebs. Simple aspiration may be adequate treatment for an initial primary spontaneous Ptx, but recurrence typically requires thoracoscopic intervention. Secondary spontaneous Ptx occurs in the setting of underlying lung disease, most commonly chronic obstructive pulmonary disease. Chest tube placement is typically required for secondary spontaneous Ptx, and pleurodesis (with pleural abrasion or a sclerosing agent) should be considered.

Traumatic Ptx usually requires chest tube placement. Iatrogenic Ptx can occur from transthoracic needle biopsy, thoracentesis, placement of a central venous catheter, or transbronchial biopsy. Treatment with O_2 or aspiration is often adequate for iatrogenic Ptx, but chest tube placement may be required. Tension Ptx can result from trauma or mechanical ventilation. Positive pleural pressure in mechanical ventilation can rapidly lead to a tension Ptx with reduced cardiac output. Urgent treatment is required, either with a chest tube or, if not immediately available, with a large-bore needle inserted into the pleural space through the second anterior intercostal space.

MEDIASTINAL DISEASE

Mediastinitis Mediastinitis can be an acute or chronic process. Acute mediastinitis can result from esophageal perforation or after cardiac surgery with median sternotomy. Esophageal perforation can occur spontaneously or iatrogenically; surgical exploration of the mediastinum, repair of the esophageal perforation, and drainage of the pleural space and mediastinum are required. Mediastinitis after median sternotomy typically presents with wound drainage and is diagnosed by mediastinal needle aspiration. Treatment requires drainage, debridement, and IV antibiotics.

Chronic mediastinitis can cause a spectrum of disease ranging from granulomatous inflammation of lymph nodes to fibrosing mediastinitis. Chronic mediastinitis is commonly caused by Tb and histoplasmosis; other etiologies are also possible, including sarcoidosis and silicosis. Granulomatous inflammation is usually asymptomatic. Fibrosing mediastinitis causes symptoms related to compression of mediastinal structures, such as the superior vena cava, esophagus, or large airways. Fibrosing mediastinitis is very difficult to treat.

Mediastinal Masses Different types of mediastinal masses are found in the anterior, middle, and posterior mediastinal compartments. The most common mass lesions in the anterior mediastinum are thymomas, lymphomas, teratomas, and thyroid lesions. In the middle mediastinum, vascular masses, enlarged lymph nodes (e.g., metastatic cancer or granulomatous disease), and bronchogenic or pleuropericardial cysts are found. Posterior mediastinal masses include neurogenic tumors, gastroenteric cysts, and esophageal diverticula.

CT scans are invaluable for evaluating mediastinal masses. Barium swallow studies can assist in evaluating posterior mediastinal masses. Biopsy procedures are typically required to diagnose mediastinal masses; needle biopsy procedures (e.g., percutaneous or bronchoscopy), mediastinoscopy, and thoracoscopy are potential options.

For a more detailed discussion, see Light RW: Disorders of the Pleura and Mediastinum, Chap. 257, p. 1658, in HPIM-17.

143 Disorders of Ventilation

ALVEOLAR HYPOVENTILATION

Exists when arterial P_{CO_2} increases above the normal 37–43 mmHg. In most clinically important chronic hypoventilation syndromes, Pa_{CO_2} is 50–80 mmHg.

TABLE 143-1	CHRONIC HYPOVENTILATION SYNDROMES	
Mechanism	**Site of Defect**	**Disorder**
Impaired respiratory drive	Peripheral and central chemoreceptors	Carotid body dysfunction, trauma
	Brainstem respiratory neurons	Prolonged hypoxia
		Metabolic alkalosis
		Bulbar poliomyelitis, encephalitis
		Brainstem infarction, hemorrhage, trauma
		Brainstem demyelination, degeneration
		Chronic drug administration
		Primary alveolar hypoventilation syndrome
Defective respiratory neuromuscular system	Spinal cord and peripheral nerves	High cervical trauma
		Poliomyelitis
		Motor neuron disease
	Respiratory muscles	Peripheral neuropathy
		Myasthenia gravis
		Muscular dystrophy
		Chronic myopathy
Impaired ventilatory apparatus	Chest wall	Kyphoscoliosis
		Fibrothorax
		Thoracoplasty
		Ankylosing spondylitis
		Obesity-hypoventilation
	Airways and lungs	Laryngeal and tracheal stenosis
		Obstructive sleep apnea
		Cystic fibrosis
		Chronic obstructive pulmonary disease

Source: EA Phillipson: HPIM-17, p. 1661.

Cause Alveolar hypoventilation is always (1) a defect in the metabolic respiratory control system, (2) a defect in the respiratory neuromuscular system, or (3) a defect in the ventilatory apparatus (Table 143-1).

Disorders associated with impaired respiratory drive, defects in respiratory neuromuscular system, and upper airway obstruction produce an increase in Pa_{CO_2}, despite normal lungs, because of a decrease in overall minute ventilation.

Disorders of chest wall, lower airways, and lungs produce an increase in Pa_{CO_2}, despite a normal or increased minute ventilation.

Increased Pa_{CO_2} leads to respiratory acidosis, compensatory increase in HCO_3^-, and decrease in Pa_{O_2}.

Hypoxemia may induce secondary polycythemia, pulmonary hypertension, right heart failure. Gas exchange worsens during sleep, resulting in morning headache, impaired sleep quality, fatigue, daytime somnolence, mental confusion.

HYPOVENTILATION SYNDROMES

Primary Alveolar Cause unknown; rare; thought to arise from defect in metabolic respiratory control system; key diagnostic finding is chronic respiratory acidosis without respiratory muscle weakness or impaired ventilatory mechanics. Some pts respond to respiratory stimulants and supplemental O_2.

Neuromuscular Several primary neuromuscular disorders produce chronic hypoventilation (Table 143-1). Hypoventilation usually develops gradually, but acute, superimposed respiratory loads (e.g., viral bronchitis with airways obstruction) may precipitate respiratory failure. Diaphragm weakness is a common feature, with orthopnea and paradoxical abdominal movement in supine posture. Testing reveals low maximum voluntary ventilation and reduced maximal inspiratory and expiratory pressures. Therapy involves treatment of underlying condition. Many pts benefit from mechanical ventilatory assistance at night (often through nasal mask) or the entire day (typically through tracheostomy).

Obesity-Hypoventilation Massive obesity imposes a mechanical load on the respiratory system. Small percentage of morbidly obese pts develop hypercapnia, hypoxemia, and ultimately polycythemia, pulmonary hypertension, and right heart failure. Most pts have mild to moderate airflow obstruction. Treatment includes weight loss, smoking cessation, and pharmacologic respiratory stimulants such as progesterone. Nocturnal mask ventilation may minimize nocturnal hypoxemia and treats coexisting sleep-disordered breathing.

HYPERVENTILATION

Increased ventilation, causing $Pa_{CO_2} < 37$ mmHg. Causes include lesions of the CNS, metabolic acidosis, anxiety, drugs (e.g., salicylates), hypoxemia, hypoglycemia, hepatic coma, and sepsis. Hyperventilation may also occur with some types of lung disease, particularly interstitial disease and pulmonary edema.

For a more detailed discussion, see Phillipson EA: Disorders of Ventilation, Chap. 258, p. 1661.

144 Sleep Apnea

By convention, apnea is defined as cessation of airflow for >10 s. Hypopnea is defined as reduction in airflow resulting in arousal from sleep or oxygen desaturation. Minimum number of apneic or hypopneic events per night for diagnosis is uncertain, but most pts have at least 10–15/h of sleep. Prevalence estimates vary depending on threshold for diagnosis (events/h) and on definition of hypopnea (degree of desaturation required), but conservative figures are 10% of working-age men and 4% of women.

Some pts have *central apnea* with transient loss of neural drive to respiratory muscles during sleep. Vast majority have primarily *obstructive apnea* with oc-

TABLE 144-1 MANAGEMENT OF OBSTRUCTIVE SLEEP APNEA (OSA)

Mechanism	Mild to Moderate OSA	Moderate to Severe OSA
↑ Upper airway muscle tone	Avoidance of alcohol, sedatives	
↑ Upper airway lumen size	Weight reduction Avoidance of supine posture Oral prosthesis	Uvulopalatopharyngoplasty
↓ Upper airway subatmospheric pressure	Improved nasal patency	Nasal continuous positive airway pressure
Bypass occlusion		Tracheostomy

Source: EA Phillipson: HPIM-16, p. 1575.

clusion in the upper airway. Snoring is frequent. Sleep plays a permissive role in collapse of upper airway. Alcohol and sedatives exacerbate the condition.

SYMPTOMS

These include snoring, excessive daytime sleepiness, memory loss, depression, and impotence. Sleepiness increases risk of automobile accidents. Nocturnal hypoxia, a consequence of apnea, may contribute to systemic hypertension, arrhythmias, and right ventricular hypertrophy.

Most pts have structural narrowing of upper airway. Obesity is frequent, but many pts have normal body habitus. Most pts have obstruction at nasal or palatal level. Mandibular deformities (retrognathia) also predispose.

DIAGNOSIS

This requires overnight observation of the pt. The definitive test for obstructive sleep apnea is overnight polysomnography, including sleep staging and respiratory monitoring.

R𝗑 Sleep Apnea (See Table 144-1)

Therapy is directed at increasing upper airway size, increasing upper airway tone, and minimizing upper airway collapsing pressures. Weight loss often reduces disease severity but infrequently obviates the need for other therapy. Majority of pts with severe sleep apnea require nasal continuous positive airway pressure (nasal C-PAP). Mandibular positioning device (dental) may treat pts with mild or moderate disease. Surgery (uvulopalatopharyngoplasty) is usually reserved for pts who fail other therapies.

For a more detailed discussion, see Douglas, NJ: Sleep Apnea, Chap. 259, p. 1665, in HPIM-17.

145 Approach to the Patient with Renal Disease

The approach to renal disease begins with recognition of particular syndromes on the basis of findings such as presence or absence of azotemia, proteinuria, hypertension, edema, abnormal urinalysis, electrolyte disorders, abnormal urine volumes, or infection (Table 145-1).

ACUTE RENAL FAILURE (See Chap. 146)

Clinical syndrome is characterized by a rapid, severe decrease in glomerular filtration rate (GFR) [rise in serum creatinine and blood urea nitrogen (BUN)], usually with reduced urine output. Extracellular fluid expansion leads to edema, hypertension, and occasionally acute pulmonary edema. Hyperkalemia, hyponatremia, and acidosis are common. Etiologies include ischemia; nephrotoxic injury due to drugs, toxins, or endogenous pigments; sepsis; severe renovascular disease; glomerulonephritis (GN); interstitial nephritis, particularly allergic interstitial nephritis due to medications; thrombotic microangiopathy; or conditions related to pregnancy. Prerenal and postrenal failure are potentially reversible causes.

Rapidly Progressive Glomerulonephritis Defined as a >50% reduction in renal function, occurring over weeks to months. Broadly classified into three major subtypes on the basis of renal biopsy findings and pathophysiology: (1) immune complex–associated, e.g., in systemic lupus erythematosus (SLE); (2) "pauci-immune," associated with antineutrophil cytoplasmic antibodies (ANCA) specific for myeloperoxidase or proteinase-3; and (3) associated with anti–glomerular basement (anti-GBM) antibodies, e.g., in Goodpasture's syndrome.

Pts are initially nonoliguric and may have recent flulike symptoms (myalgias, low-grade fevers, etc.); later, oliguric renal failure with uremic symptoms supervenes. Hypertension is common, particularly in poststreptococcal GN. Symptoms of associated disorders may be prominent, e.g., arthritis/arthralgias in SLE or vasculitis. Pulmonary manifestations in ANCA- and anti-GBM-associated rapidly progressive GN range from asymptomatic infiltrates to life-threatening pulmonary hemorrhage. Urinalysis typically shows hematuria, proteinuria, and red blood cell (RBC) casts; however, while highly specific for GN, RBC casts are not a particularly sensitive finding.

Acute Glomerulonephritis (See Chap. 150) Often called nephritic syndrome, classically caused by poststreptococcal GN. An acute illness with sudden onset of hematuria, edema, hypertension, oliguria, and elevated BUN and creatinine. Mild pulmonary congestion may be present. An antecedent or concurrent infection or multisystem disease may be causative, or glomerular disease may exist alone. Hematuria, proteinuria, and pyuria are usually present, and RBC casts confirm the diagnosis. Serum complement may be decreased in certain conditions.

TABLE 145-1 INITIAL CLINICAL AND LABORATORY DATABASE FOR DEFINING MAJOR SYNDROMES IN NEPHROLOGY

Syndromes	Important Clues to Diagnosis	Common Findings
Acute or rapidly progressive renal failure	Anuria Oliguria Documented recent decline in GFR	Hypertension, pulmonary edema, peripheral edema, hematuria, proteinuria, pyuria
Acute nephritis	Hematuria, RBC casts Azotemia, oliguria Edema, hypertension	Proteinuria Pyuria Circulatory congestion
Chronic renal failure	Azotemia for >3 months Symptoms or signs of uremia Shrunken, echogenic kidneys on ultrasound Anemia, hyperparathyroidism	Hematuria, proteinuria Edema, hypertension Hyperkalemia, acidosis, hypocalcemia, anemia
Nephrotic syndrome	Proteinuria >3.5 g per 1.73 m^2 per 24 h Hypoalbuminemia Hyperlipidemia Lipiduria	Edema
Asymptomatic urinary abnormalities	Hematuria Proteinuria (below nephrotic range) Sterile pyuria, casts	
Urinary tract infection	Bacteriuria >10^5 colonies per mL Other infectious agent documented in urine Pyuria, leukocyte casts Frequency, urgency Bladder tenderness, flank tenderness	Hematuria Mild azotemia Mild proteinuria Fever
Renal tubule defects	Electrolyte (Na$^+$, K$^+$, Mg^{2+}, phosphate, or Ca^{2+}) or solute (glucose, uric acid, amino acid) disorders Polyuria, nocturia Symptoms or signs of renal osteodystrophy Structurally abnormal kidneys, e.g., cysts	Hematuria "Tubular" proteinuria Enuresis Electrolyte or acid-base disorders
Hypertension	Systolic/diastolic hypertension	Moderate proteinuria Azotemia
Nephrolithiasis	Previous history of stone passage or removal Previous history of stone seen by x-ray Renal colic	Hematuria Pyuria Frequency, urgency
Urinary tract obstruction	Azotemia, oliguria, anuria Polyuria, nocturia, urinary retention Slowing of urinary stream Large prostate, large kidneys Flank tenderness, full bladder after voiding	Hematuria Pyuria Enuresis, dysuria

Note: GFR, glomerular filtration rate; RBC, red blood cell.
Source: Modified from FL Coe, BM Brenner: HPIM-14.

CHRONIC RENAL FAILURE   (See Chap. 147)

Progressive permanent loss of renal function over months to years does not cause symptoms of uremia until GFR is reduced to about 10–15% of normal. Hypertension may occur early. Later, manifestations include anorexia, nausea, vomiting, dysgeusia, insomnia, weight loss, weakness, paresthesia, bleeding, serositis, anemia, acidosis, hypocalcemia, hyperphosphatemia, and hyperkalemia. Common causes include diabetes mellitus, severe hypertension, glomerular disease, urinary tract obstruction, vascular disease, polycystic kidney disease, and interstitial nephritis. Indications of chronicity include longstanding azotemia, anemia, hyperphosphatemia, hypocalcemia, shrunken kidneys, renal osteodystrophy by x-ray, or findings on renal biopsy (extensive glomerular sclerosis, arteriosclerosis, and/or tubulointerstitial fibrosis).

NEPHROTIC SYNDROME   (See Chap. 150)

Defined as heavy albuminuria (>3.5 g/d in the adult) with or without edema, hypoalbuminemia, hyperlipidemia, and varying degrees of renal insufficiency. Can be idiopathic or due to drugs, infections, neoplasms, or multisystem or hereditary diseases. Complications include severe edema, thromboembolic events, infection, and protein malnutrition.

ASYMPTOMATIC URINARY ABNORMALITIES

Hematuria may be due to neoplasms, stones, infection at any level of the urinary tract, sickle cell disease, or analgesic abuse. Renal parenchymal causes are suggested by RBC casts, proteinuria, and/or dysmorphic RBCs in urine. Pattern of gross hematuria may be helpful in localizing site. Hematuria with minimal or low-grade proteinuria is most commonly due to thin basement membrane nephropathy or IgA nephropathy. Modest *proteinuria* may be an isolated finding due to fever, exertion, congestive heart failure (CHF), or upright posture; renal causes include early stages of diabetes nephropathy, amyloidosis, or other causes of glomerular disease. *Pyuria* can be caused by urinary tract infection (UTI), interstitial nephritis, GN, or renal transplant rejection. "Sterile" pyuria is associated with UTI treated with antibiotics, glucocorticoid therapy, acute febrile episodes, cyclophosphamide therapy, pregnancy, renal transplant rejection, genitourinary trauma, prostatitis, cystourethritis, tuberculosis and other mycobacterial infections, fungal infection, *Haemophilus influenzae*, anaerobic infection, fastidious bacteria, and bacterial L forms.

URINARY TRACT INFECTION   (See Chap. 152)

Generally defined as >10^5 bacteria per mL of urine. Levels between 10^2 and 10^5/mL may indicate infection but are usually due to poor sample collection, especially if mixed flora are present. Adults at risk are sexually active women or anyone with urinary tract obstruction, vesicoureteral reflux, bladder catheterization, neurogenic bladder (associated with diabetes mellitus), or primary neurologic diseases. Prostatitis, urethritis, and vaginitis may be distinguished by quantitative urine culture. Flank pain, nausea, vomiting, fever, and chills indicate kidney infection, i.e., pyelonephritis. UTI is a common cause of sepsis, especially in the elderly and institutionalized.

RENAL TUBULAR DEFECTS   (See Chap. 151)

Generally inherited, these include anatomic defects (polycystic kidneys, medullary cystic disease, medullary sponge kidney) detected in the evaluation of hematuria, flank pain, infection, or renal failure of unknown cause. Isolated or generalized defects of renal tubular salt, solute, acid, and water transport can also occur. The Fanconi syndrome is characterized by multiple defects in proximal tubular solute transport; cardinal features include generalized aminoaciduria, glycosuria with a normal serum glucose, and phosphaturia. The Fanconi syndrome can also encompass a proximal renal tubular acidosis, hypouricemia, hypokalemia, polyuria, hypovitaminosis D and hypocalcemia, and low-molecular-weight proteinuria. This syndrome can be hereditary (e.g., in Dent's disease and cystinosis) or acquired, the latter due to drugs (ifosfamide, tenofovir, valproic acid), toxins (aristolochic acid), heavy metals, multiple myeloma, or amyloidosis. Hereditary hypokalemic alkalosis is typically caused by defects in ion transport by the thick ascending limb (Bartter's syndrome) and the distal convoluted tubule (Gitelman's syndrome); similar acquired defects can occur after exposure to aminoglycosides or cisplatin. Nephrogenic diabetes insipidus and renal tubular acidosis are caused by defects in distal tubular water and acid transport, respectively; these also have both hereditary and acquired forms.

HYPERTENSION   (See Chap. 124)

Blood pressure >140/90 mmHg affects 20% of the U.S. adult population; when inadequately controlled, it is an important cause of cerebrovascular accident, myocardial infarction, and CHF and can contribute to the development of renal failure. Hypertension is usually asymptomatic until cardiac, renal, or neurologic symptoms appear; retinopathy or left ventricular hypertrophy (S4 heart sound, electrocardiographic or echocardiographic evidence) may be the only clinical sequelae. In most cases hypertension is idiopathic and becomes evident between ages 25 and 45. Secondary hypertension is generally suggested by the following clinical scenarios: (1) severe or refractory hypertension, (2) a sudden increase in blood pressure over prior values, (3) onset prior to puberty, or (4) age <30 in a nonobese, non-African-American patient with a negative family history. Clinical clues may suggest specific causes. Hypokalemia suggests renovascular hypertension or primary hyperaldosteronism; paroxysmal hypertension with headache, diaphoresis, and palpitations can occur in pheochromocytoma.

NEPHROLITHIASIS   (See Chap. 154)

Causes colicky pain, UTI, hematuria, dysuria, or unexplained pyuria. Stones may be found on routine x-ray of kidneys, ureter, and bladder (KUB); however, noncontrast helical CT, with 5-mm CT cuts, will pick up stones not detected by KUB x-ray and will furthermore assess for the presence of obstruction. Most are radiopaque Ca stones and are associated with high levels of urinary Ca, and/or oxalate excretion, and/or low levels of urinary citrate excretion. Staghorn calculi are large, branching, radiopaque stones within the renal pelvis due to recurrent infection. Uric acid stones are radiolucent. Urinalysis may reveal hematuria, pyuria, or pathologic crystals.

URINARY TRACT OBSTRUCTION   (See Chap. 155)

Causes variable symptoms depending on the underlying etiology and whether obstruction is acute or chronic, unilateral or bilateral, complete or partial. It is an important, reversible cause of unexplained renal failure. Upper tract obstruction may be silent or produce flank pain, hematuria, and renal infection. Bladder symptoms or prostatism may be present in lower tract obstruction. Functional consequences include polyuria, anuria, nocturia, acidosis, hyperkalemia, and hypertension. A flank or suprapubic mass may be found on physical exam; an obstructed, enlarged bladder is typically dull to percussion.

For a more detailed discussion, see Part 12: Disorders of the Kidney and Urinary Tract, p. 1741, in HPIM-17; and Coe FL, Brenner BM: Approach to the Patient with Disease of the Kidneys and Urinary Tract, p. 1495, in HPIM-14.

146 Acute Renal Failure

DEFINITION

Acute renal failure (ARF) or acute kidney injury (AKI), defined as a measurable increase in the serum creatinine (Cr) concentration [usually relative increase of 50% or absolute increase by 44–88 μmol/L (0.5–1.0 mg/dL)], occurs in ~5–7% of hospitalized pts. It is associated with a substantial increase in in-hospital mortality and morbidity. ARF can be anticipated in some clinical circumstances (e.g., after radiocontrast exposure or major surgery), and there are no specific pharmacologic therapies proven helpful at preventing or reversing the condition. Maintaining optimal renal perfusion and intravascular volume appears to be important in most clinical circumstances; important cofactors in ARF include hypovolemia and drugs that interfere with renal perfusion and/or glomerular filtration [nonsteroidal anti-inflammatory drugs (NSAIDs), angiotensin-converting enzyme (ACE) inhibitors, and angiotensin receptor blockers].

DIFFERENTIAL DIAGNOSIS

The separation into three broad categories (prerenal, intrinsic renal, and postrenal failure) is of considerable clinical utility (Table 146-1). *Prerenal failure* is most common among hospitalized pts. It may result from true volume depletion (e.g., diarrhea, vomiting, GI or other hemorrhage) or "effective circulatory volume" depletion, i.e., reduced renal perfusion in the setting of adequate or excess blood volume. Reduced renal perfusion may be seen in congestive heart failure (CHF) (due to reduced cardiac output and/or potent vasodilator therapy), hepatic cirrhosis (due most likely to peripheral vasodilation and arteriovenous shunting), nephrotic syndrome and other states of severe hypoproteinemia [total serum protein <54 g/L (<5.4 g/dL)], and renovascular disease (because of fixed stenosis at the level of the main renal artery or large branch vessels). Several drugs can reduce renal perfusion, most notably NSAIDs. ACE inhibitors and angiotensin II receptor antagonists may reduce glomerular filtration rate but do not tend to reduce renal perfusion.

Causes of *intrinsic renal failure* depend on the clinical setting. Among hospitalized patients, especially on surgical services or in intensive care units, acute tubular necrosis (ATN) is the most common diagnosis. A well-defined ischemic event or toxic exposure (e.g., aminoglycoside therapy) may lead to in-hospital ATN. Alternatively, patients may be admitted to the hospital with ATN associated with rhabdomyolysis; common predisposing factors include alcoholism, hypokalemia, and various drugs (e.g., statins). Allergic interstitial nephritis, usually due to antibiotics (e.g., penicillins, cephalosporins, sulfa drugs, quinolones, and rifampin), or NSAIDs, may also be responsible. Radiographic contrast dyes may cause ARF in patients with pre-existing kidney disease; the risk is substantially

TABLE 146-1 COMMON CAUSES OF ACUTE RENAL FAILURE

Prerenal

Volume depletion
    Blood loss
    GI fluid loss (e.g., vomiting, diarrhea)
    Overzealous diuretic use
Volume overload with reduced renal perfusion
    Congestive heart failure
        Low-output with systolic dysfunction
        "High-output" (e.g., anemia, thyrotoxicosis)
    Hepatic cirrhosis
    Severe hypoproteinemia
Renovascular disease
Drugs
    NSAIDs, cyclosporine, amphotericin B, ACE inhibitors, ARBs
Other
    Hypercalcemia, "third spacing" (e.g., pancreatitis, systemic inflammatory response), hepatorenal syndrome

Intrinsic

Acute tubular necrosis (ATN)
    Hypotension or shock, prolonged prerenal azotemia, postoperative sepsis syndrome, rhabdomyolysis, hemolysis, drugs
    Radiocontrast, aminoglycosides, cisplatin
Other tubulointerstitial disease
    Allergic interstitial nephritis
    Pyelonephritis (bilateral, or unilateral in single functional kidney)
    Heavy metal poisoning
Atheroembolic disease—after vascular procedures, thrombolysis, or anticoagulation
Glomerulonephritis
    (1) ANCA-associated: Wegener's granulomatosis, idiopathic pauci-immune GN, PAN
    (2) Anti-GBM disease; isolated or with pulmonary involvement (Goodpasture's syndrome)
    (3) Immune complex–mediated
    Subacute bacterial endocarditis, SLE, cryoglobulinemia (with or without hepatitis C infection), postinfectious GN (classically poststreptococcal)
IgA nephropathy and Henoch-Schönlein purpura
Glomerular endotheliopathies
Thrombotic microangiopathy, malignant hypertension, scleroderma, antiphospholipid syndrome, preeclampsia

Postrenal (Urinary Tract Obstruction)

Bladder neck obstruction, bladder calculi
Prostatic hypertrophy
Ureteral obstruction due to compression
    Pelvic or abdominal malignancy, retroperitoneal fibrosis
Nephrolithiasis
Papillary necrosis with obstruction

Note: NSAIDs, nonsteroidal anti-inflammatory drugs; ACE, angiotensin-converting enzyme; ARBs, angiotensin receptor blockers; ANCA, antineutrophil cytoplasmic antibody; GN, glomerulonephritis; PAN, polyarteritis nodosa; GBM, glomerular basement membrane; SLE, systemic lupus erythematosus.

higher in diabetics with chronic kidney disease. Coronary angiography, other vascular procedures, thrombolysis, or anticoagulation may lead to atheroemboli, which cause ARF due to both hemodynamic and inflammatory effects; livedo reticularis, embolic phenomena with preserved peripheral pulses, and eosinophilia are important clues to this diagnosis. Acute glomerulonephritis (Chap. 150) and thrombotic microangiopathies (Chap. 153) may also cause ARF. Thrombotic microangiopathies can be clinically subdivided into renal-limited forms [e.g., *E. coli*–associated hemolytic uremic syndrome (HUS)] and systemic forms [e.g., thrombotic thrombocytopenic purpura (TTP)]. A variety of drugs can cause thrombotic microangiopathies, including calcineurin inhibitors (cyclosporine and tacrolimus), quinine, antiplatelet agents (e.g., ticlopidine), and chemotherapeutics (e.g., mitomycin C and gemcitabine). Important associated disorders include HIV infection, bone marrow transplantation, systemic lupus erythematosus (SLE), and antiphospholipid syndrome.

Postrenal failure is due to urinary tract obstruction, which is also more common among ambulatory rather than hospitalized pts. More common in men than women, it is most often caused by ureteral or urethral blockade. Occasionally, stones, sloughed renal papillae, or malignancy (primary or metastatic) may cause more proximal obstruction.

CHARACTERISTIC FINDINGS AND DIAGNOSTIC WORKUP

All pts with ARF manifest some degree of azotemia [increased blood urea nitrogen (BUN) and Cr]. Other clinical features depend on the etiology of renal disease. Pts with *prerenal azotemia* due to volume depletion usually demonstrate orthostatic hypotension, tachycardia, low jugular venous pressure, and dry mucous membranes. Pts with prerenal azotemia and CHF may show jugular venous distention, an S_3 gallop, and peripheral and pulmonary edema. Therefore, the physical exam is critical in the workup of pts with prerenal ARF. In general, the BUN/Cr ratio tends to be high (>20:1), more so with volume depletion and CHF than with cirrhosis. The uric acid may also be disproportionately elevated in noncirrhotic prerenal states (due to increased proximal tubular absorption). Urine chemistries tend to show low urine [Na^+] (<10–20 mmol/L, <10 with hepatorenal syndrome) and a fractional excretion of sodium (FE_{Na}) of <1% (Table 146-2). The urinalysis (UA) typically shows hyaline and a few granular casts, without cells or cellular casts. Renal ultrasonography is usually normal.

Pts with *intrinsic renal disease* present with varying complaints. Glomerulonephritis (GN) is often accompanied by hypertension and mild to moderate edema (associated with Na retention and proteinuria, and sometimes with hematuria). An antecedent prodromal illness and/or prominent extrarenal symptoms and signs may occur if GN occurs in the context of a systemic illness, e.g., vasculitis or SLE; these may include hemoptysis or pulmonary hemorrhage (vasculitis and Goodpasture's syndrome), arthralgias/arthritis (vasculitis or SLE), serositis (SLE), and unexplained sinusitis (vasculitis). The urine chemistries may be indistinguishable from those in pts with prerenal failure; in fact, some pts with GN have renal hypoperfusion (due to glomerular inflammation and ischemia) with resultant hyperreninemia leading to acute volume expansion and hypertension. The urine sediment can be very helpful in these cases. Red blood cell (RBC), white blood cell (WBC), and cellular casts are characteristic of GN; RBC casts are rarely seen in other conditions (i.e., they are highly specific). In the setting of inflammatory nephritis (GN or interstitial nephritis, see below), there may be increased renal echogenicity on ultrasonography. Unlike pts with GN, pts with interstitial diseases are less likely to have hypertension or proteinuria; a notable exception is NSAID-associated acute interstitial nephri-

TABLE 146-2 URINE DIAGNOSTIC INDICES IN DIFFERENTIATION OF PRERENAL VERSUS INTRINSIC RENAL AZOTEMIA

Diagnostic Index	Typical Findings	
	Prerenal Azotemia	Intrinsic Renal Azotemia
Fractional excretion of sodium (%)[a] $U_{Na} \times P_{Cr}/P_{Na} \times U_{Cr} \times 100$	<1	>1
Urine sodium concentration (mmol/L)	<10	>20
Urine creatinine to plasma creatinine ratio	>40	>20
Urine urea nitrogen to plasma urea nitrogen ratio	>8	<3
Urine specific gravity	>1.018	<1.015
Urine osmolality (mosmol/kg H_2O)	>500	<300
Plasma BUN/creatinine ratio	>20	<10–15
Renal failure index $U_{Na}/U_{Cr}/P_{Cr}$	<1	>1
Urinary sediment	Hyaline casts	Muddy brown granular casts

[a]Most sensitive indices.
Note: U_{Na}, urine sodium concentration; P_{Cr}, plasma creatinine concentration; P_{Na}, plasma sodium concentration; U_{Cr}, urine creatinine concentration; BUN, blood urea nitrogen.

tis, which can be accompanied by proteinuria due to an associated minimal-change glomerular lesion. Hematuria and pyuria may present on UA; the classic sediment finding in allergic interstitial nephritis is a predominance (>10%) of urinary eosinophils with Wright's or Hansel's stain. WBC casts may also be seen, particularly in cases of pyelonephritis.

The UA of patients with ischemic or toxic ATN will characteristically contain pigmented "muddy-brown" granular casts and casts containing tubular epithelial cells. The FE_{Na} is typically >1% in ATN but may be <1% in patients with milder, nonoliguric ATN (e.g., from rhabdomyolysis) and in patients with underlying "prerenal" disorders such as CHF or cirrhosis.

Pts with *postrenal ARF* due to urinary tract obstruction are usually less severely ill than pts with prerenal or intrinsic renal disease, and their presentation may be delayed until azotemia is markedly advanced [BUN >54 μmol/L (150 mg/dL), Cr >1060–1325 μmol/L (12–15 mg/dL)]. An associated impairment of urinary concentrating ability often "protects" the pt from complications of volume overload. Urinary electrolytes typically show a FE_{Na} >1%, and microscopic examination of the urinary sediment is usually bland. Ultrasonography is the key diagnostic tool. More than 90% of pts with postrenal ARF show obstruction of the urinary collection system on ultrasound (e.g., dilated ureter, calyces); false negatives include hyperacute obstruction and encasement of the ureter and/or kidney by tumor, functionally obstructing urinary outflow without structural dilation.

℞ **Acute Renal Failure**

Treatment should focus on providing etiology-specific supportive care. For example, pts with prerenal failure due to GI fluid loss may experience relatively rapid correction of ARF after the administration of IV fluid to expand volume. The same treatment in prerenal pts with CHF would be counterproductive; in this case, treatment of the underlying disease with vasodilators and/or inotropic agents would more likely be of benefit.

There are relatively few intrinsic renal causes of ARF for which there is safe and effective therapy. GN associated with vasculitis or SLE may respond to high-dose glucocorticoids and cytotoxic agents (e.g., cyclophosphamide); plasmapheresis and plasma exchange may be useful in other selected circumstances (e.g., Goodpasture's syndrome and HUS/TTP, respectively). Antibiotic therapy may be sufficient for the treatment of ARF associated with pyelonephritis or endocarditis. There are conflicting data regarding the utility of glucocorticoids in allergic interstitial nephritis. Many practitioners advocate their use with clinical evidence of progressive renal insufficiency despite discontinuation of the offending drug, or with biopsy evidence of potentially reversible, severe disease.

The treatment of urinary tract obstruction often involves consultation with a urologist. Interventions as simple as Foley catheter placement or as complicated as multiple ureteral stents and/or nephrostomy tubes may be required.

DIALYSIS FOR ARF AND RECOVERY OF RENAL FUNCTION

Most cases of community- and hospital-acquired ARF resolve with conservative supportive measures, time, and patience. If nonprerenal ARF continues to progress, dialysis must be considered. The traditional indications for dialysis—volume overload refractory to diuretic agents; hyperkalemia; encephalopathy not otherwise explained; pericarditis, pleuritis, or other inflammatory serositis; and severe metabolic acidosis, compromising respiratory or circulatory function—can seriously compromise recovery from acute nonrenal illness. Therefore, dialysis should generally be provided in advance of these complications. The inability to provide requisite fluids for antibiotics, inotropes and other drugs, and/or nutrition should also be considered an indication for dialysis.

Dialytic options for ARF include (1) intermittent hemodialysis (IHD), (2) peritoneal dialysis (PD), and (3) continuous renal replacement therapy (CRRT, i.e., continuous arteriovenous or venovenous hemodiafiltration). Most pts are treated with IHD. It is unknown whether conventional thrice-weekly hemodialysis is sufficient or more frequent treatments are required. Few centers rely on PD for management of ARF (risks include infection associated with intraperitoneal catheter insertion and respiratory compromise due to abdominal distention). At some centers, CRRT is prescribed only in pts intolerant of IHD, usually because of hypotension; other centers use it as the modality of choice for pts in intensive care units. Hybrid hemodialysis techniques, such as slow low-efficiency dialysis (SLED), may be used in centers less familiar with CRRT.

For a more detailed discussion, see Liu KD, Chertow GM: Acute Renal Failure, Chap. 273, p. 1752, in HPIM-17.

147 Chronic Kidney Disease and Uremia

EPIDEMIOLOGY

The prevalence of chronic kidney disease (CKD), generally defined as a long-standing, irreversible impairment of kidney function, is substantially greater than the number of pts with end-stage renal disease (ESRD), now ≥300,000 in the United States. There is a spectrum of disease related to decrements in renal function; clinical and therapeutic issues differ greatly depending on whether the glomerular filtration rate (GFR) reduction is moderate (stage 3 CKD, 30–59 mL/min per 1.73 m^2) (Table 58-1), severe (stage 4 CKD, 15–29 mL/min per 1.73 m^2), or "end-stage renal disease" (stage 5 CKD, <15 mL/min per 1.73 m^2). Dialysis is usually required to control symptoms of uremia with GFR < 10 mL/min per 1.73 m^2. Common causes of CKD are outlined in Table 147-1.

DIFFERENTIAL DIAGNOSIS

The first step in the differential diagnosis of CKD is establishing its chronicity, i.e., disproving a major acute component. The two most common means of determining disease chronicity are the history and prior laboratory data (if available) and the renal ultrasound, which is used to measure kidney size. In general, kidneys that have shrunk (<10–11.5 cm, depending on body size) are more likely affected by chronic disease. While reasonably specific (few false positives), reduced kidney size is only a moderately sensitive marker for CKD, i.e., there are several relatively common conditions in which kidney disease may be chronic without any reduction in renal size. Diabetic nephropathy, HIV-associated nephropathy, and infiltrative diseases such as multiple myeloma may in fact be associated with relatively large kidneys despite chronicity. Renal biopsy, although rarely performed in patients with CKD, is a more reliable means of proving chronicity; a predominance of glomerulosclerosis or interstitial fibrosis argues strongly for chronic disease. Hyperphosphatemia and other metabolic derangements are not reliable indicators in distinguishing acute from chronic disease.

Once chronicity has been established, clues from the physical exam, laboratory panel, and urine sediment evaluation can be used to determine etiology. A detailed Hx will identify important comorbid conditions, such as diabetes, HIV

TABLE 147-1   COMMON CAUSES OF CHRONIC RENAL FAILURE

Diabetic nephropathy
Hypertensive nephrosclerosis[a]
Glomerulonephritis
Renovascular disease (ischemic nephropathy)
Polycystic kidney disease
Reflux nephropathy and other congenital renal diseases
Interstitial nephritis, including analgesic nephropathy
HIV-associated nephropathy
Transplant allograft failure ("chronic rejection")

---

[a]Often diagnosis of exclusion; very few pts undergo renal biopsy; may be occult renal disease with hypertension.

seropositivity, or peripheral vascular disease. The family Hx is paramount in the workup of autosomal dominant polycystic kidney disease or hereditary nephritis (Alport's syndrome). An occupational Hx may reveal exposure to environmental toxins or culprit drugs (including over-the-counter agents, such as analgesics or Chinese herbs).

Physical exam may demonstrate abdominal masses (i.e., polycystic kidneys), diminished pulses or femoral/carotid bruits (i.e., atherosclerotic peripheral vascular disease), or an abdominal bruit (i.e., renovascular disease). The Hx and exam may also yield important data regarding severity of disease. The presence of foreshortened fingers (due to resorption of the distal phalangeal tufts) and/or subcutaneous nodules may be seen with advanced CKD and secondary hyperparathyroidism. Excoriations (uremic pruritus), pallor (anemia), muscle wasting, and a nitrogenous fetor are all signs of advanced CKD, as are pericarditis, pleuritis, and asterixis, complications of particular concern that usually prompt the initiation of dialysis.

Laboratory Findings   Serum and urine laboratory findings typically provide additional information useful in determining the etiology and severity of CKD. Heavy proteinuria (>3.5 g/d), hypoalbuminemia, hypercholesterolemia, and edema suggest nephrotic syndrome (Chap. 150). Diabetic nephropathy, membranous nephropathy, focal segmental glomerulosclerosis, minimal change disease, amyloid, and HIV-associated nephropathy are principal causes. Proteinuria may decrease slightly with decreasing GFR but rarely to normal levels. Hyperkalemia and metabolic acidosis may complicate all forms of CKD eventually but can be more prominent in pts with interstitial renal diseases.

THE UREMIC SYNDROME

The culprit toxin(s) responsible for the uremic syndrome remain elusive. The serum creatinine (Cr) is the most common laboratory surrogate of renal function. GFR can be estimated using serum Cr–based equations derived from the Modification of Diet in Renal Disease Study. This "eGFR" is now reported with serum Cr by most clinical laboratories in the United States and is the basis for the National Kidney Foundation classification of chronic kidney disease (Table 58-1).

Uremic symptoms tend to develop with serum Cr > 530–710 μmol/L (> 6–8 mg/dL) or Cr_{Cl} < 10 mL/min, although these values vary widely. Uremia is thus a clinical diagnosis made in patients with CKD. Symptoms of advanced uremia include anorexia, weight loss, dyspnea, fatigue, pruritus, sleep and taste disturbance, and confusion and other forms of encephalopathy. Key findings on physical exam include hypertension, jugular venous distention, pericardial and/or pleural friction rub, muscle wasting, asterixis, excoriations, and ecchymoses. Laboratory abnormalities may include hyperkalemia, hyperphosphatemia, metabolic acidosis, hypocalcemia, hyperuricemia, anemia, and hypoalbuminemia. Most of these abnormalities eventually resolve with initiation of dialysis or renal transplantation (Chaps. 148 and 149) or with appropriate drug therapies (see below).

Rx Chronic Kidney Disease and Uremia

Hypertension complicates many forms of CKD and warrants aggressive treatment to reduce the risk of stroke and potentially to slow the progression of CKD (see below). Volume overload contributes to hypertension in many cases, and potent diuretic agents are frequently required. Anemia can be reversed with recombinant human erythropoietin (rHuEPO); 2000–6000 units SC once or twice weekly can increase Hb concentrations toward the normal range in most pts. Iron deficiency and/or other causes of anemia can reduce the response to rHuEPO and should be investigated if present. Iron supplementation is often required; many patients require parenteral iron therapy.

Hyperphosphatemia can be controlled with judicious restriction of dietary phosphorus and the use of postprandial phosphate binders, either calcium-based salts (calcium carbonate or acetate) or nonabsorbed agents (e.g., sevelamer). Hyperkalemia should be controlled with dietary potassium restriction. Sodium polystyrene sulfonate (Kayexalate) can be used in refractory cases, although dialysis should be considered if the potassium is >6 mmol/L on repeated occasions. If these conditions cannot be conservatively controlled, dialysis should be instituted (Chap. 148). It is also advisable to begin dialysis if severe anorexia, weight loss, and/or hypoalbuminemia develop, as it has been definitively shown that outcomes for dialysis pts with malnutrition are particularly poor.

SLOWING PROGRESSION OF RENAL DISEASE

Prospective clinical trials have explored the roles of blood pressure control and dietary protein restriction on the rate of progression of renal failure. Control of hypertension is of benefit, although angiotensin-converting enzyme (ACE) inhibitors and angiotensin receptor blockers (ARBs) may exert unique beneficial effects, most likely due to their effects on intrarenal hemodynamics. The effects of ACE inhibitors and ARBs are most pronounced in pts with diabetic nephropathy and in those without diabetes but with significant proteinuria (>1 g/d). Diuretics and other antihypertensive agents are often required, in addition to ACE inhibitors and ARBs, to optimize hypertension control and attenuate disease progression; diuretics may also help control serum $[K^+]$. Dietary protein restriction may offer an additional benefit, particularly in these same subgroups.

For a more detailed discussion, see Bargman JM, Skorecki K: Chronic Kidney Disease, Chap. 274, p. 1761, in HPIM-17.

148 Dialysis

OVERVIEW

Initiation of dialysis usually depends on a combination of the pt's symptoms, comorbid conditions, and laboratory parameters. Unless a living donor is identified, transplantation is deferred by necessity, due to the scarcity of cadaveric donor organs (median waiting time, 3–6 years at most transplant centers). Dialytic options include hemodialysis and peritoneal dialysis (PD). Roughly 85% of U.S. pts are started on hemodialysis.

Absolute indications for dialysis include severe volume overload refractory to diuretic agents, severe hyperkalemia and/or acidosis, encephalopathy not otherwise explained, and pericarditis or other serositis. Additional indications for dialysis include symptomatic uremia (Chap. 147) (e.g., intractable fatigue, anorexia, dysgeusia, nausea, vomiting, pruritus, difficulty maintaining attention and concentration) and protein-energy malnutrition/failure to thrive without other overt cause. No absolute serum creatinine, blood urea nitrogen, creatinine or urea clearance, or glomerular filtration rate (GFR) is used as an absolute cutoff for requiring dialysis, although most individuals experience, or will soon develop, symptoms and complications when the GFR is below ~10 mL/min.

HEMODIALYSIS

This requires direct access to the circulation, either via a native arteriovenous fistula (the preferred method of vascular access), usually at the wrist (a "Brescia-Cimino" fistula); an arteriovenous graft, usually made of polytetrafluoroethylene; a large-bore intravenous catheter; or a subcutaneous device attached to intravascular catheters. Blood is pumped though hollow fibers of an artificial kidney (the "dialyzer") and bathed with a solution of favorable chemical composition (isotonic, free of urea and other nitrogenous compounds, and generally low in potassium). Dialysate [K^+] is varied from 0 to 4 mM, depending on predialysis [K^+] and the clinical setting. Dialysate [Ca^{2+}] is typically 2.5 mg/dL (1.25 mM), [HCO_3^-] typically 35 meq/L, and dialysate [Na+] 140 mM; these can also be modified, depending on the clinical situation. Most pts undergo dialysis thrice weekly, usually for 3–4 h. The efficiency of dialysis is largely dependent on the duration of dialysis, blood flow rate, dialysate flow rate, and surface area of the dialyzer.

Complications of hemodialysis are outlined in Table 148-1. Many of these relate to the process of hemodialysis as an intense, intermittent therapy. In contrast to the native kidney or to PD, both major dialytic functions (i.e., clearance of solutes and fluid removal, or "ultrafiltration") are accomplished over relatively short time periods. The rapid flux of fluid can cause hypotension, even without a pt reaching "dry weight." Hemodialysis-related hypotension is common in diabetic pts whose neuropathy prevents the compensatory responses (vasoconstriction and tachycardia) to intravascular volume depletion. Occasionally, confusion or other central nervous system symptoms will occur. The dialysis "disequilibrium syndrome" refers to the development of headache, confusion, and rarely seizures, in association with rapid solute removal early in the pt's dialysis history, before adaptation to the procedure; this complication is largely avoided by an incremental induction of chronic dialytic therapy in uremic patients, starting with treatments of short duration, lower blood flows, and lower dialysate flow rates.

PERITONEAL DIALYSIS

PD does not require direct access to the circulation; rather, it obligates placement of a peritoneal catheter that allows infusion of a dialysate solution into the abdominal cavity; this allows transfer of solutes (i.e., urea, potassium, other uremic molecules) across the peritoneal membrane, which serves as the "artifi-

TABLE 148-1 COMPLICATIONS OF HEMODIALYSIS	
Hypotension	Dialysis-related amyloidosis
Accelerated vascular disease	Protein-energy malnutrition
Rapid loss of residual renal function	Hemorrhage
Access thrombosis	Dyspnea/hypoxemia[a]
Access or catheter sepsis	Leukopenia[a]

[a]Particularly with first use of conventional modified cellulosic dialyzer.

TABLE 148-2	**COMPLICATIONS OF PERITONEAL DIALYSIS**
Peritonitis	Dialysis-related amyloidosis
Hyperglycemia	Insufficient clearance due to vascular disease or
Hypertriglyceridemia	other factors
Obesity	Uremia secondary to loss of residual renal function
Hypoproteinemia	

cial kidney." This solution is similar to that used for hemodialysis, except that it must be sterile, and it uses lactate, rather than bicarbonate, to provide base equivalents. PD is far less efficient at cleansing the bloodstream than hemodialysis and therefore requires a much longer duration of therapy. Pts generally have the choice of performing their own "exchanges" (2–3 L of dialysate, 4–5 times during daytime hours) or using an automated device at night. Compared with hemodialysis, PD offers the major advantages of (1) independence and flexibility, and (2) a more gentle hemodynamic profile.

Complications are outlined in Table 148-2. Peritonitis is the most important complication. The clinical presentation typically consists of abdominal pain and cloudy dialysate; peritoneal fluid leukocyte count is typically >100/μL, 50% neutrophils. In addition to the negative effects of the systemic inflammatory response, protein loss is magnified severalfold during the peritonitis episode. If severe or prolonged, an episode of peritonitis may prompt removal of the peritoneal catheter or even discontinuation of the modality (i.e., switch to hemodialysis). Gram-positive organisms (especially *Staphylococcus aureus* and other *Staphylococcus* spp.) predominate; *Pseudomonas* or fungal (usually *Candida*) infections tend to be more resistant to medical therapy and typically obligate catheter removal. Antibiotic administration may be intravenous or intraperitoneal when intensive therapy is required.

For a more detailed discussion, see Liu KD, Chertow GM: Dialysis in the Treatment of Renal Failure: Chap. 275, p. 1772, in HPIM-17.

149 Renal Transplantation

With the advent of more potent and well-tolerated immunosuppressive regimens and further improvements in short-term graft survival, renal transplantation remains the treatment of choice for most pts with end-stage renal disease. Results are best with living-related transplantation, in part because of optimized tissue matching and in part because waiting time can be minimized; ideally, these patients are transplanted prior to the onset of symptomatic uremia or indications for dialysis. Many centers now perform living-unrelated donor (e.g., spousal) transplants. Graft survival in these cases is far superior to that observed with cadaveric transplants, although less favorable than with living-related transplants. Factors that influence graft survival are outlined in Table 149-1. Contraindications to renal transplantation are outlined in Table 149-2.

TABLE 149-1 SOME FACTORS THAT INFLUENCE GRAFT SURVIVAL IN RENAL TRANSPLANTATION

HLA mismatch	↓
Presensitization (preformed antibodies)	↓
Pretransplant blood transfusion	↑
Very young or older donor age	↓
Female donor sex	↓
African-American donor race (compared with Caucasian)	↓
Older recipient age	↑
African-American recipient race (compared with Caucasian)	↓
Prolonged cold ischemia time	↓
Large recipient body size	↓

REJECTION

Immunologic rejection is the major hazard to the short-term success of renal transplantation. Rejection may be (1) hyperacute (immediate graft dysfunction due to presensitization) or (2) acute (sudden change in renal function occurring within weeks to months). Rejection is usually detected by a rise in serum creatinine but may also lead to hypertension, fever, reduced urine output, and occasionally graft tenderness. A percutaneous renal transplant biopsy confirms the diagnosis. Treatment usually consists of a "pulse" of methylprednisolone (500–1000 mg/d for 3 days). In refractory or particularly severe cases, 7–10 days of a monoclonal antibody directed at human T lymphocytes may be given.

IMMUNOSUPPRESSION

Maintenance immunosuppressive therapy usually consists of a three-drug regimen, with each drug targeted at a different stage in the immune response. The calcineurin inhibitors cyclosporine and tacrolimus are the cornerstones

TABLE 149-2 CONTRAINDICATIONS TO RENAL TRANSPLANTATION

Absolute Contraindications

Active glomerulonephritis
Active bacterial or other infection
Active or very recent malignancy
HIV infection
Hepatitis B surface antigenemia
Severe degrees of comorbidity (e.g., advanced atherosclerotic vascular disease)

Relative Contraindications

Age > 70 years
Severe psychiatric disease
Moderately severe degrees of comorbidity
Hepatitis C infection with chronic hepatitis or cirrhosis
Noncompliance with dialysis or other medical therapy
Primary renal diseases
Primary focal sclerosis with prior recurrence in transplant
Multiple myeloma
Amyloid
Oxalosis

of immunosuppressive therapy. The most potent of orally available agents, cal-cineurin inhibitors have vastly improved short-term graft survival. Side effects of cyclosporine include hypertension, hyperkalemia, resting tremor, hirsutism, gingival hypertrophy, hyperlipidemia, hyperuricemia and gout, and a slowly progressive loss of renal function with characteristic histopathologic patterns (also seen in exposed recipients of heart and liver transplants). While the side effect profile of tacrolimus is generally similar to cyclosporine, there is a higher risk of hyperglycemia, a lower risk of hypertension, and occasional hair loss rather than hirsutism.

Prednisone is frequently used in conjunction with cyclosporine, at least for the first several months following successful graft function. Side effects of prednisone include hypertension, glucose intolerance, Cushingoid features, os-teoporosis, hyperlipidemia, acne, and depression and other mood disturbances.

Mycophenolate mofetil has proved more effective than azathioprine in combi-nation therapy with calcineurin inhibitors and prednisone. The major side effects of mycophenolate mofetil are gastrointestinal (diarrhea is most common); leuko-penia (and thrombocytopenia to a lesser extent) develops in a fraction of patients.

Sirolimus is a newer immunosuppressive agent often used in combination with other drugs, particularly when calcineurin inhibitors are reduced or elimi-nated. Side effects include hyperlipidemia and oral ulcers.

OTHER COMPLICATIONS

Infection and neoplasia are important complications of renal transplantation. Infection is common in the heavily immunosuppressed host (e.g., cadaveric transplant recipient with multiple episodes of rejection requiring steroid pulses or monoclonal antibody treatment). The culprit organism depends in part on characteristics of the donor and recipient and timing following transplantation. In the first month, bacterial organisms predominate. After 1 month, there is a significant risk of systemic infection with cytomegalovirus (CMV), particularly in recipients without prior exposure whose donor was CMV positive. Prophy-lactic use of ganciclovir or valacyclovir can reduce the risk of CMV disease. Later on, there is a substantial risk of fungal and related infections, especially in pts who are unable to taper prednisone to <20–30 mg/d. Daily low-dose tri-methoprim-sulfamethoxazole is effective at reducing the risk of *Pneumocystis carinii* infection.

The polyoma group of DNA viruses (BK, JC, SV40) can be activated by im-munosuppression. Reactivation of BK is associated with a typical pattern of re-nal inflammation, BK nephropathy, which can lead to loss of the allograft; therapy typically involves reduction of immunosuppression to aid in clearance of the reactivated virus.

Epstein-Barr virus–associated lymphoproliferative disease is the most im-portant neoplastic complication of renal transplantation, especially in pts who receive polyclonal (antilymphocyte globulin, used at some centers for induction of immunosuppression) or monoclonal antibody therapy. Non-Hodgkin's lym-phoma and squamous cell carcinoma of the skin are also more common in this population.

For a more detailed discussion, see Carpenter CB, Milford EL, Sayegh MH: Transplantation in the Treatment of Renal Failure, Chap. 276, p. 1776, in HPIM-17.

150 Glomerular Diseases

ACUTE GLOMERULONEPHRITIS (GN)

Often called the "nephritic syndrome." Characterized by development, over days, of azotemia, hypertension, edema, hematuria, proteinuria, and sometimes oliguria. Salt and water retention are due to reduced glomerular filtration rate (GFR) and may result in circulatory congestion. Red blood cell (RBC) casts on urinalysis confirm Dx. Proteinuria is usually <3 g/d. Most forms of acute GN are mediated by humoral immune mechanisms. Clinical course depends on underlying lesion (Table 150-1).

Acute Poststreptococcal GN This is the prototype and most common cause in childhood. Nephritis develops 1–3 weeks after pharyngeal or cutaneous infection with "nephritogenic" strains of group A β-hemolytic streptococci. Dx depends on a positive pharyngeal or skin culture (if available), positive titers for antistreptococcal antigens (ASO, anti-DNAse, or antihyaluronidase), and hypocomplementemia. Renal biopsy reveals diffuse proliferative GN. Treatment consists of correction of fluid and electrolyte imbalance. In most cases the disease is self-limited, although the prognosis is less favorable and urinary abnormalities are more likely to persist in adults.

Postinfectious GN May follow other bacterial, viral, and parasitic infections. Examples are bacterial endocarditis, sepsis, hepatitis B, and pneumococcal pneumonia. Features are milder than with poststreptococcal GN. Control of primary infection usually produces resolution of GN.

TABLE 150-1 CAUSES OF ACUTE GLOMERULONEPHRITIS

I. Infectious diseases
    A. Poststreptococcal glomerulonephritis[a]
    B. Nonstreptococcal postinfectious glomerulonephritis
        1. Bacterial: infective endocarditis, "shunt nephritis," sepsis, pneumococcal pneumonia, typhoid fever, secondary syphilis, meningococcemia
        2. Viral: hepatitis B, infectious mononucleosis, mumps, measles, varicella, vaccinia, echovirus, and coxsackievirus
        3. Parasitic: malaria, toxoplasmosis
II. Multisystem diseases: SLE, vasculitis, Henoch-Schönlein purpura, Goodpasture's syndrome
III. Primary glomerular diseases: mesangiocapillary glomerulonephritis, Berger's disease (IgA nephropathy), "pure" mesangial proliferative glomerulonephritis
IV. Miscellaneous: Guillain-Barré syndrome, irradiation of Wilms' tumor, self-administered diphtheria-pertussis-tetanus vaccine, serum sickness

[a]Most common cause.
Note: SLE, systemic lupus erythematosus.
Source: RJ Glassock, BM Brenner: HPIM-13.

RAPIDLY PROGRESSIVE GLOMERULONEPHRITIS (GN)

Defined as a subacute reduction in GFR of >50%, with evidence of a proliferative GN; causes overlap with those of acute GN (Table 150-2). Broadly classified into three major subtypes on the basis of renal biopsy findings and pathophysiology: (1) immune complex–associated, e.g., in systemic lupus erythematosus (SLE); (2) "pauci-immune," associated with antineutrophil cytoplasmic antibodies (ANCA); and (3) associated with anti–glomerular basement (anti-GBM) antibodies, e.g., in Goodpasture's syndrome. All three forms will typically have a proliferative, crescentic GN by light microscopy but differ in the results of the immunofluorescence and electron microscopy components of the renal biopsy.

TABLE 150-2   **CAUSES OF RAPIDLY PROGRESSIVE GLOMERULONEPHRITIS**

I. Infectious diseases
   A. Poststreptococcal glomerulonephritis[a]
   B. Infective endocarditis
   C. Occult visceral sepsis
   D. Hepatitis B infection (with vasculitis and/or cryoglobulinemia)
   E. HIV infection (?)
   F. Hepatitis C infection (with cryoglobulinemia, membranoproliferative glomerulonephritis)
II. Multisystem diseases
   A. Systemic lupus erythematosus
   B. Henoch-Schönlein purpura
   C. Systemic necrotizing vasculitis (including Wegener's granulomatosis)
   D. Goodpasture's syndrome
   E. Essential mixed (IgG/IgM) cryoglobulinemia
   F. Malignancy
   G. Relapsing polychondritis
   H. Rheumatoid arthritis (with vasculitis)
III. Drugs
   A. Penicillamine
   B. Hydralazine
   C. Allopurinol (with vasculitis)
   D. Rifampin
IV. Idiopathic or primary glomerular disease
   A. Idiopathic crescentic glomerulonephritis
      1. Type I—with linear deposits of Ig (anti-GBM antibody–mediated)
      2. Type II—with granular deposits of Ig (immune complex–mediated)
      3. Type III—with few or no immune deposits of Ig ("pauci-immune")
      4. Antineutrophil cytoplasmic antibody–induced,? forme fruste of vasculitis
      5. Immunotactoid glomerulonephritis
      6. Fibrillary glomerulonephritis
   B. Superimposed on another primary glomerular disease
      1. Mesangiocapillary (membranoproliferative) glomerulonephritis (especially type II)
      2. Membranous glomerulonephritis
      3. Berger's disease (IgA nephropathy)

---

[a]Most common cause.
Note: GBM, glomerular basement membrane.
Source: RJ Glassock, BM Brenner: HPIM-13.

SLE (Lupus) Renal involvement is due to deposition of circulating immune complexes. Clinical features of SLE with or without renal involvement include arthralgias, "butterfly" skin rash, serositis, alopecia (hair loss), and central nervous system disease. Nephrotic syndrome with renal insufficiency is common. Renal biopsy reveals mesangial, focal, or diffuse GN and/or membranous nephropathy. Diffuse GN, the most common finding in renal biopsy series, is characterized by an active sediment, severe proteinuria, and progressive renal insufficiency and may have an ominous prognosis. Pts have a positive antinuclear antibody test, anti-dsDNA antibodies, and hypocomplementemia. Treatment includes glucocorticoids and cytotoxic agents. Oral or IV monthly cyclophosphamide is most commonly employed, typically for a period of 6 months. Mycophenolate mofetil or azathioprine may be used for longer-term therapy.

Antineutrophil Cytoplasmic Antibody (ANCA)-Associated, Pauci-Immune GN

May be renal-limited (idiopathic pauci-immune GN) or associated with systemic vasculitis (Wegener's granulomatosis or microscopic polyarteritis nodosa). Defining characteristic is the presence of circulating ANCA. These are detected by immunofluorescence of alcohol-fixed neutrophils; a "perinuclear" pattern (pANCA) is usually due to antibodies against myeloperoxidase (MPO), whereas a "cytoplasmic" pattern (cANCA) is almost always due to reactivity against proteinase-3 (PR3). Confirmatory enzyme-linked immunosorbent assay testing against the MPO and PR3 antigens is mandatory, since the pANCA pattern can be caused by antibodies against other neutrophil components, e.g., lactoferrin; these do not have the same consistent relationship to vasculitis and pauci-immune GN. The anti-MPO or anti-PR3 titer does not always correlate with disease activity.

Patients typically have a prodromal, "flulike" syndrome, which may encompass myalgias, fever, arthralgias, anorexia, and weight loss. There may be associated cutaneous, pulmonary, upper respiratory (sinusitis), or neurologic (mononeuritis monoplex) complications of associated systemic vasculitis. In particular, pulmonary necrotizing capillaritis can lead to hemoptysis and pulmonary hemorrhage.

Standard therapy for ANCA-associated RPGN should include steroids and cyclophosphamide. Some centers will also utilize plasmapheresis in the initial management of patients with a severe pulmonary-renal syndrome or to stave off dialysis in patients with severe renal impairment.

Anti-Glomerular Basement Membrane Disease

Caused by antibodies against the $\alpha 3$ NCI (noncollagenous) domain of type IV collagen; circulating anti-GBM antibody and linear immunofluorescence on renal biopsy establish the Dx. Patients may have isolated GN; Goodpasture's syndrome encompasses GN and lung hemorrhage. Plasma exchange may produce remission. Severe lung hemorrhage is treated with IV glucocorticoids (e.g., 1 g/d × 3 days). Approximately 10–15% will also have ANCA against MPO, some with evidence of vasculitis, e.g., leukocytoclastic vasculitis in the skin.

Henoch-Schönlein Purpura

A generalized vasculitis causing IgA nephropathy, purpura, arthralgias, and abdominal pain; occurs mainly in children. Renal involvement is manifested by hematuria and proteinuria. Serum IgA is increased in half of pts. Renal biopsy is useful for prognosis. Treatment is symptomatic.

NEPHROTIC SYNDROME (NS)

Characterized by albuminuria (>3.5 g/d) and hypoalbuminemia (<30 g/L) and accompanied by edema, hyperlipidemia, and lipiduria. Complications include renal

TABLE 150-3	CAUSES OF NEPHROTIC SYNDROME (NS)
Systemic Causes (25%)	Glomerular Disease (75%)
Diabetes mellitus, SLE, amyloidosis, HIV-associated nephropathy	Membranous (40%)
Drugs: gold, penicillamine, probenecid, street heroin, captopril, NSAIDs	Minimal change disease (15%)
Infections: bacterial endocarditis, hepatitis B, shunt infections, syphilis, malaria, hepatic schistosomiasis	Focal glomerulosclerosis (15%)
Malignancy: multiple myeloma, light chain deposition disease, Hodgkin's and other lymphomas, leukemia, carcinoma of breast, GI tract	Membranoproliferative GN (7%)
	Mesangioproliferative GN (5%)
	Immunotactoid and fibrillary GN

Note: SLE, systemic lupus erythematosus; NSAIDs, nonsteroidal anti-inflammatory drugs; GN, glomerulonephritis.
Source: Modified from RJ Glassock, BM Brenner: HPIM-13.

vein thrombosis and other thromboembolic events, infection, vitamin D deficiency, protein malnutrition, and drug toxicities due to decreased protein binding.

In adults, the most common cause of nephritic syndrome is diabetes. A minority of cases are secondary to SLE, amyloidosis, drugs, neoplasia, or other disorders (Table 150-3). By exclusion, the remainder are idiopathic. Renal biopsy is required to make the diagnosis and determine therapy in idiopathic NS.

Minimal Change Disease Causes about 10–15% of idiopathic NS in adults, but 70–90% of NS in children. Blood pressure is normal; GFR is normal or slightly reduced; urinary sediment is benign or may show few RBCs. Protein selectivity is variable in adults. Recent upper respiratory infection, allergies, or immunizations are present in some cases; nonsteroidal anti-inflammatory drugs can cause minimal change disease with interstitial nephritis. Acute renal failure may rarely occur, particularly among elderly persons. Renal biopsy shows only foot process fusion on electron microscopy. Remission of proteinuria with glucocorticoids carries a good prognosis; cytotoxic therapy may be required for relapse. Progression to renal failure is uncommon. Focal sclerosis has been suspected in some cases refractory to steroid therapy.

Membranous GN Characterized by subepithelial IgG deposits; accounts for ~30% of adult NS. Pts present with edema and nephrotic proteinuria. Blood pressure, GFR, and urine sediment are usually normal at initial presentation. Hypertension, mild renal insufficiency, and abnormal urine sediment develop later. Renal vein thrombosis is relatively common, more so than with other forms of nephrotic syndrome. Underlying diseases such as SLE, hepatitis B, and solid tumors and exposure to such drugs as high-dose captopril or penicillamine should be sought. Some pts progress to end-stage renal disease (ESRD); however, 20–33% may experience a spontaneous remission. Male gender, older age, hypertension, and persistence of significant proteinuria (>6 g/d) are associated with a higher risk of progressive disease. Optimal immunosuppressive therapy is controversial. Glucocorticoids alone are ineffective. Cytotoxic agents may promote complete or partial remission in some pts, as may cyclosporine. Anti-CD20 antibody therapy with rituximab has recently shown considerable promise, consistent with a role for B cells and antibody production in the pathophysiology. Reduction of proteinuria with angiotensin-converting enzyme (ACE) inhibitors and/or angiotensin receptor blockers (ARBs) is also an important mainstay of therapy.

Focal Glomerulosclerosis (FGS)   Can be primary or secondary. Primary tends to be more acute, similar to minimal change disease in abruptness of nephrotic syndrome, but with added features of hypertension, renal insufficiency, and hematuria. Involves fibrosis of portions of some (primarily juxtamedullary) glomeruli and is found in ~33% of pts with NS; African Americans are disproportionately affected (causing ~50% of NS). HIV-associated nephropathy (HIVAN) and collapsing nephropathy have similar pathologic features; both tend to be more rapidly progressive than typical cases. The frequency and severity of HIVAN has decreased with highly active antiretroviral therapy (HAART).

Treatment typically begins with an extended course of steroids; fewer than half undergo remission. Cyclosporine is an evolving therapy for maintenance of remission and for steroid-resistant patients. As in other glomerulopathies, reduction of proteinuria with ACE inhibitors and/or ARBs is also an important component of therapy. Finally, primary FGS may recur after renal transplant, when it may lead to loss of the allograft.

Secondary FGS can occur in the late stages of any form of kidney disease associated with nephron loss (e.g., remote GN, pyelonephritis, vesicoureteral reflux). Typically responds to ACE inhibition and blood pressure control. No benefit of glucocorticoids in secondary FGS. Clinical history, kidney size, biopsy findings, and associated conditions usually allow differentiation of primary vs. secondary causes.

Membranoproliferative Glomerulonephritis (MPGN)   Mesangial expansion and proliferation extend into the capillary loop. Two ultrastructural variants exist. In MPGN I, subendothelial electron-dense deposits are present, C3 is deposited in a granular pattern indicative of immune-complex pathogenesis, and IgG and the early components of complement may or may not be present. In MPGN II, the lamina densa of the GBM is transformed into an electron-dense character, as is the basement membrane in Bowman's capsule and tubules. C3 is found irregularly in the GBM. Small amounts of Ig (usually IgM) are present, but early components of complement are absent. Serum complement levels are decreased. MPGN affects young adults. Blood pressure and GFR are abnormal, and the urine sediment is active. Some have acute nephritis or hematuria. Similar lesions occur in SLE and hemolytic-uremic syndrome. Infection with hepatitis C virus (HCV) has been linked to MPGN. Treatment with interferon α and ribavirin has resulted in remission of renal disease in some cases, depending on HCV serotype. Glucocorticoids, cytotoxic agents, antiplatelet agents, and plasmapheresis have been used with limited success. MPGN may recur in allografts.

Diabetic Nephropathy   The most common cause of NS. Pathologic changes include diffuse and/or nodular glomerulosclerosis, nephrosclerosis, chronic pyelonephritis, and papillary necrosis. Clinical features include proteinuria, hypertension, azotemia, and bacteriuria. Although prior duration of diabetes mellitus (DM) is variable, in type 1 DM proteinuria may develop 10–15 years after onset, progress to NS, and then lead to renal failure over 3–5 years. Other complications of DM are common; retinopathy is nearly universal. Treatment with ACE inhibitors delays the onset of nephropathy and should be instituted in all pts tolerant to that class of drug.

If a cough develops in a pt treated with an ACE inhibitor, an ARB is the next best choice; although long-term studies are lacking, many authorities advocate adding ARBs to ACE inhibitors in patients with persistent, significant proteinuria. If hyperkalemia develops and cannot be controlled with (1) optimizing glucose

TABLE 150-4   **EVALUATION OF NEPHROTIC SYNDROME**

24-h urine for protein; creatinine clearance
Serum albumin, cholesterol, complement
Urine protein electrophoresis
Rule out SLE, diabetes mellitus
Review drug exposure
Renal biopsy
Consider malignancy (in elderly pt with membranous GN or minimal change
   disease)
Consider renal vein thrombosis (if membranous GN or symptoms of pulmonary
   embolism are present)

Note: SLE, systemic lupus erythematosus; GN, glomerulonephritis.

control, (2) loop diuretics, or (3) occasional polystyrene sulfonate (Kayexalate), then tight control of blood pressure with alternative agents is warranted. Modest restriction of dietary protein may also slow decline of renal function.

Evaluation of NS is shown in Table 150-4.

ASYMPTOMATIC URINARY ABNORMALITIES

Proteinuria in the nonnephrotic range and/or hematuria unaccompanied by edema, reduced GFR, or hypertension can be due to multiple causes (Table 150-5).

TABLE 150-5   **GLOMERULAR CAUSES OF ASYMPTOMATIC
                     URINARY ABNORMALITIES**

I. Hematuria with or without proteinuria
   A. Primary glomerular diseases
      1. Berger's disease (IgA nephropathy)[a]
      2. Mesangiocapillary glomerulonephritis
      3. Other primary glomerular hematurias accompanied by "pure" mesan-
         gial proliferation, focal and segmental proliferative glomerulonephritis,
         or other lesions
      4. "Thin basement membrane" disease (? forme fruste of Alport's syndrome)
   B. Associated with multisystem or hereditary diseases
      1. Alport's syndrome and other "benign" familial hematurias
      2. Fabry's disease
      3. Sickle cell disease
   C. Associated with infections
      1. Resolving poststreptococcal glomerulonephritis
      2. Other postinfectious glomerulonephritides
II. Isolated nonnephrotic proteinuria
   A. Primary glomerular diseases
      1. "Orthostatic" proteinuria
      2. Focal and segmental glomerulosclerosis
      3. Membranous glomerulonephritis
   B. Associated with multisystem or heredofamilial diseases
      1. Diabetes mellitus
      2. Amyloidosis
      3. Nail-patella syndrome

[a]Most common.
Source: RJ Glassock, BM Brenner: HPIM-13.

TABLE 150-6 SEROLOGIC FINDINGS IN SELECTED MULTISYSTEM DISEASES CAUSING GLOMERULAR DISEASE

Disease	C3	Ig	FANA	Anti-dsDNA	Anti-GBM	Cryo-Ig	CIC	ANCA
SLE	↓	↑IgG	+++	++	−	++	+++	±
Goodpasture's syndrome	−	−	−	−	+++	−	±	+ (10–15%)
Henoch-Schönlein purpura	−	↑ IgA	−	−	−	±	++	−
Polyarteritis	↓↑	↑ IgG	+	±	−	++	+++	+++
Wegener's granulomatosis	↓↑	↑ IgA, IgE	−	−	−	±	++	+++
Cryoglobulinemia	↓	± ↓↑ IgG IgA, IgD IgE	−	−	−	+++	++	−
Multiple myeloma	−	↑ IgM	−	−	−	+	−	−
Waldenström's macroglobulinemia	−	↑ IgM	−	−	−	−	−	−
Amyloidosis	−	± Ig	−	−	−	−	−	−

Note: C3, complement component 3; Ig, immunoglobulin levels; FANA, fluorescent antinuclear antibody assay; anti-dsDNA, antibody to double-stranded (native) DNA; anti-GBM, antibody to glomerular basement membrane antigens; cryo-Ig, cryoimmunoglobulin; CIC, circulating immune complexes; ANCA, antineutrophil cytoplasmic antibody; SLE, systemic lupus erythematosus; −, normal; +, occasionally slightly abnormal; ++, often abnormal; +++, severely abnormal.

Source: RJ Glassock, BM Brenner: HPIM-13.

Thin Basement Membrane Nephropathy　Also known as benign familial hematuria, may cause up to 25% of isolated, sustained hematuria without proteinuria. Diffuse thinning of the glomerular basement membrane on renal biopsy, with minimal other changes. May be hereditary, caused in some instances by defects in type IV collagen. Patients have persistent glomerular hematuria, with minimal proteinuria. The renal prognosis is controversial but appears to be relatively benign.

IgA Nephropathy　Another very common cause of recurrent hematuria of glomerular origin; is most frequent in young men. Episodes of macroscopic hematuria are present with flulike symptoms, without skin rash, abdominal pain, or arthritis. Renal biopsy shows diffuse mesangial deposition of IgA, often with lesser amounts of IgG, nearly always by C3 and properdin but not by C1q or C4. Prognosis is variable; 50% develop ESRD within 25 years; men with hypertension and heavy proteinuria are at highest risk. Glucocorticoids and other immunosuppressive agents have not proved successful. A randomized clinical trial of fish oil supplementation suggested a modest therapeutic benefit. Rarely recurs in allografts.

Chronic Glomerulonephritis　Characterized by persistent urinary abnormalities, slow progressive impairment of renal function, symmetrically contracted kidneys, moderate to heavy proteinuria, abnormal urinary sediment (especially RBC casts), and x-ray evidence of normal pyelocalyceal systems. The time to progression to ESRD is variable, hastened by uncontrolled hypertension and infections. Control of blood pressure is of paramount importance and is the most important factor influencing the pace of progression. While ACE inhibitors and ARBs may be the most effective agents, additional agents should be added if blood pressure is not optimally controlled with ACE inhibitors alone. Diuretics, nondihydropyridine calcium antagonists, and β-adrenergic blockers have been successfully used in a variety of clinical settings.

Glomerulopathies Associated with Multisystem Disease　(See Table 150-6)

For a more detailed discussion, see Lewis JB, Neilson EG: Glomerular Diseases, Chap. 277, p. 1782, in HPIM-17.

151　Renal Tubular Disease

Tubulointerstitial diseases constitute a diverse group of acute and chronic, hereditary and acquired disorders involving the renal tubules and supporting structures (Table 151-1). Functionally, they may result in a wide variety of physiologic phenotypes, including nephrogenic diabetes insipidus (DI) with polyuria, non-anion-gap metabolic acidosis, salt-wasting, and hypo- or hyperkalemia. Azotemia is common, owing to associated glomerular fibrosis and/or ischemia. Compared with glomerulopathies, proteinuria and hematuria are less dramatic, and hypertension is less common. The functional consequences of tubular dysfunction are outlined in Table 151-2.

TABLE 151-1	PRINCIPAL CAUSES OF TUBULOINTERSTITIAL DISEASE OF THE KIDNEY

Toxins

Exogenous toxins	Metabolic toxins
Analgesic nephropathy[a]	Acute uric acid nephropathy
Lead nephropathy	Gouty nephropathy[a]
Chinese herb nephropathy	Hypercalcemic nephropathy
Balkan endemic nephropathy	Hypokalemic nephropathy
Miscellaneous nephrotoxins (e.g., antibiotics, cyclosporine, radiographic contrast media, heavy metals)[a,b]	Miscellaneous metabolic toxins (e.g., hyperoxaluria, cystinosis, Fabry's disease)

Neoplasia

Lymphoma
Leukemia
Multiple myeloma (cast nephropathy, AL amyloidosis)

Immune Disorders

Acute (allergic) interstitial nephritis[a,b]	Transplant rejection
Sjögren's syndrome	HIV-associated nephropathy
Amyloidosis	

Vascular Disorders

Arteriolar nephrosclerosis[a]	Sickle cell nephropathy
Atheroembolic disease	Acute tubular necrosis[a,b]

Hereditary Renal Diseases

Disorders associated with renal failure	Hereditary tubular disorders
Autosomal dominant polycystic kidney disease	Bartter's syndrome (hereditary hypokalemic alkalosis)
Autosomal recessive polycystic kidney disease	Gitelman's syndrome (hereditary hypokalemic alkalosis)
Medullary cystic kidney disease	Pseudohypoaldosteronism type I (hypotension/salt wasting and hyperkalemia)
Hereditary nephritis (Alport's syndrome)	Pseudohypoaldosteronism type II (hereditary hypertension and hyperkalemia)
	Liddle's syndrome (hypertension and hypokalemia)
	Hereditary hypomagnesemia
	Hereditary nephrogenic diabetes insipidus
	X-linked (AVP receptor dysfunction)
	Autosomal (aquaporin-2 dysfunction)

(continued)

TABLE 151-1	PRINCIPAL CAUSES OF TUBULOINTERSTITIAL DISEASE OF THE KIDNEY (CONTINUED)

Infectious Injury

Acute pyelonephritis[a,b]
Chronic pyelonephritis

Miscellaneous Disorders

Chronic urinary tract obstruction[a]
Vesicoureteral reflux[a]
Radiation nephritis

[a]Common.
[b]Typically acute.

ACUTE INTERSTITIAL NEPHRITIS (AIN)

Drugs are a leading cause of this type of renal failure, usually identified by a gradual rise in the serum creatinine at least several days after the institution of therapy, occasionally accompanied by fever, eosinophilia, rash, and arthralgias. The onset of renal dysfunction may be very rapid in pts who have previously been sensitized to the offending agent; this is particularly true for rifampin, for which intermittent or interrupted therapy appears to be associated with the development of AIN. In addition to azotemia, there may be evidence of tubular dysfunction (e.g., hyperkalemia, metabolic acidosis). Urinalysis may show hematuria, pyuria, white cell casts, and eosinophiluria on Hansel's or Wright's stain; notably, however, eosinophiluria is not specific for AIN, occurring in other causes of acute renal failure, including atheroemboli.

TABLE 151-2	TRANSPORT DYSFUNCTION IN TUBULOINTERSTITIAL DISEASE

Defect	Cause(s)
Reduced GFR[a]	Obliteration of microvasculature and obstruction of tubules
Fanconi syndrome	Damage to proximal tubular reabsorption of solutes, primarily glucose, amino acids, and phosphate; may also exhibit hypouricemia, proximal tubular acidosis, low-molecular-weight proteinuria
Hyperchloremic acidosis[a]	1. Reduced ammonia production (CKD) or excretion (hyperkalemia)
	2. Inability to acidify the collecting duct fluid (distal renal tubular acidosis)
	3. Proximal bicarbonate wasting (proximal RTA)
Polyuria, isothenuria[a]	Damage to medullary tubules (thick ascending limb and/or collecting duct) and vasculature
Hypokalemic alkalosis	Damage or hereditary dysfunction of the thick ascending limb or distal convoluted tubule (Bartter's and Gitelman's syndromes)
Hyperkalemia[a]	Potassium secretory defects including aldosterone resistance
Salt wasting	Distal tubular damage with impaired sodium reabsorption

[a]Common.
Note: GFR, glomerular filtration rate; CKD, chronic kidney disease; RTA, renal tubular acidosis.

TABLE 151-3 **CAUSES OF ACUTE INTERSTITIAL NEPHRITIS**

Drugs (70%, antibiotics in one-third)
   Antibiotics
      Methicillin, nafcillin, oxacillin
      Rifampin
      Penicillins, cephalosporins
      Ciprofloxacin
      Sulfamethoxazole and other sulfonamides
   Proton pump inhibitors, e.g., omeprazole
   H_2 blockers, e.g., cimetidine
   Allopurinol
   5-aminosalicylates
   NSAIDS, including COX-2 inhibitors
Infections (16%)
   Leptospirosis, *Legionella*, streptococcal, tuberculosis
Tubulointerstitial nephritis and uveitis syndrome (TINU) (5%)
Idiopathic (8%)
Sarcoidosis (1%)

Note: NSAIDs, nonsteroidal anti-inflammatory drugs; COX-2, cyclooxygenase 2.

Drugs that commonly cause AIN are listed in Table 151-3. Some drugs have a particular predilection for causing AIN, e.g., nafcillin; however, less frequent causes may be apparent only from case reports, such that a detailed history and literature review may be required to make the association with AIN. Many drugs, nonsteroidal anti-inflammatory drugs (NSAIDs) in particular, may elicit a glomerular lesion with similarity to minimal change disease, in addition to AIN; these pts typically have nephrotic-range proteinuria, versus the modest proteinuria typically associated with tubulointerstitial disease.

Renal dysfunction in drug-associated AIN usually improves after withdrawal of the offending drug, but complete recovery may be delayed and incomplete. In uncontrolled studies, glucocorticoids have been shown to promote earlier recovery of renal function and reduce fibrosis; this therapy is generally reserved to avoid or reduce the duration of dialytic therapy in pts who fail to respond to medication withdrawal.

AIN may also occur in the context of systemic infections, classically leptospirosis, *Legionella* infection, and streptococcal bacterial infection. Finally, the tubulointerstitial nephritis and uveitis syndrome (TINU) is another increasingly recognized form of AIN. In addition to uveitis, which may precede or follow the AIN in pts with TINU, systemic symptoms and signs are common, e.g., weight loss, fever, malaise, arthralgias, and an elevated erythrocyte sedimentation rate. The renal disease is typically self-limited; those with progressive disease are often treated with prednisone.

CHRONIC INTERSTITIAL NEPHRITIS (IN)

Analgesic nephropathy is an important cause of chronic kidney disease that results from the cumulative (in quantity and duration) effects of combination analgesic agents, usually phenacetin and aspirin. It is thought to be a more common cause of end-stage renal disease (ESRD) in Australia/New Zealand than elsewhere owing to the larger per capita ingestion of analgesic agents in that region of the world. Transitional cell carcinoma may develop. Analgesic nephropathy should be suspected in pts with a history of chronic headache or back pain with chronic kidney disease (CKD) that is otherwise unexplained. Manifestations include papillary necrosis, calculi, sterile pyuria, and azotemia.

A severe form of chronic tubulointerstitial fibrosis has been associated with the ingestion of Chinese herbal medicines, typically employed as part of a dieting regimen; Balkan endemic nephropathy (BEN), geographically restricted to pts from this region of southeastern Europe, shares many similarities with Chinese herbal nephropathy. These disorders are thought to be caused by exposure to aristolochic acid and/or other plant, endemic (in BEN), and medical toxins (the appetite suppressants fenfluramine and diethylpropion, in Chinese herbal nephropathy). Like analgesic nephropathies, these syndromes are both characterized by a high incidence of genitourinary malignancy.

Metabolic causes of chronic IN include hypercalcemia (with nephrocalcinosis), oxalosis (primary or secondary, e.g., with intestinal disease and hyperabsorption of dietary oxalate), hypokalemia, and hyperuricemia or hyperuricosuria. The renal pathology associated with chronic hypokalemia includes a relatively specific proximal tubular vacuolization, interstitial nephritis, and renal cysts; both chronic and acute renal failure have been described. Chronic IN can occur in association with several systemic diseases, including sarcoidosis, Sjögren's syndrome, and following radiation or chemotherapy exposure (e.g., ifosfamide, cisplatin).

MONOCLONAL IMMUNOGLOBULINS AND RENAL DISEASE

Monoclonal immunoglobulins are associated with a wide variety of renal manifestations (Table 151-4), of which myeloma-associated cast nephropathy is the most common. The physiochemical characteristics of the monoclonal immunoglobulin light or heavy chains determine the clinical phenotype in individual pts, most commonly cast nephropathy, light chain deposition disease, and AL amy-

TABLE 151-4	RENAL DISEASES ASSOCIATED WITH MONOCLONAL IMMUNOGLOBULINS
Disease	**Notes**
Cast nephropathy	Most common cause of CKD in myeloma
	Tubular obstruction with light chains
	Interstitial inflammation
	Acute or chronic renal failure
Light chain deposition disease	Nephrotic syndrome, chronic renal failure
	~40% have associated myeloma
Heavy chain deposition disease	Nephrotic syndrome, chronic renal failure
AL amyloidosis	Nephrotic syndrome, cardiac/endocrine/neuropathic involvement
	~10% have associated myeloma
	Renal tubular dysfunction (RTA, nephrogenic DI, etc.)
Hypercalcemia	With myeloma
Hyperviscosity syndrome	With Waldenström's macroglobulinemia
Fanconi syndrome	Glucosuria, aminoaciduria, phosphaturia, ± hypouricemia, proximal RTA, etc.

Note: CKD, chronic kidney disease; RTA, renal tubular acidosis; DI, diabetes insipidus.

loidosis. In cast nephropathy, filtered light chains aggregate and cause tubular obstruction, tubular damage, and interstitial inflammation. Pts can present with chronic renal dysfunction or with acute renal failure; important predisposing factors in acute cast nephropathy include hypercalcemia and volume depletion.

Diagnosis of cast nephropathy relies on the detection of monoclonal light chains in serum and/or urine, typically by protein electrophoresis and immunofixation. Dipstick analysis of the urine for protein is classically negative in cast nephropathy, despite the excretion of up to several grams a day of light chain protein; light chains are not detected by this screening test, which tests only for albuminuria. In contrast, the glomerular deposition of light chains in light chain deposition disease or AL amyloidosis can result in nephrotic-range proteinuria (Table 151-4), with strongly *positive* urine dipstick for protein.

Management of cast nephropathy encompasses aggressive hydration, treatment of hypercalcemia if present, and chemotherapy for the associated multiple myeloma. Some experts advocate the use of plasmapheresis for pts with acute renal failure and high levels of serum or urine monoclonal light chains; however, a recent negative randomized trial has reduced the enthusiasm for the routine employment of plasmapheresis in this setting.

Filtered light chains and multiple other low-molecular-weight proteins are also endocytosed and metabolized by the proximal tubule. Rarely, specific light chains generate crystalline depositions within proximal tubule cells, causing a Fanconi syndrome; again, this property appears to be caused by the specific physicochemical characteristics of the associated light chains. Fanconi syndrome or dysfunction of the distal nephron (hyperkalemic acidosis or nephrogenic DI) may also complicate renal amyloidosis.

POLYCYSTIC KIDNEY DISEASE

Autosomal dominant polycystic kidney disease (ADPKD) is the most common life-threatening monogenic genetic disorder, caused by autosomal dominant mutations in the *PKD1* and *PKD2* genes; it is a quantitatively important cause of ESRD. Autosomal recessive polycystic disease is a less much common cause of renal failure, typically presenting in infancy; hepatic involvement is much more prominent. The massive renal cysts in ADPKD can lead to progressive CKD, episodic flank pain, hematuria (often gross), hypertension, and/or urinary tract infection. The kidneys are often palpable and occasionally of very large size. Hepatic cysts and intracranial aneurysms may also be present; pts with ADPKD and a family history of ruptured intracranial aneurysms should undergo presymptomatic screening. Other common extrarenal features include diverticulosis and mitral valve prolapse.

The expression of ADPKD is highly variable, with the age of onset of ESRD ranging from childhood to old age. The renal phenotype is much milder in pts with mutations in *PKD1*, who on average develop ESRD approximately 15 years earlier than those with *PKD2* mutations. Indeed, some pts with ADPKD discover the disease incidentally in late adult life, having had mild to moderate hypertension earlier.

The diagnosis is usually made by ultrasonography. In a 15- to 29-year-old at-risk individual from a family with ADPKD, the presence of at least two renal cysts (unilateral or bilateral) is sufficient for diagnosis. Notably, however, renal cysts are a common ultrasound finding in older pts without ADPKD, particularly those with CKD. Therefore, in at-risk individuals 30–59 years of age, the presence of at least two cysts in each kidney is required for the diagnosis; this increases to four cysts in each kidney for those older than 60. Conversely, the absence of at least two cysts in each kidney excludes the diagnosis of ADPKD in at-risk individuals between the ages of 30 and 59.

Hypertension is common in ADPKD, often in the absence of an apparent reduction in glomerular filtration rate. Activation of the renin-angiotensin system appears to play a dominant role; angiotensin-converting enzyme inhibitors or angiotensin receptor blockers are the recommended antihypertensive agents, with a target bp of 120/80 mmHg. Promising treatment modalities for halting progression of CKD in ADPKD include vasopressin antagonists and inhibitors of CFTR (the transport protein defective in cystic fibrosis), which dramatically reduce cyst enlargement and renal progression in animal models.

Urinary tract infections are also common in ADPKD. In particular, pts may develop cyst infections, often with negative urine cultures and an absence of pyuria. Pts with an infected cyst may have a discrete area of tenderness, as opposed to the more diffuse discomfort of pyelonephritis; however, clinical distinction between these two possibilities can be problematic. Many commonly utilized antibiotics, including penicillins and aminoglycosides, fail to penetrate cysts and are ineffective; therapy of kidney infections in ADPKD should utilize an antibiotic that is known to penetrate cysts (e.g., quinolones), guided initially by local antimicrobial susceptibility patterns.

RENAL TUBULAR ACIDOSIS (RTA)

This describes a number of pathophysiologically distinct entities of tubular function whose common feature is the presence of a non-anion-gap metabolic acidosis. Diarrhea, CKD, and RTA together constitute the vast majority of cases of non-anion-gap metabolic acidosis. Pts with earlier stages of CKD (Table 57-1) typically develop a non-anion-gap acidosis, with a superimposed increase in the anion gap at later stages (Chap. 2). Acidosis may develop at an earlier stage of CKD in those with prominent injury to the distal nephron, as for example in reflux nephropathy.

Distal Hypokalemic (Type 1) RTA Pts are unable to acidify the urine despite systemic acidosis; the urinary anion gap is positive, reflective of a decrease in ammonium excretion (Chap. 2). Distal hypokalemic RTA may be inherited (both autosomal dominant and autosomal recessive) or acquired due to autoimmune and inflammatory diseases (e.g., Sjögren's syndrome, sarcoidosis), urinary tract obstruction, or amphotericin B therapy. Chronic type I RTA is typically associated with hypercalciuria and osteomalacia, a consequence of the long-term buffering of acidosis by bone.

Proximal (Type II) RTA There is a defect in bicarbonate reabsorption, usually associated with features of Fanconi syndrome; glycosuria, aminoaciduria, phosphaturia, and uricosuria (indicating proximal tubular dysfunction). Isolated proximal RTA is caused by hereditary dysfunction of the basolateral sodium-bicarbonate cotransporter. Fanconi syndrome may be inherited or acquired due to myeloma, chronic IN (e.g., Chinese herbal nephropathy), or drugs (e.g., ifosfamide, tenofovir). Treatment requires large doses of bicarbonate, which may aggravate hypokalemia, and repletion of phosphorus to prevent bone disease.

Type IV RTA This may be due to hyporeninemic hypoaldosteronism or to resistance of the distal nephron to aldosterone. Hyporeninemic hypoaldosteronism is typically associated with volume expansion and most commonly seen in elderly and/or diabetic pts with CKD. The hyperkalemia associated with NSAIDs and cyclosporine is at least partially due to hyporeninemic hypoaldosteronism. Pts with hyporeninemic hypoaldosteronism are typically hyperkalemic; they may also exhibit a mild non-anion-gap acidosis, with urine pH <5.5 and a positive urinary anion gap. Acidosis often improves with reduction in serum [K⁺], e.g., with Kayexalate therapy; hyperkalemia appears to interfere with medullary concentration of ammonium by the renal countercurrent mechanism. Should reduction in serum [K⁺] not improve acidosis, pts should be treated with oral bicarbonate or citrate. Finally, various forms of distal tubular injury and tubulointerstitial disease, e.g., interstitial nephritis, are associated with distal insensitivity to aldosterone; urine pH is classically >5.5, again with a positive urinary anion gap.

For a more detailed discussion, see Yu ASL, Brenner BM: Tubulo-interstitial Diseases of the Kidney, Chap. 279, p. 1806, in HPIM-17.

152 Urinary Tract Infections

ACUTE INFECTIONS: URETHRITIS, CYSTITIS, AND PYELONEPHRITIS

Epidemiology Urinary tract infections (UTIs) are classified epidemiologically as catheter-associated (nosocomial) and non-catheter-associated (community-acquired). Community-acquired UTIs result in >7 million office visits annually in the United States. Most cases involve sexually active young women. UTIs are rare among men <50 years of age. Asymptomatic bacteriuria is common among young women but is most frequently documented in elderly men and women, with rates up to 50% in some studies.

Etiology Uncomplicated community-acquired UTIs—defined as those not associated with calculi, obstruction, or urologic manipulation—are caused by *Escherichia coli* in ~80% of cases; other gram-negative rods, including *Proteus*, *Klebsiella*, and occasionally *Enterobacter* species, cause smaller proportions of cases. Gram-positive etiologic agents of UTI include *Staphylococcus saprophyticus*, which causes 10–15% of acute UTIs in young women, and enterococci. *E. coli, Proteus, Klebsiella, Enterobacter, Serratia*, and *Pseudomonas* cause recurrent infections and UTIs associated with urologic manipulation, calculi, or obstruction. *Proteus* and *Klebsiella* predispose to stone formation and are isolated more often from pts with calculi. *Staphylococcus epidermidis* is a common cause of catheter-associated UTI.

Pathogenesis Most UTIs result when bacteria gain access to the bladder via the urethra. Some strains of bacteria (e.g., *E. coli, Proteus*) are uropathogenic. These strains have virulence genes that increase the likelihood of UTI (e.g., genes encoding fimbriae that mediate attachment to uroepithelial cells). Upper tract disease occurs when bacteria ascend from the bladder. Women prone to infections are colonized with enteric gram-negative bacilli in the periurethral area and distal urethra prior to bacteriuria. Alterations of the normal vaginal flora (e.g., due to antibiotic treatment, other genital infections, or contraceptive use) contribute to UTIs. Other risk factors include female gender, sexual activity, pregnancy, genitourinary obstruction, neurogenic bladder dysfunction, and vesiculoureteral reflux. Hematogenous infection of the kidney is less common and occurs most often in debilitated pts or in the setting of staphylococcal bacteremia or candidemia.

Clinical Presentations

- Cystitis: Pts have dysuria, frequency, urgency, and suprapubic pain. Urine is cloudy, malodorous, and sometimes bloody. Systemic signs are usually absent. Approximately one-third of pts may have silent upper tract disease.
- Acute pyelonephritis: Symptoms develop quickly over an interval lasting from hours to a day. Pts are febrile with shaking chills and can have nausea, vomiting, and diarrhea. Symptoms of cystitis may be absent. Marked tenderness may be evident on deep pressure in one or both costovertebral angles or on deep abdominal palpation.
- Urethritis: Women with dysuria, frequency, and pyuria but no growth on bacterial urine cultures may have urethritis due to sexually transmitted pathogens such as *Chlamydia trachomatis*, *Neisseria gonorrhoeae*, or herpes simplex virus (Chap. 90). Pts with hematuria, suprapubic pain, an abrupt onset of illness, an illness duration of <3 days, and a history of UTIs along with a urine culture yielding low counts of *E. coli or S. saprophyticus* usually have cystitis.
- Catheter-associated UTIs (Chap. 85): Most of these infections cause minimal symptoms and no fever; they often resolve after catheter removal. Treatment without catheter removal usually fails. Bacteriuria should be ignored unless the pt develops symptoms or is at high risk for bacteremia.

Diagnosis

- Urine cultures should be performed for all pts with suspected upper tract infections, for those with complicating factors, and when the diagnosis of cystitis is in question. Most symptomatic pts have $\geq 10^5$ bacteria/mL of urine. Bacteriuria from suprapubic aspirates or $\geq 10^2$ bacteria/mL of urine obtained via catheterization is significant.
- The presence of bacteria in Gram-stained uncentrifuged urine indicates infection and correlates with $\geq 10^5$ bacteria/mL in urine cultures.
- Urinalysis: Pyuria is a highly sensitive indicator of infection. Leukocyte esterase "dipstick" positivity is useful when microscopy is not available. Pyuria without bacteriuria may indicate infection with unusual organisms such as *C. trachomatis* or *Mycobacterium tuberculosis* or may be due to noninfectious causes such as calculi. Leukocyte casts are pathognomonic of acute pyelonephritis.

R_X Acute Infections: Urethritis, Cystitis, and Pyelonephritis

Underlying Principles

- Except in acute uncomplicated cystitis in women, a quantitative urine culture with susceptibility testing should precede empirical treatment.
- Factors predisposing to infection should be identified and corrected if possible.
- Relief of clinical symptoms does not always indicate bacteriologic cure.
- Each course of treatment should be classified as a cure or a failure, and recurrent infections should be classified as early (developing within 2 weeks of the end of therapy) or late and as same-strain or different-strain.

- Lower-tract infections usually require only short courses of treatment. Early recurrences may be due to upper-tract foci of infection, while late infections usually represent reinfection.
- Most community-acquired infections are due to antibiotic-sensitive strains, despite increasing antibiotic resistance.
- Antibiotic-resistant infections should be suspected in pts with recurrent infections, instrumentation, or recent hospitalization.

Specific Recommendations

See Table 152-1 for antibiotic choices. Asymptomatic bacteriuria in non-catheterized pts should not be treated unless the pt is pregnant or has other medical conditions such as neutropenia, renal transplantation, or obstruction. Pregnant women should be screened for asymptomatic bacteriuria in the first trimester. Acute pyelonephritis in pregnancy should be managed with hospitalization and parenteral antibiotic therapy. Urologic evaluation should be considered in pts with relapsing infection, a history of childhood infection, stones, or painless hematuria and in women with recurrent pyelonephritis. Most men with UTIs should have a urologic evaluation. Anyone with signs or symptoms of obstruction or stones should undergo prompt urologic evaluation.

Prognosis   Repeated symptomatic UTIs with obstructive uropathy, neurogenic bladder, structural renal disease, or diabetes progress to chronic renal disease with high frequency.

Prevention   Women experiencing symptomatic UTIs ≥3 times a year are candidates for long-term administration of low-dose antibiotics. These women should avoid spermicide use and should void after intercourse. Trimethoprim-sulfamethoxazole (TMP-SMX; 80/400 mg), trimethoprim (100 mg), or nitrofurantoin (50 mg) daily or thrice weekly is effective. Alternatively, if UTIs are temporally related to sexual intercourse, the same regimens prevent infection if given only after intercourse.

PAPILLARY NECROSIS

- Papillary necrosis is an infection of the renal pyramids in association with vascular disease of the kidney or urinary tract obstruction. Acute renal failure with oliguria or anuria can occur.
- Risk factors include diabetes, sickle cell disease, alcoholism, and vascular disease.
- Hematuria, flank or abdominal pain, chills, and fever are common symptoms.

EMPHYSEMATOUS PYELONEPHRITIS

- Emphysematous pyelonephritis is seen in diabetic pts in concert with urinary obstruction and chronic infection.
- This disease is characterized by a rapidly progressive course, fever, leukocytosis, renal parenchymal necrosis, and the accumulation of fermentative gases in kidney and perinephric tissues.
- The syndrome is caused most often by *E. coli* and less commonly by other Enterobacteriaceae.

TABLE 152-1 TREATMENT REGIMENS FOR BACTERIAL URINARY TRACT INFECTIONS

Condition	Characteristic Pathogens	Mitigating Circumstances	Recommended Empirical Treatment[a]
Acute uncomplicated cystitis in women	*Escherichia coli, Staphylococcus saprophyticus, Proteus mirabilis, Klebsiella pneumoniae*	None	3-Day regimens: oral TMP-SMX, TMP, quinolone; 7-day regimen: macrocrystalline nitrofurantoin[b]
		Diabetes, symptoms for >7 d, recent UTI, use of diaphragm, age >65 years	Consider 7-day regimen: oral TMP-SMX, TMP, quinolone[b]
		Pregnancy	Consider 7-day regimen: oral amoxicillin, macrocrystalline nitrofurantoin, cefpodoxime proxetil, or TMP-SMX[b]
Acute uncomplicated pyelonephritis in women	*E. coli, P. mirabilis, S. saprophyticus*	Mild to moderate illness, no nausea or vomiting: outpt therapy	Oral[c] quinolone for 7–14 d (initial dose given IV if desired); or single-dose ceftriaxone (1 g) or gentamicin (3–5 mg/kg) IV followed by oral TMP-SMX[b] for 14 d
		Severe illness or possible urosepsis: hospitalization required	Parenteral[d] quinolone, gentamicin (± ampicillin), ceftriaxone, or aztreonam until defervescence; then oral[c] quinolone, cephalosporin, or TMP-SMX for 14 d

| Complicated UTI in men and women | E. coli, Proteus, Klebsiella, Pseudomonas, Serratia, enterococci, staphylococci | Mild to moderate illness, no nausea or vomiting: outpt therapy | Oral[c] quinolone for 10–14 d |
| | | Severe illness or possible urosepsis: hospitalization required | Parenteral[d] ampicillin and gentamicin, quinolone, ceftriaxone, aztreonam, ticarcillin/clavulanate, or imipenem-cilastatin until defervescence; then oral[c] quinolone or TMP-SMX for 10–21 d |

[a]Treatments listed are those to be prescribed before the etiologic agent is known; Gram's staining can be helpful in the selection of empirical therapy. Such therapy can be modified once the infecting agent has been identified. Fluoroquinolones should not be used in pregnancy. TMP-SMX, although not approved for use in pregnancy, has been widely used. Gentamicin should be used with caution in pregnancy because of its possible toxicity to eighth-nerve development in the fetus.

[b]Multiday oral regimens for cystitis are as follows: TMP-SMX, 160/800 mg q12h; TMP, 100 mg q12h; norfloxacin, 400 mg q12h; ciprofloxacin, 250 mg q12h; ofloxacin, 200 mg q12h; levofloxacin, 250 mg/d; lomefloxacin, 400 mg/d; enoxacin, 400 mg q12h; macrocrystalline nitrofurantoin, 100 mg qid; amoxicillin, 250 mg q8h; cefpodoxime proxetil, 100 mg q12h.

[c]Oral regimens for pyelonephritis and complicated UTI are as follows: TMP-SMX, 160/800 mg q12h; ciprofloxacin, 500 mg q12h; ofloxacin, 200–300 mg q12h; lomefloxacin, 400 mg/d; enoxacin, 400 mg q12h; levofloxacin, 250 mg q12h; amoxicillin, 500 mg q8h; cefpodoxime proxetil, 200 mg q12h.

[d]Parenteral regimens are as follows: ciprofloxacin, 400 mg q12h; ofloxacin, 400 mg q12h; levofloxacin, 500 mg/d; gentamicin, 1 mg/kg q8h; ceftriaxone, 1–2 g/d; ampicillin, 1 g q6h; imipenem-cilastatin, 250–500 mg q6–8h; ticarcillin/clavulanate, 3.2 g q8h; aztreonam, 1 g q8–12h.

Note: TMP-SMX, trimethoprim-sulfamethoxazole.

PROSTATITIS

ACUTE BACTERIAL PROSTATITIS

Acute bacterial prostatitis occurs spontaneously in young men but is associated with indwelling catheters in older men. Pts have fever, chills, dysuria, and a tense or boggy, tender prostate. Prostatic massage can cause bacteremia and should be avoided. Gram's staining and culture of urine identify the etiologic agent. *E. coli* or *Klebsiella* causes most non-catheter-associated cases, while catheter-associated cases are caused by a broader spectrum of pathogens. Third-generation cephalosporins, fluoroquinolones, or aminoglycosides are efficacious.

CHRONIC BACTERIAL PROSTATITIS

Chronic bacterial prostatitis is an uncommon entity. The diagnosis is suggested by a pattern of relapsing UTI in middle-aged men. Symptoms are lacking between episodes, and the prostate feels normal on examination. Some pts have obstructive symptoms or perineal pain. *E. coli*, *Klebsiella*, *Proteus*, or other uropathogenic bacteria can be cultured from expressed prostatic secretions or postmassage urine. Antibiotics relieve acute symptoms, but antibiotic penetration into an uninflamed prostate is poor, and relapse is common. Fluoroquinolones are the most effective agents but must be given for at least 12 weeks. Prolonged courses of low-dose antimicrobial agents may suppress symptoms and keep bladder urine sterile.

CHRONIC PELVIC PAIN SYNDROME

Chronic pelvic pain syndrome is characterized by the symptoms of prostatitis with few clinical signs and no bacterial growth in cultures. In sexually active young men, a sexually transmitted disease is likely. Some pts improve with 4–6 weeks of treatment with erythromycin, doxycycline, TMP-SMX, or a fluoroquinolone, but controlled trials are lacking.

For a more detailed discussion, see Stamm WE: Urinary Tract Infections, Pyelonephritis, and Prostatitis, Chap. 282, p. 1820, in HPIM-17.

153 Renovascular Disease

Ischemic injury to the kidney depends on the rate, site, severity, and duration of vascular compromise. Manifestations range from painful infarction to acute renal failure (ARF), impaired glomerular filtration rate (GFR), hematuria, or tubular dysfunction. Renal ischemia of any etiology may cause renin-mediated hypertension.

ACUTE OCCLUSION OF A RENAL ARTERY

Can be due to thrombosis or embolism (from valvular disease, endocarditis, mural thrombi, or atrial arrhythmias) or to intraoperative occlusion, e.g., during endovascular repair of abdominal aortic aneurysms.

Thrombosis of Renal Arteries Large renal infarcts cause pain, vomiting, nausea, hypertension, fever, proteinuria, hematuria, and elevated lactate dehydrogenase (LDH) and aspartate aminotransferase. In unilateral lesion, renal functional loss depends on contralateral function. IV pyelogram or radionuclide scan shows unilateral hypofunction; ultrasound is typically normal until scarring develops. Renal arteriography establishes diagnosis. With occlusions of large arteries, surgery may be the initial therapy; anticoagulation should be used for occlusions of small arteries. Pts should be evaluated for a thrombotic diathesis, e.g., antiphospholipid syndrome.

Renal Atheroembolism Usually arises when aortic or coronary angiography or surgery causes cholesterol embolization of small renal vessels in a pt with diffuse atherosclerosis. May also be spontaneous or associated with thrombolysis, or rarely may occur after the initiation of anticoagulation (e.g., with warfarin). Renal insufficiency may develop suddenly, a few days or weeks after a procedure or intervention, or gradually; the pace may alternatively be progressive or "stuttering," with punctuated drops in GFR. Associated findings can include retinal ischemia with cholesterol emboli visible on funduscopic examination, pancreatitis, neurologic deficits (especially confusion), livedo reticularis, peripheral embolic phenomena (e.g., gangrenous toes with palpable pedal pulses), abdominal pain from mesenteric emboli, and hypertension (sometimes malignant). Systemic symptoms may also occur, including fever, myalgias, headache, and weight loss. Peripheral eosinophilia, eosinophiluria, and hypocomplementemia may be observed, mimicking other forms of acute and subacute renal injury. Indeed, atheroembolic renal disease is the "great imitator" of clinical nephrology, presenting in rare instances with malignant hypertension, with nephrotic syndrome, or with what looks like rapidly progressive glomerulonephritis with an "active" urinary sediment; the diagnosis is made by history, clinical findings, and/or the renal biopsy.

Renal biopsy is usually successful in detecting the cholesterol emboli in the renal microvasculature, which are seen as needle-shaped clefts after solvent fixation of the biopsy specimen; these emboli are typically associated with an exuberant intravascular inflammatory response.

There is no specific therapy, and pts have a poor overall prognosis due to the associated burden of atherosclerotic vascular disease. However, there is often a partial improvement in renal function several months after the onset of renal impairment.

RENAL VEIN THROMBOSIS

This occurs in a variety of settings, including pregnancy, oral contraceptive use, trauma, nephrotic syndrome (especially membranous nephropathy; see Chap. 150), dehydration (in infants), extrinsic compression of the renal vein (lymph nodes, aortic aneurysm, tumor), and invasion of the renal vein by renal cell carcinoma. Definitive Dx is established by selective renal renography. Thrombolytic therapy may be effective. Oral anticoagulants (warfarin) are usually prescribed for longer–term therapy.

RENAL ARTERY STENOSIS AND ISCHEMIC NEPHROPATHY (See Table 153-1)

Main cause of renovascular hypertension. Due to (1) atherosclerosis (two-thirds of cases; usually men age >60 years, advanced retinopathy, history or findings of generalized atherosclerosis, e.g., femoral bruits) or (2) fibromuscular dysplasia (one-third of cases; usually white women age <45 years, brief history of hypertension). Renal hypoperfusion due to renal artery stenosis (RAS) activates

TABLE 153-1   CLINICAL FINDINGS ASSOCIATED WITH RENAL ARTERY STENOSIS

Hypertension
    Abrupt onset of hypertension before the age of 50 years (suggestive of fibro-
       muscular dysplasia)
    Abrupt onset of hypertension at or after the age of 50 years (suggestive of ath-
       erosclerotic renal artery stenosis)
    Accelerated or malignant hypertension; can sometimes be associated with
       polydipsia and hyponatremia
    Refractory hypertension (not responsive to therapy with ≥3 drugs)
Renal abnormalities
    Unexplained azotemia (suggestive of atherosclerotic renal artery stenosis)
    Azotemia induced by treatment with an angiotensin-converting enzyme
       inhibitor
    Unilateral small kidney
    Unexplained hypokalemia
Other findings
    Abdominal bruit, flank bruit, or both
    Severe retinopathy
    Carotid, coronary, or peripheral vascular disease
    Unexplained congestive heart failure or acute pulmonary edema

Source: From RD Safian, SC Textor: Am J Kidney Dis 36:1089, 2000, reprinted with permission.

the renin-angiotensin-aldosterone (RAA) axis. Suggestive clinical features include onset of hypertension <30 or >50 years of age, abdominal or femoral
bruits, hypokalemic alkalosis, moderate to severe retinopathy, acute onset of
hypertension or malignant hypertension, recurrent episodes of acute, otherwise
unexplained pulmonary edema (typically with bilateral RAS or RAS in a solitary kidney), and hypertension resistant to medical therapy. Malignant hypertension (Chap. 124) may also be caused by renal vascular occlusion. Pts,
particularly those with bilateral atherosclerotic disease, may develop chronic
kidney disease (ischemic nephropathy). Although the incidence is difficult to
assess, ischemic nephropathy is clearly a major cause of end-stage renal disease
(ESRD) in those over 50.

Nitroprusside, labetalol, or calcium antagonists are generally effective in
lowering bp acutely; inhibitors of the RAA axis [e.g., angiotensin-converting
enzyme (ACE) inhibitors, angiotensin II receptor blockers] are the most effective long-term treatment.

The "gold standard" in diagnosis of renal artery stenosis is conventional arteriography. Magnetic resonance angiography (MRA) has been used in many
centers, given the risk of radiographic contrast nephropathy in pts with renal insufficiency; however, the newly appreciated risk of nephrogenic systemic fibrosis (NSF) in pts with renal insufficiency, attributed to gadolinium-containing
MRI contrast agents, has dramatically restricted this practice in most institutions. In pts with normal renal function and hypertension, the captopril (or enal-
aprilat) renogram may be used as a screening test. Lateralization of renal
function [accentuation of the difference between affected and unaffected (or
"less affected") sides] is suggestive of significant vascular disease. Test results
may be falsely negative in the presence of bilateral disease.

Medical therapy is advocated for most pts with renal artery stenosis, such
that investigation of suspected RAS should be reserved for those in whom an
intervention is anticipated. Medical management of atherosclerotic RAS should
include lifestyle modification and management of dyslipidemia (Fig. 153-1).
Intervention should be reserved for the following scenarios: (1) progressive, un-

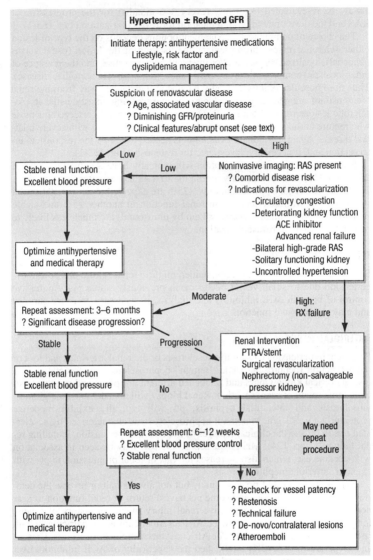

FIGURE 153-1 Management of pts with renal artery stenosis and/or ischemic nephropathy. ACE, angiotensin-converting enzyme; GFR, glomerular filtration rate; PTRA, percutaneous transluminal renal angioplasty; RAS, renal artery stenosis. *[From Textor SC: Renovascular hypertension and ischemic nephropathy, in* The Kidney, *8th Ed, Brenner BM (ed). Philadelphia, Saunders 2008; with permission.]*

explained renal failure, particularly in the setting of improved blood pressure control (i.e., with reduced renal perfusion); (2) poorly controlled hypertension despite multiple agents; (3) malignant hypertension; and/or (4) recurrent episodes of acute, otherwise unexplained pulmonary edema. Notably, pts should always be re-evaluated frequently (every 3–6 months) for the progression of RAS and the development of an indication for revascularization (Fig. 153-1).

The choice of nonmedical management options depends on the type of lesion (atherosclerotic versus fibromuscular), the location of the lesion (ostial versus nonostial), localized surgical and/or interventional expertise, and the presence of other localized comorbidities (i.e., aortic aneurysm or severe aortoiliac disease). Thus fibromuscular lesions, typically located at a distance away from the renal artery ostium, are generally amenable to percutaneous angioplasty; ostial atherosclerotic lesions require stenting. Surgery is more commonly reserved for those who require aortic surgery, but it may be appropriate for those with severe bilateral disease. Again, periodic re-evaluation is needed to follow the response to intervention and, if necessary, investigate for restenosis (Fig. 153-1).

Pts who respond to vascularization will typically have a reduction in bp of 25–30 mmHg systolic, generally within the first 48 h or so after the procedure. For those with renal dysfunction, only ~25% are expected to demonstrate renal improvement, with deterioration in renal function in another 25% and stable function in ~50%. Small kidneys (<8 cm by ultrasound) are much less likely to respond favorably to revascularization.

SCLERODERMA

Scleroderma renal crisis can cause sudden oliguric renal failure and severe hypertension due to small-vessel occlusion in previously stable pts. Aggressive control of bp with ACE inhibitors and dialysis, if necessary, improve survival and may restore renal function.

ARTERIOLAR NEPHROSCLEROSIS

Persistent hypertension causes arteriosclerosis of the renal arterioles and loss of renal function (nephrosclerosis). "Benign" nephrosclerosis is associated with loss of cortical kidney mass and thickened afferent arterioles and mild to moderate impairment of renal function. Renal biopsy will also demonstrate glomerulosclerosis and interstitial nephritis; pts will typically exhibit moderate proteinuria, i.e., <1 g/d. Malignant nephrosclerosis is characterized by accelerated rise in bp and the clinical features of malignant hypertension, including renal failure (Chap. 124). Malignant nephrosclerosis may be seen in association with cocaine use, which also increases the risk of renal progression in pts with "benign" arteriolar nephrosclerosis.

Aggressive control of bp can usually but not always halt or reverse the deterioration of renal function, and some pts have a return of renal function to near normal. Risk factors for progressive renal injury include a history of severe, longstanding hypertension; however, African Americans are at particularly high risk of progressive renal injury. The African American Study of Kidney Disease and Hypertension (AASK) established the superiority of ACE inhibitors over beta blockers or calcium channel blockers, with respect to progression of kidney disease.

THROMBOTIC MICROANGIOPATHIES

The thrombotic microangiopathies (TMAs) are classically subdivided into two general syndromes: thrombotic thrombocytopenic purpura (TTP) and hemolytic uremic syndrome (HUS). TMAs are thus broadly characterized by the presence of ARF, microangiopathic hemolytic anemia, thrombocytopenia, and neurologic dysfunction. Pts with TTP may suffer from the classic pentad of microangiopathic hemolytic anemia, fever, thrombocytopenia, neurologic symp-

TABLE 153-2 CAUSES OF THROMBOTIC MICROANGIOPATHY

Genetic
  TTP: deficiency of ADAMTS13 (vWF protease)
  HUS: deficiency of complement factor H, complement factor I, membrane
    cofactor protein
Idiopathic
  TTP: acquired antibodies to ADAMTS13 (vWF protease)
  HUS: acquired antibodies to complement factor H, complement factor I,
    membrane cofactor protein
Infectious
  Bacterial: *Escherichia coli* O157:H7, *Shigella*, *Salmonella*, *Campylobacter*, etc.
  Viral: HIV, CMV, EBV, etc.
Drug-related
  Calcineurin inhibitors: tacrolimus and cyclosporine
  Antiplatelet agents: ticlopidine, clopidogrel
  Quinine
  Chemotherapy: mitomycin C, gemcitabine, cisplatin
  OKT3 monoclonal antibody
  Angiogenesis/VEGF inhibitors: bevacizumab, sunitinib, sorafenib
Autoimmune
  Antiphospholipid antibody syndrome
  SLE, vasculitis
Miscellaneous
  Post–bone marrow transplantation
  Disseminated malignancy
  Pregnancy

Note: TTP, thrombotic thrombocytopenic purpura; ADAMTS13, a disintegrin-like and metalloprotease with thrombospondin type I motif-13; vWF, von Willebrand factor; HUS, hemolytic uremic syndrome; CMV, cytomegalovirus; EBV, Epstein-Barr virus; VEGF, vascular endothelial growth factor; SLE, systemic lupus erythematosus.

toms and signs, and renal dysfunction. Extrarenal symptoms are in contrast less prominent or common, but not unheard of, in postdiarrheal HUS.

The major causes of TMA are listed in Table 153-2; the common pathogenic pathway is endothelial injury. In idiopathic and familial TTP, pts have a marked deficiency in the ADAMTS13 protease, leading to accumulation of ultra-large, unprocessed von Willebrand Factor (vWF) polymers, platelet aggregation, and TMA. In contrast, postdiarrheal HUS is associated with presence of a bacterial toxin (Shiga toxin or verotoxin) that causes endothelial injury; children and the elderly are particularly susceptible. Pts with atypical or nondiarrheal HUS may in turn have inherited or acquired deficiencies in membrane-associated regulatory proteins of the alternative complement pathway, enhancing endothelial sensitivity to complement.

Laboratory evaluation will usually reveal evidence of a microangiopathic hemolytic anemia, although this may be absent in certain causes, e.g., antiphospholipid antibody syndrome. The reticulocyte count should be elevated, along with an increase in the red cell distribution width. Hemolysis should increase levels of LDH and decrease circulating haptoglobin, with a negative Coomb's test. Examination of the peripheral smear is key, since the presence of schistocytes will help establish the diagnosis. Specific diagnostic tests—e.g., HIV testing, antiphospholipid antibody screens—may be useful in the differential diagnosis. Measurement of vWF protease activity promises considerable diagnostic and therapeutic utility; however, at this point, this is not routinely available in a time frame suitable for routine clinical use. Renal biopsy will classically demonstrate fibrin- and/or vWF-positive thrombi in arterioles and glomeruli, endothelial injury, and widening of the subendothelial space leading to a "double contour" appearance of the glomerular capillaries.

Treatment of TMA depends on the underlying pathogenesis. Idiopathic TTP is due to the presence of circulating antibody inhibitors of ADAMTS13 and thus responds to plasma exchange, combining plasmapheresis (removal of antibody) and infusion of fresh-frozen plasma (repletion with native ADAMTS13/vWF protease).

TOXEMIAS OF PREGNANCY

Preeclampsia is characterized by hypertension, proteinuria, edema, consumptive coagulopathy, sodium retention, hyperuricemia, and hyperreflexia; eclampsia is the further development of seizures. Glomerular swelling and/or ischemia causes renal insufficiency. Coagulation abnormalities and ARF may occur. Treatment consists of bed rest, sedation, control of neurologic manifestations with magnesium sulfate, control of hypertension with vasodilators and other antihypertensive agents proven safe in pregnancy, and delivery of the infant.

VASCULITIS

Renal complications are frequent and severe in polyarteritis nodosa, hypersensitivity angiitis, Wegener's granulomatosis, and other forms of vasculitis (Chap. 168). Therapy is directed toward the underlying disease.

SICKLE CELL NEPHROPATHY

The hypertonic and relatively hypoxic renal medulla coupled with slow blood flow in the vasa recta favors sickling. Papillary necrosis, cortical infarcts, functional tubule abnormalities (nephrogenic diabetes insipidus), glomerulopathy, nephrotic syndrome, and, rarely, ESRD may be complications.

For a more detailed discussion, see Badr KF, Brenner BM: Vascular Injury to the Kidney, Chap. 280, p. 1811, in HPIM-17.

154 Nephrolithiasis

Renal calculi are common, affecting ~1% of the population, and recurrent in more than half of pts. Stone formation begins when urine becomes supersaturated with insoluble components due to (1) low urinary volume, (2) excessive or insufficient excretion of selected compounds, or (3) other factors (e.g., urinary pH) that diminish solubility. Approximately 75% of stones are Ca-based (the majority Ca oxalate; also Ca phosphate and other mixed stones), 15% struvite (magnesium-ammonium-phosphate), 5% uric acid, and 1% cystine, reflecting the metabolic disturbance(s) from which they arise.

SIGNS AND SYMPTOMS

Stones in the renal pelvis may be asymptomatic or cause hematuria alone; with passage, obstruction may occur at any site along the collecting system. Obstruction related to the passing of a stone leads to severe pain, often radiating to the groin, sometimes accompanied by intense visceral symptoms (i.e., nausea, vomiting, diaphoresis, light-headedness), hematuria, pyuria, urinary tract infection (UTI), and, rarely, hydronephrosis. In contrast, staghorn calculi, associated with recurrent UTI with urea-splitting organisms (*Proteus, Klebsiella, Providencia, Morganella*, and others), may be completely asymptomatic, presenting with loss of renal function.

STONE COMPOSITION

Most stones are composed of Ca oxalate. These may be associated with hypercalciuria and/or hyperoxaluria. Hypercalciuria can be seen in association with a very high-Na diet, loop diuretic therapy, distal (type I) renal tubular acidosis (RTA), sarcoidosis, Cushing's syndrome, aldosterone excess, or conditions associated with hypercalcemia (e.g., primary hyperparathyroidism, vitamin D excess, milk-alkali syndrome), or it may be idiopathic.

Hyperoxaluria may be seen with intestinal (especially ileal) malabsorption syndromes (e.g., inflammatory bowel disease, pancreatitis), due to reduced intestinal secretion of oxalate and/or the binding of intestinal Ca by fatty acids within the bowel lumen, with enhanced absorption of free oxalate and hyperoxaluria. Ca oxalate stones may also form due to (1) a deficiency of urinary citrate, an inhibitor of stone formation that is underexcreted with metabolic acidosis; and (2) hyperuricosuria (see below). Ca phosphate stones are much less common and tend to occur in the setting of an abnormally high urinary pH (7–8), usually in association with a complete or partial distal RTA.

Struvite stones form in the collecting system when infection with urea-splitting organisms is present. Struvite is the most common component of staghorn calculi and obstruction. Risk factors include previous UTI, nonstruvite stone disease, urinary catheters, neurogenic bladder (e.g., with diabetes or multiple sclerosis), and instrumentation.

Uric acid stones develop when the urine is saturated with uric acid in the presence of an acid urine pH; pts typically have underlying metabolic syndrome and insulin resistance, associated with a relative defect in ammoniagenesis and urine pH that is <5.4 and often <5.0. Pts with myeloproliferative disorders (esp. after treatment with chemotherapy), gout, acute and chronic renal failure, and following cyclosporine therapy often develop hyperuricemia and hyperuricosuria and are at risk for stones if the urine volume diminishes. Hyperuricosuria without hyperuricemia may be seen in association with certain drugs (e.g., probenecid, high-dose salicylates).

Cystine stones are the result of a rare inherited defect in renal and intestinal transport of several dibasic amino acids; the overexcretion of cystine (cysteine disulfide), which is relatively insoluble, leads to nephrolithiasis. Stones begin in childhood and are a rare cause of staghorn calculi; they occasionally lead to end-stage renal disease. Cystine stones are more likely to form in acidic urinary pH.

WORKUP

Although some have advocated a complete workup after a first stone episode, others would defer that evaluation until there has been evidence of recurrence or if there is no obvious cause (e.g., low fluid intake during the summer months with obvious dehydration). Table 154-1 outlines a reasonable workup for an outpatient with an uncomplicated kidney stone. On occasion, a stone is recov-

TABLE 154-1 WORKUP FOR AN OUTPATIENT WITH A RENAL STONE

1. Dietary and fluid intake history
2. Careful medical history and physical examination, focusing on systemic diseases
3. Noncontrast helical CT, with 5-mm CT cuts
4. Routine UA; presence of crystals, hematuria, measurement of urine pH
5. Serum chemistries: BUN, Cr, uric acid, calcium, phosphate, chloride, bicarbonate, PTH
6. Timed urine collections (at least 1 day during week, 1 day on weekend): Cr, Na, K, urea nitrogen, uric acid, calcium, phosphate, oxalate, citrate, pH

Note: UA, urinalysis; BUN, blood urea nitrogen; Cr, creatinine; PTH, parathyroid hormone.

ered and can be analyzed for content, yielding important clues to pathogenesis and management. For example, a predominance of Ca phosphate suggests underlying distal RTA or hyperparathyroidism.

℞ Nephrolithiasis

Treatment of renal calculi is often empirical, based on odds (Ca oxalate stones most common), clinical Hx, and/or the metabolic workup. An increase in fluid intake to at least 2.5–3 L/d is perhaps the single most effective intervention, regardless of the type of stone. Conservative recommendations for pts with Ca oxalate stones (i.e., low-salt, low-fat, moderate-protein diet) are thought to be healthful in general and therefore advisable in pts whose condition is otherwise uncomplicated. In contrast to prior assumptions, dietary calcium intake does not contribute to stone risk; rather, dietary calcium may help to reduce oxalate absorption and reduce stone risk. Table 154-2 outlines stone-specific therapies for pts with complex or recurrent nephrolithiasis.

TABLE 154-2 SPECIFIC THERAPIES FOR NEPHROLITHIASIS

Stone Type	Dietary Modifications	Other
Calcium oxalate	Increase fluid intake Moderate sodium intake Moderate oxalate intake Moderate protein intake Moderate fat intake	Citrate supplementation (calcium or potassium salts > sodium) Cholestyramine or other therapy for fat malabsorption Thiazides if hypercalciuric Allopurinol if hyperuricosuric
Calcium phosphate	Increase fluid intake Moderate sodium intake	Thiazides if hypercalciuric Treat hyperparathyroidism if present Alkali for distal renal tubular acidosis
Struvite	Increase fluid intake; same as calcium oxalate if evidence of calcium oxalate nidus for struvite	Methenamine and vitamin C or daily suppressive antibiotic therapy (e.g., trimethoprim-sulfamethoxazole)
Uric acid	Increase fluid intake Moderate dietary protein intake	Allopurinol Alkali therapy (K^+ citrate) to raise urine pH to 6.0–6.5
Cystine	Increase fluid intake	Alkali therapy Penicillamine

Note: Sodium excretion correlates with calcium excretion.

For a more detailed discussion, see Asplin JR, Coe FL, Favus MJ: Nephrolithiasis, Chap. 281, p. 1815, in HPIM-17

155 Urinary Tract Obstruction

Urinary tract obstruction (UTO), a potentially reversible cause of renal failure (RF), should be considered in all cases of acute or abrupt worsening of chronic RF. Consequences depend on duration and severity and whether the obstruction is unilateral or bilateral. UTO may occur at any level from collecting tubule to urethra. It is preponderant in women (pelvic tumors), elderly men (prostatic disease), diabetic pts (papillary necrosis), pts with neurologic diseases (spinal cord injury or multiple sclerosis, with neurogenic bladder), and individuals with retroperitoneal lymphadenopathy or fibrosis, vesicoureteral reflux, nephrolithiasis, or other causes of functional urinary retention (e.g., anticholinergic drugs).

CLINICAL MANIFESTATIONS

Pain can occur in some settings (obstruction due to stones) but is not common. In men, there is frequently a history of prostatism. Physical exam may reveal an enlarged bladder by percussion over the lower abdominal wall. Other findings depend on the clinical scenario. Prostatic hypertrophy can be determined by digital rectal examination. A bimanual examination in women may show a pelvic or rectal mass. The workup of pts with RF suspected of having UTO is shown in Fig. 155-1. Laboratory studies may show marked elevations of blood urea nitrogen and creatinine; if the obstruction has been of sufficient duration, there may be evidence of tubulointerstitial disease (e.g., hyperkalemia, non-anion-gap metabolic acidosis, mild hypernatremia). Urinalysis is most often benign or with a small number of cells; heavy proteinuria is rare. An obstructing stone may be visualized on abdominal radiography or helical noncontrast CT with 5-mm cuts.

Ultrasonography can be used to assess the degree of hydronephrosis and the integrity of the renal parenchyma; CT or IV urography may be required to localize the level of obstruction. Calyceal dilation is commonly seen; it may be absent with hyperacute obstruction, upper tract encasement by tumor or retroperitoneal fibrosis, or indwelling staghorn calculi. Kidney size may indicate the duration of obstruction. It should be noted that unilateral obstruction may be prolonged and severe (ultimately leading to loss of renal function in the obstructed kidney), with no hint of abnormality on physical exam and laboratory survey.

℞ Treatment

Management of acute RF associated with UTO is dictated by (1) the level of obstruction (upper vs. lower tract), and (2) the acuity of the obstruction and its clinical consequences, including renal dysfunction and infection. Benign causes of UTO, including bladder outlet obstruction and nephrolithiasis, should be ruled out because conservative management, including Foley cathe-

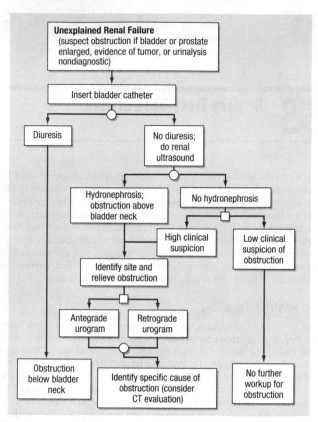

FIGURE 155-1 Diagnostic approach for urinary tract obstruction in unexplained renal failure. Circles represent diagnostic procedures and squares indicate clinical decisions based on available data.

ter placement and IV fluids, respectively, will usually relieve the obstruction in most cases.

Among more seriously ill pts, ureteral obstruction due to tumor is the most common and concerning cause of UTO. If technically feasible, ureteral obstruction due to tumor is best managed by cystoscopic placement of a ureteral stent. Otherwise, the placement of nephrostomy tubes with external drainage may be required. IV antibiotics should also be given if there are signs of pyelonephritis or urosepsis. Fluid and electrolyte status should be carefully monitored after obstruction is relieved. There may be a physiologic natriuresis/diuresis related to volume overload. However, there may be an "inappropriate" natriuresis/diuresis related to (1) elevated urea nitrogen, leading to an osmotic diuresis; and (2) acquired nephrogenic diabetes insipidus. Hypernatremia, sometimes of a severe degree, may develop.

For a more detailed discussion, see Seifter JL, Brenner BM: Urinary Tract Obstruction, Chap. 283, p. 1827, in HPIM-17.

156 Peptic Ulcer and Related Disorders

PEPTIC ULCER DISEASE (PUD)

PUD occurs most commonly in duodenal bulb (duodenal ulcer, DU) and stomach (gastric ulcer, GU). It may also occur in esophagus, pyloric channel, duodenal loop, jejunum, Meckel's diverticulum. PUD results when "aggressive" factors (gastric acid, pepsin) overwhelm "defensive" factors involved in mucosal resistance (gastric mucus, bicarbonate, microcirculation, prostaglandins, mucosal "barrier"), and from effects of *Helicobacter pylori*.

Causes and Risk Factors   **General**   *H. pylori* is a spiral urease-producing organism that colonizes gastric antral mucosa in up to 100% of persons with DU and 80% with GU. It is also found in normals (increasing prevalence with age) and in those of low socioeconomic status. *H. pylori* is invariably associated with histologic evidence of active chronic gastritis, which over years can lead to atrophic gastritis and gastric cancer. The other major cause of ulcers (those not due to *H. pylori*) is nonsteroidal anti-inflammatory drugs (NSAIDs). Fewer than 1% are due to gastrinoma (Zollinger-Ellison syndrome). Other risk factors and associations: hereditary (? increased parietal cell number), smoking, hypercalcemia, mastocytosis, blood group O (antigens may bind *H. pylori*). Unproven: stress, coffee, alcohol.

Duodenal Ulcer   Mild gastric acid hypersecretion resulting from (1) increased release of gastrin, presumably due to (a) stimulation of antral G cells by cytokines released by inflammatory cells and (b) diminished production of somatostatin by D cells, both resulting from *H. pylori* infection; and (2) an exaggerated acid response to gastrin due to an increased parietal cell mass resulting from gastrin stimulation. These abnormalities reverse rapidly with eradication of *H. pylori*. However, a mildly elevated maximum gastric acid output in response to exogenous gastrin persists in some pts long after eradication of *H. pylori*, suggesting that gastric acid hypersecretion may be, in part, genetically determined. *H. pylori* may also result in elevated serum pepsinogen levels. Mucosal defense in duodenum is compromised by toxic effects of *H. pylori* infection on patches of gastric metaplasia that result from gastric acid hypersecretion or rapid gastric emptying. Other risk factors include glucocorticoids, NSAIDs, chronic renal failure, renal transplantation, cirrhosis, chronic lung disease.

Gastric Ulcer   *H. pylori* is also principal cause. Gastric acid secretory rates are usually normal or reduced, possibly reflecting earlier age of infection by *H. pylori* than in DU pts. Gastritis due to reflux of duodenal contents (including bile) may play a role. Chronic salicylate or NSAID use may account for 15–30% of GUs and increase risk of associated bleeding, perforation.

Clinical Features   **Duodenal Ulcer**   Burning epigastric pain 90 min to 3 h after meals, often nocturnal, relieved by food.

Gastric Ulcer   Burning epigastric pain made worse by or unrelated to food; anorexia, food aversion, weight loss (in 40%). Great individual variation. Similar symptoms may occur in persons without demonstrated peptic ulcers ("nonulcer dyspepsia"); less responsive to standard therapy.

Complications   Bleeding, obstruction, penetration causing acute pancreatitis, perforation, intractability.

Diagnosis   Duodenal Ulcer   Upper endoscopy or upper GI barium radiography.

Gastric Ulcer   Upper endoscopy preferable to exclude possibility that ulcer is malignant (brush cytology, ≥6 pinch biopsies of ulcer margin). Radiographic features suggesting malignancy: ulcer within a mass, folds that do not radiate from ulcer margin, a large ulcer (>2.5–3 cm).

Detection of *H. pylori*   Detection of antibodies in serum (inexpensive, preferred when endoscopy is not required); rapid urease test of antral biopsy (when endoscopy is required). Urea breath test generally used to confirm eradication of *H. pylori*, if necessary. The fecal antigen test is sensitive, specific, and inexpensive (Table 156-1).

Rx   Peptic Ulcer Disease

MEDICAL
Objectives: pain relief, healing, prevention of complications, prevention of recurrences. For GU, exclude malignancy (follow endoscopically to healing). Dietary restriction unnecessary with contemporary drugs; discontinue NSAIDs; smoking may prevent healing and should be stopped. Eradication of *H. pylori* markedly reduces rate of ulcer relapse and is indicated for all DUs and GUs associated with *H. pylori* (Table 156-2). Sequential therapy is most effective in

TABLE 156-1   TESTS FOR DETECTION OF *H. PYLORI*

Test	Sensitivity/ Specificity, %	Comments
Invasive (Endoscopy/Biopsy Required)		
Rapid urease	80–95/95–100	Simple; false negative with recent use of PPIs, antibiotics, or bismuth compounds
Histology	80–90/>95	Requires pathology processing and staining; provides histologic information
Culture	–/–	Time-consuming, expensive, dependent on experience; allows determination of antibiotic susceptibility
Noninvasive		
Serology	>80/>90	Inexpensive, convenient; not useful for early follow-up
Urea breath test	>90/>90	Simple, rapid; useful for early follow-up; false negative with recent therapy (see rapid urease test); exposure to low-dose radiation with 14-C test
Stool antigen	>90/>90	Inexpensive, convenient; not established for eradication but promising

Note: PPI, proton pump inhibitor.

TABLE 156-2 REGIMENS RECOMMENDED FOR ERADICATION OF *H. PYLORI* INFECTION

Drug	Dose
Triple Therapy	
1. Bismuth subsalicylate *plus*	2 tablets qid
Metronidazole *plus*	250 mg qid
Tetracycline[a]	500 mg qid
2. Ranitidine bismuth citrate *plus*	400 mg bid
Tetracycline *plus*	500 mg bid
Clarithromycin *or* metronidazole	500 mg bid
3. Omeprazole (lansoprazole) *plus*	20 mg bid (30 mg bid)
Clarithromycin *plus*	250 or 500 mg bid
Metronidazole[b] *or*	500 mg bid
Amoxicillin[c]	1 g bid
Quadruple Therapy	
Omeprazole (lansoprazole)	20 mg (30 mg) daily
Bismuth subsalicylate	2 tablets qid
Metronidazole	250 mg qid
Tetracycline	500 mg qid
Sequential Therapy	
Pantoprazole	40 mg bid days 1–10
Amoxicillin	1 g bid days 1–5
Clarithromycin	500 mg bid days 6–10
Tinidazole	500 mg bid days 6–10

[a]Alternative: use prepacked Helidac.
[b]Alternative: use prepacked Prevpac.
[c]Use either metronidazole or amoxicillin, but not both.

the treatment-naïve patient. Acid suppression is generally included in regimen. Standard drugs (H_2 receptor blockers, sucralfate, antacids) heal 80–90% of DUs and 60% of GUs in 6 weeks; healing is more rapid with omeprazole (20 mg/d).

SURGERY

Used for complications (persistent or recurrent bleeding, obstruction, perforation) or, uncommonly, intractability (first screen for surreptitious NSAID use and gastrinoma). For DU, see Table 156-3. For GU, perform subtotal gastrectomy.

TABLE 156-3 SURGICAL TREATMENT OF DUODENAL ULCER

Operation	Recurrence Rate	Complication Rate
Vagotomy + antrectomy (Billroth I or II)[a]	1%	Highest
Vagotomy and pyloroplasty	10%	Intermediate
Parietal cell (proximal gastric, superselective) vagotomy	≥10%	Lowest

[a]Billroth I, gastroduodenostomy; Billroth II, gastrojejunostomy.

Complications of Surgery

(1) Obstructed afferent loop (Billroth II), (2) bile reflux gastritis, (3) dumping syndrome (rapid gastric emptying with abdominal distress + postprandial vasomotor symptoms), (4) postvagotomy diarrhea, (5) bezoar, (6) anemia (iron, B_{12}, folate malabsorption), (7) malabsorption (poor mixing of gastric contents, pancreatic juices, bile; bacterial overgrowth), (8) osteomalacia and osteoporosis (vitamin D and Ca malabsorption), (9) gastric remnant carcinoma.

APPROACH TO THE PATIENT WITH PEPTIC ULCER DISEASE

Optimal approach is uncertain. Serologic testing for *H. pylori* and treating, if present, may be cost-effective. Other options include trial of acid-suppressive therapy, endoscopy only in treatment failures, or initial endoscopy in all cases.

GASTROPATHIES

Erosive Gastropathies Hemorrhagic gastritis, multiple gastric erosions may be caused by aspirin and other NSAIDs (lower risk with newer agents, e.g., nabumetone and etodolac, which do not inhibit gastric mucosal prostaglandins) or severe stress (burns, sepsis, trauma, surgery, shock, or respiratory, renal, or liver failure). Pt may be asymptomatic or experience epigastric discomfort, nausea, hematemesis, or melena. Diagnosis is made by upper endoscopy.

Rx Erosive Gastropathies

Removal of offending agent and maintenance of O_2 and blood volume as required. For prevention of stress ulcers in critically ill pts, hourly oral administration of liquid antacids (e.g., Maalox 30 mL), IV H_2 receptor antagonist (e.g., cimetidine, 300-mg bolus + 37.5–50 mg/h IV), or both is recommended to maintain gastric pH > 4. Alternatively, sucralfate slurry, 1 g PO q6h, can be given; does not raise gastric pH and may thus avoid increased risk of aspiration pneumonia associated with liquid antacids. Pantoprazole can be administered IV to suppress gastric acid in the critically ill. Misoprostol, 200 µg PO qid, or profound acid suppression (e.g., famotidine, 40 mg PO bid) can be used with NSAIDs to prevent NSAID-induced ulcers.

Chronic Gastritis Identified histologically by an inflammatory cell infiltrate dominated by lymphocytes and plasma cells with scant neutrophils. In its early stage, the changes are limited to the lamina propria (*superficial gastritis*). When the disease progresses to destroy glands, it becomes *atrophic gastritis*. The final stage is *gastric atrophy*, in which the mucosa is thin and the infiltrate sparse. Chronic gastritis can be classified based on predominant site of involvement.

Type A Gastritis This is the body-predominant and less common form. Generally asymptomatic, common in elderly; autoimmune mechanism may be associated with achlorhydria, pernicious anemia, and increased risk of gastric cancer (value of screening endoscopy uncertain). Antibodies to parietal cells present in >90%.

Type B Gastritis This is antral-predominant disease and caused by *H. pylori*. Often asymptomatic but may be associated with dyspepsia. Atrophic gastritis, gastric atrophy, gastric lymphoid follicles, and gastric B cell lymphomas may occur. Infection early in life or in setting of malnutrition or low gastric acid output is associated with gastritis of entire stomach (including body) and increased risk of gastric cancer. Eradication of *H. pylori* (Table 156-2) not routinely recommended unless PUD or gastric mucosa-associated lymphoid tissue (MALT) lymphoma is present.

Specific Types of Gastropathy or Gastritis Alcoholic gastropathy (submucosal hemorrhages), Ménétrier's disease (hypertrophic gastropathy), eosinophilic gastritis, granulomatous gastritis, Crohn's disease, sarcoidosis, infections (tuberculosis, syphilis, fungi, viruses, parasites), pseudolymphoma, radiation, corrosive gastritis.

ZOLLINGER-ELLISON (Z-E) SYNDROME (GASTRINOMA)

Consider when ulcer disease is severe, refractory to therapy, associated with ulcers in atypical locations, or associated with diarrhea. Tumors are usually pancreatic or in duodenum (submucosal, often small), may be multiple, slowly growing; >60% malignant; 25% associated with MEN 1, i.e., multiple endocrine neoplasia type 1 (gastrinoma, hyperparathyroidism, pituitary neoplasm), often duodenal, small, multicentric, less likely to metastasize to liver than pancreatic gastrinomas but often metastasize to local lymph nodes.

Diagnosis **Suggestive** Basal acid output > 15 mmol/h; basal/maximal acid output > 60%; large mucosal folds on endoscopy or upper GI radiograph.

Confirmatory Serum gastrin > 1000 ng/L or rise in gastrin of 200 ng/L following IV secretin and, if necessary, rise of 400 ng/L following IV calcium (Table 156-4).

Differential Diagnosis **Increased Gastric Acid Secretion** Z-E syndrome, antral G cell hyperplasia or hyperfunction (? due to *H. pylori*), postgastrectomy retained antrum, renal failure, massive small bowel resection, chronic gastric outlet obstruction.

Normal or Decreased Gastric Acid Secretion Pernicious anemia, chronic gastritis, gastric cancer, vagotomy, pheochromocytoma.

℞ Zollinger-Ellison Syndrome

Omeprazole, beginning at 60 mg PO q A.M. and increasing until maximal gastric acid output is <10 mmol/h before next dose, is drug of choice during evaluation and in pts who are not surgical candidates; dose can often be reduced over time. Radiolabeled octreotide scanning has emerged as the most sensitive test for detecting primary tumors and metastases; may be supplemented

TABLE 156-4 DIFFERENTIAL DIAGNOSTIC TESTS

		Gastrin Response to	
Condition	Fasting Gastrin	IV Secretin	Food
DU	N (≤150 ng/L)	NC	Slight ↑
Z-E	↑↑↑	↑↑↑	NC
Antral G (gastrin) cell hyperplasia	↑	↑, NC	↑↑↑

Note: DU, duodenal ulcer; N, normal; NC, no change; Z-E, Zollinger-Ellison syndrome.

by endoscopic ultrasonography. Exploratory laparotomy with resection of primary tumor and solitary metastases is done when possible. In pts with MEN 1, tumor is often multifocal and unresectable; treat hyperparathyroidism first (hypergastrinemia may improve). For unresectable tumors, parietal cell vagotomy may enhance control of ulcer disease by drugs. Chemotherapy is used for metastatic tumor to control symptoms (e.g., streptozocin, 5-fluorouracil, doxorubicin, or interferon α); 40% partial response rate.

For a more detailed discussion, see Del Valle J: Peptic Ulcer Disease and Related Disorders, Chap. 287, p. 1855, in HPIM-17.

157 Inflammatory Bowel Diseases

Inflammatory bowel diseases (IBD) are chronic inflammatory disorders of unknown etiology involving the GI tract. Peak occurrence is between ages 15 and 30 and between ages 60 and 80, but onset may occur at any age. Epidemiologic features are shown in Table 157-1. Pathogenesis of IBD involves activation of immune cells by unknown inciting agent (? microorganism, dietary component, bacterial or self-antigen) leading to release of cytokines and inflammatory mediators. Genetic component suggested by increased risk in first-degree relatives of pts with IBD and concurrence of type of IBD, location of Crohn's disease, and clinical course. Reported associations include HLA-DR2 in Japanese patients with ulcerative colitis and a Crohn's disease–related gene called *CARD15* on chromosome 16p. *CARD15* mutations may account for 10% of CD risk. Other potential pathogenic factors include serum antineutrophil cytoplasmic antibodies (ANCA) in 70% of pts with ulcerative colitis (also in 5–10% of Crohn's disease pts) and antibodies to *Saccharomyces cerevisiae* (ASCA) in 60–70% of Crohn's disease pts (also in 10–15% of ulcerative colitis pts and 5% of normal controls). Granulomatous angiitis (vasculitis) may occur in Crohn's disease. Acute flares may be pre-

TABLE 157-1	**EPIDEMIOLOGY OF IBD**	
	Ulcerative Colitis	**Crohn's Disease**
Incidence (North America) per person-years	2.2–14.3/100,000	3.1–14.6/100,000
Age of onset	15–30 & 60–80	15–30 & 60–80
Ethnicity	Jewish > Non-Jewish Caucasian > African American > Hispanic > Asian	
Male:female ratio	1:1	1.1–1.8:1
Smoking	May prevent disease	May cause disease
Oral contraceptives	No increased risk	Odds ratio 1.4
Appendectomy	Protective	Not protective
Monozygotic twins	6% concordance	58% concordance
Dizygotic twins	0% concordance	4% concordance

cipitated by infections, nonsteroidal anti-inflammatory drugs (NSAIDs), stress. Onset of ulcerative colitis often follows cessation of smoking.

ULCERATIVE COLITIS (UC)

Pathology Colonic mucosal inflammation; rectum almost always involved, with inflammation extending continuously (no skip areas) proximally for a variable extent; histologic features include epithelial damage, inflammation, crypt abscesses, loss of goblet cells.

Clinical Manifestations Bloody diarrhea, mucus, fever, abdominal pain, tenesmus, weight loss; spectrum of severity (majority of cases are mild, limited to rectosigmoid). In severe cases dehydration, anemia, hypokalemia, hypoalbuminemia.

Complications Toxic megacolon, colonic perforation; cancer risk related to extent and duration of colitis; often preceded by or coincident with dysplasia, which may be detected on surveillance colonoscopic biopsies.

Diagnosis Sigmoidoscopy/colonoscopy: mucosal erythema, granularity, friability, exudate, hemorrhage, ulcers, inflammatory polyps (pseudopolyps). Barium enema: loss of haustrations, mucosal irregularity, ulcerations.

CROHN'S DISEASE (CD)

Pathology Any part of GI tract, usually terminal ileum and/or colon; transmural inflammation, bowel wall thickening, linear ulcerations, and submucosal thickening leading to cobblestone pattern; discontinuous (skip areas); histologic features include transmural inflammation, granulomas (often absent), fissures, fistulas.

Clinical Manifestations Fever, abdominal pain, diarrhea (often without blood), fatigue, weight loss, growth retardation in children; acute ileitis mimicking appendicitis; anorectal fissures, fistulas, abscesses. Clinical course falls into three broad patterns: (1) inflammatory, (2) stricturing, and (3) fistulizing.

Complications Intestinal obstruction (edema vs. fibrosis); rarely toxic megacolon or perforation; intestinal fistulas to bowel, bladder, vagina, skin, soft tissue, often with abscess formation; bile salt malabsorption leading to cholesterol gallstones and/or oxalate kidney stones; intestinal malignancy; amyloidosis.

Diagnosis Sigmoidoscopy/colonoscopy, barium enema, upper GI and small-bowel series: nodularity, rigidity, ulcers that may be deep or longitudinal, cobblestoning, skip areas, strictures, fistulas. CT may show thickened, matted bowel loops or an abscess.

DIFFERENTIAL DIAGNOSIS

Infectious Enterocolitis *Shigella, Salmonella, Campylobacter, Yersinia* (acute ileitis), *Plesiomonas shigelloides, Aeromonas hydrophila, Escherichia coli* serotype O157:H7, *Gonorrhea, Lymphogranuloma venereum, Clostridium difficile* (pseudomembranous colitis), tuberculosis, amebiasis, cytomegalovirus, AIDS.

Others Ischemic bowel disease, appendicitis, diverticulitis, radiation enterocolitis, bile salt–induced diarrhea (ileal resection), drug-induced colitis (e.g., NSAIDs), bleeding colonic lesion (e.g., neoplasm), irritable bowel syndrome (no bleeding), microscopic (lymphocytic) or collagenous colitis (chronic watery diarrhea)—normal colonoscopy, but biopsies show superficial colonic epithelial inflammation and, in collagenous colitis, a thick subepithelial layer of collagen; response to aminosalicylates and glucocorticoids variable.

EXTRAINTESTINAL MANIFESTATIONS OF UC AND CD

1. *Joint*: Peripheral arthritis—parallels activity of bowel disease; ankylosing spondylitis and sacroiliitis (associated with HLA-B27)—activity independent of bowel disease.
2. *Skin*: Erythema nodosum, aphthous ulcers, pyoderma gangrenosum, cutaneous Crohn's disease.
3. *Eye*: Episcleritis, iritis, uveitis.
4. *Liver*: Fatty liver, "pericholangitis" (intrahepatic sclerosing cholangitis), primary sclerosing cholangitis, cholangiocarcinoma, chronic hepatitis.
5. *Others*: Autoimmune hemolytic anemia, phlebitis, pulmonary embolus (hypercoagulable state).

℞ Inflammatory Bowel Diseases See Fig. 157-1

Supportive

Antidiarrheal agents (diphenoxylate and atropine, loperamide) in mild disease; IV hydration and blood transfusions in severe disease; parenteral nutrition or defined enteral formulas—effective as primary therapy in CD, although high relapse rate when oral feeding is resumed; should not replace drug therapy; important role in preoperative preparation of malnourished pt; emotional support.

Sulfasalazine and Aminosalicylates

Active component of sulfasalazine is 5-aminosalicylic acid (5-ASA) linked to sulfapyridine carrier; useful in colonic disease of mild to moderate severity (1–1.5 g PO qid); efficacy in maintaining remission demonstrated only for UC (500 mg PO qid). Toxicity (generally due to sulfapyridine component): dose-related—nausea, headache, rarely hemolytic anemia—may resolve when drug dose is lowered; idiosyncratic—fever, rash, neutropenia, pancreatitis, hepatitis, etc.; miscellaneous—oligospermia. Newer aminosalicylates are as effective as sulfasalazine but with fewer side effects. Enemas containing 4 g of 5-ASA (mesalamine) may be used in distal UC, 1 nightly retained qhs until remission, then q2hs or q3hs. Suppositories containing 500 mg of 5-ASA may be used in proctitis.

Glucocorticoids

Useful in severe disease and ileal or ileocolonic CD. Prednisone, 40–60 mg PO qd, then taper; IV hydrocortisone, 100 mg tid or equivalent, in hospitalized pts; IV adrenocorticotropic hormone drip (120 U qd) may be preferable in first attacks of UC. Nightly hydrocortisone retention enemas in proctosigmoiditis. Numerous side effects make long-term use problematic.

Immunosuppressive Agents

Azathioprine, 6-mercaptopurine—50 mg PO qd up to 2.0 or 1.5 mg/kg qd, respectively. Useful as steroid-sparing agents and in intractable or fistulous CD (may require 2- to 6-month trial before efficacy seen). Toxicity—immunosuppression, pancreatitis, ? carcinogenicity. Avoid in pregnancy.

Metronidazole

Appears effective in colonic CD (500 mg PO bid) and refractory perineal CD (10–20 mg/kg PO qd). Toxicity—peripheral neuropathy, metallic taste, ? car-

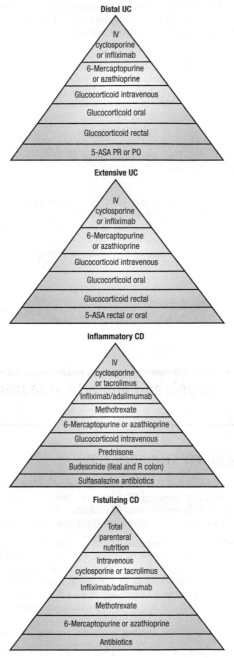

Distal UC

IV cyclosporine or infliximab

6-Mercaptopurine or azathioprine

Glucocorticoid intravenous

Glucocorticoid oral

Glucocorticoid rectal

5-ASA PR or PO

Extensive UC

IV cyclosporine or infliximab

6-Mercaptopurine or azathioprine

Glucocorticoid intravenous

Glucocorticoid oral

Glucocorticoid rectal

5-ASA rectal or oral

Inflammatory CD

IV cyclosporine or tacrolimus

Infliximab/adalimumab

Methotrexate

6-Mercaptopurine or azathioprine

Glucocorticoid intravenous

Prednisone

Budesonide (Ileal and R colon)

Sulfasalazine antibiotics

Fistulizing CD

Total parenteral nutrition

Intravenous cyclosporine or tacrolimus

Infliximab/adalimumab

Methotrexate

6-Mercaptopurine or azathioprine

Antibiotics

FIGURE 157-1 Medical management of IBD.

cinogenicity. Avoid in pregnancy. Other antibiotics (e.g., ciprofloxacin 500 mg PO bid) may be of value in terminal ileal and perianal CD, and broad-spectrum IV antibiotics are indicated for fulminant colitis and abscesses.

Others

Cyclosporine [potential value in a dose of 4 (mg/kg)/d IV for 7–14 days in severe UC and possibly intractable Crohn's fistulas]; experimental—methotrexate, chloroquine, fish oil, nicotine, others. Infliximab [monoclonal antibody to tumor necrosis factor (TNF)] 5 mg/kg IV induces responses in 65% (complete in 33%) of CD pts refractory to 5-ASA, glucocorticoids, and 6-mercaptopurine. In UC, 27–49% of patients respond.

Adalimumab is a humanized version of the anti-TNF antibody that is less likely to elicit neutralizing antibodies in the pt. Pegylated versions of anti-TNF antibody may be used once monthly.

Surgery

UC: Colectomy (curative) for intractability, toxic megacolon (if no improvement with aggressive medical therapy in 24–48 h), cancer, dysplasia. Ileal pouch—anal anastomosis is operation of choice in UC but contraindicated in CD and in elderly. CD: Resection for fixed obstruction (or stricturoplasty), abscesses, persistent symptomatic fistulas, intractability.

For a more detailed discussion, see Friedman S, Blumberg RS: Inflammatory Bowel Disease, Chap. 289, p. 1886, in HPIM-17.

158 Colonic and Anorectal Diseases

IRRITABLE BOWEL SYNDROME (IBS)

Characterized by altered bowel habits, abdominal pain, and absence of detectable organic pathology. Most common GI disease in clinical practice. Three types of clinical presentations: (1) spastic colon (chronic abdominal pain and constipation), (2) alternating constipation and diarrhea, or (3) chronic, painless diarrhea.

Pathophysiology Visceral hyperalgesia to mechanoreceptor stimuli is common. Reported abnormalities include altered colonic motility at rest and in response to stress, cholinergic drugs, cholecystokinin; altered small-intestinal motility; enhanced visceral sensation (lower pain threshold in response to gut distention); and abnormal extrinsic innervation of the gut. Pts presenting with IBS to a physician have an increased frequency of psychological disturbances—depression, hysteria, obsessive-compulsive disorder. Specific food intolerances and malabsorption of bile acids by the terminal ileum may account for a few cases.

Clinical Manifestations Onset often before age 30; females:males = 2:1. Abdominal pain and irregular bowel habits. Additional symptoms often include abdominal distention, relief of abdominal pain with bowel movement, increased

TABLE 158-1	DIAGNOSTIC CRITERIA FOR IRRITABLE BOWEL SYNDROME[a]

Recurrent abdominal pain or discomfort[b] at least 3 days per month in the last 3 months associated with *two or more* of the following:
1. Improvement with defecation
2. Onset associated with a change in frequency of stool
3. Onset associated with a change in form (appearance) of stool

[a]Criteria fulfilled for the last 3 months with symptom onset at least 6 months prior to diagnosis.
[b]Discomfort means an uncomfortable sensation not described as pain. In pathophysiology research and clinical trials, a pain/discomfort frequency of at least 2 days a week during screening evaluation is required for subject eligibility.
Source: Adapted from Longstreth GF et al: Functional bowel disorders. Gastroenterology 130:1480, 2006; with permission.

frequency of stools with pain, loose stools with pain, mucus in stools, and sense of incomplete evacuation. Associated findings include pasty stools, ribbony or pencil-thin stools, heartburn, bloating, back pain, weakness, faintness, palpitations, urinary frequency.

Diagnosis IBS is a diagnosis of exclusion. Rome criteria for diagnosis are shown in Table 158-1. Consider sigmoidoscopy and barium radiographs to exclude inflammatory bowel disease or malignancy; consider excluding giardiasis, intestinal lactase deficiency, hyperthyroidism.

℞ Irritable Bowel Syndrome (Table 158-2)

Reassurance and supportive physician-pt relationship, avoidance of stress or precipitating factors, dietary bulk (fiber, psyllium extract, e.g., Metamucil 1 tbsp daily or bid); for diarrhea, trials of loperamide (2-mg tabs PO q A.M. then 1 PO after each loose stool to a maximum of 8/d, then titrate), diphenoxylate (Lomotil) (up to 2-mg tabs PO qid), or cholestyramine (up to 1-gram packet mixed in water PO qid); for pain, anticholinergics (e.g., dicyclomine HCl 10–40 mg PO qid) or hyoscyamine as Levsin 1–2 PO q4h prn. Amitriptyline 25–50 mg PO qhs or other antidepressants in low doses may relieve pain. Selective serotonin reuptake inhibitors such as paroxetine are being evaluated in constipation-dominant pts, and serotonin receptor antagonists such as alosetron are being evaluated in diarrhea-dominant pts. Psychotherapy, hypnotherapy of possible benefit in severe refractory cases.

DIVERTICULAR DISEASE

Herniations or saclike protrusions of the mucosa through the muscularis at points of nutrient artery penetration; possibly due to increased intraluminal pressure, low-fiber diet; most common in sigmoid colon.

Clinical Presentation

1. *Asymptomatic* (detected by barium enema or colonoscopy).
2. *Pain*: Recurrent left lower quadrant pain relieved by defecation; alternating constipation and diarrhea. Diagnosis by barium enema.
3. *Diverticulitis*: Pain, fever, altered bowel habits, tender colon, leukocytosis. Best confirmed and staged by CT after opacification of bowel. (In pts who recover with medical therapy, perform elective barium enema or colonoscopy in 4–6 weeks to exclude cancer.) Complications: pericolic abscess, perfo-

TABLE 158-2 **POSSIBLE DRUGS FOR A DOMINANT SYMPTOM IN IBS**

Symptom	Drug	Dose
Diarrhea	Loperamide	2–4 mg when necessary/maximum 12 g/d
	Cholestyramine resin	4 g with meals
	Alosetron[a]	0.5–1 mg bid (for severe IBS, women)
Constipation	Psyllium husk	3–4 g bid with meals, then adjust
	Methylcellulose	2 g bid with meals, then adjust
	Calcium polycarbophil	1 g qd to qid
	Lactulose syrup	10–20 g bid
	70% sorbitol	15 mL bid
	Polyethylene glycol 3350	17 g in 250 mL water qd
	Lubiprostone (Amitiza)	24 mg bid
	Magnesium hydroxide	30–60 mL qd
Abdominal pain	Smooth-muscle relaxant	qd to qid ac
	Tricyclic antidepressants	Start 25–50 mg hs, then adjust
	Selective serotonin reuptake inhibitors	Begin small dose, increase as needed

[a]Available only in the United States.
Source: Adapted from Longstreth GF et al: Functional bowel disorders. Gastroenterology 130:1480, 2006; with permission.

ration, fistula (to bladder, vagina, skin, soft tissue), liver abscess, stricture. Frequently require surgery or, for abscesses, percutaneous drainage.
4. *Hemorrhage*: Usually in absence of diverticulitis, often from ascending colon and self-limited. If persistent, manage with mesenteric arteriography and intraarterial infusion of vasopressin, or surgery (Chap. 55).

℞ Diverticular Disease

Pain
High-fiber diet, psyllium extract (e.g., Metamucil 1 tbsp PO qd or bid), anticholinergics (e.g., dicyclomine HCl 10–40 mg PO qid).

Diverticulitis
NPO, IV fluids, antibiotics for 7–10 d (e.g., trimethoprim/sulfamethoxazole or ciprofloxacin and metronidazole; add ampicillin to cover enterococci in nonresponders); for ambulatory pts, ampicillin/clavulanate (clear liquid diet); surgical resection in refractory or frequently recurrent cases, young persons (<age 50), immunosuppressed pts, or when there is inability to exclude cancer.

Pts who have had at least two documented episodes and those who respond slowly to medical therapy should be offered surgical options to achieve removal of the diseased colonic segment, controlling sepsis, eliminating obstructions or fistulas, and restoring intestinal continuity.

INTESTINAL PSEUDOOBSTRUCTION

Recurrent attacks of nausea, vomiting, and abdominal pain and distention mimicking mechanical obstruction; may be complicated by steatorrhea due to bacterial overgrowth.

Causes *Primary*: Familial visceral neuropathy, familial visceral myopathy, idiopathic. *Secondary*: Scleroderma, amyloidosis, diabetes, celiac disease, parkinsonism, muscular dystrophy, drugs, electrolyte imbalance, postsurgical.

℞ Intestinal Pseudoobstruction

For acute attacks: intestinal decompression with long tube. Oral antibiotics for bacterial overgrowth (e.g., metronidazole 250 mg PO tid, tetracycline 500 mg PO qid, or ciprofloxacin 500 mg bid 1 week out of each month, usually in an alternating rotation of at least two antibiotics). Avoid surgery. In refractory cases, consider long-term parenteral hyperalimentation.

VASCULAR DISORDERS (SMALL AND LARGE INTESTINE)

Mechanisms of Mesenteric Ischemia   (1) Occlusive: embolus (atrial fibrillation, valvular heart disease); arterial thrombus (atherosclerosis); venous thrombosis (trauma, neoplasm, infection, cirrhosis, oral contraceptives, antithrombin-III deficiency, protein S or C deficiency, lupus anticoagulant, factor V Leiden mutation, idiopathic); vasculitis (systemic lupus erythematosus, polyarteritis, rheumatoid arthritis, Henoch-Schönlein purpura); (2) nonocclusive: hypotension, heart failure, arrhythmia, digitalis (vasoconstrictor).

Acute Mesenteric Ischemia   Periumbilical pain out of proportion to tenderness; nausea, vomiting, distention, GI bleeding, altered bowel habits. Abdominal x-ray shows bowel distention, air-fluid levels, thumbprinting (submucosal edema) but may be normal early in course. Peritoneal signs indicate infarcted bowel requiring surgical resection. Early celiac and mesenteric arteriography is recommended in all cases following hemodynamic resuscitation (avoid vasopressors, digitalis). Intraarterial vasodilators (e.g., papaverine) can be administered to reverse vasoconstriction. Laparotomy indicated to restore intestinal blood flow obstructed by embolus or thrombosis or to resect necrotic bowel. Postoperative anticoagulation indicated in mesenteric venous thrombosis, controversial in arterial occlusion.

Chronic Mesenteric Insufficiency   "Abdominal angina": dull, crampy periumbilical pain 15–30 min after a meal and lasting for several hours; weight loss; occasionally diarrhea. Evaluate with mesenteric arteriography for possible bypass graft surgery.

Ischemic Colitis   Usually due to nonocclusive disease in pts with atherosclerosis. Severe lower abdominal pain, rectal bleeding, hypotension. Abdominal x-ray shows colonic dilatation, thumbprinting. Sigmoidoscopy shows submucosal hemorrhage, friability, ulcerations; rectum often spared. Conservative management (NPO, IV fluids); surgical resection for infarction or postischemic stricture.

COLONIC ANGIODYSPLASIA

In persons over age 60, vascular ectasias, usually in right colon, account for up to 40% of cases of chronic or recurrent lower GI bleeding. May be associated with aortic stenosis. Diagnosis is by arteriography (clusters of small vessels, early and prolonged opacification of draining vein) or colonoscopy (flat, bright red, fernlike lesions). For bleeding, treat by colonoscopic electro- or laser coagulation, band ligation, arteriographic embolization, or, if necessary, right hemicolectomy (Chap. 55).

ANORECTAL DISEASES

Hemorrhoids Due to increased hydrostatic pressure in hemorrhoidal venous plexus (associated with straining at stool, pregnancy). May be external, internal, thrombosed, acute (prolapsed or strangulated), or bleeding. Treat pain with bulk laxative and stool softeners (psyllium extract, dioctyl sodium sulfosuccinate 100–200 mg/d), sitz baths 1–4 per day, witch hazel compresses, analgesics as needed. Bleeding may require rubber band ligation or injection sclerotherapy. Operative hemorrhoidectomy in severe or refractory cases.

Anal Fissures Medical therapy as for hemorrhoids. Relaxation of the anal canal with nitroglycerin ointment (0.2%) applied tid or botulinum toxin type A up to 20 U injected into the internal sphincter on each side of the fissure. Internal anal sphincterotomy in refractory cases.

Pruritus Ani Often of unclear cause; may be due to poor hygiene, fungal or parasitic infection. Treat with thorough cleansing after bowel movement, topical glucocorticoid, antifungal agent if indicated.

Anal Condylomas (Genital Warts) Wartlike papillomas due to sexually transmitted papillomavirus. Treat with cautious application of liquid nitrogen or podophyllotoxin or with intralesional interferon-α. Tend to recur. May be prevented by vaccination with Gardasil.

For a more detailed discussion, see Owyang C: Irritable Bowel Syndrome, Chap. 290, p. 1899; Gearhart SL: Diverticular Disease and Common Anorectal Disorders, Chap. 291, p. 1903; and Gearhart SL: Mesenteric Vascular Insufficiency, Chap. 292, p. 1910, in HPIM-17.

159 Cholelithiasis, Cholecystitis, and Cholangitis

CHOLELITHIASIS

There are two major types of gallstones: cholesterol and pigment stones. Cholesterol gallstones contain >50% cholesterol monohydrate. Pigment stones have <20% cholesterol and are composed primarily of calcium bilirubinate. In the United States, 80% of stones are cholesterol and 20% pigment.

Epidemiology One million new cases of cholelithiasis per year in the United States. Predisposing factors include demographic/genetics (increased prevalence in North American Indians), obesity, weight loss, female sex hormones, age, ileal disease, pregnancy, type IV hyperlipidemia, and cirrhosis.

Symptoms and Signs Many gallstones are "silent," i.e., present in asymptomatic patients. Symptoms occur when stones produce inflammation or obstruction of the cystic or common bile ducts. Major symptoms: (1) biliary colic—a severe steady ache in the RUQ or epigastrium that begins suddenly; often occurs 30–90 min after meals, lasts for several hours, and occasionally radiates to the right scapula or back; (2) nausea, vomiting. Physical exam may be normal or show epigastric or RUQ tenderness.

Laboratory Occasionally, mild and transient elevations in bilirubin [<85 µmol/L (<5 mg/dL)] accompany biliary colic.

Imaging Only 10% of cholesterol gallstones are radiopaque. Ultrasonography is best diagnostic test. The oral cholecystogram has been largely replaced by ultrasound but may be used to assess the patency of the cystic duct and gallbladder emptying function (Table 159-1).

Differential Diagnosis Includes peptic ulcer disease (PUD), gastroesophageal reflux, irritable bowel syndrome, and hepatitis.

Complications Cholecystitis, pancreatitis, cholangitis.

℞ Cholelthiasis

In asymptomatic patients, risk of developing complications requiring surgery is small. Elective cholecystectomy should be reserved for: (1) symptomatic patients (i.e., biliary colic despite low-fat diet); (2) persons with previous complications of cholelithiasis (see below); and (3) presence of an underlying condition predisposing to an increased risk of complications (calcified or porcelain gallbladder). Patients with gallstones > 3 cm or with an anomalous gallbladder containing stones should also be considered for surgery. Laparoscopic cholecystectomy is minimally invasive and is the procedure of choice for most patients undergoing elective cholecystectomy. Oral dissolution agents (ursodeoxycholic acid) partially or completely dissolve small radiolucent stones in 50% of selected patients within 6–24 months. Because of the frequency of stone recurrence and the effectiveness of laparoscopic surgery, the role of oral dissolution therapy has been reduced to selected patients who are not candidates for elective cholecystectomy.

ACUTE CHOLECYSTITIS

Acute inflammation of the gallbladder is usually caused by cystic duct obstruction by an impacted stone. Inflammatory response is evoked by: (1) mechanical inflammation from increased intraluminal pressure; (2) chemical inflammation from release of lysolecithin; (3) bacterial inflammation, which plays a role in 50–85% of patients with acute cholecystitis.

Etiology 90% calculous; 10% acalculous. Acalculous cholecystitis associated with higher complication rate and associated with acute illness (i.e., burns, trauma, major surgery), fasting, hyperalimentation leading to gallbladder stasis, vasculitis, carcinoma of gallbladder or common bile duct, some gallbladder infections (*Leptospira, Streptococcus, Salmonella,* or *Vibrio cholerae*), but in >50% of cases an underlying explanation is not found.

Symptoms and Signs (1) Attack of bilary colic (RUQ or epigastric pain) that progressively worsens; (2) nausea, vomiting, anorexia; and (3) fever. Examination typically reveals RUQ tenderness; palpable RUQ mass found in 20% of pts. *Murphy's sign* is present when deep inspiration or cough during palpation of the RUQ produces increased pain or inspiratory arrest.

TABLE 159-1	DIAGNOSTIC EVALUATION OF THE BILE DUCTS

Diagnostic Advantages	Diagnostic Limitations
Hepatobiliary Ultrasound	
Rapid	Bowel gas
Simultaneous scanning of GB, liver, bile ducts, pancreas	Massive obesity
	Ascites
Accurate identification of dilated bile ducts	Barium
Not limited by jaundice, pregnancy	Partial bile duct obstruction
Guidance for fine-needle biopsy	Poor visualization of distal CBD
Computed Tomography	
Simultaneous scanning of GB, liver, bile ducts, pancreas	Extreme cachexia
	Movement artifact
Accurate identification of dilated bile ducts, masses	Ileus
	Partial bile duct obstruction
Not limited by jaundice, gas, obesity, ascites	
High-resolution image	
Guidance for fine-needle biopsy	
Magnetic Resonance Cholangiopancreatography	
Useful modality for visualizing pancreatic and biliary ducts	Cannot offer therapeutic intervention
Has excellent sensitivity for bile duct dilatation, biliary stricture, and intraductal abnormalities	High cost
Can identify pancreatic duct dilatation or stricture, pancreatic duct stenosis, and pancreas divisum	
Endoscopic Retrograde Cholangiopancreatography	
Simultaneous pancreatography	Gastroduodenal obstruction
Best visualization of distal biliary tract	? Roux en Y biliary-enteric anastomosis
Bile or pancreatic cytology	
Endoscopic sphincterotomy and stone removal	
Biliary manometry	
Percutaneous Transhepatic Cholangiogram	
Extremely successful when bile ducts dilated	Nondilated or sclerosed ducts
Best visualization of proximal biliary tract	
Bile cytology/culture	
Percutaneous transhepatic drainage	
Endoscopic Ultrasound	
Most sensitive method to detect ampullary stones	

Laboratory   Mild leukocytosis; serum bilirubin, alkaline phosphatase, and AST may be mildly elevated.

Imaging   Ultrasonography is useful for demonstrating gallstones and occasionally a phlegmonous mass surrounding the gallbladder. Radionuclide scans (HIDA, DIDA, DISIDA, etc.) may identify cystic duct obstruction.

Differential Diagnosis   Includes acute pancreatitis, appendicitis, pyelonephritis, peptic ulcer disease, hepatitis, and hepatic abscess.

Complications   Empyema, hydrops, gangrene, perforation, fistulization, gallstone ileus, porcelain gallbladder.

Acute Cholecystitis

No oral intake, nasogastric suction, IV fluids and electrolytes, analgesia (meperidine or NSAIDS), and antibiotics (ureidopenicillins, ampicillin sulbactam, ciprofloxacin, third-generation cephalosporins; anaerobic coverage should be added if gangrenous or emphysematous cholecystitis is suspected; imipenem/meropenem cover the spectrum of bacteria causing ascending cholangitis but should be reserved for the most life-threatening infections when other antibiotics have failed). Acute symptoms will resolve in 70% of patients. Optimal timing of surgery depends on patient stabilization and should be performed as soon as feasible. Urgent cholecystectomy is appropriate in most patients with a suspected or confirmed complication. Delayed surgery is reserved for patients with high risk of emergent surgery and where the diagnosis is in doubt.

CHRONIC CHOLECYSTITIS

Etiology   Chronic inflammation of the gallbladder; almost always associated with gallstones. Results from repeated acute/subacute cholecystitis or prolonged mechanical irritation of gallbladder wall.

Symptoms and Signs   May be asymptomatic for years, may progress to symptomatic gallbladder disease or to acute cholecystitis, or present with complications.

Laboratory   Tests are usually normal.

Imaging   Ultrasonography preferred; usually shows gallstones within a contracted gallbladder (Table 159-1).

Differential Diagnosis   Peptic ulcer disease, esophagitis, irritable bowel syndrome.

Chronic Cholecystitis

Surgery indicated if patient is symptomatic.

CHOLEDOCHOLITHIASIS/CHOLANGITIS

Etiology   In patients with cholelithiasis, passage of gallstones into common bile duct (CBD) occurs in 10–15%; increases with age. At cholecystectomy, undetected stones are left behind in 1–5% of pts.

Symptoms and Signs   Choledocholithiasis may present as an incidental finding, biliary colic, obstructive jaundice, cholangitis, or pancreatitis. Cholangitis usually presents as fever, RUQ pain, and jaundice (*Charcot's triad*).

Laboratory   Elevations in serum bilirubin, alkaline phosphatase, and aminotransferases. Leukocytosis usually accompanies cholangitis; blood cultures are frequently positive. Amylase is elevated in 15% of cases.

Imaging   Diagnosis usually made by cholangiography either preoperatively by endoscopic retrograde cholangiopancreatography (ERCP) or intraoperatively at the time of cholecystectomy. Ultrasonography may reveal dilated bile ducts but is not sensitive for detecting CBD stones (Table 159-1).

Differential Diagnosis   Acute cholecystitis, renal colic, perforated viscus, pancreatitis.

Complications   Cholangitis, obstructive jaundice, gallstone-induced pancreatitis, and secondary biliary cirrhosis.

Rx Choledocholithiasis/Cholangitis

Laparoscopic cholecystectomy and ERCP have decreased the need for choledocholithotomy and T-tube drainage of the bile ducts. When CBD stones are suspected prior to laparoscopic cholecystectomy, preoperative ERCP with endoscopic palpillotomy and stone extraction is the preferred approach. CBD stones should be suspected in gallstone pts with (1) history of jaundice or pancreatitis, (2) abnormal LFT, and (3) ultrasound evidence of a dilated common bile duct or stones in the duct. Cholangitis treated like acute cholecystitis; no oral intake, hydration, analgesia, and antibiotics are the mainstays; stones should be removed surgically or endoscopically.

PRIMARY SCLEROSING CHOLANGITIS (PSC)

PSC is a sclerosing, inflammatory, and obliterative process involving the biliary tree.

Etiology   Associations: inflammatory bowel disease (75% of cases of PSC—especially ulcerative colitis), AIDS, rarely retroperitoneal fibrosis.

Symptoms and Signs   Pruritus, RUQ pain, jaundice, fever, weight loss, and malaise. 44% may be asymptomatic at diagnosis. May progress to cirrhosis with portal hypertension.

Laboratory   Evidence of cholestasis (elevated bilirubin and alkaline phosphatase) common.

Radiology/Endoscopy   Transhepatic or endoscopic cholangiograms reveal stenosis and dilation of the intra- and extrahepatic bile ducts.

Differential Diagnosis   Cholangiocarcinoma, Caroli's disease (cystic dilation of bile ducts), *Fasciola hepatica* infection, echinococcosis, and ascariasis.

Rx Primary Sclerosing Cholangitis

No satisfactory therapy. Cholangitis should be treated as outlined above. Cholestyramine may control pruritus. Supplemental vitamin D and calcium may retard bone loss. Glucocorticoids, methotrexate, and cyclosporine have not been shown to be effective. Urodeoxycholic acid improves liver tests, but has not been shown to affect survival. Surgical relief of biliary obstruction may be appropriate but has a high complication rate. Liver transplantation should be considered in pts with end-stage cirrhosis. Median survival: 9–12 years after diagnosis, with age, bilirubin level, histologic stage, and splenomegaly being predictors of survival.

For a more detailed discussion, see Greenberger NJ, Paumgartner G: Diseases of the Gallbladder and Bile Ducts, Chap. 305, p. 1991, in HPIM-17.

160 Pancreatitis

ACUTE PANCREATITIS

The pathologic spectrum of acute pancreatitis varies from *interstitial pancreatitis*, which is usually a mild and self-limited disorder, to *necrotizing pancreatitis,* in which the degree of pancreatic necrosis correlates with the severity of the attack and its systemic manifestations.

Etiology   Most common causes in the United States are cholelithiasis and alcohol. Others are listed in Table 160-1.

Clinical Features   Can vary from mild abdominal pain to shock. *Common symptoms*: (1) steady, boring midepigastric pain radiating to the back that is frequently increased in the supine position; (2) nausea, vomiting.

Physical exam: (1) low-grade fever, tachycardia, hypotension; (2) erythematous skin nodules due to subcutaneous fat necrosis; (3) basilar rales, pleural effusion (often on the left); (4) abdominal tenderness and rigidity, diminished bowel sounds, palpable upper abdominal mass; (5) Cullen's sign: blue discoloration in the periumbilical area due to hemoperitoneum; (6) Turner's sign: blue-red-purple or green-brown discoloration of the flanks due to tissue catabolism of hemoglobin.

Laboratory

1. *Serum amylase*: Large elevations (>3 × normal) virtually assure the diagnosis if salivary gland disease and intestinal perforation/infarction are excluded. However, normal serum amylase does not exclude the diagnosis of acute pancreatitis, and the degree of elevation does not predict severity of pancreatitis. Amylase levels typically return to normal in 48–72 h.
2. *Urinary amylase–creatinine clearance ratio*: no more sensitive or specific than blood amylase levels.
3. *Serum lipase* level: increases in parallel with amylase level and measurement of both tests increases the diagnostic yield.
4. *Other tests*: *Hypocalcemia* occurs in ~25% of patients. *Leukocytosis* (15,000–20,000/μL) occurs frequently. *Hypertriglyceridemia* occurs in 15–20% of cas-

| TABLE 160-1 | CAUSES OF ACUTE PANCREATITIS |

Common Causes

Gallstones (including microlithiasis)
Alcohol (acute and chronic alcoholism)
Hypertriglyceridemia
Endoscopic retrograde cholangiopancreatography (ERCP), especially after biliary manometry
Trauma (especially blunt abdominal trauma)
Postoperative (abdominal and nonabdominal operations)
Drugs (azathioprine, 6-mercaptopurine, sulfonamides, estrogens, tetracycline, valproic acid, anti-HIV medications)
Sphincter of Oddi dysfunction

Uncommon Causes

Vascular causes and vasculitis (ischemic-hypoperfusion states after cardiac surgery)
Connective tissue disorders and thrombotic thrombocytopenic purpura (TTP)
Cancer of the pancreas
Hypercalcemia
Periampullary diverticulum
Pancreas divisum
Hereditary pancreatitis
Cystic fibrosis
Renal failure

Rare Causes

Infections (mumps, coxsackievirus, cytomegalovirus, echovirus, parasites)
Autoimmune (e.g., Sjögren's syndrome)

Causes to Consider in Patients with Recurrent Bouts of Acute Pancreatitis without an Obvious Etiology

Occult disease of the biliary tree or pancreatic ducts, especially microlithiasis, sludge
Drugs
Hypertriglyceridemia
Pancreas divisum
Pancreatic cancer
Sphincter of Oddi dysfunction
Cystic fibrosis
Idiopathic

es and can cause a spuriously normal serum amylase level. *Hyperglycemia* is common. *Serum bilirubin, alkaline phosphatase*, and *aspartame aminotransferase* can be transiently elevated. *Hypoalbuminemia* and marked elevations of *serum lactic dehydrogenase* (LDH) are associated with an increased mortality rate. *Hypoxemia* is present in 25% of patients. Arterial pH < 7.32 may spuriously elevate serum amylase.

Imaging

1. *Abdominal radiographs* are abnormal in 30–50% of patients but are not specific for pancreatitis. Common findings include total or partial ileus ("sentinel loop") and the "colon cut-off sign," which results from isolated distention of the transverse colon. Useful for excluding diagnoses such as intestinal perforation with free air.

TABLE 160-2	**RISK FACTORS THAT ADVERSELY AFFECT SURVIVAL IN ACUTE PANCREATITIS**

Severe Acute Pancreatitis

1. Associated with organ failure and/or local complications such as necrosis
2. Clinical manifestations
   a. Obesity BMI > 30
   b. Hemoconcentration (hematocrit > 44%)
   c. Age > 70
3. Organ failure[a]
   a. Shock
   b. Pulmonary insufficiency (P_{O_2} < 60)
   c. Renal failure (CR > 2.0 mg%)
   d. GI bleeding
4. ≥ 3 Ransom criteria (not fully utilizable until 48 h)
5. Apache II score > 8 (cumbersome)

[a]Usually declares itself shortly after onset.

2. *Ultrasound* often fails to visualize the pancreas because of overlying intestinal gas but may detect gallstones, pseudocysts, mass lesions, or edema or enlargement of the pancreas.
3. *CT* can confirm diagnosis of pancreatitis (edematous pancreas) and is useful for predicting and identifying late complications. Contrast-enhanced dynamic CT is indicated for clinical deterioration, the presence of risk factors that adversely affect survival (Table 160-2), or other features of serious illness.

Differential Diagnosis Intestinal perforation (especially peptic ulcer), cholecystitis, acute intestinal obstruction, mesenteric ischemia, renal colic, myocardial ischemia, aortic dissection, connective tissue disorders, pneumonia, and diabetic ketoacidosis.

℞ Acute Pancreatitis

Most (90%) cases subside over a period of 3–7 days. Conventional measures: (1) analgesics, such as meperidine; (2) IV fluids and colloids; (3) no oral alimentation. The benefit of antibiotic prophylaxis in necrotizing acute pancreatitis remains controversial. Current recommendation is use of an antibiotic such as imipenem-cilastatin, 500 mg tid for 2 weeks. Not effective: cimetidine (or related agents), H_2 blockers, protease inhibitors, glucocorticoids, nasogastric suction, glucagon, peritoneal lavage, and anticholinergic medications. Precipitating factors (alcohol, medications) must be eliminated. In mild or moderate pancreatitis, a clear liquid diet can usually be started after 3–6 days. Patients with severe gallstone-induced pancreatitis often benefit from early (<3 days) papillotomy.

Complications It is important to identify patients who are at risk of poor outcome. Risk factors that adversely affect survival in acute pancreatitis are listed in Table 160-2. Fulminant pancreatitis requires aggressive fluid support and meticulous management. Mortality is largely due to infection.

Systemic Shock, GI bleeding, common duct obstruction, ileus, splenic infarction or rupture, DIC, subcutaneous fat necrosis, ARDS, pleural effusion, acute renal failure, sudden blindness.

Local

1. Sterile or infected *pancreatic necrosis*—necrosis may become secondarily infected in 40–60% of patients, typically within 1–2 weeks after the onset of pancreatitis. Most frequent organisms: gram-negative bacteria of alimentary origin, but intraabdominal *Candida* infection increasing in frequency. Necrosis can be visualized by contrast-enhanced dynamic CT, with infection diagnosed by CT-guided needle aspiration. Laparotomy with removal of necrotic material and adequate drainage should be considered for patients with sterile acute necrotic pancreatitis, if patient continues to deteriorate despite conventional therapy. Infected pancreatic necrosis requires aggressive surgical debridement and antibiotics.

2. *Pancreatic pseudocysts* develop over 1–4 weeks in 15% of patients. Abdominal pain is the usual complaint, and a tender upper abdominal mass may be present. Can be detected by abdominal ultrasound or CT. In patients who are stable and uncomplicated, treatment is supportive; pseudocysts that are >5 cm in diameter and persist for >6 weeks should be considered for drainage. In patients with an expanding pseudocyst or one complicated by hemorrhage, rupture, or abscess, surgery should be performed.

3. *Pancreatic abscess*—ill-defined liquid collection of pus that evolves over 4–6 weeks. Can be treated surgically or in selected cases by percutaneous drainage.

4. *Pancreatic ascites* and *pleural effusions* are usually due to disruption of the main pancreatic duct. Treatment involves nasogastric suction and parenteral alimentation for 2–3 weeks. If medical management fails, pancreatography followed by surgery should be performed.

CHRONIC PANCREATITIS

Chronic pancreatitis may occur as recurrent episodes of acute inflammation superimposed upon a previously injured pancreas or as chronic damage with pain and malabsorption.

Etiology Chronic alcoholism is most frequent cause of pancreatic exocrine insufficiency in U.S. adults; in 25% of adults, etiology is unknown. Other causes are listed in Table 160-3.

Symptoms and Signs *Pain* is cardinal symptom. Weight loss, steatorrhea, and other signs and symptoms of malabsorption common. Physical exam often unremarkable.

Laboratory No specific laboratory test for chronic pancreatitis. Serum amylase and lipase levels are often normal. Serum bilirubin and alkaline phosphatase may be elevated. Steatorrhea (fecal fat concentration $\geq 9.5\%$) late in the course. The bentiromide test, a simple, effective test of pancreatic exocrine function, may be helpful. D-Xylose urinary excretion test is usually normal. Impaired glucose tolerance is present in >50% of pts. Secretin stimulation test is a relatively sensitive test for pancreatic exocrine deficiency.

Imaging *Plain films* of the abdomen reveal pancreatic calcifications in 30–60%. *Ultrasound* and *CT scans* may show dilation of the pancreatic duct. *ERCP* and endoscopic ultrasound (*EUS*) provide information about the main pancreatic and smaller ducts.

Differential Diagnosis Important to distinguish from pancreatic carcinoma; may require radiographically guided biopsy.

TABLE 160-3	**CHRONIC PANCREATITIS AND PANCREATIC EXOCRINE INSUFFICIENCY: TIGAR-O CLASSIFICATION SYSTEM**

Toxic-metabolic
- Alcoholic
- Tobacco smoking
- Hypercalcemia
- Hyperlipidemia
- Chronic renal failure
- Medications—phenacetin abuse
- Toxins—organotin compounds (e.g., DBTC)

Idiopathic
- Early onset
- Late onset
- Tropical

Genetic
- Hereditary pancreatitis
- Cationic trypsinogen
- CFTR mutations
- SPINK1 mutations

Autoimmune
- Isolated autoimmune CP
- Autoimmune CP associated with
  - Sjögren's syndrome
  - Inflammatory bowel disease
  - Primary biliary cirrhosis

Recurrent and severe acute pancreatitis
- Postnecrotic (severe acute pancreatitis)
- Recurrent acute pancreatitis
- Vascular diseases/ischemia
- Postirradiation

Obstructive
- Pancreas divisum
- Sphincter of Oddi disorders (controversial)
- Duct obstruction (e.g., tumor)
- Preampullary duodenal wall cysts
- Posttraumatic pancreatic duct scars

CP, chronic pancreatitis; TIGAR-O, toxic-metabolic, idiopathic, genetic, autoimmune, recurrent and severe acute pancreatitis, obstructive.

℞ Chronic Pancreatitis

Aimed at controlling pain and malabsorption. Intermittent attacks treated like acute pancreatitis. Alcohol and large, fatty meals must be avoided. Narcotics for severe pain, but subsequent addiction is common. Patients unable to maintain adequate hydration should be hospitalized, while those with milder symptoms can be managed on an ambulatory basis. Surgery may control pain if there is a ductal stricture. Subtotal pancreatectomy may also control pain but at the cost of exocrine insufficiency and diabetes. Malabsorption is managed with a low-fat diet and pancreatic enzyme replacement. Because pancreatic enzymes are inactivated by acid, agents that reduce acid production (e.g., omeprazole or sodium bicarbonate) may improve their efficacy (but should not be given with enteric-coated preparations). Insulin may be necessary to control serum glucose.

Complications Vitamin B_{12} malabsorption in 40% of alcohol-induced and all cystic fibrosis cases. Impaired glucose tolerance. Nondiabetic retinopathy due to vitamin A and/or zinc deficiency. GI bleeding, icterus, effusions, subcutaneous fat necrosis, and bone pain occasionally occur. Increased risk for pancreatic carcinoma. Narcotic addiction common.

For a more detailed discussion, see Toskes PP, Greenberger NJ: Approach to the Patient with Pancreatic Disease, Chap. 306, p. 2001; Greenberger NJ, Toskes PP: Acute and Chronic Pancreatitis, Chap. 307, p. 2005, in HPIM-17.

161 Acute Hepatitis

VIRAL HEPATITIS

Acute viral hepatitis is a systemic infection affecting the liver predominantly. Clinically characterized by malaise, nausea, vomiting, diarrhea, and low-grade fever followed by dark urine, jaundice, and tender hepatomegaly; may be subclinical and detected on basis of elevated aspartate and alanine aminotransferase (AST and ALT) levels. Hepatitis B may be associated with immune-complex phenomena, including arthritis, serum sickness–like illness, glomerulonephritis, and a polyarteritis nodosa–like vasculitis. Hepatitis-like illnesses may be caused not only by hepatotropic viruses (A, B, C, D, E) but also by other viruses (Epstein-Barr, CMV, coxsackievirus, etc.), alcohol, drugs, hypotension and ischemia, and biliary tract disease (Table 161-1).

Hepatitis A (HAV)   27-nm picornavirus (hepatovirus) with single-stranded RNA genome.

Clinical Course   See Fig. 161-1.

Outcome   Recovery within 6–12 months, usually with no clinical sequelae; a small proportion will have one or two apparent clinical and serologic relapses; in some cases, pronounced cholestasis suggesting biliary obstruction may occur; rare fatalities (fulminant hepatitis), no chronic carrier state.

Diagnosis   IgM anti-HAV in acute or early convalescent serum sample.

Epidemiology   Fecal-oral transmission; endemic in underdeveloped countries; food-borne and waterborne epidemics; outbreaks in day-care centers, residential institutions.

Prevention   *After exposure*: immune globulin 0.02 mL/kg IM within 2 weeks to household and institutional contacts (not casual contacts at work). *Before exposure*: inactivated HAV vaccine 1 mL IM (unit dose depends on formulation); half dose to children; repeat at 6–12 months; target travelers, military recruits, animal handlers, day-care personnel, laboratory workers, patients with chronic liver disease, especially hepatitis C.

Hepatitis B (HBV)   42-nm hepadnavirus with outer surface coat (HBsAg), inner nucleocapsid core (HBcAg), DNA polymerase, and partially double-stranded DNA genome of 3200 nucleotides. Circulating form of HBcAg is HBeAg, a marker of viral replication and infectivity. Multiple serotypes and genetic heterogeneity.

Clinical Course   See Fig. 161-2.

Outcome   Recovery >90%, fulminant hepatitis (<1%), chronic hepatitis or carrier state (only 1–2% of immunocompetent adults; higher in neonates, elderly, immunocompromised), cirrhosis, and hepatocellular carcinoma (especially following chronic infection beginning in infancy or early childhood) (see Chap. 163).

Diagnosis   HBsAg in serum (acute or chronic infection); IgM anti-HBc (early anti-HBc indicative of acute or recent infection). Most sensitive test is detection of HBV DNA in serum; not generally required for routine diagnosis.

TABLE 161-1 THE HEPATITIS VIRUSES

	HAV	HBV	HCV	HDV	HEV
Viral Properties					
Size, nm	27	42	~55	~36	~32
Nucleic acid	RNA	DNA	RNA	RNA	RNA
Genome length, kb	7.5	3.2	9.4	1.7	7.5
Classification	Picornavirus	Hepadnavirus	Flavivirus-like	—	Calicivirus-like or alpha-virus-like
Incubation, days	15–45	30–180	15–160	21–140	14–63
Transmission					
Fecal-oral	+++	—	—	—	+++
Percutaneous	Rare	+++	+++	+++	—
Sexual	?	++	Uncommon	++	—
Perinatal	—	+++	Uncommon	+	—
Clinical Features					
Severity	Usually mild	Moderate	Mild	May be severe	Usually mild
Chronic infection	No	1–10%; up to 90% in neonates	80–90%	Common	No
Carrier state	No	Yes	Yes	Yes	No
Fulminant hepatitis	0.1%	1%	Rare	Up to 20% in superinfection	10–20% in pregnant women
Hepatocellular carcinoma	No	Yes	Yes	?	No
Prophylaxis	Ig; vaccine	HBIg; vaccine	None	None (HBV vaccine for susceptibles)	None

Note: HAV, hepatitis A virus; HBV, hepatitis B virus; HCV, hepatitis C virus; HDV, hepatitis D virus; HEV, hepatitis E virus; Ig, immune globulin; + +, sometimes; + + +, often; ?, possibly.

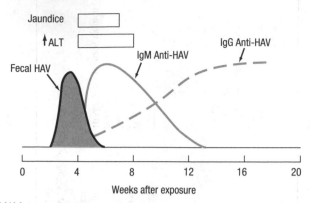

FIGURE 161-1 Scheme of typical clinical and laboratory features of HAV. (*Reproduced from JL Dienstag, HPIM-17, p. 1932.*)

Epidemiology Percutaneous (needle stick), sexual, or perinatal transmission. Endemic in sub-Saharan Africa and Southeast Asia, where up to 20% of population acquire infection, usually early in life.

Prevention *After exposure in unvaccinated persons*: hepatitis B immune globulin (HBIg) 0.06 mL/ kg IM immediately after needle stick to within 14 days of sexual exposure in combination with vaccine series. For perinatal exposure (HbsAg+ mother) HBIg 0.05 mL in the thigh immediately after birth with the vaccine series started within the first 12 h of life. *Before exposure*: recombinant hepatitis B vaccine IM (dose depends on formulation as well as adult or pediatric and hemodialysis); at 0, 1, and 6 months; deltoid, not gluteal injection. Has been targeted to high-risk groups (e.g., health workers, persons with multiple sexual partners, IV drug users, hemodialysis pts, hemophiliacs, household and sexual contacts of HBsAg carriers, persons travelling in endemic areas, unvaccinated children < 18). Universal vaccination of all children is now recommended in the United States.

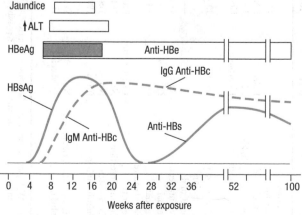

FIGURE 161-2 Scheme of typical clinical and laboratory features of HBV. (*Reproduced from JL Dienstag, HPIM-17, p. 1934.*)

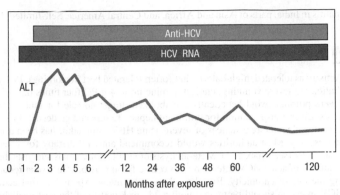

FIGURE 161-3 Scheme of typical laboratory features during acute hepatitis C progressing to chronicity. HCV RNA is the first detectable event, preceding ALT elevation and the appearance of anti-HCV. (*Reproduced from JL Dienstag, HPIM-17, p. 1937.*)

Hepatitis C (HCV) Caused by flavi-like virus with RNA genome of >9000 nucleotides (similar to yellow fever virus, dengue virus); genetic heterogeneity. Incubation period 7–8 weeks.

Clinical Course Often clinically mild and marked by fluctuating elevations of serum aminotransferase levels; >50% likelihood of chronicity, leading to cirrhosis in >20%.

Diagnosis Anti-HCV in serum. Current third-generation immunoassay incorporates proteins from the core, NS3, and NS5 regions. The most sensitive indicator of HCV infection is HCV RNA (Fig. 161-3).

Epidemiology HCV accounts for >90% of transfusion-associated hepatitis cases. IV drug use accounts >50% of reported cases of hepatitis C. Little evidence for frequent sexual or perinatal transmission.

Prevention Exclusion of paid blood donors, testing of donated blood for anti-HCV. Anti-HCV detected by enzyme immunoassay in blood donors with normal ALT is often falsely positive (30%); result should be confirmed by HCV RNA in serum.

Hepatitis D (HDV, Delta Agent) Defective 37-nm RNA virus that requires HBV for its replication; either co-infects with HBV or superinfects a chronic HBV carrier. Enhances severity of HBV infection (acceleration of chronic hepatitis to cirrhosis, occasionally fulminant acute hepatitis).

Diagnosis Anti-HDV in serum (acute hepatitis D—often in low titer, is transient; chronic hepatitis D—in higher titer, is sustained).

Epidemiology Endemic among HBV carriers in Mediterranean Basin, where it is spread predominantly by nonpercutaneous means. In nonendemic areas (e.g., northern Europe, United States) HDV is spread percutaneously among HbsAg+ IV drug users or by transfusion in hemophiliacs and to a lesser extent among HbsAg+ men who have sex with men.

Prevention Hepatitis B vaccine (noncarriers only).

Hepatitis E (HEV) Caused by 29- to 32-nm agent thought to be related to caliciviruses. Enterically transmitted and responsible for waterborne epidemics of hepatitis in India, parts of Asia and Africa, and Central America. Self-limited illness with high (10–20%) mortality rate in pregnant women.

Rx Viral Hepatitis

Activity as tolerated, high-calorie diet (often tolerated best in morning), IV hydration for severe vomiting, cholestyramine up to 4 g PO four times daily for severe pruritus, avoid hepatically metabolized drugs; no role for glucocorticoids. Liver transplantation for fulminant hepatic failure and grades III–IV encephalopathy. In rare instances of severe acute HBV, lamivudine has been used successfully. Most authorities would recommend antiviral therapy for severe acute HBV (see Chap. 162). Meta-analysis of small clinical trials suggests that treatment of acute HCV infection with α-interferon may be effective at reducing the rate of chronicity. Based on these data, many experts feel that acute HCV infection should be treated with a 24-week course of the best available regimens currently used to treat chronic HCV infection (see Chap. 162).

TOXIC AND DRUG-INDUCED HEPATITIS

Dose-Dependent (Direct Hepatotoxins)   Onset is within 48 h, predictable, necrosis around terminal hepatic venule–e.g., carbon tetrachloride, benzene derivatives, mushroom poisoning, acetaminophen, or microvesicular steatosis (e.g., tetracyclines, valproic acid).

Idiosyncratic   Variable dose and time of onset; small number of exposed persons affected; may be associated with fever, rash, arthralgias, eosinophilia. In many cases, mechanism may actually involve toxic metabolite, possibly determined on genetic basis—e.g., isoniazid, halothane, phenytoin, methyldopa, carbamazepine, diclofenac, oxacillin, sulfonamides.

Rx Toxic and Drug-Induced Hepatitis

Supportive as for viral hepatitis; withdraw suspected agent, and include use of gastric lavage and oral administration of charcoal or cholestyramine. Liver transplantation if necessary. In acetaminophen overdose, more specific therapy is available in the form of sulfhydryl compounds (e.g., N-acetylcysteine). These agents appear to act by providing a reservoir of sulfhydryl groups to bind the toxic metabolites or by stimulating synthesis of hepatic glutathione. Therapy should be begun within 8 h of ingestion, but may be effective even if given as late as 24–36 h after overdose.

ACUTE HEPATIC FAILURE

Massive hepatic necrosis with impaired consciousness occurring within 8 weeks of the onset of illness.

Causes   Infections [viral, including HAV, HBV, HCV (rarely), HDV, HEV; bacterial, rickettsial, parasitic], drugs and toxins, ischemia (shock), Budd-Chiari syndrome, idiopathic chronic active hepatitis, acute Wilson's disease, microvesicular fat syndromes (Reye's syndrome, acute fatty liver of pregnancy).

Clinical Manifestations   Neuropsychiatric changes—delirium, personality change, stupor, coma; cerebral edema—suggested by profuse sweating, hemodynamic instability, tachyarrhythmias, tachypnea, fever, papilledema, decerebrate rigidity (though all may be absent); deep jaundice, coagulopathy, bleeding, renal failure, acid-base disturbance, hypoglycemia, acute pancreatitis, cardiorespiratory failure, infections (bacterial, fungal).

Adverse Prognostic Indicators Age <10 or >40, certain causes (e.g., halothane, hepatitis C), duration of jaundice >7 d before onset of encephalopathy, serum bilirubin > 300 μmol/L (>18 mg/dL), coma (survival <20%), rapid reduction in liver size, respiratory failure, marked prolongation of PT, factor V level < 20%. In acetaminophen overdose, adverse prognosis is suggested by blood pH < 7.30, serum creatinine > 266 μmol/L (>3 mg/dL), markedly prolonged PT.

℞ Acute Hepatic Failure

Endotracheal intubation often required. Monitor serum glucose—IV D10 or D20 as necessary. Prevent GI bleeding with H_2-receptor antagonists and antacids (maintain gastric pH ≥ 3.5). In many centers intracranial pressure is monitored—more sensitive than CT in detecting cerebral edema. Value of dexamethasone for cerebral edema unclear; IV mannitol may be beneficial. Liver transplantation should be considered in pts with grades III–IV encephalopathy and other adverse prognostic indicators.

For a more detailed discussion, see Dienstag JL: Acute Viral Hepatitis, Chap. 298, p. 1932, and Dienstag JL: Toxic and Drug-Induced Hepatitis, Chap. 299, p. 1949, in HPIM-17.

162 Chronic Hepatitis

A group of disorders characterized by a chronic inflammatory reaction in the liver for at least 6 months.

OVERVIEW

Etiology Hepatitis B virus (HBV), hepatitis C virus (HCV), hepatitis D virus (HDV, delta agent), drugs (methyldopa, nitrofurantoin, isoniazid, dantrolene), autoimmune hepatitis, Wilson's disease, hemochromatosis, α_1-antitrypsin deficiency.

Histologic Classification Chronic hepatitis can be classified by *grade* and *stage*. The grade is a histologic assessment of necrosis and inflammatory activity and is based on examination of the liver biopsy. The stage of chronic hepatitis reflects the level of disease progression and is based on the degree of fibrosis (see Table 300-2, p. 1956, HPIM-17).

Presentation Wide clinical spectrum ranging from asymptomatic serum aminotransferase elevations to apparently acute, even fulminant, hepatitis. Common

TABLE 162-1 **COMPARISON OF INTERFERON (PEG IFN), LAMIVUDINE, ADEFOVIR, AND ENTECAVIR THERAPY FOR CHRONIC HEPATITIS B[a]**

Feature	PEG IFN[b]
Route of administration	Subcutaneous injection
Duration of therapy[c]	48–52 weeks
Tolerability	Poorly tolerated
HBeAg loss 1 year	29–30%
HBeAg seroconversion	
1 year Rx	18–20%
>1 year Rx	NA
HBeAg seroconversion if ALT >5 × normal	Not reported
Log_{10} HBV DNA reduction (mean copies/mL)	
HBeAg-reactive	4.5
HBeAg-negative	4.1
HBV DNA PCR negative (<300–400 copies/mL; <1,000 copies/mL for adefovir) end of year 1	
HBeAg-reactive	10–25%
HBeAg-negative	63%
ALT normalization at end of year 1	
HBeAg-reactive	39%
HBeAg-negative	34–38%
HBsAg loss during year 1	0–7%
HBsAg loss after therapy	3–7% after 6 months
Histologic improvement (≥2 point reduction in HAI) at year 1	
HBeAg-reactive	38% 6 months after
HBeAg-negative	48% 6 months after
Viral resistance	None
Durability of response 4–6 months after therapy[f]	
HBeAg-reactive	Limited data
HBeAg-negative	36%
Cost (U.S. $) for 1 year	~$18,000

[a]Generally, these comparisons are based on data on each drug tested individually versus placebo in registration clinical trials. With rare exception, these comparisons are not based on head-to-head testing of these drugs, hence relative advantages and disadvantages should be interpreted cautiously.

[b]Although standard interferon α administered daily or three times a week is approved as therapy for chronic hepatitis B, it has been supplanted by pegylated interferon (PEG IFN), which is administered once a week and is more effective. Standard interferon has no advantages over PEG IFN.

[c]Duration of therapy in clinical efficacy trials; use in clinical practice may vary.

[d]Because of a computer-generated randomization error that resulted in misallocation of drug versus placebo during the second year of clinical-trial treatment, the frequency of HBeAg serconversion beyond the first year is an estimate (Kaplan-Meier analysis) based on the small subset in whom adefovir was administered correctly.

symptoms include fatigue, malaise, anorexia, low-grade fever; jaundice is frequent in severe disease. Some pts may present with complications of cirrhosis: ascites, variceal bleeding, encephalopathy, coagulopathy, and hypersplenism. In chronic HBV or HCV and autoimmune hepatitis, extrahepatic features may predominate.

Lamivudine	Adefovir	Entecavir
Oral	Oral	Oral
≥52 weeks	≥48 weeks	≥48 weeks
Well tolerated	Well tolerated; creatinine monitoring recommended	Well tolerated
20–33%	23%	22%
16–21%	12%	21%
Up to 50% @ 5 years	43% @ 3 years[d]	31% @ 2 years
>50%	21%	Not reported
5.5	Median 3.5–5	6.9
4.4–4.7	Median 3.5–3.9	5.0
36–40%	12–21%	69% (80% @ 2 years)
39–73%	51% (79% @ 3 years)	90%
41–75%	58% (81% @ year 3)	78%
62–79%	48% (69% @ year 3)	78%
0–4%	0% (1–2% @ 2 years)	2% (5% @ 2 years)
23% after 2 years	Not reported	Not reported
51–62%	53%	62%
61–66%	64%	70%
15–30% @ 1 year	None @ 1 year	None @ 2 years[e]
70% @ 5 years	29% @ 5 years	
70–80%	91%	82%
23–35%	Low	48%
~$2,500	~$6,500	~$8,700[g]

[e]7% during a year of therapy (9% during two years) in lamivudine-resistant patients.
[f]In HBeAg-reactive patients, durability of HBeAg seroconversion; in HBeAg-negative patients, durability of virologic (HBV DNA undetectable by PCR) and biochemical (normal ALT) response.
[g]~17,400 for lamivudine-refractory patients.
Note: ALT, alanine aminotransferase; HAI, histologic activity index; HBeAg, hepatitis B e antigen; HBsAg, hepatitis B surface antigen; HBV, hepatitis B virus; NA, not applicable; Rx, therapy; PCR, polymerase chain reaction.

CHRONIC HEPATITIS B

Follows up to 1–2% of cases of acute hepatitis B in immunocompetent hosts; more frequent in immunocompromised hosts. Spectrum of disease: asymptomatic antigenemia, chronic hepatitis, cirrhosis, hepatocellular cancer; early phase

TABLE 162-2   RECOMMENDATIONS FOR TREATMENT OF CHRONIC HEPATITIS B

HBeAg Status	Clinical	HBV DNA (copies/mL)	ALT	Recommendation
HBeAg-reactive	[a]			
	Chronic hepatitis	<10^5	Normal (≤2 × ULN)[b]	No treatment; monitor
		≥10^5	Normal (≤2 × ULN)[b, c]	No treatment; current treatment of limited benefit (Some suggest liver biopsy and treating if abnormal)
	Chronic hepatitis	≥10^5	Elevated (>2 × ULN)[b]	Treat[d]
	Cirrhosis compensated	+ or —[e]	Normal or elevated	Treat[e] with oral agents,[f] not PEG IFN
	Cirrhosis decompensated	+ or —[e]	Normal or elevated	Treat[e] with oral agents,[g] not PEG IFN; refer for liver transplantation
HBeAg-negative	[a]			
	Chronic hepatitis	<10^4 or 10^{5h}	Normal (≤2 × ULN)[b]	Inactive carrier; treatment not necessary
	Chronic hepatitis	≥10^4 or 10^{5h}	Normal	Consider liver biopsy; treat if biopsy abnormal
	Cirrhosis compensated	≥10^4 or 10^{5h} (>2 × ULN)[b]	Elevated	Treat[i]
		+ or —	Elevated or normal	Treat with oral agents,[j] not PEG IFN (some authorities recommend either following or treating for HBV DNA <10^4 copies/mL)

| Cirrhosis decompensated | + or – | Treat with oral agents;[j] not PEG IFN (some authorities would follow without therapy for undetectable HBV DNA; refer for liver transplantation) |

[a] Liver disease tends to be mild or inactive clinically; most such patients do not undergo liver biopsy.

[b] In some guidelines, ALT categories are normal or elevated; in others, ALT categories are ≤ or > 2 times the upper limit of normal.

[c] Typical pattern in childhood-acquired infection, common in Asian populations.

[d] Any of the oral drugs (lamivudine, adefovir, entecavir) or PEG IFN can be used as first-line therapy (see text); although still used extensively in some countries as first-line therapy, lamivudine has been supplanted in some parts of the world. The oral agents, but not PEG IFN, should be used for interferon-refractory/intolerant and immunocompromised patients. PEG IFN is administered weekly by subcutaneous injection for a year; the oral agents are administered daily for at least a year and continued indefinitely or until at least 6 months after HBeAg seroconversion.

[e] Treating or monitoring without therapy are options for patients with HBV DNA $<10^4$ or $<10^5$ copies/mL.

[f] Some authorities would observe without treatment if HBV DNA is undetectable ($<10^4$ copies/mL), while others would treat regardless of the HBV DNA status. Lamivudine monotherapy is not an attractive choice because of its resistance profile.

[g] Some authorities recommend treating regardless of HBV DNA status, while others suggest referring for liver transplantation, without treatment, for those with undetectable

Elevated or normal

HBV DNA ($<10^5$ copies/mL). Lamivudine is a less attractive choice because of its resistance profile. Because the emergence of resistance can lead to loss of antiviral benefit and further deterioration in decompensated cirrhosis, some authorities recommend combination therapy (e.g., lamivudine or entecavir plus adefovir) for patients with decompensated cirrhosis.

[h] Some authorities rely on a cutoff of 10^4 copies/mL, while others choose 10^5 copies/mL.

[i] Because HBeAg seroconversion is not an option, the goal of therapy is to suppress HBV DNA and maintain a normal ALT. Although any of the oral agents or PEG IFN can be used as first-line therapy, lamivudine is less favored because of its resistance profile and the need, in the vast majority of cases, for long-term therapy. PEG IFN is administered by subcutaneous injection weekly for a year (caution is warranted in relying on a 6-month posttreatment interval to define a sustained response; the majority of such responses are lost thereafter). Adefovir and entecavir are administered daily, usually indefinitely or, until, as occurs very rarely, virologic and biochemical responses are accompanied by an HBsAg seroconversion.

[j] Low-resistance regimen favored (i.e., adefovir or entecavir, not lamivudine) indefinitely.

Note: ALT, alanine aminotransferase; HBeAg, hepatitis B e antigen; HBsAg, hepatitis B surface antigen; HBV, hepatitis B virus; ULN, upper limits of normal; PEG IFN, peglyated interferon.

often associated with continued symptoms of hepatitis, elevated aminotransferase levels, presence in serum of HBeAg and HBV DNA, and presence in liver of replicative form of HBV; later phase in some pts may be associated with clinical and biochemical improvement, disappearance of HBeAg and HBV DNA and appearance of anti-HBeAg in serum, and integration of HBV DNA into host hepatocyte genome. In Mediterranean and European countries as well as in Asia, a frequent variant is characterized by readily detectable HBV DNA, but without HBeAg (anti-HBeAg-reactive). Most of these cases are due to a mutation in the pre-C region of the HBV genome that prevents HBeAg synthesis (may appear during course of chronic wild-type HBV infection as a result of immune pressure and may also account for some cases of fulminant hepatitis B). Chronic hepatitis B ultimately leads to cirrhosis in 25–40% of cases (particularly in pts with HDV superinfection or the pre-C mutation) and hepatocellular carcinoma in many of these pts (particularly when chronic infection is acquired early in life).

Extrahepatic Manifestations (Immune Complex-Mediated) Rash, urticaria, arthritis, polyarteritis nodosa–like vasculitis, polyneuropathy, glomerulonephritis.

 Chronic Hepatitis B

There are currently five approved drugs for the treatment of chronic HBV: interferon-α, pegylated interferon, lamivudine, adefovir dipivoxil, and entecavir (see Table 162-1). Table 162-2 summarizes recommendations for treatment of chronic HBV.

CHRONIC HEPATITIS C

Follows 50–70% of cases of transfusion-associated and sporadic hepatitis C. Clinically mild, often waxing and waning aminotransferase elevations; mild chronic hepatitis on liver biopsy. Extrahepatic manifestations include cryoglobulinemia, porphyria cutanea tarda, membranoproliferative glomerulonephritis, and lymphocytic sialadenitis. Diagnosis confirmed by detecting anti-HCV in serum. May lead to cirrhosis in ≥20% of cases after 20 years.

 Chronic Hepatitis C

Therapy should be considered in pts with biopsy evidence of at least moderate chronic hepatitis (portal or bridging fibrosis) and HCV RNA in serum. The current therapy of choice for chronic HCV infection is a combination of pegylated interferon-α and the guanosine nucleoside analogue ribavirin (see Table 162-3). The dosage and duration of therapy depend on viral genotype (see Table 162-4). Monitoring of HCV plasma RNA is useful in assessing response to therapy. The failure to achieve a 2-log drop in HCV RNA by week 12 of therapy ("early virologic response") makes it unlikely that further therapy will result in a sustained virologic response. Thus, it is recommended that HCV RNA be measured at baseline and after 12 weeks of therapy. The current consensus view is that therapy can be stopped if an early virologic response is not achieved; however, some experts feel that histologic benefit may occur even in the absence of a virologic response.

TABLE 162-3	PEGYLATED INTERFERON-α2A AND α2B FOR CHRONIC HEPATITIS C	
	PEG IFN-α2b	PEG IFN-α2a
PEG size	12 kDa linear	40 kDa branched
Elimination half-life	54 h	65 h
Clearance	725 mL/h	60 mL/h
Best dose monotherapy[a]	1.0 μg/kg (weight-based)	180 μg
Best dose combination therapy	1.5 μg/kg (weight-based)	180 μg
Storage	Room temperature	Refrigerated
Ribavirin dose		
Genotype 1	800 mg[b]	1000–1200 mg[c]
Genotype 2/3	800 mg	800 mg
Duration of therapy		
Genotype 1	48 weeks	48 weeks
Genotype 2/3	48 weeks[d]	24 weeks
Efficacy of combination Rx[e]	54%	56%
Genotype 1	42%	46–51%
Genotype 2/3	82%	76–78%

[a]Reserved for patients in whom ribavirin is contraindicated or not tolerated.

[b]In the registration trial for PEG IFN-α2b plus ribavirin, the optimal regimen was 1.5 μg of PEG IFN plus 800 mg of ribavirin; however, a post hoc analysis of this study suggested that higher ribavirin doses are better. In addition, data from the study of PEG IFN-α2a supported weight-based dosing, 1000 mg (for patients weighing <75 kg) and 1200 mg (for patients weighing ≥75 kg) for genotype 1. Therefore, the higher ribavirin doses are recommended for both types of PEG IFN in patients with genotype 1.

[c]1000 mg for patients weighing <75 kg; 1200 mg for patients weighing ≥75 kg.

[d]In the registration trial for PEG IFN-α2b plus ribavirin, all patients were treated for 48 weeks; however, data from other trials of standard interferons and the other PEG IFN demonstrated that 24 weeks suffices for patients with genotypes 2 and 3. For patients with genotype 3 who have advanced fibrosis/cirrhosis and/or high-level HCV RNA, a full 48 weeks is preferable.

[e]To date, direct, head-to-head comparisons of the two PEG IFNs have not been reported. Attempts to compare the two PEG IFN preparations based on the results of registration clinical trials are confounded by differences between trials of the two agents in methodological details (different ribavirin doses, different methods for recording depression and other side effects) and study-population composition (different proportion with bridging fibrosis/cirrhosis, proportion from the United States versus international, mean weight, proportion with genotype 1, and proportion with high-level HCV RNA).

Note: HCV RNA, hepatitis C virus RNA; PEG, polyethylene glycol; PEG IFN, pegylated interferon.

HEPATITIS A

Although hepatitis A rarely causes fulminant hepatic failure, it may do so more frequently in pts with chronic liver disease—especially those with chronic hepatitis B or C. The hepatitis A vaccine is immunogenic and well tolerated in pts with chronic hepatitis. Thus, pts with chronic liver disease, especially those with chronic hepatitis B or C, should be vaccinated against hepatitis A.

AUTOIMMUNE HEPATITIS

Classification   *Type I*: classic autoimmune hepatitis, anti-smooth-muscle and/ or antinuclear antibodies (ANA). *Type II*: associated with anti-liver/kidney mi-

TABLE 162-4 **INDICATIONS AND RECOMMENDATIONS FOR ANTIVIRAL THERAPY OF CHRONIC HEPATITIS C**

Standard Indications for Therapy
Detectable HCV RNA (with or without elevated ALT)
Portal/bridging fibrosis or moderate to severe hepatitis on liver biopsy

Retreatment Recommended
Relapsers after a previous course of standard interferon monotherapy or combination standard interferon/ribavirin therapy
    A course of PEG IFN plus ribavirin
Nonresponders to a previous course of standard IFN monotherapy or combination standard IFN/ribavirin therapy
    A course of PEG IFN plus ribavirin—more likely to achieve a sustained virologic response in Caucasian patients without previous ribavirin therapy, with low baseline HCV RNA levels, with a 2-$\log_{10}$ reduction in HCV RNA during previous therapy, with genotypes 2 and 3, and without reduction in ribavirin dose.

Antiviral Therapy Not Recommended Routinely but Management Decisions Made on an Individual Basis
Children (age <18 years)
Age >60
Mild hepatitis on liver biopsy

Long-Term Maintenance Therapy Recommended
Cutaneous vasculitis and glomerulonephritis associated with chronic hepatitis C

Long-Term Maintenance Therapy Being Assessed in Clinical Trials
Relapsers
Nonresponders

Antiviral Therapy Not Recommended
Decompensated cirrhosis
Pregnancy (teratogenicity of ribavirin)

Therapeutic Regimens
First-line treatment: PEG IFN subcutaneously once a week plus daily ribavirin orally
    HCV genotypes 1 and 4–48 weeks of therapy
    PEG IFN-α2a 180 μg weekly plus ribavirin 1,000 mg/d (weight <75 kg) to 1200 mg/d (weight ≥75 kg) or
    PEG IFN-α2b 1.5 μg/kg weekly plus ribavirin 800 mg/d (the dose used in registration clinical trials, but the higher, weight-based ribavirin doses above are recommended for both types of PEG IFN)
    HCV genotypes 2 and 3–24 weeks of therapy
    PEG IFN-α2a 180 μg weekly plus ribavirin 800 mg/d or
    PEG IFN-α2b 1.5 μg/kg weekly plus ribavirin 800 mg/d (for patients with genotype 3 who have advanced fibrosis and/or high-level HCV RNA, a full 48 weeks of therapy may be preferable)
Alternative regimen: PEG IFN (α2a 180 μg or α2b 1.0 μg/kg) subcutaneously once a week (primarily for patients in whom ribavirin is contraindicated or not tolerated) for 24 (genotypes 2 and 3) or 48 (genotypes 1 and 4) weeks
For HCV-HIV co-infected patients: 48 weeks, regardless of genotype, of weekly PEG IFN-α2a (180 μg) or PEG IFN-α2b (1.5 μg/kg) plus a daily ribavirin dose of at least 600–800 mg, up to full weight-based 1000–1200 mg dosing if tolerated
(continued)

TABLE 162-4	INDICATIONS AND RECOMMENDATIONS FOR ANTIVIRAL THERAPY OF CHRONIC HEPATITIS C (CONTINUED)

Features Associated with Reduced Responsiveness
Genotype 1
High-level HCV RNA (>2 million copies/mL or >800,000 IU/mL)
Advanced fibrosis (bridging fibrosis, cirrhosis)
Long-duration disease
Age >40
High HCV quasispecies diversity
Immunosuppression
African American
Obesity
Hepatic steatosis
Reduced adherence (lower drug doses and reduced duration of therapy)

Note: ALT, alanine aminotransferase; HCV, hepatitis C virus; IFN, interferon; PEG IFN, pegylated interferon; IU, international units (1 IU/mL is equivalent to ~2.5 copies/mL).

crosomal (anti-LKM) antibodies, which are directed against cytochrome P450IID6 (seen primarily in southern Europe). *Type III* patients lack ANA and anti-LKM, have antibodies reactive with hepatocyte cytokeratins; clinically similar to type I. Criteria have been suggested by an international group for establishing a diagnosis of autoimmune hepatitis.

Clinical Manifestations Classic autoimmune hepatitis (type I): 80% women, third to fifth decades. Abrupt onset (acute hepatitis) in a third. Insidious onset in two-thirds: progressive jaundice, anorexia, hepatomegaly, abdominal pain, epistaxis, fever, fatigue, amenorrhea. Leads to cirrhosis; >50% 5-year mortality if untreated.

Extrahepatic Manifestations Rash, arthralgias, keratoconjunctivitis sicca, thyroiditis, hemolytic anemia, nephritis.

Serologic Abnormalities Hypergammaglobulinemia, positive rheumatoid factor, smooth-muscle antibody (40–80%), ANA (20–50%), antimitochondrial antibody (10–20%), false-positive anti-HCV enzyme immunoassay but usually not HCV RNA, atypical pANCA. Type II: anti-LKM antibody.

℞ Autoimmune Hepatitis

Indicated for symptomatic disease with biopsy evidence of severe chronic hepatitis (bridging necrosis), marked aminotransferase elevations (5- to 10-fold), and hypergammaglobulinemia. Prednisone or prednisolone 30–60 mg/d PO tapered to 10–15 mg/d over several weeks; often azathioprine 50 mg/d PO is also administered to permit lower glucocorticoid doses and avoid steroid side effects. Monitor liver function tests (LFTs) monthly. Symptoms may improve rapidly, but biochemical improvement may take weeks or months and subsequent histologic improvement (to lesion of mild chronic hepatitis or normal biopsy) up to 18–24 months. Therapy should be continued for at least 12–18 months. Relapse occurs in at least 50% of cases (re-treat). For frequent relapses, consider maintenance therapy with low-dose glucocorticoids or azathioprine 2 (mg/kg)/d.

For a more detailed discussion, see Dienstag JL: Chronic Hepatitis, Chap. 300, p. 1955, in HPIM-17.

163 Cirrhosis and Alcoholic Liver Disease

CIRRHOSIS

Cirrhosis is defined histopathologically and has a variety of causes, clinical features, and complications. In cirrhosis, there is the development of liver fibrosis to the point that there is architectural distortion with the formation of regenerative nodules, which results in decreased liver function.

Causes (See Table 163-1)

Clinical Manifestations May be absent, with cirrhosis being incidentally found at surgery.

Symptoms Anorexia, nausea, vomiting, diarrhea, vague RUQ pain, fatigue, weakness, fever, jaundice, amenorrhea, impotence, infertility.

Signs Spider telangiectases, palmar erythema, jaundice, scleral icterus, parotid and lacrimal gland enlargement, clubbing, Dupuytren's contracture, gynecomastia, testicular atrophy, hepatosplenomegaly, ascites, gastrointestinal bleeding (e.g., varices), hepatic encephalopathy.

Laboratory Findings Anemia (microcytic due to blood loss, macrocytic due to folate deficiency; hemolytic called *Zieve's syndrome*), pancytopenia (hypersplenism), prolonged PT, rarely overt DIC; hyponatremia, hypokalemic alkalosis, glucose disturbances, hypoalbuminemia.

Diagnostic Studies Depend on clinical setting. Serum: HBsAg, anti-HBc, anti-HBs, anti-HCV, anti-HDV, Fe, total iron-binding capacity, ferritin, antimitochondrial antibody (AMA), smooth-muscle antibody (SMA), anti-liver/kidney microsomal (anti-LKM) antibody, ANA, ceruloplasmin, α_1 antitrypsin (and pi typing); abdominal ultrasound with doppler study, CT or MRI (may show cirrhotic liver, splenomegaly, collaterals, venous thrombosis). Definitive diagnosis often depends on liver biopsy (percutaneous, transjugular, or open).

Complications (See Table 163-2 and Chaps. 55, 56, and 164) The Child-Pugh scoring system has been used to predict the severity of cirrhosis and the risk of complications (see Table 163-3).

TABLE 163-1 CAUSES OF CIRRHOSIS

Alcoholism	Cardiac cirrhosis
Chronic viral hepatitis	Inherited metabolic liver disease
Hepatitis B	Hemochromatosis
Hepatitis C	Wilson's disease
Autoimmune hepatitis	α_1-Antitrypsin deficiency
Nonalcoholic steatohepatitis	Cystic fibrosis
Biliary cirrhosis	Cryptogenic cirrhosis
Primary biliary cirrhosis	
Primary sclerosing cholangitis	
Autoimmune cholangiopathy	

TABLE 163-2	COMPLICATIONS OF CIRRHOSIS

Portal hypertension	Coagulopathy
Gastroesophageal varices	Factor deficiency
Portal hypertensive gastropathy	Fibrinolysis
Splenomegaly, hypersplenism	Thrombocytopenia
Ascites	Bone disease
Spontaneous bacterial peritonitis	Osteopenia
Hepatorenal syndrome	Osteoporosis
Type 1	Osteomalacia
Type 2	Hematologic abnormalities
Hepatic encephalopathy	Anemia
Hepatopulmonary syndrome	Hemolysis
Portopulmonary hypertension	Thrombocytopenia
Malnutrition	Neutropenia

ALCOHOLIC LIVER DISEASE

Excessive alcohol use can cause: fatty liver, alcoholic hepatitis, cirrhosis. Alcoholic cirrhosis accounts for about 40% of the deaths due to cirrhosis. History of excessive alcohol use often denied. Severe forms (hepatitis, cirrhosis) associated with ingestion of 160 g/d for 10–20 years; women more susceptible than men and develop advanced liver disease with less alcohol intake. Hepatitis B and C may be cofactors in the development of liver disease. Malnutrition may contribute to development of cirrhosis.

Fatty Liver Often presents as asymptomatic hepatomegaly and mild elevations in biochemical liver tests. Reverses on withdrawal of ethanol; does not lead to cirrhosis.

Alcoholic Hepatitis Clinical presentation ranges from asymptomatic to severe liver failure with jaundice, ascites, GI bleeding, and encephalopathy. Typically anorexia, nausea, vomiting, fever, jaundice, tender hepatomegaly. Occasional

TABLE 163-3	CHILD-PUGH CLASSIFICATION OF CIRRHOSIS

Factor	Units	1	2	3
Serum bilirubin	μmol/L	<34	34–51	>51
	mg/dL	<2.0	2.0–3.0	>3.0
Serum albumin	g/L	>35	30–35	<30
	g/dL	>3.5	3.0–3.5	<3.0
Prothrombin time	Seconds prolonged	0–4	4–6	>6
	INR	<1.7	1.7–2.3	>2.3
Ascites		None	Easily controlled	Poorly controlled
Hepatic encephalopathy		None	Minimal	Advanced

Note: The Child-Pugh score is calculated by adding the scores of the five factors and can range from 5–15. Child-Pugh class is either A (a score of 5–6), B (7–9), or C (10 or above). Decompensation indicates cirrhosis with a Child-Pugh score of 7 or more (class B). This level has been the accepted criterion for listing for liver transplantation.

cholestatic picture mimicking biliary obstruction. Aspartate aminotransferase (AST) usually <400 U/L and more than twofold higher than alanine aminotransferase (ALT). Bilirubin and WBC may be elevated. Diagnosis defined by liver biopsy findings: hepatocyte swelling, alcoholic hyaline (Mallory bodies), infiltration of PMNs, necrosis of hepatocytes, pericentral venular fibrosis.

Other Metabolic Consequences of Alcoholism Increased NADH/NAD ratio leads to lactic acidemia, ketoacidosis, hyperuricemia, hypoglycemia. Hypomagnesemia, hypophosphatemia. Also mitochondrial dysfunction, induction of microsomal enzymes resulting in altered drug metabolism, lipid peroxidation leading to membrane damage, hypermetabolic state; many features of alcoholic hepatitis are attributable to toxic effects of acetaldehyde and cytokines (interleukins 1 and 6, and TNF, released because of impaired detoxification of endotoxin).

Adverse Prognostic Factors Critically ill patients with alcoholic hepatitis have 30-day mortality rates >50%. Severe alcoholic hepatitis characterized by: PT > 5 × above control, bilirubin > 137 μmmol/L (>8 mg/dL), hypoalbuminemia, azotemia. A discriminant function can be calculated as 4.6 × (patient's PT in seconds) (control PT in seconds) + serum bilirubin (mg/dL). Values ≥32 are associated with poor prognosis. Ascites, variceal hemorrhage, encephalopathy, hepatorenal syndrome predict a poor prognosis.

℞ Alcoholic Liver Disease

Abstinence is essential; 8500–12,500 kJ (2000–3000 kcal) diet with 1 g/kg protein (less if encephalopathy). Daily multivitamin, thiamine 100 mg, folic acid 1 mg. Correct potassium, magnesium, and phosphate deficiencies. Transfusions of packed red cells, plasma as necessary. Monitor glucose (hypoglycemia in severe liver disease). Prednisone 40 mg/d or prednisolone 32 mg/d PO for 1 month may be beneficial in severe alcoholic hepatitis with encephalopathy (in absence of GI bleeding, renal failure, infection). Pentoxifylline demonstrated improved survival and led to the inclusion of this agent as an alternative to glucocorticoids in the treatment of severe alcoholic hepatitis. Liver transplantation may be an option in carefully selected cirrhotic pts who have been abstinent >6 months.

PRIMARY BILIARY CIRRHOSIS

PBC is a progressive nonsuppurative destructive intrahepatic cholangitis. Strong female predominance, median age of 50 years. Presents as asymptomatic elevation in alkaline phosphatase (better prognosis) or with pruritus, progressive jaundice, consequences of impaired bile excretion, and ultimately cirrhosis and liver failure.

Clinical Manifestations Pruritus, fatigue, jaundice, xanthelasma, xanthomata, osteoporosis, steatorrhea, skin pigmentation, hepatosplenomegaly, portal hypertension; elevations in serum alkaline phosphatase, bilirubin, cholesterol, and IgM levels.

Associated Diseases Sjögren's syndrome, collagen vascular diseases, thyroiditis, glomerulonephritis, pernicious anemia, renal tubular acidosis.

Diagnosis Antimitochondrial antibodies (AMA) in 90% (directed against enzymes of the pyruvate dehydrogenase complex and other 2-oxo-acid dehydrogenase mitochondrial enzymes). Liver biopsy most important in AMA-negative PBC.

Biopsies identify 4 stages: stage 1—destruction of interlobular bile ducts, granulomas; stage 2—ductular proliferation; stage 3—fibrosis; stage 4—cirrhosis.

Prognosis Correlates with age, serum bilirubin, serum albumin, prothrombin time, edema.

Rx Primary Biliary Cirrhosis

Urodeoxycholic acid 13–15 mg/kg per day has been shown to improve the biochemical and histologic features of disease. Response is greatest when given early. Cholestyramine 4 g PO with meals for pruritus; in refractory cases consider rifampin, naltrexone, plasmapheresis. Calcium, vitamin D, and bisphosphonates are given for osteoporosis. Liver transplantation for end-stage disease.

LIVER TRANSPLANTATION

Consider in the absence of contraindications for chronic, irreversible, progressive liver disease or fulminant hepatic failure when no alternative therapy is available (see Table 163-4).

Contraindications (See Table 163-5)

Selection of Donor Matched for ABO blood group compatibility and liver size (reduced-size grafts may be used, esp. in children). Should be negative for HIV, HBV, and HCV. Living-donor transplant has gained increased popularity with transplantation of the right hepatic lobe from a healthy adult donor to an adult. Living-donor transplant of the left lobe accounts for one-third of all liver transplants in children.

TABLE 163-4 INDICATIONS FOR LIVER TRANSPLANTATION	
Children	Adults
Biliary atresia	Primary biliary cirrhosis
Neonatal hepatitis	Secondary biliary cirrhosis
Congenital hepatic fibrosis	Primary sclerosing cholangitis
Alagille's disease[a]	Autoimmune hepatitis
Byler's disease[b]	Caroli's disease[c]
α_1-Antitrypsin deficiency	Cryptogenic cirrhosis
Inherited disorders of metabolism	Chronic hepatitis with cirrhosis
Wilson's disease	Hepatic vein thrombosis
Tyrosinemia	Fulminant hepatitis
Glycogen storage diseases	Alcoholic cirrhosis
Lysosomal storage diseases	Chronic viral hepatitis
Protoporphyria	Primary hepatocellular malignancies
Crigler-Najjar disease type I	Hepatic adenomas
Familial hypercholesterolemia	Nonalcoholic steatohepatitis
Primary hyperoxaluria type I	Familial amyloid polyneuropathy
Hemophilia	

[a]Arteriohepatic dysplasia, with paucity of bile ducts, and congenital malformations, including pulmonary stenosis.
[b]Intrahepatic cholestasis, progressive liver failure, mental and growth retardation.
[c]Multiple cystic dilatations of the intrahepatic biliary tree.

TABLE 163-5   CONTRAINDICATIONS TO LIVER TRANSPLANTATION

Absolute	Relative
Uncontrolled extrahepatobiliary infection	Age >70
	Prior extensive hepatobiliary surgery
Active, untreated sepsis	Portal vein thrombosis
Uncorrectable, life-limiting congenital anomalies	Renal failure
Active substance or alcohol abuse	Previous extrahepatic malignancy (not including nonmelanoma skin cancer)
Advanced cardiopulmonary disease	Severe obesity
Extrahepatobiliary malignancy (not including nonmelanoma skin cancer)	Severe malnutrition/wasting
	Medical noncompliance
Metastatic malignancy to the liver	HIV seropositivity
Cholangiocarcinoma	Intrahepatic sepsis
AIDS	Severe hypoxemia secondary to right-to-left intrapulmonary shunts (P_{O_2} < 50 mmHg)
Life-threatening systemic diseases	
	Severe pulmonary hypertension (mean PA pressure >35 mmHg)
	Uncontrolled psychiatric disorder

Immunosuppression   Various combinations of tacrolimus or cyclosporine and glucocorticoids, sirolimus, mycophenolate mofetil, or OKT3 (monoclonal anti-thymocyte globulin).

Medical Complications after Transplantation   Liver graft dysfunction (primary nonfunction, acute or chronic rejection, ischemia, hepatic artery thrombosis, biliary obstruction or leak, recurrence of primary disease); infections (bacterial, viral, fungal, opportunistic); renal dysfunction; neuropsychiatric disorders, cardiovascular instability, pulmonary compromise.

Success Rate   Currently, 5-year survival rates exceed 60%; less for certain conditions (e.g., chronic hepatitis B, hepatocellular carcinoma).

> For a more detailed discussion, see Bacon BR: Cirrhosis and Its Complications, Chap. 302, p. 1971; Mailliard ME, Sorrell MF: Alcoholic Liver Disease, Chap. 301, p. 1969; Dienstag JL, Chung RT: Liver Transplantation, Chap. 304, p. 1983, in HPIM-17.

164   Portal Hypertension

Portal hypertension is defined as elevation of the hepatic venous pressure gradient to >5 mmHg, which occurs as a consequence of cirrhosis (see Chap. 163). It is caused by increased intrahepatic resistance to the passage of blood flow through the liver due to cirrhosis together with increased splanchnic blood flow due to vasodilatation within the splanchnic vascular bed.

TABLE 164-1	CLASSIFICATION OF PORTAL HYPERTENSION

Prehepatic
  Portal vein thrombosis
  Splenic vein thrombosis
  Massive splenomegaly (Banti's syndrome)
Hepatic
  Presinusoidal
    Schistosomiasis
    Congenital hepatic fibrosis
  Sinusoidal
    Cirrhosis—many causes
    Alcoholic hepatitis
  Postsinusoidal
    Hepatic sinusoidal obstruction (venoocclusive syndrome)
Posthepatic
  Budd-Chiari syndrome
  Inferior vena caval webs
  Cardiac causes
    Restrictive cardiomyopathy
    Constrictive pericarditis
    Severe congestive heart failure

Classification   See Table 164-1.

Consequences   The three primary complications of portal hypertension are (1) gastroesophageal varices with hemorrhage, (2) ascites (see Chap. 56), (3) hypersplenism.

ESOPHAGOGASTRIC VARICES

About one-third of patients with cirrhosis have varices, and one-third of patients with varices will develop bleeding. Bleeding is a life-threatening complication; risk of bleeding correlates with: variceal size and location, the degree of portal hypertension (portal venous pressure >12 mmHg), and the severity of cirrhosis, e.g., Child-Pugh classification (see Table 163-3).

Diagnosis   *Esophagogastroscopy*: procedure of choice for evaluation of upper GI hemorrhage in pts with known or suspected portal hypertension. *Celiac* and *mesenteric arteriography* are alternatives when massive bleeding prevents endoscopy and to evaluate portal vein patency (portal vein may also be studied by ultrasound with Doppler and MRI).

Rx Esophogastric Varices

See Chap. 54 for general measures to treat GI bleeding.

CONTROL OF ACUTE BLEEDING
Choice of approach depends on clinical setting and availability.

1. Endoscopic intervention is employed as first-line treatment to control bleeding acutely. Endoscopic variceal ligation (EVL) is used to control acute bleeding in >90% of cases. EVL is less successful when varices extend into proximal stomach. Some endoscopists will use variceal injection (sclerotherapy) as initial therapy, particularly when bleeding is vigorous.

2. Vasoconstricting agents: somatostatin or octreotide (50–100 µg/h by continuous infusion).
3. Balloon tamponade (Blakemore-Sengstaken or Minnesota tube). Can be used when endoscopic therapy is not immediately available or in pts who need stabilization prior to endoscopic therapy. Complications—obstruction of pharynx, asphyxiation, aspiration, esophageal ulceration. Generally reserved for massive bleeding, failure of vasopressin and/or endoscopic therapy.
4. Transjugular intrahepatic portosystemic shunt (TIPS)—portacaval shunt placed by interventional radiologic technique, reserved for failure of other approaches; risk of hepatic encephalopathy (20–30%), shunt stenosis or occlusion (30–60%), infection.

PREVENTION OF RECURRENT BLEEDING
1. EVL should be repeated until obliteration of all varices is accomplished.
2. Propranolol or nadolol—nonselective beta blockers that act as portal venous antihypertensives; may decrease the risk of variceal hemorrhage and mortality due to hemorrhage.
3. TIPS—regarded as useful "bridge" to liver transplantation in pt who has failed pharmacologic therapy and is awaiting a donor liver.
4. Portosystemic shunt surgery used less commonly with the advent of TIPS; could be considered for pts with good hepatic synthetic function.

PREVENTION OF INITIAL BLEED
For pts at high risk of variceal bleeding, consider prophylaxis with EVL and/or nonselective beta blockers.

HEPATIC ENCEPHALOPATHY

An alteration in mental status and cognitive function occurring in the presence of liver failure; may be acute and reversible or chronic and progressive.

Clinical Features Confusion, slurred speech, change in personality that can include being violent and hard to manage to being sleepy and difficult to arouse, asterixis (flapping tremor). Can progress to coma; initially responsive to noxious stimuli, later unresponsive.

Pathophysiology Gut-derived neurotoxins that are not removed by the liver because of vascular shunting and decreased hepatic mass reach the brain and cause the symptoms of hepatic encephalopathy. Ammonia levels are typically elevated in encephalopathy, but the correlation between the severity of liver disease and height of ammonia levels is often poor. Other compounds that may contribute include false neurotransmitters and mercaptans.

Precipitants GI bleeding, azotemia, constipation, high-protein meal, hypokalemic alkalosis, CNS depressant drugs (e.g., benzodiazepines and barbiturates), hypoxia, hypercarbia, sepsis.

℞ Hepatic Encephalopathy

Remove precipitants; correct electrolyte imbalances. Lactulose (nonabsorbable dissacharide) results in colonic acidification and diarrhea and is the mainstay of treatment; goal is to produce 2–3 soft stools per day. Poorly absorbed antibiotics are often used in patients who do not tolerate lactulose, with alternating administration of neomycin and metronidazole being used to reduce the individual side effects of each. Rifaximin has recently also been used; zinc supplementation is sometimes helpful. Liver transplantation when otherwise indicated.

For a more detailed discussion, see Bacon BR: Cirrhosis and Its Complications, Chap. 302, p.1971; in HPIM-17.

SECTION 12   ALLERGY, CLINICAL IMMUNOLOGY, AND RHEUMATOLOGY

165   Diseases of Immediate Type Hypersensitivity

Definition   These diseases result from IgE-dependent release of mediators from sensitized basophils and mast cells on contact with appropriate antigen (allergen). Associated disorders include anaphylaxis, allergic rhinitis, urticaria, asthma, and eczematous (atopic) dermatitis. Atopic allergy implies a familial tendency to the development of these disorders singly or in combination.

Pathophysiology   IgE binds to the surface of mast cells and basophils through a high-affinity receptor. Cross-linking of this IgE by antigen causes cellular activation with subsequent release of preformed and newly synthesized mediators including histamine, prostaglandins, leukotrienes (C_4, D_4, and E_4, collectively known as *slow-reacting substance of anaphylaxis—SRS-A*), acid hydrolases, neutral proteases, proteoglycans, and cytokines (Fig. 165-1). The mediators have been implicated in many pathophysiologic events associated with immedi-

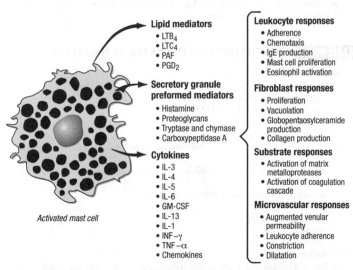

Lipid mediators
- LTB_4
- LTC_4
- PAF
- PGD_2

Secretory granule preformed mediators
- Histamine
- Proteoglycans
- Tryptase and chymase
- Carboxypeptidase A

Cytokines
- IL-3
- IL-4
- IL-5
- IL-6
- GM-CSF
- IL-13
- IL-1
- INF–γ
- TNF–α
- Chemokines

Activated mast cell

Leukocyte responses
- Adherence
- Chemotaxis
- IgE production
- Mast cell proliferation
- Eosinophil activation

Fibroblast responses
- Proliferation
- Vacuolation
- Globopentaosylceramide production
- Collagen production

Substrate responses
- Activation of matrix metalloproteases
- Activation of coagulation cascade

Microvascular responses
- Augmented venular permeability
- Leukocyte adherence
- Constriction
- Dilatation

FIGURE 165-1 Bioactive mediators of three categories generated by IgE-dependent activation of murine mast cells can elicit common but sequential target cell effects leading to acute and sustained inflammatory responses. LT, leukotriene; PAF, platelet-activating factor; PGD_2, prostaglandin D_2; IL, interleukin; GM-CSF, granulocyte-macrophage colony-stimulating factor; INF, interferon; TNF, tumor necrosis factor.

ate type hypersensitivity, such as vasodilatation, increased vasopermeability, smooth-muscle contraction, and chemotactic attraction of neutrophils and other inflammatory cells. The clinical manifestations of each allergic reaction depend largely on the anatomic site(s) and time course of mediator release.

URTICARIA AND ANGIOEDEMA

Definition May occur together or separately. *Urticaria* involves only the superficial dermis and presents as circumscribed wheals with raised serpiginous borders and blanched centers; wheals may coalesce. *Angioedema* involves deeper layers of skin and may include subcutaneous tissue. The classification of urticaria-angioedema focuses on mechanisms that elicit clinical disease and can be useful for differential diagnosis (see Table 165-1).

Pathophysiology Characterized by massive edema formation in the dermis (and subcutaneous tissue in angioedema). Presumably the edema is due to increased vasopermeability caused by mediator release from mast cells or other cell populations.

Diagnosis History, with special attention to possible offending exposures and/ or ingestion as well as the duration of lesions. Vasculitic urticaria typically persists >72 h, whereas conventional urticaria often has a duration <48 h.

- Skin testing to food and/or inhalant antigens.
- Physical provocation, e.g., challenge with vibratory or cold stimuli.
- Laboratory exam: complement levels, ESR (neither an elevated ESR nor hypocomplementemia is observed in IgE-mediated urticaria or angioedema); C1 inhibitor (C1INH) testing for deficiency of C1INH antigen (type 1) or a nonfunctional protein (type 2) if history suggests hereditary angioedema; cryoglobulins, hepatitis B antigen, and antibody studies; autoantibody screen.
- Skin biopsy may be necessary.

TABLE 165-1 CLASSIFICATION OF URTICARIA AND/OR ANGIOEDEMA

1. IgE-dependent
   a. Specific antigen sensitivity (pollens, foods, drugs, fungi, molds, Hymenoptera venom, helminths)
   b. Physical: dermographism, cold, solar
   c. Autoimmune
2. Bradykinin-mediated
   a. Hereditary angioedema: C1 inhibitor deficiency: null (type 1) and dysfunctional (type 2)
   b. Acquired angioedema: C1 inhibitor deficiency: anti-idiotype and anti-C1 inhibitor
   c. Angiotensin-converting enzyme inhibitors
3. Complement-mediated
   a. Necrotizing vasculitis
   b. Serum sickness
   c. Reactions to blood products
4. Nonimmunologic
   a. Direct mast cell–releasing agents (opiates, antibiotics, curare, D-tubocurarine, radiocontrast media)
   b. Agents that alter arachidonic acid metabolism (aspirin and nonsteroidal anti-inflammatory agents, azo dyes, and benzoates)
5. Idiopathic

Differential Diagnosis   Atopic dermatitis, contact sensitivity, cutaneous mastocytosis (urticaria pigmentosa), systemic mastocytosis.

Prevention   Identification and avoidance of offending agent(s), if possible.

R_x Urticaria and Angioedema

- H_1 antihistamines may be helpful: e.g., chlorpheniramine up to 24 mg PO daily; diphenhydramine 25–50 mg PO qid; hydroxyzine 40–200 mg PO daily; cyproheptadine 8–32 mg PO daily; or the nonsedating class, e.g., loratidine 10 mg PO daily; fexofenadine up to 180 mg PO daily; cetirizine 5–10 mg PO daily.
- H_2 antihistamines: e.g., ranitidine 150 mg PO bid may add benefit.
- Leukotriene receptor antagonists can be add-on therapy: e.g., montelukast 10 mg daily or zafirlukast 20 mg bid.
- Topical glucocorticoids are of no value in the management of urticaria and/ or angioedema. Because of their long-term toxicity, systemic glucocorticoids should not be used in the treatment of idiopathic, allergen-induced, or physical urticaria.

ALLERGIC RHINITIS

Definition   An inflammatory condition of the nose characterized by sneezing, rhinorrhea, and obstruction of nasal passages; may be associated with conjunctival and pharyngeal itching, lacrimation, and sinusitis. Seasonal allergic rhinitis is commonly caused by exposure to pollens, especially from grasses, trees, weeds, and molds. Perennial allergic rhinitis is frequently due to contact with house dust (containing dust mite antigens) and animal danders.

Pathophysiology   Deposition of pollens and other allergens on nasal mucosa of sensitized individuals results in IgE-dependent triggering of mast cells with subsequent release of mediators that cause development of mucosal hyperemia, swelling, and fluid transudation. Inflammation of nasal mucosal surface probably allows penetration of allergens deeper into tissue, where they contact perivenular mast cells. Obstruction of sinus ostia may result in development of secondary sinusitis, with or without bacterial infection.

Diagnosis   Accurate history of symptoms correlated with time of seasonal pollenation of plants in a given locale; special attention must be paid to other potentially sensitizing antigens such as pets.

- Physical examination: nasal mucosa may be boggy or erythematous; nasal polyps may be present; conjunctivae may be inflamed or edematous; manifestations of other allergic conditions (e.g., asthma, eczema) may be present.
- Skin tests to inhalant and/or food antigens.
- Nasal smear may reveal large numbers of eosinophils; presence of neutrophils may suggest infection.
- Total and specific serum IgE (as assessed by immunoassay) may be elevated.

Differential Diagnosis   Vasomotor rhinitis, URI, irritant exposure, pregnancy with nasal mucosal edema, rhinitis medicamentosa, nonallergic rhinitis with eosinophilia, rhinitis due to use of α-adrenergic agents.

Prevention   Identification and avoidance of offending antigen(s).

℞ Allergic Rhinitis

- Older antihistamines (e.g., chlorpheniramine, diphenhydramine) are effective but cause sedation and psychomotor impairment including reduced hand-eye coordination and impaired automobile driving skills. Newer antihistamines (e.g., fexofenadine, loratadine, desloradine, cetirizine, and azelastine) are equally effective but are less sedating and more H_1 specific.
- Oral sympathomimetics, e.g., pseudoephedrine 30–60 mg PO qid; may aggravate hypertension; combination antihistamine/decongestant preparations may balance side effects and provide improved pt convenience.
- Topical vasoconstrictors—should be used sparingly due to rebound congestion and chronic rhinitis associated with prolonged use.
- Topical nasal glucocorticoids, e.g., beclomethasone, 2 sprays in each nostril bid, or fluticasone, 2 sprays in each nostril once daily.
- Topical nasal cromolyn sodium, 1–2 sprays in each nostril qid.
- Montelukast 10 mg PO daily is approved for seasonal and perennial rhinitis.
- Hyposensitization therapy, if more conservative therapy is unsuccessful.

SYSTEMIC MASTOCYTOSIS

Definition A systemic disorder characterized by mast cell hyperplasia; generally recognized in bone marrow, skin, GI mucosa, liver, and spleen. Classified as (1) indolent, (2) associated with concomitant hematologic disorder, (3) aggressive, (4) mastocytic leukemia, and (5) mast cell sarcoma.

Pathophysiology and Clinical Manifestations The clinical manifestations of systemic mastocytosis are due to tissue occupancy by the mast cell mass, the tissue response to that mass (fibrosis), and the release of bioactive substances acting both locally (urticaria pigmentosa, crampy abdominal pain, gastritis, peptic ulcer) and at distal sites (headache, pruritus, flushing, vascular collapse). Clinical manifestations may be aggravated by alcohol, use of narcotics (e.g., codeine), ingestion of NSAIDs.

Diagnosis Although the diagnosis of mastocytosis may be suspected on the basis of clinical and laboratory findings, it can be established only by tissue biopsy (usually bone marrow biopsy). The diagnostic criteria for systemic mastocytosis are shown in Table 165-2. Laboratory studies that can help support a diagnosis of systemic mastocytosis include measurement of urinary or blood le-

TABLE 165-2 DIAGNOSTIC CRITERIA FOR SYSTEMIC MASTOCYTOSIS[a]

Major: Multifocal dense infiltrates of mast cells in bone marrow or other extra-cutaneous tissues with confirmation by immunodetection of tryptase or metachromasia

Minor: Abnormal mast cell morphology with a spindle shape and/or multilobed or eccentric nucleus

Aberrant mast cell surface phenotype with expression of CD25 and CD2 (IL-2 receptor) in addition to C117 (c-*kit*)

Detection of codon 816 mutation in peripheral blood cells, bone marrow cells, or lesional tissue

Total serum tryptase (mostly alpha) >20 ng/mL

[a]Diagnosis requires either major and one minor or three minor criteria.

vels of mast cell products such as histamine, histamine metabolites, prostaglandin D_2 (PGD_2) metabolites, or mast cell tryptase. Other studies including bone scan, skeletal survey, GI contrast studies may be helpful. Other flushing disorders (e.g., carcinoid syndrome, pheochromocytoma) should be excluded.

R̲x̲ Systemic Mastocystosis

- H_1 and H_2 antihistamines.
- Proton pump inhibitors for gastric hypersecretion.
- Oral cromolyn sodium for diarrhea and abdominal pain.
- NSAIDs (in nonsensitive pts) may help by blocking PGD_2 production.
- Systemic glucocorticoids may help but frequently are associated with complications.
- Hydroxyurea to reduce mast cell lineage progenitors may have merit in aggressive systemic mastocystosis.
- Chemotherapy for frank leukemias.

> For a more detailed discussion, see Austen KF: Allergies, Anaphylaxis, and Systemic Mastocytosis, Chap. 311, p. 2061, in HPIM-17.

166 Primary Immune Deficiency Diseases

DEFINITION

Disorders involving the cell-mediated (T cell) or antibody-mediated (B cell) pathways of the immune system; some disorders may manifest abnormalities of both pathways. Pts are prone to development of recurrent infections and, in certain disorders, lymphoproliferative neoplasms. *Primary disorders* may be congenital or acquired; some are familial in nature. *Secondary disorders* are not caused by intrinsic abnormalities of immune cells but may be due to infection (such as in AIDS; see HPIM-17, Chap. 182), treatment with cytotoxic drugs, radiation therapy, or lymphoreticular malignancies. Pts with disorders of antibody formation are chiefly prone to infection caused by pyogenic bacteria such as *Streptococcus pneumoniae*, *Haemophilus*, *Staphylococcus aureus*, and *Giardia*. Individuals with T cell defects are generally susceptible to infections with viruses, fungi, and protozoa.

DIAGNOSIS   See Table 166-1

CLASSIFICATION

SEVERE COMBINED IMMUNODEFICIENCY (SCID)

Congenital (autosomal recessive or X-linked); affected infants rarely survive beyond 1 year without treatment. Dysfunction of both cell mediated and humoral immunity.

TABLE 166-1   **LABORATORY EVALUATION OF HOST DEFENSE STATUS**

Initial Screening Assays[a]

Complete blood count with differential smear
Serum immunoglobulin levels: IgM, IgG, IgA, IgD, IgE

Other Readily Available Assays

Quantification of blood mononuclear cell populations by immunofluorescence assays employing monoclonal antibody markers[b]
- T cells: CD3, CD4, CD8, TCR$\alpha\beta$, TCR$\gamma\delta$
- B cells: CD19, CD20, CD21, Ig(μ, δ, γ, α, κ, λ), Ig-associated molecules (α, β)
- Activation markers: HLA-DR, CD25, CD80 (B cells), CD154 (T cells)
- NK cells: CD16/CD56
- Monocytes: CD15

T cell functional evaluation
1. Delayed hypersensitivity skin tests (PPD, *Candida*, histoplasmin, tetanus toxoid)
2. Proliferative response to mitogens (anti-CD3 antibody, phytohemagglutinin, concanavalin A) and allogeneic cells (mixed lymphocyte response)
3. Cytokine production

B cell functional evaluation
1. Natural or commonly acquired antibodies: isohemagglutinins; antibodies to common viruses (influenza, rubella, rubeola) and bacterial toxins (diphtheria, tetanus)
2. Response to immunization with protein (tetanus toxoid) and carbohydrate (pneumococcal vaccine, *H. influenzae B* vaccine) antigens
3. Quantitative IgG subclass determinations

Complement
1. CH$_{50}$ assays (classic and alternative pathways)
2. C3, C4, and other components

Phagocyte function
1. Reduction of nitroblue tetrazolium
2. Chemotaxis assays
3. Bactericidal activity

[a]Together with a history and physical examination, these tests will identify more than 95% of patients with primary immunodeficiencies.
[b]The menu of monoclonal antibody markers may be expanded or contracted to focus on particular clinical questions.

Genetic deficiencies in Orail and CD45 may lead to a T$^-$B$^+$NK$^+$ SCID phenotype.

Recombinase activating gene (RAG) deficiency: Autosomal recessive; severe lymphopenia involving B and T cells. Some cases due to mutations in the *RAG-1* or *RAG-2* genes, the combined activities of which are needed for V(D)J recombination of the T and B cell antigen receptors.

Function-loss mutations in the *DNA-dependent tyrosine kinase, Artemis, ligase IV,* or *Cernunnos* genes may cause SCID as they encode essential enzymes for the V(D)J rearrangement process.

Adenosine deaminase (ADA) deficiency: About half of pts with autosomal recessive SCID are deficient in ADA, due to mutations in the *ADA* gene.

X-linked SCID: Characterized by an absence of peripheral T cells and natural killer (NK) cells. B lymphocytes are present in normal numbers but are functionally defective. These pts have a mutation in the gene that encodes the gamma chain common to the interleukin (IL) -2, -4, -7, -9, -15 receptors, thus disrupting the action of these important lymphokines. The same phenotype seen in X-linked SCID can be inherited as an autosomal recessive disease due to mutations in the JAK3 protein kinase gene. This enzyme associates with the common gamma chain of the receptors for IL-2, -4, -9, and -15 and is a key element in the signal transduction pathways used by these receptors.

 Severe Combined Immunodeficiency

Bone marrow transplantation is useful in some SCID pts.

T CELL IMMUNODEFICIENCY

DiGeorge's syndrome: Maldevelopment of organs derived embryologically from third and fourth pharyngeal pouches (including thymus); associated with congenital cardiac defects, parathyroid hypoplasia with hypocalcemic tetany, abnormal facies, thymic aplasia; serum Ig levels may be normal, but specific IgG and IgA antibody responses are impaired.

T cell receptor (TCR) complex deficiency: Immunodeficiencies due to inherited mutations of the CD3γ and CD3ε components of the TCR complex have been identified. CD3γ mutations result in a selective defect in CD8 T cells, whereas CD3ε mutations lead to a preferential reduction in CD4 T cells.

MHC class II deficiency: Antigen-presenting cells from pts with this rare disorder fail to express the class II molecules DP, DQ, and DR on their surface, which results in limited development of CD4+ T cells in the thymus and defective interaction of CD4 T cells and antigen-presenting cells in the periphery. Affected pts experience recurrent bronchopulmonary infections, chronic diarrhea, and severe viral infections.

Inherited deficiency of purine nucleoside phosphorylase: Functions in same salvage pathway as ADA; cellular dysfunction may be related to intracellular accumulation of purine metabolites.

Ataxia-telangiectasia: Autosomal recessive disorder caused by mutation in the *ATM* gene (gene product involved in DNA repair). Clinical manifestations include cerebellar ataxia, oculocutaneous telangiectasia, immunodeficiency; not all pts have immunodeficiency; lymphomas common; IgG subclasses may be abnormal.

The nude syndrome: This is the counterpart to the *nude* mouse and is caused by a mutation in the *whn* gene resulting in impairment of hair follicle and epithelial thymic development. The phenotype is characterized by congenital baldness, nail dystrophy, and severe T cell immunodeficiency.

Zap70 kinase deficiency: This tyrosine kinase is a pivotal component of the T cell receptor complex. Mutations in this gene result in a T cell immunodeficiency manifested by recurrent opportunistic infections that begin in the first year of life.

 T Cell Immunodeficiency

Treatment for T cell disorders is complex and largely investigational. Live vaccines and blood transfusions containing viable T cells should be assiduously avoided. Preventive therapy for *Pneumocystis jiroveci* pneumonia should be considered in selected pts with severe T cell deficiency.

IMMUNOGLOBULIN DEFICIENCY SYNDROMES

X-linked agammaglobulinemia: Due to a mutation in the *Bruton's tyrosine kinase (Btk)* gene. Marked deficiency of circulating B lymphocytes; all Ig classes low;

recurrent sinopulmonary infections are the most frequent clinical problem. Mycoplasma infections can cause arthritis in some patients and chronic viral encephalitis sometimes associated with dermatomyositis can be a fatal complication.

Autosomal agammaglobulinemia: This can result from mutations in a variety of genes required for B lineage differentiation.

Transient hypogammaglobulinemia of infancy: This occurs between 3 and 6 months of age as maternally derived IgG levels decline.

Isolated IgA deficiency: Most common immunodeficiency; the majority of affected individuals do not have increased infections; antibodies against IgA may lead to anaphylaxis during transfusion of blood or plasma; may be associated with deficiencies of IgG subclasses; often familial.

IgG subclass deficiencies: Total serum IgG may be normal, yet some individuals may be prone to recurrent sinopulmonary infections due to selective deficiencies of certain IgG subclasses.

Common variable immunodeficiency: Heterogeneous group of syndromes characterized by panhypogammaglobulinemia, deficiency of IgG and IgA, or selective IgG deficiency and recurrent sinopulmonary infections; associated conditions include chronic giardiasis, intestinal malabsorption, atrophic gastritis with pernicious anemia, benign lymphoid hyperplasia, lymphoreticular neoplasms, arthritis, and autoimmune diseases.

X-linked immunodeficiency with hyper IgM: In most pts this syndrome results from genetic mutation in the gene encoding CD40 ligand, a transmembrane protein expressed by activated T cells and necessary for normal T and B cell cooperation, germinal center formation, and immunoglobulin isotype switching. Pts exhibit normal or increased serum IgM with low or absent IgG and IgA and recurrent sinopulmonary infections; pts also exhibit T lymphocyte abnormalities with increased susceptibility to infection with opportunistic pathogens (*P. jiroveci, Cryptosporidium*). Associated conditions include neutropenia and hepatobiliary tract disease.

℞ Immunoglobulin Deficiency Syndromes

Intravenous immunoglobulin administration (only for pts who have recurrent bacterial infections and are deficient in IgG):
- Starting dose 400–500 mg/kg given every 3–4 weeks
- Adjust dose to keep trough IgG level > 500 mg/dL
- Usually done in outpatient setting
- Decision to treat based on severity of clinical symptoms and response to antigenic challenge

MISCELLANEOUS IMMUNODEFICIENCY SYNDROMES

- Mucocutaneous candidiasis
- Interferon gamma receptor deficiency
- Interleukin 12 receptor deficiency
- X-linked lymphoproliferative syndrome
- Immunodeficiency with thymoma
- Wiskott-Aldrich syndrome
- Hyper-IgE syndrome
- Metabolic abnormalities associated with immunodeficiency

For a more detailed discussion, see Cooper MD, Schroeder HW Jr: Primary Immune Deficiency Diseases, Chap. 310, p. 2053, in HPIM-17.

167 SLE, RA, and Other Connective Tissue Diseases

CONNECTIVE TISSUE DISEASE

Definition Heterogeneous disorders that share certain common features, including inflammation of skin, joints, and other structures rich in connective tissue; as well as altered patterns of immunoregulation, including production of autoantibodies and abnormalities of cell-mediated immunity. While distinct clinical entities can be defined, manifestations may vary considerably from one patient (pt) to the next, and overlap of clinical features between and among specific diseases can occur.

SYSTEMIC LUPUS ERYTHEMATOSUS (SLE)

Definition and Pathogenesis Disease of unknown etiology in which tissues and cells undergo damage mediated by tissue-binding autoantibodies and immune complexes. Genetic, environmental, and sex hormonal factors are likely of pathogenic importance. T and B cell hyperactivity, production of autoantibodies with specificity for nuclear antigenic determinants, and abnormalities of T cell function occur.

Clinical Manifestations 90% of pts are women, usually of child-bearing age; more common in blacks than whites. Course of disease is often characterized by periods of exacerbation and relative quiescence. May involve virtually any organ system and have a wide range of disease severity. Common features include:

- *Constitutional*—fatigue, fever, malaise, weight loss
- *Cutaneous*—rashes (especially malar "butterfly" rash), photosensitivity, vasculitis, alopecia, oral ulcers
- *Arthritis*—inflammatory, symmetric, nonerosive
- *Hematologic*—anemia (may be hemolytic), neutropenia, thrombocytopenia, lymphadenopathy, splenomegaly, venous or arterial thrombosis
- *Cardiopulmonary*—pleuritis, pericarditis, myocarditis, endocarditis
- *Nephritis*—classification is primarily histologic (see Table 313-2, p. 2077, in HPIM-17)
- *GI*—peritonitis, vasculitis
- *Neurologic*—organic brain syndromes, seizures, psychosis, cerebritis

Drug-Induced Lupus A clinical and immunologic picture similar to spontaneous SLE may be induced by drugs; in particular: procainamide, hydralazine, isoniazid, chlorpromazine, methyldopa, minocycline, anti-TNF agents. Features are predominantly constitutional, joint, and pleuropericardial; CNS and renal disease are rare. All pts have antinuclear antibodies (ANA); antihistone antibodies may be present, but antibodies to dsDNA and hypocomplementemia are uncommon. Most pts improve following withdrawal of offending drug.

Evaluation

- Hx and physical exam
- Presence of ANA is a cardinal feature, but a (+) ANA is not specific for SLE. Laboratory assessment should include: CBC, ESR, ANA and ANA

subtypes (antibodies to dsDNA, ssDNA, Sm, Ro, La, histone), complement levels (C3, C4, CH50), serum immunoglobulins, VDRL, PT, PTT, anticardiolipin antibody, lupus anticoagulant, UA.
- Appropriate radiographic studies
- ECG
- Consideration of renal biopsy if evidence of glomerulonephritis

Diagnosis   Made in the presence of four or more published criteria (Table 313-3, p. 2077, in HPIM-17).

℞ Systemic Lupus Erythematosus

Choice of therapy is based on type and severity of disease manifestations. Goals are to control acute, severe flares and to develop maintenance strategies where symptoms are suppressed to an acceptable level. Treatment choices depend on (1) whether disease is life-threatening or likely to cause organ damage; (2) whether manifestations are reversible; and (3) the best approach to prevent complications of disease and treatment (see Fig. 313-2, p. 2078, and Table 313-5, p. 2080, in HPIM-17).

CONSERVATIVE THERAPIES FOR NON-LIFE-THREATENING DISEASE
- *NSAIDs* (e.g., ibuprofen 400–800 mg three to four times a day). Must consider renal, GI, and cardiovascular complications.
- *Antimalarials* (hydroxychloroquine 400 mg/d)—may improve constitutional, cutaneous, articular manifestations. Ophthalmologic evaluation required before and during Rx to rule out ocular toxicity.

TREATMENTS FOR LIFE-THREATENING SLE
- *Systemic glucocorticoids*.
- *Cytotoxic/immunosuppressive agents*—added to glucocorticoids to treat serious SLE.
  1. Cyclophosphamide—administered as IV pulse 7–25 mg/kg every 4 weeks. Daily oral dosing 1.5–3.0 mg/kg per day can also be used but has a greater risk of urinary bladder toxicity.
  2. Mycophenolate mofetil—2–3g/d; efficacy data limited to nephritis.
  3. Azathioprine—may be effective but is slower in inducing therapeutic response.
- *Anticoagulation*—may be indicated in pts with thrombotic complications.

RHEUMATOID ARTHRITIS (RA)

Definition and Pathogenesis   A chronic multisystem disease of unknown etiology characterized by persistent inflammatory synovitis, usually involving peripheral joints in a symmetric fashion. Although cartilaginous destruction, bony erosions, and joint deformity are hallmarks, the course of RA can be quite variable. An association with HLA-DR4 has been noted; both genetic and environmental factors may play a role in initiating disease. The propagation of RA is an immunologically mediated event in which joint injury occurs from synovial hyperplasia; lymphocytic infiltration of synovium; and local production of cytokines and chemokines by activated lymphocytes, macrophages, and fibroblasts.

Clinical Manifestations   RA occurs in ~0.8% of the population; women affected 3 times more often than men; prevalence increases with age, onset most frequent in fourth and fifth decades.

Articular manifestations—typically a symmetric polyarthritis of peripheral joints with pain, tenderness, and swelling of affected joints; morning stiffness is common; PIP and MCP joints frequently involved; joint deformities may develop after persistent inflammation.

Extraarticular manifestations:

Cutaneous—rheumatoid nodules, vasculitis

Pulmonary—nodules, interstitial disease, bronchiolitis obliterans–organizing pneumonia (BOOP), pleural disease, Caplan's syndrome [sero (+) RA associated with pneumoconiosis]

Ocular—keratoconjunctivitis sicca, episcleritis, scleritis

Hematologic—anemia, Felty's syndrome (splenomegaly and neutropenia)

Cardiac—pericarditis, myocarditis

Neurologic—myelopathies secondary to cervical spine disease, entrapment, vasculitis.

Evaluation

- Hx and physical exam with careful examination of all joints.
- Rheumatoid factor (RF) is present in >66% of pts; its presence correlates with severe disease, nodules, extraarticular features.
- Antibodies to cyclic citrullinated protein (anti-CCP) have similar sensitivity but higher specificity than RF; may be most useful in early RA; presence most common in pts with aggressive disease with a tendency for developing bone erosions.
- Other laboratory data: CBC, ESR.
- Synovial fluid analysis—useful to rule out crystalline disease, infection.
- Radiographs—juxtaarticular osteopenia, joint space narrowing, marginal erosions. Chest x-ray should be obtained.

Diagnosis Not difficult in pts with typical established disease. May be confusing early. Classification criteria were developed for investigational purposes, but may be useful (Table 314-1, p. 2089, in HPIM-17).

Differential Diagnosis Gout, SLE, psoriatic arthritis, infectious arthritis, osteoarthritis, sarcoid.

Rx Rheumatoid Arthritis

Goals: lessen pain, reduce inflammation, improve/maintain function, prevent long-term joint damage, control of systemic involvement. Increasing trend to treat RA more aggressively earlier in disease course (Fig. 167-1).

- Pt education on disease, joint protection
- Physical and occupational therapy—strengthen periarticular muscles, consider assistive devices.
- Aspirin or NSAIDs.
- Intraarticular glucocorticoids.
- Systemic glucocorticoids.
- Disease-modifying antirheumatic drugs (DMARDs)—e.g., methotrexate; IM gold compounds; hydroxychloroquine; sulfasalazine; D-penicillamine. Each agent has individual toxicities—pt education and monitoring required. Have been used in combination but with increased toxicity.
- Biologic therapy—TNF modulatory agents (etanercept, infliximab, adalimumab) effective at controlling RA in many pts and can slow the rate of progression of radiographic joint damage and decrease disability; carries potential for serious infection and individual toxicities. IL-1 receptor an-

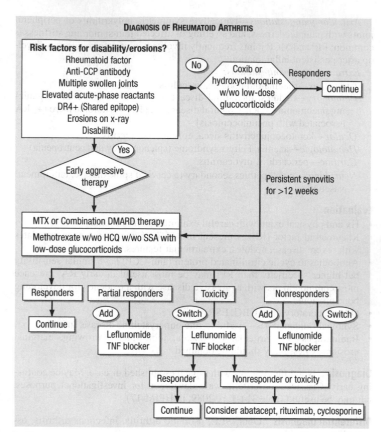

FIGURE 167-1 Algorithm for the medical management of rheumatoid arthritis. Coxib, COX-2 inhibitors; DMARD, disease-modifying anti-rheumatic drug; CCP, cyclic citrullinated polypeptide; MTX, methotrexate; SSA, sulfasalazine; TNF, tumor necrosis factor.

tagonist (anakinra) can improve the signs and symptoms of RA. Rituximab, a chimeric antibody directed to CD20 that depletes mature B cells, has been approved for RA patients who have failed anti-TNF therapy. Abatacept (CTLA4-Ig)—inhibits T cell activation, can be given with or without methotrexate, and is usually given in those who have failed or have contraindications to anti-TNF therapy.

- Immunosuppressive therapy—e.g., azathioprine, leflunomide, cyclosporine, and cyclophosphamide. Generally reserved for pts who have failed DMARDs and biologics.
- Surgery—may be considered for severe functional impairment due to deformity.

SYSTEMIC SCLEROSIS (SCLERODERMA, SSC)

Definition and Pathogenesis Systemic sclerosis (SSc) is a multisystem disorder characterized by thickening of the skin (scleroderma) and distinctive involvement of multiple internal organs (chiefly GI tract, lungs, heart, and kidney). Pathogenesis unclear; involves immunologic mechanisms leading to vascular endothelial damage and activation of fibroblasts.

Clinical Manifestations

- *Cutaneous*—edema followed by fibrosis of the skin (chiefly extremities, face, trunk); telangiectasis; calcinosis; Raynaud's phenomenon
- *Arthralgias and/or arthritis*
- *GI*—esophageal hypomotility; intestinal hypofunction
- *Pulmonary*—fibrosis, pulmonary hypertension, alveolitis
- *Cardiac*—pericarditis, cardiomyopathy, conduction abnormalities
- *Renal*—hypertension; renal crisis/failure

Two distinct subsets can be identified:

1. *Diffuse cutaneous SSc*—rapid development of symmetric skin thickening of proximal and distal extremity, face, and trunk. At high risk for development of visceral disease early in course.
2. *Limited cutaneous SSc*—often have long-standing Raynaud's phenomenon before other features appear; skin involvement limited to fingers (sclerodactyly), extremity distal to elbows, and face; associated with better prognosis; a subset of limited SSc has features of *CREST syndrome* (*c*alcinosis, *R*aynaud's, *e*sophageal dysmotility, *s*clerodactyly, *t*elangiectasias).

Evaluation

- Hx and physical exam with particular attention to blood pressure (heralding feature of renal disease).
- Laboratories: ESR, ANA (anticentromere pattern associated with limited SSc), specific antibodies may include antitopoisomerase I (Scl-70), UA
- Radiographs: CXR, barium swallow if indicated, hand x-rays may show distal tuft resorption and calcinosis.
- Additional studies: ECG, echo, PFT, consider skin biopsy.

℞ **Systemic Sclerosis**

- Education regarding warm clothing, smoking cessation, antireflux measures
- Calcium channel blockers (e.g., nifedipine) useful for Raynaud's phenomenon. Other agents with potential benefit include sildenafil, losartan, nitroglycerin paste, fluoxetine, bosantan, digital sympathectomy.
- ACE inhibitors—particularly important for controlling hypertension and limiting progression of renal disease.
- Antacids, H2 antagonists, omeprazole, and metoclopramide may be useful for esophageal reflux.
- D-Penicillamine—controversial benefit to reduce skin thickening and prevent organ involvement; no advantages to using doses >125 mg every other day.
- Glucocorticoids—no efficacy in slowing progression of SSc; indicated for inflammatory myositis or pericarditis; high doses early in disease may be associated with development of renal crisis.
- Cyclophosphamide—improves lung function and survival in pts with alveolitis.
- Epoprostenol (prostacyclin) and bosentan (endothelin-1 receptor antagonist)—may improve cardiopulmonary hemodynamics in pts with pulmonary hypertension.

MIXED CONNECTIVE TISSUE DISEASE (MCTD)

Definition Syndrome characterized by a combination of clinical features similar to those of SLE, SSc, polymyositis, and RA; unusually high titers of circulating antibodies to a nuclear ribonucleoprotein (RNP) are found. It is controversial whether MCTD is a truly distinct entity or a subset of SLE or SSc.

Clinical Manifestations Raynaud's phenomenon, polyarthritis, swollen hands or sclerodactyly, esophageal dysfunction, pulmonary fibrosis, inflammatory myopathy. Renal involvement occurs in about 25%. Laboratory abnormalities include high-titer ANAs, very high titers of antibody to RNP, positive rheumatoid factor in 50% of pts.

Evaluation Similar to that for SLE and SSc.

 Mixed Connective Tissue Disease

Few published data. Treat based upon manifestations with similar approach to that used if feature occurred in SLE/SSc/polymyositis/RA.

SJÖGREN'S SYNDROME

Definition An immunologic disorder characterized by progressive lymphocytic destruction of exocrine glands most frequently resulting in symptomatic eye and mouth dryness; can be associated with extraglandular manifestations; predominantly affects middle-age females; may be primary or secondary when it occurs in association with other autoimmune diseases.

Clinical Manifestations
- *Constitutional*—fatigue
- *Sicca symptoms*—keratoconjunctivitis sicca (KCS) and xerostomia
- *Dryness of other surfaces*—nose, vagina, trachea, skin
- *Extraglandular features*—arthralgia/arthritis, Raynaud's, lymphadenopathy, interstitial pneumonitis, vasculitis (usually cutaneous), nephritis, lymphoma.

Evaluation
- Hx and physical exam—with special attention to oral, ocular, lymphatic exam and presence of other autoimmune disorders.
- Presence of autoantibodies is a hallmark of disease (ANA, RF, anti-Ro, anti-La)
- Other laboratories—ESR; CBC; renal, liver, and thyroid function tests; serum protein electrophoresis (SPEP) (hypergammaglobulinemia or monoclonal gammopathy common); UA.
- Ocular studies—to diagnose and quantitate KCS; Schirmer's test, Rose bengal staining.
- Oral exam—unstimulated salivary flow, dental exam.
- Labial salivary gland biopsy—demonstrates lymphocytic infiltration and destruction of glandular tissue.

Diagnosis Criteria often include: KCS, xerostomia, (+) serologic features of autoimmunity. Positive lip biopsy considered necessary in some series—should be performed in setting of objective KCS/xerostomia with negative serologies.

Sjögren's Syndrome

- Regular follow-up with dentist and ophthalmologist.
- Dry eyes-artificial tears, ophthalmic lubricating ointments, local stimulation with cyclic adenosine monophosphate or cyclosporine drops.
- Xerostomia-frequent sips of water, sugarless candy.
- Pilocarpine or cevimeline—may help sicca manifestations.
- Hydroxychloroquine—may help arthralgias.
- Glucocorticoids—not effective for sicca Sx but may have role in treatment of extraglandular manifestations.

For a more detailed discussion, see Hahn BH: Systemic Lupus Erythematosus, Chap. 313, p. 2075; Lipsky PE: Rheumatoid Arthritis, Chap. 314, p. 2083; Varga J: Systemic Sclerosis (Scleroderma) and Related Disorders, Chap. 316, p. 2096; Moutsopoulos HM: Sjögren's Syndrome, Chap. 317, p. 2107, in HPIM-17.

168 Vasculitis

DEFINITION AND PATHOGENESIS

A clinicopathologic process characterized by inflammation of and damage to blood vessels, compromise of vessel lumen, and resulting ischemia. Clinical manifestations depend on size and location of affected vessel. Most vasculitic syndromes appear to be mediated by immune mechanisms. May be primary or sole manifestation of a disease or secondary to another disease process. Unique vasculitic syndromes can differ greatly with regards to clinical features, disease severity, histology, and treatment.

PRIMARY VASCULITIS SYNDROMES

Wegener's Granulomatosis   Granulomatous vasculitis of upper and lower respiratory tracts together with glomerulonephritis; upper airway lesions affecting the nose and sinuses can cause purulent or bloody nasal discharge, mucosal ulceration, septal perforation, and cartilaginous destruction (saddlenose deformity). Lung involvement may be asymptomatic or cause cough, hemoptysis, dyspnea; eye involvement may occur; glomerulonephritis can be rapidly progressive, asymptomatic, and lead to renal failure.

Churg-Strauss Syndrome (Allergic Angiitis and Granulomatosis)   Granulomatous vasculitis of multiple organ systems, particularly the lung; characterized by asthma, peripheral eosinophilia, eosinophilic tissue infiltration; glomerulonephritis can occur.

Polyarteritis Nodosa (PAN)   Medium-sized muscular arteries involved; frequently associated with arteriographic aneurysms; commonly affects renal arteries, liver, GI tract, peripheral nerves, skin, heart; can be associated with hepatitis B.

Microscopic Polyangiitis Small-vessel vasculitis that can affect the glomerulus and lungs; medium-sized vessels may also be affected.

Giant Cell Arteritis (Temporal Arteritis) Inflammation of medium- and large-sized arteries; primarily involves temporal artery but systemic and large vessel involvement may occur; symptoms include headache, jaw/tongue claudication, scalp tenderness, fever, musculoskeletal symptoms (polymyalgia rheumatica); sudden blindness from involvement of optic vessels is a dreaded complication.

Takayasu's Arteritis Vasculitis of the large arteries with strong predilection for aortic arch and its branches; most common in young women; presents with inflammatory or ischemic symptoms in arms and neck, systemic inflammatory symptoms, aortic regurgitation.

Henoch-Schönlein Purpura Characterized by involvement of skin, GI tract, kidneys; more common in children; may recur after initial remission.

Essential Mixed Cryoglobulinemia Majority of cases are associated with hepatitis C where an aberrant immune response leads to formation of cryoglobulin; characterized by cutaneous vasculitis, arthritis, peripheral neuropathy, and glomerulonephritis.

Idiopathic Cutaneous Vasculitis Cutaneous vasculitis is defined broadly as inflammation of the blood vessels of the dermis; due to underlying disease in >70% of cases (see "Secondary Vasculitis Syndromes," below) with 30% occurring idiopathically.

Miscellaneous Vasculitic Syndromes

- Kawasaki disease (mucocutaneous lymph node syndrome)
- Isolated vasculitis of the central nervous system
- Behçet's syndrome
- Cogan's syndrome
- Polyangiitis overlap syndrome

SECONDARY VASCULITIS SYNDROMES

- Drug-induced vasculitis
- Serum sickness
- Vasculitis associated with infection, malignancy, rheumatic disease

EVALUATION (See Fig. 168-1)

- Thorough Hx and physical exam—special reference to ischemic manifestations and systemic inflammatory signs/symptoms.
- Laboratories—important in assessing organ involvement: CBC with differential, ESR, renal function tests, UA. Should also be obtained to rule out other diseases: ANA, rheumatoid factor, anti-GBM, hepatitis B/C serologies, HIV.
- Antineutrophil cytoplasmic autoantibodies (ANCA)—associated with Wegener's granulomatosis, microscopic polyangiitis, and some patients with Churg-Strauss syndrome; presence of ANCA is adjunctive and should not be used in place of biopsy as a means of diagnosis or to guide treatment decisions.
- Radiographs—CXR should be performed even in the absence of symptoms.
- Diagnosis—can usually be made only by arteriogram or biopsy of affected organ(s).

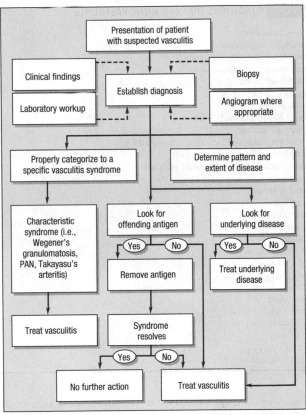

FIGURE 168-1 Algorithm for the approach to a pt with suspected diagnosis of vasculitis. PAN, polyarteritis nodosa.

DIFFERENTIAL DIAGNOSIS

Guided by organ manifestations. In many instances includes infections and neoplasms, which must be ruled out prior to beginning immunosuppressive therapy. Consideration must also be given for diseases that can mimic vasculitis (Table 168-1).

Rx Vasculitis

Therapy is based on the specific vasculitic syndrome and the severity of its manifestations. Immunosuppressive therapy should be avoided in disease that rarely results in irreversible organ system dysfunction or that usually does not respond to such agents (e.g., isolated cutaneous vasculitis). Antiviral agents play an important role in treating vasculitis occurring with hepatitis B or C. Glucocorticoids alone may control giant cell arteritis and Takayasu's arteritis. Cytotoxic agents are particularly important in syndromes with life-threatening organ system involvement, especially active glomerulonephritis. Frequently used agents:

TABLE 168-1	CONDITIONS THAT CAN MIMIC VASCULITIS

Infectious diseases
  Bacterial endocarditis
  Disseminated gonococcal infection
  Pulmonary histoplasmosis
  Coccidioidomycosis
  Syphilis
  Lyme disease
  Rocky Mountain spotted fever
  Whipple's disease
Coagulopathies/thrombotic microangiopathies
  Antiphospholipid antibody syndrome
  Thrombotic thrombocytopenic purpura
Neoplasms
  Atrial myxoma
  Lymphoma
  Carcinomatosis
Drug toxicity
  Cocaine
  Amphetamines
  Ergot alkaloids
  Methysergide
  Arsenic
Sarcoidosis
Atheroembolic disease
Goodpasture's syndrome
Amyloidosis
Migraine
Cryofibrinogenemia

- Prednisone 1 (mg/kg)/d initially, then tapered; convert to alternate-day regimen and discontinue.
- Cyclophosphamide 2 (mg/kg)/d, adjusted to avoid severe leukopenia. Morning administration with a large amount of fluid is important in minimizing bladder toxicity. Treatment should be limited to 3–6 months followed by transition to maintenance therapy with methotrexate or azathioprine. Pulsed intravenous cyclophosphamide (1 g/m^2 per month) is less effective but may be considered in selected pts who cannot tolerate daily dosing.
- Methotrexate in weekly doses up to 25 mg/week may be used to induce remission in Wegener's granulomatosis pts who do not have immediately life-threatening disease or cannot tolerate cyclophosphamide. It may also be used for maintaining remission after induction with cyclophosphamide. Cannot be used in renal insufficiency or chronic liver disease.
- Azathioprine 2 (mg/kg)/d. Less effective in treating active disease but useful in maintaining remission after induction with cyclophosphamide.
- Plasmapheresis may have an adjunctive role in rapidly progressive glomerulonephritis.

For a more detailed discussion, see Langford CA, Fauci AS: The Vasculitis Syndromes, Chap. 319, p. 2119; in HPIM-17.

169 Ankylosing Spondylitis

DEFINITION

Chronic and progressive inflammatory disease of the axial skeleton with sacro-iliitis (usually bilateral) as its hallmark. Peripheral joints and extraarticular structures may also be affected. Most frequently presents in young men in second or third decade; strong association with histocompatibility antigen HLA-B27. In Europe, also known as *Marie-Strumpell* or *Bechterew's disease*.

CLINICAL MANIFESTATIONS

- *Back pain and stiffness*—not relieved by lying down, often present at night forcing pt to leave bed, worse in the morning, improves with activity, insidious onset, duration >3 months (often called symptoms of "inflammatory" back pain).
- *Extraaxial arthritis*—hip and shoulders 25–35%, other peripheral joint involvement up to 30%, usually asymmetric.
- *Chest pain*—from involvement of thoracic skeleton and muscular insertions.
- *Extra/juxtaarticular pain*—due to "enthesitis": inflammation at insertion of tendons and ligaments into bone; frequently affects greater trochanter, iliac crests, ischial tuberosities, tibial tubercles, heels.
- *Extraarticular findings*—include acute anterior uveitis in about 20% of pts, aortitis, aortic insufficiency, GI inflammation, cardiac conduction defects, amyloidosis, bilateral upper lobe pulmonary fibrosis.
- *Constitutional symptoms*—fever, fatigue, weight loss may occur.
- *Neurologic complications*—related to spinal fracture/dislocation (can occur with even minor trauma), atlantoaxial subluxation, cauda equina syndrome.

PHYSICAL EXAMINATION

- Tenderness over involved joints
- Diminished chest expansion
- Diminished anterior flexion of lumbar spine (Schober test)

EVALUATION

- Erythrocyte sedimentation rate (ESR) and C-reactive protein elevated in majority.
- Mild anemia.
- Rheumatoid factor and ANA negative.
- HLA-B27 may be helpful in pts with inflammatory back Sx but negative x-rays.
- Radiographs: early may be normal. Sacroiliac joints: usually symmetric; bony erosions with "pseudowidening" followed by fibrosis and ankylosis. Spine: squaring of vertebrae; syndesmophytes; ossification of annulus fibrosis and anterior longitudinal ligament causing "bamboo spine." Sites of enthesitis may ossify and be visible on x-ray. MRI is procedure of choice when plain radiographs do not reveal sacroiliac abnormalities and can show early intraarticular inflammation, cartilage changes, and bone marrow edema.

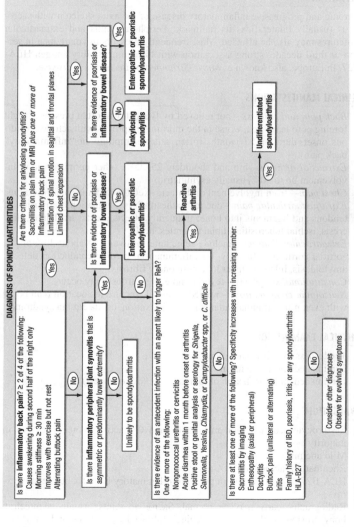

DIAGNOSIS OF SPONDYLOARTHRITIDES

Is there **inflammatory back pain?** ≥ 2 of 4 of the following:
- Causes awakening during second half of the night only
- Morning stiffness ≥ 30 min
- Improves with exercise but not rest
- Alternating buttock pain

↓ No

Is there **inflammatory peripheral joint synovitis** that is asymmetric or predominantly lower extremity?

↓ No

Unlikely to be spondyloarthritis

Yes →

Are there criteria for ankylosing spondylitis?
- Sacroiliitis on plain film or MRI *plus one or more of*
- Inflammatory back pain
- Limitation of spinal motion in sagittal and frontal planes
- Limited chest expansion

Yes → Is there evidence of psoriasis or inflammatory bowel disease?

No → **Ankylosing spondylitis**

Yes → **Enteropathic or psoriatic spondyloarthritis**

No → Is there evidence of psoriasis or inflammatory bowel disease?

Yes → **Enteropathic or psoriatic spondyloarthritis**

No → Is there evidence of an antecedent infection with an agent likely to trigger ReA?
One or more of the following:
- Nongonococcal urethritis or cervicitis
- Acute diarrhea within 1 month before onset of arthritis
- Positive stool or genital analysis or serology for *Shigella, Salmonella, Yersinia, Chlamydia,* or *Campylobacter* spp. or *C. difficile*

Yes → **Reactive arthritis**

No → Is there at least one or more of the following? Specificity increases with increasing number:
- Sacroiliitis by imaging
- Enthesopathy (axial or peripheral)
- Dactylitis
- Buttock pain (unilateral or alternating)
- Iritis
- Family history of IBD, psoriasis, iritis, or any spondyloarthritis
- HLA-B27

Yes → **Undifferentiated spondyloarthritis**

No → Consider other diagnoses
Observe for evolving symptoms

FIGURE 169-1 Algorithm for diagnosis of the spondyloarthritides.

DIAGNOSIS

Modified New York criteria widely used: radiographic evidence of sacroiliitis plus one of: (1) Hx of inflammatory back pain symptoms, (2) lumbar motion limitation, (3) limited chest expansion.

Differential Diagnosis Spondyloarthropathy associated with reactive arthritis, psoriatic arthritis, enteropathic arthritis (Fig. 169-1). Diffuse idiopathic skeletal hyperostosis.

Rx Ankylosing Spondylitis

- Exercise program to maintain posture and mobility is important.
- TNF modulatory agents (etanercept, infliximab, adalimumab) have been found to suppress disease activity and improve function.
- NSAIDs (e.g., indomethacin 75 mg slow-release daily or bid) useful in most pts.
- Sulfasalazine 2–3 g/d is of modest benefit, primarily for peripheral arthritis.
- Methotrexate, widely used but has not been of proven benefit.
- No documented therapeutic role for systemic glucocorticoids.
- Intraarticular glucocorticoids for persistent enthesitis or peripheral synovitis; ocular glucocorticoids for uveitis with systemic immunosuppression required in some cases; surgery for severely affected or deformed joints.

For a more detailed discussion, see Taurog JD: The Spondyloarthritides, Chap. 318, p. 2109, in HPIM-17.

170 Psoriatic Arthritis

DEFINITION

Psoriatic arthritis is a chronic inflammatory arthritis that affects 5–30% of persons with psoriasis. Some pts, especially those with spondylitis, will carry the HLA-B27 histocompatibility antigen. Onset of psoriasis usually precedes development of joint disease; approximately 15–20% of pts develop arthritis prior to onset of skin disease. Nail changes are seen in 90% of patients with psoriatic arthritis.

PATTERNS OF JOINT INVOLVEMENT

There are 5 patterns of joint involvement in psoriatic arthritis (Table 170-1).

EVALUATION

- Negative tests for rheumatoid factor.
- Hypoproliferative anemia, elevated erythrocyte sedimentation rate (ESR).
- Hyperuricemia may be present.
- HIV should be suspected in fulminant disease.

TABLE 170-1	PATTERNS OF JOINT INVOLVEMENT IN PSORIATIC ARTHRITIS

- *Asymmetric oligoarthritis*: often involves distal interphalangeal/proximal interphalangeal (DIP/PIP) joints of hands and feet, knees, wrists, ankles; "sausage digits" may be present, reflecting tendon sheath inflammation.
- *Symmetric polyarthritis* (40%): resembles rheumatoid arthritis except rheumatoid factor is negative, absence of rheumatoid nodules.
- *Predominantly DIP joint involvement* (15%): high frequency of association with psoriatic nail changes.
- *"Arthritis mutilans"* (3–5%): aggressive, destructive form of arthritis with severe joint deformities and bony dissolution.
- *Spondylitis and/or sacroiliitis*: axial involvement is present in 20–40% of pts with psoriatic arthritis; may occur in absence of peripheral arthritis.

- Inflammatory synovial fluid and biopsy without specific findings.
- Radiographic features include erosion at joint margin, bony ankylosis, tuft resorption of terminal phalanges, "pencil-in-cup" deformity (bone proliferation at base of distal phalanx with tapering of proximal phalanx), axial skeleton with asymmetric sacroiliitis, asymmetric nonmarginal syndesmophytes.

DIAGNOSIS

Suggested by: pattern of arthritis and inflammatory nature, absence of rheumatoid factor, radiographic characteristics, presence of skin and nail changes of psoriasis (see Fig. 169-1).

℞ Psoriatic Arthritis

- Coordinated therapy is directed at the skin and joints.
- Pt education, physical and occupational therapy.
- TNF modulatory agents (etanercept, infliximab, adalimumab) can improve skin and joint disease and delay radiographic progression.
- Alefacept in combination with methotrexate can benefit skin and joint disease.
- NSAIDs.
- Intraarticular steroid injections—useful in some settings. Systemic glucocorticoids should rarely be used as may induce rebound flare of skin disease upon tapering.
- Efficacy of gold salts and antimalarials controversial.
- Methotrexate 15–25 mg/week and sulfasalazine 2–3 g/d have clinical efficacy but do not halt joint erosion.
- Leflunomide may be of benefit for skin and joint disease.

For a more detailed discussion, see Taurog JD: The Spondyloarthritides, Chap. 318, p. 2109, in HPIM-17.

171 Reactive Arthritis

DEFINITION

Reactive arthritis refers to acute nonpurulent arthritis complicating an infection elsewhere in the body. The term has been used primarily to refer to spondyloarthritides following enteric or urogenital infections occurring predominantly in HLA-B27-positive individuals. The triad of arthritis, conjunctivitis, and nongonococcal urethritis was once known by the eponym of *Fiessenger-Leroy-Reiter syndrome*, which is now of historic interest only.

PATHOGENESIS

Up to 85% of pts possess the HLA-B27 alloantigen. It is thought that in individuals with appropriate genetic background, reactive arthritis may be triggered by an enteric infection with any of several *Shigella, Salmonella, Yersinia*, and *Campylobacter* species; by genitourinary infection with *Chlamydia trachomatis*; and possibly by other agents.

CLINICAL MANIFESTATIONS

The sex ratio following enteric infection is 1:1; however, genitourinary-acquired reactive arthritis is predominantly seen in young males. In a majority of cases Hx will elicit Sx of genitourinary or enteric infection 1–4 weeks prior to onset of other features.

Constitutional—fatigue, malaise, fever, weight loss.
Arthritis—usually acute, asymmetric, oligoarticular, involving predominantly lower extremities; sacroiliitis may occur.
Enthesitis—inflammation at insertion of tendons and ligaments into bone; dactylitis or "sausage digit," plantar fasciitis, and Achilles tendinitis common.
Ocular features—conjunctivitis, usually minimal; uveitis, keratitis, and optic neuritis rarely present.
Urethritis—discharge intermittent and may be asymptomatic.
Other urogenital manifestations—prostatitis, cervicitis, salpingitis.
Mucocutaneous lesions—painless lesions on glans penis (*circinate balanitis*) and oral mucosa in approximately a third of pts; *keratoderma blenorrhagica*: cutaneous vesicles that become hyperkerotic, most common on soles and palms.
Uncommon manifestations—pleuropericarditis, aortic regurgitation, neurologic manifestations, secondary amyloidosis.

Reactive arthritis is associated with and may be the presenting sign and Sx of HIV.

EVALUATION

- Pursuit of triggering infection by culture, serology, or molecular methods as clinically suggested.
- Rheumatoid factor and ANA negative.
- Mild anemia, leukocytosis, elevated ESR may be seen.
- HLA-B27 may be helpful in atypical cases.
- HIV screening should be performed in all pts.

- Synovial fluid analysis—often very inflammatory; negative for crystals or infection.
- Radiographs—erosions may be seen with new periosteal bone formation, ossification of entheses, sacroiliitis (often unilateral).

DIFFERENTIAL DIAGNOSIS

Includes septic arthritis (gram +/–), gonococcal arthritis, crystalline arthritis, psoriatic arthritis (see Fig. 169-1).

℞ Reactive Arthritis

- Controlled trials have failed to demonstrate any benefit of antibiotics in reactive arthritis. Prompt antibiotic treatment of acute chlamydial urethritis may prevent subsequent reactive arthritis.
- NSAIDs (e.g., indomethacin 25–50 mg PO tid) benefit most pts.
- Intraarticular glucocorticoids.
- Sulfasalazine up to 3 g/d in divided doses may help some pts with persistent arthritis.
- Cytotoxic therapy, such as azathioprine [1–2 (mg/kg)/d] or methotrexate (7.5–15 mg/week) may be considered for debilitating disease refractory to other modalities; contraindicated in HIV disease.
- Uveitis may require therapy with ocular or systemic glucocorticoids

OUTCOME

Prognosis is variable; 30–60% will have recurrent or sustained disease, with 15–25% developing permanent disability.

For a more detailed discussion, see Taurog JD: The Spondyloarthritides, Chap. 318, p. 2109, in HPIM-17.

172 Osteoarthritis

DEFINITION

Osteoarthritis (OA) is a disorder characterized by progressive joint failure in which all structures of the joint have undergone pathologic change. The pathologic sine qua non of OA is hyaline articular cartilage loss accompanied by increasing thickness and sclerosis of the subchondral bone plate, outgrowth of osteophytes at the joint margin, stretching of the articular capsule, and weakness of the muscles bridging the joint. There are numerous pathways that lead to OA, but the initial step is often joint injury in the setting of a failure of protective mechanisms.

EPIDEMIOLOGY

OA is the most common type of arthritis. The prevalence of OA correlates strikingly with age and it is much more common in women than in men. Joint vulnerability and joint loading are the two major risk factors contributing to OA. These are influenced by factors that include age, female sex, race, genetic factors, nutritional factors, joint trauma, previous damage, malalignment, proprioceptive deficiencies, and obesity.

PATHOGENESIS

The earliest changes of OA may begin in cartilage. The 2 major components of cartilage are type 2 collagen, which provides tensile strength, and aggrecan, a proteoglycan. OA cartilage is characterized by gradual depletion of aggrecan, unfurling of the collagen matrix, and loss of type 2 collagen, which leads to increased vulnerability.

CLINICAL MANIFESTATIONS

OA can affect almost any joint, but usually occurs in weight-bearing and frequently used joints such as the knee, hip, spine, and hands. The hand joints that are typically affected are the DIP, PIP, or first carpometacarpal (thumb base); metacarpophalangeal joint involvement is rare.

Symptoms

- Use-related pain affecting one or a few joints (rest and nocturnal pain less common)
- Stiffness after rest or in morning may occur but is usually brief (<30 min)
- Loss of joint movement or functional limitation
- Joint instability
- Joint deformity
- Joint crepitation ("crackling")

Physical Examination

- Chronic monarthritis or asymmetric oligo/polyarthritis
- Firm or "bony" swellings of the joint margins, e.g., Heberden's nodes (hand DIP) or Bouchard's nodes (hand PIP)
- Mild synovitis with a cool effusion can occur but is uncommon
- Crepitance—audible creaking or crackling of joint on passive or active movement
- Deformity, e.g., OA of knee may involve medial, lateral, or patellofemoral compartments resulting in varus or valgus deformities
- Restriction of movement, e.g., limitation of internal rotation of hip
- Objective neurologic abnormalities may be seen with spine involvement (may affect intervertebral disks, apophyseal joints, and paraspinal ligaments)

EVALUATION

- Routine lab work usually normal.
- ESR usually normal but may be elevated in patients who have synovitis.
- Rheumatoid factor, ANA studies negative.
- Joint fluid is straw-colored with good viscosity; fluid WBCs < 1000/μL; of value in ruling out crystal-induced arthritis, inflammatory arthritis, or infection.
- Radiographs may be normal at first but as disease progresses may show joint space narrowing, subchondral bone sclerosis, subchondral cysts, and osteophytes. Erosions are distinct from those of rheumatoid and psoriatic

arthritis as they occur subchondrally along the central portion of the joint surface.

DIAGNOSIS

Usually established on basis of pattern of joint involvement. Radiographic features, normal laboratory tests, and synovial fluid findings can be helpful if signs suggest an inflammatory arthritis.

Differential Diagnosis Osteonecrosis, Charcot joint, rheumatoid arthritis, psoriatic arthritis, crystal-induced arthritides.

℞ Osteoarthritis

- Treatment goal—alleviate pain and minimize loss of physical function.
- Nonpharmacotherapy strategies aimed at altering loading across the painful joint—includes patient education, weight reduction, appropriate use of cane and other supports, isometric exercises to strengthen muscles around affected joints, bracing/orthotics to correct malalignment.
- Topical capsaicin cream may help relieve hand or knee pain.
- Acetaminophen, salicylates, NSAIDs, COX-2 inhibitors—must weigh individual risks and benefits.
- Tramadol—may be considered in patients whose symptoms are inadequately controlled with NSAIDs; as it is a synthetic opioid agonist, habituation is a potential concern.
- Intraarticular glucocorticoids—may provide symptomatic relief but typically short-lived.
- Intraarticular hyaluronin—can be given for symptomatic knee and hip OA but it is controversial whether they have efficacy beyond placebo.
- Glucosamine and chondroitin—although widely sold, is not FDA approved for use in OA. Proof of efficacy has not been established.
- Systemic glucocorticoids have no place in the treatment of OA.
- Arthroscopic debridement and lavage—can be helpful in the subgroup of patients with knee OA in whom disruption of the meniscus causes mechanical symptoms such as locking or buckling. In patients who do not have mechanical symptoms, this modality appears to be of no greater benefit than placebo.
- Joint replacement surgery may be considered in patients with advanced OA who have intractable pain and loss of function in whom aggressive medical management has failed.

For a more detailed discussion, see Felson DT: Osteoarthritis, Chap. 326, p. 2158, in HPIM-17.

173 Gout, Pseudogout, and Related Diseases

GOUT

DEFINITION

Gout is a metabolic disease most often affecting middle-aged to elderly men and postmenopausal women. Hyperuricemia is the biologic hallmark of gout. When present, plasma and extracellular fluids become supersaturated with uric acid, which, under the right conditions, may crystallize and result in a spectrum of clinical manifestations that may occur singly or in combination.

PATHOGENESIS

Uric acid is the end product of purine nucleotide degradation; its production is closely linked to pathways of purine metabolism, with the intracellular concentration of 5-phosphoribosyl-1-pyrophosphate (PRPP) being the major determinant of the rate of uric acid biosynthesis. Uric acid is excreted primarily by the kidney through mechanisms of glomerular filtration, tubular secretion, and reabsorption. Hyperuricemia may thus arise in a wide range of settings that cause overproduction or reduced excretion of uric acid or a combination of the two (see Table 353-2, p. 2445; HPIM-17).

Acute Gouty Arthritis Monosodium urate (MSU) crystals present in the joint are phagocytosed by leukocytes; release of inflammatory mediators and lysosomal enzymes leads to recruitment of additional phagocytes into the joint and to synovial inflammation.

CLINICAL MANIFESTATIONS

Acute arthritis—most frequent early clinical manifestation of gout. Usually initially affects one joint, but may be polyarticular in later episodes. The first metatarsophalangeal joint (*podagra*) is often involved. Acute gout frequently begins at night with dramatic pain, swelling, warmth, and tenderness. Attack will generally subside spontaneously after 3–10 days. Although some patients may have a single attack, most patients have recurrent episodes with intervals of varying length with no symptoms between attacks. Acute gout may be precipitated by: dietary excess, trauma, surgery, excessive ethanol ingestion, hypouricemic therapy, and serious medical illnesses such as myocardial infarction and stroke.

Chronic arthritis–a proportion of gout patients may have a chronic nonsymmetric synovitis; may rarely be the only manifestation. Can also present with periarticular *tophi* (aggregates of MSU crystals surrounded by a giant cell inflammatory reaction). Occurs in the setting of long-standing gout.

Extraarticular tophi—often occur in olecranon bursa, helix and anthelix of ears, ulnar surface of forearm, Achilles tendon.

Tenosynovitis

Urate nephropathy—deposition of MSU crystals in interstitium and pyramids. Can cause chronic renal insufficiency.

Acute uric acid nephropathy—reversible cause of acute renal failure due to precipitation of urate in the tubules; patients receiving cytotoxic treatment for neoplastic disease are at risk.

Uric acid nephrolithiasis—responsible for 10% of renal stones in the United States.

DIAGNOSIS

- Synovial fluid analysis—should be performed to confirm gout even when clinical appearance is strongly suggestive; joint aspiration and demonstration of both intracellular and extracellular needle-shaped negatively birefringent MSU crystals by polarizing microscopy. Gram stain and culture should be performed on all fluid to rule out infection. MSU crystals can also be demonstrated in chronically involved joints or tophaceous deposits.
- Serum uric acid—normal levels do not rule out gout.
- Urine uric acid—excretion of >800 mg/d on regular diet in the absence of drugs suggests overproduction.
- Screening for risk factors or sequelae—urinalysis; serum creatinine, liver function tests, glucose and lipids; complete blood counts.
- If overproduction is suspected, measurement of erythrocyte hypoxanthine guanine phosphoribosyl transferase (HGPRT) and PRPP levels may be indicated.
- Joint x-rays—may demonstrate cystic changes, erosions with sclerotic margins in advanced chronic arthritis.
- If renal stones suggested, abdominal flat plate (stones often radiolucent), possibly IVP.
- Chemical analysis of renal stones.

Differential Diagnosis Septic arthritis, reactive arthritis, calcium pyrophosphate deposition disease (CPPD), rheumatoid arthritis.

 Gout

Asymptomatic Hyperuricemia

As only ~5% of hyperuricemic pts develop gout, treatment of asymptomatic hyperuricemia is not indicated. Exceptions are patients about to receive cytotoxic therapy for neoplasms.

Acute Gouty Arthritis

Treatment is given for symptomatic relief only since attacks are self-limited and will resolve spontaneously. Toxicity of therapy must be considered in each pt.

- Analgesia
- NSAIDs—Rx of choice when not contraindicated.
- Colchicine—generally only effective within first 24 h of attack; overdose has potentially life-threatening side effects; use is contraindicated in pts with renal insufficiency, cytopenias, LFTs > 2 × normal, sepsis. PO—0.6 mg qh until patient improves, has GI side effects, or maximal dose of 4 mg is reached. IV administration—dangerous and best avoided; if used, give no more than 2 mg over 24 h and no further drug for 7 days following; IV must never be given in a patient who has received PO colchicine.
- Intraarticular glucocorticoids—septic arthritis must be ruled out prior to injection.
- Systemic glucocorticoids—brief taper may be considered in patients with a polyarticular gouty attack for whom other modalities are contraindicated and where articular or systemic infection has been ruled out.

Uric Acid–Lowering Agents

Indications for initiating uric acid–lowering therapy include recurrent frequent acute gouty arthritis, polyarticular gouty arthritis, tophaceous gout, renal stones, prophylaxis during cytotoxic therapy. Should not start during an acute attack. Initiation can precipitate an acute flare; consider concomitant PO colchicine 0.6 mg qd until uric acid < 5.0 mg/dL, then discontinue.

1. *Allopurinol*: Decreases uric acid synthesis by inhibiting xanthine oxidase. Must be dose-reduced in renal insufficiency. Has significant side effects and drug interactions.

2. *Uricosuric drugs* (probenecid, sulfinpyrazone): Increases uric acid excretion by inhibiting its tubular reabsorption; ineffective in renal insufficiency; should not be used in these settings: age > 60, renal stones, tophi, increased urinary uric acid excretion, cytotoxic therapy prophylaxis.

CPPD DEPOSITION DISEASE (PSEUDOGOUT)

DEFINITION AND PATHOGENESIS

CPPD disease is characterized by acute and chronic inflammatory joint disease, usually affecting older individuals. The knee and other large joints most commonly affected. Calcium deposits in articular cartilage (*chondrocalcinosis*) may be seen radiographically; these are not always associated with symptoms.

CPPD is most often idiopathic but can be associated with other conditions (Table 173-1).

Crystals are thought not to form in synovial fluid but are probably shed from articular cartilage into joint space, where they are phagocytosed by neutrophils and incite an inflammatory response.

CLINICAL MANIFESTATIONS

• *Acute CCPD arthritis ("pseudogout")*—knee is most frequently involved, but polyarticular in $^2/_3$ of cases; involved joint is erythematous, swollen, warm, and painful. Most patients have evidence of chondrocalcinosis.

TABLE 173-1	CONDITIONS ASSOCIATED WITH CALCIUM PYROPHOSPHATE DIHYDRATE DISEASE

Aging
Disease-associated
   Primary hyperparathyroidism
   Hemochromatosis
   Hypophosphatasia
   Hypomagnesemia
   Chronic gout
   Postmeniscectomy
Epiphyseal dysplasias
Hereditary: Slovakian-Hungarian, Spanish, Spanish-American (Argentinian,[a] Colombian, and Chilean), French,[a] Swedish, Dutch, Canadian, Mexican-American, Italian-American,[a] German-American, Japanese, Tunisian, Jewish, English[a]

[a]Mutations in the *ANKH* gene.

- *Chronic arthropathy*—progressive degenerative changes in multiple joints; can resemble osteoarthritis (OA). Joint distribution may suggest CPPD with common sites including knee, wrist, MCP, hips, and shoulders.
- *Symmetric proliferative synovitis*—seen in familial forms with early onset; clinically similar to RA.
- *Intervertebral disk and ligament calcification*
- *Spinal stenosis*

DIAGNOSIS

- Synovial fluid analysis—demonstration of calcium pyrophosphate dihydrate crystals that appear as short blunt rods, rhomboids, and cuboids with weak positive birefringence by polarizing microscopy
- Radiographs may demonstrate chondrocalcinosis and degenerative changes (joint space narrowing, subchondral sclerosis/cysts).
- Secondary causes of CPPD should be considered in patients <50 years old.

Differential Diagnosis OA, RA, gout, septic arthritis.

Rx Pseudogout

- NSAIDs
- Intraarticular injection of glucocorticoids
- Colchicine is variably effective.

CALCIUM APATITE DEPOSITION DISEASE

Apatite is the primary mineral of normal bone and teeth. Abnormal accumulation can occur in a wide range of clinical settings (Table 173-2). Apatite is an important factor in *Milwaukee shoulder*, a destructive arthropathy of the elderly that occurs in the shoulders and knees. Apatite crystals are small; clumps may stain purplish on Wright's stain and bright red with alizarin red S. Definitive

TABLE 173-2 **CONDITIONS ASSOCIATED WITH APATITE DEPOSITION DISEASE**

Aging
Osteoarthritis
Hemorrhagic shoulder effusions in the elderly (Milwaukee shoulder)
Destructive arthropathy
Tendinitis, bursitis
Tumoral calcinosis (sporadic cases)
Disease-associated
    Hyperparathyroidism
    Milk-alkali syndrome
    Renal failure/long-term dialysis
    Connective tissue diseases (e.g., systemic sclerosis, idiopathic myositis, SLE)
    Heterotopic calcification following neurologic catastrophes (e.g., stroke, spinal cord injury)
Heredity
    Bursitis, arthritis
    Tumoral calcinosis
    Fibrodysplasia ossificans progressiva

Note: SLE, systemic lupus erythematosus.

identification requires electron microscopy or x-ray diffraction studies. Radiographic appearance resembles CPPD disease. *Treatment*: NSAIDs, repeated aspiration, and rest of affected joint.

CALCIUM OXALATE DEPOSITION DISEASE

CaOx crystals may be deposited in joints in primary oxalosis (rare) or secondary oxalosis (a complication of end-stage renal disease). Clinical syndrome similar to gout and CPPD disease. *Treatment*: marginally effective.

> For a more detailed discussion, see Wortmann RL: Disorders of Purine and Pyrimidine Metabolism, Chap. 353, p. 2444; and Schumacher HR, Chen LX: Gout and Other Crystal-Associated Arthropathies, Chap. 327, p. 2165, in HPIM-17.

174 Other Musculoskeletal Disorders

ENTEROPATHIC ARTHRITIS

Both peripheral and axial arthritis may be associated with the inflammatory bowel diseases (IBD) of ulcerative colitis or Crohn's disease. The arthritis can occur after or before the onset of intestinal symptoms. Peripheral arthritis is episodic, asymmetric, and most frequently affects knee and ankle. Attacks usually subside within several weeks and characteristically resolve completely without residual joint damage. Enthesitis (inflammation at insertion of tendons and ligaments into bone) can occur with manifestations of "sausage digit," Achilles tendinitis, plantar fasciitis. Axial involvement can manifest as spondylitis and/or sacroiliitis (often symmetric). Laboratory findings are nonspecific; rheumatoid factor (RF) absent; only 30–70% HLA-B27 positive; radiographs of peripheral joints usually normal; axial involvement is often indistinguishable from ankylosing spondylitis (see Fig. 169-1).

℞ Enteropathic Arthritis

Directed at underlying IBD; NSAIDs may alleviate joint symptoms but can precipitate flares of IBD; sulfasalazine may benefit peripheral arthritis; treatment of Crohn's disease with infliximab or adalimumab has improved arthritis.

Whipple's Disease Characterized by arthritis in up to 75% of patients that usually precedes appearance of other symptoms. Usually oligo- or polyarticular, symmetric, transient but may become chronic. Joint manifestations respond to antibiotic therapy.

NEUROPATHIC JOINT DISEASE

Also known as *Charcot's joint*, this is a severe destructive arthropathy that occurs in joints deprived of pain and position sense; may occur in diabetic neuropathy, tabes dorsalis, syringomyelia, amyloidosis, spinal cord or peripheral nerve injury. Distribution depends on the underlying joint disease. Joint effusions are usually noninflammatory but can be hemorrhagic. Radiographs can reveal either bone resorption or new bone formation with bone dislocation and fragmentation.

 Neuropathic Joint Disease

Stabilization of joint; surgical fusion may improve function.

RELAPSING POLYCHONDRITIS

An idiopathic disorder characterized by recurrent inflammation of cartilaginous structures. Cardinal manifestations include ear and nose involvement with floppy ear and saddlenose deformities, inflammation and collapse of tracheal and bronchial cartilaginous rings, asymmetric episodic nondeforming polyarthritis. Other features can include scleritis, conjunctivitis, iritis, keratitis, aortic regurgitation, glomerulonephritis, and other features of systemic vasculitis. Onset is frequently abrupt, with the appearance of 1–2 sites of cartilaginous inflammation. Diagnosis is made clinically and may be confirmed by biopsy of affected cartilage.

 Relapsing Polychondritis

Glucocorticoids (prednisone 40–60 mg/d with subsequent taper) may suppress acute features and reduce the severity/frequency of recurrences. Cytotoxic agents should be reserved for unresponsive disease or for patients who require high glucocorticoid doses. When airway obstruction is severe, tracheostomy is required.

HYPERTROPHIC OSTEOARTHROPATHY

Syndrome consisting of periosteal new bone formation, digital clubbing, and arthritis. Most commonly seen in association with lung carcinoma but also occurs with chronic lung or liver disease; congenital heart, lung, or liver disease in children; and idiopathic and familial forms. Symptoms include burning and aching pain most pronounced in distal extremities. Radiographs show periosteal thickening with new bone formation of distal ends of long bones.

 Hypertrophic Osteoarthropathy

Identify and treat associated disorder; aspirin, NSAIDs, other analgesics, vagotomy, or percutaneous nerve block may help to relieve symptoms.

FIBROMYALGIA

A common disorder characterized by chronic widespread musculoskeletal pain, aching, stiffness, paresthesia, disturbed sleep, and easy fatigability along with multiple tender points. More common in women than men. Diagnosis is made clinically; evaluation reveals soft tissue tender points but no objective joint abnormalities by exam, laboratory, or radiograph.

 Fibromyalgia

Benzodiazepines or tricyclics for sleep disorder, local measures (heat, massage, injection of tender points), NSAIDs.

POLYMYALGIA RHEUMATICA (PMR)

Clinical syndrome characterized by aching and morning stiffness in the shoulder girdle, hip girdle, or neck for >1 month, elevated ESR, and rapid response to low-dose prednisone (15 mg qd). Rarely occurs before age 50; more common in women. PMR can occur in association with giant cell (temporal) arteritis, which requires treatment with higher doses of prednisone. Evaluation should include a careful history to elicit Sx suggestive of giant cell arteritis (Chap. 169); ESR; labs to rule out other processes usually include RF, ANA, CBC, CPK, serum protein electrophoresis; and renal, hepatic, and thyroid function tests.

 PMR

Patients rapidly improve on prednisone, 10–20 mg qd, but may require treatment over months to years.

OSTEONECROSIS (AVASCULAR NECROSIS)

Caused by death of cellular elements of bone, believed to be due to impairment in blood supply. Frequent associations include glucocorticoid treatment, connective tissue disease, trauma, sickle cell disease, embolization, alcohol use. Commonly involved sites include femoral and humeral heads, femoral condyles, proximal tibia. Hip disease is bilateral in >50% of cases. Clinical presentation is usually the abrupt onset of articular pain. Early changes are not visible on plain radiograph and are best seen by MRI; later stages demonstrate bone collapse ("crescent sign"), flattening of articular surface with joint space loss.

 Osteonecrosis

Limited weight-bearing of unclear benefit; NSAIDs for Sx. Surgical procedures to enhance blood flow may be considered in early-stage disease but are of controversial efficacy; joint replacement may be necessary in late-stage disease for pain unresponsive to other measures.

PERIARTICULAR DISORDERS

Bursitis Inflammation of the thin-walled bursal sac surrounding tendons and muscles over bony prominences. The subacromial and greater trochanteric bursae are most commonly involved.

℞ Bursitis

Prevention of aggravating conditions, rest, NSAIDs, and local glucocorticoid injections.

Tendinitis   May involve virtually any tendon but frequently affects tendons of the rotator cuff around shoulder, especially the supraspinatus. Pain is dull and aching but becomes acute and sharp when tendon is squeezed below acromion.

℞ Tendinitis

NSAIDs, glucocorticoid injection, and physical therapy may be beneficial. The rotator cuff tendons or biceps tendon may rupture acutely, frequently requiring surgical repair.

Calcific Tendinitis   Results from deposition of calcium salts in tendon, usually supraspinatus. The resulting pain may be sudden and severe.

Adhesive Capsulitis ("Frozen Shoulder")   Results from conditions that enforce prolonged immobility of shoulder joint. Shoulder is painful and tender to palpation, and both active and passive range of motion is restricted.

℞ Adhesive Capsulitis

Spontaneous improvement may occur; NSAIDs, local injections of glucocorticoids, and physical therapy may be helpful.

For a more detailed discussion, see Taurog JD: The Spondyloarthritides, Chap. 318, p. 2109; Langford CA, Gilliland BC: Fibromyalgia, Chap. 329, p. 2175; Langford CA, Gilliland BC: Arthritis Associated with Systemic Disease, and Other Arthritides, Chap. 330, p. 2177; Langford CA, Gilliland BC: Periarticular Disorders of the Extremities, Chap. 331, p. 2184; and Langford CA, Gilliland BC: Relapsing Polychondritis, Chap. 321, p. 2133, in HPIM-17.

175   Sarcoidosis

DEFINITION

An inflammatory multisystem disease characterized by the presence of noncaseating granulomas of unknown etiology.

PATHOPHYSIOLOGY

The cause of sarcoid is unknown, and current evidence suggests that the triggering of an inflammatory response by an unidentified antigen in a genetically susceptible host is involved. The granuloma is the pathologic hallmark of sarcoidosis. The initial inflammatory response is an influx of T helper cells and an accumulation of activated monocytes. This leads to an increased release of cytokines and the formation of a granuloma. The granuloma may resolve or lead to chronic disease, including fibrosis.

CLINICAL MANIFESTATIONS

In 10–20% of cases, sarcoidosis may first be detected as asymptomatic hilar adenopathy. Sarcoid manifests clinically in organs where it affects function or where it is readily observed. *Löfgren's syndrome* consists of hilar adenopathy, erythema nodosum, acute arthritis presenting in one or both ankles spreading to involve other joints, and uveitis.

Disease manifestations of sarcoid include:

- *Lung*—most commonly involved organ; 90% of patients with sarcoidosis will have abnormal CXR some time during course. Features include: hilar adenopathy, alveolitis, interstitial pneumonitis; airways may be involved and cause obstruction to airflow; pleural disease and hemoptysis are uncommon.
- *Lymph nodes*—intrathoracic nodes enlarged in 75–90% of patients. Extrathoracic lymph nodes affected in 15%.
- *Skin*—25% will have skin involvement; lesions include erythema nodosum, plaques, maculopapular eruptions, subcutaneous nodules, and *lupus pernio* (indurated blue-purple shiny lesions on face, fingers, and knees).
- *Eye*—uveitis in 30%; may progress to blindness.
- *Upper respiratory tract*—nasal mucosa involved in up to 20%, larynx 5%.
- *Bone marrow and spleen*—mild anemia and thrombocytopenia may occur.
- *Liver*—involved on biopsy in 60–90%; rarely important clinically.
- *Kidney*—parenchymal disease <5%, nephrolithiasis secondary to abnormalities of calcium metabolism.
- *Nervous system*—occurs in 5–10%; cranial/peripheral neuropathy, chronic meningitis, pituitary involvement, space-occupying lesions, seizures.
- *Heart*—disturbances of rhythm and/or contractility, pericarditis.
- *Musculoskeletal*—bone lesions involving cortical bone seen in 3–13%, consisting of cysts in areas of expanded bone or lattice-like changes; dactylitis; joint involvement occurs in 25–50% with chronic mono- or oligoarthritis of knee, ankle, proximal interphalangeal joints.
- *Constitutional symptoms*—fever, weight loss, anorexia, fatigue.
- *Other organ systems*—endocrine/reproductive, exocrine glands, GI.

EVALUATION

- Hx and physical exam to rule out exposures and other causes of interstitial lung disease.
- CBC, Ca^{2+}, LFTs, ACE, PPD and control skin tests.
- CXR and/or chest CT, ECG, PFTs.
- Biopsy of lung or other affected organ.
- Bronchoalveolar lavage and gallium scan of lungs may help decide when treatment is indicated and may help to follow therapy; however, these are not uniformly accepted.

DIAGNOSIS

Made on basis of clinical, radiographic, and histologic findings. Biopsy of lung or other affected organs is mandatory to establish diagnosis before starting ther-

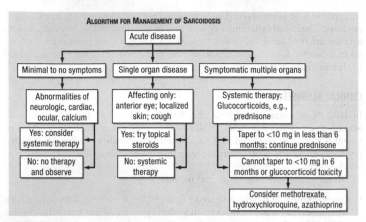

FIGURE 175-1 The management of acute sarcoidosis is based on level of symptoms and extent of organ involvement. In patients with mild symptoms, no therapy may be needed unless specified manifestations are noted.

apy. Transbronchial lung biopsy usually adequate to make the diagnosis. No blood findings are diagnostic. Differential diagnosis includes neoplasms, infections, HIV, other granulomatous processes.

℞ Sarcoidosis

As sarcoidosis may remit spontaneously, treatment is largely based upon the level of symptoms and extent of organ involvement (Figs. 175-1 and 175-2). When systemic therapy is indicated, glucocorticoids are the mainstay of therapy. Other immunomodulatory agents have been used in refractory or severe cases or when prednisone cannot be tapered.

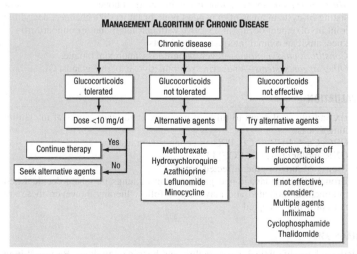

FIGURE 175-2 Approach to chronic disease is based on whether glucocorticoid therapy is tolerated or not.

OUTCOME

Sarcoidosis is usually a self-limited, non-life-threatening disease. Overall, 50% of pts with sarcoid have some permanent organ dysfunction; death directly due to disease occurs in 5% of cases usually related to lung, cardiac, neurologic, or liver involvement. Respiratory tract abnormalities cause most of the morbidity and mortality related to sarcoid.

For a more detailed discussion, see Baughman RP, Lower EE: Sarcoidosis, Chap. 322, p. 2135, in HPIM-17.

176 Amyloidosis

DEFINITION

Amyloidosis is a term for a group of diseases that are due to the extracellular deposition of insoluble polymeric protein fibrils in organs and tissues. Clinical manifestations depend on anatomic distribution and intensity of amyloid protein deposition and range from local deposition with little significance to involvement of virtually any organ system with severe pathophysiologic consequences.

CLASSIFICATION

Amyloid diseases are defined by the biochemical nature of the protein in the fibril deposits and are classified according to whether they are systemic or localized, acquired or inherited, and by their clinical patterns. The accepted nomenclature is *AX* where *A* indicates amyloidosis and *X* is the protein in the fibril (see Table 324-1, p. 2145, in HPIM-17):

- AL (immunoglobulin light chains): *Primary amyloidosis*; most common form of systemic amyloidosis; arises from a clonal B cell disorder, usually multiple myeloma.
- AA (serum amyloid A): *Secondary amyloidosis;* can occur in association with almost any chronic inflammatory state [e.g., RA, SLE, familial Mediterranean fever (FMF), Crohn's disease] or chronic infections.
- AF (familial amyloidoses): number of different types that are dominantly transmitted in association with a mutation that enhances protein misfolding and fibril formation; most commonly due to transthyretin.
- $A\beta_2M$: composed of β_2 microglobulin; occurs in end-stage renal disease of long duration.
- Localized or organ-limited amyloidoses: most common form is $A\beta$ found in Alzheimer's disease derived from abnormal proteolytic processing of the amyloid precursor protein.

CLINICAL MANIFESTATIONS

Clinical features are varied and depend entirely on biochemical nature of the fibril protein. Frequent sites of involvement:

- *Kidney*—seen with AA and AL; proteinuria, nephrosis, azotemia.
- *Liver*—occurs in AA, AL, and AF; hepatomegaly.
- *Skin*—characteristic of AL but can be seen in AA; raised waxy papules.
- *Heart*—common in AL and AF; CHF, cardiomegaly, arrhythmias.
- *GI*—common in all types; GI obstruction or ulceration, hemorrhage, protein loss, diarrhea, macroglossia, disordered esophageal motility.
- *Joints*—usually AL, frequently with myeloma; periarticular amyloid deposits, "shoulder pad sign": firm amyloid deposits in soft tissue around the shoulder, symmetric arthritis of shoulders, wrists, knees, hands.
- *Nervous system*—prominent in AF; peripheral neuropathy, postural hypotension, dementia. Carpal tunnel syndrome may occur in AL and A_2M.
- *Respiratory*—lower airways can be affected in AL; localized amyloid can cause obstruction along upper airways.

DIAGNOSIS

Diagnosis relies on the identification of fibrillar deposits in tissues and typing of the amyloid (Fig. 176-1). Congo red staining of abdominal fat will demonstrate amyloid deposits in >80% of patients with systemic amyloid.

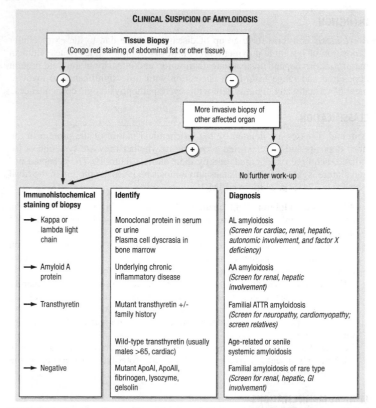

FIGURE 176-1 Algorithm for the diagnosis of amyloidosis and determination of type: Clinical suspicion: unexplained nephropathy, cardiomyopathy, neuropathy, enteropathy, arthropathy, and macroglossia. ApoAI, apolipoprotein AI, ApoAII, apolipoprotein AII, GI, gastrointestinal.

PROGNOSIS

Outcome is variable and depends on type of amyloidosis and organ involvement. Average survival of AL amyloid is ~12 months; prognosis is poor when associated with myeloma. Cardiac dysfunction associated with death in 75% of patients.

℞ Amyloidosis

For AL most effective treatment is high-dose intravenous melphalan followed by autologous stem-cell transplantation. Only 50% are eligible for such aggressive treatment and peritransplant mortality is higher than for other hematologic diseases because of impaired organ function. In patients who are not candidates for hematopoietic cell transplant, cyclic melphalan and glucocorticoids can decrease the plasma cell burden, but produces remission in only a few percent of patients with a minimal improvement in survival (median 2 years). Treatment of AA is directed towards controlling the underlying inflammatory condition. Colchicine (1–2 mg/d) may prevent acute attacks in FMF and thus may block amyloid deposition. One study found that eprodisate slowed the decline of renal function in AA, but had no significant effect on progression to end-stage renal disease or risk of death. In certain of the forms of AF, genetic counseling is important and liver transplantation is a successful form of therapy.

For a more detailed discussion, see Seldin DC, Skinner M: Amyloidosis, Chap. 324, p. 2145, in HPIM-17.

177   Disorders of the Anterior Pituitary and Hypothalamus

The anterior pituitary is often referred to as the "master gland" because, together with the hypothalamus, it orchestrates the complex regulatory functions of multiple other glands (Fig. 177-1). The anterior pituitary produces six major hormones: (1) prolactin (PRL); (2) growth hormone (GH); (3) adrenocorticotropin hormone (ACTH); (4) luteinizing hormone (LH); (5) follicle-stimulating hormone (FSH); and (6) thyroid-stimulating hormone (TSH). Pituitary hormones are secreted in a pulsatile manner, reflecting intermittent stimulation by specific hypothalamic-releasing factors. Each of these pituitary hormones elicits specific responses in peripheral target glands. The hormonal products of these peripheral glands, in turn, exert feedback control at the level of the hypothalamus and pituitary to modulate pituitary function. Disorders of the pituitary include neoplasms that lead to mass effects and clinical syndromes due to excess or deficiency of one or more pituitary hormones.

PITUITARY TUMORS

Pituitary adenomas are benign monoclonal tumors that arise from one of the five anterior pituitary cell types and may cause clinical effects from either overproduction of a pituitary hormone or compressive effects on surrounding structures, including the hypothalamus, pituitary, or both. Tumors secreting prolactin are most common and have a greater prevalence in women than in men. GH- and ACTH-secreting tumors each account for about 10–15% of pituitary tumors. About one-third of all adenomas are clinically nonfunctioning and produce no distinct clinical hypersecretory syndrome. Adenomas are classified as microadenomas (<10 mm) or macroadenomas (≥10 mm). Other entities that can present as a sellar mass include craniopharyngiomas, Rathke's cleft cysts, sella chordomas, meningiomas, pituitary metastases, and gliomas.

Clinical Features   Symptoms from mass effects include headache; visual loss through compression of the optic chiasm superiorly (classically a bitemporal hemianopsia); and diplopia, ptosis, ophthalmoplegia, and decreased facial sensation from cranial nerve compression laterally. Pituitary stalk compression from the tumor may also result in mild hyperprolactinemia. Symptoms of hypopituitarism or hormonal excess may be present as well (see below).

Pituitary apoplexy is an endocrine emergency that typically presents with features that include severe headache, bilateral visual changes, ophthalmoplegia, and, in severe cases, cardiovascular collapse and loss of consciousness. It may result in hypotension, severe hypoglycemia, CNS hemorrhage, and death. Patients with no evident visual loss or impaired consciousness can usually be observed and managed conservatively with high-dose glucocorticoids; surgical decompression should be considered when these features are present.

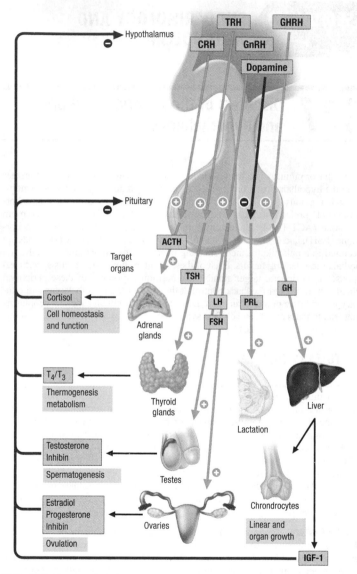

FIGURE 177-1 Diagram of pituitary axes. Hypothalamic hormones regulate anterior pituitary tropic hormones that, in turn, determine target gland secretion. Peripheral hormones feed back to regulate hypothalamic and pituitary hormones. TRH, thyrotropin-releasing hormone; for other abbreviations, see text.

Diagnosis Sagittal and coronal T1-weighted MRI images with specific pituitary cuts should be obtained before and after administration of gadolinium. In patients with lesions close to the optic chiasm, visual field assessment that uses perimetry techniques should be performed. Initial hormonal evaluation is listed in Table 177-1.

TABLE 177-1 INITIAL HORMONAL EVALUATION OF PITUITARY ADENOMAS

Pituitary Hormone	Test for Hyperfunction	Test for Deficiency
Prolactin	Prolactin	
Growth hormone	Insulin-like growth factor I (IGF-I)	IGF-I, GH stimulation tests
ACTH	24-h urinary free cortisol *or* 1-mg overnight dexamethasone suppression test	8 A.M. serum cortisol *or* ACTH stimulation test
Gonadotropins	FSH, LH	Testosterone in men Menstrual history in women
TSH	TSH, free T_4	TSH, free T_4
Other	α-subunit	

In pituitary apoplexy, CT or MRI of the pituitary may reveal signs of sellar hemorrhage, with deviation of the pituitary stalk and compression of pituitary tissue.

℞ Pituitary Tumors

Pituitary surgery is indicated for mass lesions that impinge on surrounding structures or to correct hormonal hypersecretion (see below). Transsphenoidal surgery, rather than transfrontal resection, is the desired surgical approach for most patients. The goal is selective resection of the pituitary mass lesion without damage to the normal pituitary tissue, to decrease the likelihood of hypopituitarism. Transient or permanent diabetes insipidus, hypopituitarism, CSF rhinorrhea, visual loss, and oculomotor palsy may occur postoperatively. Tumor invasion outside of the sella is rarely amenable to surgical cure, but debulking procedures may relieve tumor mass effects and reduce hormonal hypersecretion. Radiation may be used as an adjunct to surgery, but >50% of patients develop hormonal deficiencies within 10 years, usually due to hypothalamic damage. Prolactin-, GH-, and TSH-secreting tumors may also be amenable to medical therapy.

PITUITARY HORMONE HYPERSECRETION SYNDROMES

HYPERPROLACTINEMIA

Prolactin is unique among the pituitary hormones in that the predominant central control mechanism is inhibitory, reflecting dopamine-mediated suppression of prolactin release. Prolactin acts to induce and maintain lactation and decrease reproductive function and drive [via suppression of gonadotropin-releasing hormone (GnRH), gonadotropins, and gonadal steroidogenesis].

Etiology Physiologic elevation of prolactin occurs in pregnancy and lactation. Otherwise, prolactin-secreting pituitary adenomas (prolactinomas) are the most common cause of prolactin levels > 100 μg/L. Less pronounced hyperprolactinemia is commonly caused by medications [chlorpromazine, perphenazine, haloperidol, metoclopramide, opiates, H_2 antagonists, amitriptyline, selective serotonin reuptake inhibitors (SSRIs), verapamil, estrogens], pituitary stalk damage (tumors, lymphocytic hypophysitis, granulomas, trauma, irradiation), primary hypothyroidism, or renal failure. Nipple stimulation may also cause acute prolactin increases.

Clinical Features In women, amenorrhea, galactorrhea, and infertility are the hallmarks of hyperprolactinemia. In men, symptoms of hypogonadism (Chap. 183) or mass effects are the usual presenting symptoms, and galactorrhea is uncommon.

Diagnosis Fasting, morning prolactin levels should be measured; when clinical suspicion is high, measurement of levels on several different occasions may be required. If hyperprolactinemia is present, non-neoplastic causes should be excluded (e.g., pregnancy test, hypothyroidism, medications).

℞ Hyperprolactinemia

If the patient is taking a medication that is known to cause hyperprolactinemia, the drug should be withdrawn, if possible. A pituitary MRI should be performed if the underlying cause of prolactin elevation is unknown. Resection of hypothalamic or sellar mass lesions can reverse hyperprolactinemia due to stalk compression. Medical therapy with a dopamine agonist is indicated in microprolactinomas for control of symptomatic galactorrhea, restoration of gonadal function, or when fertility is desired. Alternatively, estrogen replacement may be indicated if fertility is not desired. Dopamine agonist therapy for macroprolactinomas generally results in both adenoma shrinkage and reduction of prolactin levels. Cabergoline (initial dose 0.5 mg a week, usual dose 0.5–1 mg twice a week) or bromocriptine (initial dose 0.625–1.25 mg qhs, usual dose 2.5 PO three times a day) are the two most frequently used dopamine agonists. These medications should initially be taken at bedtime with food, followed by gradual dose increases, to reduce the side effects of nausea and postural hypotension. Other side effects include constipation, nasal stuffiness, dry mouth, nightmares, insomnia, or vertigo; decreasing the dose usually alleviates these symptoms. Dopamine agonists may also precipitate or worsen underlying psychiatric conditions. Spontaneous remission of microadenomas, presumably caused by infarction, occurs in up to 30% of patients. Surgical debulking may be required for macroprolactinomas that do not respond to medical therapy.

Women with microprolactinomas who become pregnant should discontinue bromocriptine therapy, as the risk for significant tumor growth during pregnancy is low. In those with macroprolactinomas, visual field testing should be performed at each trimester. A pituitary MRI should be performed if severe headache and/or visual defects occur.

ACROMEGALY

Etiology GH hypersecretion is primarily the result of pituitary adenomas; extrapituitary causes of acromegaly are rare.

Clinical Features In children, GH hypersecretion prior to long bone epiphyseal closure results in gigantism. The presentation of acromegaly in adults is usually indolent. Patients may note a change in facial features, widened teeth spacing, deepening of the voice, snoring, increased shoe or glove size, ring tightening, hyperhidrosis, oily skin, arthropathy, and carpal tunnel syndrome. Frontal bossing, mandibular enlargement with prognathism, macroglossia, an enlarged thyroid, skin tags, thick heel pads, and hypertension may be present on examination. Associated conditions include cardiomyopathy, left ventricular hypertrophy, diastolic dysfunction, sleep apnea, diabetes mellitus, colon polyps, and colonic malignancy. Overall mortality is increased approximately threefold.

Diagnosis   Insulin-like growth factor type I (IGF-I) levels are a useful screening measure, with elevation suggesting acromegaly. Due to the pulsatility of GH, measurement of a single random GH level is not useful for screening. The diagnosis of acromegaly is confirmed by demonstrating the failure of GH suppression to <1 μg/L within 1–2 h of a 75-g oral glucose load.

℞ Acromegaly

GH levels are not normalized by surgery alone in many patients with macroadenomas; somatostatin analogues provide adjunctive medical therapy that suppresses GH secretion with modest effects on tumor size. Octreotide (50 μg SC three times a day) is used for initial therapy. Once tolerance of side effects (nausea, abdominal discomfort, diarrhea, flatulence) is established, patients may be changed to long-acting depot formulations (20–30 mg IM every 2–4 weeks). The GH receptor antagonist pegvisomant can be added in patients who do not respond to somatostatin analogues. Pituitary irradiation may also be required as adjuvant therapy but has a high rate of late hypopituitarism.

CUSHING'S DISEASE   See Chap. 180

NONFUNCTIONING AND GONADOTROPIN-PRODUCING ADENOMAS

These tumors usually present with symptoms of one or more hormonal deficiencies or mass effect. They typically produce small amounts of intact gonadotropins (usually FSH) as well as uncombined and LHβ and FSHβ subunits. Surgery is indicated for mass effects or hypopituitarism; asymptomatic small adenomas may be followed with regular MRI and visual field testing. Diagnosis is based on immunohistochemical analysis of resected tumor tissue.

TSH-SECRETING ADENOMAS

TSH-producing adenomas are rare but often large and locally invasive when they occur. Patients present with goiter and hyperthyroidism, and/or sella mass effects. Diagnosis is based on elevated serum free T_4 levels in the setting of inappropriately normal or high TSH secretion and MRI evidence of pituitary adenoma. Surgery is indicated and is usually followed by somatostatin analogue therapy to treat residual tumor. Thyroid ablation or antithyroid drugs can be used to reduce thyroid hormone levels.

HYPOPITUITARISM

Etiology   A variety of disorders may cause deficiencies of one or more pituitary hormones. These disorders may be congenital, traumatic (pituitary surgery, cranial irradiation, head injury), neoplastic (large pituitary adenoma, parasellar mass, craniopharyngioma, metastases, meningioma), infiltrative (hemochromatosis, lymphocytic hypophysitis, sarcoidosis, histiocytosis X), vascular (pituitary apoplexy, postpartum necrosis, sickle cell disease), or infectious (tuberculous, fungal, parasitic).

TABLE 177-2 HORMONE REPLACEMENT THERAPY FOR ADULT HYPOPITUITARISM[a]

Trophic Hormone Deficit	Hormone Replacement
ACTH	Hydrocortisone (10–20 mg A.M.; 5–10 mg P.M.)
	Cortisone acetate (25 mg A.M.; 12.5 mg P.M.)
	Prednisone (5 mg A.M.; 2.5 mg P.M.)
TSH	L-Thyroxine (0.075–0.15 mg daily)
FSH/LH	Males
	Testosterone enanthate (200 mg IM every 2 weeks)
	Testosterone gel (5–10 g/d)
	Females
	Conjugated estrogen (0.625–1.25 mg qd for 25 days)
	Progesterone (5–10 mg qd) on days 16–25
	Estradiol skin patch (0.5 mg, every other day)
	For fertility: Menopausal gonadotropins, human chorionic gonadotropins
GH	Adults: Somatotropin (0.1–1.25 mg SC qd)
	Children: Somatotropin [0.02–0.05 (mg/kg per day)]
Vasopressin	Intranasal desmopressin (5–20 μg twice daily)
	Oral 300–600 μg qd

[a]All doses shown should be individualized for specific patients and should be reassessed during stress, surgery, or pregnancy. Male and female fertility requirements should be managed as discussed in Chaps. 183 and 184.
Note: For abbreviations, see text.

Clinical Features   Hormonal abnormalities after cranial irradiation may occur 5–15 years later, with GH deficiency occurring first, followed sequentially by gonadotropin, TSH, and ACTH deficiency.

Each hormone deficiency is associated with specific findings:

- GH: growth disorders in children; increased intraabdominal fat, reduced lean body mass, hyperlipidemia, reduced bone mineral density, and social isolation in adults
- FSH/LH: menstrual disorders and infertility in women (Chap. 184); hypogonadism in men (Chap. 183)
- ACTH: features of hypocortisolism (Chap. 180) without mineralocorticoid deficiency
- TSH: growth retardation in children, features of hypothyroidism in children and adults (Chap. 179)

Diagnosis   Biochemical diagnosis of pituitary insufficiency is made by demonstrating low or inappropriately normal levels of pituitary hormones in the setting of low target hormone levels. Initial testing should include an 8 A.M. cortisol level, TSH and free T_4, IGF-I, testosterone in men, assessment of menstrual cycles in women, and prolactin level. Provocative tests may be required to assess pituitary reserve for individual hormones. Adult GH deficiency is diagnosed by demonstrating a subnormal GH response to a standard provocative test (insulin tolerance test, L-arginine + GHRH). Acute ACTH deficiency may be diagnosed by a subnormal response in an insulin tolerance test, metyrapone test, or corticotropin-releasing hormone (CRH) stimulation test. Standard ACTH (cosyntropin) stimulation tests may be normal in acute ACTH deficiency; with adrenal atrophy, the cortisol response to cosyntropin is blunted.

Rx Hypopituitarism

Hormonal replacement should aim to mimic physiologic hormone production. Effective dose schedules are outlined in Table 177-2. GH therapy, particularly when excessive, may be associated with fluid retention, joint pain, and carpal tunnel syndrome. Glucocorticoid replacement should always precede levothyroxine therapy to avoid precipitation of adrenal crisis. Patients requiring glucocorticoid replacement should wear a medical alert bracelet and should be instructed to take additional doses during stressful events such as acute illness, dental procedures, trauma, and acute hospitalization.

For a more detailed discussion, see Melmed S, Jameson JL: Disorders of the Anterior Pituitary and Hypothalamus, Chap. 333, p. 2195, in HPIM-17.

178 Diabetes Insipidus and SIADH

The neurohypophysis, or posterior pituitary gland, produces two hormones: (1) arginine vasopressin (AVP), also known as antidiuretic hormone (ADH), and (2) oxytocin. AVP acts on the renal tubules to induce water retention, leading to concentration of the urine. Oxytocin stimulates postpartum milk letdown in response to suckling. Clinical syndromes may result from deficiency or excess of AVP.

DIABETES INSIPIDUS

Etiology Diabetes insipidus (DI) results from abnormalities of AVP production from the hypothalamus or AVP action in the kidney. AVP deficiency is characterized by production of large amounts of dilute urine. In *central DI*, insufficient AVP is released in response to physiologic stimuli. Causes include acquired (head trauma; neoplastic or inflammatory conditions affecting the posterior pituitary), congenital, and genetic disorders, but almost half of cases are idiopathic. In *gestational DI*, increased metabolism of plasma AVP by an aminopeptidase produced by the placenta leads to a deficiency of AVP during pregnancy. *Primary polydipsia* results in secondary insufficiencies of AVP due to inhibition of AVP secretion by excessive fluid intake. *Nephrogenic DI* can be genetic or acquired from drug exposure (lithium, demeclocycline, amphotericin B), metabolic conditions (hypercalcemia), or renal damage.

Clinical Features Symptoms include polyuria, excessive thirst, and polydipsia, with a 24-h urine output of >50 (mL/kg)/day and a urine osmolality that is less than that of serum (<300 mosmol/kg; specific gravity <1.010). Clinical or laboratory signs of dehydration, including hypernatremia, occur only if the pt simultaneously has a thirst defect or does not have access to water. Other etiologies of hypernatremia are described in Chap. 2.

Diagnosis DI must be differentiated from other etiologies of polyuria (Chap. 57). Unless an inappropriately dilute urine is present in the setting of serum hyperosmolality, a fluid deprivation test is used to make the diagnosis of DI. This test should be started in the morning, and body weight, plasma osmolality, sodium concentration, and urine volume and osmolality should be measured hourly. The test should be stopped when body weight decreases by 5% or plasma osmolality/sodium exceed the upper limit of normal. If the urine osmolality is <300 mosmol/kg with serum hyperosmolality, desmopressin (0.03 µg/kg SC) should be administered with repeat measurement of urine osmolality 1–2 h later. An increase of >50% indicates severe pituitary DI, whereas a smaller or absent response suggests nephrogenic DI. Measurement of AVP levels before and after fluid deprivation may be required to diagnose partial DI. Occasionally, hypertonic saline infusion may be required if fluid deprivation does not achieve the requisite level of hypertonic dehydration.

 Diabetes Insipidus

Pituitary DI can be treated with desmopressin (DDAVP) subcutaneously (1–2 µg once or twice per day), via nasal spray (10–20 µg two or three times a day), or orally (100–400 µg two or three times a day), with recommendations

TABLE 178-1	CAUSES OF SYNDROME OF INAPPROPRIATE ANTIDIURETIC HORMONE (SIADH)
Neoplasms	Neurologic
Carcinomas	Guillain-Barré syndrome
Lung	Multiple sclerosis
Duodenum	Delirium tremens
Pancreas	Amyotrophic lateral sclerosis
Ovary	Hydrocephalus
Bladder, ureter	Psychosis
Other neoplasms	Peripheral neuropathy
Thymoma	Congenital malformations
Mesothelioma	Agenesis corpus callosum
Bronchial adenoma	Cleft lip/palate
Carcinoid	Other midline defects
Gangliocytoma	Metabolic
Ewing's sarcoma	Acute intermittent porphyria
Head trauma	Pulmonary
Infections	Asthma
Pneumonia, bacterial or viral	Pneumothorax
Abscess, lung or brain	Positive-pressure respiration
Cavitation (aspergillosis)	Drugs
Tuberculosis, lung or brain	Vasopressin or DDAVP
Meningitis, bacterial or viral	Chlorpropamide
Encephalitis	Oxytocin, high dose
AIDS	Vincristine
Vascular	Carbamazepine
Cerebrovascular occlusions,	Nicotine
hemorrhage	Phenothiazines
Cavernous sinus thrombosis	Cyclophosphamide
	Tricyclic antidepressants
	Monoamine oxidase inhibitors
	Serotonin reuptake inhibitors

to drink to thirst. Symptoms of nephrogenic DI may be ameliorated by treatment with a thiazide diuretic and/or amiloride in conjunction with a low-sodium diet, or with prostaglandin synthesis inhibitors (e.g., indomethacin).

SYNDROME OF INAPPROPRIATE ANTIDIURETIC HORMONE (SIADH)

Etiology   Excessive or inappropriate production of AVP predisposes to hyponatremia, reflecting water retention. The evaluation of hyponatremia is described in Chap. 2. Etiologies of SIADH include neoplasms, lung infections, CNS disorders, and drugs (Table 178-1).

Clinical Features   If hyponatremia develops gradually, it may be asymptomatic. However, if it develops acutely, symptoms of water intoxication may include mild headache, confusion, anorexia, nausea, vomiting, coma, and convulsions. Laboratory findings include low BUN, creatinine, uric acid, and albumin; serum Na < 130 mmol/L and plasma osmolality < 270 mmol/kg; urine is almost always hypertonic to plasma, and urinary Na^+ is usually >20 mmol/L.

℞ SIADH

Fluid intake should be restricted to 500 mL less than urinary output. In patients with severe symptoms or signs, hypertonic (3%) saline can be infused at ≤0.05 mL/kg body weight IV per minute, with hourly sodium levels measured until Na increases by 12 mmol/L or to 130 mmol/L, whichever occurs first. However, if the hyponatremia has been present for >24–48 h and is corrected too rapidly, saline infusion has the potential to produce central pontine myelinolysis. Demeclocycline (150–300 mg PO three or four times a day) or fludrocortisone (0.05–0.2 mg PO twice a day) may be required to manage chronic SIADH.

For a more detailed discussion, see Robertson GL: Disorders of the Neurohypophysis, Chap. 334, p. 2217, in HPIM-17.

179   Thyroid Gland Disorders

Disorders of the thyroid gland result primarily from autoimmune processes that stimulate the overproduction of thyroid hormones (*thyrotoxicosis*) or cause glandular destruction and underproduction of thyroid hormones (*hypothyroidism*). *Neoplastic processes* in the thyroid gland can lead to benign nodules or thyroid cancer.

Thyroidal production of the hormones thyroxine (T_4) and triiodothyronine (T_3) is controlled via a classic endocrine feedback loop (see Fig. 177-1). Some T_3 is secreted by the thyroid, but most is produced by deiodination of T_4 in peripheral tissues. Both T_4 and T_3 are bound to carrier proteins [thyroid-binding globulin

(TBG), transthyretin, and albumin] in the circulation. Increased levels of total T_4 and T_3 with normal free levels are seen in states of increased carrier proteins (pregnancy, estrogens, cirrhosis, hepatitis, and inherited disorders). Conversely, decreased total T_4 and T_3 levels with normal free levels are seen in severe systemic illness, chronic liver disease, and nephrosis.

HYPOTHYROIDISM

Etiology   Deficient thyroid hormone secretion can be due to thyroid failure (primary hypothyroidism) or, less commonly, pituitary or hypothalamic disease (secondary hypothyroidism) (Table 179-1). Transient hypothyroidism may occur in silent or subacute thyroiditis. *Subclinical* (or *mild*) *hypothyroidism* is a state of normal thyroid hormone levels and mild elevation of TSH; despite the name, some pts may have minor symptoms. With higher TSH levels and low free T_4 levels, symptoms become more readily apparent in *clinical* (or *overt*) *hypothyroidism*. In areas of iodine sufficiency, autoimmune disease and iatrogenic causes are most common.

Clinical Features   Symptoms of hypothyroidism include lethargy, dry hair and skin, cold intolerance, hair loss, difficulty concentrating, poor memory, constipation, mild weight gain with poor appetite, dyspnea, hoarse voice, muscle cramping, and menorrhagia. Cardinal features on examination include bradycardia, mild diastolic hypertension, prolongation of the relaxation phase of deep tendon reflexes, and cool peripheral extremities. Goiter may be palpated, or the thyroid may be atrophic and nonpalpable. Carpal tunnel syndrome may

---

TABLE 179-1   CAUSES OF HYPOTHYROIDISM

Primary
   Autoimmune hypothyroidism: Hashimoto's thyroiditis, atrophic thyroiditis
   Iatrogenic: ^{131}I treatment, subtotal or total thyroidectomy, external irradiation of neck for lymphoma or cancer
   Drugs: iodine excess (including iodine-containing contrast media and amiodarone), lithium, antithyroid drugs, *p*-aminosalicylic acid, interferon-α and other cytokines, aminoglutethimide
   Congenital hypothyroidism: absent or ectopic thyroid gland, dyshormonogenesis, TSH-R mutation
   Iodine deficiency
   Infiltrative disorders: amyloidosis, sarcoidosis, hemochromatosis, scleroderma, cystinosis, Riedel's thyroiditis
Transient
   Silent thyroiditis, including postpartum thyroiditis
   Subacute thyroiditis
   Withdrawal of thyroxine treatment in individuals with an intact thyroid
   After ^{131}I treatment or subtotal thyroidectomy for Graves' disease
Secondary
   Hypopituitarism: tumors, pituitary surgery or irradiation, infiltrative disorders, Sheehan's syndrome, trauma, genetic forms of combined pituitary hormone deficiencies
   Isolated TSH deficiency or inactivity
   Bexarotene treatment
   Hypothalamic disease: tumors, trauma, infiltrative disorders, idiopathic

---

Note: TSH, thyroid-stimulating hormone; TSH-R, TSH receptor.

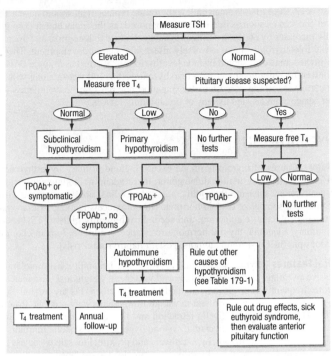

FIGURE 179-1 Evaluation of hypothyroidism. TPOAb+, thyroid peroxidase antibodies present; TPOAb−, thyroid peroxidase antibodies not present.

be present. Cardiomegaly may be present due to pericardial effusion. The most extreme presentation is a dull, expressionless face, sparse hair, periorbital puffiness, large tongue, and pale, doughy, cool skin. The condition may progress into a hypothermic, stuporous state (*myxedema coma*) with respiratory depression. Factors that predispose to myxedema coma include cold exposure, trauma, infection, and administration of narcotics.

Diagnosis Decreased serum T_4 is common to all varieties of hypothyroidism. An elevated TSH is a sensitive marker of primary hypothyroidism. A summary of the investigations used to determine the existence and cause of hypothyroidism is provided in Fig. 179-1. Thyroid peroxidase (TPO) antibodies are increased in >90% of pts with autoimmune-mediated hypothyroidism. Elevated cholesterol, increased creatine phosphokinase, and anemia may be present; bradycardia, low-amplitude QRS complexes, and flattened or inverted T waves may be present on ECG.

R̲x̲ Hypothyroidism

Adult pts <60 years without evidence of heart disease may be started on 50–100 μg of levothyroxine (T_4) daily. In the elderly or in pts with known coronary artery disease, the starting dose of levothyroxine is 12.5–25 μg/d. The dose should be adjusted in 12.5- to 25-μg increments every 6–8 weeks on the basis of TSH levels, until a normal TSH level is achieved. The usual daily replacement dose is 1.6 (µg/kg)/d. Women on levothyroxine replacement should have a TSH level checked as soon as pregnancy is diagnosed, as the replacement dose typically increases by 30–50% during pregnancy. Failure to recognize and treat maternal hypothyroidism may adversely affect fetal neural development. Therapy for myxedema coma should include levothyroxine (500 µg) as a single IV bolus followed by daily treatment with levothyroxine (50–100 µg/d), along with hydrocortisone (50 mg every 6 h) for impaired adrenal reserve, ventilatory support, space blankets, and therapy of precipitating factors.

THYROTOXICOSIS

Etiology   Causes of thyroid hormone excess include primary hyperthyroidism (Graves' disease, toxic multinodular goiter, toxic adenoma, iodine excess); thyroid destruction (subacute thyroiditis, silent thyroiditis, amiodarone, radiation); extrathyroidal sources of thyroid hormone (thyrotoxicosis factitia, struma ovarii, functioning follicular carcinoma); and secondary hyperthyroidism [TSH-secreting pituitary adenoma, thyroid hormone resistance syndrome, human chorionic gonadotropin (hCG)-secreting tumors, gestational thyrotoxicosis].

Clinical Features   Symptoms include nervousness, irritability, heat intolerance, excessive sweating, palpitations, fatigue and weakness, weight loss with increased appetite, frequent bowel movements, and oligomenorrhea. Pts are anxious, restless, and fidgety. Skin is warm and moist, and fingernails may separate from the nail bed (Plummer's nails). Eyelid retraction and lid lag may be present. Cardiovascular findings include tachycardia, systolic hypertension, systolic murmur, and atrial fibrillation. A fine tremor, hyperreflexia, and proximal muscle weakness may also be present. Long-standing thyrotoxicosis may lead to osteopenia.

In Graves' disease, the thyroid is usually diffusely enlarged to two to three times its normal size, and a bruit or thrill may be present. Infiltrative ophthalmopathy (with variable degrees of proptosis, periorbital swelling, and ophthalmoplegia) and dermopathy (pretibial myxedema) may also be found. In subacute thyroiditis, the thyroid is exquisitely tender and enlarged with referred pain to the jaw or ear, and sometimes accompanied by fever and preceded by an upper respiratory tract infection. Solitary or multiple nodules may be present in toxic adenoma or toxic multinodular goiter.

Thyrotoxic crisis, or thyroid storm, is rare, presents as a life-threatening exacerbation of hyperthyroidism, and can be accompanied by fever, delirium, seizures, arrhythmias, coma, vomiting, diarrhea, and jaundice.

Diagnosis   Investigations used to determine the existence and causes of thyrotoxicosis are summarized in Fig. 179-2. Serum TSH is a sensitive marker of thyrotoxicosis caused by Graves' disease, autonomous thyroid nodules, thyroiditis, and exogenous levothyroxine treatment. Associated laboratory abnormalities include elevation of bilirubin, liver enzymes, and ferritin. Radionuclide uptake may be required to distinguish the various etiologies: high uptake in Graves' disease and nodular disease vs. low uptake in thyroid destruction, iodine excess, and extrathyroidal sources of thyroid hormone. The ESR is elevated in subacute thyroiditis.

℞ Thyrotoxicosis

Graves' disease may be treated with antithyroid drugs or radioiodine; subtotal thyroidectomy is rarely indicated. The main antithyroid drugs are methima-

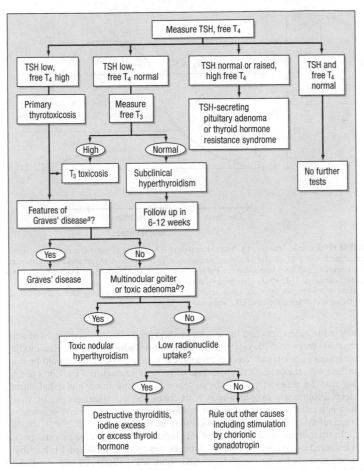

FIGURE 179-2 Evaluation of thyrotoxicosis. [a]Diffuse goiter, positive TPO antibodies, ophthalmopathy, dermopathy; [b]can be confirmed by radionuclide scan.

zole or carbimazole (10–20 mg two to three times a day initially, titrated to 2.5–10 mg/d) and propylthiouracil (100–200 mg every 8 h initially, titrated to 50 mg once or twice a day). Thyroid function tests should be checked 3–4 weeks after initiation of treatment, with adjustments to maintain a normal free T_4 level. The common side effects are rash, urticaria, fever, and arthralgia (1–5% of pts). Rare but major side effects include hepatitis, an SLE-like syndrome, and agranulocytosis (<1%). All pts should be given written instructions regarding the symptoms of possible agranulocytosis (sore throat, fever, mouth ulcers) and the need to stop treatment pending a complete blood count to confirm that agranulocytosis is not present. Propranolol (20–40 mg every 6 h) or longer acting beta blockers such as atenolol (50 mg/d) may be useful to control adrenergic symptoms. Anticoagulation with warfarin should be considered in all pts with atrial fibrillation. Radioiodine can also be used as initial treatment or in pts who do not undergo remission after a 1- to 2-year trial of antithyroid drugs. Antecedent treatment with antithyroid drugs should be con-

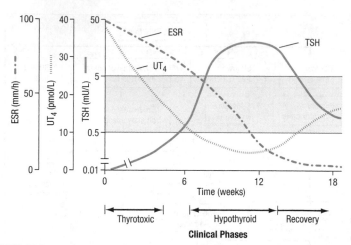

FIGURE 179-3 Clinical course of subacute thyroiditis. The release of thyroid hormones is initially associated with a thyrotoxic phase and suppressed TSH levels. A hypothyroid phase then ensues, with T_4 and TSH levels that are initially low, but gradually increase. During the recovery phase, increased TSH levels combined with resolution of thyroid follicular injury leads to normalization of thyroid function, often several months after the beginning of the illness. ESR, erythrocyte sedimentation rate; UT_4, unbound T_4.

sidered in elderly pts and those with cardiac problems, with cessation of antithyroid drugs 3–5 days prior to radioiodine administration. Radioiodine treatment is contraindicated in pregnancy; instead, symptoms should be controlled with the lowest effective dose of propylthiouracil (PTU). Corneal drying may be relieved with artificial tears and taping the eyelids shut during sleep. Progressive exophthalmos with chemosis, ophthalmoplegia, or vision loss is treated with large doses of prednisone (40–80 mg/d) and ophthalmologic referral; orbital decompression may be required.

In thyroid storm, large doses of PTU (600-mg loading dose) should be administered orally, per nasogastric tube, or per rectum, followed 1 h later by 5 drops saturated solution of KI (SSKI) q6h. PTU (200–300 mg every 6 h) should be continued, along with propranolol (40–60 mg PO q4h or 2 mg IV every 4 h) and dexamethasone (2 mg every 6 h). Any underlying precipitating cause should be identified and treated.

Radioiodine is the treatment of choice for toxic nodules. Subacute thyroiditis should be treated with NSAIDs and beta blockade to control symptoms, with monitoring of the TSH and free T_4 levels every 4 weeks. The clinical course of subacute thyroiditis is summarized in Fig. 179-3. Transient levothyroxine replacement (50–100 µg/d) may be required if the hypothyroid phase is prolonged. Silent thyroiditis (or postpartum thyroiditis if within 3–6 months of delivery) should be treated with beta blockade during the thyrotoxic phase and levothyroxine in the hypothyroid phase, with withdrawal after 6–9 months to assess recovery.

SICK EUTHYROID SYNDROME

Any acute, severe illness can cause abnormalities of circulating thyroid hormone levels or TSH, even in the absence of underlying thyroid disease. Therefore, the routine testing of thyroid function should be avoided in acutely ill pts unless a thyroid disorder is strongly suspected. The most common pattern in sick euthyroid syndrome is a decrease in total and free T_3 levels, with normal levels of TSH and T_4. More ill pts may additionally have a fall in total T_4 levels, with normal free T_4 levels. TSH levels may range from <0.1 to >20 mU/L, with normalization after recovery from illness. Unless there is historic or clinical evidence of hypothyroidism, thyroid hormone should not be administered and thyroid function tests should be repeated after recovery.

AMIODARONE

Amiodarone treatment is associated with (1) acute, transient changes in thyroid function, (2) hypothyroidism, or (3) thyrotoxicosis. There are two major forms of amiodarone-induced thyrotoxicosis (AIT). Type 1 AIT is associated with an underlying thyroid abnormality (preclinical Graves' disease or nodular goiter). Thyroid hormone synthesis becomes excessive as a result of increased iodine exposure. Type 2 AIT occurs in pts with no intrinsic thyroid abnormalities and is the result of destructive thyroiditis. Differentiation between type 1 and type 2 AIT may be difficult as the high iodine load interferes with thyroid scans. The drug should be stopped, if possible, with administration of high-dose antithyroid drugs in type 1 AIT or potassium perchlorate (200 mg every 6 h) in type 1 and glucocorticoids in type 2 AIT.

NONTOXIC GOITER

Goiter refers to an enlarged thyroid gland (>20–25 g) and is more common in women than men. Biosynthetic defects, iodine deficiency, autoimmune disease, and nodular diseases can lead to goiter. If thyroid function is preserved, most goiters are asymptomatic. Substernal goiter may obstruct the thoracic inlet and should be evaluated with respiratory flow measurements and CT or MRI in pts with obstructive signs or symptoms (difficulty swallowing, tracheal compression, or plethora). Thyroid function tests should be performed in all pts with goiter to exclude thyrotoxicosis or hypothyroidism. Ultrasound is not generally indicated in the evaluation of diffuse goiter, unless a nodule is palpable on physical exam.

Iodine or thyroid hormone replacement induces variable regression of goiter in iodine deficiency. Radioiodine reduces goiter size by about 50% in the majority of pts. Surgery is rarely indicated for diffuse goiter but may be required to alleviate compression in pts with nontoxic multinodular goiter.

TOXIC MULTINODULAR GOITER AND TOXIC ADENOMA

TOXIC MULTINODULAR GOITER (MNG)

In addition to features of goiter, the clinical presentation of toxic MNG includes subclinical hyperthyroidism or mild thyrotoxicosis. The pt is usually elderly and may present with atrial fibrillation or palpitations, tachycardia, nervousness, tremor, or weight loss. Recent exposure to iodine, from contrast dyes or other sources, may precipitate or exacerbate thyrotoxicosis; this may be prevented by prior administration of an antithyroid drug. The TSH level is low. T_4 may be normal or minimally increased; T_3 is often elevated to a greater degree than T_4. Thyroid scan shows heterogeneous uptake with multiple regions of increased and decreased uptake; 24-h uptake of radioiodine may not be increased.

Cold nodules in a multinodular goiter should be evaluated in the same way as solitary nodules (see below). Antithyroid drugs, often in combination with beta blockers, can normalize thyroid function and improve clinical features of thyrotoxicosis but do not induce remission. A trial of radioiodine should be considered before subjecting pts, many of whom are elderly, to surgery.

TOXIC ADENOMA

A solitary, autonomously functioning thyroid nodule is referred to as *toxic adenoma*. A thyroid scan provides a definitive diagnostic test, demonstrating focal uptake in the hyperfunctioning nodule and diminished uptake in the remainder of the gland, as activity of the normal thyroid is suppressed. Radioiodine ablation (e.g., 10–29.9 mCi ^{131}I) is usually the treatment of choice.

THYROID NEOPLASMS

Etiology   Thyroid neoplasms may be benign (adenomas) or malignant (carcinomas). Carcinomas of the follicular epithelium include papillary, follicular, and anaplastic thyroid cancer. Papillary thyroid cancer is the most common type of thyroid cancer. It tends to be multifocal and to invade locally. Follicular thyroid cancer is difficult to diagnose via fine-needle aspiration (FNA) because the distinction between benign and malignant follicular neoplasms rests largely on evidence of invasion into vessels, nerves, or adjacent structures. It tends to spread hematogenously, leading to bone, lung, and CNS metastases. Anaplastic carcinoma is rare, highly malignant, and rapidly fatal. Thyroid lymphoma often arises in the background of Hashimoto's thyroiditis and occurs in the setting of a rapidly expanding thyroid mass. Medullary thyroid carcinoma arises from parafollicular (C) cells and may occur sporadically or as a familial disorder, sometimes in association with multiple endocrine neoplasia type 2.

Clinical Features   Features suggesting carcinoma include recent or rapid growth of a nodule or mass, history of neck irradiation, lymph node involvement, hoarseness, and fixation to surrounding tissues. Glandular enlargement may result in compression and displacement of the trachea or esophagus and obstructive symptoms. Age <20 or >45, male sex, and larger nodule size are associated with a worse prognosis.

Diagnosis   An approach to the evaluation of a solitary nodule is outlined in Fig. 179-4.

℞ Thyroid Neoplasms

Benign nodules should be monitored via serial examination.

Follicular adenomas cannot be distinguished from follicular carcinomas on the basis of cytologic analysis of FNA specimens. The extent of surgical resection (lobectomy vs. near-total thyroidectomy) should be discussed prior to surgery.

Near-total thyroidectomy is required for papillary and follicular carcinoma and should be performed by a surgeon who is highly experienced in the procedure. If risk factors and pathologic features indicate the need for radioiodine treatment, the pt should be treated for several weeks postoperatively with liothyronine (25 µg two to three times a day), followed by withdrawal for an additional 2 weeks, in preparation for postsurgical radioablation of remnant tissue. A therapeutic dose of ^{131}I is administered when the TSH level > 50 IU/L. Subsequent levothyroxine suppression of TSH to a low, but detectable, level

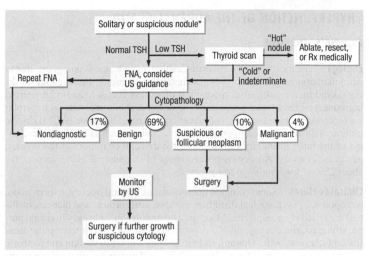

FIGURE 179-4 Approach to the patient with a thyroid nodule. US, ultrasound; FNA, fine-needle aspiration.

should be attempted in pts with a high risk of recurrence, and to 0.1–0.5 IU/L in those with a low risk of recurrence. Follow-up scans and thyroglobulin levels should be performed at regular intervals after either thyroid hormone withdrawal or administration of recombinant human TSH.

The management of medullary thyroid carcinoma is surgical, as these tumors do not take up radioiodine. Testing for the *RET* mutation should be performed. Elevated serum calcitonin provides a marker of residual or recurrent disease.

For a more detailed discussion, see Jameson JL, Weetman AP: Disorders of the Thyroid Gland, Chap. 335, p. 2244, in HPIM-17.

180 Adrenal Gland Disorders

The adrenal cortex produces three major classes of steroids: (1) glucocorticoids, (2) mineralocorticoids, and (3) adrenal androgens. Clinical syndromes may result from deficiencies or excesses of these hormones. The adrenal medulla produces catecholamines, with excess leading to pheochromocytoma (Chap. 124).

HYPERFUNCTION OF THE ADRENAL GLAND

CUSHING'S SYNDROME

Etiology The most common cause of Cushing's syndrome is iatrogenic, due to administration of glucocorticoids for therapeutic reasons. Endogenous Cushing's syndrome results from production of excess cortisol (and other steroid hormones) by the adrenal cortex. The major cause is bilateral adrenal hyperplasia secondary to hypersecretion of adrenocorticotropic hormone (ACTH) by the pituitary (Cushing's disease) or from ectopic sources such as small cell carcinoma of the lung; medullary carcinoma of the thyroid; or tumors of the thymus, pancreas, or ovary. Adenomas or carcinoma of the adrenal gland account for about 25% of Cushing's syndrome cases.

Clinical Features Some common manifestations (central obesity, hypertension, osteoporosis, psychological disturbances, acne, amenorrhea, and diabetes mellitus) are relatively nonspecific. More specific findings include easy bruising, purple striae, proximal myopathy, fat deposition in the face and interscapular areas (moon facies and buffalo hump), and virilization. Thin, fragile skin and plethoric moon facies may also be found. Hypokalemia and metabolic alkalosis are prominent, particularly with ectopic production of ACTH.

Diagnosis The diagnosis of Cushing's syndrome requires demonstration of increased cortisol production and abnormal cortisol suppression in response to dexamethasone. For initial screening, measurement of 24-h urinary free cortisol, the 1-mg overnight dexamethasone test [8 A.M. plasma cortisol < 1.8 µg/dL (50 nmol/L)] or late night salivary cortisol measurement is appropriate. Repeat testing or performance of more than one screening test may be required. Definitive diagnosis is established in equivocal cases by inadequate suppression of urinary [<10 µg/d (25 nmol/d)] or plasma cortisol [<5 µg/dL (140 nmol/L)] after 0.5 mg dexamethasone every 6 h for 48 h. This test may also be combined with corticotropin-releasing hormone (CRH) testing to rule out pseudo-Cushing's states. Once the diagnosis of Cushing's syndrome is established, further biochemical testing is required to localize the source. Low levels of plasma ACTH levels suggest an adrenal adenoma or carcinoma; inappropriately normal or high plasma ACTH levels suggest a pituitary or ectopic source. In 95% of ACTH-producing pituitary microadenomas, cortisol production is suppressed by high-dose dexamethasone (2 mg every 6 h for 48 h), and MRI of the pituitary should be obtained. However, because up to 10% of ectopic sources of ACTH may also suppress after high-dose dexamethasone testing, inferior petrosal sinus sampling may be required to distinguish pituitary from peripheral sources of ACTH. Imaging of the chest and abdomen is required to localize the source of ectopic ACTH production. Pts with chronic alcoholism and depression may have false-positive results in testing for Cushing's syndrome. Similarly, pts with acute illness may have abnormal laboratory test results, since major stress disrupts the normal regulation of ACTH secretion.

℞ Cushing's Syndrome

Therapy of adrenal adenoma or carcinoma requires surgical excision; stress doses of glucocorticoids must be given pre- and postoperatively. Metastatic and unresectable adrenal carcinomas are treated with mitotane in doses gradually increased to 6 g/d in three or four divided doses. Transsphenoidal surgery can be curative for pituitary microadenomas that secrete ACTH, though radiation may be used when cure is not achieved (see Chap. 177). On occasion, debulking of lung carcinoma or resection of carcinoid tumors can result in remission of ectopic Cushing's syndrome. If the source of ACTH cannot be resected, bilateral total adrenalectomy or medical management with ketoconazole (600–1200 mg/d), metyrapone (2–3 g/d), or mitotane (2–3 mg/d) may relieve manifestations of cortisol excess. Patients with unresectable pituitary adenomas who have bilateral adrenalectomy are at risk for Nelson's syndrome (pituitary adenoma enlargement).

ALDOSTERONISM

Etiology Aldosteronism is caused by hypersecretion of the adrenal mineralocorticoid aldosterone. *Primary aldosteronism* refers to an adrenal cause and can be due to either an adrenal adenoma or bilateral adrenal hyperplasia. The term *secondary aldosteronism* is used when an extraadrenal stimulus is present, as in renal artery stenosis or diuretic therapy.

Clinical Features Most pts with primary hyperaldosteronism have headaches and diastolic hypertension. Edema is characteristically absent, unless congestive heart failure or renal disease is present. Hypokalemia, caused by urinary potassium losses, may cause muscle weakness and fatigue, though potassium levels may be normal in mild primary aldosteronism. Hypernatremia and metabolic alkalosis may also occur.

Diagnosis The diagnosis is suggested by hypertension that is associated with persistent hypokalemia in a nonedematous pt who is not receiving potassium-wasting diuretics. In pts receiving potassium-wasting diuretics, the diuretic should be discontinued and potassium supplements should be administered for 1–2 weeks. If hypokalemia persists after supplementation, screening using a serum aldosterone and plasma renin activity should be performed. A ratio of serum aldosterone (in ng/dL) to plasma renin activity (in ng/mL per hour) >30 and an absolute level of aldosterone >15 ng/dL suggest primary aldosteronism. Failure to suppress plasma aldosterone (to <5 ng/dL after 500 mL/h of normal saline × 4 h) or urinary aldosterone after saline or sodium loading (to <10 μg/d on day 3 of 200 mmol/d Na PO + fludrocortisone 0.2 mg twice daily × 3 days) confirms primary hyperaldosteronism. Localization should then be undertaken with a high-resolution CT scan of the adrenal glands. If the CT scan is negative, bilateral adrenal vein sampling may be required to diagnose a unilateral aldosterone-producing adenoma. Secondary hyperaldosteronism is associated with elevated plasma renin activity.

℞ Aldosteronism

Surgery can be curative in pts with adrenal adenoma but is not effective for adrenal hyperplasia, which is managed with sodium restriction and spironolactone (25–100 mg twice daily) or eplerenone (25–50 mg twice daily). Secondary aldosteronism is treated with salt restriction and correction of the underlying cause.

SYNDROMES OF ADRENAL ANDROGEN EXCESS

See Chap. 184 for discussion of hirsutism and virilization.

HYPOFUNCTION OF THE ADRENAL GLAND

Primary adrenal insufficiency is due to failure of the adrenal gland, whereas *secondary adrenal insufficiency* is due to failure of ACTH production or release.

ADDISON'S DISEASE

Etiology   Addison's disease occurs when >90% of adrenal tissue is destroyed surgically, by granulomatous disease (tuberculosis, histoplasmosis, coccidioidomycosis, cryptococcosis), or via autoimmune mechanisms (alone, or in type I or type II polyglandular autoimmune syndromes). Bilateral tumor metastases, bilateral hemorrhage, CMV, HIV, amyloidosis, sarcoidosis, and adrenoleukodystrophy are rare causes.

Clinical Features   Manifestations include fatigue, weakness, anorexia, nausea and vomiting, weight loss, abdominal pain, cutaneous and mucosal pigmentation, salt craving, hypotension, and, occasionally, hypoglycemia. Routine laboratory parameters may be normal, or serum Na can be reduced and serum K increased. Extracellular fluid depletion accentuates hypotension.

Diagnosis   The best screening test is the cortisol response 60 min after 250 µg ACTH (cosyntropin) IV or IM. Cortisol levels should exceed 18 µg/dL 30–60 min after the ACTH. If the response is abnormal, then primary and secondary deficiency may be distinguished by measurement of aldosterone from the same blood samples. In secondary, but not primary, adrenal insufficiency, the aldosterone increment from baseline will be normal (≥5 ng/dL). Furthermore, in primary adrenal insufficiency, plasma ACTH is elevated, whereas in secondary adrenal insufficiency, plasma ACTH values are low or inappropriately normal. Pts with recent onset or partial pituitary insufficiency may have a normal response to the rapid ACTH stimulation test. In these pts, alternative testing (metyrapone test or insulin tolerance testing) may be used for diagnosis.

℞ Addison's Disease

Hydrocortisone, at 20–30 mg/d divided into $^2/_3$ in the morning and $^1/_3$ in the afternoon, is the mainstay of glucocorticoid replacement. Some pts benefit from doses administered three times daily, and other glucocorticoids may be given at equivalent doses. Mineralocorticoid supplementation is usually needed for primary adrenal insufficiency, with administration of 0.05–0.1 mg fludrocortisone PO qd and maintenance of adequate Na intake. Doses should be titrated to normalize Na and K levels and to maintain normal bp without postural changes. Measurement of plasma renin levels may also be useful in titrating the dose. All pts with adrenal insufficiency should be instructed in the parenteral self-administration of steroids and should be registered with a medical alert system. During periods of intercurrent illness, the dose of hydrocortisone should be doubled. During adrenal crisis, high-dose hydrocortisone (10 mg/h continuous IV or 100-mg bolus IV three times a day) should be administered along with normal saline. Thereafter, if the patient is improving and is afebrile, the dose can be tapered by 20–30% daily to usual replacement doses.

HYPOALDOSTERONISM

Isolated aldosterone deficiency accompanied by normal cortisol production occurs with hyporeninism, as an inherited biosynthetic defect, postoperatively fol-

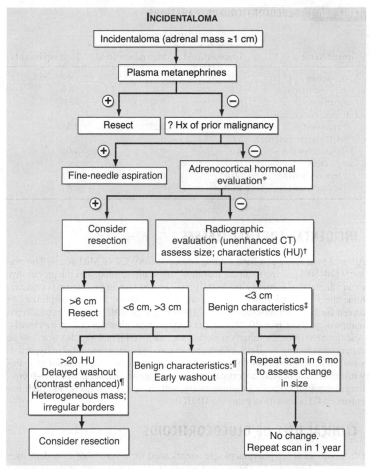

FIGURE 180-1 Incidentaloma. *Adrenocortical hormonal evaluation: Dexamethasone suppression test in all patients; plasma renin activity/aldosterone ratio for hypertensives; sex steroid (DHEA sulfate, estradiol) for clinical signs in females and males, respectively. †Hounsfield units (HU): a measurement of x-ray attenuation or lipid content of neoplasms. A lipid-rich mass (<10 HU) is diagnostic of a benign cortical adenoma. ‡Benign characteristics: homogeneous mass, smooth borders, HU <10. ¶Benign adrenal adenomas are also characterized by earlier washout of contrast enhancement than other neoplasms.

lowing removal of aldosterone-secreting adenomas, and during protracted heparin therapy. Hyporeninemic hypoaldosteronism is seen most commonly in adults with mild renal failure and diabetes mellitus in association with disproportionate hyperkalemia. Oral fludrocortisone (0.05–0.15 mg/d PO) restores electrolyte balance if salt intake is adequate. In pts with hypertension, mild renal insufficiency, or congestive heart failure, an alternative approach is to reduce salt intake and to administer furosemide.

TABLE 180-1 GLUCOCORTICOID PREPARATIONS

Generic Name	Relative Potency Glucocorticoid	Relative Potency Mineralocorticoid	Dose Equivalent
Short-acting			
Hydrocortisone	1.0	1.0	20.0
Cortisone	0.8	0.8	25.0
Intermediate-acting			
Prednisone	4.0	0.25	5.0
Methylprednisolone	5.0	0	4.0
Triamcinolone	5.0	0	4.0
Long-acting			
Dexamethasone	30.0	0	0.75
Betamethasone	25.0	0	0.6

INCIDENTAL ADRENAL MASSES

Adrenal masses are common findings on abdominal CT or MRI scans. The majority (70–80%) of such "incidentalomas" are nonfunctional, and the probability of an adrenal carcinoma is low (<0.01%). The first step in evaluation is to determine the functional status by measurement of plasma free metanephrines to screen for pheochromocytoma (Fig. 180-1). In a pt with a known extraadrenal malignancy, there is a 30–50% chance that the incidentaloma is a metastasis. Additional hormonal evaluation should include overnight 1-mg dexamethasone suppression testing in all pts, plasma renin activity/aldosterone ratio in hypertensives, DHEAS in women with signs of androgen excess, and estradiol in males with feminization. Adrenocortical cancer is suggested by large size (>4–6 cm), irregular margins, tumor inhomogeneity, soft tissue calcifications, and high unenhanced CT attenuation values (>10 HU).

CLINICAL USES OF GLUCOCORTICOIDS

Glucocorticoids are pharmacologic agents used for a variety of disorders such as asthma, rheumatoid arthritis, and psoriasis. The almost certain development of complications (weight gain, hypertension, Cushingoid facies, diabetes mellitus, osteoporosis, myopathy, increased intraocular pressure, ischemic bone necrosis, infection, and hypercholesterolemia) must be weighed against the potential therapeutic benefits of glucocorticoid therapy. These side effects can

TABLE 180-2 A CHECKLIST FOR USE PRIOR TO THE ADMINISTRATION OF GLUCOCORTICOIDS IN PHARMACOLOGIC DOSES

Presence of tuberculosis or other chronic infection (chest x-ray, tuberculin test)
Evidence of glucose intolerance, history of gestational diabetes mellitus, or high risk for type 2 diabetes mellitus
Evidence of preexisting osteoporosis (bone density assessment in organ transplant recipients or postmenopausal patients)
History of peptic ulcer, gastritis, or esophagitis (stool guaiac test)
Evidence of hypertension, cardiovascular disease, or hypertriglyceridemia
History of psychological disorders

be minimized by a careful choice of steroid preparations (Table 180-1), alternate-day or interrupted therapy; the use of topical steroids, i.e., inhaled, intranasal, or dermal whenever possible; the judicious use of non-steroid therapies; monitoring of caloric intake; and instituting measures to minimize bone loss. Pts should be evaluated for the risk of complications before the initiation of glucocorticoid therapy (Table 180-2). Higher doses of glucocorticoids may be required during periods of stress, since the adrenal gland may atrophy in the setting of exogenous glucocorticoids. In addition, following long-term use, glucocorticoids should be tapered with the dual goals of allowing the pituitary-adrenal axis to recover and the avoidance of underlying disease flare.

For a more detailed discussion, see Williams GH, Dluhy RG: Disorders of the Adrenal Cortex, Chap. 336, p. 2247, in HPIM-17.

181 Obesity

Obesity is a state of excess adipose tissue mass. Obesity should not be defined by body weight alone, as muscular individuals may be overweight by arbitrary standards without having increased adiposity. The most widely used method to classify weight status and risk of disease is the *body mass index* (BMI), which is equal to weight/height^2 in kg/m^2 (Table 181-1). At a similar BMI, women have more body fat than men. Furthermore, regional fat distribution may influence the risks associated with obesity. Central obesity (high ratio of the circumference of the waist to the circumference of the hips, >0.9 in women and 1.0 in men) is independently associated with a higher risk for diabetes mellitus and cardiovascular disease.

ETIOLOGY

Obesity can result from increased energy intake, decreased energy expenditure, or a combination of the two. Excess accumulation of body fat is the consequence of environmental and genetic factors; social factors and economic conditions also

TABLE 181-1 **CLASSIFICATION OF WEIGHT STATUS AND RISK OF DISEASE**

	BMI (kg/m^2)	Obesity Class	Risk of Disease
Underweight	<18.5		
Healthy weight	18.5–24.9		
Overweight	25.0–29.9		Increased
Obesity	30.0–34.9	I	High
Obesity	35.0–39.9	II	Very high
Extreme obesity	≥40	III	Extremely high

Source: Adapted from National Institutes of Health, National Heart, Lung, and Blood Institute: *Clinical Guidelines on the Identification, Evaluation, and Treatment of Overweight and Obesity in Adults.* U.S. Department of Health and Human Services, Public Health Service, 1998.

represent important influences. The susceptibility to obesity is polygenic in nature, and 30–50% of the variability in total fat stores is believed to be genetically determined. Secondary causes of obesity include hypothalamic injury, hypothyroidism, Cushing's syndrome, and hypogonadism. Drug-induced weight gain is also common in those who use antidiabetes agents (insulin, sulfonylureas, thiazolidinediones), glucocorticoids, psychotropic agents, mood stabilizers (lithium), antidepressants (tricyclics, monoamine oxidase inhibitors, paroxetine, mirtazapine), or antiepileptic drugs (valproate, gabapentin, carbamazepine). Insulin-secreting tumors can cause overeating.

CLINICAL FEATURES

Obesity has major adverse effects on health. Increased mortality from obesity is primarily due to cardiovascular disease, hypertension, gall bladder disease, diabetes mellitus, and certain forms of cancer. The incidence of endometrial cancer and postmenopausal breast cancer, prostate cancer, and colorectal cancer in both men and women is increased with obesity. Sleep apnea in severely obese individuals poses serious health risks. Obesity is also associated with an increased incidence of steatohepatitis, osteoarthritis, and gout.

Rx Obesity

Obesity is a chronic medical condition that requires ongoing treatment and lifestyle modifications. Treatment is important because of the associated health risks but is made difficult by a limited repertoire of effective therapeutic options. Weight regain after weight loss is common with all forms of nonsurgical therapy. The urgency and selection of treatment modalities should be based on the BMI and a risk assessment.

Diet, exercise, and behavior therapy are recommended for all pts with a BMI $\geq$ 25 kg/m^2. Behavior modification including group counseling, diet diaries, and changes in eating patterns should be initiated. Food-related behaviors should be monitored carefully (avoid cafeteria-style settings, eat small and frequent meals, eat breakfast). A deficit of 7500 kcal will produce a weight loss of approximately 1 kg. Therefore, eating 100 kcal/d less for a year should cause a 5-kg weight loss, and a deficit of 1000 kcal/d should cause a loss of ~1 kg per week. Physical activity should be increased to a minimum of 150 min of moderate intensity physical activity per wk.

Pharmacotherapy may be added to a lifestyle program for pts with a BMI $\geq$ 30 kg/m^2 or $\geq$ 27 kg/m^2 with concomitant obesity-related diseases. Sibutramine is a central reuptake inhibitor of both norepinephrine and serotonin that produces a 5–9% weight loss at 12 months, though it increases heart rate and bp in some pts. Orlistat is an inhibitor of intestinal lipase that causes modest weight loss (9–10% at 12 months with lifestyle measures) due to drug-induced fat malabsorption. Metformin tends to decrease body weight in pts with obesity and type 2 diabetes mellitus.

Surgery should be considered for pts with severe obesity (BMI $\geq$ 40 kg/m^2) or moderate obesity (BMI $\geq$ 35 kg/m^2) associated with a serious medical condition, repeated failures of other therapeutic approaches, at eligible weight for >3 years, capable of tolerating surgery, without addictions or major psychopathology. Weight-loss surgeries are either restrictive (limiting the amount of food the stomach can hold and slowing gastric emptying), such as laparoscopic adjustable silicone gastric banding, or restrictive-malabsorptive, such as Roux-en-Y

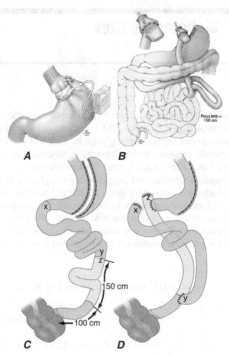

FIGURE 181-1 Bariatric surgical procedures. Examples of operative interventions used for surgical manipulation of the gastrointestinal tract. *A.* Laparoscopic gastric band (LAGB). *B.* The Roux-en-Y gastric bypass. *C.* Biliopancreatic diversion with duodenal switch. *D.* Biliopancreatic diversion. (*From ML Kendrick, GF Dakin, Surgical approches to obesity. Mayo Clinic Proc 815:518, 2006; with permission.*)

gastric bypass (Fig. 181-1). These procedures generally produce a 30–35% weight loss that is maintained in nearly 60% of pts at 5 yrs. Procedures with a malabsorptive component require lifelong supplementation of micronutrients (iron, folate, calcium, vitamins B_{12} and D) and are associated with a risk of islet cell hyperplasia and hypoglycemia.

For a more detailed discussion, see Flier JS, Maratos-Flier E: Biology of Obesity, Chap. 74, p. 462 and Kushner RF: Evaluation and Management of Obesity, Chap. 75, p. 468, in HPIM-17.

182 Diabetes Mellitus

ETIOLOGY

Diabetes mellitus (DM) comprises a group of metabolic disorders that share the common phenotype of hyperglycemia. DM is currently classified on the basis of the pathogenic process that leads to hyperglycemia. Type 1 DM is characterized by insulin deficiency and a tendency to develop ketosis, whereas type 2 DM is a heterogeneous group of disorders characterized by variable degrees of insulin resistance, impaired insulin secretion, and excessive hepatic glucose production. Other specific types include DM caused by genetic defects [maturity-onset diabetes of the young (MODY)], diseases of the exocrine pancreas (chronic pancreatitis, cystic fibrosis, hemochromatosis), endocrinopathies (acromegaly, Cushing's syndrome, glucagonoma, pheochromocytoma, hyperthyroidism), drugs (nicotinic acid, glucocorticoids, thiazides, protease inhibitors), and pregnancy (gestational DM).

DIAGNOSIS

Criteria for the diagnosis of DM include one of the following:

- Fasting plasma glucose ≥ 7.0 mmol/L (≥126 mg/dL)
- Symptoms of diabetes plus a random blood glucose concentration ≥ 11.1 mmol/L (≥200 mg/dL)
- 2-h plasma glucose ≥ 11.1 mmol/L (≥200 mg/dL) during a 75-g oral glucose tolerance test.

These criteria should be confirmed by repeat testing on a different day, unless unequivocal hyperglycemia is present.

Two intermediate categories have also been designated:

- Impaired fasting glucose (IFG) for a fasting plasma glucose level of 5.6–6.9 mmol/L (100–125 mg/dL)
- Impaired glucose tolerance (IGT) for plasma glucose levels of 7.8–11.1 mmol/L (140–199 mg/dL) 2 h after a 75-g oral glucose load

Individuals with IFG or IGT do not have DM but are at substantial risk for developing type 2 DM and cardiovascular disease in the future. The hemoglobin A_{1c} (HbA_{1c}) level is useful for monitoring responses to therapy but is not recommended for screening or diagnosis of DM.

Screening with a fasting plasma glucose level is recommended every 3 years for individuals over the age of 45, as well as for younger individuals who are overweight (body mass index ≥ 25 kg/m^2) and have one or more additional risk factors (Table 182-1).

The *metabolic syndrome*, the *insulin resistance syndrome*, and *syndrome X* are terms used to describe a commonly found constellation of metabolic derangements that includes insulin resistance (with or without diabetes), hypertension, dyslipidemia, central or visceral obesity, and endothelial dysfunction and is associated with accelerated cardiovascular disease (Chap. 125).

CLINICAL FEATURES

Common presenting symptoms of DM include polyuria, polydipsia, weight loss, fatigue, weakness, blurred vision, frequent superficial infections, and poor

TABLE 182-1 CRITERIA FOR TESTING FOR PRE-DIABETES AND DIABETES IN ASYMPTOMATIC INDIVIDUALS[a]

Risk Factors
- First-degree relative with diabetes
- Physical inactivity
- Race/ethnicity (e.g., African American, Latino, Native American, Asian American, Pacific Islander)
- Previously identified IFG or IGT
- History of GDM or delivery of baby >4 kg (>9 lb)
- Hypertension (blood pressure ≥ 140/90 mmHg)
- HDL cholesterol level ≤ 0.90 mmol/L (35 mg/dL) and/or a triglyceride level ≥ 2.82 mmol/L (250 mg/dL)
- Polycystic ovary syndrome or acanthosis nigricans
- History of vascular disease

[a]Testing should be considered in all adults at age 45 and adults <45 y with BMI ≥ 25 kg/m2 and one or more of the following risk factors for diabetes.
Note: BMI, body mass index; IFG, impaired fasting glucose; IGT, impaired glucose tolerance; GDM, gestational diabetes mellitus; HDL, high-density lipoprotein.
Source: Adapted from American Diabetes Association, 2008.

wound healing. A complete medical history should be obtained with special emphasis on weight, exercise, smoking, ethanol use, family history of DM, and risk factors for cardiovascular disease. In a patient with established DM, assessment of prior diabetes care, HbA$_{1c}$ levels, self-monitoring blood glucose results, frequency of hypoglycemia, and pt's knowledge about DM should be obtained. Special attention should be given on physical exam to retinal exam, orthostatic bp, foot exam (including vibratory sensation and monofilament testing), peripheral pulses, and insulin injection sites. Acute complications of DM that may be seen on presentation include diabetic ketoacidosis (DKA) and hyperglycemic hyperosmolar state (Chap. 25).

The chronic complications of DM are listed below:

- Ophthalmologic: nonproliferative or proliferative diabetic retinopathy, macular edema
- Renal: proteinuria, end-stage renal disease (ESRD), type IV renal tubular acidosis
- Neurologic: distal symmetric polyneuropathy, polyradiculopathy, mononeuropathy, autonomic neuropathy
- Gastrointestinal: gastroparesis, diarrhea, constipation
- Genitourinary: cystopathy, erectile dysfunction, female sexual dysfunction
- Cardiovascular: coronary artery disease, congestive heart failure, peripheral vascular disease, stroke
- Lower extremity: foot deformity (hammer toe, claw toe, Charcot foot), ulceration, amputation

℞ Diabetes Mellitus

Optimal treatment of DM requires more than plasma glucose management. Comprehensive diabetes care should also detect and manage DM-specific complications and modify risk factors for DM-associated diseases. The pt with type 1 or type 2 DM should receive education about nutrition, exercise, care of diabetes during illness, and medications to lower the plasma glucose.

TABLE 182-2 PHARMACOKINETICS OF INSULIN PREPARATIONS

Preparation	Time of Action		
	Onset, h	Peak, h	Effective Duration, h
Short-acting, subcutaneous			
Lispro	<0.25	0.5–1.5	3–4
Aspart	<0.25	0.5–1.5	3–4
Glulisine	<0.25	0.5–1.5	3–4
Regular	0.5–1.0	2–3	4–6
Short-acting, inhaled			
Inhaled regular insulin	<0.25	0.5–1.5	4–6
Long-acting			
NPH	1–4	6–10	10–16
Detemir	1–4	—[a]	12–20
Glargine	1–4	—[a]	24
Insulin Combinations			
75/25–75% protamine lispro, 25% lispro	<0.25	1.5 h[b]	Up to 10–16
70/30–70% protamine aspart, 30% aspart	<0.25	1.5 h[b]	Up to 10–16
50/50–50% protamine lispro, 50% lispro	<0.25	1.5 h[b]	Up to 10–16
70/30–70% NPH, 30% regular insulin	0.5–1	Dual	10–16
50/50–50% NPH, 50% regular insulin	0.5–1	Dual	10–16

[a]Glargine has minimal peak activity; detemir has some peak activity at 6–14 h.
[b]Dual: two peaks; one at 2–3 h; the second several hours later.
Source: Adapted from JS Skyler, *Therapy for Diabetes Mellitus and Related Disorders*, American Diabetes Association, Alexandria, VA, 2004.

In general, the target HbA$_{1c}$ level should be <7.0%, though individual considerations (age, ability to implement a complex treatment regimen, and presence of other medical conditions) should also be taken into account. Intensive therapy reduces long-term complications but is associated with more frequent and more severe hypoglycemic episodes. Goal preprandial capillary plasma glucose levels should be 5.0–7.2 mmol/L (90–130 mg/dL) and postprandial levels should be <10.0 mmol/L (<180 mg/dL) 1–2 hr after a meal.

In general, pts with type 1 DM require 0.5–1.0 U/kg per day of insulin divided into multiple doses. Combinations of insulin preparations with different times of onset and duration of action should be used (Table 182-2). Preferred regimens include injection of glargine at bedtime with preprandial lispro, glulisine, or insulin aspart or continuous subcutaneous insulin using an infusion device.

Pts with type 2 DM may be managed with diet and exercise alone or in conjunction with oral glucose-lowering agents, insulin, or a combination of oral agents and insulin. The classes of oral glucose-lowering agents and dosing regimens are listed in Table 182-3. In addition, exenatide is an injectable DPP-IV inhibitor that may be used in combination with metformin or sulfonylureas. A reasonable treatment algorithm for initial therapy proposes metformin as initial therapy because of its efficacy (1–2% decrease in HbA$_{1c}$), known side-effect profile, and relatively low cost (Fig. 182-1). Metformin has

TABLE 182-3 ORAL GLUCOSE-LOWERING AGENTS

Agent	Daily Dose, mg	Doses/d	Contraindications
Biguanide			Cr > 133 μmol/L (1.5 mg/dL) (men); >124 μmol/L (1.4 mg/dL) (women); CHF; liver disease
Metformin	500–2500	1–3	
Sulfonylureas			Renal/liver disease
Glimepiride	1–8	1	
Glipizide	2.5–40	1–2	
Glipizide (ext. release)	5–10	1	
Glyburide	1.25–20	1–2	
Glyburide (micronized)	0.75–12	1–2	
Non-sulfonylurea secretagogue			Renal/liver disease
Repaglinide	0.5–16	1–4	
Netaglinide	180–360	1–3	
α-Glucosidase inhibitor			IBD, liver disease, or Cr > 177 μmol/L (2.0 mg/dL)
Acarbose	25–300	1–3	
Miglitol	25–300	1–3	
Thiazolidinedione			Liver disease, CHF
Rosiglitazone	2–8	1–2	
Pioglitazone	15–45	1	
DPP-IV inhibitor			↓ Dose with renal failure
Sitagliptin	100	1	

the advantage that it promotes mild weight loss, lowers insulin levels, improves the lipid profile slightly, and does not cause hypoglycemia when used as monotherapy, though it is contraindicated in renal insufficiency, congestive heart failure, any form of acidosis, liver disease, or severe hypoxia, and should be temporarily discontinued in pts who are seriously ill or receiving radiographic contrast material. Combinations of two oral agents may be used with additive effects, with stepwise addition of bedtime insulin or a third oral agent if adequate control is not achieved. As endogenous insulin production falls, multiple injections of long-acting and short-acting insulin may be required, as in type 1 DM. Individuals who require >1 U/kg per day of long-acting insulin should be considered for combination therapy with an insulin-sensitizing agent such as metformin or a thiazolidinedione.

The morbidity and mortality of DM-related complications can be greatly reduced by timely and consistent surveillance procedures (Table 182-4). A routine urinalysis may be performed as an initial screen for diabetic nephropathy. If it is positive for protein, quantification of protein on a 24-h urine collection should be performed. If the urinalysis is negative for protein, a spot collection for microalbuminuria should be performed (present if 30–300 μg/mg creatinine on two of three tests within a 3- to 6-month period). A resting ECG should be performed in adults, with more extensive cardiac testing for high-risk pts. Therapeutic goals to prevent complications of DM include management of proteinuria with ACE inhibitor therapy, bp control (<130/80 mmHg if no proteinuria, <125/75 if proteinuria), and dyslipidemia manage-

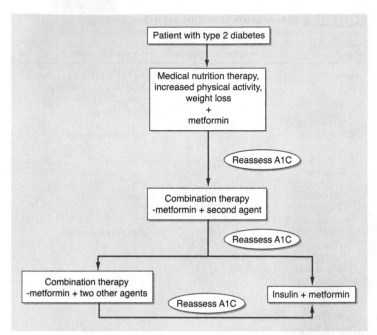

FIGURE 182-1 Glycemic management of type 2 diabetes. Agents that can be combined with metformin include insulin secretagogues, thiazolidinediones, α-glucosidase inhibitors, DPP-IV inhibitors, and exenatide.

ment [LDL < 2.6 mmol/L (<100 mg/dL) HDL > 1.1 mmol/L (>40 mg/dL) in men and >1.38 mmol/L (50 mg/dL) in women, triglycerides < 1.7 mmol/L (<150 mg/dL)]. In addition, any diabetic over 40 yrs should take a statin, regardless of the LDL cholesterol, and in those with existing cardiovascular disease, the LDL target should be <1.8 mmol/L (70 mg/dL).

MANAGEMENT OF THE HOSPITALIZED PATIENT
The goals of diabetes management during hospitalization are near-normal glycemic control, avoidance of hypoglycemia, and transition back to the outpatient

TABLE 182-4	**GUIDELINES FOR ONGOING MEDICAL CARE FOR PATIENTS WITH DIABETES**

- Self-monitoring of blood glucose (individualized frequency)
- HbA$_{1c}$ testing (2–4 times/year)
- Patient education in diabetes management (annual)
- Medical nutrition therapy and education (annual)
- Eye examination (annual)
- Foot examination (1–2 times/year by physician; daily by patient)
- Screening for diabetic nephropathy (annual urine microalbumin)
- Blood pressure measurement (quarterly)
- Lipid profile and serum creatinine (annual)
- Influenza/pneumococcal immunizations
- Consider antiplatelet therapy

diabetes treatment regimen. Pts with type 1 DM undergoing general anesthesia and surgery, or with serious illness, should receive continuous insulin, either through an IV insulin infusion or by SC administration of a reduced dose of long-acting insulin. Short-acting insulin alone is insufficient to prevent the onset of diabetic ketoacidosis. Oral hypoglycemic agents should be discontinued in pts with type 2 DM at the time of hospitalization. Either regular insulin infusion (0.05–0.15 U/kg per hour) or a reduced dose (by 30–50%) of long-acting insulin and short-acting insulin (held, or reduced by 30–50%), with infusion of a solution of 5% dextrose, should be administered when pts are NPO for a procedure. A regimen of long- and short-acting SC insulin should be used in type 2 pts who are eating. Those with DM undergoing radiographic procedures with contrast dye should be well hydrated before and after dye exposure, and the serum creatinine should be monitored after the procedure.

For a more detailed discussion, see Powers AC: Diabetes Mellitus, Chap. 338, p. 2275, in HPIM-17.

183 Disorders of the Male Reproductive System

The testes produce sperm and testosterone. Inadequate production of sperm can occur in isolation or in the presence of androgen deficiency, which impairs spermatogenesis secondarily.

ANDROGEN DEFICIENCY

Etiology Androgen deficiency can be due to either testicular failure (*primary hypogonadism*) or hypothalamic-pituitary defects (*secondary hypogonadism*).

Primary hypogonadism is diagnosed when testosterone levels are low and gonadotropin levels [luteinizing hormone (LH) and follicle-stimulating hormone (FSH)] are high. Klinefelter's syndrome is the most common cause and is due to the presence of one or more extra X chromosomes, usually a 47,XXY karyotype. Acquired primary testicular failure usually results from viral orchitis but may be due to trauma, cryptorchidism, radiation damage, or systemic diseases such as amyloidosis, Hodgkin's disease, sickle cell disease, or granulomatous diseases. Testicular failure can occur as a part of a polyglandular autoimmune failure syndrome in which multiple primary endocrine deficiencies coexist. Malnutrition, AIDS, renal failure, liver disease, myotonic dystrophy, paraplegia, and toxins such as alcohol, marijuana, heroin, methadone, lead, and antineoplastic and chemotherapeutic agents can also cause testicular failure. Testosterone synthesis may be blocked by ketoconazole, and testosterone action may be diminished by competition at the androgen receptor by spironolactone and cimetidine.

Secondary hypogonadism is diagnosed when levels of both testosterone and gonadotropins are low (*hypogonadotropic hypogonadism*). Kallmann's syndrome is due to impairment of the synthesis and/or release of gonadotropin-releasing hormone (GnRH) and is characterized by low levels of LH and FSH, and anosmia. Other individuals present with idiopathic congenital GnRH deficiency without anosmia. Critical illness, Cushing's syndrome, adrenal hypoplasia congenita, hemochromatosis, and hyperprolactinemia (due to pituitary adenomas or drugs such as phenothiazines) are other causes of isolated hypogonadotropic hypogonadism. Destruction of the pituitary gland by tumors, infection, trauma, or metastatic disease causes hypogonadism in conjunction with disturbances in the production of other pituitary hormones (see Chap. 177).

Clinical Features   The history should focus on developmental stages such as puberty and growth spurts, as well as androgen-dependent events such as early morning erections, frequency and intensity of sexual thoughts, and frequency of masturbation or intercourse. The physical examination should focus on secondary sex characteristics such as hair growth in the face, axilla, chest, and pubic regions; gynecomastia; testicular volume; prostate; and height and body proportions. Eunuchoidal proportions are defined as an arm span >2 cm greater than height and suggest that androgen deficiency occurred prior to epiphyseal fusion. Normal testicular size ranges from 3.5–5.5 cm in length, which corresponds to a volume of 12–25 mL. The presence of varicocele should be sought by palpation of the testicular veins with the patient standing. Patients with Klinefelter's syndrome have small (1–2 mL), firm testes.

A morning total testosterone level <6.93 nmol/L (<200 ng/dL), in association with symptoms, suggests testosterone deficiency. A level of >12.13 nmol/L (>350 ng/dL) makes the diagnosis of androgen deficiency unlikely. In men with testosterone levels between 6.93 and 12.13 nmol/L (200 and 350 ng/dL), the total testosterone level should be repeated and a free testosterone level should be measured. In older men and in patients with other clinical states that are associated with alterations in sex hormone–binding globulin levels, a direct measurement of free testosterone by equilibrium dialysis can be useful in unmasking testosterone deficiency. When androgen deficiency has been confirmed by low testosterone concentrations, LH should be measured to classify the patient as having primary (high LH) or secondary (low or inappropriately normal LH) hypogonadism. In men with primary hypogonadism of unknown cause, a karyotype should be performed to exclude Klinefelter's syndrome. Measurement of a prolactin level and MRI scan of the hypothalamic-pituitary region should be considered in men with secondary hypogonadism. Gynecomastia in the absence of androgen deficiency should be further evaluated (Fig. 183-1).

Rx   Androgen Deficiency

Treatment of hypogonadal men with androgens restores normal male secondary sexual characteristics (beard, body hair, external genitalia), male sexual drive, and masculine somatic development (hemoglobin, muscle mass). Administration of gradually increasing doses of testosterone is recommended for disorders in which hypogonadism occurred prior to puberty. Testosterone levels in the normal range may be achieved through daily application of transdermal testosterone patches (5–10 mg/d) or gel (50–100 mg/d) or parenteral administration of a long-acting testosterone ester (100–200 mg testosterone enanthate at 1- to 3-week intervals). Prostate cancer, severe symptoms of lower urinary tract obstruction, baseline hematocrit > 50%, severe sleep apnea, and class IV congestive heart failure are contraindications for androgen replacement.

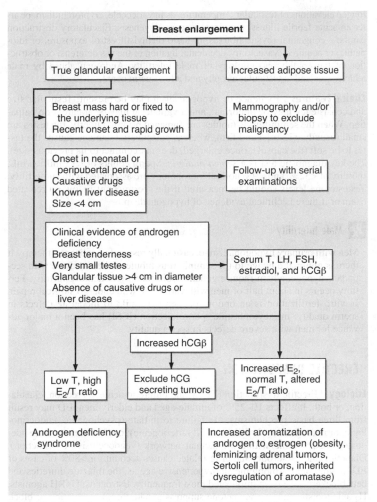

FIGURE 183-1 Evaluation of gynecomastia. T, testosterone; LH, luteinizing hormone; FSH, follicle-stimulating hormone; hCGβ, human chorionic gonadotropin β; E2, 17β-estradiol.

MALE INFERTILITY

Etiology Male infertility plays a role in 25% of infertile couples (couples who fail to conceive after 1 year of unprotected intercourse). Known causes of male infertility include primary hypogonadism (30–40%), disorders of sperm transport (10–20%), and secondary hypogonadism (2%), with an unknown etiology in up to half of men with suspected male factor infertility (see Fig. 184-3). Impaired spermatogenesis occurs with testosterone deficiency but may also be present without testosterone deficiency. Y chromosome microdeletions and substitutions, viral orchitis, tuberculosis, STDs, radiation, chemotherapeutic agents, and environmental toxins have all been associated with isolated impaired spermatogenesis. Prolonged elevations of testicular temperature, as in varicocele, cryptorchidism, or after an acute febrile illness, may impair spermatogenesis. Ejaculatory obstruction can be a congenital (cystic fibrosis, in utero diethylstilbestrol exposure, or idiopathic) or acquired (vasectomy, accidental ligation of the vas deferens, or obstruction of the epididymis) etiology of male infertility. Androgen abuse by male athletes can lead to testicular atrophy and a low sperm count.

Clinical Features   Evidence of hypogonadism may be present. Testicular size and consistency may be abnormal, and a varicocele may be apparent on palpation. When the seminiferous tubules are damaged prior to puberty, the testes are small (usually <12 mL) and firm, whereas postpubertal damage causes the testes to be soft (the capsule, once enlarged, does not contract to its previous size). The key diagnostic test is a *semen analysis*. Sperm counts of <13 million/mL, motility of <32%, and <9% normal morphology are associated with subfertility. Testosterone levels should be measured if the sperm count is low on repeated exam or if there is clinical evidence of hypogonadism.

℞ Male Infertility

Men with primary hypogonadism occasionally respond to androgen therapy if there is minimal damage to the seminiferous tubules, whereas those with secondary hypogonadism require gonadotropin therapy to achieve fertility. Fertility occurs in about half of men with varicocele who undergo surgical repair. In vitro fertilization is an option for men with mild to moderate defects in sperm quality; intracytoplasmic sperm injection (ICSI) has been a major advance for men with severe defects in sperm quality.

ERECTILE DYSFUNCTION

Etiology   Erectile dysfunction (ED) is the failure to achieve erection, ejaculation, or both. It affects 10–25% of middle-aged and elderly men. ED may result from three basic mechanisms: (1) failure to initiate (psychogenic, endocrinologic, or neurogenic); (2) failure to fill (arteriogenic); or (3) failure to store adequate blood volume within the lacunar network (venoocclusive dysfunction). Diabetic, atherosclerotic, and drug-related causes account for >80% of cases of ED in older men. Among the antihypertensive agents, the thiazide diuretics and beta blockers have been implicated most frequently. Estrogens, GnRH agonists, H_2 antagonists, and spironolactone suppress gonadotropin production or block androgen action. Antidepressant and antipsychotic agents—particularly neuroleptics, tricyclics, and selective serotonin reuptake inhibitors—are associated with erectile, ejaculatory, orgasmic, and sexual desire difficulties. Recreational drugs, including ethanol, cocaine, and marijuana, may also cause ED. Any disorder that affects the sacral spinal cord or the autonomic fibers to the penis may lead to ED.

Clinical Features   Men with sexual dysfunction may complain of loss of libido, inability to initiate or maintain an erection, ejaculatory failure, premature ejaculation, or inability to achieve orgasm. Initial questions should focus on the onset of symptoms, the presence and duration of partial erections, and the progression of ED. A history of nocturnal or early morning erections is useful for distinguishing physiologic from psychogenic ED. Relevant risk factors should be identified, such as diabetes mellitus, coronary artery disease, lipid disorders, hypertension, peripheral vascular disease, smoking, alcoholism, and endocrine or

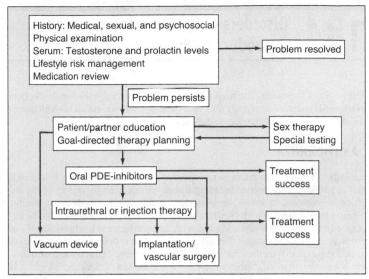

FIGURE 183-2 Algorithm for the evaluation and management of patients with ED.

neurologic disorders. The patient's surgical history should be explored, with an emphasis on bowel, bladder, prostate, or vascular procedures. Evaluation includes a detailed general as well as genital physical exam. Penile abnormalities (Peyronie's disease), testicular size, and gynecomastia should be noted. Peripheral pulses should be palpated, and bruits should be sought. Neurologic exam should assess anal sphincter tone, perineal sensation, and bulbocavernosus reflex. Serum testosterone and prolactin should be measured. Penile arteriography, electromyography, or penile Doppler ultrasound is occasionally performed.

 Erectile Dysfunction

An approach to the evaluation and treatment of ED is summarized in Fig. 183-2. Correction of the underlying disorders or discontinuation of responsible medications should be attempted. Oral inhibitors of PDE-5 (sildenafil, tadalafil, and vardenafil) enhance erections after sexual stimulation, with an onset of approximately 60–120 min. They are contraindicated in men receiving any form of nitrate therapy and should be avoided in those with congestive heart failure. Vacuum constriction devices or injection of alprostadil into the urethra or corpora cavernosa may also be effective. The insertion of penile prosthesis is rarely indicated.

For a more detailed discussion, see Bhasin S, Jameson JL: Disorders of the Testes and Male Reproductive System, Chap. 340, p. 2310; Hall JE: The Female Reproductive System: Infertility and Contraception, Chap. 341, p. 2324; McVary KT: Sexual Dysfunction, Chap. 49, p. 296, in HPIM-17.

184 Disorders of the Female Reproductive System

The pituitary hormones, luteinizing hormone (LH) and follicle-stimulating hormone (FSH), stimulate ovarian follicular development and result in ovulation at about day 14 of the 28-day menstrual cycle.

AMENORRHEA

Etiology *Amenorrhea* refers to the absence of menstrual periods. It is classified as *primary*, if menstrual bleeding has never occurred by age 15 in the absence of hormonal treatment, or *secondary*, if menstrual periods are absent for >3 months in a woman with previous periodic menses. Pregnancy should be excluded in women of childbearing age with amenorrhea, even when history and physical exam are not suggestive. *Oligoamenorrhea* is defined as a cycle length of >35 days or <10 menses per year. Both the frequency and amount of bleeding are irregular in oligoamenorrhea. Frequent or heavy irregular bleeding is termed *dysfunctional uterine bleeding* if anatomic uterine lesions or a bleeding diathesis have been excluded.

The causes of primary and secondary amenorrhea overlap, and it is generally more useful to classify disorders of menstrual function into disorders of the uterus and outflow tract and disorders of ovulation (Fig. 184-1).

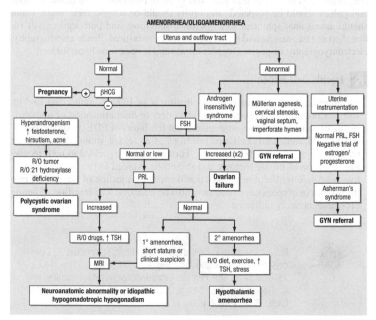

FIGURE 184-1 Algorithm for evaluation of amenorrhea. β-hCG, human chorionic gonadotropin; PRL, prolactin; FSH, follicle-stimulating hormone; TSH, thyroid-stimulating hormone.

Anatomic defects of the outflow tract that prevent vaginal bleeding include absence of vagina or uterus, imperforate hymen, transverse vaginal septae, and cervical stenosis.

Women with amenorrhea and low FSH levels usually have hypogonadotropic hypogonadism due to disease of either the hypothalamus or the pituitary. Hypothalamic causes include Kallmann's syndrome or Sheehan's syndrome, hypothalamic lesions (craniopharyngiomas and other tumors, tuberculosis, sarcoidosis, metastatic tumors), hypothalamic trauma or irradiation, rigorous exercise, eating disorders, stressful events, and chronic debilitating diseases (end-stage renal disease, malignancy, malabsorption). Disorders of the pituitary can lead to amenorrhea by two mechanisms: direct interference with gonadotropin secretion or inhibition of gonadotropin secretion via excess prolactin (Chap. 177).

Women with amenorrhea and high FSH levels have ovarian failure, which may be due to Turner's syndrome, pure gonadal dygenesis, premature ovarian failure, the resistant-ovary syndrome, and chemotherapy or radiation therapy for malignancy. The diagnosis of premature ovarian failure is applied to women who cease menstruating before age 40.

Polycystic ovarian syndrome (PCOS) is characterized by the presence of clinical or biochemical hyperandrogenism (hirsutism, acne, male pattern baldness) in association with amenorrhea or oligomenorrhea. Metabolic changes, including insulin resistance, and infertility are often present; these features are worsened with coexistent obesity. Additional disorders with a similar presentation include excess androgen production from adrenal or ovarian tumors, adult-onset congenital adrenal hyperplasia, and thyroid disorders.

Diagnosis The initial evaluation involves careful physical exam including assessment of hyperandrogenism, serum or urine human chorionic gonadotropin (hCG), and serum FSH levels (Fig. 184-1). Anatomic defects are usually diagnosed by physical exam, though hysterosalpingography or direct visual examination by hysteroscopy may be required. Chromosomal analysis should be performed when gonadal dysgenesis is suspected. The diagnosis of PCOS is based on the coexistence of chronic anovulation and androgen excess, after ruling out other etiologies for these features. The evaluation of hyperprolactinemia is described in Chap. 177. In the absence of a known etiology for hypogonadotropic hypogonadism, MRI of the pituitary-hypothalamic region should be performed when gonadotropins are low or inappropriately normal.

℞ Amenorrhea

Disorders of the outflow tract are managed surgically. Decreased estrogen production, whether from ovarian failure or hypothalamic/pituitary disease, should be treated with cyclic estrogens, either in the form of oral contraceptives or conjugated estrogens (0.625–1.25 mg/d PO) and medroxyprogesterone acetate (2.5 mg/d PO or 5–10 mg during the last 5 days of the month). PCOS may be treated with medications to induce periodic withdrawal menses (medroxyprogesterone acetate 5–10 mg or prometrium 200 mg daily for 10–14 days of each month, or oral contraceptive agents) and weight reduction, along with treatment of hirsutism (see below). Individuals with PCOS may benefit from insulin-sensitizing drugs and should be screened for diabetes mellitus.

PELVIC PAIN

Etiology Pelvic pain may be associated with normal or abnormal menstrual cycles and may originate in the pelvis or be referred from another region of

	Acute	Chronic
TABLE 184-1 CAUSES OF PELVIC PAIN		
Cyclic pelvic pain		Premenstrual symptoms
		Mittelschmerz
		Dysmenorrhea
		Endometriosis
Noncyclic pelvic pain	Pelvic inflammatory disease	Pelvic congestion syndrome
	Ruptured or hemorrhagic ovarian cyst or ovarian torsion	Adhesions and retroversion of the uterus
	Ectopic pregnancy	Pelvic malignancy
	Endometritis	Vulvodynia
	Acute growth or degeneration of uterine myoma	History of sexual abuse

the body. A high index of suspicion must be entertained for extrapelvic disorders that refer to the pelvis, such as appendicitis, diverticulitis, cholecystitis, intestinal obstruction, and urinary tract infections. A thorough history including the type, location, radiation, and status with respect to increasing or decreasing severity can help to identify the cause of acute pelvic pain. Associations with vaginal bleeding, sexual activity, defecation, urination, movement, or eating should be sought. Determination of whether the pain is acute versus chronic and cyclic versus noncyclic will direct further investigation (Table 184-1).

Acute Pelvic Pain Pelvic inflammatory disease most commonly presents with bilateral lower abdominal pain. Unilateral pain suggests adnexal pathology from rupture, bleeding, or torsion of ovarian cysts, or, less commonly, neoplasms of the ovary, fallopian tubes, or paraovarian areas. Ectopic pregnancy is associated with right- or left-sided lower abdominal pain, vaginal bleeding, and menstrual cycle abnormalities, with clinical signs appearing 6–8 weeks after the last normal menstrual period. Orthostatic signs and fever may be present. Uterine pathology includes endometritis and degenerating leiomyomas.

Chronic Pelvic Pain Many women experience lower abdominal discomfort with ovulation (*mittelschmerz*), characterized as a dull, aching pain at midcycle that lasts minutes to hours. In addition, ovulatory women may experience somatic symptoms during the few days prior to menses, including edema, breast engorgement, and abdominal bloating or discomfort. A symptom complex of cyclic irritability, depression, and lethargy is known as *premenstrual syndrome* (PMS). Severe or incapacitating cramping with ovulatory menses in the absence of demonstrable disorders of the pelvis is termed *primary dysmenorrhea*. *Secondary dysmenorrhea* is caused by underlying pelvic pathology such as endometriosis, adenomyosis, or cervical stenosis.

Diagnosis Evaluation includes a history, pelvic exam, hCG measurement, tests for chlamydial and gonococcal infections, and pelvic ultrasound. Laparoscopy or laparotomy is indicated in some cases of pelvic pain of undetermined cause.

Rx Pelvic Pain

Primary dysmenorrhea is best treated with NSAIDs or oral contraceptive agents. Infections should be treated with the appropriate antibiotics. Symptoms from PMS may improve with selective serotonin reuptake inhibitor (SSRI) therapy. The majority of unruptured ectopic pregnancies are treated with methotrexate. Surgery may be required for structural abnormalities.

HIRSUTISM

Etiology *Hirsutism*, defined as excessive male-pattern hair growth, affects ~10% of women. It may be familial or caused by PCOS, ovarian or adrenal neoplasms, congenital adrenal hyperplasia, Cushing's syndrome, hyperprolactinemia, acromegaly, pregnancy, and drugs (androgens, oral contraceptives containing androgenic progestins). Other drugs, such as minoxidil, phenytoin, diazoxide, and cyclosporine, can cause excessive growth of non-androgen-dependent vellus hair, leading to hypertrichosis.

Clinical Features An objective clinical assessment of hair distribution and quantity is central to the evaluation. A commonly used method to grade hair growth is the Ferriman-Gallwey score (see Fig. 50-1, p. 302, in HPIM-17). Associated manifestations of androgen excess include acne and male-pattern balding (androgenic alopecia). *Virilization*, on the other hand, refers to the state in which androgen levels are sufficiently high to cause deepening of the voice, breast atrophy, increased muscle bulk, clitoromegaly, and increased libido. Historic elements include menstrual history and the age of onset, rate of progression, and distribution of hair growth. Sudden development of hirsutism, rapid progression, and virilization suggest an ovarian or adrenal neoplasm.

Diagnosis An approach to testing for androgen excess is depicted in Fig. 184-2. PCOS is a relatively common cause of hirsutism. The dexamethasone androgen-suppression test (0.5 mg PO every 6 h × 4 days, with free testosterone levels obtained before and after administration of dexamethasone) may distinguish ovarian from adrenal overproduction. Incomplete suppression suggests ovarian androgen excess. Congenital adrenal hyperplasia due to 21-hydroxylase deficiency can be excluded by a 17-hydroxyprogesterone level that is <6 nmol/L (<2 µg/L) either in the morning during the follicular phase or 1 h after administration of 250 µg of cosyntropin. CT may localize an adrenal mass, and ultrasound will identify an ovarian mass, if evaluation suggests these possibilities.

Rx Hirsutism

Nonpharmacologic treatments include (1) bleaching; (2) depilatory such as shaving and chemical treatments; and (3) epilatory such as plucking, waxing, electrolysis, and laser therapy. Pharmacologic therapy includes oral contraceptives with a low androgenic progestin and spironolactone (100–200 mg/d PO), often in combination. Glucocorticoids (dexamethasone, 0.25–0.5 mg at bedtime, or prednisone, 5–10 mg at bedtime) are the mainstay of treatment in pts with congenital adrenal hyperplasia. Attenuation of hair growth with pharmacologic therapy is typically not evident until 6 months after initiation of medical treatment and therefore should be used in conjunction with nonpharmacologic treatments.

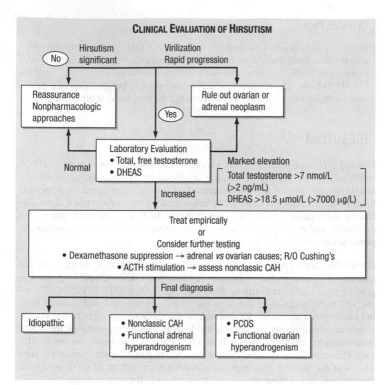

FIGURE 184-2 Algorithm for the evaluation and differential diagnosis of hirsutism. ACTH, adrenocorticotropic hormone; CAH, congenital adrenal hyperplasia; DHEAS, sulfated form of dehydroepiandrosterone; GnRH, gonadotropin-releasing hormone; PCOS, polycystic ovarian syndrome.

MENOPAUSE

Etiology *Menopause* is defined as the final episode of menstrual bleeding and occurs at a median age of 51 years. It is the consequence of depletion of ovarian follicles or of oophorectomy. The onset of *perimenopause*, when fertility wanes and menstrual irregularity increases, precedes the final menses by 2–8 years.

Clinical Features The most common menopausal symptoms are vasomotor instability (hot flashes and night sweats), mood changes (nervousness, anxiety, irritability, and depression), insomnia, and atrophy of the urogenital epithelium and skin. FSH levels are elevated to ≥40 IU/L with estradiol levels that are <30 pg/mL.

℞ Menopause

During the perimenopause, low-dose combined oral contraceptives may be of benefit. The rational use of postmenopausal hormone therapy requires balancing the potential benefits and risks. Short-term therapy (<5 years) may be beneficial in controlling symptoms of menopause, as long as no contraindications exist. These include unexplained vaginal bleeding, active liver disease, venous thromboembolism, history of endometrial cancer (except stage I without deep invasion), breast cancer, preexisting cardiovascular disease, and diabetes. Hypertriglyceridemia (>400 mg/dL) and active gallbladder disease are relative contraindications. Alternative therapies for symptoms include venlafaxine, fluoxetine, paroxetine, gabapentin, clonidine, vitamin E, or soy-based products. Vaginal estradiol tablets may be used for genitourinary symptoms. Long-term therapy (≥5 years) should be carefully considered, particularly in light of alternative therapies for osteoporosis (bisphosphonates, raloxifene) and of the risks of venous thromboembolism and breast cancer. Estrogens should be given in the minimal effective doses (conjugated estrogen, 0.625 mg/d PO; micronized estradiol, 1.0 mg/d PO; or transdermal estradiol, 0.05–1.0 mg once or twice a week). Women with an intact uterus should be given estrogen in combination with a progestin (medroxyprogesterone either cyclically, 5–10 mg/d PO for days 15–25 each month, or continuously, 2.5 mg/d PO) to avoid the increased risk of endometrial carcinoma seen with unopposed estrogen use.

CONTRACEPTION

The most widely used methods for fertility control include (1) barrier methods, (2) oral contraceptives, (3) intrauterine devices, (4) long-acting progestins, (5) sterilization, and (6) abortion.

Oral contraceptive agents are widely used for both prevention of pregnancy and control of dysmenorrhea and anovulatory bleeding. Combination oral contraceptive agents contain synthetic estrogen (ethinyl estradiol or mestranol) and synthetic progestins. Low-dose norgestimate and third-generation progestins (desogestrel, gestodene, drosperinone) have a less androgenic profile; levonorgestrel appears to be the most androgenic of the progestins and should be avoided in pts with hyperandrogenic symptoms. The three major formulation types include fixed-dose estrogen-progestin, phasic estrogen-progestin, and progestin only.

Despite overall safety, oral contraceptive users are at risk for venous thromboembolism, hypertension, and cholelithiasis. Risks for myocardial infarction and stroke are increased with smoking and aging. Side effects, including breakthrough bleeding, amenorrhea, breast tenderness, and weight gain, are often responsive to a change in formulation.

Absolute contraindications to the use of oral contraceptives include previous thromboembolic disorders, cerebrovascular or coronary artery disease, carcinoma of the breasts or other estrogen-dependent neoplasia, liver disease, hypertriglyceridemia, heavy smoking with age over 35, undiagnosed uterine bleeding, or known or suspected pregnancy. Relative contraindications include hypertension and anticonvulsant drug therapy.

New methods include a weekly contraceptive patch, a monthly contraceptive injection, and a monthly vaginal ring. Long-term progestins may be administered in the form of Depo-Provera.

Emergency contraceptive pills, containing progestin only or estrogen and progestin, can be used within 72 h of unprotected intercourse for prevention of pregnancy. Both Plan B and Preven are emergency contraceptive kits specifically designed for postcoital contraception. In addition, certain oral contraceptive pills may be dosed within 72 h for emergency contraception (Ovral, 2 tabs, 12 h apart; Lo/Ovral, 4 tabs, 12 h apart). Side effects include nausea, vomiting, and breast soreness. Mifepristone (RU486) may also be used, with fewer side effects.

INFERTILITY

Etiology   *Infertility* is defined as the inability to conceive after 12 months of unprotected sexual intercourse. The causes of infertility are outlined in Fig. 184-3. Male infertility is discussed in Chap. 183.

Clinical Features   The initial evaluation includes discussion of the appropriate timing of intercourse, semen analysis in the male, confirmation of ovulation in the female, and, in the majority of situations, documentation of tubal patency in the female. Abnormalities in menstrual function constitute the most common cause of female infertility (Fig. 184-1). A history of regular, cyclic, predictable, spontaneous menses usually indicates ovulatory cycles, which may be confirmed by urinary ovulation predictor kits, basal body temperature graphs, or plasma progesterone measurements during the luteal phase of the cycle. An FSH level < 10 IU/mL on day 3 of the cycle predicts adequate ovarian oocyte reserve. Tubal disease can be evaluated by obtaining a hysterosalpingogram or by diagnostic laparoscopy. Endometriosis may be suggested by history and exam but is often clinically silent and can only be excluded definitively by laparoscopy.

℞ Infertility

The treatment of infertility should be tailored to the problems unique to each couple. Treatment options include expectant management, clomiphene citrate with or without intrauterine insemination (IUI), gonadotropins with or without IUI, and in vitro fertilization (IVF). In specific situations, surgery, pulsatile GnRH therapy, intracytoplasmic sperm injection (ICSI), or assisted reproductive technologies with donor egg or sperm may be required.

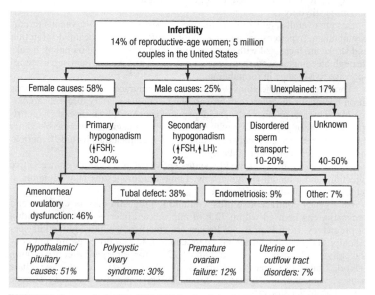

FIGURE 184-3 Causes of infertility, FSH, follicle-stimulating hormone; LH, luteinizing hormone.

For a more detailed discussion, see Ehrmann DA: Hirsutism and Virilization, Chap. 50, p. 301; Hall JE: Menstrual Disorders and Pelvic Pain, Chap. 51, p. 304; Hall JE: The Female Reproductive System: Infertility and Contraception, Chap. 341, p. 2324; and Manson JE, Bassuk SS: The Menopause Transition and Postmenopausal Hormone Therapy, Chap. 342, p. 2334, in HPIM-17.

185 Hypercalcemia and Hypocalcemia

HYPERCALCEMIA

Hypercalcemia from any cause can result in fatigue, depression, mental confusion, anorexia, nausea, constipation, renal tubular defects, polyuria, a short QT interval, and arrhythmias. CNS and GI symptoms can occur at levels of serum calcium >2.9 mmol/L (>11.5 mg/dL), and nephrocalcinosis and impairment of renal function occur when serum calcium is >3.2 mmol/L (>13 mg/dL). Severe hypercalcemia, usually defined as >3.7 mmol/L (>15 mg/dL), can be a medical emergency, leading to coma and cardiac arrest.

Etiology The regulation of the calcium homeostasis is depicted in Fig. 185-1. The causes of hypercalcemia are listed in Table 185-1. Hyperparathyroidism and malignancy account for 90% of cases.

Primary hyperparathyroidism is a generalized disorder of bone metabolism due to increased secretion of parathyroid hormone (PTH) by an adenoma (81%) or carcinoma (4%) in a single gland, or by parathyroid hyperplasia (15%). Familial hyperparathyroidism may be part of multiple endocrine neoplasia type 1 (MEN 1), which also includes pituitary and pancreatic islet tumors, or of MEN 2A, in which hyperparathyroidism occurs with pheochromocytoma and medullary carcinoma of the thyroid.

Hypercalcemia associated with malignancy is often severe and difficult to manage. Mechanisms for this include release of PTH-related protein (PTHrP) in lung, kidney, and squamous cell carcinoma; local bone destruction in myeloma and breast carcinoma; activation of lymphocytes leading to release of IL-1 and TNF in myeloma and lymphoma; or an increased synthesis of $1,25(OH)_2D$ in lymphoma.

Several other conditions have been associated with hypercalcemia. These include: sarcoidosis and other granulomatous diseases, which lead to increased synthesis of $1,25(OH)_2D$; vitamin D intoxication from chronic ingestion of large vitamin doses (50–100 × physiologic requirements); lithium therapy, which results in hyperfunctioning of the parathyroid glands; and familial hypocalciuric hypercalcemia (FHH) due to autosomal dominant inheritance of a mutation in the calcium-sensing receptor, which results in inappropriate secretion of PTH and enhanced renal calcium resorption. Severe secondary hyperparathyroidism may also complicate end-stage renal disease. Progression to tertiary hyperthyroidism occurs when PTH hypersecretion becomes autonomous and is no longer responsive to medical therapy.

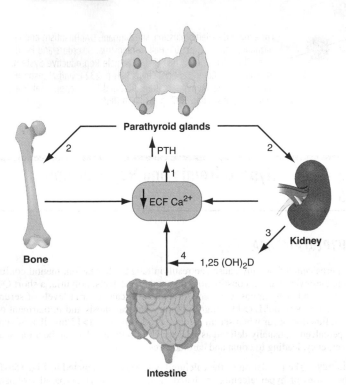

FIGURE 185-1 Feedback mechanisms maintaining extracellular calcium concentrations within a narrow, physiologic range [8.9–10.1 mg/dL (2.2–2.5 mM)]. A decrease in extracellular (ECF) calcium (Ca^{2+}) triggers an increase in parathyroid hormone (PTH) secretion (1) via activation of the calcium sensor receptor on parathyroid cells. PTH, in turn, results in increased tubular reabsorption of calcium by the kidney (2) and resorption of calcium from bone (2) and also stimulates renal 1,25(OH)$_2$D production (3). 1,25(OH)$_2$D, in turn, acts principally on the intestine to increase calcium absorption (4). Collectively, these homeostatic mechanisms serve to restore serum calcium levels to normal.

Clinical Features Most pts with hyperparathyroidism are asymptomatic, even when the disease involves the kidneys and the skeletal system. Pts frequently have hypercalciuria and polyuria, and calcium can be deposited in the renal parenchyma or form calcium oxalate stones. The characteristic skeletal lesion is osteopenia or, rarely, the more severe disorder osteitis fibrosa cystica. Increased bone resorption primarily involves cortical rather than trabecular bone. Hypercalcemia may be intermittent or sustained, and serum phosphate is usually low but may be normal.

Diagnosis Primary hyperparathyroidism is confirmed by demonstration of an inappropriately high PTH level for the degree of hypercalcemia. Hypercalciuria helps to distinguish this disorder from FHH, in which PTH levels are usually in the normal range and the urine calcium level is low. Levels of PTH are low in hypercalcemia of malignancy (Table 185-2).

TABLE 185-1	CLASSIFICATION OF CAUSES OF HYPERCALCEMIA

I. Parathyroid-related
    A. Primary hyperparathyroidism
        1. Solitary adenomas
        2. Multiple endocrine neoplasia
    B. Lithium therapy
    C. Familial hypocalciuric hypercalcemia
II. Malignancy-related
    A. Solid tumor with humoral mediation of hypercalcemia (lung, kidney)
    B. Solid tumor with metastases (breast)
    C. Hematologic malignancies (multiple myeloma, lymphoma, leukemia)
III. Vitamin D–related
    A. Vitamin D intoxication
    B. ↑ $1,25(OH)_2D$; sarcoidosis and other granulomatous diseases
    C. Idiopathic hypercalcemia of infancy
IV. Associated with high bone turnover
    A. Hyperthyroidism
    B. Immobilization
    C. Thiazides
    D. Vitamin A intoxication
V. Associated with renal failure
    A. Severe secondary hyperparathyroidism
    B. Aluminum intoxication
    C. Milk-alkali syndrome

Source: JT Potts Jr: HPIM-16, p. 2252.

℞ Hypercalcemia

The type of treatment is based on the severity of the hypercalcemia and the nature of the associated symptoms. Table 185-3 shows general recommendations that apply to therapy of severe hypercalcemia [levels of >3.2 mmol/L (>13 mg/dL)] from any cause.

TABLE 185-2	DIFFERENTIAL DIAGNOSIS OF HYPERCALCEMIA: LABORATORY CRITERIA

	Blood[a]			
	Ca	P_i	$1,25(OH)_2D$	iPTH
Primary hyperparathyroidism	↑	↓	↑↔	↑(↔)
Malignancy-associated hypercalcemia:				
Humoral hypercalcemia	↑↑	↓	↓↔	↓
Local destruction (osteolytic metastases)	↑	↔	↓↔	↓

[a]Symbols in parentheses refer to values rarely seen in the particular disease.
Note: P_i, inorganic phosphate; iPTH, immunoreactive parathyroid hormone.
Source: JT Potts Jr: HPIM-12, p. 1911.

TABLE 185-3 THERAPIES FOR SEVERE HYPERCALCEMIA

Treatment	Onset of Action	Duration of Action	Advantages	Disadvantages
Hydration with saline (≤6 L/d)	Hours	During infusion	Rehydrates; rapid action	Volume overload; electrolyte disturbance
Forced diuresis (furosemide q1–2h along with aggressive hydration)	Hours	During treatment	Rapid action	Monitoring required to avoid dehydration
Pamidronate 30–90 mg IV over 4 h	1–2 days	10–14 days	High potency; prolonged action	Fever in 20% ↓ Ca, ↓ phosphate, ↓ Mg
Zolendronate 4–8 mg IV over 15 min	1–2 days	>3 weeks	High potency; prolonged action; rapid infusion	Minor: Fever; rare ↓ Ca, ↓ phosphate
Calcitonin (2–8 U/kg SC 6–12 h)	Hours	1–2 days	Rapid onset	Limited effect; tachyphylaxis
Glucocorticoids (prednisone 10–25 mg PO qid)	Days	Days–weeks	Useful in myeloma, lymphoma, breast CA, sarcoid, vitamin D intox	Effects limited to certain disorders; glucocorticoid side effects
Dialysis	Hours	During use–2 days	Useful in renal failure; immediate effect	Complex procedure

In pts with severe primary hyperparathyroidism, surgical parathyroidectomy should be performed promptly. Asymptomatic disease may not require surgery; usual surgical indications include age <50, nephrolithiasis, urine Ca > 400 mg/d, reduced creatinine clearance, reduction in bone mass (T score <–2.5), or serum calcium > 0.25 mmol/L (>1 mg/dL) above the normal range. A minimally invasive approach may be used if preoperative localization via sestamibi scans with SPECT or neck ultrasound demonstrates a solitary adenoma and intraoperative PTH assays are available. Otherwise, neck exploration is required. Postoperative management requires close monitoring of calcium and phosphorus. Calcium supplementation is given for symptomatic hypocalcemia.

Hypercalcemia of malignancy is managed by treating the underlying tumor. Adequate hydration and parenteral bisphosphonates can be used to reduce calcium levels.

No therapy is recommended for FHH. Secondary hyperparathyroidism should be treated with phosphate restriction, the use of nonabsorbable antacids or sevelamer, and calcitriol. Tertiary hyperparathyroidism requires parathyroidectomy.

HYPOCALCEMIA

Chronic hypocalcemia is less common than hypercalcemia but is usually symptomatic and requires treatment. Symptoms include peripheral and perioral paresthesia, muscle spasms, carpopedal spasm, laryngeal spasm, seizure, and respiratory arrest. Increased intracranial pressure and papilledema may occur with long-standing hypocalcemia, and other manifestations may include irritability, depression, psychosis, intestinal cramps, and chronic malabsorption. Chvostek's and Trousseau's signs are frequently positive, and the QT interval is prolonged. Both hypomagnesemia and alkalosis lower the threshold for tetany.

Etiology Transient hypocalcemia often occurs in critically ill pts with burns, sepsis, and acute renal failure; following transfusion with citrated blood; or with medications such as protamine and heparin. Hypoalbuminemia can reduce serum calcium below normal, although ionized calcium levels remain normal. A simplified correction is sometimes used to assess whether the serum calcium concentration is abnormal when serum proteins are low. The correction is to add 0.2 mmol/L (0.8 mg/dL) to the serum calcium level for every 10 g/L (1 g/dL) by which the serum albumin level is below 40 g/L (4.0 g/dL). Alkalosis increases calcium binding to proteins, and in this setting direct measurements of ionized calcium should be used.

The causes of hypocalcemia can be divided into those in which PTH is absent (hereditary or acquired hypoparathyroidism, hypomagnesemia), PTH is ineffective (chronic renal failure, vitamin D deficiency, intestinal malabsorption, pseudohypoparathyroidism), or PTH is overwhelmed (severe, acute hyperphosphatemia in tumor lysis, acute renal failure, or rhabdomyolysis; hungry bone syndrome postparathyroidectomy). The cause of hypocalcemia associated with acute pancreatitis is unclear.

℞ Hypocalcemia

Symptomatic hypocalcemia may be treated with intravenous calcium gluconate (bolus of 1–2 g IV over 10–20 minutes followed by infusion of 10 ampules of 10% calcium gluconate diluted in 1 L D_5W infused at 30–100 mL/h). Management of chronic hypocalcemia requires an oral calcium preparation, usually with a vitamin D preparation (Chap. 186). Hypoparathyroidism requires administration of calcium (1–3 g/d) and calcitriol (0.25–1 µg/d), adjusted according to serum calcium levels and urinary excretion. Restoration of magnesium stores may be required to reverse hypocalcemia in the setting of severe hypomagnesemia.

HYPOPHOSPHATEMIA

Mild hypophosphatemia is not usually associated with clinical symptoms. In severe hypophosphatemia, pts may have muscle weakness, numbness, paresthesia, and confusion. Rhabdomyolysis may develop during rapidly progressive hypophosphatemia. Respiratory insufficiency can result from diaphragm muscle weakness.

Etiology The causes of hypophosphatemia include: decreased intestinal absorption (vitamin D deficiency, phosphorus-binding antacids, malabsorption); urinary losses (hyperparathyroidism, vitamin D deficiency, hyperglycemic states, X-linked hypophosphatemic rickets, oncogenic osteomalacia, alcoholism, or certain toxins); and shifts of phosphorus from extracellular to intracellular compartments (administration of insulin in diabetic ketoacidosis or by hyperalimentation or refeeding in a malnourished pt).

Rx Hypophosphatemia

Mild hypophosphatemia can be replaced orally with milk, carbonated beverages, or Neutraphos or K-phos (up to 2 g/d in divided doses). For severe hypophosphatemia [0.5 mmol/L; (<1.5 mg/dL)], IV phosphate may be administered at initial doses of 0.4–0.8 mmol/kg of elemental phosphorus over 6 h. Hypocalcemia should be corrected first, and the dose reduced 50% in hypercalcemia. Serum calcium and phosphate levels should be measured every 6–12 h; a serum calcium × phosphate level >50 must be avoided.

HYPERPHOSPHATEMIA

In adults, hyperphosphatemia is defined as a level >1.8 mmol/L (>5.5 mg/dL). The most common causes are acute and chronic renal failure, but it may also be seen in hypoparathyroidism, vitamin D intoxication, acidosis, rhabdomyolysis, and hemolysis. In addition to treating the underlying disorder, dietary phosphorus intake should be limited. Oral aluminum phosphate binders or sevalamer may be used, and hemodialysis should be considered in severe cases.

HYPOMAGNESEMIA

Muscle weakness, prolonged PR and QT intervals, and cardiac arrhythmias are the most common manifestations of hypomagnesemia. Magnesium is important for effective PTH secretion as well as the renal and skeletal responsiveness to PTH. Therefore, hypomagnesemia is often associated with hypocalcemia.

Etiology Hypomagnesemia generally results from a derangement in renal or intestinal handling of magnesium and is classified as primary (hereditary) or secondary (acquired). Secondary causes are much more common, with renal losses being due to volume expansion, hypercalcemia, osmotic diuresis, loop diuretics, alcohol, aminoglycosides, cisplatin, cyclosporine, and amphotericin B, and gastrointestinal losses most commonly resulting from vomiting and diarrhea.

℞ Hypomagnesemia

For mild deficiency, oral replacement in divided doses totaling 20–30 mmol/d (40–60 meq/d) is effective, though diarrhea may result. Parenteral magnesium administration is usually needed for serum levels <0.5 mmol/L (<1.2 mg/dL), with a continuous infusion of magnesium chloride IV to deliver 50 mmol/d over a 24-h period (dose reduced by 50–75% in renal failure). Therapy may be required for several days. Other electrolyte disturbances should be treated simultaneously. Patients with associated seizures or acute arrhythmias can be given 1–2 g of magnesium sulfate IV over 5–10 min.

HYPERMAGNESEMIA

Hypermagnesemia is rare but can be seen in renal failure when pts are taking magnesium-containing antacids, laxatives, enemas, or infusions, or in acute rhabdomyolysis. The most readily detectable clinical sign of hypermagnesemia is the disappearance of deep tendon reflexes, but hypotension, paralysis of respiratory muscles, complete heart block, and cardiac arrest can occur. Treatment includes stopping the preparation, dialysis against a low magnesium bath, or, if associated with life-threatening complications, 100–200 mg of elemental calcium IV over 1–2 h.

For a more detailed discussion, see Bringhurst FR, Demay MB, Krane SM, Kronenberg HM: Bone and Mineral Metabolism in Health and Disease, Chap. 346, p. 2365; Khosla S: Hypercalcemia and Hypocalcemia, Chap. 47, p. 285-287; and Potts JT Jr: Diseases of the Parathyroid Gland and Other Hyper- and Hypocalcemic Disorders, Chap. 347, p. 2377, in HPIM-17.

186 Osteoporosis and Osteomalacia

OSTEOPOROSIS

Osteoporosis is defined as a reduction in bone mass (or density) or the presence of fragility fracture. It is defined operationally as a bone density that falls 2.5 SD below the mean for a young normal individual (a T-score of <–2.5). Those with a T-score of <1.0 have low bone density and are at increased risk for osteoporosis. The most common sites for osteoporosis-related fractures are the vertebrae, hip, and distal radius.

Etiology   Low bone density may result from low peak bone mass or increased bone loss. Risk factors for an osteoporotic fracture are listed in Table 186-1,

TABLE 186-1   **RISK FACTORS FOR OSTEOPOROSIS FRACTURE**

Nonmodifiable	Estrogen deficiency
Personal history of fracture as an adult	Early menopause (<45 years) or bilateral ovariectomy
History of fracture in first-degree relative	Prolonged premenopausal amen-orrhea (>1 year)
Female sex	Low calcium intake
Advanced age	Alcoholism
Caucasian race	Impaired eyesight despite adequate correction
Dementia	
Potentially modifiable	Recurrent falls
Current cigarette smoking	Inadequate physical activity
Low body weight [<58 kg (127 lb)]	Poor health/frailty

and diseases associated with osteoporosis are listed in Table 186-2. Certain drugs, primarily glucocorticoids, cyclosporine, cytotoxic drugs, anticonvulsants, aluminum, and heparin, also have detrimental effects on the skeleton.

Clinical Features   Pts with multiple vertebral crush fractures may have height loss, kyphosis, and secondary pain from altered biomechanics of the back. Thoracic fractures can be associated with restrictive lung disease, whereas lumbar fractures are sometimes associated with abdominal symptoms or nerve compres-

TABLE 186-2   **DISEASES ASSOCIATED WITH AN INCREASED RISK OF GENERALIZED OSTEOPOROSIS IN ADULTS**

Hypogonadal states	Hematologic disorders/malignancy
Turner's syndrome	Multiple myeloma
Klinefelter's syndrome	Lymphoma and leukemia
Anorexia nervosa	Malignancy-associated parathyroid hormone–related (PTHrP) production
Hypothalamic amenorrhea	Mastocytosis
Hyperprolactinemia	Hemophilia
Other primary or secondary hypogonadal states	Thalassemia
Endocrine disorders	Selected inherited disorders
Cushing's syndrome	Osteogenesis imperfecta
Hyperparathyroidism	Marfan's syndrome
Thyrotoxicosis	Hemochromatosis
Type 1 diabetes mellitus	Hypophosphatasia
Acromegaly	Glycogen storage diseases
Adrenal insufficiency	Homocystinuria
Nutritional and gastrointestinal disorders	Ehlers-Danlos syndrome
Malnutrition	Porphyria
Parenteral nutrition	Menkes' syndrome
Malabsorption syndromes	Epidermolysis bullosa
Gastrectomy	Other disorders
Severe liver disease, especially biliary cirrhosis	Immobilization
	Chronic obstructive pulmonary disease
Pernicious anemia	Pregnancy and lactation
Rheumatologic disorders	Scoliosis
Rheumatoid arthritis	Multiple sclerosis
Ankylosing spondylitis	Sarcoidosis
	Amyloidosis

TABLE 186-3	FDA-APPROVED INDICATIONS FOR BMD TESTS[a]

Estrogen-deficient women at clinical risk of osteoporosis

Vertebral abnormalities on x-ray suggestive of osteoporosis (osteopenia, vertebral fracture)

Glucocorticoid treatment equivalent to ≥7.5 mg of prednisone, or duration of therapy >3 months

Primary hyperparathyroidism

Monitoring response to an FDA-approved medication for osteoporosis

Repeat BMD evaluations at >23-month intervals, or more frequently, if medically justified

---

[a]Criteria adapted from the 1998 Bone Mass Measurement Act.

Note: BMD, bone mineral density.

---

sion leading to sciatica. Dual-energy x-ray absorptiometry has become the standard for measuring bone density. The U.S. Preventive Health Services Task Force recommends that women aged 65 and older be screened routinely for osteoporosis, and at age 60 for women with increased risk. Criteria approved for Medicare reimbursement of bone mass measurement are summarized in Table 186-3. A general laboratory evaluation includes complete blood count, serum and 24-h urine calcium, 25(OH)D level, and renal and hepatic function tests. Further testing is based on clinical suspicion and may include thyroid-stimulating hormone (TSH), urinary free cortisol, parathyroid hormone (PTH), serum and urine electrophoresis, and testosterone levels (in men). Transglutaminase Ab testing may identify asymptomatic celiac disease. Markers of bone resorption (e.g., urine cross-linked *N*-telopeptide) may be helpful in detecting an early response to antiresorptive therapy if measured prior to and 4–6 months after initiating therapy.

℞ Osteoporosis

Treatment involves the management of acute fractures, modifying risk factors, and treating any underlying disorders that lead to reduced bone mass. Treatment decisions are based on an individual's risk factors, but active treatment is generally recommended if the T-score is ≤2.5. Oral calcium (1–1.5 g/d of elemental calcium in divided doses), vitamin D (400–800 IU/d), exercise, and smoking cessation should be initiated in all patients with osteoporosis. Bisphosphonates (alendronate, 70 mg PO weekly; risedronate, 35 mg PO weekly; ibandronate, 150 mg PO monthly or 3 mg IV every 3 mo; zoledronic acid, 5 mg IV annually) augment bone density and decrease fracture rates. Oral bisphosphonates are poorly absorbed and should be taken in the morning on an empty stomach with 0.25 L (8 oz) of tap water. Estrogen decreases the rate of bone reabsorption, but therapy should be considered carefully in the context of increased risks of cardiovascular disease and breast cancer. Raloxifene (60 mg/d PO), a selective estrogen receptor modulator, increases bone density and decreases total and LDL cholesterol without stimulating endometrial hyperplasia, though it may precipitate hot flashes. PTH(1-34) induces bone formation and may be administered as a daily injection for a maximum of 2 years.

OSTEOMALACIA

Etiology   Defective mineralization of the organic matrix of bone results in *osteomalacia*. Osteomalacia is caused by inadequate intake or malabsorption of vitamin D (chronic pancreatic insufficiency, gastrectomy, malabsorption) and disorders of vitamin D metabolism (anticonvulsant therapy, chronic renal failure).

Clinical Features Skeletal deformities may be overlooked until fractures occur after minimal trauma. Symptoms include diffuse skeletal pain and bony tenderness and may be subtle. Proximal muscle weakness may mimic primary muscle disorders. A decrease in bone density is usually associated with loss of trabeculae and thinning of the cortices. Characteristic x-ray findings are radiolucent bands (Looser's zones or pseudofractures) ranging from a few millimeters to several centimeters in length, usually perpendicular to the surface of the femur, pelvis, and scapula. Changes in serum calcium, phosphorus, 25(OH)D, and 1,25(OH)$_2$D levels vary depending on the cause. However, modest vitamin D deficiency leads to compensatory secondary hyperparathyroidism characterized by increased levels of PTH and alkaline phosphatase and relatively low levels of ionized calcium. 1,25-Dihydroxyvitamin D levels may be preserved, reflecting upregulation of 1α-hydroxylase activity.

R_x Osteomalacia

In osteomalacia due to vitamin D deficiency [serum 25(OH)D < 50 nmol/L (<20 ng/mL)], vitamin D$_2$ (ergocalciferol) is given orally in doses of 50,000 IU weekly for 8 weeks, followed by maintenance therapy with 800 IU daily. Osteomalacia due to malabsorption requires larger doses of vitamin D (up to 100,000 IU/d or 250,000 IU IM biannually). In pts taking anticonvulsants, concurrent vitamin D should be administered in doses that maintain the serum calcium and 25(OH)D levels in the normal range. Calcitriol (0.25–0.5 μg/d PO) is effective in treating hypocalcemia or osteodystrophy caused by chronic renal failure. Vitamin D deficiency should always be repleted in conjunction with calcium supplementation (1.5–2.0 g of elemental calcium daily). Serum and urinary calcium measurements are efficacious for monitoring resolution of vitamin D deficiency, with a goal 24-h urinary calcium excretion of 100–250 mg/24 h.

For a more detailed discussion, see Bringhurst FR, Demay MB, Krane SM, Kronenberg HM: Bone and Mineral Metabolism in Health and Disease, Chap. 346, p. 2365; and Lindsay R, Cosman F: Osteoporosis, Chap. 333, p. 2397, in HPIM-17.

187 Hypercholesterolemia and Hypertriglyceridemia

Hyperlipoproteinemia may be characterized by hypercholesterolemia, isolated hypertriglyceridemia, or both (Table 187-1). Diabetes mellitus, obesity, ethanol consumption, oral contraceptives, glucocorticoids, renal disease, hepatic disease, and hypothyroidism can cause secondary hyperlipoproteinemias or worsen underlying hyperlipoproteinemic states.

Standard lipoprotein analysis assesses total cholesterol, HDL, and triglycerides with a calculation of LDL levels using the equation: LDL = total choles-

TABLE 187-1 CHARACTERISTICS OF COMMON HYPERLIPIDEMIAS

Lipid Phenotype	Plasma Lipid Levels, mmol/L (mg/dL)	Lipoproteins Elevated	Phenotype	Clinical Signs
Isolated Hypercholesterolemia				
Familial hypercholesterolemia	Heterozygotes: total chol = 7–13 (275–500)	LDL	IIa	Usually develop xanthomas in adulthood and vascular disease at 30–50 years
	Homozygotes: total chol > 13 (>500)	LDL	IIa	Usually develop xanthomas and vascular disease in childhood
Familial defective apo B100	Heterozygotes: total chol = 7–13 (275–500)	LDL	IIa	
Polygenic hypercholesterolemia	Total chol = 6.5–9.0 (250–350)	LDL	IIa	Usually asymptomatic until vascular disease develops; no xanthomas
Isolated Hypertriglyceridemia				
Familial hypertriglyceridemia	TG = 2.8–8.5 (250–750) (plasma may be cloudy)	VLDL	IV	Asymptomatic; may be associated with increased risk of vascular disease
Familial lipoprotein lipase deficiency	TG > 8.5 (>750) (plasma may be milky)	Chylomicrons	I, V	May be asymptomatic; may be associated with pancreatitis, abdominal pain, hepatosplenomegaly
Familial apo CII deficiency	TG > 8.5 (>750) (plasma may be milky)	Chylomicrons	I, V	As above
Hypertriglyceridemia and Hypercholesterolemia				
Combined hyperlipidemia	TG = 2.8–8.5 (250–750) Total chol = 6.5–13.0 (250–500)	VLDL, LDL	IIb	Usually asymptomatic until vascular disease develops; familial form may also present as isolated high TG or an isolated high LDL cholesterol
Dysbetalipoproteinemia	TG = 2.8–5.6 (250–500) Total chol = 6.5–13.0 (250–500)	VLDL, IDL; LDL normal	III	Usually asymptomatic until vascular disease develops; may have palmar or tuboeruptive xanthomas

Note: Total chol, the sum of free and esterified cholesterol; LDL, low-density lipoprotein; TG, triglycerides; VLDL, very low density lipoproteins; IDL, intermediate-density lipoprotein. *Source:* From HN Ginsberg, IJ Goldberg: HPIM-15, p. 2250.

terol HDL triglycerides/5. The LDL cholesterol concentration can be estimated using this method only if triglycerides are <4.0 mmol/L (<350 mg/dL). Both LDL and HDL cholesterol levels are temporarily decreased for several weeks after myocardial infarction or acute inflammatory states but can be accurately measured if blood is obtained within 8 h of the event.

ISOLATED HYPERCHOLESTEROLEMIA

Elevated levels of fasting plasma total cholesterol [>5.2 mmol/L (>200 mg/dL)] in the presence of normal levels of triglycerides are almost always associated with increased concentrations of plasma LDL cholesterol. A rare individual with markedly elevated HDL cholesterol may also have increased plasma total cholesterol levels. Elevations of LDL cholesterol can result from single-gene defects, polygenic disorders, or from the secondary effects of other disease states.

FAMILIAL HYPERCHOLESTEROLEMIA (FH)

FH is a codominant genetic disorder that is due to mutations in the gene for the LDL receptor. Plasma LDL levels are elevated at birth and remain so throughout life. In untreated heterozygous adults, total cholesterol levels range from 7.1–12.9 mmol/L (275–500 mg/dL). Plasma triglyceride levels are typically normal, and HDL cholesterol levels are normal or reduced. Heterozygotes, especially men, are prone to accelerated atherosclerosis and premature coronary artery disease (CAD). *Tendon xanthomas* (most commonly of the Achilles tendons and the extensor tendons of the knuckles), *tuberous xanthomas* (softer, painless nodules on the ankles and buttocks), and *xanthelasmas* (deposits on the eyelids) are common.

FAMILIAL DEFECTIVE APO B-100

This autosomal dominant disorder impairs the synthesis and/or function of apo B-100, thereby reducing the affinity for the LDL receptor, slowing LDL catabolism, and causing a phenocopy of FH.

POLYGENIC HYPERCHOLESTEROLEMIA

Most moderate hypercholesterolemia [<9.1 mmol/L (<350 mg/dL)] arises from an interaction of multiple genetic defects and environmental factors such as diet, age, and exercise. Plasma HDL and triglyceride levels are normal, and xanthomas are not present.

 Isolated Hypercholesterolemia

An algorithm for the evaluation and treatment of hypercholesterolemia is displayed in Fig. 187-1. Therapy for all of these disorders includes restriction of dietary cholesterol and HMG-CoA reductase inhibitors. Cholesterol absorption inhibitors and bile acid sequestrants or nicotinic acid may also be required (Table 187-2).

ISOLATED HYPERTRIGLYCERIDEMIA

The diagnosis of hypertriglyceridemia is made by measuring plasma lipid levels after an overnight fast. Hypertriglyceridemia in adults is defined as a triglyceride level > 2.3 mmol/L (> 200 mg/dL). An isolated increase in plasma

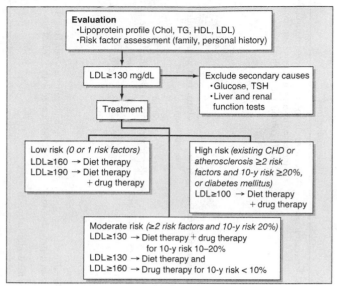

A

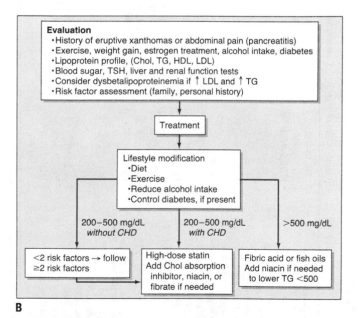

B

FIGURE 187-1 Algorithms for the evaluation and treatment of hypercholesterolemia (*A*) and hypertriglyceridemia (*B*). Statin, HMG-CoA reductase inhibitor; Chol, cholesterol; HDL, high-density lipoprotein; LDL, low-density lipoprotein; TG, triglyceride; TSH, thyroid-stimulating hormone; CHD, coronary heart disease.

TABLE 187-2 HYPOLIPIDEMIC DRUGS

Drugs	Lipoprotein Class Affected	Common Side Effects	Contraindications
HMG-CoA reductase inhibitors Lovastatin 20–80 mg/d Pravastatin 40–80 mg qhs Simvastatin 20–80 mg qhs Fluvastatin 20–80 mg qhs Atorvastatin 10–80 mg qhs Rosuvastatin 10–40 mg qhs	↓ LDL 18–55% ↓ TG 7–30% ↑ HDL 5–15%	Myalgias, arthralgias, ↑ transaminases, dyspepsia	Acute or chronic liver disease of myositis increased by impaired renal function and in combination with a fibrate
Cholesterol absorption inhibitors Ezetimibe 10 mg qd	↓ LDL 18% ↓ TG 8%	↑ Transaminases	
Bile acid sequestrant Cholestyramine 4–32 g qd Cholestipol 5–40 g qd Colesevelam 3750–4375 mg qd	↓ LDL 15–30% ↓ TG 10% ↑ HDL 3–5%	Constipation, gastric discomfort, nausea	Biliary tract obstruction, gastric outlet obstruction
Nicotinic acid Immediate release 100 mg tid, gradual increase to 1 g tid Sustained release 250 mg–1.5 g bid Extended release 500 mg–2 g qhs	↓ LDL 5–25% ↓ TG 20–50% ↑ HDL 15–35%	Flushing (may be relieved by aspirin), hepatic dysfunction, nausea, diarrhea, glucose intolerance, hyperuricemia	Peptic ulcer disease, hepatic disease, gout
Fibric acid derivatives Gemfibrozil 600 mg bid Fenofibrate 145 mg qd Fish oils 3–6 g qd	↑ or ↓ LDL ↓ TG 20–50% ↑ HDL 10–20% ↓ TG 5–10%	↓ Absorption of other drugs ↑ Gallstones, dyspepsia, hepatic dysfunction, myalgia Dyspepsia, diarrhea, fishy odor to breath	Hepatic or biliary disease, renal insufficiency associated with ↑ risk of myositis

Note: LDL, low-density lipoprotein; VLDL, very low density lipoprotein; TG, triglycerides; HDL, high-density lipoprotein; LPL, lipoprotein lipase; CPK, creative phosphokinase.

triglycerides indicates that chylomicrons and/or very low density lipoprotein (VLDL) are increased. Plasma is usually clear when triglyceride levels are <4.5 mmol/L (<400 mg/dL) and cloudy when levels are higher due to VLDL (and/or chylomicron) particles becoming large enough to scatter light. When chylomicrons are present, a creamy layer floats to the top of plasma after refrigeration for several hours. Tendon xanthomas and xanthelasmas do not occur with isolated hypertriglyceridemia, but *eruptive xanthomas* (small orange-red papules) can appear on the trunk and extremities and *lipemia retinalis* (orange-yellow retinal vessels) may be seen when the triglyceride levels are >11.3 mmol/L (>1000 mg/dL). Pancreatitis is associated with these high concentrations.

FAMILIAL HYPERTRIGLYCERIDEMIA

In this autosomal dominant disorder, increased plasma VLDL causes elevated plasma triglyceride concentrations. Obesity, hyperglycemia, and hyperinsulinemia are characteristic, and diabetes mellitus, ethanol consumption, oral contraceptives, and hypothyroidism may exacerbate the condition. The diagnosis is suggested by the triad of elevated plasma triglycerides [2.8–11.3 mmol/L (250–1000 mg/dL)], normal or only mildly increased cholesterol levels [<6.5 mmol/L (<250 mg/dL)], and reduced plasma HDL. The identification of other first-degree relatives with hypertriglyceridemia is useful in making the diagnosis. Familial dysbetalipoproteinemia and familial combined hyperlipidemia should be ruled out, as these two conditions are associated with accelerated atherosclerosis.

LIPOPROTEIN LIPASE DEFICIENCY

This rare autosomal recessive disorder results from the absence or deficiency of lipoprotein lipase, which in turn impairs the metabolism of chylomicrons. Accumulation of chylomicrons in plasma causes recurrent bouts of pancreatitis, usually beginning in childhood, and hepatosplenomegaly is present. Accelerated atherosclerosis is not a feature.

APO CII DEFICIENCY

This rare autosomal recessive disorder is due to the absence of apo CII, an essential cofactor for lipoprotein lipase. As a result, chylomicrons and triglycerides accumulate and cause manifestations similar to those in lipoprotein lipase deficiency.

 Isolated Hypertriglyceridemia

An algorithm for the evaluation and treatment of hypertriglyceridemia is displayed in **Fig. 187-1**. All pts with hypertriglyceridemia should be placed on a fat-free diet with fat-soluble vitamin supplementation. In those with familial hypertriglyceridemia, fibric acid derivatives should be administered if dietary measures fail (**Table 187-2**).

HYPERCHOLESTEROLEMIA AND HYPERTRIGLYCERIDEMIA

Elevations of both triglycerides and cholesterol are caused by elevations in both VLDL and LDL or in VLDL remnant particles.

FAMILIAL COMBINED HYPERLIPIDEMIA (FCHL)

This inherited disorder, present in 1/200 persons, can cause different lipoprotein abnormalities in affected individuals, including hypercholesterolemia (elevated LDL), hypertriglyceridemia (elevated triglycerides and VLDL), or both. Atherosclerosis is accelerated. A mixed dyslipidemia [plasma triglycerides 2.3–9.0 mmol/L (200–800 mg/dL), cholesterol levels 5.2–10.3 mmol/L (200–400 mg/dL) and HDL levels <10.3 mmol/L (<40 mg/dL) in men and <12.9 mmol/L (<50 mg/dL) in women] and a family history of hyperlipidemia and/or premature cardiovascular disease suggests the diagnosis of FCHL. Many of these patients also have the metabolic syndrome (Chap. 125). All pts should restrict dietary cholesterol and fat and avoid alcohol and oral contraceptives; patients with diabetes should be treated aggressively. An HMG-CoA reductase inhibitor is usually required, and many patients will require a second drug (cholesterol absorption inhibitor, niacin, or fibrate) for optimal control.

DYSBETALIPOPROTEINEMIA

This rare disorder is associated with homozygosity for apo E2, but the development of disease requires additional environmental and/or genetic factors. Plasma cholesterol [6.5–13.0 mmol/L (250–500 mg/dL)] and triglycerides [2.8–5.6 mmol/L (250–500 mg/dL)] are increased due to accumulation of VLDL and chylomicron remnant particles. Patients usually present in adulthood with xanthomas and premature coronary and peripheral vascular disease. Cutaneous xanthomas are distinctive, in the form of *palmar* and *tuberoeruptive xanthomas*. Triglycerides and cholesterol are both elevated. Diagnosis is established by lipoprotein electrophoresis or a ratio of VLDL (by centrifugation) to total plasma triglycerides of >0.3. If present, hypothyroidism and diabetes mellitus should be treated, dietary modifications should be instituted, and HMG-CoA reductase inhibitors, fibrates, and/or niacin may be necessary.

PREVENTION OF THE COMPLICATIONS OF ATHEROSCLEROSIS

The National Cholesterol Education Program guidelines (Fig. 187-1) are based on plasma LDL levels and estimations of other risk factors. The goal in pts with the highest risk (known coronary heart or other atherosclerotic disease, 10-year Framingham Heart Study risk for coronary heart disease >20%, or diabetes mellitus) is to lower LDL cholesterol to <2.6 mmol/L (<100 mg/dL). In pts with very high risk, clinical trials suggest additional benefit by reducing LDL cholesterol to <1.8 mmol/L (<70 mg/dL). The goal is an LDL cholesterol <3.4 mmol/L (<130 mg/dL) in pts with two or more risk factors for atherosclerotic heart disease and a 10-year absolute risk of 10–20%, though a treatment goal of <2.6 mmol/L (<100 mg/dL) can be considered. The intensity of LDL-lowering drug treatment in high- and moderately high-risk pts should achieve at least a 30% reduction in LDL levels. Risk factors include (1) men > age 45, women > age 55 or after menopause; (2) family history of early CAD (<55 years in a male parent or sibling and <65 years in a female parent or sibling); (3) hypertension (even if it is controlled with medications); (4) cigarette smoking (>10 cigarettes/day); and (5) HDL cholesterol < 1.0 mmol/L (<40 mg/dL). Therapy begins with a low-fat diet, but pharmacologic intervention is often required (Table 187-2).

For a more detailed discussion, see Rader DJ, Hobbs HH: Disorders of Lipoprotein Metabolism, Chap. 350, p. 2416; in HPIM-17.

188 Hemochromatosis, Porphyrias, and Wilson's Disease

HEMOCHROMATOSIS

Hemochromatosis is a disorder of iron storage that results in increased intestinal iron absorption with Fe deposition and damage to many tissues. The classic clinical constellation of hemochromatosis is a patient presenting with bronze skin, diabetes, cardiac conduction abnormalities, and liver disease. Two major causes of hemochromatosis exist: hereditary (due to inheritance of mutant *HFE* genes) and secondary iron overload (usually the result of disordered erythropoiesis). Alcoholic liver disease and chronic excessive Fe ingestion may also be associated with a moderate increase in hepatic Fe and elevated body Fe stores.

Clinical Features   Early symptoms include weakness, lassitude, weight loss, a bronze pigmentation or darkening of skin, abdominal pain, and loss of libido. Hepatomegaly occurs in 95% of pts, sometimes in the presence of normal LFTs. Other signs include spider angiomas, splenomegaly, arthropathy, ascites, cardiac arrhythmias, CHF, loss of body hair, palmar erythema, gynecomastia, and testicular atrophy. Diabetes mellitus occurs in about 65%, usually in pts with family history of diabetes. Adrenal insufficiency, hypothyroidism, and hypoparathyroidism rarely occur.

Diagnosis   Serum Fe, percent transferrin saturation, and serum ferritin levels are increased. In an otherwise-healthy person, a fasting serum transferrin saturation > 50% is abnormal and suggests homozygosity for hemochromatosis. In most untreated pts with hemochromatosis, the serum ferritin level is also greatly increased. If either the percent transferrin saturation or the serum ferritin level is abnormal, genetic testing for hemochromatosis should be performed. All first-degree relatives of pts with hemochromatosis should be tested for the C282Y and H63D mutations. Liver biopsy may be required in affected individuals to evaluate possible cirrhosis or to quantify tissue iron. An algorithm for evaluating pts with possible hemochromatosis is shown in **Fig. 188-1**. Death in untreated pts results from cardiac failure (30%), cirrhosis (25%), and hepatocellular carcinoma (30%); the latter may develop despite adequate Fe removal.

R_x Hemochromatosis

Therapy involves removal of excess body Fe, usually by intermittent phlebotomy, and supportive treatment of damaged organs. Since 1 unit of blood contains ~250 mg Fe, and since ≥25 g of Fe must be removed, phlebotomy is performed weekly for 1–2 years. Less frequent phlebotomy is then used to maintain serum Fe at <27 μmol/L (<150 μg/dL). Chelating agents such as deferoxamine (infused SC using a portable pump) remove 10–20 mg iron per day, a fraction of that mobilized by weekly phlebotomy. Chelation therapy is indicated, however, when phlebotomy is inappropriate, such as with anemia or hypoproteinemia. Alcohol consumption should be eliminated.

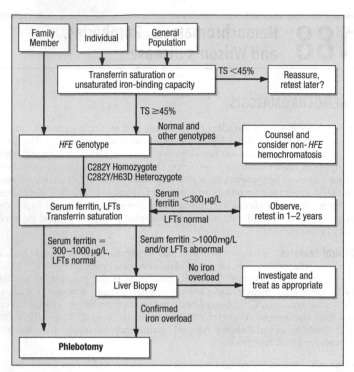

FIGURE 188-1 Algorithm for screening for *HFE*-associated hemochromatosis. LFT, liver function tests; TS, transferrin saturation. (*From EJ Eijkelkamp et al., Can J Gastroenterol 14, No. 2, 2000; with permission.*)

PORPHYRIAS

The porphyrias are inherited or acquired disturbances in heme biosynthesis. Each disorder causes a unique pattern of overproduction, accumulation, and excretion of intermediates of heme synthesis. These disorders are classified as either hepatic or erythropoietic, depending on the primary site of overproduction and accumulation of the porphyrin precursor or porphyrin. The major manifestations of the hepatic porphyrias are neurologic (neuropathic abdominal pain, neuropathy, and mental disturbances), whereas the erythropoietic porphyrias characteristically cause cutaneous photosensitivity. Laboratory testing is required to confirm or exclude the various types of porphyria. However, a definite diagnosis requires demonstration of the specific enzyme deficiency or gene defect.

ACUTE INTERMITTENT PORPHYRIA

This is an autosomal dominant disorder with variable expressivity. Manifestations include colicky abdominal pain, vomiting, constipation, port-wine colored urine, and neurologic and psychiatric disturbances. Acute attacks rarely occur before puberty and may last from days to months. Photosensitivity does not occur. Clinical and biochemical manifestations may be precipitated by barbiturates, anticonvulsants, estrogens, oral contraceptives, alcohol, or low-calorie diets. Diagnosis is established by demonstrating elevation of urinary porphobilinogen (PBG) and γ-aminolevulinic acid (ALA) during an acute attack.

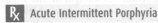 **Acute Intermittent Porphyria**

As soon as possible after the onset of an attack, 3–4 mg of heme, in the form of heme arginate, heme albumin, or hematin, should be infused daily for 4 days. Administration of IV glucose at rates up to 20 g/h or parenteral nutrition, if oral feeding is not possible for long periods, can be effective in acute attacks. Narcotic analgesics may be required during acute attacks for abdominal pain, and phenothiazines are useful for nausea, vomiting, anxiety, and restlessness. Treatment between attacks involves adequate nutritional intake, avoidance of drugs known to exacerbate the disease, and prompt treatment of other intercurrent diseases or infections.

PORPHYRIA CUTANEA TARDA

This is the most common porphyria and is characterized by cutaneous photosensitivity and, usually, hepatic disease. It is due to deficiency (inherited or acquired) of hepatic uroporphyrinogen decarboxylase. Photosensitivity causes facial pigmentation, increased fragility of skin, erythema, and vesicular and ulcerative lesions, typically involving face, forehead, and forearms. Neurologic manifestations are not observed. Contributing factors include excess alcohol, iron, and estrogens. Pts with liver disease are at risk for hepatocellular carcinoma. Plasma and urine uroporphyrin and 7-carboxylate porphyrin are increased.

Porphyria Cutanea Tarda

Avoidance of precipitating factors, including abstinence from alcohol, estrogens, iron supplements, and other exacerbating drugs, is the first line of therapy. A complete response can almost always be achieved by repeated phlebotomy (every 1–2 weeks) until hepatic iron is reduced. Chloroquine or hydroxychloroquine may be used in low doses (e.g., 125 mg chloroquine phosphate twice weekly) to promote porphyrin excretion in pts unable to undergo or unresponsive to phlebotomy.

ERYTHROPOIETIC PORPHYRIA

In erythropoietic porphyria, porphyrins from bone marrow erythrocytes and plasma are deposited in the skin and lead to cutaneous photosensitivity. Skin photosensitivity usually begins in childhood. The skin manifestations differ from those of other porphyrias, in that vesicular lesions are uncommon. Redness, swelling, burning, and itching can develop within minutes of sun exposure and resemble angioedema. Symptoms may seem out of proportion to the visible skin lesions. Chronic skin changes may include lichenification, leathery pseudovesicles, labial grooving, and nail changes. Liver function is usually normal, but liver disease and gallstones may occur. Protoporphyrin levels are increased in bone marrow, circulating erythrocytes, plasma, bile, and feces. Urinary levels are normal. Diagnosis is confirmed by identifying a mutation in the ferrochelatase gene.

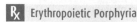 Erythropoietic Porphyria

Oral β-carotene (120–180 mg/d) improves tolerance to sunlight in many patients. The dosage may be adjusted to maintain serum carotene levels between 10 and 15 μmol/L (600–800 μg/dL). Cholestyramine or activated charcoal may promote fecal excretion of protoporphyrin. Transfusions or intravenous heme therapy may be beneficial.

WILSON'S DISEASE

Wilson's disease is an inherited disorder of copper metabolism, resulting in the toxic accumulation of copper in the liver, brain, and other organs. Individuals with Wilson's disease have mutations in the *ATP7B* gene.

Clinical Features Hepatic disease may present as hepatitis, cirrhosis, or hepatic decompensation. In other pts, neurologic or psychiatric disturbances are the first clinical sign and are always accompanied by Kayser-Fleischer rings (corneal deposits of copper). Dystonia, incoordination, or tremor may be present, and dysarthria and dysphagia are common. Autonomic disturbances may also be present. Microscopic hematuria is common. In about 5% of pts, the first manifestation may be primary or secondary amenorrhea or repeated spontaneous abortions.

Diagnosis Serum ceruloplasmin levels are often low, and urine copper levels are elevated. The "gold standard" for diagnosis is an elevated copper level on liver biopsy.

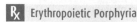 Wilson's Disease

Hepatitis or cirrhosis without decompensation should be treated with zinc (50 mg PO three times a day). For pts with hepatic decompensation, trientene (500 mg PO twice a day) plus zinc (separated by at least 1 h) is recommended, though liver transplantation should be considered for severe hepatic decompensation. For initial neurologic therapy, trientine and zinc are recommended for 8 weeks, followed by therapy with zinc alone. Tetrathiomolybdate is an alternative therapeutic option available in the future. Penicillamine is no longer first-line therapy. Zinc treatment does not require monitoring for toxicity, and 24-h urine copper can be followed for a therapeutic response. Trientine may induce bone marrow suppression and proteinuria, and free serum copper levels (adjusting total serum copper for ceruloplasmin copper) must be followed for a therapeutic response. Anticopper therapy must be lifelong.

For a more detailed discussion, see Powell LW: Hemochromatosis, Chap. 351, p. 2429; Desnick RJ and Astrin KH: The Porphyrias, Chap. 352, p. 2434; Brewer GJ: Wilson Disease, Chap. 354, p. 2449; in HPIM-17.

189 The Neurologic Examination

MENTAL STATUS EXAM

- *The bare minimum: During the interview, look for difficulties with communication and determine whether the pt has recall and insight into recent and past events.*

The goal of the mental status exam is to evaluate attention, orientation, memory, insight, judgment, and grasp of general information. Attention is tested by asking the pt to respond every time a specific item recurs in a list. Orientation is evaluated by asking about the day, date, and location. Memory can be tested by asking pt to immediately recall a sequence of numbers and by testing recall of a series of objects after defined times (e.g., 5 and 15 min). More remote memory is evaluated by assessing pt's ability to provide a cogent chronologic history of the illness or personal life events. Recall of historic events or dates of current events can be used to assess knowledge. Evaluation of language function should include assessment of spontaneous speech, naming, repetition, reading, writing, and comprehension. Additional tests such as ability to draw

TABLE 189-1 THE MINI-MENTAL STATUS EXAMINATION

	Points
Orientation	
Name: season/date/day/month/year	5 (1 for each name)
Name: hospital floor/town/state/country	5 (1 for each name)
Registration	
Identify three objects by name and ask patient to repeat	3 (1 for each object)
Attention and calculation	
Serial 7s; subtract from 100 (e.g., 93–86–79–72–65)	5 (1 for each subtraction)
Recall	
Recall the three objects presented earlier	3 (1 for each object)
Language	
Name pencil and watch	2 (1 for each object)
Repeat "No ifs, ands, or buts"	1
Follow a 3-step command (e.g., "Take this paper, fold it in half, and place it on the table")	3 (1 for each command)
Write "close your eyes" and ask patient to obey written command	1
Ask patient to write a sentence	1
Ask patient to copy a design (e.g., intersecting pentagons)	1
TOTAL	30

TABLE 189-2 MUSCLES THAT MOVE JOINTS

	Muscle	Nerve	Segmental Innervation
Shoulder	Supraspinatus	Suprascapular n.	C5,6
	Deltoid	Axillary n.	C5,6
Forearm	Biceps	Musculocutaneous n.	C5,6
	Brachioradialis	Radial n.	C5,6
	Triceps	Radial n.	C6,7,8
	Ext. carpi radialis	Radial n.	C5,6
	Ext. carpi ulnaris	P. interosseous n.	C7,8
	Ext. digitorum	P. interosseous n.	C7,8
	Supinator	P. interosseous n.	C6,7
	Flex. carpi radialis	Median n.	C6,7
	Flex. carpi ulnaris	Ulnar n.	C7,8,T1
	Pronator teres	Median n.	C6,7
Wrist	Ext. carpi ulnaris	Ulnar n.	C7,8,T1
	Flex. carpi radialis	Median n.	C6,7
Hand	Lumbricals	Median + ulnar n.	C8,T1
	Interossei	Ulnar n.	C8,T1
	Flex. digitorum	Median + A. interosseous n.	C7,C8,T1
Thumb	Opponens pollicis	Median n.	C8,T1
	Ext. pollicis	P. interosseous n.	C7,8
	Add. pollicis	Median n.	C8,T1
	Abd. pollicis	Ulnar n.	C8,T1
	Flex. pollicis br.	Ulnar n.	C8,T1
Thigh	Iliopsoas	Femoral n.	L1,2,3
	Glutei	Sup. + inf. gluteal n.	L4,L5,S1,S2
	Quadriceps	Femoral n.	L2,3,4
	Adductors	Obturator n.	L2,3,4
	Hamstrings	Sciatic n.	L5,S1,S2
Foot	Gastrocnemius	Tibial n.	S1,S2
	Tibialis ant.	Deep peroneal n.	L4,5
	Peronei	Deep peroneal n.	L5,S1
	Tibialis post.	Tibial n.	L4,5
Toes	Ext. hallucis l.	Deep peroneal n.	L5,S1

and copy, perform calculations, interpret proverbs or logic problems, identify right vs. left, name and identify body parts, etc., are also important.

A useful screening examination of cognitive function is the mini-mental status examination (MMSE) (Table 189-1).

CRANIAL NERVE (CN) EXAM

- *The bare minimum: Check the fundi, visual fields, pupil size and reactivity, extraocular movements, and facial movements.*

CN I Occlude each nostril sequentially and ask pt to gently sniff and identify a mild test stimulus, such as soap, toothpaste, coffee, or lemon oil.

CN II Check visual acuity with and without correction using a Snellen chart (distance) and Jaeger's test type (near). Map visual fields (VFs) by confrontation testing in each quadrant of visual field for each eye individually. The best method is to sit facing pt (2–3 ft apart), have pt cover one eye gently and fix uncov-

Function

Abduction of upper arm
Abduction of upper arm
Flexion of the supinated forearm
Forearm flexion with arm between pronation and supination
Extension of forearm
Extension and abduction of hand at the wrist
Extension and adduction of hand at the wrist
Extension of fingers at the MCP joints
Supination of the extended forearm
Flexion and abduction of hand at the wrist
Flexion and adduction of hand at the wrist
Pronation of the forearm
Extension/adduction at the wrist
Flexion/abduction at the wrist
Extension of fingers at PIP joint with the MCP joint extended and fixed
Abduction/adduction of the fingers
Flexion of the fingers
Touching the base of the 5th finger with thumb
Extension of the thumb
Adduction of the thumb
Abduction of the thumb
Flexion of the thumb
Flexion of the thigh
Abduction, extension, and internal rotation of the leg
Extension of the leg at the knee
Adduction of the leg
Flexion of the leg at the knee
Plantar flexion of the foot
Dorsiflexion of the foot
Eversion of the foot
Inversion of the foot
Dorsiflexion of the great toe

---

ered eye on examiner's nose. A small white object (e.g., a cotton-tipped applicator) is then moved slowly from periphery of field toward center until seen. Pt's VF should be mapped against examiner's for comparison. Formal perimetry and tangent screen exam are essential to identify and delineate small defects. Optic fundi should be examined with an ophthalmoscope, and the color, size, and degree of swelling or elevation of the optic disc recorded. The retinal vessels should be checked for size, regularity, AV nicking at crossing points, hemorrhage, exudates, and aneurysms. The retina, including the macula, should be examined for abnormal pigmentation and other lesions.

CNs III, IV, VI   Describe size, regularity, and shape of pupils; reaction (direct and consensual) to light; and convergence (pt follows an object as it moves closer). Check for lid drooping, lag, or retraction. Ask pt to follow your finger as you move it horizontally to left and right and vertically with each eye first fully adducted then fully abducted. Check for failure to move fully in particular directions and for presence of regular, rhythmic, involuntary oscillations of eyes

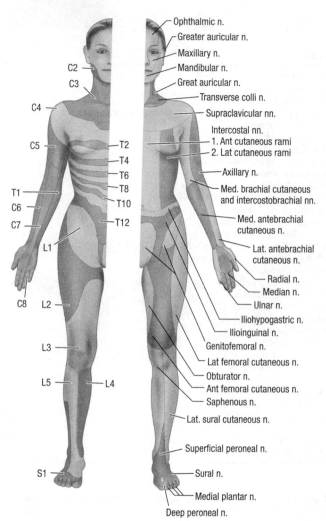

FIGURE 189-1 Anterior view of dermatomes (*left*) and cutaneous areas (*right*) supplied by individual peripheral nerves. (*Modified from MB Carpenter and J Sutin, in Human Neuroanatomy, 8th ed, Baltimore, Williams & Wilkins, 1983.*)

(nystagmus). Test quick voluntary eye movements (saccades) as well as pursuit (e.g., follow the finger).

CN V   Feel the masseter and temporalis muscles as pt bites down and test jaw opening, protrusion, and lateral motion against resistance. Examine sensation over entire face as well as response to touching each cornea lightly with a small wisp of cotton.

CN VII   Look for asymmetry of face at rest and with spontaneous as well as emotion-induced (e.g., laughing) movements. Test eyebrow elevation, forehead

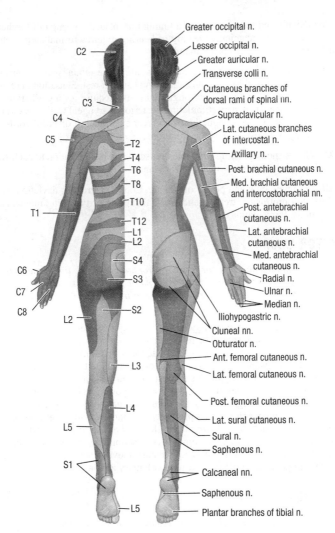

FIGURE 189-2 Posterior view of dermatomes (*left*) and cutaneous areas (*right*) supplied by individual peripheral nerves. (*Modified from MB Carpenter and J Sutin, in Human Neuroanatomy, 8th ed, Baltimore, Williams & Wilkins, 1983.*)

wrinkling, eye closure, smiling, frowning; check puff, whistle, lip pursing, and chin muscle contraction. Observe for differences in strength of lower and upper facial muscles. Taste on the anterior two-thirds of tongue can be affected by lesions of the seventh CN proximal to the chorda tympani. Test taste for sweet (sugar), salt, sour (lemon), and bitter (quinine) using a cotton-tipped applicator moistened in appropriate solution and placed on lateral margin of protruded tongue halfway back from tip.

CN VIII   Check ability to hear tuning fork, finger rub, watch tick, and whispered voice at specified distances with each ear. Check for air vs. mastoid bone conduction (Rinne) and lateralization of a tuning fork placed on center of forehead (Weber). Accurate, quantitative testing of hearing requires formal audiometry. Remember to examine tympanic membranes.

CNs IX, X Check for symmetric elevation of palate-uvula with phonation ("ahh"), as well as position of uvula and palatal arch at rest. Sensation in region of tonsils, posterior pharynx, and tongue may also require testing. Pharyngeal ("gag") reflex is evaluated by stimulating posterior pharyngeal wall on each side with a blunt object (e.g., tongue blade). Direct examination of vocal cords by laryngoscopy is necessary in some situations.

CN XI Check shoulder shrug (trapezius muscle) and head rotation to each side (sternocleidomastoid muscle) against resistance.

CN XII Examine bulk and power of tongue. Look for atrophy, deviation from midline with protrusion, tremor, and small flickering or twitching movements (fibrillations, fasciculations).

MOTOR EXAM

- *The bare minimum: Look for muscle atrophy and check limb tone. Assess upper limb strength by checking for pronator drift and strength of wrist or finger reflexes. Test for lower limb strength by asking pt to walk normally and on heels and toes.*

Power should be systematically tested for major movements at each joint (Table 189-2). Strength should be recorded using a reproducible scale (e.g., 0 = no movement, 1 = flicker or trace of contraction with no associated movement at a joint, 2 = movement present but cannot be sustained against gravity, 3 = movement against gravity but not against applied resistance, 4 = movement against some degree of resistance, and 5 = full power; values can be supplemented with + and – signs to provide additional gradations). Speed of movement, ability to relax contractions promptly, and fatigue with repetition should all be noted. Loss in bulk and size of muscle (atrophy) should be noted, as well as the presence of irregular involuntary contraction (twitching) of groups of muscle fibers (fasciculations). Any involuntary movements should be noted at rest, during maintained posture, and with voluntary action.

REFLEXES

- *The bare minimum: Tap the biceps, patellar, and Achilles reflexes.*

Important muscle-stretch reflexes to test routinely and the spinal cord segments involved in their reflex arcs include biceps (C5, 6); brachioradialis (C5, 6); triceps (C7, 8); patellar (L3, 4); and Achilles (S1, 2). A common grading scale is 0 = absent, 1 = present but diminished, 2 = normal, 3 = hyperactive, and 4 = hyperactive with clonus (repetitive rhythmic contractions with maintained stretch). The plantar reflex should be tested by using a blunt-ended object such as the point of a key to stroke the outer border of the sole of the foot from the heel toward the base of the great toe. An abnormal response (Babinski sign) is extension (dorsiflexion) of the great toe at the metatarsophalangeal joint. In some cases this may be associated with abduction (fanning) of other toes and variable degrees of flexion at ankle, knee, and hip. Normal response is plantar flexion of the toes. Superficial abdominal and anal reflexes are important in certain situations; unlike muscle stretch reflexes, these cutaneous reflexes disappear with CNS lesions.

TABLE 189-3 **FINDINGS HELPFUL FOR LOCALIZATION WITHIN THE NERVOUS SYSTEM**

	Signs
Cerebrum	Abnormal mental status or cognitive impairment
	Seizures
	Unilateral weakness[a] and sensory abnormalities including head and limbs
	Visual field abnormalities
	Movement abnormalities (e.g., diffuse incoordination, tremor, chorea)
Brainstem	Isolated cranial nerve abnormalities (single or multiple)
	"Crossed" weakness[a] and sensory abnormalities of head and limbs, e.g., weakness of right face and left arm and leg
Spinal cord	Back pain or tenderness
	Weakness[a] and sensory abnormalities sparing the head
	Mixed upper and lower motor neuron findings
	Sensory level
	Sphincter dysfunction
Spinal roots	Radiating limb pain
	Weakness[b] or sensory abnormalities following root distribution (see Figs. 189-1 and 189-2)
	Loss of reflexes
Peripheral nerve	Mid or distal limb pain
	Weakness[b] or sensory abnormalities following nerve distribution (see Figs. 189-1 and 189-2)
	"Stocking or glove" distribution of sensory loss
	Loss of reflexes
Neuromuscular junction	Bilateral weakness including face (ptosis, diplopia, dysphagia) and proximal limbs
	Increasing weakness with exertion
	Sparing of sensation
Muscle	Bilateral proximal or distal weakness
	Sparing of sensation

[a]Weakness along with other abnormalities having an "upper motor neuron" pattern, i.e., spasticity, weakness of extensors > flexors in the upper extremity and flexors > extensors in the lower extremity, hyperreflexia.
[b]Weakness along with other abnormalities having a "lower motor neuron" pattern, i.e., flaccidity and hyporeflexia.

SENSORY EXAM

- *The bare minimum: Ask whether the pt can feel light touch and the temperature of a cool object in each distal extremity. Check double simultaneous stimulation using light touch on the hands.*

For most purposes it is sufficient to test sensation to pinprick, touch, position, and vibration in each of the four extremities (Figs. 189-1 and 189-2). Specific problems often require more thorough evaluation. Patients with cerebral lesions may have abnormalities in "discriminative sensation" such as the ability to perceive double simultaneous stimuli, to localize stimuli accurately, to identify closely approximated stimuli as separate (two-point discrimination), to identify objects by touch alone (stereognosis), or to judge weights, evaluate texture, or identify letters or numbers written on the skin surface (graphesthesia).

COORDINATION AND GAIT

- *The bare minimum: Test rapid alternating movements of the fingers and feet, and the finger-to-nose maneuver. Observe the patient while he or she is walking along a straight line.*

The ability to move the index finger accurately from the nose to the examiner's outstretched finger and the ability to slide the heel of each foot from the knee down the shin are tests of coordination. Additional tests (drawing objects in the air, following a moving finger, tapping with index finger against thumb or alternately against each individual finger) may also be useful. The ability to stand with feet together and eyes closed (Romberg test), to walk a straight line (tandem walk), and to turn should all be observed.

THE NEUROLOGIC METHOD AND LOCALIZATION

The clinical data obtained from the neurologic examination coupled with a careful history are interpreted to arrive at an anatomic localization that best explains the clinical findings (Table 189-3) and to select the diagnostic tests most likely to be informative in order to define the pathophysiology of the anatomic lesion.

For a more detailed discussion, see Lowenstein DH, Martin JB, Hauser SL: Approach to the Patient with Neurologic Disease, Chap. 361, p. 2484, in HPIM-17

190 Neuroimaging

The clinician caring for pts with neurologic symptoms is faced with an expanding number of imaging options. MRI is more sensitive than CT for detection of many lesions affecting the nervous system, particularly those of the spinal cord, cranial nerves, and posterior fossa structures. Diffusion MR, a sequence that detects reduction of microscopic motion of water, is the most sensitive technique for detecting acute ischemic stroke and is useful in the detection of encephalitis, abscesses, and prion diseases. CT, however, can be quickly obtained and is widely available, making it a pragmatic choice for initial evaluation of pts with suspected acute stroke (especially when coupled with CT angiography and perfusion CT), hemorrhage, and intracranial or spinal trauma. CT is also more sensitive than MRI for visualizing fine osseous detail and is indicated in the initial evaluation of conductive hearing loss as well as lesions affecting the skull base and calvarium. MRI and CT-myelography have replaced conventional myelography for evaluation of disease of the spinal cord and canal. An increasing number of interventional neuroradiologic techniques are available including embolization, coiling, and stenting of vascular structures as well as spine interventions such as discography, selective nerve root injection, and epidural injection. Conventional angiography is now reserved for patients in whom small-

TABLE 190-1 GUIDELINES FOR THE USE OF CT, ULTRASOUND, AND MRI

Condition	Recommended Technique
Hemorrhage	
Acute parenchymal	CT, MR
Subacute/chronic	MRI
Subarachnoid hemorrhage	CT, CTA, lumbar puncture → angiography
Aneurysm	Angiography > CTA, MRA
Ischemic infarction	
Hemorrhagic infarction	CT or MRI
Bland infarction	MRI > CT, CTA, angiography
Carotid or vertebral dissection	MRI/MRA
Vertebral basilar insufficiency	CTA, MRI/MRA
Carotid stenosis	CTA > Doppler ultrasound, MRA
Suspected mass lesion	
Neoplasm, primary or metastatic	MRI + contrast
Infection/abscess	MRI + contrast
Immunosuppressed with focal findings	MRI + contrast
Vascular malformation	MRI +/– angiography
White matter disorders	MRI
Demyelinating disease	MRI +/– contrast
Dementia	MRI > CT
Trauma	
Acute trauma	CT (noncontrast)
Shear injury/chronic hemorrhage	MRI
Headache/migraine	CT (noncontrast) / MRI
Seizure	
First time, no focal neurologic deficits	?CT as screen +/– contrast
Partial complex/refractory	MRI with coronal T2W imaging
Cranial neuropathy	MRI with contrast
Meningeal disease	MRI with contrast
Spine	
Low back pain	
No neurologic deficits	MRI or CT after 4 weeks
With focal deficits	MRI > CT
Spinal stenosis	MRI or CT
Cervical spondylosis	MRI or CT myelography
Infection	MRI + contrast, CT
Myelopathy	MRI + contrast > myelography
Arteriovenous malformation	MRI, myelography/angiography

Note: MRA, MR angiography; CTA, CT angiography; T2W, T2-weighted.

vessel detail is essential for diagnosis or for whom interventional therapies are planned. Guidelines for initial selection of neuroimaging studies are shown in Table 190-1.

For a more detailed discussion, see Dillon WP: Neuroimaging in Neurologic Disorders, Chap. 362, p. 2489, in HPIM-17.

191 Seizures and Epilepsy

A *seizure* is a paroxysmal event due to abnormal, excessive, hypersynchronous discharges from an aggregate of CNS neurons. *Epilepsy* is diagnosed when there are recurrent seizures due to a chronic, underlying process.

APPROACH TO THE PATIENT WITH SEIZURE

Seizure Classification

This is essential for diagnosis, therapy, and prognosis (Table 191-1). Seizures are partial (or focal) or generalized: *partial seizures* originate in a localized area of cortex and *generalized seizures* involve diffuse regions of the brain in a bilaterally symmetric fashion. *Simple-partial seizures* do not affect consciousness and may have motor, sensory, autonomic, or psychic symptoms. *Complex-partial seizures* include alteration in consciousness coupled with automatisms (e.g., lip smacking, chewing, aimless walking, or other complex motor activities).

Generalized seizures may occur as a primary disorder or result from secondary generalization of a partial seizure. *Tonic-clonic seizures* (grand mal) cause sudden loss of consciousness, loss of postural control, tonic muscular contraction producing teeth-clenching and rigidity in extension (tonic phase), followed by rhythmic muscular jerking (clonic phase). Tongue-biting and incontinence may occur during the seizure. Recovery of consciousness is typically gradual over many minutes to hours. Headache and confusion are common postictal phenomena. In *absence seizures* (petit mal) there is sudden, brief impairment of consciousness without loss of postural control. Events rarely last longer than 5–10 s but can recur many times per day. Minor motor symptoms are common, while complex automatisms and clonic activity are not. Other types of generalized seizures include tonic, atonic, and myoclonic seizures.

Etiology

Seizure type and age of pt provide important clues to etiology (Table 191-2).

TABLE 191-1 CLASSIFICATION OF SEIZURES

1. **Partial seizures**
    a. Simple partial seizures (with motor, sensory, autonomic, or psychic signs)
    b. Complex partial seizures
    c. Partial seizures with secondary generalization
2. **Primarily generalized seizures**
    a. Absence (petit mal)
    b. Tonic-clonic (grand mal)
    c. Tonic
    d. Atonic
    e. Myoclonic
3. **Unclassified seizures**
    a. Neonatal seizures
    b. Infantile spasms

TABLE 191-2 **CAUSES OF SEIZURES**

Neonates (<1 month)	Perinatal hypoxia and ischemia
	Intracranial hemorrhage and trauma
	Acute CNS infection
	Metabolic disturbances (hypoglycemia, hypocalcemia, hypomagnesemia, pyridoxine deficiency)
	Drug withdrawal
	Developmental disorders
	Genetic disorders
Infants and children (>1 mo and <12 years)	Febrile seizures
	Genetic disorders (metabolic, degenerative, primary epilepsy syndromes)
	CNS infection
	Developmental disorders
	Trauma
	Idiopathic
Adolescents (12–18 years)	Trauma
	Genetic disorders
	Infection
	Brain tumor
	Illicit drug use
	Idiopathic
Young adults (18–35 years)	Trauma
	Alcohol withdrawal
	Illicit drug use
	Brain tumor
	Idiopathic
Older adults (>35 years)	Cerebrovascular disease
	Brain tumor
	Alcohol withdrawal
	Metabolic disorders (uremia, hepatic failure, electrolyte abnormalities, hypoglycemia)
	Alzheimer's disease and other degenerative CNS diseases
	Idiopathic

Note: CNS, central nervous system.

CLINICAL EVALUATION

Careful history is essential since diagnosis of seizures and epilepsy is often based solely on clinical grounds. Differential diagnosis (Table 191-3) includes syncope or psychogenic seizures (pseudoseizures). General exam includes search for infection, trauma, toxins, systemic illness, neurocutaneous abnormalities, and vascular disease. A number of drugs lower the seizure threshold (Table 191-4). Asymmetries in neurologic exam suggest brain tumor, stroke, trauma, or other focal lesions. An algorithmic approach is shown in Fig. 191-1.

LABORATORY EVALUATION

Routine blood studies are indicated to identify the more common metabolic causes of seizures such as abnormalities in electrolytes, glucose, calcium, or magnesium, and hepatic or renal disease. A screen for toxins in blood and urine should be obtained. A lumbar puncture is indicated if there is any suspicion of CNS infection such as meningitis or encephalitis; it is mandatory in HIV-infected patients even in the absence of symptoms or signs suggesting infection.

TABLE 191-3   DIFFERENTIAL DIAGNOSIS OF SEIZURES

Syncope
   Vasovagal syncope
   Cardiac arrhythmia
   Valvular heart disease
   Cardiac failure
   Orthostatic hypotension
Psychological disorders
   Psychogenic seizure
   Hyperventilation
   Panic attack
Metabolic disturbances
   Alcoholic blackouts
   Delirium tremens
   Hypoglycemia
   Hypoxia
   Psychoactive drugs (e.g.,
     hallucinogens)
Migraine
   Confusional migraine
   Basilar migraine

Transient ischemic attack (TIA)
   Basilar artery TIA
Sleep disorders
   Narcolepsy/cataplexy
   Benign sleep myoclonus
Movement disorders
   Tics
   Nonepileptic myoclonus
   Paroxysmal choreoathetosis
Special considerations in children
   Breath-holding spells
   Migraine with recurrent abdominal
     pain and cyclic vomiting
   Benign paroxysmal vertigo
   Apnea
   Night terrors
   Sleepwalking

Electroencephalography (EEG)   All pts should be evaluated as soon as possible with an EEG, which measures electrical activity of the brain by recording from electrodes placed on the scalp. The presence of electrographic seizure activity during the clinically evident event, i.e., abnormal, repetitive, rhythmic activity

TABLE 191-4   DRUGS AND OTHER SUBSTANCES THAT CAN CAUSE SEIZURES

Alkylating agents (e.g., busulfan,
   chlorambucil)
Antimalarials (chloroquine,
   mefloquine)
Antimicrobials/antivirals
   β-Lactam and related compounds
   Quinolones
   Acyclovir
   Isoniazid
   Ganciclovir
Anesthetics and analgesics
   Meperidine
   Tramadol
   Local anesthetics
Dietary supplements
   Ephedra (ma huang)
   Gingko
Immunomodulatory drugs
   Cyclosporine
   OKT3 (monoclonal antibodies to
     T cells)
   Tacrolimus
   Interferons

Psychotropics
   Antidepressants
   Antipsychotics
   Lithium
Radiographic contrast agents
Theophylline
Sedative-hypnotic drug withdrawal
   Alcohol
   Barbiturates (short-acting)
   Benzodiazepines (short-acting)
Drugs of abuse
   Amphetamine
   Cocaine
   Phencyclidine
   Methylphenidate
Flumazenil[a]

[a]In benzodiazepine-dependent patients.

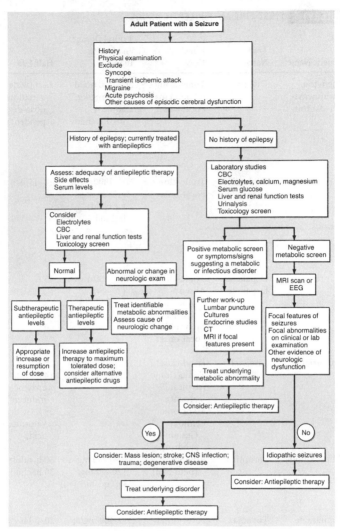

FIGURE 191-1 Evaluation of the adult patient with a seizure. CBC, complete blood count; CT, computed tomography; MRI, magnetic resonance imaging; EEG, electroencephalogram; CNS, central nervous system.

having an abrupt onset and termination, establishes the diagnosis. The absence of electrographic seizure activity does not exclude a seizure disorder, however. The EEG is always abnormal during generalized tonic-clonic seizures. Continuous monitoring for prolonged periods may be required to capture the EEG abnormalities. The EEG can show abnormal discharges during the interictal period that support the diagnosis of epilepsy, and is useful for classifying seizure disorders and determining prognosis.

TABLE 191-5   FIRST-LINE ANTIEPILEPTIC DRUGS

Generic Name	Trade Name	Principal Uses	Typical Dosage and Dosing Intervals	Half-Life
Phenytoin (diphenyl-hydantoin	Dilantin	Tonic-clonic (grand mal) Focal-onset	300–400 mg/d (3–6 mg/kg, adult; 4–8 mg/kg, child) qd-bid	24 h (wide variation, dose-dependent)
Carbamazepine	Tegretol Carbatrol	Tonic-clonic Focal-onset	600–1800 mg/d (15–35 mg/kg, child) bid-qid	10–17 h
Valproic acid	Depakene Depakote	Tonic-clonic Absence Atypical absence Myoclonic Focal-onset	750–2000 mg/d (20–60 mg/kg) bid-qid	15 h
Lamotrigine	Lamictal	Focal-onset Tonic-clonic Atypical absence Myoclonic Lennox-Gastaut syndrome	150–500 mg/d bid	25 h 14 h (with enzyme-inducers) 59 h (with valproic acid)
Ethosuximide	Zarontin	Absence (petit mal)	750–1250 mg/d (20–40 mg/kg) qd-bid	60 h, adult 30 h, child
Topiramate	Topamax	Focal-onset Tonic-clonic Lennox-Gastaut syndrome	200–400 mg/d; bid	20–30 h
Oxcarbazepine	Trileptal	Focal-onset	900–2400 mg/d (30–45 mg/kg, child); bid	10–17 h (for active metabolite)

aPhenytoin, carbamazepine, phenobarbital.

Therapeutic Range	Adverse Effects		Drug Interactions
	Neurologic	Systemic	
10–20 μg/mL	Dizziness Diplopia Ataxia Incoordination Confusion	Gum hyperplasia Lymphadenopathy Hirsutism Osteomalacia Facial coarsening Skin rash	Level increased by isoniazid, sulfonamides, fluoxetine Level decreased by enzyme-inducing drugs[a] Altered folate metabolism
6–12 μg/μL	Ataxia Dizziness Diplopia Vertigo	Aplastic anemia Leukopenia Gastrointestinal irritation Hepatotoxicity Hyponatremia	Level decreased by enzyme-inducing drugs[a] Level increased by erythromycin propoxyphene, isoniazid, cimetidine, fluoxetine
50–150 μg/μL	Ataxia Sedation Tremor	Hepatotoxicity Thrombocytopenia Gastrointestinal irritation Weight gain Transient alopecia Hyperammonemia	Level decreased by enzyme-inducing drugs[a]
Not established	Dizziness Diplopia Sedation Ataxia Headache	Skin rash Stevens-Johnson syndrome	Level decreased by enzyme-inducing drugs[a] Level increased by valproic acid
40–100 μg/μL	Ataxia Lethargy Headache	Gastrointestinal irritation Skin rash Bone marrow suppression	—
Not established	Psychomotor slowing Sedation Speech or language problems Fatigue Paresthesias	Renal stones (avoid use with other carbonic anhydrase inhibitors) Glaucoma Weight loss Hypohydrosis	Level decreased by enzyme-inducing drugs[a]
Not established	Fatigue Ataxia Dizziness Diplopia Vertigo Headache	See carbamazepine	Level decreased by enzyme-inducing drugs[a] May increase phenytoin

TABLE 191-6 **SELECTION OF ANTIEPILEPTIC DRUGS**

Primary Generalized Tonic-Clonic	Partial[a]	Absence	Atypical Absence, Myoclonic, Atonic
First-Line			
Valproic acid	Carbamazepine	Valproic acid	Valproic acid
Lamotrigine	Phenytoin	Ethosuximide	Lamotrigine
Topiramate	Lamotrigine		Topiramate
	Oxcarbazepine		
	Valproic acid		
Alternatives			
Zonisamide[b]	Levetiracetam[b]	Lamotrigine	Clonazepam
Phenytoin	Topiramate	Clonazepam	Felbamate
Carbamazepine	Tiagabine[b]		
Oxcarbazepine	Zonisamide[b]		
Phenobarbital	Gabapentin[b]		
Primidone	Phenobarbital		
Felbamate	Primidone		
	Felbamate		

[a]Includes simple partial, complex partial, and secondarily generalized seizures.
[b]As adjunctive therapy.

Brain Imaging All patients with unexplained new-onset seizures should have a brain imaging study (MRI or CT) to search for an underlying structural abnormality; the only exception may be children who have an unambiguous history and examination suggestive of a benign, generalized seizure disorder such as absence epilepsy. Newer MRI methods, such as fluid-attenuated inversion recovery (FLAIR), have increased the sensitivity for detection of abnormalities of cortical architecture, including hippocampal atrophy associated with mesial temporal sclerosis, and abnormalities of neuronal migration.

℞ **Seizures and Epilepsy**

Acutely, the pt should be placed in semiprone position with head to the side to avoid aspiration. Tongue blades or other objects should not be forced between clenched teeth. Oxygen should be given via face mask. Reversible metabolic disorders (e.g., hypoglycemia, hyponatremia, hypocalcemia, drug or alcohol withdrawal) should be promptly corrected. Treatment of status epilepticus is discussed in Chap. 23.

Longer-term therapy includes treatment of underlying conditions, avoidance of precipitating factors, prophylactic therapy with antiepileptic medications or surgery, and addressing various psychological and social issues. Choice of antiepileptic drug therapy depends on a variety of factors including seizure type, dosing schedule, and potential side effects (Tables 191-5 and 191-6). Therapeutic goal is complete cessation of seizures without side effects using a single drug (monotherapy) and a dosing schedule that is easy for the pt to follow. If ineffective, medication should be increased to maximal tolerated dose based primarily on clinical response rather than serum levels. If unsuccessful, a second drug should be added, and when control is obtained, the first drug can be slowly tapered. Some pts will require polytherapy with two or more drugs, although monotherapy should be the goal. Pts with certain epilepsy syndromes (e.g., temporal lobe epilepsy) are often refractory to medical therapy and benefit from surgical excision of the seizure focus.

 For a more detailed discussion, see Lowenstein DH: Seizures and Epilepsy, Chap. 363, p. 2498, in HPIM-17.

192 Alzheimer's Disease and Other Dementias

DEMENTIA

Dementia is an acquired deterioration in cognitive ability that impairs the successful performance of activities of daily living. Memory is the most common cognitive ability lost with dementia; 10% of persons over age 70 and 20–40% of individuals over age 85 have clinically identifiable memory loss. Other mental faculties are also affected in dementia, such as language, visuospatial ability, calculation, judgment, and problem solving. Neuropsychiatric and social deficits develop in many dementia syndromes, resulting in depression, withdrawal, hallucinations, delusions, agitation, insomnia, and disinhibition. Dementia is chronic and usually progressive.

Diagnosis The mini-mental status examination (MMSE) is a useful screening test for dementia (Table 189-1). A score of <24 points (out of 30) indicates a need for more detailed cognitive and physical assessment. In some patients with early cognitive disorders, the MMSE may be normal and more detailed neuropsychologic testing will be required.

APPROACH TO THE PATIENT WITH DEMENTIA

Differential Diagnosis
Dementia has many causes (Table 192-1). It is essential to exclude treatable etiologies; in one study, the most common potentially reversible diagnoses were depression, hydrocephalus, and alcohol dependence. The major degenerative dementias can usually be distinguished by distinctive symptoms, signs, and neuroimaging features (Table 192-2).

History
A subacute onset of confusion may represent delirium and should trigger the search for intoxication, infection, or metabolic derangement (Chap. 17). An elderly person with slowly progressive memory loss over several years is likely to have Alzheimer's disease (AD). A change in personality, disinhibition, gain of weight, or food obsession suggests frontotemporal dementia (FTD), not AD; apathy, loss of executive function, progressive abnormalities in speech, or relative sparing of memory also suggests FTD. Dementia with

TABLE 192-1 **DIFFERENTIAL DIAGNOSIS OF DEMENTIA**

Most Common Causes of Dementia

Alzheimer's disease
Vascular dementia
   Multi-infarct
   Diffuse white matter disease
   (Binswanger's)

Alcoholism[a]
Parkinson's disease
Drug/medication intoxication[a]

Less Common Causes of Dementia

Vitamin deficiencies
   Thiamine (B_1): Wernicke's en-
   cephalopathy[a]
   B_{12} (pernicious anemia)[a]
   Nicotinic acid (pellagra)[a]
Endocrine and other organ failure
   Hypothyroidism[a]
   Adrenal insufficiency and Cush-
   ing's syndrome[a]
   Hypo- and hyperparathyroidism[a]
   Renal failure[a]
   Liver failure[a]
   Pulmonary failure[a]
Chronic infections
   HIV
   Neurosyphilis[a]
   Papovavirus (progressive multifo-
   cal leukoencephalopathy)
   Prion (Creutzfeldt-Jakob and
   Gerstmann-Sträussler-Schein-
   ker diseases)
   Tuberculosis, fungal, and protozoal[a]
   Whipple's disease[a]
Head trauma and diffuse brain damage
   Dementia pugilistica
   Chronic subdural hematoma[a]
   Postanoxia
   Postencephalitis
   Normal-pressure hydrocephalus[a]
Neoplastic
   Primary brain tumor[a]
   Metastatic brain tumor[a]
   Paraneoplastic limbic encephalitis

Toxic disorders
   Drug, medication, and narcotic poi-
   soning[a]
   Heavy metal intoxication[a]
   Dialysis dementia (aluminum)
   Organic toxins
Psychiatric
   Depression (pseudodementia)[a]
   Schizophrenia[a]
   Conversion reaction[a]
Degenerative disorders
   Huntington's disease
   Pick's disease
   Dementia with Lewy bodies
   Progressive supranuclear palsy
   (Steel-Richardson syndrome)
   Multisystem degeneration (Shy-
   Drager syndrome)
   Hereditary ataxias (some forms)
   Motor neuron disease [amyotrophic
   lateral sclerosis (ALS); some forms]
   Frontotemporal dementia
   Cortical basal degeneration
   Multiple sclerosis
   Adult Down's syndrome with
   Alzheimer's
   ALS–Parkinson's–Dementia complex
   of Guam
Miscellaneous
   Sarcoidosis[a]
   Vasculitis[a]
   CADASIL etc
   Acute intermittent porphyria[a]
   Recurrent nonconvulsive seizures[a]
Additional conditions in children or
   adolescents
      Hallervorden-Spatz disease
      Subacute sclerosing panencephalitis
      Metabolic disorders (e.g., Wilson's
      and Leigh's diseases, leukodystro-
      phies, lipid storage diseases, mito-
      chondrial mutations)

[a]Potentially reversible dementia.

TABLE 192-2 CLINICAL DIFFERENTIATION OF THE MAJOR DEMENTIAS

Disease	First Symptom	Mental Status	Neuropsychiatry	Neurology	Imaging
AD	Memory loss	Episodic memory loss	Initially normal	Initially normal	Entorhinal cortex and hippocampal atrophy
FTD	Apathy; poor judgment/insight, speech/language; hyperorality	Frontal/executive; language; spares drawing	Apathy, disinhibition, hyperorality, euphoria, depression	Due to PSP/CBD overlap; vertical gaze palsy, axial rigidity, dystonia, alien hand	Frontal and/or temporal atrophy; spares posterior parietal lobe
DLB	Visual hallucinations, REM sleep disorder, delirium, Capgras' syndrome, parkinsonism	Drawing and frontal/executive; spares memory; delirium prone	Visual hallucinations, depression, sleep disorder, delusions	Parkinsonism	Posterior parietal atrophy; hippocampi larger than in AD
CJD	Dementia, mood, anxiety, movement disorders	Variable, frontal/executive, focal cortical, memory	Depression, anxiety	Myoclonus, rigidity, parkinsonism	Cortical ribboning and basal ganglia or thalamus hyperintensity on diffusion/flare MRI
Vascular	Often but not always sudden; variable; apathy, falls, focal weakness	Frontal/executive, cognitive slowing; can spare memory	Apathy, delusions, anxiety	Usually motor slowing, spasticity; can be normal	Cortical and/or subcortical infarctions, confluent white matter disease

Note: AD, Alzheimer's disease; FTD, frontotemporal dementia; PSP, progressive supranuclear palsy; CBD, cortical basal degeneration; DLB, dementia with Lewy bodies; CJD, Creutzfeldt-Jakob disease.

997

Lewy bodies (DLB) is suggested by the early presence of visual hallucinations, parkinsonism, delirium, or a sleep disorder.

A history of stroke suggests vascular dementia, which may also occur with hypertension, atrial fibrillation, peripheral vascular disease, and diabetes. Rapid progression of dementia with myoclonus suggests a prion disease such as Creutzfeldt-Jakob disease. Gait disturbance is prominent with vascular dementia, Parkinson's disease, or normal-pressure hydrocephalus. Multiple sex partners or intravenous drug use should trigger search for an infection, especially in persons with HIV. A history of head trauma could indicate chronic subdural hematoma, dementia pugilistica, or normal-pressure hydrocephalus. Alcoholism may suggest malnutrition and thiamine deficiency. A history of gastric surgery may result in loss of intrinsic factor and vitamin B_{12} deficiency. A careful review of medications, especially of sedatives and tranquilizers, may raise the issue of drug intoxication. A family history of dementia is found in Huntington's disease, familial AD, or familial FTD. Insomnia or weight loss is often seen with pseudodementia due to depression, which can also be caused by the recent death of a loved one.

Examination
It is essential to document the dementia, look for other signs of nervous system involvement, and search for clues of a systemic disease that might be responsible for the cognitive disorder. AD does not affect motor systems until late in the course. In contrast, FTD patients often develop axial rigidity, supranuclear gaze palsy, or features of amyotrophic lateral sclerosis. In DLB, initial symptoms may be the new onset of a parkinsonian syndrome (resting tremor, cogwheel rigidity, bradykinesia, and festinating gait). Unexplained falls, axial rigidity, and gaze deficits suggest progressive supranuclear palsy (PSP).

Focal neurologic deficits may occur in vascular dementia or brain tumor. Dementia with a myelopathy and peripheral neuropathy suggests vitamin B_{12} deficiency. A peripheral neuropathy could also indicate an underlying vitamin deficiency or metal intoxication. Dry cool skin, hair loss, and bradycardia suggest hypothyroidism. Confusion associated with repetitive stereotyped movements may indicate ongoing seizure activity. Hearing impairment or visual loss may produce confusion and disorientation misinterpreted as dementia. Such sensory deficits are common in the elderly.

Choice of Diagnostic Studies
A reversible or treatable cause must not be missed, yet no single etiology is common; thus a screen must employ multiple tests, each of which has a low yield. Table 192-3 lists most screening tests for dementia. Guidelines recommend the routine measurement of thyroid function, a vitamin B_{12} level, and a neuroimaging study (CT or MRI). Lumbar puncture need not be done routinely but is indicated if infection is a consideration. An EEG is rarely helpful except to suggest a prion disease or an underlying nonconvulsive seizure disorder. Brain biopsy is not advised except to diagnose vasculitis, potentially treatable neoplasms, unusual infections, or systemic disorders such as sarcoid.

ALZHEIMER'S DISEASE

Most common cause of dementia; affects 4 million persons in the United States. Cost > $50 billion/year.

TABLE 192-3	EVALUATION OF THE PATIENT WITH DEMENTIA

Routine Evaluation	Optional Focused Tests	Occasionally Helpful Tests
History	Psychometric testing	EEG
Physical examination	Chest x-ray	Parathyroid function
Laboratory tests	Lumbar puncture	Adrenal function
Thyroid function (TSH)	Liver function	Urine heavy metals
Vitamin B_{12}	Renal function	RBC sedimentation rate
Complete blood count	Urine toxin screen	Angiogram
Electrolytes	HIV	Brain biopsy
CT/MRI	Apolipoprotein E	SPECT
	RPR or VDRL	PET

Diagnostic Categories

Reversible Causes	Irreversible/Degenerative Dementias	Psychiatric Disorders
Examples	Examples	Depression
Hypothyroidism	Alzheimer's	Schizophrenia
Thiamine deficiency	Frontotemporal dementia	Conversion reaction
Vitamin B_{12} deficiency	Huntington's	
Normal-pressure hydrocephalus	Dementia with Lewy bodies	
Subdural hematoma	Vascular	
Chronic infection	Leukoencephalopathies	
Brain tumor	Parkinson's	
Drug intoxication		

Associated Treatable Conditions

Depression	Agitation	
Seizures	Caregiver "burnout"	
Insomnia	Drug side effects	

Note: PET, positron emission tomography; RPR, rapid plasma reagin (test); SPECT, single photon emission CT; VDRL, Venereal Disease Research Laboratory (test for syphilis).

Clinical Manifestations Pts present with subtle recent memory loss, then develop slowly progressive dementia with impairment spreading to language and visuospatial deficits. Memory loss is often not recognized initially, in part due to preservation of social graces until later phases; impaired activities of daily living (keeping track of finances, appointments) draw attention of friends/family. Disorientation, poor judgment, poor concentration, aphasia, and apraxia are increasingly evident as the disease progresses. Pts may be frustrated or unaware of deficit. In end-stage AD, pts become rigid, mute, incontinent, and bedridden. Help may be needed with the simplest tasks, such as eating, dressing, and toilet function. Often, death results from malnutrition, secondary infections, pulmonary emboli, or heart disease. Typical duration is 8–10 years, but the course can range from 1 to 25 years.

Pathogenesis Risk factors for AD are old age, positive family history. Pathology: neuritic plaques composed in part of Aβ amyloid, derived from amyloid precursor protein (APP); neurofibrillary tangles composed of abnormally phosphorylated tau protein. The apolipoprotein E (apo E) ε4 allele accelerates age of onset of AD and is associated with sporadic and late-onset familial cases. Apo E testing is not indicated as a predictive test. Rare genetic causes of AD are Down's syndrome and mutations in APP, presenilin I, and presenilin II genes; all appear to increase production of Aβ amyloid. Genetic testing available for presenilin mutations.

℞ Alzheimer's Disease

AD cannot be cured, and no highly effective drug exists. The focus is on judicious use of cholinesterase inhibitor drugs; symptomatic management of behavioral problems; and building rapport with the pt, family members, and other caregivers.

Donepezil, rivastigmine, galantamine, tacrine (tetrahydroaminoacridine), and memantine are approved by the FDA for treatment of AD. With the exception of memantine, their action is inhibition of cholinesterase, with a resulting increase in cerebral levels of acetylcholine. Memantine appears to act by blocking overexcited N-methyl-D-aspartate (NMDA) channels. These compounds are only modestly efficacious and offer little or no benefit in the late stages of AD; they are associated with improved caregiver ratings of patients' functioning and with an apparent decreased rate of decline in cognitive test scores over periods of up to 3 years. Donepezil (Aricept), 5–10 mg/d PO, has the advantages of few side effects and single daily dosage. Dosing of memantine begins at 5mg/d with gradual increases (over 1 month) to 10 mg twice a day.

The antioxidants selegiline, α-tocopherol (vitamin E), or both slowed institutionalization and progression to death of AD in one study. Because vitamin E is less toxic than selegiline and is inexpensive; the dose is 1000 IU twice a day. However, its beneficial effects are likely to be small; these high doses of vitamin E have potential cardiovascular complications, dampening enthusiasm for this treatment. There is no role for hormone replacement therapy in prevention of AD in women, and no benefit has been found in the treatment of established AD with estrogen. Prospective studies are examining the role of NSAIDs, statins, insulin regulation, and lowering of serum homocysteine. Other experimental approaches target amyloid either through diminishing its production or promoting clearance by passive immunization with monoclonal antibodies.

Depression, common in early stages of AD, may respond to antidepressant or cholinesterase inhibitors. Selective serotonin reuptake inhibitors (SSRIs) are often used due to their low anticholinergic side effects. Management of behavioral problems in conjunction with family and caregivers is essential. Mild sedation may help insomnia. Control of agitation usually involves antipsychotic medications, but recent trials have questioned the efficacy of this approach; in addition, all of the antipsychotics carry a black box warning in the elderly and should be used with caution. Notebooks and posted daily reminders can function as memory aids in early stages. Kitchens, bathrooms, and bedrooms need evaluation for safety. Pts must eventually stop driving. Caregiver burnout is common; nursing home placement may be necessary. Local and national support groups (Alzheimer's Disease and Related Disorders Association) are valuable resources.

OTHER CAUSES OF DEMENTIA

Vascular Dementia Typically follows a pattern of either multiple strokelike episodes (multi-infarct dementia) or diffuse white matter disease (leukoaraiosis,

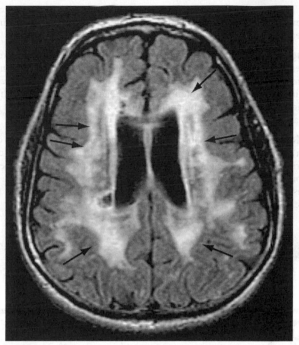

FIGURE 192-1 Diffuse white matter disease (Binswanger's disease). Axial T2-weighted MR image through the lateral ventricles reveals multiple areas of abnormal high signal intensity involving the periventricular white matter as well as the corona radiata and lentiform nuclei (arrows). While seen in some individuals with normal cognition, this appearance is more pronounced in patients with dementia of a vascular etiology.

subcortical arteriosclerotic encephalopathy, Binswanger's disease) (Fig. 192-1). Unlike AD, focal neurologic signs (e.g., hemiparesis) may be apparent at presentation. Treatment focuses on underlying causes of atherosclerosis; anticholinesterase compounds are being studied for treatment of the dementia.

Frontotemporal Dementia   Responsible for 10% of all cases of dementia. Extremely heterogeneous; presents with combinations of disinhibition, dementia, apraxia, parkinsonism, and motor neuron disease. May be sporadic or inherited; some familial cases due to mutations of tau or progranulin genes. Treatment is symptomatic; no therapies known to slow progression or improve cognitive symptoms. Many of the behaviors that accompany FTD such as depression, hyperorality, compulsions, and irritability can be helped with SSRIs.

Dementia with Lewy Bodies   Characterized by visual hallucinations, parkinsonism, fluctuating alertness, and falls. Dementia can precede or follow the appearance of parkinsonism. Lewy bodies are intraneuronal cytoplasmic inclusions. Anticholinesterase compounds, exercise programs to maximize motor function, antidepressants to treat depressive syndromes, and possibly antipsychotics in low doses to alleviate psychosis may be helpful.

Normal-Pressure Hydrocephalus (NPH)   Uncommon; presents as a gait disorder (ataxic or apractic), dementia, and urinary incontinence. Gait improves in some pts following ventricular shunting; dementia and incontinence do not improve. The diagnosis is difficult to make, and the clinical picture may overlap with several other causes of dementia including AD; historically many individuals treated for NPH have suffered from other dementias.

Huntington's Disease   Chorea, behavioral disturbance, and a frontal/executive disorder (Chap. 43). Typical onset fourth to fifth decade but can present at almost any age. Autosomal dominant inheritance due to expanded trinucleotide repeat in gene encoding the protein huntingtin. Diagnosis confirmed with genetic testing coupled with genetic counseling. Symptomatic treatment of movements and behaviors; SSRIs may help depression.

Creutzfeldt-Jakob Disease (CJD)   Prion disorders such as CJD are rare (~1 per million). CJD is a rapidly progressive disorder with dementia, focal cortical signs, rigidity, and myoclonus; death in <1 year from first symptom. The markedly abnormal periodic discharges on EEG and cortical and basal ganglia abnormalities on diffusion-weighted MR are unique diagnostic features. No proven treatments exist.

For a more detailed discussion, see Bird TD, Miller BL: Dementia, Chap. 365, p. 2536, in HPIM-17.

193   Parkinson's Disease

CLINICAL FEATURES

Parkinsonism consists of tremor, rigidity, bradykinesia, and characteristic abnormalities of gait and posture; may occur with many disorders. Parkinson's disease (PD) is idiopathic parkinsonism without evidence of more widespread neurologic involvement. PD afflicts >1 million individuals in the United States (~1% of those >55 years). Peak age of onset in the 60s (range is 35–85); course progressive over 10–25 years. Tremor ("pill rolling" of hands) at rest (4–6 Hz); worsens with stress. A faster (7–8 Hz) "action tremor" may also occur when the hands are held against gravity. Presentation with tremor confined to one limb or side of body is common. Other findings: rigidity ("cogwheeling"—increased ratchet-like resistance to passive limb movements), bradykinesia (slowness of voluntary movements), fixed expressionless face (facial masking) with reduced frequency of blinking, hypophonic voice, drooling, impaired rapid alternating movements, micrographia (small handwriting), reduced arm swing, and flexed "stooped" posture with walking, shuffling gait, difficulty initiating or stopping walking, en-bloc turning (multiple small steps required to turn), retropulsion (tendency to fall backwards). Non-motor aspects of PD include depression and anxiety, cognitive impairment, sleep disturbances, sensation of inner restlessness, loss of smell (*anosmia*), and disturbances of autonomic function. In advanced PD, intellectual and behavioral deterioration, aspiration pneumonia, and bedsores (due to immobility) common. Normal muscular strength, deep tendon reflexes, and sensory exam. Diagnosis based upon history and examination; neuroimaging, EEG, and CSF studies usually normal for age.

TABLE 193-1 **HISTORY AND EXAMINATION FEATURES SUGGESTING DIAGNOSES OTHER THAN PARKINSON'S DISEASE**

Symptoms/Signs	Alternative Diagnosis to Consider
History	
Falls as the first symptom	PSP
Exposure to neuroleptics	Drug-induced parkinsonism
Onset prior to age 40	If PD, think genetic causes
Associated unexplained liver disease	Wilson's disease
Early hallucinations	Lewy body dementia
Sudden onset of parkinsonian symptoms	Vascular parkinsonism
Physical Exam	
Dementia as first symptom	Dementia with Lewy bodies
Prominent orthostasis	MSA-p
Early dysarthria	MSA-c
Lack of tremor	Various Parkinson's-plus syndromes
High frequency (8–10 Hz) symmetric tremor	Essential tremor

Note: PSP, progressive supranuclear palsy; MSA, multiple system atrophy.

PATHOPHYSIOLOGY

Degeneration of pigmented pars compacta neurons of the substantia nigra in the midbrain resulting in lack of dopaminergic input to striatum; accumulation of eosinophilic intraneural inclusion granules (Lewy bodies). Cause of cell death is unknown, but it may result from generation of free radicals and oxidative stress. Rare genetic forms of parkinsonism exist (~5% of cases); most common are mutations in α-synuclein or parkin genes. Early age of onset suggests a possible genetic cause of PD, although one genetic form (*LLRK2*) causes PD in the same age range as sporadic PD.

DIFFERENTIAL DIAGNOSIS (See Table 193-1)

Features of parkinsonism may occur with: depression (paucity of vocal inflection and facial movement); essential tremor (high-frequency tremor with limbs held against gravity, head tremor, improves with alcohol, often family history); normal-pressure hydrocephalus (apraxic gait, urinary incontinence, dementia); Wilson's disease (early age of onset, Kayser-Fleischer rings, low serum ceruloplasmin); Huntington's disease (family history, chorea, dementia); multiple system atrophy (early urinary incontinence, orthostatic hypotension, dysarthria); dementia with Lewy bodies (early hallucinations, behavioral disturbances); progressive supranuclear palsy (early imbalance and falls, vertical gaze paresis).

℞ Parkinson's Disease

Goals are to maintain function and avoid drug-induced complications. Brady-kinesia, tremor, rigidity, and abnormal posture respond early in illness; cognitive symptoms, hypophonia, autonomic dysfunction, and balance difficulties respond poorly.

Initiation of Therapy

Dopaminomimetic therapy initiated when symptoms interfere with quality of life. The ideal first-line agent depends on the age and cognitive status of the patient. In early PD, dopamine agonist monotherapy is well tolerated and reduces risk of later treatment-related complications such as motor fluctuations and dyskinesias (which occur in 50% of pts treated >5 years with levodopa); agonists often lead to cognitive sideeffects (hallucinations) in the elderly and therefore levodopa may be a better initial choice in these patients. Dopamine agonist monotherapy requires higher doses than needed when agonist is used to supplement levodopa (Table 193-2); slow titration necessary to avoid side effects. Most pts require addition of levodopa or another agent within 1–3 years of initiating dopamine agonist monotherapy.

Motor fluctuations are the exaggerated ebb and flow of parkinsonian signs between doses of medications. *Dyskinesias* refer to choreiform and dystonic movements that can occur as a peak dose effect or at the beginning or end of the dose.

Dopamine Agonists

Compared to levodopa, they are longer acting and thus provide a more uniform stimulation of dopamine receptors. They are effective as monotherapeutic agents and as adjuncts to carbidopa/levodopa therapy. They can also be used in combination with anticholinergics and amantadine. Side effects include nausea, postural hypotension, psychiatric symptoms, daytime sedation, and occasional sleep attacks. Pergolide is a dopamine agonist removed from the U.S. market due to its association with asymptomatic valvular heart disease. Table 193-2 provides a guide to the doses and uses of these agents.

Carbidopa/Levodopa Formulations

Available in regular, immediate release (IR) formulations (Sinemet, Atamet and others; 10/100 mg, 25/100 mg, and 25/250 mg), controlled release (CR) formulations (Sinemet CR 25/100 mg, 50/200 mg), and more recently as Stalevo (Table 193-2). The latter combines IR carbidopa/levodopa with 200 mg of entacapone (see below). Carbidopa blocks peripheral levodopa decarboxylation into dopamine and thus symptoms of nausea and orthostasis often associated with the initiation of levodopa. Initial target doses of these medications are summarized in table. Gradual dose escalation recommended; initiation of dosing at mealtimes will reduce nausea.

Levodopa Augmentation

Selegiline is a selective and irreversible monoamine oxidase (MAO) B inhibitor with a modest symptomatic effect when used as monotherapy or as an adjunct to carbidopa/levodopa. Typically, selegiline is used as initial therapy (5 mg with breakfast and lunch) or is added to alleviate tremor or levodopa-associated wearing off; a side effect is insomnia. Two more potent MAO-B inhibitors with once-daily dosing were recently introduced, rasagiline (0.5–1 mg/d) and zydis selegiline (1.25–2.5 mg/d in the morning). The potential role of these drugs as neuroprotective therapies remains controversial.

The catechol *O*-methyltransferase (COMT) inhibitors entacapone and tolcapone offer yet another strategy to augment the effects of levodopa by blocking the enzymatic degradation of levodopa and dopamine. Entacapone is preferred to tolcapone (hepatic and hematologic side effects). When used with carbidopa/levodopa, these agents alleviate wearing-off symptoms and increase time a pt remains "on" (i.e., well medicated) during the day. Common side effects are GI and hyperdopaminergic, including increased dyskinesias. The dose of entacapone is 200 mg coadministered with each dose of carbidopa/levodopa.

Anticholinergics and amantadine are useful adjuncts. Anticholinergics (trihexyphenidyl, 2–5 mg three times a day; benztropine, 0.5–2 mg three times a day) are particularly useful for controlling rest tremor and dystonia, and amantadine can reduce drug-induced dyskinesias by up to 70%. The mecha-

TABLE 193-2 LEVODOPA FORMULATIONS AND DOPAMINE AGONISTS USED IN PARKINSON'S DISEASE

Agents	LD Dose Equivalency	Available Strengths (mg)	Initial Dosing	Comments
Carbidopa/Levodopa (Typical Initial Strength)				
Carbidopa/levodopa IR 25/100	100 mg (levodopa anchor dose)	10/100 25/100 25/250	25/100; 0.5–1 tab tid	Usual range = 300–800 mg/d with typical schedules being q8h to q3h.
Carbidopa/levodopa CR 50/200	150 mg	25/100 50/200	50/200; 1 tab bid to tid	Increased bioavailability with food. Splitting the tablet negates the CR properties. Usual schedule is q8h to q4h.
Carbidopa/levodopa/entacapone 25/100/200	120 mg	12.5/50/200 25/100/200 37.5/150/200	25/100/200; 1 tab bid to tid	Do not split tablets. May combine with Sinemet IR. Usual schedule is q8h to q4h.
Parcopa 25/100	100 mg	25/100 25/250	25/100; 1 tab tid	Can be used as regular or supplemental rescue doses in cases of regular dose failure. Orally dissolved without water.

(continued)

TABLE 193-2 LEVODOPA FORMULATIONS AND DOPAMINE AGONISTS USED IN PARKINSON'S DISEASE (CONTINUED)

Dopamine Agonists	DA Equivalent to Above LD Anchor Dose	Available Strengths (mg)	Approximate Target Doses			Other Considerations
			Initial Dosing	Monotherapy	As Adjuncts to LD	
Non-ergot alkaloids						
Pramipexole	1 mg	0.125, 0.25, 1, 1.5	0.125 mg tid	1.5–4.5 mg/d	0.375–3.0 mg/d	Renal metabolism; dose adjustments needed in renal insufficiency. Occasionally associated with "sleep attacks."
Ropinirole	5 mg	0.25, 0.5, 1, 2, 3, 4, 5	0.25 mg tid	12–24 mg/d	6–16 mg/d	Hepatic metabolism; potential drug-drug interactions. Occasionally associated with "sleep attacks."
Ropinirole extended release	Availability pending.					
Rotigotine		2, 4, 6	2 mg/24 h	6 mg/d	2–6 mg/d	Available as transdermal patch.
Ergot alkaloids						
Bromocriptine	2 mg	2.5, 5.0	1.25 mg bid to tid	7.5–15 mg/d	3.75–7.5 mg/d	Rare reports of pulmonary and retroperitoneal fibrosis. Relative incidence of sleep attacks not well studied.
Pergolide	Removed from U.S. market in 2007. See text.					
Cabergoline	Used in select cases of PD in Europe. Not approved for the treatment of PD in the U.S.					

Note: Equivalency doses are approximations based on clinical experience, may not be accurate in individual patients, and are not intended to correlate with the in vitro binding affinities of these compounds.

Abbreviations: DA, dopamine agonist; IR, immediate release; CR, controlled release; LD, levodopa (with carbidopa). Carbidopa/levodopa/entacapone = Stalevo.

nism of action of amantadine (100 mg twice daily) is unknown; it has anticholinergic, dopaminomimetic, and glutamate antagonist properties. In older patients, it may aggravate confusion and psychosis.

Surgical Treatments

In refractory cases, surgical treatment of PD should be considered. The use of ablation (e.g., pallidotomy or thalamotomy) has decreased greatly since the introduction of deep-brain stimulation. The selection of suitable patients for surgery is most important, since in general patients with atypical Parkinson's do not have a favorable response. The indications for surgery are (1) a diagnosis of idiopathic PD, (2) a clear response to levodopa, (3) significant intractable tremor, and/or (4) drug-induced dyskinesias and wearing off. Contraindications to surgery include atypical PD, cognitive impairment, major psychiatric illness, substantial medical comorbidities, and advanced age (a relative factor). Symptoms not responding to levodopa are unlikely to benefit from surgery.

For a more detailed discussion, see Delong MR, Juncos JL: Parkinson's Disease and Other Extrapyramidal Movement Disorders, Chap. 366, p. 2549, in HPIM-17.

194 Ataxic Disorders

CLINICAL PRESENTATION

Symptoms and signs may include gait impairment, nystagmus, dysarthria (scanning speech), impaired limb coordination, intention tremor (i.e., with movement), hypotonia. *Differential diagnosis*: Unsteady gait associated with vertigo can resemble gait instability of cerebellar disease but produces a sensation of movement, dizziness, or light-headedness. Sensory disturbances can also simulate cerebellar disease; with sensory ataxia, imbalance dramatically worsens when visual input is removed (Romberg sign). Bilateral proximal leg weakness can also rarely mimic cerebellar ataxia.

APPROACH TO THE PATIENT WITH ATAXIA

Causes are best grouped by determining whether ataxia is symmetric or focal and by the time course (Table 194-1). Also important to distinguish whether ataxia is present in isolation or is part of a multisystem neurologic disorder. Acute symmetric ataxia is usually due to medications, toxins, viral infection, or a postinfectious syndrome (especially varicella). Subacute or chronic symmetric ataxia can result from hypothyroidism, vitamin deficiencies, infections (Lyme disease, tabes dorsalis, prions), alcohol, other toxins, or an inherited condition (see below). An immune-mediated progressive ataxia is associated with antigliadin antibodies; biopsy of the small intestine may reveal villous atrophy of gluten enteropathy. Progressive nonfamilial cerebellar ataxia after age 45 suggests a paraneoplastic syndrome, either

TABLE 194-1 ETIOLOGY OF CEREBELLAR ATAXIA

	Symmetric and Progressive Signs			Focal and Ipsilateral Cerebellar Signs		
Acute (Hours to Days)	Subacute (Days to Weeks)	Chronic (Months to Years)	Acute (Hours to Days)	Subacute (Days to Weeks)	Chronic (Months to Years)	
Intoxication: alcohol, lithium, diphenyl-hydantoin, barbiturates (positive history and toxicology screen) Acute viral cerebellitis (CSF supportive of acute viral infection) Postinfection syndrome	Intoxication: mercury, solvents, gasoline, glue; cytotoxic chemotherapeutic drugs Alcoholic-nutritional (vitamin B_1 and B_{12} deficiency) Lyme disease	Paraneoplastic syndrome Anti-gliadin antibody syndrome Hypothyroidism Inherited diseases Tabes dorsalis (tertiary syphilis) Phenytoin toxicity	Vascular: cerebellar infarction, hemorrhage, or subdural hematoma Infectious: cerebellar abscess (mass lesion on MRI/CT, history in support of lesion)	Neoplastic: cerebellar glioma or metastatic tumor (positive for neoplasm on MRI/CT) Demyelinating: multiple sclerosis (history, CSF, and MRI are consistent) AIDS-related multifocal leukoencephalopathy (positive HIV test and CD4+ cell count for AIDS)	Stable gliosis secondary to vascular lesion or demyelinating plaque (stable lesion on MRI/CT older than several months) Congenital lesion: Chiari or Dandy-Walker malformations (malformation noted on MRI/CT)

Abbreviations: CSF, cerebrospinal fluid; CT, computed tomography; MRI, magnetic resonance imaging.

subacute cortical cerebellar degeneration (ovarian, breast, lung, Hodgkin's) or opsoclonus-myoclonus (neuroblastoma, breast, lung).

Unilateral ataxia suggests a focal lesion in the ipsilateral cerebellar hemisphere or its connections. An important cause of acute unilateral ataxia is stroke. Mass effect from cerebellar hemorrhage or swelling from cerebellar infarction can compress brainstem structures, producing altered consciousness and ipsilateral pontine signs (small pupils, lateral gaze or sixth nerve paresis, facial weakness); limb ataxia may not be prominent. Other diseases producing asymmetric or unilateral ataxia include tumors, multiple sclerosis, progressive multifocal leukoencephalopathy (immunodeficiency states), and congenital malformations.

INHERITED ATAXIAS

May be autosomal dominant, autosomal recessive, or mitochondrial (maternal inheritance); more than 30 disorders recognized (see Table 368-2, HPIM-17). Friedreich's ataxia is most common; autosomal recessive, onset before age 25; ataxia with areflexia, upgoing toes, vibration and position sense deficits, cardiomyopathy, hammer toes, scoliosis; linked to expanded trinucleotide repeat in the intron of gene encoding frataxin; a second form of hereditary ataxia is associated with vitamin E deficiency. Common dominantly inherited ataxias are spinocerebellar ataxia (SCA) 1 (olivopontocerebellar atrophy; "ataxin-1" gene) (Fig. 194-1) and SCA3 (Machado-Joseph disease); both may manifest as ataxia with brainstem and/or extrapyramidal signs; SCA3 may also have dystonia and amyotrophy; genes for each disorder contain unstable trinucleotide repeats in coding region.

EVALUATION

Diagnostic approach is determined by the nature of the ataxia (Table 194-1). For symmetric ataxias, drug and toxicology screens; vitamin B_1, B_{12}, and E levels;

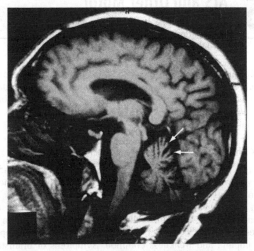

FIGURE 194-1 Sagittal MRI of the brain of a 60-year-old-man with gait ataxia and dysarthria due to SCA1, illustrating cerebellar atrophy (*arrows*).

thyroid function tests; antibody tests for syphilis and Lyme infection; anti-gliadin antibodies; paraneoplastic antibodies (see Chap. 82); and CSF studies often indicated. Genetic testing is available for many inherited ataxias. For unilateral or asymmetric ataxias, brain MRI or CT scan is the initial test of choice.

Rx Ataxia

The most important goal is to identify treatable entities including hypothyroidism, vitamin deficiency, and infectious causes. Parainfectious ataxia can be treated with glucocorticoids. Ataxia with anti-gliadin antibodies and gluten enteropathy may improve with a gluten-free diet. Paraneoplastic disorders are often refractory to therapy, but some pts improve following removal of the tumor or immunotherapy (Chap. 82). Vitamins B_1 and B_{12} should be administered to pts with deficient levels. The deleterious effects of diphenylhydantoin and alcohol on the cerebellum are well known, and these exposures should be avoided in pts with ataxia of any cause. There is no proven therapy for any of the autosomal dominant ataxias; family and genetic counseling are important. There is preliminary evidence that idebenone, a free-radical scavenger, can improve myocardial hypertrophy in Friedreich's ataxia; there is no evidence that it improves neurologic function. Iron chelators and antioxidant drugs are potentially harmful in Friedreich pts as they may increase heart muscle injury. Cerebellar hemorrhage and other mass lesions of the posterior fossa may require emergent surgical treatment to prevent fatal brainstem compression.

For a more detailed discussion, see Rosenberg RN: Ataxic Disorders, Chap. 368, p. 2565, in HPIM-17.

195 ALS and Other Motor Neuron Diseases

Amyotrophic lateral sclerosis (ALS) is the most important of the motor neuron diseases (Table 195-1). ALS is caused by degeneration of motor neurons at all levels of the CNS, including anterior horns of the spinal cord, brainstem motor nuclei, and motor cortex. Familial ALS (FALS) represents 5–10% of the total and is inherited usually as an autosomal dominant disorder.

CLINICAL FEATURES

Onset is usually midlife, with most cases progressing to death in 3–5 years. Presentation is variable depending on whether upper motor or lower motor neurons are more prominently involved initially.

Common initial symptoms are weakness, muscle wasting, stiffness and cramping, and twitching in muscles of hands and arms, often first in the intrinsic hand muscles. Legs are less severely involved than arms, with complaints of leg stiffness, cramping, and weakness common. Symptoms of brainstem involvement include dysphagia, which may lead to aspiration pneumonia and compromised energy intake; there may be prominent wasting of the tongue leading to

TABLE 195-1 SPORADIC MOTOR NEURON DISEASES

Chronic

Upper and lower motor neurons
   Amyotrophic lateral sclerosis
Predominantly upper motor neurons
   Primary lateral sclerosis
Predominantly lower motor neurons
   Multifocal motor neuropathy with conduction block
   Motor neuropathy with paraproteinemia or cancer
   Motor-predominant peripheral neuropathies
Other
   Associated with other degenerative disorders
Secondary motor neuron disorders (see Table 195-2)

Acute

Poliomyelitis
Herpes zoster
Coxsackie virus

difficulty in articulation (dysarthria), phonation, and deglutition. Weakness of ventilatory muscles leads to respiratory insufficiency. Additional features that characterize ALS are preservation of intellect, lack of sensory abnormalities, pseudobulbar palsy (e.g., involuntary laughter, crying), and absence of bowel or bladder dysfunction.

PATHOPHYSIOLOGY

Pathologic hallmark is death of lower motor neurons (consisting of anterior horn cells in the spinal cord and their brainstem homologues innervating bulbar muscles) and upper, or corticospinal, motor neurons (originating in layer five of the motor cortex and descending via the pyramidal tract to synapse with lower motor neurons). Although at onset ALS may involve selective loss of function of only upper or lower motor neurons, it ultimately causes progressive loss of both; the absence of clear involvement of both motor neuron types should call into question the diagnosis of ALS.

LABORATORY EVALUATION

EMG provides objective evidence of extensive muscle denervation not confined to the territory of individual peripheral nerves and nerve roots. CSF is usually normal. Muscle enzymes (e.g., CK) may be elevated.

Several types of secondary motor neuron disorders that resemble ALS are treatable (Table 195-2); therefore all pts should have a careful search for these disorders.

MRI or CT-myelography is often required to exclude compressive lesions of the foramen magnum or cervical spine. When involvement is restricted to lower motor neurons only, another important entity is multifocal motor neuropathy with conduction block (MMCB). A diffuse, lower motor axonal neuropathy mimicking ALS sometimes evolves in association with hematopoietic disorders such as lymphoma or multiple myeloma; an M-component in serum should prompt consideration of a bone marrow biopsy. Lyme disease may also cause an axonal, lower motor neuropathy. Other treatable disorders that occasionally mimic ALS are chronic lead poisoning and thyrotoxicosis.

TABLE 195-2	ETIOLOGY AND INVESTIGATION OF MOTOR NEURON DISORDERS
Diagnostic Category	**Investigations**
Structural lesions	MRI scan of head (including fora-
Parasagittal or foramen magnum tumors	men magnum), cervical spine[a]
Cervical spondylosis	
Chiari malformation or syrinx	
Spinal cord arteriovenous malformation	
Infections	CSF exam, culture[a]
Bacterial—tetanus, Lyme	Lyme antibody titer[a]
Viral—poliomyelitis, herpes zoster	Antiviral antibody titers
Retroviral myelopathy	HTLV-I titers
Intoxications, physical agents	
Toxins—lead, aluminum, others	24-h urine for heavy metals[a]
Drugs—strychnine, phenytoin	Serum for lead level[a]
Electric shock, x-irradiation	
Immunologic mechanisms	Complete blood count[a]
Plasma cell dyscrasias	Sedimentation rate[a]
Autoimmune polyradiculoneuropathy	Protein immunoelectrophoresis[a]
Motor neuropathy with conduction	Anti-GM1 antibodies[a]
block	
Paraneoplastic	Anti-Hu antibody
Paracarcinomatous/lymphoma	MRI scan, bone marrow biopsy
Metabolic	
Hypoglycemia	Fasting blood sugar (FBS), routine
	chemistries including calcium[a]
Hyperparathyroidism	PTH, calcium, phosphate
Hyperthyroidism	Thyroid function[a]
Deficiency of folate, vitamin B_{12}, vitamin E	Vitamin B_{12}, vitamin E, folate levels[a]
Malabsorption	24-h stool fat, carotene,
	prothrombin time
Mitochondrial dysfunction	Fasting lactate, pyruvate, ammonia
	Consider mtDNA analysis
Hereditary biochemical disorders	
Superoxide dismutase 1 gene mutation	White blood cell DNA analysis
Androgen receptor defect (Kennedy's	Abnormal CAG insert in andro-
disease)	gen receptor gene
Hexosaminidase deficiency	Lysosomal enzyme screen
Infantile (α-glucosidase deficiency/	α-Glucosidase level
Pompe's disease)	
Hyperlipidemia	Lipid electrophoresis
Hyperglycinuria	Urine and serum amino acids
Methylcrotonylglycinuria	CSF amino acids

[a]Denotes studies that should be obtained in all cases.
Note: CSF, cerebrospinal fluid; HTLV, human T cell lymphotropic virus; PTH, parathyroid hormone.

Pulmonary function studies may aid in management of ventilation. Swallowing evaluation identifies those at risk for aspiration. Genetic testing is available for superoxide dismutase 1 (SOD1) (20% of FALS) and for rare mutations in other genes.

℞ Amyotrophic Lateral Sclerosis

There is no treatment capable of arresting the underlying pathologic process in ALS. The drug riluzole produces modest lengthening of survival; in one trial the survival rate at 18 months with riluzole (100 mg/d) was similar to placebo at 15 months. It may act by diminishing glutamate release and thereby decreasing excitotoxic neuronal cell death. Side effects of riluzole include nausea, dizziness, weight loss, and elevation of liver enzymes. Clinical trials of several other agents are in progress, including insulin-like growth factor (IGF-1), ceftriaxone, and antisense oligonucleotides (ASO) that diminish expression of mutant SOD1 protein in transgenic ALS mice and rats.

A variety of rehabilitative aids may substantially assist ALS patients. Footdrop splints facilitate ambulation, and finger extension splints can potentiate grip. Respiratory support may be life-sustaining. For pts electing against long-term ventilation by tracheostomy, positive-pressure ventilation by mouth or nose provides transient (several weeks) relief from hypercarbia and hypoxia. Also beneficial are respiratory devices that produce an artificial cough; these help to clear airways and prevent aspiration pneumonia. When bulbar disease prevents normal chewing and swallowing, gastrostomy is helpful in restoring normal nutrition and hydration. Speech synthesizers can augment speech when there is advanced bulbar palsy.

Web-based information on ALS is offered by the Muscular Dystrophy Association (*www.mdausa.org*) and the Amyotrophic Lateral Sclerosis Association (*www.alsa.org*).

For a more detailed discussion, see Brown RH Jr: Amyotrophic Lateral Sclerosis and Other Motor Neuron Diseases, Chap. 369, p. 2572, in HPIM-17.

196 Autonomic Nervous System Disorders

The autonomic nervous system (ANS) (Fig. 196-1) innervates the entire neuraxis and permeates all organ systems. It regulates blood pressure (bp), heart rate, sleep, and bladder and bowel function. It operates automatically, so that its full importance becomes recognized only when ANS function is compromised, resulting in dysautonomia.

Key features of the ANS are summarized in Table 196-1. Responses to sympathetic or parasympathetic activation often have opposite effects; partial activation of both systems allows for simultaneous integration of multiple body functions.

Consider disorders of autonomic function in the differential diagnosis of pts with impotence, bladder dysfunction (urinary frequency, hesitancy, or incontinence), diarrhea, constipation, impaired lacrimation, or altered sweating (hyperhidrosis or hypohidrosis).

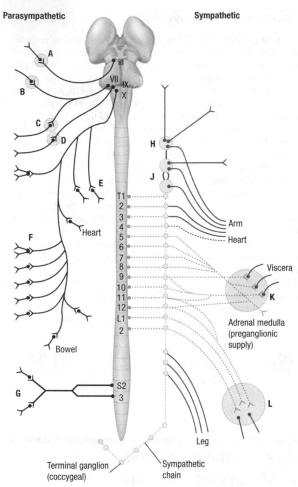

Parasympathetic

Sympathetic

Heart

Arm
Heart

Viscera

K

Adrenal medulla
(preganglionic
supply)

L

Bowel

Leg

Terminal ganglion
(coccygeal)

Sympathetic
chain

Parasympathetic system
from cranial nerves III, VII, IX, X
and from sacral nerves 2 and 3

A Ciliary ganglion
B Sphenopalatine
(pterygopalatine) ganglion
C Submandibular ganglion
D Otic ganglion
E Vagal ganglion cells
in the heart wall
F Vagal ganglion cells in
bowel wall
G Pelvic ganglia

Sympathetic system
from T1–L2
Preganglionic fibers   ··········
Postganglionic fibers   ————

H Superior cervical ganglion
J Middle cervical ganglion and
inferior cervical (stellate)
ganglion including T1
ganglion
K Coeliac and other
abdominal ganglia
L Lower abdominal
sympathetic ganglia

FIGURE 196-1 Schematic representation of the autonomic nervous system. (*From M. Moskowitz:
Clin Endocrinol Metab 6:77, 1977.*)

TABLE 196-1 FUNCTIONAL CONSEQUENCES OF NORMAL ANS ACTIVATION

	Sympathetic	Parasympathetic
Heart rate	Increased	Decreased
Blood pressure	Increased	Mildly decreased
Bladder	Increased sphincter tone	Voiding (decreased tone)
Bowel motility	Decreased motility	Increased
Lung	Bronchodilation	Bronchoconstriction
Sweat glands	Sweating	—
Pupils	Dilation	Constriction
Adrenal glands	Catecholamine release	—
Sexual function	Ejaculation, orgasm	Erection
Lacrimal glands	—	Tearing
Parotid glands	—	Salivation

Orthostatic hypotension (OH) is perhaps the most disabling feature of autonomic dysfunction. Syncope results when the drop in bp impairs cerebral perfusion (Chap. 39). Other manifestations of impaired baroreflexes are supine hypertension, a heart rate that is fixed regardless of posture, postprandial hypotension, and an excessively high nocturnal bp. Many patients with OH have a preceding diagnosis of hypertension. The most common causes of OH are not neurologic in origin; these must be distinguished from the neurogenic causes.

APPROACH TO THE PATIENT WITH AUTONOMIC NERVOUS SYSTEM DISORDERS

The first step in the evaluation of symptomatic OH is the exclusion of treatable causes. The history should include a review of medications that may cause OH (e.g., diuretics, antihypertensives, antidepressants, phenothiazines, ethanol, narcotics, insulin, dopamine agonists, barbiturates, and calcium channel blocking agents); the precipitation of OH by medications may also be the first sign of an underlying autonomic disorder. The history may reveal an underlying cause for symptoms (e.g., diabetes, Parkinson's disease) or specific underlying mechanisms (e.g., cardiac pump failure, reduced intravascular volume). The relationship of symptoms to meals (splanchnic pooling), standing on awakening in the morning (intravascular volume depletion), ambient warming (vasodilatation), or exercise (muscle arteriolar vasodilatation) should be sought.

Physical exam includes measurement of supine and standing pulse and bp. OH is defined as a sustained drop in systolic ($\geq$20 mmHg) or diastolic ($\geq$10 mmHg) bp within 3 min of standing up. In nonneurogenic causes of OH (such as hypovolemia), the bp drop is accompanied by a compensatory increase in heart rate of >15 beats/min. A clue to neurogenic OH is aggravation or precipitation of OH by autonomic stressors (such as a meal, hot tub/hot bath, and exercise). Neurologic evaluation should include a mental status exam (to exclude neurodegenerative disorders), cranial nerve exam (impaired downgaze in progressive supranuclear palsy), pupils (Horner's or Adie's pupils), motor tone (Parkinson's), and sensory exam (polyneuropathies). In pts without a clear initial diagnosis, follow-up exams and laboratory evaluations over 1 to 2 years may reveal the underlying cause.

Autonomic Testing

Autonomic function tests are helpful when the history and physical exam findings are inconclusive. Heart rate variation with deep breathing is a measure of vagal function. The Valsalva maneuver measures changes in heart rate and bp while a constant expiratory pressure of 40 mmHg is maintained for 15 s. The Valsalva ratio is the maximum heart rate during the maneuver divided by the minimum heart rate following the maneuver; the ratio reflects cardiovagal function. Tilt-table beat-to-beat bp measurements in the supine, 70° tilt, and tilt-back positions can be used to evaluate orthostatic failure in bp control in pts with unexplained syncope. Most pts with syncope do not have autonomic failure; the tilt-table test can be used to diagnose vasovagal syncope with high sensitivity, specificity, and reproducibility.

Other tests of autonomic function include the quantitative sudomotor axon reflex test (QSART) and the thermoregulatory sweat test (TST). The QSART provides quantitative measure of regional autonomic function mediated by ACh-induced sweating. The TST provides a qualitative measure of sweating in response to a standardized elevation of body temperature. For a more complete discussion of autonomic function tests, see Chap. 370, HPIM-17.

DISORDERS OF THE AUTONOMIC NERVOUS SYSTEM

Autonomic disorders may occur with a large number of disorders of the central and/or peripheral nervous systems (Table 196-2). Diseases of the CNS may cause ANS dysfunction at many levels, including hypothalamus, brainstem, or spinal cord.

Multiple system atrophy (MSA) is a progressive neurodegenerative disorder comprising autonomic failure (OH and/or a neurogenic bladder are required for diagnosis) combined with either parkinsonism (MSA-p) or cerebellar signs (MSA-c), often along with progressive cognitive dysfunction. Dysautonomia is also common in advanced Parkinson's disease (Chap. 193).

Spinal cord injury may be accompanied by autonomic hyperreflexia affecting bowel, bladder, sexual, temperature-regulation, or cardiovascular functions. Dangerous increases or decreases in body temperature may result from the inability to experience the sensory accompaniments of heat or cold exposure below the level of the injury. Markedly increased autonomic discharge (autonomic dysreflexia) can be elicited by stimulation of the bladder, skin, or muscles. Bladder distention from palpation, catheter insertion, catheter obstruction, or urinary infection is a common and correctable trigger of autonomic dysreflexia.

Peripheral neuropathies affecting the small myelinated and unmyelinated fibers of the sympathetic and parasympathetic nerves are the most common cause of chronic autonomic insufficiency (Chap. 203). Autonomic involvement in *diabetes mellitus* typically begins ~10 years after the onset of diabetes and slowly progresses. Diabetic enteric neuropathy may result in gastroparesis, nausea and vomiting, malnutrition, achlorhydria, and bowel incontinence. Impotence, urinary incontinence, pupillary abnormalities, and OH may occur as well. Prolongation of the QT interval increases the risk of sudden death. Autonomic neuropathy occurs in both sporadic and familial forms of *amyloidosis*. Pts typically present with distal, painful polyneuropathy. *Alcoholic polyneuropathy* produces symptoms of autonomic failure only when the neuropathy is severe. Attacks of *acute intermittent porphyria* (AIP) are associated with tachycardia, sweating, urinary retention, and hypertension. Blood pressure fluctuation and cardiac arrhythmias can be severe in *Guillain-Barré syndrome*. Autoimmune au-

TABLE 196-2 **CLASSIFICATION OF CLINICAL AUTONOMIC DISORDERS**

I. Autonomic disorders with brain involvement
   A. Associated with multisystem degeneration
      1. Multisystem degeneration: autonomic failure clinically prominent
         a. Multiple system atrophy (MSA)
         b. Parkinson's disease with autonomic failure
         c. Diffuse Lewy body disease (some cases)
      2. Multisystem degeneration: autonomic failure clinically not usually prominent
         a. Parkinson's disease
         b. Other extrapyramidal disorders (inherited spinocerebellar atrophies, progressive supranuclear palsy, corticobasal degeneration, Machado-Joseph disease)
   B. Unassociated with multisystem degeneration
      1. Disorders mainly due to cerebral cortex involvement
         a. Frontal cortex lesions causing urinary/bowel incontinence
         b. Partial complex seizures
      2. Disorders of the limbic and paralimbic circuits
         a. Shapiro's syndrome (agenesis of corpus callosum, hyperhidrosis, hypothermia)
         b. Autonomic seizures
      3. Disorders of the hypothalamus
         a. Wernicke-Korsakoff syndrome
         b. Diencephalic syndrome
         c. Neuroleptic malignant syndrome
         d. Serotonin syndrome
         e. Fatal familial insomnia
         f. Antidiuretic hormone (ADH) syndromes (diabetes insipidus, inappropriate ADH)
         g. Disturbances of temperature regulation (hyperthermia, hypothermia)
         h. Disturbances of sexual function
         i. Disturbances of appetite
         j. Disturbances of BP/HR and gastric function
         k. Horner's syndrome
      4. Disorders of the brainstem and cerebellum
         a. Posterior fossa tumors
         b. Syringobulbia and Arnold-Chiari malformation
         c. Disorders of BP control (hypertension, hypotension)
         d. Cardiac arrhythmias
         e. Central sleep apnea
         f. Baroreflex failure
         g. Horner's syndrome
II. Autonomic disorders with spinal cord involvement
   A. Traumatic quadriplegia
   B. Syringomyelia
   C. Subacute combined degeneration
   D. Multiple sclerosis
   E. Amyotrophic lateral sclerosis
   F. Tetanus
   G. Stiff-man syndrome
   H. Spinal cord tumors

(continued)

TABLE 196-2	CLASSIFICATION OF CLINICAL AUTONOMIC DISORDERS (CONTINUED)

III. Autonomic neuropathies
   A. Acute/subacute autonomic neuropathies
      1. Subacute autoimmune autonomic neuropathy (panautonomic neuropathy, pandysautonomia)
         a. Subacute paraneoplastic autonomic neuropathy
         b. Guillain-Barré syndrome
         c. Botulism
         d. Porphyria
         e. Drug induced autonomic neuropathies
         f. Toxic autonomic neuropathies
   B. Chronic peripheral autonomic neuropathies
      1. Distal small fiber neuropathy
      2. Combined sympathetic and parasympathetic failure
         a. Amyloid
         b. Diabetic autonomic neuropathy
         c. Autoimmune autonomic neuropathy (paraneoplastic and idiopathic)
         d. Sensory neuronopathy with autonomic failure
         e. Familial dysautonomia (Riley-Day syndrome)

Note: BP, blood pressure; HR, heart rate.

tonomic neuropathy presents as the subacute development of autonomic failure featuring OH, enteric neuropathy (gastroparesis, ileus, constipation/diarrhea), loss of sweating, sicca complex, and a tonic pupil. Onset may follow a viral infection; serum antibodies to the ganglionic ACh receptor (A_3 AChR) are diagnostic, and some pts appear to respond to immunotherapy. Rare patients develop *dysautonomia* as a paraneoplastic disorder (Chap. 82). There are five known hereditary sensory and autonomic neuropathies (*HSAN I–V*).

Botulism is associated with blurred vision, dry mouth, nausea, unreactive pupils, urinary retention, and constipation. *Postural orthostatic tachycardia syndrome* (POTS) presents with symptoms of orthostatic intolerance (not OH), including shortness of breath, light-headedness, and exercise intolerance accompanied by an increase in heart rate but no drop in bp. *Primary hyperhidrosis* affects 0.6–1.0% of the population; the usual symptoms are excessive sweating of the palms and soles. Onset is in adolescence, and symptoms tend to improve with age. Although not dangerous, this condition is socially embarrassing; treatment with either sympathectomy or local injection of botulinum toxin is often effective.

COMPLEX REGIONAL PAIN SYNDROME (REFLEX SYMPATHETIC DYSTROPHY—RSD)

Complex regional pain syndrome (CRPS) type I is a regional pain syndrome that usually develops after tissue trauma. *Allodynia* (the perception of a nonpainful stimulus as painful), *hyperpathia* (an exaggerated pain response to a painful stimulus), and *spontaneous pain* occur. The symptoms are unrelated to the severity of the initial trauma and are not confined to the distribution of a single peripheral nerve. CRPS type II is a regional pain syndrome that develops after injury to a peripheral nerve, usually a major nerve trunk. Spontaneous pain initially develops within the territory of the affected nerve but eventually may spread outside the nerve distribution.

TABLE 196-3 **INITIAL TREATMENT OF ORTHOSTATIC HYPOTENSION (OH)**

Patient education: mechanisms and stressors of OH
High-salt diet (10–20 g/d)
High-fluid intake (2 L/D)
Elevate head of bed 10 cm (4 in.)
Maintain postural stimuli
Learn physical countermaneuvers
Compression garments
Correct anemia

Early mobilization with physical therapy or a brief course of glucocorticoids may be helpful for CRPS type I. Other treatments include the use of adrenergic blockers, NSAIDs, calcium channel blockers, phenytoin, opioids, and calcitonin. Stellate ganglion blockade is a commonly used invasive therapeutic technique that often provides temporary pain relief, but the efficacy of repetitive blocks is uncertain.

R_X Autonomic Nervous System Disorders

Of particular importance is the removal of drugs or amelioration of underlying conditions that cause or aggravate the autonomic symptom. For instance, OH can be related to angiotensin-converting enzyme inhibitors, calcium channel blocking agents, tricyclic antidepressants, levodopa, alcohol, or insulin. Nonpharmacologic approaches are summarized in Table 196-3. Adequate intake of salt and fluids to produce a voiding volume between 1.5 and 2.5 L of urine (containing >170 meq of Na^+) each 24 h is essential. Sleeping with the head of the bed elevated will minimize the effects of supine nocturnal hypertension. Prolonged recumbency should be avoided. Pts are advised to sit with legs dangling over the edge of the bed for several minutes before attempting to stand in the morning. Compressive garments such as compression stockings and abdominal binders may be helpful if they can be tolerated. Anemia should be corrected, if necessary, with erythropoietin; the increased intravascular volume that accompanies the rise in hematocrit can exacerbate supine hypertension. Postprandial OH may respond to frequent, small, low-carbohydrate meals.

If these measures are not sufficient, drug treatment might be necessary. Midodrine is a directly acting α_1 agonist that does not cross the blood-brain barrier. The dose is 5–10 mg orally three times a day, but some pts respond best to a decremental dose (e.g., 15 mg on awakening, 10 mg at noon, and 5 mg in the afternoon). Midodrine should not be taken after 6 P.M. Side effects include pruritus, uncomfortable piloerection, and supine hypertension. Pyridostigmine appears to improve OH without aggravating supine hypertension by enhancing ganglionic transmission (maximal when orthostatic, minimal supine). Fludrocortisone (0.1–0.3 mg PO twice daily) will reduce OH, but it aggravates supine hypertension. Susceptible patients may develop fluid overload, congestive heart failure, supine hypertension, or hypokalemia.

For a more detailed discussion, see Low PA, Engstrom JW: Disorders of the Autonomic Nervous System, Chap. 370, p. 2576, in HPIM-17.

197 Trigeminal Neuralgia, Bell's Palsy, and Other Cranial Nerve Disorders

Disorders of vision and ocular movement are discussed in Chaps. 41 and 61; dizziness and vertigo in Chap. 40; and disorders of hearing in Chap. 61.

FACIAL PAIN OR NUMBNESS [TRIGEMINAL NERVE (V)]

(See Fig. 197-1)

Trigeminal Neuralgia (Tic Douloureux) Frequent, excruciating paroxysms of pain in lips, gums, cheek, or chin (rarely in ophthalmic division of fifth nerve) lasting seconds to minutes. Typically presents in middle or old age. Pain is often stimulated at trigger points. Sensory deficit cannot be demonstrated. Must be distinguished from other forms of facial pain arising from diseases of jaw, teeth, or sinuses. Rare causes are herpes zoster or a tumor. Onset in young adulthood or if bilateral raises the possibility of multiple sclerosis (Chap. 200).

℞ Trigeminal Neuralgia

Carbamazepine is effective in 50–75% of cases. Begin at 100 mg single daily dose taken with food and advance by 100 mg every 1–2 days until substantial (50%) pain relief occurs. Most pts require 200 mg four times a day; doses > 1200 mg daily usually provide no additional benefit. For nonresponders, phenytoin (300–400 mg/d) or baclofen (5–20 mg three to four times a day) can be tried. When medications fail, surgical lesions (heat or gamma

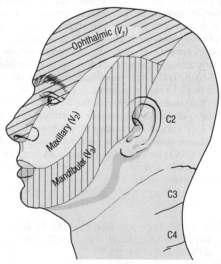

FIGURE 197-1 The three major sensory divisions of the trigeminal nerve consist of the ophthalmic, maxillary, and mandibular nerves.

knife radiosurgery) can be effective; in some centers, microvascular decompression recommended if a tortuous blood vessel is found in posterior fossa near trigeminal nerve.

Trigeminal Neuropathy   Usually presents as facial sensory loss or weakness of jaw muscles. Causes are varied (Table 197-1), including tumors of middle cranial fossa or trigeminal nerve, metastases to base of skull, or lesions in cavernous sinus (affecting first and second divisions of fifth nerve) or superior orbital fissure (affecting first division of fifth nerve).

FACIAL WEAKNESS [FACIAL NERVE (VII)]   (See Figure 197-2)

Look for hemifacial weakness that includes muscles of forehead and orbicularis oculi. If lesion is in middle ear portion, taste is lost over the anterior two-thirds of tongue and there may be hyperacusis; if lesion is at internal auditory meatus, there may be involvement of auditory and vestibular nerves; pontine lesions usually affect abducens nerve and often corticospinal tract. Peripheral nerve lesions with incomplete recovery may produce continuous contractions of affected musculature (*facial myokymia*); contraction of all facial muscles on attempts to move one group selectively (*synkinesis*); hemifacial spasms; or anomalous tears when facial muscles activated as in eating (*crocodile tears*).

Bell's Palsy   Most common form of idiopathic facial paralysis; affects 1 in 60 persons over a lifetime. Association with herpes simplex virus type 1. Weakness evolves over 12–48 h, sometimes preceded by retroaural pain. Hyperacusis may be present. Full recovery within several weeks or months in 80%; incomplete paralysis in first week is the most favorable prognostic sign.

Diagnosis can be made clinically in pts with (1) a typical presentation, (2) no risk factors or preexisting symptoms for other causes of facial paralysis, (3) no lesions of herpes zoster in the external ear canal, and (4) a normal neurologic examination with the exception of the facial nerve. In uncertain cases, an ESR, testing for diabetes mellitus, a Lyme titer, angiotensin-converting enzyme level, and chest x-ray for possible sarcoidosis, a lumbar puncture for possible Guillain-Barré syndrome, or MRI scanning may be indicated.

TABLE 197-1   TRIGEMINAL NERVE DISORDERS

Nuclear (brainstem) lesions	Peripheral nerve lesions
Multiple sclerosis	Nasopharyngeal carcinoma
Stroke	Trauma
Syringobulbia	Guillain-Barré syndrome
Glioma	Sjögren's syndrome
Lymphoma	Collagen-vascular diseases
Preganglionic lesions	Sarcoidosis
Acoustic neuroma	Leprosy
Meningioma	Drugs (stilbamidine, trichloroethylene)
Metastasis	Idiopathic trigeminal neuropathy
Chronic meningitis	
Cavernous carotid aneurysm	
Gasserian ganglion lesions	
Trigeminal neuroma	
Herpes zoster	
Infection (spread from otitis media or mastoiditis)	

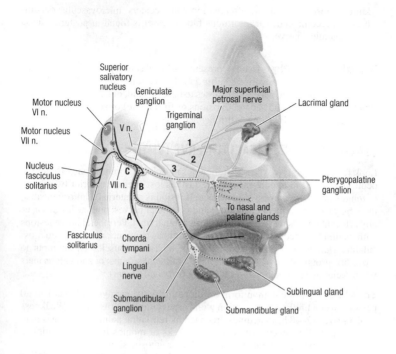

FIGURE 197-2 The facial nerve. A, B, and C denote lesions of the facial nerve at the stylomastoid foramen, distal and proximal to the geniculate ganglion, respectively. Green lines indicate the parasympathetic fibers, red lines indicate motor fibers, and purple lines indicate visceral afferent fibers (taste).

℞ Bell's Palsy

Protect the eye with paper tape to depress the upper eyelid during sleep. Prednisone (60–80 mg/d over 5 days, tapered off over the next 5 days) when started early appears to shorten the recovery period and modestly improve functional outcome. A recently published trial found no added benefit of acyclovir compared to prednisolone alone; the value of valacyclovir (usual dose 1000 mg/d for 5–7 days) is not known.

Other Facial Nerve Disorders *Ramsay Hunt syndrome* is caused by herpes zoster infection of geniculate ganglion; distinguished from Bell's palsy by a vesicular eruption in pharynx and external auditory canal, and by frequent involvement of eighth cranial nerve. *Acoustic neuromas* often compress the seventh nerve. *Infarcts, demyelinating lesions of multiple sclerosis,* and *tumors* are common pontine causes. *Bilateral facial weakness* may occur in Guillain-Barré syndrome, sarcoidosis, Lyme disease, and leprosy. *Hemifacial spasm* may occur with Bell's palsy, irritative lesions (e.g., acoustic neuroma, basilar artery aneurysm, an aberrant vessel compressing the nerve), or as an idiopathic disorder. *Blepharospasm* consists of involuntary recurrent spasms of both eyelids, usually occurring in the elderly and sometimes with associated facial spasm. May subside spontaneously. Hemifacial spasm or blepharospasm can be treated by injection of botulinum toxin into the orbicularis oculi.

OTHER CRANIAL NERVE DISORDERS

Disorders of the Sense of Smell   Olfactory nerve (I) disorders are due to interference with access of the odorant to the olfactory neuroepithelium (transport loss), injury to receptor region (sensory loss), or damage to central olfactory pathways (neural loss). The causes of olfactory disorders are summarized in Table 197-2); most common are head trauma in young adults and viral infections in older adults. More than half of people over age 60 suffer from olfactory dysfunction that is idiopathic (*presbyosmia*). Patients often present with a complaint of loss of the sense of taste even though their taste thresholds may be within normal limits.

Rx Disorders of the Sense of Smell

Therapy for allergic rhinitis, bacterial rhinitis and sinusitis, polyps, neoplasms, and structural abnormalities of the nasal cavities is usually successful in restoring the sense of smell. There is no proven treatment for sensorineural olfactory losses; fortunately, spontaneous recovery often occurs. Cases due to exposure to cigarette smoke and other airborne toxic chemicals can recover if the insult is discontinued.

Glossopharyngeal Neuralgia   This form of neuralgia involves the ninth (glossopharyngeal) and sometimes portions of the tenth (vagus) cranial nerves. Paroxysmal, intense pain in tonsillar fossa of throat that may be precipitated by swallowing. There is no demonstrable sensory and motor deficit. Other diseases affecting this nerve include herpes zoster or compressive neuropathy due to tumor or aneurysm in region of jugular foramen (when associated with vagus and accessory nerve palsies).

TABLE 197-2   CAUSES OF OLFACTORY DYSFUNCTION

Transport Losses	Neural Losses
Allergic rhinitis	AIDS
Bacterial rhinitis and sinusitis	Alcoholism
Congenital abnormalities	Alzheimer's disease
Nasal neoplasms	Cigarette smoke
Nasal polyps	Depression
Nasal septal deviation	Diabetes mellitus
Nasal surgery	Drugs/toxins
Viral infections	Huntington's chorea
Sensory Losses	Hypothyroidism
Drugs	Kallmann's syndrome
Neoplasms	Malnutrition
Radiation therapy	Neoplasms
Toxin exposure	Neurosurgery
Viral infections	Parkinson's disease
	Trauma
	Vitamin B_{12} deficiency
	Zinc deficiency

℞ Glossopharyngeal Neuralgia

Medical therapy is similar to that for trigeminal neuralgia, and carbamazepine is generally the first choice. If drug therapy is unsuccessful, surgical procedures (including microvascular decompression, if vascular compression is evident, or rhizotomy of glossopharyngeal and vagal fibers in the jugular bulb) are frequently successful.

Dysphagia and Dysphonia Lesions of the vagus nerve (X) may be responsible. Unilateral lesions produce drooping of soft palate, loss of gag reflex, and "curtain movement" of lateral wall of pharynx with hoarse, nasal voice. Etiologies include neoplastic and infectious processes of the meninges, tumors and vascular lesions in the medulla, motor neuron disease (e.g., ALS), or compression of the recurrent laryngeal nerve by intrathoracic processes. Aneurysm of the aortic arch, an enlarged left atrium, and tumors of the mediastinum and bronchi are much more frequent causes of an isolated vocal cord palsy than are intracranial disorders. A substantial number of cases of recurrent laryngeal palsy remain idiopathic.

With laryngeal palsy, first determine the site of the lesion. If intramedullary, there are usually other brainstem signs. If extramedullary, the glossopharyngeal (IX) and spinal accessory (XI) nerves are frequently involved (jugular foramen syndrome). If extracranial in the retroparotid space, there may be combinations of ninth, tenth, eleventh, and twelfth cranial nerve palsies and a Horner syndrome. If there is no sensory loss over the palate and pharynx and no palatal weakness or dysphagia, lesion is below the origin of the pharyngeal branches, which leave the vagus nerve high in the cervical region; the usual site of disease is then the mediastinum.

Neck Weakness Isolated involvement of the accessory (XI) nerve can occur anywhere along its route, resulting in paralysis of the sternocleidomastoid and trapezius muscles. More commonly, involvement occurs in combination with deficits of the ninth and tenth cranial nerves in the jugular foramen or after exit from the skull. An idiopathic form of accessory neuropathy, akin to Bell's palsy, has been described; most pts recover.

Tongue Paralysis The hypoglossal (XII) nerve supplies the ipsilateral muscles of the tongue. The nucleus of the nerve or its fibers of exit may be involved by intramedullary lesions such as tumor, poliomyelitis, or most often motor neuron disease. Lesions of the basal meninges and the occipital bones (platybasia, invagination of occipital condyles, Paget's disease) may compress the nerve in its extramedullary course or in the hypoglossal canal. Isolated lesions of unknown cause can occur. Atrophy and fasciculation of the tongue develop weeks to months after interruption of the nerve.

MULTIPLE CRANIAL NERVE PALSIES

APPROACH TO THE PATIENT WITH MULTIPLE CRANIAL NERVE PALSIES

First determine whether the process is within the brainstem or outside it. Lesions on the surface of the brainstem tend to involve adjacent cranial nerves in succession with only late and slight involvement of long sensory and motor pathways. The opposite is true of processes within the brainstem. In-

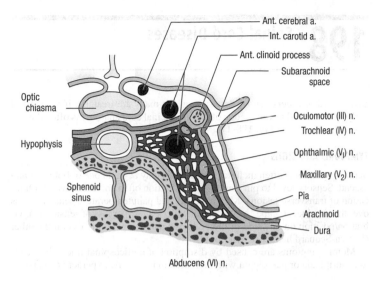

FIGURE 197-3 Anatomy of the cavernous sinus in coronal section, illustrating the location of the cranial nerves in relation to the vascular sinus, internal carotid artery (which loops anteriorly to the section), and surrounding structures.

volvement of multiple cranial nerves outside of the brainstem may be due to diabetes, trauma, infectious and noninfectious (especially carcinomatous) causes of meningitis; granulomatous diseases including sarcoidosis, tuberculosis, and Wegener's granulomatosis; tumors; and enlarging saccular aneurysms. A purely motor disorder without atrophy raises a question of myasthenia gravis. *Facial diplegia* is common in Guillain-Barré syndrome. *Ophthalmoplegia* may occur with Guillain-Barré syndrome (Fisher variant) or Wernicke's disease.

The *cavernous sinus syndrome* (Fig. 197-3) is frequently life-threatening. It often presents as orbital or facial pain; orbital swelling and chemosis; fever; oculomotor neuropathy; and trigeminal neuropathy affecting the ophthalmic (V_1) and occasionally maxillary (V_2) divisions. Cavernous sinus thrombosis, often secondary to infection from orbital cellulitis or sinusitis, is the most frequent cause; other etiologies include aneurysm of the carotid artery, a carotid-cavernous fistula (orbital bruit may be present), meningioma, nasopharyngeal carcinoma, other tumors, or an idiopathic granulomatous disorder (Tolosa-Hunt syndrome). In infectious cases, prompt administration of broad-spectrum antibiotics, drainage of any abscess cavities, and identification of the offending organism is essential. Anticoagulant therapy may benefit cases of primary thrombosis. Repair or occlusion of the carotid artery may be required for treatment of fistulas or aneurysms. The Tolosa-Hunt syndrome generally responds to glucocorticoids.

For a more detailed discussion, see Beal MF, Hauser SL: Trigeminal Neuralgia, Bell's Palsy, and Other Cranial Nerve Disorders, Chap. 371, p. 2583; and Lalwani AK: Disorders of Smell, Taste, and Hearing, Chap. 30, p. 196, in HPIM-17.

198 Spinal Cord Diseases

Spinal cord disorders can be devastating, but many are treatable if recognized early (**Table 198-1**). Knowledge of relevant spinal cord anatomy is often the key to correct diagnosis (**Fig. 198-1**).

SYMPTOMS AND SIGNS

Sensory symptoms often include paresthesias; may begin in one or both feet and ascend. Sensory level to pin sensation or vibration often correlates well with location of transverse lesions. May have isolated pain/temperature sensation loss over the shoulders ("cape" or "syringomyelic" pattern) or loss of sensation to vibration/position on one side of the body and pain/temperature loss on the other (Brown-Séquard hemicord syndrome).

Motor symptoms are caused by disruption of corticospinal tracts that leads to quadriplegia or paraplegia with increased muscle tone, hyperactive deep ten-

---

TABLE 198-1 **TREATABLE SPINAL CORD DISORDERS**

Compressive
Epidural, intradural, or intramedullary neoplasm
Epidural abscess
Epidural hemorrhage
Cervical spondylosis
Herniated disc
Posttraumatic compression by fractured or displaced vertebra or hemorrhage
Vascular
Arteriovenous malformation
Antiphospholipid syndrome and other hypercoagulable states
Inflammatory
Multiple sclerosis
Neuromyelitis optica
Transverse myelitis
Sarcoidosis
Vasculitis
Infectious
Viral: VZV, HSV-1 and -2, CMV, HIV, HTLV-I, others
Bacterial and mycobacterial: *Borrelia*, *Listeria*, syphilis, others
Mycoplasma pneumoniae
Parasitic: schistosomiasis, toxoplasmosis
Developmental
Syringomyelia
Meningomyelocoele
Tethered cord syndrome
Metabolic
Vitamin B$_{12}$ deficiency (subacute combined degeneration)
Copper deficiency

Note: VZV, varicella-zoster virus; HSV, herpes simplex virus; CMV, cytomegalovirus; HTLV, human T cell lymphotropic virus.

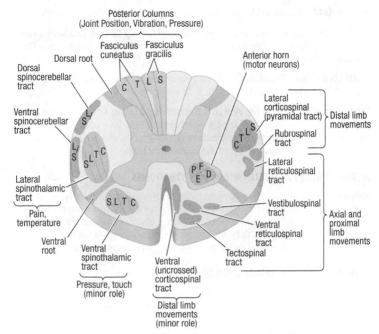

FIGURE 198-1 Transverse section through the spinal cord, composite representation, illustrating the principal ascending (*left*) and descending (*right*) pathways. The lateral and ventral spinothalamic tracts ascend contralateral to the side of the body that is innervated. C, cervical; T, thoracic; L, lumbar; S, sacral; P, proximal; D, distal; F, flexors; E, extensors.

don reflexes, and extensor plantar responses. With acute severe lesions there may be initial flaccidity and areflexia (spinal shock).

Autonomic dysfunction includes primarily urinary retention; should raise suspicion of spinal cord disease when associated with back or neck pain, weakness, and/or a sensory level.

Pain may be present. Midline back pain is of localizing value; interscapular pain may be first sign of midthoracic cord compression; radicular pain may mark site of more laterally placed spinal lesion; pain from lower cord (conus medullaris) lesion may be referred to low back.

SPECIFIC SIGNS BY SPINAL CORD LEVEL

Approximate indicators of level of lesion include the location of a sensory level, a band of hyperalgesia/hyperpathia at the upper end of the sensory disturbance, identification of isolated atrophy or fasciculations, or lost tendon reflex at a specific spinal cord segment.

Lesions Near the Foramen Magnum   Weakness of the ipsilateral shoulder and arm, followed by weakness of ipsilateral leg, then contralateral leg, then contralateral arm, with respiratory paralysis.

Cervical Cord   Best localized by noting pattern of motor weakness and areflexia; shoulder (C5), biceps (C5-6), brachioradialis (C6), triceps/finger and wrist extensors (C7), finger flexors (C8).

Thoracic Cord Localized by identification of a sensory level on the trunk.

Lumbar Cord Upper lumbar cord lesions paralyze hip flexion and knee extension, whereas lower lumbar lesions affect foot and ankle movements, knee flexion, and thigh extension.

Sacral Cord (Conus Medullaris) Saddle anesthesia, early bladder/bowel dysfunction, impotence; muscle strength is largely preserved.

Cauda Equina (Cluster of Nerve Roots Derived from Lower Cord) Lesions below spinal cord termination at the L1 vertebral level produce a flaccid, areflexic, asymmetric paraparesis with bladder/bowel dysfunction and sensory loss below L1; pain is common and projected to perineum or thighs.

INTRAMEDULLARY AND EXTRAMEDULLARY SYNDROMES

Spinal cord disorders may be intramedullary (arising from within the substance of the cord) or extramedullary (compressing the cord or its blood supply). Extramedullary lesions often produce radicular pain, early corticospinal signs, and sacral sensory loss. Intramedullary lesions produce poorly localized burning pain, less prominent corticospinal signs, and often spare perineal/sacral sensation.

ACUTE AND SUBACUTE SPINAL CORD DISEASES (See Chap. 21)

1. *Neoplastic spinal cord compression* (see Chap. 21): Most are epidural in origin, resulting from metastases to the adjacent spinal bones (Fig. 198-2). Almost any tumor can be responsible: breast, lung, prostate, lymphoma, and plasma cell dyscrasias most frequent. Thoracic cord most commonly involved. Initial symptom is usually back pain, worse when recumbent, with local tenderness preceding other symptoms by many weeks. Spinal cord compression due to metastases is a medical emergency; in general, therapy will not reverse paralysis of >48 h duration.

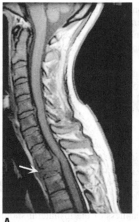
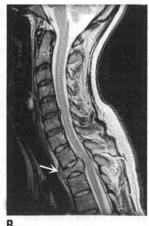

A **B**

FIGURE 198-2 Epidural spinal cord compression due to breast carcinoma. Sagittal T1-weighted (*A*) and T2-weighted (*B*) MRI scans through the cervicothoracic junction reveal an infiltrated and collapsed second thoracic vertebral body with posterior displacement and compression of the upper thoracic spinal cord. The low-intensity bone marrow signal in *A* signifies replacement by tumor.

2. *Spinal epidural abscess*: Triad of fever, localized spinal pain, and myelopathy (progressive weakness and bladder symptoms); once neurologic signs appear, cord compression rapidly progresses.
3. *Spinal epidural hematoma*: Presents as focal or radicular pain followed by variable signs of a spinal cord or cauda equina disorder.
4. *Acute disk herniation*: Cervical and thoracic disk herniations are less common than lumbar.
5. *Spinal cord infarction*: Anterior spinal artery infarction produces paraplegia or quadriplegia, sensory loss affecting pain/temperature but sparing vibration/position sensation (supplied by posterior spinal arteries), and loss of sphincter control. Onset sudden or evolving over minutes or a few hours. Associated conditions: aortic atherosclerosis, dissecting aortic aneurysm, hypotension. Therapy is directed at the predisposing condition.
6. *Immune-mediated myelopathies*: Acute transverse myelopathy (ATM) occurs in 1% of pts with SLE; associated with antiphospholipid antibodies. Sjögren's and Behçet's syndromes, mixed connective tissue disease, and p-ANCA vasculitis are other causes. Sarcoid can produce ATM with large edematous swelling of the spinal cord. Demyelinating diseases, either neuromyelitis optica (NMO) or multiple sclerosis, can also present as ATM; glucocorticoids, consisting of IV methylprednisolone followed by oral prednisone, are indicated for moderate to severe symptoms and refractory cases may respond to plasma exchange (Chap. 200). Treatment with anti-CD20 monoclonal Ab may protect against relapses in NMO. Other cases of ATM are idiopathic.
7. *Infectious myelopathies*: Herpes zoster is the most common viral agent, but herpes simplex virus types 1 and 2, EBV, CMV, and rabies virus are also well-described; in cases of suspected viral myelitis, antivirals may be appropriately started pending laboratory confirmation. Bacterial and mycobacterial causes are less common. Schistosomiasis is an important cause worldwide.

CHRONIC MYELOPATHIES

1. *Spondylitic myelopathies*: One of the most common causes of gait difficulty in the elderly. Presents as neck and shoulder pain with stiffness, radicular arm pain, and progressive spastic paraparesis with paresthesias and loss of vibration sense; in advanced cases, urinary incontinence may occur. A tendon reflex in the arms is often diminished at some level. Diagnosis is best made by MRI. Treatment is surgical (Chap. 36).
2. *Vascular malformations*: An important treatable cause of progressive or episodic myelopathy. May occur at any level; diagnosis is made by contrast-enhanced MRI (Fig 198-3) confirmed by selective spinal angiography. Treatment is embolization with occlusion of the major feeding vessels.
3. *Retrovirus-associated myelopathies*: Infection with HTLV-I may produce a slowly progressive spastic paraparesis with variable pain, sensory loss, and bladder disturbance; diagnosis is made by demonstration of specific serum antibody. Treatment is symptomatic. A progressive vacuolar myelopathy may also result from HIV infection.
4. *Syringomyelia*: Cavitary expansion of the spinal cord resulting in progressive myelopathy; may be an isolated finding or associated with protrusion of cerebellar tonsils into cervical spinal canal (Chiari type 1). Classic presentation is loss of pain/temperature sensation in the neck, shoulders, forearms, or hands with areflexic weakness in the upper limbs and progressive spastic paraparesis; cough headache, facial numbness, or thoracic kyphoscoliosis may occur. Diagnosis is made by MRI; treatment is surgical and often unsatisfactory.

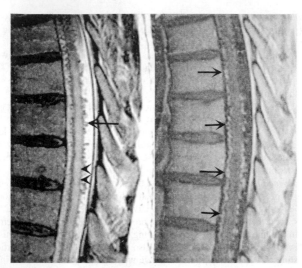

FIGURE 198-3 Arteriovenous malformation. Sagittal MR scans of the thoracic spinal cord: T2 fast spin-echo technique (*left*) and T1 post-contrast image (*right*). On the T2-weighted image (*left*), abnormally high signal intensity is noted in the central aspect of the spinal cord (*arrowheads*). Numerous punctate flow voids indent the dorsal and ventral spinal cord (*arrow*). These represent the abnormally dilated venous plexus supplied by the dural arteriovenous fistula. After contrast administration (*right*), multiple, serpentine, enhancing veins (*arrows*) on the ventral and dorsal aspect of the thoracic spinal cord are visualized, diagnostic of arteriovenous malformation. This patient was a 54-year-old man with a 4-year history of progressive paraparesis.

5. *Multiple sclerosis*: Spinal cord involvement is common, and is a major cause of disability in progressive forms of MS (Chap. 200).

6. *Subacute combined degeneration (vitamin B_{12} deficiency)*: Paresthesias in hands and feet, early loss of vibration/position sense, progressive spastic/ataxic weakness, and areflexia due to associated peripheral neuropathy; mental changes ("megaloblastic madness") and optic atrophy may be present along with a serum macrocytic anemia. Diagnosis is confirmed by a low serum B_{12} level, elevated levels of homocysteine and methylmalonic acid, and in uncertain cases, a positive Schilling test. Treatment is vitamin replacement.

7. *Hypocuric myelopathy*: Clinically nearly identical to subacute combined degeneration (above). Low levels of serum copper and usually ceruloplasmin make the diagnosis. Some cases idiopathic and others follow GI procedures that hinder absorption. Treatment is oral copper supplementation.

8. *Tabes dorsalis (tertiary syphilis)*: May present as lancinating pains, gait ataxia, bladder disturbances, and visceral crises. Cardinal signs are areflexia in the legs, impaired vibration/position sense, Romberg sign, and Argyll Robertson pupils, which fail to constrict to light but react to accommodation.

9. *Familial spastic paraplegia*: Progressive spasticity and weakness in the legs occurring on a familial basis; may be autosomal dominant, recessive, or X-linked. Over 20 different loci identified.

10. *Adrenomyeloneuropathy*: X-linked disorder that is a variant of adrenoleukodystrophy. Usually affected males have a history of adrenal insufficiency and then develop a progressive spastic paraparesis. Female heterozygotes may develop a slower progressive myelopathy without adrenal insufficiency. Diagnosis made by elevated very long chain fatty acids in serum. No

therapy is clearly effective although bone marrow transplantation and nutritional supplements have been tried.

COMPLICATIONS

Bladder dysfunction with risk of urinary tract infection; bowel dysmotility; pressure sores; in high cervical cord lesions, mechanical respiratory failure; paroxysmal hypertension or hypotension with volume changes; severe hypertension and bradycardia in response to noxious stimuli or bladder or bowel distention; venous thrombosis and pulmonary embolism.

For a more detailed discussion, see Hauser SL, Ropper AH: Diseases of the Spinal Cord, Chap. 372, p. 2588, in HPIM-17.

199 Tumors of the Nervous System

APPROACH TO THE PATIENT WITH TUMOR OF THE NERVOUS SYSTEM

Clinical Presentation

Brain tumors present with (1) progressive focal neurologic deficits, (2) seizures, or (3) "nonfocal" neurologic disorders (headache, dementia, personality change, gait disorder). Nonfocal disorders due to increased intracranial pressure (ICP), hydrocephalus, or diffuse tumor spread. Elevated ICP suggested by papilledema, impaired lateral gaze, headache that intensifies with recumbency. Stroke-like onset may reflect hemorrhage into tumor. Brain tumors may be large at presentation if located in clinically silent region (i.e., prefrontal) or slow-growing; diencephalic, frontal, or temporal lobe tumors may present as psychiatric disorder. Systemic symptoms (malaise, anorexia, weight loss, fever) suggest metastatic rather than primary brain tumor.

Evaluation

Primary brain tumors have no serologic features of malignancy such as an elevated ESR or tumor-specific antigens, unlike metastases. Neuroimaging (CT or MRI) reveals mass effect (volume of neoplasm and surrounding edema) and contrast enhancement (breakdown of blood-brain barrier). CSF exam is limited to diagnosis of possible meningitis or meningeal metastases but may cause brain herniation if mass effect or hydrocephalus present.

℞ Tumors of the Nervous System

Symptomatic Treatment

Glucocorticoids (dexamethasone 12–20 mg/d in divided doses PO or IV) to temporarily reduce edema; prophylaxis with anticonvulsants (phenytoin, carbamazepine, or valproic acid) for tumors involving cortex or hippocampus, although no good data support this practice. Low-dose subcutaneous heparin for immobile pts.

PRIMARY INTRACRANIAL TUMORS

Astrocytomas Most common primary intracranial neoplasm. Only known risk factors are ionizing radiation and uncommon hereditary syndromes (neurofibromatosis, tuberous sclerosis). Prognosis poor if age >65 years, poor baseline functional status, high-grade tumor. Difficult to treat; infiltration along white matter pathways prevents total resection. Imaging studies (Fig. 199-1) fail to indicate full tumor extent. Surgery for tissue diagnosis and to control mass effect; aggressive resection may correlate with survival, especially in younger pts. Mean survival ranges from 93 months for low-grade tumors to 5 months for high-grade tumors. Radiation therapy (RT) prolongs survival and improves quality of life. Systemic chemotherapy with temozolomide, an orally administered alkylating agent, is marginally effective, often employed as adjunct to RT for high-grade gliomas. An alternative approach to chemotherapy of high-grade gliomas is direct implantation of chemotherapy wafers into the resection cavity at the time of surgery. Role of stereotaxic radiosurgery (single dose, highly focused radiation—gamma knife) unclear; most useful for tumors <4 cm in diameter. Interstitial brachytherapy (stereotaxic implantation of radioactive beads) reserved for tumor recurrence; associated with necrosis of normal brain tissue. For low-grade astrocytoma, optimal management is uncertain; resection with or without RT most often employed.

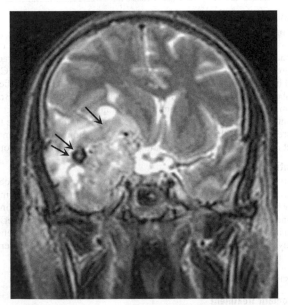

FIGURE 199-1 Malignant astrocytoma (glioblastoma). Coronal proton density–weighted MR scan through the temporal lobes demonstrates a heterogeneous right temporal lobe mass (*arrows*) compressing the third and lateral ventricles. The area of hypointense signal (*double arrows*) indicates either hemorrhage or calcification. Heterogeneous MR signal intensity is typical of glioblastoma.

Oligodendrogliomas Supratentorial, often with areas of calcification; some have a mixture of astrocytic and oligodendroglial cells. As oligodendroglial component increases in these mixed tumors, so does long-term survival. For low-grade, median survival is 7-8 years with a substantial number of pts with prolonged survival (>10 years). For high-grade tumors, median survival ~5 years. Total surgical resection often possible; chemotherapy response improved when deletions of chromosomes 1p and 19q present.

Ependymomas Derived from ependymal cells; highly cellular. Location—spinal canal more than intracranial in adults. If total excision possible, 5-year disease-free survival >80%; postoperative RT used if complete excision not possible.

Primitive Neuro-Ectodermal Tumors (PNET) Half in posterior fossa; highly cellular; derived from neural precursor cells. Treat with surgery and RT. Aggressive treatment can result in prolonged survival, although half of adult pts will relapse within 5 years of treatment.

Primary CNS Lymphomas B cell malignancy; most occur in immunosuppressed pts (organ transplantation, AIDS). May present as a single mass lesion (immunocompetent pts) or as multiple mass lesions or meningeal disease (immunosuppressed pts). Slit-lamp exam necessary to exclude ocular involvement. Prognosis generally poor. Dramatic, transient responses occur with glucocorticoids. In immunocompetent pts, chemotherapy (rituximab, high-dose methotrexate often along with other agents such as vincristine and procarbazine), and RT may increase survival to ≥3 years; AIDS-related cases survive ≤3 months.

Meningiomas Extraaxial mass attached to dura; dense and uniform contrast enhancement is diagnostic (Fig. 199-2). Total surgical resection of benign meningiomas is curative. With subtotal resection, local RT reduces recurrence to <10%. Small, asymptomatic meningiomas may be followed radiologically without surgery. Treat rare aggressive meningiomas with excision and RT.

Schwannomas Vestibular schwannomas present as progressive, unexplained unilateral hearing loss. MRI reveals dense, uniformly enhancing tumor at the cerebellopontine angle. Surgical excision may preserve hearing.

TUMORS METASTATIC TO THE NERVOUS SYSTEM

Hematogenous spread most common. Skull metastases rarely invade CNS; may compress adjacent brain or cranial nerves or obstruct intracranial venous sinuses. Primary tumors that commonly metastasize to the nervous system are listed in Table 199-1. Brain metastases are well demarcated by MRI and enhance with gadolinium. Ring enhancement is nonspecific; differential diagnosis includes brain abscess, radiation necrosis, toxoplasmosis, granulomas, tuberculosis, sarcoidosis, demyelinating lesions, primary brain tumors, CNS lymphoma, stroke, hemorrhage, and trauma. CSF cytology is unnecessary—intraparenchymal metastases rarely shed cells into CSF. One-third of pts presenting with brain metastasis have unknown primary (ultimately small cell lung cancer, melanoma most frequent); primary tumor never identified in 30%. Screen for occult cancer: examine skin and thyroid gland; blood carcinoembryonic antigen (CEA) and liver function tests; CT of chest, abdomen, and pelvis. Further imaging studies unhelpful if above studies negative. Biopsy of primary tumor or accessible brain metastasis is needed to plan treatment. Treatment is palliative—glucocorticoids, anticonvulsants, RT, or surgery may improve quality of life. Whole-brain RT is often given, because multiple microscopic tumor deposits are likely throughout the brain; stereotaxic radiosurgery is of benefit in pts with four or fewer metas-

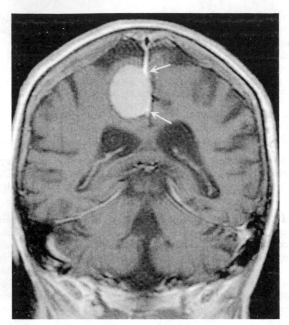

FIGURE 199-2 Meningioma. Coronal postcontrast T1-weighted MR image demonstrates an enhancing extraaxial mass arising from the falx cerebri (*arrows*). There is a "dural tail" of contrast enhancement extending superiorly along the intrahemispheric septum.

tases demonstrated by MRI. If a single metastasis is found, it may be surgically excised followed by whole-brain RT. Systemic chemotherapy may produce dramatic responses in isolated cases.

Leptomeningeal Metastases Presents as headache, encephalopathy, cranial nerve or polyradicular symptoms. Diagnosis by CSF cytology, MRI (nodular meningeal tumor deposits or diffuse meningeal enhancement), or meningeal biopsy. Associated with hydrocephalus due to CSF pathway obstruction. Aggressive treatment (intrathecal methotrexate, focal external beam RT) produces sustained response (≥6 months) in 20% of pts.

Spinal Cord Compression from Metastases (See Chap. 21) Expansion of vertebral body metastasis posteriorly into epidural space compresses cord. Most

TABLE 199-1 FREQUENCY OF NERVOUS SYSTEM METASTASES BY COMMON PRIMARY TUMORS

Site of Primary Tumor	Brain Metastases, %	Leptomeningeal Metastases, %	Spinal Cord Compression, %
Lung	40	24	18
Breast	19	41	24
Melanoma	10	12	4
Gastrointestinal tract	7	13	6
Genitourinary tract	7		18
Other	17	10	30

common primary tumors are lung, breast, or prostate primary. Back pain (>90%) precedes development of weakness, sensory level, or incontinence. Medical emergency; early recognition of impending spinal cord compression essential to avoid devastating sequelae. Diagnosis is by spine MRI.

COMPLICATIONS OF RADIATION THERAPY

Three patterns of radiation injury after CNS RT:

1. Acute—headache, sleepiness, worse neurologic deficits during or immediately after RT. Rarely seen with current protocols. Self-limited and improves with glucocorticoids.
2. Early delayed—somnolence (children), Lhermitte's sign; within 4 months of RT. Increased T2 signal on MRI. Also self-limited and improves with glucocorticoids.
3. Late delayed—dementia or other progressive neurologic deficits; typically 8–24 months after RT. White matter abnormalities on MRI; ring-enhancing mass due to radiation necrosis. Positron emission tomography (PET) can distinguish delayed necrosis from tumor recurrence. Progressive radiation necrosis is best treated palliatively with surgical resection. Radiation injury of large arteries accelerates the development of atherosclerosis, increasing the risk of stroke years after RT. Endocrine dysfunction due to hypothalamus or pituitary gland injury can be due to delayed effects of RT. Development of a second neoplasm after RT also is a risk years after exposure.

For a more detailed discussion, see Sagar SM, Israel MA: Primary and Metastic Tumors of the Nervous System, Chap. 374, p. 2601, in HPIM-17.

200 Multiple Sclerosis (MS)

Characterized by chronic inflammation and selective destruction of CNS myelin; peripheral nervous system is spared. Pathologically, the multifocal scarred lesions of MS are termed *plaques*. Etiology is thought to be autoimmune, with susceptibility determined by genetic and environmental factors. MS affects 350,000 Americans; onset is most often in early to middle adulthood, and women are affected approximately three times as often as men.

CLINICAL FEATURES

Onset may be abrupt or insidious. Some pts have symptoms that are so trivial that they may not seek medical attention for months or years. Most common are recurrent attacks of focal neurologic dysfunction, typically lasting weeks or months, and followed by variable recovery; some pts initially present with slowly progressive neurologic deterioration. Symptoms often transiently worsen with fatigue, stress, exercise, or heat. Manifestations of MS are protean but commonly include weakness and/or sensory symptoms involving a limb, visual difficulties, abnormalities of gait and coordination, urinary urgency or frequency, and abnormal fatigue. Motor involvement can present as a heavy, stiff, weak, or clumsy limb. Localized tingling, "pins and needles," and "dead" sensations are common. Optic neuritis can result in blurring of vision, especially in the central visual field, often with associated retroorbital pain accentuated by eye movement. Involvement of the brainstem may result in diplopia, nystagmus, vertigo, or facial pain, numbness, weakness, hemispasm, or myokymia (rippling muscular contractions). Ataxia, tremor, and dysarthria may reflect disease of cerebellar pathways. Lhermitte's symptom, a momentary electric shock–like sensation evoked by neck flexion, indicates disease in the cervical spinal cord. Diagnostic criteria are listed in Table 200-1; MS mimics are summarized in Table 200-2.

PHYSICAL EXAMINATION

Abnormal signs usually more widespread than expected from the history. Check for abnormalities in visual fields, loss of visual acuity, disturbed color perception, optic pallor or papillitis, afferent pupillary defect (paradoxical dilation to direct light following constriction to consensual light), nystagmus, internuclear

---

TABLE 200-1 DIAGNOSTIC CRITERIA FOR MS

1. Examination must reveal *objective* abnormalities of the CNS.
2. Involvement must reflect predominantly disease of white matter long tracts, usually including (a) pyramidal pathways, (b) cerebellar pathways, (c) medial longitudinal fasciculus, (d) optic nerve, and (e) posterior columns.
3. Examination or history must implicate involvement of two or more areas of the CNS.
   a. MRI may be used to document a second lesion when only one site of abnormality has been demonstrable on examination. A confirmatory MRI must have either four lesions involving the white matter or three lesions if one is periventricular in location. Acceptable lesions must be >3 mm in diameter. For patients older than 50 years, two of the following criteria must also be met: (a) lesion size >5 mm, (b) lesions adjacent to the bodies of the lateral ventricles, and (c) lesion(s) present in the posterior fossa.
   b. Evoked response testing may be used to document a second lesion not evident on clinical examination.
4. The clinical pattern must consist of (a) two or more separate episodes of worsening involving different sites of the CNS, each lasting at least 24 h and occurring at least 1 month apart, or (b) gradual or stepwise progression over at least 6 months if accompanied by increased IgG synthesis or two or more oligoclonal bands. MRI may be used to document dissemination in time if a new T2 lesion or a Gd-enhancing lesion is seen 3 or more months after a clinically isolated syndrome.
5. The patient's neurologic condition could not better be attributed to another disease.

Diagnostic Categories

---

1. *Definite MS*: All five criteria fulfilled.
2. *Probable MS*: All five criteria fulfilled except (a) only one objective abnormality despite two symptomatic episodes or (b) only one symptomatic episode despite two or more objective abnormalities.
3. *At risk for MS*: Criteria 1, 2, 3, and 5 fulfilled; patient has only one symptomatic episode and one objective abnormality.

Note: CNS, central nervous system; MRI, magnetic resonance imaging; Gd, gadolinium.

TABLE 200-2 DISORDERS THAT CAN MIMIC MS
Acute disseminated encephalomyelitis (ADEM)
Antiphospholipid antibody syndrome
Behçet's disease
Cerebral autosomal dominant arteriopathy, subcortical infarcts, and leukoencephalopathy (CADASIL)
Congenital leukodystrophies (e.g., adrenoleukodystrophy, metachromatic leukodystrophy)
Human immunodeficiency virus (HIV) infection
Ischemic optic neuropathy (arteritic and nonarteritic)
Lyme disease
Mitochondrial encephalopathy with lactic acidosis and stroke (MELAS)
Neoplasms (e.g., lymphoma, glioma, meningioma)
Sarcoid
Sjögren's syndrome
Stroke and ischemic cerebrovascular disease
Syphilis
Systemic lupus erythematosus and related collagen vascular disorders
Tropical spastic paraparesis (HTLV I/II infection)
Vascular malformations (especially spinal dural AV fistulas)
Vasculitis (primary CNS or other)
Vitamin B_{12} deficiency

Note: HTLV, human T cell lymphotropic virus; AV, arteriovenous; CNS, central nervous system.

ophthalmoplegia (slowness or loss of adduction in one eye with nystagmus in the abducting eye on lateral gaze), facial numbness or weakness, dysarthria, weakness and spasticity, hyperreflexia, ankle clonus, upgoing toes, ataxia, sensory abnormalities.

DISEASE COURSE

Four general categories:

- *Relapsing-remitting MS* (RRMS) is characterized by recurrent attacks of neurologic dysfunction usually with or without recovery; between attacks, no progression of neurologic impairment is noted. Accounts for 85% of new-onset MS cases.
- *Secondary progressive MS* (SPMS) always initially presents as RRMS but evolves to be gradually progressive. The majority of RRMS eventually evolves into SPMS.
- *Primary progressive MS* (PPMS) is characterized by gradual progression of disability from onset without discrete attacks; 15% of new-onset MS cases.
- *Progressive-relapsing MS* (PRMS) is a rare form that begins with a primary progressive course, but later superimposed relapses occur.

MS is a chronic illness; 15 years after diagnosis, only 20% of pts have no functional limitation; one-third to one-half will have progressed to SPMS and will require assistance with ambulation.

LABORATORY EVALUATION

MRI reveals multifocal bright areas on T2-weighted sequences in >95% of pts, often in periventricular location; gadolinium enhancement indicates acute lesions with disruption of blood-brain barrier (Fig. 200-1). MRI also useful to ex-

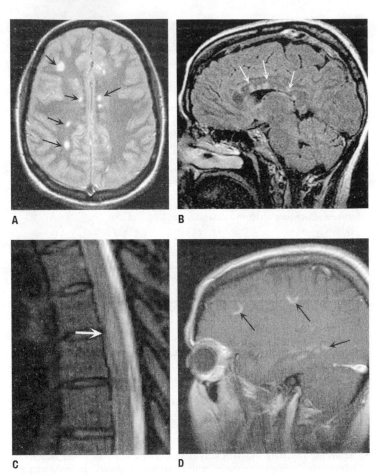

FIGURE 200-1 MRI findings in MS. *A.* Axial first-echo image from T2-weighted sequence demonstrates multiple bright signal abnormalities in white matter, typical for MS. *B.* Sagittal T2-weighted FLAIR (fluid attenuated inversion recovery) image in which the high signal of CSF has been suppressed. CSF appears dark, while areas of brain edema or demyelination appear high in signal as shown here in the corpus callosum (*arrows*). Lesions in the anterior corpus callosum are frequent in MS and rare in vascular disease. *C.* Sagittal T2-weighted fast spin echo image of the thoracic spine demonstrates a fusiform high-signal-intensity lesion in the mid thoracic spinal cord. *D.* Sagittal T1-weighted image obtained after the intravenous administration of gadolinium DPTA reveals focal areas of blood-brain barrier disruption, identified as high-signal-intensity regions (*arrows*).

clude MS mimics, although findings in MS are not completely specific for the disorder. CSF findings include mild lymphocytic pleocytosis (5–75 cells in 25%), oligoclonal bands (75–90%), elevated IgG (80%), and normal total protein level. Visual, auditory, and somatosensory evoked response tests can identify lesions that are clinically silent; one or more evoked response tests abnormal in 80–90% of pts. Urodynamic studies aid in management of bladder symptoms.

Rx Multiple Sclerosis   (See Fig. 200-2)

DISEASE-MODIFYING THERAPIES FOR RELAPSING FORMS OF MS (RRMS, SPMS WITH EXACERBATIONS)

Five treatments are available: interferon (IFN)-β1a (Avonex; 30 μg IM once a week), IFN-β1a (Rebif; 44 μg SC thrice weekly), IFN-β1b (Betaseron; 250 μg SC every other day), glatiramer acetate (Copaxone; 12 mg/d SC), and natalizumab (Tysabri; 300 mg IV every 4 weeks). Each of the first four therapies reduces annual exacerbation rates by ~30% and also reduces the development of new MRI lesions. IFN preparations that are given multiple times weekly (e.g., Rebif or Betaseron) appear to have slightly greater efficacy compared with once-weekly agents (e.g., Avonex) but are also more likely to induce neutralizing antibodies, which may reduce the clinical benefit. Natalizumab is the most effective MS agent available. It dramatically reduces the attack rate and significantly improves all measures of disease severity in MS; however, because of the development of progressive multifocal leukoencephalopathy (PML) in rare patients, it is currently used only for patients who have failed other therapies or who have particularly aggressive presentations. Regardless of which agent is chosen first, treatment should probably be altered in pts who continue to have frequent attacks (Fig. 200-2).

Side effects of IFN include flulike symptoms, local injection site reactions (with SC dosing), and mild abnormalities on routine laboratory evaluation (e.g., elevated liver function tests or lymphopenia). Rarely, more severe hepatotoxicity may occur. Side effects to IFN usually subside with time. Injection site reactions also occur with glatiramer acetate but are less severe than with IFN. Approximately 15% of pts receiving glatiramer acetate experience one or more episodes of flushing, chest tightness, dyspnea, palpitations, and anxiety.

Early treatment with a disease-modifying drug is appropriate for most MS patients. It is reasonable to delay initiating treatment in pts with (1) normal neurologic exams, (2) a single attack or a low attack frequency, and (3) a low "burden of disease" as assessed by brain MRI. Untreated pts need to be followed closely with periodic brain MRI scans; the need for therapy is reassessed if the scans reveal evidence of ongoing disease.

ACUTE RELAPSES

Acute relapses that produce functional impairment may be treated with a short course of IV methylprednisolone (1 g IV qA.M. × 3–5 days) followed by oral prednisone (60 mg qA.M. × 4; 40 mg qA.M. × 4; 20 mg qA.M. × 3). This regimen modestly reduces the severity and shortens the duration of attacks. Plasma exchange (7 exchanges: 40–60 mL/kg, every other day for 14 days) may benefit patients with fulminant attacks of demyelination (not only MS) that are unresponsive to glucocorticoids; cost is high and evidence of efficacy is only preliminary.

PROGRESSIVE SYMPTOMS

For pts with secondary progressive MS who continue to experience relapses, treatment with one of the IFNs is reasonable; however, the IFNs are ineffective against purely progressive MS symptoms. The immunosuppressant/immunomodulator drug mitoxantrone (12 mg/m² by IV infusion every 3 months) is approved in the United States for treatment of secondary progressive MS; however, the evidence for efficacy is relatively weak, and dose-related cardiac toxicity is an important concern. Methotrexate (7.5–20 mg PO once each week) or azathioprine (2–3 mg/kg per day PO) is sometimes tried, but efficacy is modest. Pulse therapy with cyclophosphamide is employed in some centers for young adults with aggressive forms of MS. Other smaller studies have examined monthly

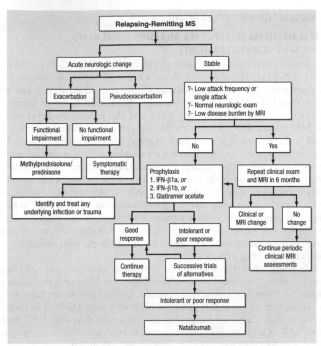

A

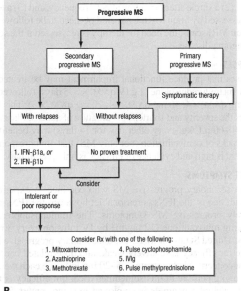

B

FIGURE 200-2 Therapeutic decision-making for MS.

pulses of intravenous immunoglobulin (IVIg) or intravenous methylpredniso-lone. For patients with PPMS, symptomatic therapy only is recommended.

SYMPTOMATIC THERAPY

Spasticity may respond to physical therapy, lioresal (20–120 mg/d), diazepam (2–40 mg/d), tizanidine (8–32 mg/d), dantrolene (25–400 mg/d), and cycloben-zaprine hydrochloride (10–60 mg/d). Dysesthesia may respond to carbamazepine (100–1200 mg/d in divided doses), phenytoin (300 mg/d), gabapentin (300–3600 mg/d), pregabalin (50–300 mg/d), or amitriptyline (50–200 mg/d). Treatment of bladder symptoms is based on the underlying pathophysiology investigated with urodynamic testing: bladder hyperreflexia is treated with evening fluid restriction and frequent voiding; if this fails, anticholinergics such as oxybutinin (5–15 mg/d) may be tried; hyporeflexia is treated with the cholinergic drug bethanecol (10–50 mg three to four times a day), and dyssynergia due to loss of coordination be-tween bladder wall and sphincter muscles is treated with anticholinergics and in-termittent catheterization. Depression should be treated aggressively.

CLINICAL VARIANTS OF MS

Neuromyelitis optica (NMO), or Devic's syndrome, consists of separate attacks of acute optic neuritis (bilateral or unilateral) and myelitis. In contrast to MS, the brain MRI is typically, but not always, normal. A focal enhancing region of swelling and cavitation, extending over three or more spinal cord segments, is typically seen on spinal MRI. A highly specific autoantibody directed against the water channel aquaporin-4 is present in the sera of more than half of patients with a clinical diagnosis of NMO. Acute attacks are usually treated with high-dose glucocorticoids as for MS exacerbations. Plasma exchange has also been used empirically for acute episodes that fail to respond to glucocorticoids. Immuno-suppressants or IFNs are sometimes used in the hope that further relapses will be prevented; preliminary evidence indicates that B cell depletion with anti-CD20 monoclonal antibody (rituximab) holds promise in preventing NMO relapses.

Acute MS (Marburg's variant) is a fulminant demyelinating process that progresses to death within 1–2 years. No controlled trials of therapy exist; high-dose glucocorticoids, plasma exchange, and cyclophosphamide have been tried, with uncertain benefit.

ACUTE DISSEMINATED ENCEPHALOMYELITIS (ADEM)

A fulminant, often devastating, demyelinating disease that has a monophasic course and may be associated with antecedent immunization or infection. Signs of disseminated neurologic disease are consistently present (e.g., hemiparesis or quad-riparesis, extensor plantar responses, lost or hyperactive tendon reflexes, sensory loss, and brainstem involvement). Fever, headache, meningismus, lethargy pro-gressing to coma, and seizures may occur. CSF pleocytosis, generally 200 cells/µl, is common. MRI may reveal extensive gadolinium enhancement of white matter in brain and spinal cord. Initial treatment is with high-dose glucocorticoids. Patients who fail to respond may benefit from a course of plasma exchange or IVIg.

For a more detailed discussion, see Hauser SL, Goodin DS: Multiple Sclerosis and Other Demyelinating Diseases, Chap. 375, p. 2611, in HPIM-17.

201 Acute Meningitis and Encephalitis

Acute infections of the nervous system include bacterial meningitis, viral meningitis, encephalitis, focal infections such as brain abscess and subdural empyema, and infectious thrombophlebitis. Key goals: emergently distinguish between these conditions, identify the pathogen, and initiate appropriate antimicrobial therapy.

APPROACH TO THE PATIENT WITH ACUTE INFECTION OF THE NERVOUS SYSTEM

(Fig. 201-1A) First identify whether infection predominantly involves the subarachnoid space (*meningitis*) or brain tissue (termed *encephalitis* when viral, *cerebritis* or *abscess* if bacterial, fungal, or parasitic). Nuchal rigidity is the pathognomonic sign of meningeal irritation and is present when the neck resists passive flexion.

Principles of management:

- Initiate empirical therapy whenever bacterial meningitis is considered.
- All pts with head trauma, immunocompromised states, known malignancies, or focal neurologic findings (including papilledema or stupor/coma) should undergo a neuroimaging study of the brain prior to LP. If bacterial meningitis is suspected, begin empirical antibiotic therapy prior to neuroimaging and LP.
- Stupor/coma, seizures, or focal neurologic deficits only rarely occur in viral ("aseptic") meningitis; pts with these symptoms should be hospitalized and treated empirically for bacterial and viral meningoencephalitis.
- Immunocompetent pts with a normal level of consciousness, no prior antimicrobial treatment, and a CSF profile consistent with viral meningitis (lymphocytic pleocytosis and a normal glucose concentration) can often be treated as outpatients. Failure of a pt with suspected viral meningitis to improve within 48 h should prompt a reevaluation including follow-up exam, repeat imaging and laboratory studies, often including a second LP.

ACUTE BACTERIAL MENINGITIS

Pathogens most frequently involved in immunocompetent adults are *Streptococcus pneumoniae* ("pneumococcus," ~50%) and *Neisseria meningitidis* ("meningococcus," ~25%). Predisposing factors for pneumococcal meningitis include infection (pneumonia, otitis, sinusitis), asplenia, hypogammaglobulinemia, complement deficiency, alcoholism, diabetes, and head trauma with CSF leak. *Listeria monocytogenes* is an important consideration in pregnant women, individuals >60 years, alcoholics, and immunocompromised individuals of all ages. Enteric gram-negative bacilli and group B streptococcus are increasingly common causes of meningitis in individuals with chronic medical conditions. *Staphylococcus aureus* and coagulase-negative staphylococci are important causes following invasive neurosurgical procedures, especially shunting procedures for hydrocephalus.

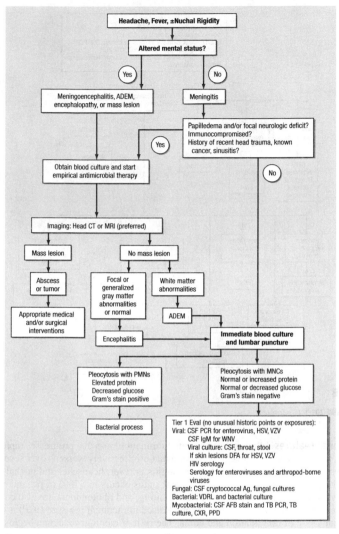

A

FIGURE 201-1 The management of patients with suspected CNS infection. ADEM, acute disseminated encephalomyelitis; CT, computed tomography; MRI, magnetic resonance imaging; PMNs, polymorphonuclear leukocytes; MNCs, mononuclear cells; CSF, cerebrospinal fluid; PCR, polymerase chain reaction; HSV, herpes simplex virus; VZV, varicella-zoster virus; WNV, West Nile virus; DFA, direct fluorescent antibody; Ag, antigen; VDRL, Venereal Disease Research Laboratory; AFB, acid-fast bacillus; TB, tuberculosis; CXR, chest x-ray; PPD, purified protein derivative; EBV, Epstein-Barr virus; CTFV, Colorado tick fever virus; HHV, human herpesvirus; LCMV, lymphocytic choriomeningitis virus. *(Continued)*

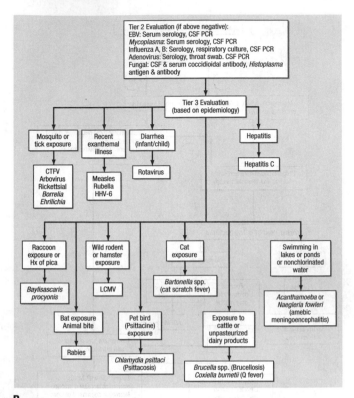

B

FIGURE 201-1 *(Continued)*

Clinical Features Presents as an acute fulminant illness that progresses rapidly in a few hours or as a subacute infection that progressively worsens over several days. The classic clinical triad of meningitis is fever, headache, and nuchal rigidity ("stiff neck"). Alteration in mental status occurs in >75% of pts and can vary from lethargy to coma. Nausea, vomiting, and photophobia are also common. Seizures occur in 20–40% of pts. Raised intracranial pressure (ICP) is the major cause of obtundation and coma. The rash of meningococcemia begins as a diffuse maculopapular rash resembling a viral exanthem but rapidly becomes petechial on trunk and lower extremities, mucous membranes and conjunctiva, and occasionally palms and soles.

Laboratory Evaluation The CSF profile is shown in Table 201-1. CSF bacterial cultures are positive in >80% of pts, and CSF Gram stain demonstrates organisms in >60%. The latex agglutination (LA) test for detection of bacterial antigens of *S. pneumoniae*, *N. meningitidis*, *Haemophilus influenzae* type b, group B streptococcus, and *Escherichia coli* K1 strains in the CSF is very useful for rapid diagnosis, especially in pts pretreated with antibiotics and when the CSF Gram stain and culture are negative; CSF bacterial PCR assays are replacing this technique. The Limulus amebocyte lysate assay rapidly detects gram-negative endotoxin in CSF and thus is useful in diagnosis of gram-negative bac-

TABLE 201-1	CEREBROSPINAL FLUID (CSF) ABNORMALITIES IN BACTERIAL MENINGITIS
Opening pressure	>180 mmH$_2$O
White blood cells	10/μL to 10,000/μL; neutrophils predominate
Red blood cells	Absent in nontraumatic tap
Glucose	<2.2 mmol/L (<40 mg/dL)
CSF/serum glucose	<0.4
Protein	>0.45 g/L (>45 mg/dL)
Gram's stain	Positive in >60%
Culture	Positive in >80%
Latex agglutination	May be positive in patients with meningitis due to *S. pneumoniae, N. meningitidis, H. influenzae* type b, *E. coli,* group B streptococci
Limulus lysate	Positive in cases of gram-negative meningitis
PCR	Detects bacterial DNA

Note: PCR, polymerase chain reaction.

terial meningitis; false-positives may occur but sensitivity approaches 100%. Petechial skin lesions, if present, should be biopsied. Blood cultures should always be obtained.

Differential Diagnosis Includes viral meningoencephalitis, especially herpes simplex virus (HSV) encephalitis (see below); rickettsial diseases such as Rocky Mountain spotted fever (immunofluorescent staining of skin lesions); focal suppurative CNS infections including subdural and epidural empyema and brain abscess (see below); subarachnoid hemorrhage (Chap. 19); and the demyelinating disease acute disseminated encephalomyelitis (ADEM, Chap. 200).

Rx Acute Bacterial Meningitis

Recommendations for empirical therapy are summarized in Table 201-2. Therapy is then modified based on results of CSF culture (Table 201-3). In general, the treatment course is 7 days for meningococcus, 14 days for pneumococcus, 21 days for gram-negative meningitis, and at least 21 days for *L. monocytogenes.*

Adjunctive therapy with dexamethasone (10 mg IV), administered 15–20 min before the first dose of an antimicrobial agent and repeated every 6 h for 4 days, improves outcome from bacterial meningitis; benefits most striking in pneumococcal meningitis. Dexamethasone may decrease the penetration of vancomycin into CSF, and thus its potential benefit should be carefully weighed when vancomycin is the antibiotic of choice.

In meningococcal meningitis, all close contacts should receive prophylaxis with rifampin [600 mg in adults (10 mg/kg in children > 1 year)] every 12 h for 2 days; rifampin is not recommended in pregnant women. Alternatively, adults can be treated with one dose of ciprofloxacin (750 mg), one dose of azithromycin (500 mg), or one IM dose of ceftriaxone (250 mg).

Prognosis Moderate or severe sequelae occur in ~25% of survivors; outcome varies with the infecting organism. Common sequelae include decreased intellectual function, memory impairment, seizures, hearing loss and dizziness, and gait disturbances.

TABLE 201-2   ANTIBIOTICS USED IN EMPIRICAL THERAPY OF BACTERIAL MENINGITIS AND FOCAL CNS INFECTIONS[a]

Indication	Antibiotic
Preterm infants to infants <1 month	Ampicillin + cefotaxime
Infants 1–3 mos	Ampicillin + cefotaxime or ceftriaxone
Immunocompetent children >3 mos and adults <55	Cefotaxime or ceftriaxone + vancomycin
Adults >55 and adults of any age with alcoholism or other debilitating illnesses	Ampicillin + cefotaxime or ceftriaxone + vancomycin
Hospital-acquired meningitis, posttraumatic or postneurosurgery meningitis, neutropenic patients, or patients with impaired cell-mediated immunity	Ampicillin + ceftazidime + vancomycin

Antimicrobial Agent	Total Daily Dose and Dosing Interval	
	Child (>1 month)	Adult
Ampicillin	200 (mg/kg)/d, q4h	12 g/d, q4h
Cefepime	150 (mg/kg)/d, q8h	6 g/d, q8h
Cefotaxime	200 (mg/kg)/d, q6h	12 g/d, q4h
Ceftriaxone	100 (mg/kg)/d, q12h	4 g/d, q12h
Ceftazidime	150 (mg/kg)/d, q8h	6 g/d, q8h
Gentamicin	7.5 (mg/kg)/d, q8h[b]	7.5 (mg/kg)/d, q8h
Meropenem	120 (mg/kg)/d, q8h	3 g/d, q8h
Metronidazole	30 (mg/kg)/d, q6h	1500–2000 mg/d, q6h
Nafcillin	100–200 (mg/kg)/d, q6h	9–12 g/d, q4h
Penicillin G	400,000 (U/kg)/d, q4h	20–24 million U/d, q4h
Vancomycin	60 (mg/kg)/d, q6h	2 g/d, q12h[b]

[a]All antibiotics are administered intravenously; doses indicated assume normal renal and hepatic function.
[b]Doses should be adjusted based on serum peak and trough levels: gentamicin therapeutic level: peak: 5–8 μg/mL; trough: <2 μg/mL; vancomycin therapeutic level: peak: 25–40 μg/mL; trough: 5–15 μg/mL.

VIRAL MENINGITIS

Presents as fever, headache, and meningeal irritation associated with a CSF lymphocytic pleocytosis. Fever may be accompanied by malaise, myalgia, anorexia, nausea and vomiting, abdominal pain, and/or diarrhea. A mild degree of lethargy or drowsiness may occur; however, a more profound alteration in consciousness should prompt consideration of alternative diagnoses, including encephalitis.

Etiology   Using a variety of diagnostic techniques, including CSF PCR, culture, and serology, a specific viral cause can be found in 75–90% of cases. The most important agents are enteroviruses, HSV type 2, and arboviruses (Table 201-4). The incidence of enteroviral and arboviral infections is greatly increased during the summer.

Diagnosis   Most important test is examination of the CSF. The typical profile is a lymphocytic pleocytosis (25–500 cells/μL), a normal or slightly elevated protein concentration [0.2–0.8 g/L (20–80 mg/dL)], a normal glucose concentration,

TABLE 201-3	ANTIMICROBIAL THERAPY OF CNS BACTERIAL INFECTIONS BASED ON PATHOGEN[a]

Organism	Antibiotic
Neisseria meningitides	
Penicillin-sensitive	Penicillin G or ampicillin
Penicillin-resistant	Ceftriaxone or cefotaxime
Streptococcus pneumoniae	
Penicillin-sensitive	Penicillin G
Penicillin-intermediate	Ceftriaxone or cefotaxime
Penicillin-resistant	(Ceftriaxone or cefotaxime) + vancomycin
Gram-negative bacilli (except *Pseudomonas* spp.)	Ceftriaxone or cefotaxime
Pseudomonas aeruginosa	Ceftazidime or cefepime or meropenem
Staphylococci spp.	
Methicillin-sensitive	Nafcillin
Methicillin-resistant	Vancomycin
Listeria monocytogenes	Ampicillin + gentamicin
Haemophilus influenzae	Ceftriaxone or cefotaxime
Streptococcus agalactiae	Penicillin G or ampicillin
Bacteroides fragilis	Metronidazole
Fusobacterium spp.	Metronidazole

[a]Doses are as indicated in Table 201-2.

TABLE 201-4	VIRUSES CAUSING ACUTE MENINGITIS AND ENCEPHALITIS IN NORTH AMERICA

Acute Meningitis

Common	Less Common
Enteroviruses (coxsackieviruses, echoviruses, and human enteroviruses 68–71)	Varicella zoster virus
	Epstein-Barr virus
Herpes simplex virus 2	Lymphocytic choriomeningitis virus
Arthropod-borne viruses	
HIV	

Acute Encephalitis

Common	Less Common
Herpesviruses	Rabies
Herpes simplex virus 1	Eastern equine encephalitis virus
Varicella zoster virus	Western equine encephalitis virus
Epstein-Barr virus	Powassan virus
Arthropod-borne viruses	Cytomegalovirus[a]
La Crosse virus	Enteroviruses[a]
West Nile virus	Colorado tick fever
St. Louis encephalitis virus	Mumps

[a]Immunocompromised host.

and a normal or mildly elevated opening pressure (100–350 mmH$_2$O). Organisms are *not* seen on Gram or acid-fast stained smears or India ink preparations of CSF. Rarely, polymorphonuclear leukocytes (PMN) predominate in the first 48 h of illness, especially with echovirus 9, West Nile virus (WNV), eastern equine encephalitis virus, or mumps. The total CSF cell count in viral meningitis is typically 25–500/μL. As a general rule, a lymphocytic pleocytosis with a low glucose concentration should suggest fungal, listerial, or tuberculous meningitis or noninfectious disorders (e.g., sarcoid, neoplastic meningitis).

CSF PCR testing is the procedure of choice for rapid, sensitive, and specific identification of enteroviruses, HSV, EBV, varicella zoster virus (VZV), human herpes virus 6 (HHV-6), and CMV. Attempts should also be made to culture virus from CSF and other sites and body fluids including blood, throat swabs, stool, and urine. Serologic studies, including those utilizing paired CSF and serum specimens, may be helpful for retrospective diagnosis; they are particularly important for diagnosis of WNV and other arbovirus etiologies.

Differential Diagnosis Consider bacterial, fungal, tuberculous, spirochetal, and other infectious causes of meningitis; parameningeal infections; partially treated bacterial meningitis; neoplastic meningitis; noninfectious inflammatory diseases including sarcoid and Behçet's disease.

R$_X$ Viral Meningitis

Supportive or symptomatic therapy is usually sufficient, and hospitalization is not required. The elderly and immunocompromised pts should be hospitalized, as should individuals in whom the diagnosis is uncertain or those with significant alterations in consciousness, seizures, or focal neurologic signs or symptoms. Severe cases of meningitis due to HSV, EBV, and VZV can be treated with IV acyclovir (10 mg/kg every 8 h for 7–14 days); for mildly affected pts, a 1-week course of oral antivirals may be appropriate. Additional supportive or symptomatic therapy can include analgesics and antipyretics. Prognosis for full recovery is excellent. Vaccination is an effective method of preventing the development of meningitis and other neurologic complications associated with poliovirus, mumps, measles, and VZV infection.

VIRAL ENCEPHALITIS

An infection of the brain parenchyma commonly associated with meningitis ("meningoencephalitis"). Clinical features are those of viral meningitis plus evidence of brain tissue involvement, commonly including altered consciousness such as behavioral changes and hallucinations; seizures; and focal neurologic findings such as aphasia, hemiparesis, involuntary movements, and cranial nerve deficits.

Etiology The same organisms responsible for aseptic meningitis are also responsible for encephalitis, although relative frequencies differ. The most common causes of sporadic encephalitis in immunocompetent adults are herpesviruses (HSV, VZV, EBV) (Table 201-4). HSV encephalitis should be considered when focal findings are present and when involvement of the inferomedial frontotemporal regions of the brain is likely (olfactory hallucinations, anosmia, bizarre behavior, or memory disturbance). Epidemics of encephalitis are usually caused by arboviruses. WNV has been responsible for the majority of arbovirus meningitis and encephalitis cases in the United States. since 2002; prominent motor manifestations, including acute poliomyelitis-like paralysis, may occur with WNV.

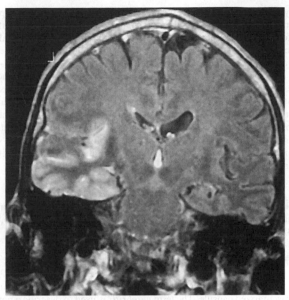

FIGURE 201-2 Coronal FLAIR magnetic resonance image from a patient with herpes simplex encephalitis. Note the area of increased signal in the right temporal lobe (left side of image) confined predominantly to the gray matter. This patient had predominantly unilateral disease; bilateral lesions are more common but may be quite asymmetric in their intensity.

Diagnosis   CSF studies are essential; typical CSF profile is similar to viral meningitis. CSF PCR tests allow for rapid and reliable diagnosis of HSV, EBV, VZV, CMV, HHV-6, and enteroviruses. CSF virus cultures are generally negative. Serologic studies also have a role for some viruses. Demonstration of WNV IgM antibodies is diagnostic of WNV encephalitis.

MRI is the neuroimaging procedure of choice and demonstrates areas of increased T2 signal. Bitemporal and orbitofrontal areas of increased signal are seen in HSV encephalitis but are not diagnostic (Fig. 201-2). The EEG may suggest seizures or show temporally predominant periodic spikes on a slow, low-amplitude background suggestive of HSV encephalitis.

Brain biopsy is now used only when CSF PCR studies fail to identify the cause, focal abnormalities on MRI are present, and progressive clinical deterioration occurs despite treatment with acyclovir and supportive therapy.

Differential Diagnosis   Includes both infectious and noninfectious causes of encephalitis, including vascular diseases; abscess and empyema; fungal (*Cryptococcus* and *Mucor*), spirochetal (*Leptospira*), rickettsial, bacterial (*Listeria*), tuberculous, and mycoplasma infections; tumors; toxic encephalopathy; SLE; and acute disseminated encephalomyelitis.

℞ Viral Encephalitis

All pts with suspected HSV encephalitis should be treated with IV acyclovir (10 mg/kg every 8 h) while awaiting diagnostic studies. Pts with a PCR-confirmed diagnosis of HSV encephalitis should receive a minimum 14-day course of therapy. Consider repeat CSF PCR after completion of acyclovir therapy; pts with a persistently positive CSF PCR for HSV after completing a standard course of acyclovir therapy should be treated for an additional 7 days, followed by a repeat CSF PCR test. Acyclovir treatment may also benefit encephalitis due to EBV and VZV. No therapy currently available for enteroviral, mumps, or measles encephalitis. Intravenous ribavirin (15–25 mg/ kg per day given in 3 divided doses) may benefit severe arbovirus encephalitis due to California encephalitis (LaCrosse) virus. CMV encephalitis should be treated with ganciclovir, foscarnet, or a combination of the two drugs; cidofovir may provide an alternative for nonresponders. No proven therapy is available for WNV encephalitis; small groups of pts have been treated with interferon, ribavirin, WNV-specific antisense oligonucleotides, and intravenous immunoglobulin preparations of Israeli origin containing high titer anti-WNV antibody.

Prognosis In HSV encephalitis treated with acyclovir, 81% survival in one series; neurologic sequelae were mild or absent in 46%, moderate in 12%, and severe in 42%.

BRAIN ABSCESS

A focal, suppurative infection within the brain parenchyma, typically surrounded by a vascularized capsule. The term *cerebritis* is used to describe a nonencapsulated brain abscess. Predisposing conditions include otitis media and mastoiditis, paranasal sinusitis, pyogenic infections in the chest or other body sites, head trauma, neurosurgical procedures, and dental infections. Many brain abscesses occur in immunocompromised hosts and are caused less often by bacteria than by fungi and parasites including *Toxoplasma gondii*, *Aspergillus* spp., *Nocardia* spp., *Candida* spp., and *Cryptococcus neoformans*. In Latin America and in immigrants from Latin America, the most common cause of brain abscess is *Taenia solium* (neurocysticercosis). In India and the Far East, mycobacterial infection (tuberculoma) remains a major cause of focal CNS mass lesions.

Clinical Features Brain abscess typically presents as an expanding intracranial mass lesion, rather than as an infectious process. The classic triad of headache, fever, and a focal neurologic deficit is present in <50% of cases.

Diagnosis MRI is better than CT for demonstrating abscesses in the early (cerebritis) stages and is superior to CT for identifying abscesses in the posterior fossa. A mature brain abscess appears on CT as a focal area of hypodensity surrounded by ring enhancement. The CT and MRI appearance, particularly of the capsule, may be altered by treatment with glucocorticoids. The distinction between a brain abscess and other focal lesions such as tumors may be facilitated with diffusion-weighted imaging (DWI) sequences in which brain abscesses typically show increased signal and low apparent diffusion coefficient.

Microbiologic diagnosis best determined by Gram stain and culture of abscess material obtained by stereotactic needle aspiration. Up to 10% of patients will also have positive blood cultures. CSF analysis contributes nothing to diagnosis or therapy, and LP increases the risk of herniation.

 Brain Abscess

Optimal therapy involves a combination of high-dose parenteral antibiotics and neurosurgical drainage. Empirical therapy of community-acquired brain abscess in an immunocompetent patient typically includes a third-generation cephalosporin (e.g., cefotaxime or ceftriaxone) and metronidazole (see Table 201-2 for antibiotic dosages). In pts with penetrating head trauma or recent neurosurgical procedures, treatment should include ceftazidime as the third-generation cephalosporin to enhance coverage of *Pseudomonas* spp. and vancomycin for coverage of resistant staphylococci. Meropenem plus vancomycin also provides good coverage in this setting.

Aspiration and drainage essential in most cases. Empirical antibiotic coverage is modified based on the results of Gram stain and culture of the abscess contents. Medical therapy alone is reserved for pts whose abscesses are neurosurgically inaccessible and for cerebritis. All pts should receive a minimum of 6–8 weeks of parenteral antibiotic therapy. Pts should receive prophylactic anticonvulsant therapy. Glucocorticoids should not be given routinely.

Prognosis   In modern series the mortality is typically <15%. Significant sequelae including seizures, persisting weakness, aphasia, or mental impairment occur in ≥20% of survivors.

PROGRESSIVE MULTIFOCAL LEUKOENCEPHALOPATHY (PML)

Clinical Features   A progressive disorder due to infection with the JC virus, a human polyoma virus; characterized pathologically by multifocal areas of demyelination of varying size distributed throughout the CNS but sparing the spinal cord and optic nerves. In addition, there are characteristic cytologic alterations in both astrocytes and oligodendrocytes. Pts often present with visual deficits (45%), typically a homonymous hemianopia, and mental impairment (38%) (dementia, confusion, personality change), weakness, and ataxia. Almost all pts have an underlying immunosuppressive disorder. More than 80% of currently diagnosed PML cases occur in patients with AIDS; it has been estimated that nearly 5% of AIDS patients will develop PML.

Diagnostic Studies   MRI reveals multifocal asymmetric, coalescing white matter lesions located periventricularly, in the centrum semiovale, in the parietal-occipital region, and in the cerebellum. These lesions have increased T2 and decreased T1 signal, are generally nonenhancing (rarely they may show ring enhancement), and are not associated with edema or mass effect. CT scans, which are less sensitive than MRI for the diagnosis of PML, often show hypodense nonenhancing white matter lesions.

The CSF is typically normal, although mild elevation in protein and/or IgG may be found. Pleocytosis occurs in <25% of cases, is predominantly mononuclear, and rarely exceeds 25 cells/μL. PCR amplification of JC virus DNA from CSF has become an important diagnostic tool. A positive CSF PCR for JC virus DNA in association with typical MRI lesions in the appropriate clinical setting is diagnostic of PML. Pts with negative CSF PCR studies may require brain biopsy for definitive diagnosis as sensitivity of this test is variable; JC virus antigen and nucleic acid can be detected by immunocytochemistry, in situ hybridization, or PCR amplification on tissue. Detection of JC virus antigen or genomic material should be considered diagnostic of PML only if accompanied by characteristic pathologic changes, since both antigen and genomic material have been found in the brains of normal pts. Serologic studies are of no utility given high basal seroprevalence level (>80%).

$\mathbf{R_x}$ Progressive Multifocal Leukoencephalopathy

No effective therapy is available. Some pts with HIV-associated PML have shown dramatic clinical gains associated with improvement in immune status following institution of highly active antiretroviral therapy (HAART).

For a more detailed discussion, see Roos KL, Tyler KL: Meningitis, Encephalitis, Brain Abscess, and Empyema, Chap. 376, p. 2621, in HPIM-17; and HPIM-17 chapters covering specific organisms or infections.

202 Chronic Meningitis

Chronic inflammation of the meninges (pia, arachnoid, and dura) can produce profound neurologic disability and may be fatal if not successfully treated. The causes are varied. Five categories of disease account for most cases of chronic meningitis:

- Meningeal infections
- Malignancy
- Noninfectious inflammatory disorders
- Chemical meningitis
- Parameningeal infections

CLINICAL FEATURES

Neurologic manifestations consist of persistent headache with or without stiff neck and hydrocephalus; cranial neuropathies; radiculopathies; and/or cognitive or personality changes (Table 202-1). The diagnosis is usually made when clinical presentation leads the physician to examine CSF for signs of inflammation; on occasion the diagnosis is made when a neuroimaging study shows contrast enhancement of the meninges.

Two clinical forms of chronic meningitis exist. In the first, symptoms are chronic and persistent, whereas in the second there are recurrent, discrete episodes with complete resolution of meningeal inflammation between episodes without specific therapy. In the latter group, likely etiologies are herpes simplex virus type 2, chemical meningitis due to leakage from a tumor, a primary inflammatory condition, or drug hypersensitivity.

APPROACH TO THE PATIENT WITH CHRONIC MENINGITIS

Once chronic meningitis is confirmed by CSF examination, effort is focused on identifying the cause (Tables 202-2 and 202-3) by (1) further analysis of the CSF, (2) diagnosis of an underlying systemic infection or noninfectious inflammatory condition, or (3) examination of meningeal biopsy tissue.

TABLE 202-1 SYMPTOMS AND SIGNS OF CHRONIC MENINGITIS

Symptoms	Signs
Chronic headache	± Papilledema
Neck or back pain	Brudzinski's or Kernig's sign of meningeal irritation
Change in personality	Altered mental status—drowsiness, inattention, disorientation, memory loss, frontal release signs (grasp, suck, snout), perseveration
Facial weakness	Peripheral seventh CN palsy
Double vision	Palsy of CNs III, IV, VI
Visual loss	Papilledema, optic atrophy
Hearing loss	Eighth CN palsy
Arm or leg weakness	Myelopathy or radiculopathy
Numbness in arms or legs	Myelopathy or radiculopathy
Sphincter dysfunction	Myelopathy or radiculopathy Frontal lobe dysfunction (hydrocephalus)
Clumsiness	Ataxia

Note: CN, cranial nerve.

Proper analysis of the CSF is essential; if the possibility of raised intracranial pressure (ICP) exists, a brain imaging study should be performed before LP. In pts with communicating hydrocephalus caused by impaired resorption of CSF, LP is safe and may lead to temporary improvement. However, if ICP is elevated because of a mass lesion, brain swelling, or a block in ventricular CSF outflow (obstructive hydrocephalus), then LP carries the potential risk of brain herniation. Obstructive hydrocephalus usually requires direct ventricular drainage of CSF.

Contrast-enhanced MRI or CT studies of the brain and spinal cord can identify meningeal enhancement, parameningeal infections (including brain abscess), encasement of the spinal cord (malignancy or inflammation and infection), or nodular deposits on the meninges or nerve roots (malignancy or sarcoidosis). Imaging studies are also useful to localize areas of meningeal disease prior to meningeal biopsy. Cerebral angiography may identify arteritis.

A meningeal biopsy should be considered in pts who are disabled, who need chronic ventricular decompression, or whose illness is progressing rapidly. The diagnostic yield of meningeal biopsy can be increased by targeting regions that enhance with contrast on MRI or CT; in one series, diagnostic biopsies most often identified sarcoid (31%) or metastatic adenocarcinoma (25%). Tuberculosis is the most common condition identified in many reports outside of the United States.

In approximately one-third of cases, the diagnosis is not known despite careful evaluation. A number of the organisms that cause chronic meningitis may take weeks to be identified by culture. It is reasonable to wait until cultures are finalized if symptoms are mild and not progressive. However, in many cases progressive neurologic deterioration occurs, and rapid treatment is required. Empirical therapy in the United States consists of antimycobacterial agents, amphotericin for fungal infection, or glucocorticoids for noninfectious inflammatory causes (most common). It is important to direct empirical therapy of lymphocytic meningitis at tuberculosis, particularly if the condition is associated with hypoglycorrhachia and sixth and other cranial nerve palsies, since untreated disease can be fatal in 4–8 weeks. Carcinomatous or lymphomatous meningitis may be difficult to diagnose initially,

TABLE 202-2 **INFECTIOUS CAUSES OF CHRONIC MENINGITIS**

Common Bacterial Causes

Partially treated suppurative meningitis
Parameningeal infection
Mycobacterium tuberculosis
Lyme disease (Bannwarth's syndrome): *Borrelia burgdorferi*
Syphilis (secondary, tertiary): *Treponema pallidum*

Uncommon Bacterial Causes

Actinomyces	*Brucella*
Nocardia	Whipple's disease: *Tropherema whippelii*

Rare Bacterial Causes

Leptospirosis; *Pseudoallescheria boydii*

Fungal Causes

Cryptococcus neoformans	*Blastomyces dermatitidis*
Coccidioides immitis	*Aspergillus* sp.
Candida sp.	*Sporothrix schenckii*
Histoplasma capsulatum	

Rare Fungal Causes

Xylohypha (formerly *Cladosporium*) *trichoides* and other dark-walled (demateaceous) fungi such as *Curvularia, Drechslera; Mucor, Pseudoallescheria boydii*

Protozoal Causes

Toxoplasma gondii
Trypanosomiasis *Trypanosoma gambiense, Trypanosoma rhodesiense*

Rare Protozoal Causes

Acanthamoeba sp.

Helminthic Causes

Cysticercosis (infection with cysts of *Taenia solium*)
Gnathostoma spinigerum
Angiostrongylus cantonensis
Baylisascaris procyonis (raccoon ascarid)

Rare Helminthic Causes

Trichinella spiralis (trichinosis); *Echinococcus* cysts; *Schistosoma* sp.

Viral Causes

Mumps	HIV (acute retroviral syndrome)
Lymphocytic choriomeningitis	Herpes simplex (HSV)
Echovirus	
Obstructive hydrocephalus usually requires direct ventricular drainage of CSF.	

TABLE 202-3   NONINFECTIOUS CAUSES OF CHRONIC MENINGITIS

Malignancy
Chemical compounds (may cause recurrent meningitis)
Primary inflammation
   CNS sarcoidosis
   Vogt-Koyanagi-Harada syndrome (recurrent meningitis)
   Isolated granulomatous angiitis of the nervous system
   Systemic lupus erythematosus
   Behçet's syndrome (recurrent meningitis)
   Chronic benign lymphocytic meningitis
   Mollaret's recurrent meningitis
   Drug hypersensitivity
   Wegener's granulomatosis
Other: multiple sclerosis, Sjögren's syndrome, and rarer forms of vasculitis (e.g.,
   Cogan's syndrome)

but the diagnosis becomes evident with time. Important causes of chronic meningitis in AIDS pts include infection with *Toxoplasma* (usually presents as intracranial abscesses), *Cryptococcus*, *Nocardia*, *Candida*, or other fungi; syphilis; and lymphoma.

For a more detailed discussion, see Koroshetz WJ, Swartz MN: Chronic and Recurrent Meningitis, Chap. 377, p. 2641, in HPIM-17.

203 Peripheral Neuropathies Including Guillain-Barré Syndrome (GBS)

APPROACH TO THE PATIENT WITH PERIPHERAL NEUROPATHY

Peripheral neuropathy (PN) refers to a peripheral nerve disorder of any cause. Nerve involvement may be single (mononeuropathy) or multiple (polyneuropathy); pathology may be axonal or demyelinating. An approach to pts with suspected neuropathy appears in Fig. 203-1.

Address the following initial questions:

1. *Is this a peripheral neuropathy?* Initial symptoms may be intermittent and examination can be normal. Patients may present with positive (e.g., paresthesias) and/or negative (e.g., numbness) symptoms (Table 203-1). In most cases polyneuropathy begins distally in the toes or feet and then spreads proximally in a stocking distribution. Ankle reflexes are lost. Only once sensory loss reaches the knees or thighs does numbness of fingers appear. Paresthesias that begin in one hand only suggest an entrapment neuropathy such as carpal tunnel syndrome. Motor symptoms usually have a

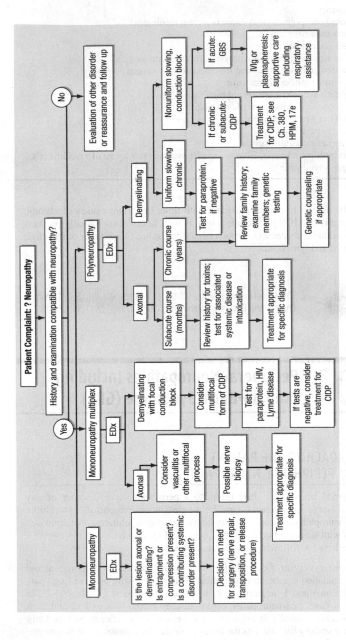

FIGURE 203-1 Approach to evaluation of peripheral neuropathies. CIDP, chronic inflammatory demyelinating polyradiculoneuropathy; EDX, electrodiagnostic studies; GBS, Guillain-Barré syndrome; IVIg, intravenous immunoglobulin.

TABLE 203-1 SYMPTOMS, SIGNS, AND TESTS IN PERIPHERAL NEUROPATHY

Large Fiber	Small Fiber	Motor	Autonomic
Symptoms			
Numbness "Pins and needles" Tingling Poor balance	Pain: burning, shock-like, stabbing, prickling, shooting, lancinating Allodynia	Cramps Weak grip Footdrop Twitching	Decreased or increased sweating Dry eyes, mouth, Erectile dysfunction Gastroparesis/diarrhea Faintness, lightheadedness
Signs			
Decreased Vibration Joint-position sense Reflexes	Decreased Pin prick Temperature sensation	Reduced Strength Reflexes	Orthostasis Unequal pupil size
Tests			
NCS-EMG Nerve biopsy LP	Skin biopsy QST Nerve biopsy	NCS-EMG	QSART Tilt table R-R interval Valsalva

Note: NCS-EMG, nerve conduction studies/electromyography; QSART, quantitative sudomotor axon reflex testing; QST, quantitative sensory test; LP, lumbar puncture.

later onset than sensory, but when pure motor symptoms are present, it may be difficult to distinguish neuropathy from muscle or neuromuscular junction disorders (which usually feature a more symmetric proximal pattern of weakness). Weakness and atrophy evolve from distal to proximal—initial toe dorsiflexion weakness may progress to bilateral foot drop, intrinsic hand muscle weakness, or (in extreme cases) impairment of muscles needed for ventilation and sphincter function.

2. *What is its distribution?* Polyneuropathy involves widespread and symmetric dysfunction of the peripheral nerves; mononeuropathy involves a single nerve usually due to trauma or compression; multiple mononeuropathies (mononeuropathy multiplex) can be a result of multiple entrapments, vasculitis, or infiltration.

3. *Which fibers are affected?* Can be classified as small-fiber sensory, large-fiber sensory, motor, and/or autonomic (Table 203-2).

4. *What is the anatomic pattern?* Clinical evaluation categorizes neuropathy as axonal, demyelinating, or neuronal (dorsal root ganglion, DRG) (Table 203-3). Electrodiagnostic tests (nerve conduction studies and electromyography, NCS-EMG) can confirm or clarify this clinical categorization.

5. *What is the time course?* Rapidly evolving neuropathies are often inflammatory; subacute evolution suggests an inflammatory, toxic, or nutritional cause; chronic neuropathies that are long-standing over years may be hereditary (Table 203-4).

6. *What is the likely etiology?* Categories of polyneuropathy include metabolic (diabetes mellitus, renal failure); infectious (HIV, Lyme disease,

TABLE 203-2 **CLASSIFICATION OF NEUROPATHY BY FIBER TYPE**

Small-fiber sensory (painful neuropathies and dissociated sensory loss)
    Hereditary sensory neuropathies (early)
    Lepromatous leprosy
    Diabetic (includes glucose intolerance) small-fiber neuropathy
    Amyloidosis
    Analphalipoproteinemia (Tangier disease)
    Fabry's disease (pain predominates)
    Dysautonomia (Riley-Day syndrome)
    HIV and antiretroviral therapy neuropathy
Large-fiber sensory (ataxic-neuropathies)
    Sjögren's syndrome
    Vitamin B_{12} neuropathy (from dorsal column involvement)
    Cisplatin neuropathy
    Pyridoxine toxicity
    Friedreich's ataxia
Small- and large-fiber: Global sensory loss
    Carcinomatous sensory neuropathy
    Hereditary sensory neuropathies (recessive and dominant)
    Diabetic sensory neuropathy
    Vacor intoxication
    Xanthomatous neuropathy of primary biliary cirrhosis (tabes dorsalis)
Motor-predominant neuropathies
    Immune neuropathies: acute (Guillain-Barré syndrome); relapsing
    Heritable motor-sensory neuropathies
    Acute intermittent porphyria
    Diphtheritic neuropathy
    Lead neuropathy
    Brachial neuritis
    Diabetic lumbosacralplexus neuropathy (diabetic amyotrophy)
Autonomic
    Acute: Acute pandysautonomic neuropathy, botulism, porphyria, GBS, vacore, amiodarone, vincristine
    Chronic: Amyloid, diabetes, Sjögren's, HSAN I and III (Riley-Day), Chagas, paraneoplastic

Note: GBS, Guillain-Barré syndrome; HSAN, hereditary sensory and autonomic neuropathy.

syphilis); immune-mediated (GBS); hereditary (Charcot-Marie-Tooth disease, CMT); toxic (medications, alcohol); vasculitic (polyarteritis nodosa, cryoglobulinemia); paraneoplastic (especially lung); nutritional (B vitamin deficiencies); and miscellaneous (celiac disease) (Table 203-5).

POLYNEUROPATHY

Diagnostic Evaluation Screening laboratory studies in a distal, symmetric polyneuropathy may include fasting blood glucose, HbA_{1C}, serum vitamin B_{12}, tests for systemic vasculitis or collagen vascular disease, serum immunoelectrophoresis, measurement of neuropathy-associated antibodies (against gangliosides such as GM1 and MAG or paraneoplastic antigens such as Hu), tests of kidney and thyroid function, and urine screen for heavy metals. Other studies are suggested by the differential diagnosis.

TABLE 203-3   CLASSIFICATION OF NEUROPATHY BY HISTOPATHOLOGY

	Demyelinating	Axonal	Neuronal
Pattern	Proximal = distal	Distal > proximal; length-dependent	Non-length-dependent; UE, LE, face
Onset	Acute/subacute	Slow evolution	Rapid
Symptoms	Paresthesia and weakness	Dysesthesias and distal weakness	Paresthesias, gait ataxia
Sensory signs	Vibration and proprioception > pain and temperature	Pain and temperature affected > vibration and proprioception	Vibration and proprioception > pain and temperature
Motor	Distal and proximal weakness	Distal weakness	Proprioceptive weakness
DTRs	Areflexia	Distal areflexia	Areflexia
NCS	Velocity affected > amplitude	Amplitudes affected > velocity	Sensory amplitudes affected; radial > sural
Nerve biopsy	Demyelination and remyelination	Axonal degeneration and regeneration	Axonal degeneration but no regeneration
Prognosis	Rapid recovery	Slow recovery	Poor recovery
Causes	GBS, diphtheria, CIDP, DM, MMN	Toxic, metabolic, HIV, CMT2, DM	Sjögren's, cisplatin, pyridoxine

Note: UE, LE, upper, lower extremities; DTRs, deep tendon reflexes; NCS, nerve conduction studies; GBS, Guillain-Barré syndrome; CIDP, chronic inflammatory demyelinating neuropathy; DM, diabetes mellitus; MMN, multifocal motor neuropathy; CMT, Charcot-Marie-Tooth.

Diagnostic tests to further characterize the neuropathy include NCS-EMG, sural nerve biopsy, muscle biopsy, and quantitative sensory testing. Diagnostic tests are more likely to be informative in pts with asymmetric, motor-predominant, rapid-onset, or demyelinating neuropathies.

Electrodiagnosis (NCS-EMG)   NCSs are carried out by stimulating motor or sensory nerves electrically at two or more sites. Electrodiagnostic (EDX) features of

TABLE 203-4   CLASSIFICATION OF NEUROPATHY BY TIME COURSE

Acute
   GBS, porphyria, toxic (triorthocresyl phosphate, vacor, thallium), diphtheria, brachial neuritis
Subacute
   Toxic (hexacarbon, acrylamid), angiopathic, nutritional, alcoholic
Chronic
   Diabetic, CIDP, paraneoplastic, paraprotein
Longstanding heritable
   CMT, Friedreich's ataxia
Recurrent
   Relapsing CIDP, porphyria, Refsum's disease, HNPP

Note: GBS, Guillain-Barré syndrome; CIDP, chronic inflammatory demyelinating neuropathy; CMT, Charcot-Marie-Tooth (disease); HNPP, hereditary neuropathy with pressure palsies.

TABLE 203-5	**POLYNEUROPATHIES (PN)**[a]
Axonal	**Demyelinative**

Acquired

Axonal	Demyelinative
Diabetes	Diabetes
Uremia	Carcinoma
B$_{12}$ deficiency	HIV infection
Critical illness	Lymphoma
HIV infection	Multiple myeloma
Lyme disease	Benign monoclonal gammopathy (IgM)
Lymphoma	Acute inflammatory demyelinating PN (AIDP)
Multiple myeloma	
Acute motor axonal neuropathy	Chronic inflammatory demyelinating PN (CIDP)
Drugs: cisplatin, hydralazine, isoniazid, metronidazole, nitrofurantoin, phenytoin, pyridoxine, vincristine	Diphtheria toxin
Toxins: arsenic, thallium, inorganic lead, organophosphates	Idiopathic
Benign monoclonal gammopathy (IgA, IgG)	
Idiopathic	

Hereditary

Axonal	Demyelinative
HMSN II[b]	HMSN I
Amyloid	HMSN III
Porphyria	Adrenomyeloneuropathy
Fabry's disease	Metachromatic leukodystrophy
Abetalipoproteinemia	Refsum's disease
Friedreich's ataxia	Hereditary liability to pressure palsies
Adrenomyeloneuropathy	
Ataxia telangiectasia	

[a]Does not include rare causes
[b]Hereditary motor and sensory neuropathy

demyelination are slowing of nerve conduction velocity (NCV), dispersion of evoked compound action potentials, conduction block (major decrease in amplitude of muscle compound action potentials on proximal stimulation of the nerve, as compared to distal stimulation), and marked prolongation of distal latencies. In contrast, axonal neuropathies are characterized by a reduced amplitude of evoked compound action potentials with relative preservation of NCV. EMG involves recording for electrical potentials from a needle electrode in muscle at rest and during voluntary contraction. EMG is most useful for distinguishing between and among myopathic and neuropathic disorders. Myopathic disorders are marked by small, short-duration, polyphasic muscle action potentials; by contrast, neuropathic disorders are characterized by muscle denervation. Denervation features a decrease in the number of motor units (e.g., an anterior horn cell, its axon, and the motor end plates and muscle fibers it innervates). In long-standing muscle denervation, motor unit potentials become large and polyphasic. This occurs as a result of collateral reinnervation of denervated muscle fibers by axonal sprouts from surviving motor axons. Other EMG features that favor denervation include fibrillations (random, unregulated firing of individual denervated muscle fibers) and fasciculations (random, spontaneous firing of motor units).

℞ Polyneuropathy

Treatment of the underlying disorder, pain management, and supportive care to protect and rehabilitate damaged tissue all need to be considered. Examples of specific therapies include tight glycemic control in diabetic neuropathy, vitamin replacement for B_{12} deficiency, and immunosuppression for vasculitis.

Pain management usually begins with tricyclic antidepressants (TCAs), duloxetine hydrochloride, or anticonvulsants such as gabapentin. Topical anesthetic agents including lidocaine and capsaicin cream can provide additional relief.

Physical and occupational therapy is important. Proper care of denervated areas prevents skin ulceration, which can lead to poor wound healing, tissue resorption, arthropathy, and ultimately amputation.

Specific Polyneuropathies

1. *Acute inflammatory demyelinating polyneuropathy (AIDP)* or *Guillain-Barré syndrome (GBS)*: an ascending, usually demyelinating, motor > sensory polyneuropathy accompanied by areflexia, motor paralysis, and elevated CSF total protein without pleocytosis. Over two-thirds are preceded by an acute respiratory or gastrointestinal infection. Maximum weakness is usually reached within 2 weeks; demyelination by EMG. Most pts are hospitalized; one-third require ventilatory assistance. 85% make a complete or near-complete recovery with supportive care. Intravenous immune globulin (IVIg) (2 g/kg divided over 5 days) or plasmapheresis (40–50 mL/kg daily for 4–5 days) significantly shortens the course. Glucocorticoids are ineffective. Variants of GBS include Fisher syndrome (ophthalmoparesis, facial diplegia, ataxia, areflexia; associated with serum antibodies to ganglioside GQ1b) and acute motor axonal neuropathy (more severe course than demyelinating GBS; antibodies to GM_1 in some cases).

2. *Chronic inflammatory demyelinating polyneuropathy (CIDP)*: a slowly progressive or relapsing polyneuropathy characterized by diffuse hyporeflexia or areflexia, diffuse weakness, elevated CSF protein without pleocytosis, and demyelination by EMG. Begin treatment when progression is rapid or walking is compromised. Initial treatment is usually IVIg; most pts require periodic retreatment at 6-week intervals. Other treatment options include plasmapheresis or glucocorticoids; immunosuppressants (azathioprine, methotrexate, cyclosporine, cyclophosphamide) used in refractory cases.

3. *Diabetic neuropathy*: typically a distal symmetric, sensorimotor, axonal polyneuropathy. A mixture of demyelination and axonal loss is frequent. Other variants include: isolated sixth or third cranial nerve palsies, asymmetric proximal motor neuropathy in the legs, truncal neuropathy, autonomic neuropathy, and an increased frequency of entrapment neuropathy (see below). The lifetime prevalence is ~55% for type 1 and 45% for type 2 diabetes.

4. *Mononeuropathy multiplex (MM)*: defined as involvement of multiple individual peripheral nerves. When an inflammatory disorder is the cause, *mononeuritis multiplex* is the term used. Both systemic (67%) and nonsystemic (33%) vasculitis may present as MM. Immunosuppressive treatment of the underlying disease (usually with glucocorticoids and cyclophosphamide) is indicated. A tissue diagnosis of vasculitis should be obtained before initiating treatment; a positive biopsy helps to justify the necessary long-term treatment with immunosuppressive medications, and pathologic confirmation is difficult after treatment has commenced.

TABLE 203-6 MONONEUROPATHIES

	Symptoms	Precipitating Activities	Examination	Electro-Diagnosis	Differential Diagnosis	Treatment
Carpal tunnel syndrome	Numbness, pain or paresthesias in fingers	Sleep or repetitive hand activity	Sensory loss in thumb, second, and third fingers Weakness in thenar muscles; inability to make a circle with thumb and index finger Tinel and Phalen signs	Slowing of sensory and motor conduction across carpal tunnel	C6 radiculopathy	Splint Surgery definitive treatment
Ulnar nerve entrapment at the elbow (UNE)	Numbness or paresthesias in ulnar aspect of hand	Elbow flexion during sleep; elbow resting on desk	Sensory loss in the little finger and ulnar half of ring finger Weakness of the interossei and thumb adductor; claw-hand	Focal slowing of nerve conduction velocity at the elbow	Thoracic outlet syndrome C8-T1 radiculopathy	Elbow pads Avoid further injury Surgery when conservative treatment fails
Ulnar nerve entrapment at the wrist	Numbness or weakness in the ulnar distribution in the hand	Unusual hand activities with tools, bicycling	Like UNE but sensory examination spares dorsum of the hand, and selected hand muscles affected	Prolongation of distal motor latency in the hand	UNE	Avoid precipitating activities

Condition	Symptoms	History	Examination	Investigation	Differential	Management
Radial neuropathy at the spiral groove	Wrist drop	Sleeping on arm after inebriation with alcohol—"Saturday night palsy"	Wrist drop with sparing of elbow extension (triceps sparing); finger and thumb extensors paralyzed; sensory loss in radial region of wrist	Early—conduction block along the spiral groove; Late—denervation in radial muscles; reduced radial SNAP	Posterior cord lesion; deltoid also weak; Posterior interosseous nerve (PIN); isolated finger drop; C7 radiculopathy	Splint; Spontaneous recovery provided no ongoing injury
Thoracic outlet syndrome	Numbness, paresthesias in medial arm, forearm, hand and fingers	Lifting heavy objects with the hand	Sensory loss resembles ulnar nerve and motor loss resembles median nerve	Absent ulnar sensory response and reduced median motor response	UNE	Surgery if correctable lesion present
Femoral neuropathy	Buckling of knee, numbness or tingling in thigh/medial leg	Abdominal hysterectomy; lithotomy position; hematoma, diabetes	Wasting and weakness of quadriceps; absent knee jerk; sensory loss in medial thigh and lower leg	EMG of quadriceps, iliopsoas, paraspinal muscles, adductor muscles	L2-4 radiculopathy; Lumbar plexopathy	Physiotherapy to strengthen quadriceps and mobilize hip joint; Surgery if needed
Obturator neuropathy	Weakness of the leg, thigh numbness	Stretch during hip surgery; pelvic fracture; childbirth	Weakness of hip adductors; sensory loss in upper medial thigh	EMG—denervation limited to hip adductors sparing the quadriceps	L3-4 radiculopathy; Lumbar plexopathy	Conservative management; Surgery if needed
Meralgia paresthetica	Pain or numbness in the anterior lateral thigh	Standing or walking; Recent weight gain	Sensory loss in the pocket of the pant distribution	Sometimes slowing of sensory response can be demonstrated across the inguinal ligament	L2 radiculopathy	Usually resolves spontaneously

(continued)

TABLE 203-6 MONONEUROPATHIES (CONTINUED)

	Symptoms	Precipitating Activities	Examination	Electro-Diagnosis	Differential Diagnosis	Treatment
Peroneal nerve entrapment at the fibular head	Footdrop	Usually an acute compressive episode identifiable; weight loss	Weak dorsiflexion, eversion of the foot. Sensory loss in the anterolateral leg and dorsum of the foot	Focal slowing of nerve conduction across fibular head. Denervation in tibialis anterior and peroneus longus muscles	L5 radiculopathy	Foot brace; remove external source of compression
Sciatic neuropathy	Flail foot and numbness in foot	Injection injury; fracture/dislocation of hip; prolonged pressure on hip (comatose patient)	Weakness of hamstring, plantar and dorsiflexion of foot; sensory loss in tibial and peroneal nerve distribution	NCS—abnormal sural, peroneal, and tibial amplitudes. EMG—denervation in sciatic nerve distribution sparing glutei and paraspinal	L5-S1 radiculopathies. Common peroneal neuropathy (partial sciatic nerve injury). LS plexopathies	Conservative follow up for partial sciatic nerve injuries. Brace and physiotherapy. Surgical exploration if needed
Tarsal tunnel syndrome	Pain and paresthesias in the sole of the foot but not in the heel	At the end of the day after standing or walking; nocturnal	Sensory loss in the sole of the foot. Tinel's sign at tarsal tunnel	Reduced amplitude in sensory or motor components of medial and planter nerves	Polyneuropathy, foot deformity, poor circulation	Surgery if no external cause identified

MONONEUROPATHY

Clinical Features Mononeuropathies are usually caused by trauma, compression, or entrapment. Sensory and motor symptoms are in the distribution of a single nerve—most commonly ulnar or median nerves in the arms or peroneal nerve in the leg. Intrinsic factors making pts more susceptible to entrapment include arthritis, fluid retention (pregnancy), amyloid, tumors, and diabetes mellitus. Clinical features favoring conservative management of median neuropathy at the wrist (carpal tunnel syndrome) or ulnar neuropathy at the elbow include sudden onset, no motor deficit, few or no sensory findings (pain or paresthesias may be present), and no evidence of axonal loss by EMG. Surgical decompression considered if chronic course, lack of response to conservative treatment, and site of entrapment is clearly defined. The most frequently encountered mononeuropathies are summarized in Table 203-6.

For a more detailed discussion, see Chaudhry V: Peripheral Neuropathy, Chap. 379, p. 2651; and Hauser SL, Asbury AK: Guillain-Barré Syndrome and Other Immune-Mediated Neuropathies, Chap. 380, p. 2667, in HPIM-17.

204 Myasthenia Gravis (MG)

An autoimmune neuromuscular disorder resulting in weakness and fatigability of skeletal muscles, due to autoantibodies directed against acetylcholine receptors (AChRs) at neuromuscular junctions (NMJs).

CLINICAL FEATURES

May present at any age. Symptoms fluctuate throughout the day and are provoked by exertion. Characteristic distribution: cranial muscles (eyelids, extraocular muscles, facial weakness, "nasal" or slurred speech, dysphagia); in 85%, limb muscles (often proximal and asymmetric) become involved. Reflexes and sensation normal. May be limited to extraocular muscles only. Complications: aspiration pneumonia (weak bulbar muscles), respiratory failure (weak chest wall muscles), exacerbation of myasthenia due to administration of drugs with neuromuscular junction blocking effects (quinolones, macrolides, aminoglycosides, procainamide, propranolol, nondepolarizing muscle relaxants).

PATHOPHYSIOLOGY

Anti-AChR antibodies reduce the number of available AChRs at the NMJ. Postsynaptic folds are flattened or "simplified," with resulting inefficient neuromuscular transmission. During repeated or sustained muscle contraction, decrease in amount of ACh released per nerve impulse ("presynaptic rundown," a normal occurrence), combined with disease-specific decrease in postsynaptic AChRs, results in pathologic fatigue. Thymus is abnormal in 75% of pts (65%

hyperplasia, 10% thymoma). Other autoimmune diseases may coexist: Hashimoto's thyroiditis, Graves' disease, rheumatoid arthritis, lupus erythematosus.

DIFFERENTIAL DIAGNOSIS

1. Lambert-Eaton syndrome (autoantibodies to calcium channels in presynaptic motor nerve terminals)—reduced ACh release; may be associated with malignancy
2. Neurasthenia—weakness/fatigue without underlying organic disorder
3. Penicillamine may cause MG; resolves weeks to months after discontinuing drug
4. Botulism—toxin inhibits presynaptic ACh release; most common form is food-borne.
5. Diplopia from an intracranial mass lesion—compression of nerves to extraocular muscles or brainstem lesions affecting cranial nerve nuclei
6. Hyperthyroidism
7. Progressive external ophthalmoplegia—seen in rare mitochondrial disorders that can be detected with muscle biopsy

LABORATORY EVALUATION

- AChR antibodies—levels do not correlate with disease severity; 85% of all MG patients positive; only 50% with pure ocular findings are positive; positive antibodies are diagnostic. Muscle-specific kinase (MuSK) antibodies present in 40% of AchR antibody-negative pts with generalized MG.
- Tensilon (edrophonium) test—a short-acting anticholinesterase—look for rapid and transient improvement of strength; false-positive (placebo response, motor neuron disease) and false-negative tests occur. Atropine IV should be on hand if symptoms such as bradycardia occur.
- EMG—low-frequency (2–4 Hz) repetitive stimulation produces rapid decrement in amplitude (>10–15%) of evoked motor responses.
- Chest CT/MRI—search for thymoma.
- Consider thyroid and other studies (e.g., ANA) for associated autoimmune disease.
- Measurements of baseline respiratory function are useful.

Rx   Myasthenia Gravis   (See Fig. 204-1)

The anticholinesterase drug pyridostigmine (Mestinon) titrated to assist pt with functional activities (chewing, swallowing, strength during exertion); usual initial dose of 30–60 mg 3–4 times daily; long-acting tablets help at night but have variable absorption so are not reliable during the day. Muscarinic side effects (diarrhea, abdominal cramps, salivation, nausea) blocked with atropine/diphenoxylate or loperamide if required. Plasmapheresis or IV immune globulin (IVIg; 400 mg/kg per day for 5 days) provides temporary boost for seriously ill pts; used to improve condition prior to surgery or during myasthenic crisis (severe exacerbation of weakness with respiratory compromise). Thymectomy improves likelihood of long-term remission in adult pts; whether it helps those with pure ocular disease or those age >55 remains unclear. Glucocorticoids are a mainstay of treatment; begin prednisone at low dose (15–25 mg/d), increase by 5 mg/d every 2–3 days until marked clinical improvement or dose of 50–60 mg/d is reached. Maintain high dose for 1–3 months, then decrease to alternate-day regimen. Immunosuppressive drugs (azathioprine, cyclosporine, mycophenolate mofetil, cyclophosphamide) may spare dose of prednisone required long-term to control symptoms. Myasthenic crisis is de-

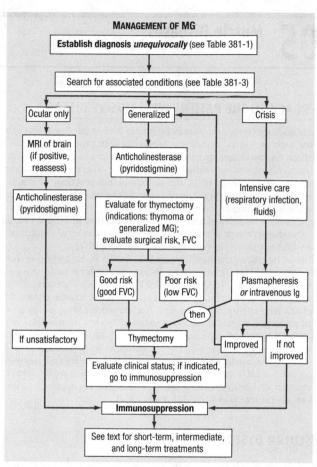

FIGURE 204-1 Algorithm for the management of myasthenia gravis. FVC, forced vital capacity.

fined as an exacerbation of weakness, usually with respiratory failure, sufficient to endanger life; expert management in an intensive care setting essential as is prompt treatment with IVIg or plasmapheresis to hasten recovery.

For a more detailed discussion, see Drachman DB: Myasthenia Gravis and Other Diseases of the Neuromuscular Junction, Chap. 381, p. 2672, in HPIM-17.

205 Muscle Diseases

APPROACH TO THE PATIENT WITH MUSCLE DISEASE

Muscle diseases (*myopathies*) may be intermittent or persistent and usually present with proximal, symmetric weakness with preserved reflexes and sensation. An associated sensory loss suggests injury to peripheral nerve or the central nervous system rather than myopathy; on occasion, disorders affecting the anterior horn cells, the neuromuscular junction, or peripheral nerves can mimic myopathy. Any disorder causing muscle weakness may be accompanied by *fatigue*, referring to an inability to maintain or sustain a force; this must be distinguished from asthenia, a type of fatigue caused by excess tiredness or lack of energy. Fatigue without abnormal clinical or laboratory findings almost never indicates a true myopathy.

Muscle disorders are usually painless; however, *myalgias*, or muscle pains, may occur. Myalgias must be distinguished from *muscle cramps*, i.e., painful muscle contractions, usually due to neurogenic disorders. A *muscle contracture* due to an inability to relax after an active muscle contraction is associated with energy failure in glycolytic disorders. *Myotonia* is a condition of prolonged muscle contraction followed by slow muscle relaxation.

A limited battery of tests can be used to evaluate a suspected myopathy. CK is the preferred muscle enzyme to measure in the evaluation of myopathies. Electrodiagnostic studies (nerve conduction studies and electromyography, NCS-EMG) are usually necessary to distinguish myopathies from neuropathies and neuromuscular junction disorders. An approach to muscle weakness is presented in Figs. 205-1 and 205-2.

MUSCULAR DYSTROPHIES

A varied group of inherited, progressive degenerations of muscle each with unique features.

DUCHENNE DYSTROPHY

X-linked recessive mutation of the dystrophin gene that affects males almost exclusively. Progressive weakness in hip and shoulder girdle muscles beginning by age 5; by age 12, the majority are nonambulatory. Survival beyond age 25 is rare. Associated problems include tendon and muscle contractures, progressive kyphoscoliosis, impaired pulmonary function, cardiomyopathy, and intellectual impairment. Palpable enlargement and firmness of some muscles. Becker dystrophy is a less severe form, with a slower course and later age of onset (5–15) but similar clinical, laboratory, and genetic features.

Laboratory findings include massive elevations (20–100 × normal) of serum CK, a myopathic pattern on EMG testing, and evidence of groups of necrotic muscle fibers with regeneration, phagocytosis, and fatty replacement of muscle on biopsy. Diagnosis is established by determination of dystrophin deficiency in muscle tissue or mutation analysis on peripheral blood leukocytes. Testing available for detecting carriers and prenatal diagnosis.

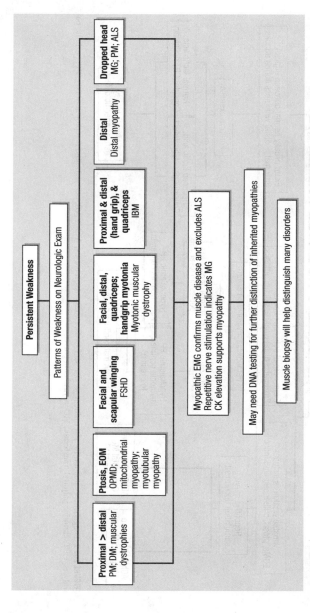

FIGURE 205-1 Diagnostic evaluation of persistent weakness. EOM, extraocular muscle; OPMD, oculopharyngeal muscular dystrophy; FSHD, facioscapulo-humeral muscular dystrophy; IBM, inclusion body myositis; DM, dermatomyositis; PM, polymyositis; MG, myasthenia gravis; ALS, amyotrophic lateral sclerosis; CK, creatinine kinase.

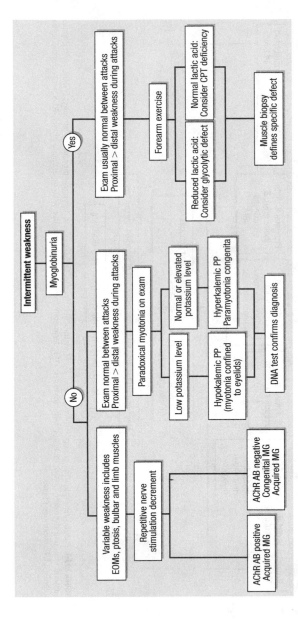

FIGURE 205-2 Diagnostic evaluation for intermittent weakness. EOMs, extraocular muscles; AChR AB, acetylcholine receptor antibody; PP, periodic paralysis; CPT, carnitine palmityl transferase; MG, myasthenia gravis.

Muscular Dystrophy

Treatment is with glucocorticoids [prednisone (0.75 mg/kg)/d]. These slow progression of disease for up to 3 years; some patients cannot tolerate this therapy due to weight gain and increased risk of fractures.

LIMB-GIRDLE DYSTROPHY

A constellation of diseases with proximal muscle weakness involving the pelvic and shoulder girdle musculature. Age of onset, rate of progression, severity of manifestations, inheritance pattern (autosomal dominant or autosomal recessive), and associated complications (e.g., cardiac, respiratory) vary with the specific subtype of disease.

MYOTONIC DYSTROPHY

Autosomal dominant disorder with genetic anticipation. Weakness typically becomes obvious in the second to third decade and initially involves the muscles of the face, neck, and distal extremities. This results in a distinctive facial appearance ("hatchet face") characterized by ptosis, temporal wasting, drooping of the lower lip, and sagging of the jaw. Myotonia manifests as a peculiar inability to relax muscles rapidly following a strong exertion (e.g., after tight hand grip) usually by the age of 5, as well as by sustained contraction of muscles following percussion (e.g., of tongue or thenar eminence).

Associated problems can include frontal baldness, posterior subcapsular cataracts, gonadal atrophy, respiratory and cardiac problems, endocrine abnormalities, intellectual impairment, and hypersomnia. Cardiac disturbances, including complete heart block, may be life-threatening. Respiratory function should be carefully followed, as chronic hypoxia may lead to cor pulmonale.

Laboratory studies show normal or mildly elevated CK, characteristic myotonia and myopathic features on EMG, and a typical pattern of muscle fiber injury on biopsy, including selective type I fiber atrophy in 50% of cases. Pts with myotonic dystrophy type 1 have an unstable region of DNA with an increased number of trinucleotide CTG repeats on chromosome 19q13.3 in a protein kinase gene. Genetic testing for early detection and prenatal diagnosis is possible.

 Myotonic Dystrophy

Phenytoin or mexiletine may help alleviate myotonia, although patients are rarely bothered by this symptom. Pacemaker insertion may be required for syncope or heart block. Orthoses may control foot drop, stabilize the ankle, and decrease falling. Excessive daytime somnolence with or without sleep apnea is not uncommon; sleep studies, noninvasive respiratory support (BiPAP), and treatment with modafinil may be beneficial.

FACIOSCAPULOHUMERAL (FSH) DYSTROPHY

An autosomal dominant, slowly progressive disorder with onset in childhood or young adulthood. Weakness involves facial (usually the initial manifestation), shoulder girdle, and proximal arm muscles and can result in atrophy of biceps, triceps, and scapular winging. Facial weakness results in inability to smile, whistle, or fully close the eyes with loss of facial expressivity. Foot drop and leg weakness may cause falls and progressive difficulty with ambulation.

Laboratory studies reveal normal or slightly elevated CK and usually myopathic features on EMG and muscle biopsy. Pts have deletions at chromosome 4q35. Genetic testing available for carrier detection and prenatal diagnosis.

℞ Facioscapulohumeral Dystrophy

Ankle-foot orthoses are helpful for foot drop. Scapular stabilization procedures may help scapular winging but may not improve function.

OCULOPHARYNGEAL DYSTROPHY (PROGRESSIVE EXTERNAL OPHTHALMOPLEGIA)

Onset in the fourth to sixth decade of ptosis, limitation of extraocular movements, and facial and cricopharyngeal weakness. Dysphagia may be life-threatening. Most pts are of French-Canadian or Spanish-American descent. Mutation in a poly-RNA binding protein responsible.

INFLAMMATORY MYOPATHIES

The most common group of acquired and potentially treatable skeletal muscle disorders. Three major forms: polymyositis (PM), dermatomyositis (DM), and inclusion body myositis (IBM). Usually present as progressive and symmetric muscle weakness; extraocular muscles spared but pharyngeal weakness (dysphagia) and head drop from neck muscle weakness common. Respiratory muscles may be affected in advanced cases. IBM is characterized by early involvement of quadriceps (leading to falls) and distal muscles; IBM may have an asymmetric pattern. Progression is over weeks or months in PM and DM, but typically over years in IBM. Skin involvement in DM may consist of a heliotrope rash (blue-purple discoloration) on the upper eyelids with edema, a flat red rash on the face and upper trunk, or erythema over knuckles (*Gottron's sign*). A variety of cancers are associated with DM. Features of each disorder are summarized in Table 205-1.

℞ Inflammatory Myopathies

Often effective for PM and DM but not for IBM.
- Step 1: Glucocorticoids (prednisone, 1 mg/kg per day for 3–4 weeks, then tapered very gradually)
- Step 2: Approximately 75% of pts require additional therapy with other immunosuppressive drugs. Azathioprine up to 3 mg/kg per day, methotrexate (7.5 mg/week gradually increasing to 25 mg/week), or mycophenolate mofetil commonly used.
- Step 3: Intravenous immunoglobulin (2 g/kg divided over 2–5 days)
- Step 4: A trial of one of the following agents: rituximab, cyclosporine, cyclophosphamide, or tacrolimus.

DISORDERS OF MUSCLE ENERGY METABOLISM

There are two principal sources of energy for skeletal muscle: fatty acids and glucose. Abnormalities in either glucose or lipid utilization can be associated with distinct clinical presentations that can range from an acute, painful syndrome that mimics polymyositis to a chronic, progressive muscle weakness simulating muscular dystrophy. Definitive diagnosis usually requires biochemical-

TABLE 205-1 FEATURES ASSOCIATED WITH INFLAMMATORY MYOPATHIES

Characteristic	Polymyositis	Dermatomyositis	Inclusion Body Myositis
Age at onset	>18 yr	Adulthood and childhood	>50 yr
Familial association	No	No	Yes, in some cases
Extramuscular manifestations	Yes	Yes	Yes
Associated conditions			
Connective tissue diseases	Yes[a]	Scleroderma and mixed connective tissue disease (overlap syndromes)	Yes, in up to 20% of cases[a]
Systemic autoimmune diseases[b]	Frequent	Infrequent	Infrequent
Malignancy	No	Yes, in up to 15% of cases	No
Viruses	Yes[c]	Unproven	Yes[c]
Drugs[d]	Yes	Yes, rarely	No
Parasites and bacteria[e]	Yes	No	No

[a]Systemic lupus erythematosus, rheumatoid arthritis, Sjögren's syndrome, systemic sclerosis, mixed connective tissue disease.
[b]Crohn's disease, vasculitis, sarcoidosis, primary biliary cirrhosis, adult celiac disease, chronic graft-versus-host disease, discoid lupus, ankylosing spondylitis, Behçet's syndrome, myasthenia gravis, acne fulminans, dermatitis herpetiformis, psoriasis, Hashimoto's disease, granulomatous diseases, agammaglobulinemia, monoclonal gammopathy, hypereosinophilic syndrome, Lyme disease, Kawasaki disease, autoimmune thrombocytopenia, hypergammaglobulinemic purpura, hereditary complement deficiency, IgA deficiency.
[c]HIV (human immunodeficiency virus) and HTLV-I (human T cell lymphotropic virus type I).
[d]Drugs include penicillamine (dermatomyositis and polymyositis), zidovudine (polymyositis), and contaminated tryptophan (dermatomyositis-like illness). Other myotoxic drugs may cause myopathy but not an inflammatory myopathy (see text for details).
[e]Parasites (protozoa, cestodes, nematodes), tropical and bacterial myositis (pyomyositis).

enzymatic studies of biopsied muscle. However, muscle enzymes, EMG, and muscle biopsy all might be abnormal and may suggest specific disorders.

Progressive muscle weakness beginning usually in the third or fourth decade can be due to the adult form of *acid maltase deficiency*. Respiratory failure is often the initial manifestation; treatment with enzyme replacement may be of benefit. Progressive weakness beginning after puberty occurs with *debranching enzyme deficiency*. *Glycolytic defects*, including *myophosphorylase deficiency* (McArdle's disease) or *phosphofructokinase deficiency*, present as exercise intolerance with myalgias. Disorders of fatty acid metabolism present with a similar picture. In adults, the most common cause is *carnitine palmitoyltransferase deficiency*. Exercise-induced cramps and myoglobinuria are common; strength is normal between the attacks. Dietary approaches (frequent meals and a low-fat high-carbohydrate diet, or a diet rich in medium-chain triglycerides) are of uncertain value.

MITOCHONDRIAL MYOPATHIES

More accurately referred to as *mitochondrial cytopathies* because multiple tissues are usually affected, these disorders result from defects in mitochondrial DNA. The clinical presentations vary greatly: muscle symptoms may include weakness, ophthalmoparesis, pain, stiffness, or may even be absent; age of onset ranges from infancy to adulthood; associated clinical presentations include ataxia, encephalopathy, seizures, strokelike episodes, and recurrent vomiting. Three groups: chronic progressive external ophthalmoplegia (CPEO), skeletal muscle–central nervous system syndromes, and pure myopathy syndromes simulating muscular dystrophy. The characteristic finding on muscle biopsy is "ragged red fibers," which are muscle fibers with accumulations of abnormal mitochondria. Genetics often show a maternal pattern of inheritance because mitochondrial genes are inherited almost exclusively from the oocyte.

PERIODIC PARALYSES

Muscle membrane excitability is affected in a group of disorders referred to as *channelopathies*. Onset is usually in childhood or adolescence. Episodes typically occur after rest or sleep, often following earlier exercise. May be due to genetic disorders of calcium [hypokalemic periodic paralysis (hypoKPP)], sodium (hyperkalemic periodic paralysis), chloride, or potassium channels. Attacks of hypoKPP are treated with potassium chloride (usually oral), and prophylaxis with acetazolamide (125–1000 mg/d in divided doses) is usually effective. Attacks of thyrotoxic periodic paralysis (usually in Asian men) resemble those of hypoKPP; attacks abate with treatment of the underlying thyroid condition.

ENDOCRINE AND METABOLIC MYOPATHIES

Abnormalities of thyroid function can cause a wide array of muscle disorders. Hypothyroidism is associated with muscle cramps, pain, and stiffness, and proximal muscle weakness occurs in one-third of pts; the relaxation phase of muscle stretch reflexes is characteristically prolonged, and serum CK is often elevated (up to 10 times normal).

Hyperthyroidism can produce proximal muscle weakness and atrophy; bulbar, respiratory, and even esophageal muscles are occasionally involved, causing dysphagia, dysphonia, and aspiration. Other neuromuscular disorders associated with hyperthyroidism include hypoKPP, myasthenia gravis, and a progressive ocular myopathy associated with proptosis (*Graves' ophthalmopathy*). Other endocrine conditions, including parathyroid, adrenal, and pituitary disorders, as well as diabetes mellitus, can also produce myopathy. Deficiencies of vitamins D and E are additional causes of muscle weakness.

DRUG-INDUCED MYOPATHIES

Drugs (including glucocorticoids, statins and other lipid-lowering agents) and toxins (e.g., alcohol) are commonly associated with myopathies (Table 205-2). In most cases, weakness is symmetric and involves proximal limb girdle muscles. Weakness, myalgia, and cramps are common symptoms. An elevated CK is often an important indication of toxicity. Diagnosis often depends on resolution of signs and symptoms with removal of offending agent.

TABLE 205-2 DRUG-INDUCED MYOPATHIES

Drugs	Major Toxic Reaction

Lipid-lowering agents
  Fibric acid derivatives
  HMG-CoA reductase
    inhibitors
  Niacin (nicotinic acid)
	Drugs belonging to all three of the major classes of lipid-lowering agents can produce a spectrum of toxicity: asymptomatic serum creatine kinase elevation, myalgias, exercised-induced pain, rhabdomyolysis, and myoglobinuria.

Glucocorticoids	Acute, high-dose glucocorticoid treatment can cause acute quadriplegic myopathy. These high doses of steroids are often combined with nondepolarizing neuromuscular blocking agents but the weakness can occur without their use. Chronic steroid administration produces predominantly proximal weakness.

Nondepolarizing neuro-
  muscular blocking
  agents
	Acute quadriplegic myopathy can occur with or without concomitant glucocorticoids.

Zidovudine	Mitochondrial myopathy with ragged red fibers.

Drugs of abuse
  Alcohol
  Amphetamines
  Cocaine
  Heroin
  Phencyclidine
  Meperidine
	All drugs in this group can lead to widespread muscle breakdown, rhabdomyolysis, and myoglobinuria.
	
	Local injections cause muscle necrosis, skin induration, and limb contractures.

Autoimmune toxic
  myopathy
  D-Penicillamine
	Use of this drug may cause polymyositis and myasthenia gravis.

Amphophilic cationic
  drugs
  Amiodarone
  Chloroquine
  Hydroxychloroquine
	All amphophilic drugs have the potential to produce painless, proximal weakness associated with autophagic vacuoles in the muscle biopsy.

Antimicrotubular drugs Colchicine	This drug produces painless, proximal weakness especially in the setting of renal failure. Muscle biopsy shows autophagic vacuoles.

For a more detailed discussion, see Brown RH Jr., Amato AA, Mendell JR: Muscular Dystrophies and Other Muscle Diseases, Chap. 382, p. 2678; Dalakas MC: Polymyositis, Dermatomyositis, and Inclusion Body Myositis, Chap. 383, p. 2696, in HPIM-17.

206 Psychiatric Disorders

Mental disorders are common in medical practice and may present either as a primary disorder or as a comorbid condition. The prevalence of mental or substance use disorders in the United States is ~30%, but only one-third of those individuals are currently receiving treatment.

Disorders of mood, thinking, and behavior may be due to a primary psychiatric diagnosis [DSM-IV (*Diagnostic and Statistical Manual*, 4th edition, American Psychiatric Association) Axis I major psychiatric disorders] or a personality disorder (DSM-IV Axis II disorders) or may be secondary to metabolic abnormalities, drug toxicities, focal cerebral lesions, seizure disorders, or degenerative neurologic disease. Any pt presenting with new onset of psychiatric symptoms must be evaluated for underlying psychoactive substance abuse and/or medical or neurologic illness. Psychiatric medications are discussed in Chap. 207. The DSM-IV-PC (Primary Care) Manual provides a synopsis of mental disorders commonly seen in medical practice.

MAJOR PSYCHIATRIC DISORDERS (AXIS I DIAGNOSES)

MOOD DISORDERS (MAJOR AFFECTIVE DISORDERS)

Mood disorders are characterized by a disturbance in the regulation of mood, behavior, and affect; subdivided into (1) depressive disorders, (2) bipolar disorders (depression plus manic or hypomanic episodes), and (3) depression in association with medical illness or alcohol and substance abuse (see Chaps. 209 and 210).

Major Depression   Clinical Features   Affects 15% of the general population at some point in life; 6–8% of all outpatients in primary care settings satisfy diagnostic criteria. Diagnosis is made when five (or more) of the following symptoms have been present for 2 weeks (at least one of the symptoms must be #1 or #2 below):

1. Depressed mood
2. Loss of interest or pleasure
3. Change in appetite or weight
4. Insomnia or hypersomnia
5. Fatigue or loss of energy
6. Psychomotor agitation or retardation
7. Feelings of worthlessness or inappropriate guilt
8. Decreased ability to concentrate and make decisions
9. Recurrent thoughts of death or suicide.

A small number of pts with major depression will have psychotic symptoms (hallucinations and delusions) with their depressed mood. Negative life events can precipitate depression, but genetic factors influence the sensitivity to these events.

Onset of a first depressive episode is typically in early adulthood, although major depression can occur at any age. Untreated episodes generally resolve spontaneously in a few months to a year; however, a sizable number of pts suffer from chronic, unremitting depression or from partial treatment response. Half of all pts experiencing a first depressive episode will go on to a recurrent course. Untreated or partially treated episodes put the pt at risk for future problems with mood disorders. Within an individual, the nature of episodes may be similar over time. A family history of mood disorder is common and tends to predict a recurrent course. Major depression can also be the initial presentation of bipolar disorder (manic depressive illness).

Suicide Approximately 4–5% of all depressed pts will commit suicide, and most will have sought help from a physician within 1 month of their death. Physicians must always inquire about suicide when evaluating a pt with depression.

Depression with Medical Illness Virtually every class of *medication* can potentially induce or worsen depression. Antihypertensive drugs, anticholesterolemic agents, and antiarrhythmic agents are common triggers of depressive symptoms. Among the antihypertensive agents, β-adrenergic blockers and, to a lesser extent, calcium channel blockers are the most likely to cause depressed mood. Iatrogenic depression should also be considered in pts receiving glucocorticoids, antimicrobials, systemic analgesics, antiparkinsonian medications, and anticonvulsants.

Between 20 and 30% of cardiac pts manifest a depressive disorder. Tricyclic antidepressants (TCAs) are contraindicated in patients with bundle branch block, and TCA-induced tachycardia is an additional concern in pts with congestive heart failure. Selective serotonin reuptake inhibitors (SSRIs) appear not to induce ECG changes or adverse cardiac events and thus are reasonable first-line drugs for patients at risk for TCA-related complications. SSRIs may interfere with hepatic metabolism of anticoagulants, however, causing increased anticoagulation.

In *cancer*, the prevalence of depression is 25%, but it occurs in 40–50% of pts with cancers of the pancreas or oropharynx. Extreme cachexia from cancer may be misinterpreted as depression. Antidepressant medications in cancer pts improve quality of life as well as mood.

Diabetes mellitus is another consideration; the severity of the mood state correlates with the level of hyperglycemia and the presence of diabetic complications. Monoamine oxidase inhibitors (MAOIs) can induce hypoglycemia and weight gain. TCAs can produce hyperglycemia and carbohydrate craving. SSRIs, like MAOIs, may reduce fasting plasma glucose, but they are easier to use and may also improve dietary and medication compliance.

Depression may also occur with *hypothyroidism* or *hyperthyroidism*, *neurologic disorders*, in *HIV*-positive individuals, and in *chronic hepatitis C infection* (depression worsens with interferon treatment). Some chronic disorders of uncertain etiology, such as *chronic fatigue syndrome* and *fibromyalgia*, are strongly associated with depression.

℞ Major Depression

Pts with suicidal ideation require treatment by a psychiatrist and may require hospitalization. Most other pts with an uncomplicated unipolar major depression (a major depression that is not part of a cyclical mood disorder, such as a bipolar disorder) can be successfully treated by a nonpsychiatric physician.

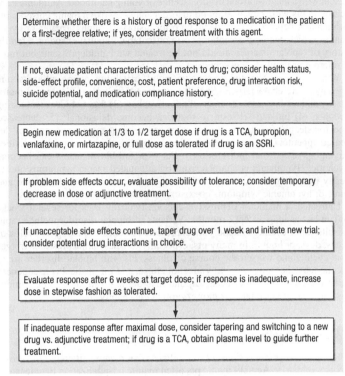

FIGURE 206-1 A guideline for the medical management of major depressive disorder. SSRI, selective serotonin reuptake inhibitor; TCA, tricyclic antidepressant.

Vigorous intervention and successful treatment appear to decrease the risk of future relapse. Pts who do not respond fully to standard treatment should be referred to a psychiatrist.

Antidepressant medications are the mainstay of treatment, although combined treatment with psychotherapy improves outcome. Symptoms are ameliorated after 6–8 weeks at a therapeutic dose in 60–70% of pts. A guideline for the medical management of depression is shown in Fig. 206-1. Once remission is achieved, antidepressants should be continued for 6–9 months. Pts must be monitored carefully after termination of treatment since relapse is common. Pts with two or more episodes of depression should be considered for indefinite maintenance treatment. Electroconvulsive therapy is generally reserved for life-threatening depression unresponsive to medication or for pts in whom the use of antidepressants is medically contraindicated. Vagus nerve stimulation (VNS) has been approved for treatment-resistant depression as well, but its degree of efficacy is controversial.

Bipolar Disorder (Manic Depressive Illness) Clinical Features A cyclical mood disorder in which episodes of major depression are interspersed with episodes of mania or hypomania; 1.5% of the population is affected. Most pts initially present with a manic episode in adolescence or young adulthood. Antidepressant therapy in pts with a cyclical mood disorder may provoke a manic episode; pts with a major depressive episode and a prior history of "highs" (mania or hypomania—which can be pleasant/euphoric or irritable/impulsive) and/or a family history of bipolar disorder should not be treated with antidepressants but must be referred promptly to a psychiatrist.

With mania, an elevated, expansive mood, irritability, angry outbursts, and impulsivity are characteristic. Specific symptoms include: (1) increased motor activity and restlessness; (2) unusual talkativeness; (3) flight of ideas and racing thoughts; (4) inflated self-esteem that can become delusional; (5) decreased need for sleep (often the first feature of an incipient manic episode); (6) decreased appetite; (7) distractability; (8) excessive involvement in risky activities (buying sprees, sexual indiscretions). Pts with full-blown mania can become psychotic. Hypomania is characterized by attenuated manic symptoms and is greatly underdiagnosed, as are "mixed episodes," where both depressive and manic or hypomanic symptoms coexist simultaneously.

Untreated, a manic or depressive episode typically lasts for several weeks but can last as long as 8–12 months. Variants of bipolar disorder include rapid and ultrarapid cycling (manic and depressed episodes occurring at cycles of weeks, days, or hours). In many pts, especially females, antidepressants trigger rapid cycling and worsen the course of illness. Pts with bipolar disorder are at risk for substance use, especially alcohol abuse, and for medical consequences of risky sexual behavior (STDs). Bipolar disorder has a strong genetic component; the concordance rate for monozygotic twins approaches 80%.

℞ Bipolar Disorder

Bipolar disorder is a serious, chronic illness that requires lifelong monitoring by a psychiatrist. Acutely manic pts often require hospitalization to reduce environmental stimulation and to protect themselves and others from the consequences of their reckless behavior. The recurrent nature of bipolar disorder necessitates maintenance treatment. Mood stabilizers (lithium, valproic acid, carbamazepine, lamotrigine) are effective for the resolution of acute episodes and for prophylaxis of future episodes.

SCHIZOPHRENIA AND OTHER PSYCHOTIC DISORDERS

Schizophrenia Clinical Features Occurs in 0.85% of the population worldwide; lifetime prevalence is ~1–1.5%. Characterized by perturbations of language, perception, thinking, social activity, affect, and volition. Pts usually present in late adolescence, often after an insidious premorbid course of subtle psychosocial difficulties. Core psychotic features last ≥6 months and include positive symptoms (such as conceptual disorganization, delusions, or hallucinations) and negative symptoms (loss of function, anhedonia, decreased emotional expression, impaired concentration, and diminished social engagement). Negative symptoms predominate in one-third and are associated with a poor long-term outcome and poor response to treatment.

Prognosis depends not on symptom severity but on the response to antipsychotic medication. A permanent remission without recurrence does occasionally occur. About 10% of schizophrenic patients commit suicide. Comorbid substance abuse is common.

R͓ₓ Schizophrenia

Hospitalization is required for acutely psychotic pts who may be dangerous to themselves or others. Conventional antipsychotic medications are effective against hallucinations, delusions, and thought disorder. The novel antipsychotic medications—clozapine, risperidone, olanzapine, quetiapine, ziprasidone, and aripiprazole—are helpful in pts unresponsive to conventional neuroleptics and may also be more useful for negative and cognitive symptoms. Drug treatment by itself is insufficient, and educational efforts directed toward families and relevant community resources are necessary to maintain stability and optimize outcomes.

Other Psychotic Disorders These include *schizoaffective disorder* (where symptoms of schizophrenia are interspersed with major mood episodes) and *schizophreniform* disorder (pts who meet the symptom requirements but not the duration requirements for schizophrenia).

ANXIETY DISORDERS

Characterized by severe, persistent anxiety or sense of dread or foreboding. Most prevalent group of psychiatric illnesses seen in the community; present in 15–20% of medical clinic patients.

Panic Disorder Occurs in 1–3% of the population; familial aggregation may occur. Onset in late adolescence or early adulthood. Initial presentation is almost always to a nonpsychiatric physician, frequently in the ER, as a possible heart attack or serious respiratory problem. The disorder is often initially unrecognized or misdiagnosed. Three quarters of pts with panic disorder will also satisfy criteria for major depression at some point.

Clinical Features Characterized by panic attacks, which are sudden, unexpected, overwhelming paroxysms of terror and apprehension with multiple associated somatic symptoms. Attacks usually reach a peak within 10 min, then slowly resolve spontaneously, occurring in an unexpected fashion. Diagnostic criteria for panic disorder include recurrent panic attacks and at least 1 month of concern or worry about the attacks or a change in behavior related to them. Panic attacks must be accompanied by at least four of the following: palpitations, sweating, trembling or shaking, dyspnea, choking, chest pain, nausea or abdominal distress, dizziness or faintness, derealization or depersonalization, fear of losing control, fear of death, paresthesias, and chills or hot flashes.

When the disorder goes unrecognized and untreated, pts often experience significant morbidity: they become afraid of leaving home and may develop anticipatory anxiety, agoraphobia, and other spreading phobias; many turn to self-medication with alcohol or benzodiazepines.

Panic disorder must be differentiated from cardiovascular and respiratory disorders. Conditions that may mimic or worsen panic attacks include hyperthyroidism, pheochromocytoma, hypoglycemia, drug ingestions (amphetamines, cocaine, caffeine, sympathomimetic nasal decongestants), and drug withdrawal (alcohol, barbiturates, opiates, minor tranquilizers).

R͓ₓ Panic Disorder

The cornerstone of drug therapy is antidepressant medication. SSRIs benefit the majority of panic disorder patients and do not have the adverse effects of the TCAs. Benzodiazepines may be used in the short term while waiting for antidepressants to take effect.

Early psychotherapeutic intervention and education aimed at symptom control enhances the effectiveness of drug treatment. Cognitive-behavioral psychotherapy (CBP) (identifying and aborting panic attacks through relaxation and breathing techniques) can be effective.

Generalized Anxiety Disorder (GAD)   Characterized by persistent, chronic anxiety; occurs in 5–6% of the population.

Clinical Features   Pts experience persistent, excessive, and/or unrealistic worry associated with muscle tension, impaired concentration, autonomic arousal, feeling "on edge" or restless, and insomnia. Pts worry excessively over minor matters, with life-disrupting effects; unlike panic disorder, complaints of shortness of breath, palpitations, and tachycardia are relatively rare. Secondary depression is common, as is social phobia and comorbid substance abuse.

R̶x̶   Generalized Anxiety Disorder

A combination of pharmacologic and psychotherapeutic interventions is most effective; complete symptom relief is rare. Benzodiazepines are the initial agents of choice when generalized anxiety is severe and acute enough to warrant drug therapy; physicians must be alert to psychological and physical dependence on benzodiazepines. Some SSRIs are also effective. A subgroup of pts respond to buspirone, a nonbenzodiazepine anxiolytic. Anticonvulsants with GABA-ergic properties (gabapentin, oxcarbazepine, tiagabine, pregabalin, divalproex) may also be effective against anxiety.

Obsessive-Compulsive Disorder (OCD)   A severe disorder present in 2–3% of the population and characterized by recurrent obsessions (persistent intrusive thoughts) and compulsions (repetitive behaviors) that impair everyday functioning. Pts are often ashamed of their symptoms; physicians must ask specific questions to screen for this disorder including asking about recurrent thoughts and behaviors.

Clinical Features   Common obsessions include thoughts of violence (such as killing a loved one), obsessive slowness for fear of making a mistake, fears of germs or contamination, and excessive doubt or uncertainty. Examples of compulsions include repeated checking to be assured that something was done properly, hand washing, extreme neatness and ordering behavior, and counting rituals, such as numbering one's steps while walking.

Onset is usually in adolescence (childhood onset is not rare); more common in males and first-born children. Comorbid conditions are common, the most frequent being depression, other anxiety disorders, eating disorders, and tics. The course of OCD is usually episodic with periods of incomplete remission; some cases may show a steady deterioration in psychosocial functioning.

R̶x̶   Obsessive-Compulsive Disorder

Clomipramine and the SSRIs (fluoxetine, fluvoxamine) are effective, but only 50–60% of pts show adequate improvement with pharmacotherapy alone. A combination of drug therapy and CBP is most effective for the majority of pts.

Posttraumatic Stress Disorder (PTSD) Occurs in a subgroup of individuals exposed to a severe life-threatening trauma. If the reaction occurs shortly after the event, it is termed *acute stress disorder*, but if the reaction is delayed and subject to recurrence, PTSD is diagnosed. Predisposing factors include a past psychiatric history and personality characteristics of extroversion and high neuroticism.

Clinical Features Individuals experience associated symptoms of detachment and loss of emotional responsivity. The pt may feel depersonalized and unable to recall specific events of the trauma, although it is reexperienced through intrusions in thought, dreams, or flashbacks. Comorbid substance abuse and other mood and anxiety disorders are common. This disorder is extremely debilitating; most pts require referral to a psychiatrist for ongoing care.

> **Rx Posttraumatic Stress Disorder**
>
> TCAs, phenelzine (an MAOI), and the SSRIs all are somewhat effective. Trazodone is frequently used at night to help with insomnia. Psychotherapeutic strategies help the pt overcome avoidance behaviors and master fear of recurrence of the trauma.

Phobic Disorders Clinical Features Recurring, irrational fears of specific objects, activities, or situations, with subsequent avoidance behavior of the phobic stimulus. Diagnosis is made only when the avoidance behavior interferes with social or occupational functioning. Affects ~10% of the population.

1. *Agoraphobia*: Fear of being in public places. May occur in absence of panic disorder, but is almost invariably preceded by that condition.
2. *Social phobia*: Persistent irrational fear of, and need to avoid, any situation where there is risk of scrutiny by others, with potential for embarrassment or humiliation. Common examples include excessive fear of public speaking and excessive fear of social engagements.
3. *Simple phobias*: Persistent irrational fears and avoidance of specific objects. Examples include fear of heights (acrophobia), blood, and closed spaces (claustrophobia).

> **Rx Phobic Disorders**
>
> Agoraphobia is treated as for panic disorder. Beta blockers (e.g., propranolol, 20–40 mg PO 2 h before the event) are particularly effective in the treatment of "performance anxiety." SSRIs are very helpful in treating social phobias. Social and simple phobias respond well to behaviorally focused psychotherapy.

Somatoform Disorders Clinical Features Pts with multiple somatic complaints that cannot be explained by a known medical condition or by the effects of substances; seen commonly in primary care practice (prevalence of 5%). In *somatization disorder*, the pt presents with multiple physical complaints referable to different organ systems. Onset is before age 30, and the disorder is persistent; pts with somatization disorder can be impulsive and demanding. In *conversion disorder*, the symptoms involve voluntary motor or sensory function. In *hypochondriasis*, the pt believes there is a serious medical illness, despite reassurance and appropriate medical evaluation. As with somatization disorder, these pts have a history of poor relationships with physicians due to their sense that they have not received adequate evaluation. Hypochondriasis can be disabling and show a waxing and waning course. In *factitious illnesses*, the pt consciously and voluntarily produces physical symptoms; the sick role is gratifying. *Munchausen's syndrome* refers to individuals with dramatic, chronic, or severe factitious illness. A variety of signs, symptoms, and diseases have been simulated in factitious illnesses; most common are chronic diarrhea, fever of unknown origin, intestinal bleeding, hematuria, seizures, hypoglycemia. In *malingering*, the fabrication of illness derives from a desire for an external gain (narcotics, disability).

℞ Somatoform Disorders

Pts with somatoform disorders are usually subjected to multiple diagnostic tests and exploratory surgeries in an attempt to find their "real" illness. This approach is doomed to failure. Successful treatment is achieved through behavior modification, in which access to the physician is adjusted to provide a consistent, sustained, and predictable level of support that is not contingent on the pt's level of presenting symptoms or distress. Visits are brief, supportive, and structured and are not associated with a need for diagnostic or treatment action. Pts may benefit from antidepressant treatment. Consultation with a psychiatrist is essential.

PERSONALITY DISORDERS (AXIS II DIAGNOSES)

Characteristic patterns of thinking, feeling, and interpersonal behavior that are relatively inflexible and cause significant functional impairment or subjective distress for the individual. Individuals with personality disorders are often regarded as "difficult patients."

DSM-IV describes three major categories of personality disorders; pts usually present with a combination of features.

CLUSTER A PERSONALITY DISORDERS

Includes individuals who are odd and eccentric and who maintain an emotional distance from others. The *paranoid* personality pt has pervasive mistrust and suspiciousness of others. The *schizoid* personality is interpersonally isolated, cold, and indifferent, while the *schizotypal* personality is eccentric and superstitious, with magical thinking and unusual perceptual experiences.

CLUSTER B PERSONALITY DISORDERS

Describes individuals whose behavior is impulsive, excessively emotional, and erratic. The *borderline* personality is impulsive and manipulative, with unpredictable and fluctuating intense moods and unstable relationships, a fear of abandonment, and occasional rage episodes. The *histrionic* pt is dramatic, engaging, seductive, and attention-seeking. The *narcissistic* pt is self-centered and has an inflated sense of self-importance combined with a tendency to devalue or demean others, while pts with *antisocial* personality disorder use other people to achieve their own ends and engage in exploitative and manipulative behavior with no sense of remorse.

CLUSTER C PERSONALITY DISORDERS

Enduring traits are anxiety and fear. The *dependent* pt fears separation, tries to engage others to assume responsibility, and often has a help-rejecting style. Pts with *compulsive* personality disorder are meticulous and perfectionistic but also inflexible and indecisive. *Avoidant* pts are anxious about social contact and have difficulty assuming responsibility for their isolation.

For a more detailed discussion, see Reus VI: Mental Disorders, Chap. 386, p. 2710, in HPIM-17.

207 Psychiatric Medications

Four major classes are commonly used in adults: (1) antidepressants, (2) anxiolytics, (3) antipsychotics, and (4) mood stabilizing agents. Nonpsychiatric physicians should become familiar with one or two drugs in each of the first three classes so that the indications, dose range, efficacy, potential side effects, and interactions with other medications are well known.

GENERAL PRINCIPLES OF USE

1. Most treatment failures are due to undermedication and impatience. For a proper medication trial to take place, an effective dose must be taken for an adequate amount of time. For antidepressants, antipsychotics, and mood stabilizers, full effects may take weeks or months to occur.
2. History of a positive response to a medication usually indicates that a response to the same drug will occur again. A family history of a positive response to a specific medication is also useful.
3. Pts who fail to respond to one drug will often respond to another in the same class; one should attempt another trial with a drug that has a different mechanism of action or a different chemical structure. Treatment failures should be referred to a psychiatrist, as should all pts with psychotic symptoms or who require mood stabilizers.
4. Avoid polypharmacy; a pt who is not responding to standard monotherapy requires referral to a psychiatrist.
5. Pharmacokinetics may be altered in the elderly, with smaller volumes of distribution, reduced renal and hepatic clearance, longer biologic half-lives, and greater potential for CNS toxicity. The rule with elderly pts is to "start low and go slow."
6. Never stop treatment abruptly; especially true for antidepressants and anxiolytics. In general, medications should be slowly tapered and discontinued over 2–4 weeks.
7. Review possible side effects each time a drug is prescribed; educate pts and family members about side effects and need for patience in awaiting a response.

ANTIDEPRESSANTS (ADs)

Useful to group according to known actions on CNS monoaminergic systems (Table 207-1). The selective serotonin reuptake inhibitors (SSRIs) have predominant effects on serotonergic neurotransmission, also reflected in side effect profile.

TABLE 207-1 ANTIDEPRESSANTS

Name	Usual Daily Dose, mg	Side Effects	Comments
SSRIs			
Fluoxetine (Prozac)	10–80	Headache; nausea and other GI effects; jitteriness; insomnia; sexual dysfunction; can affect plasma levels of other meds (except sertraline); akathisia rare	Once daily dosing, usually in A.M.; fluoxetine has very long half-life; must not be combined with MAOIs
Sertraline (Zoloft)	50–200		
Paroxetine (Paxil)	20–60		
Fluvoxamine (Luvox)	100–300		
Citalopram (Celexa)	20–60		
Escitalopram (Lexapro)	10–30		
TCAs			
Amitriptyline (Elavil)	150–300	Anticholinergic (dry mouth, tachycardia, constipation, urinary retention, blurred vision); sweating; tremor; postural hypotension; cardiac conduction delay; sedation; weight gain	Once daily dosing, usually qhs; blood levels of most TCAs available; can be lethal in O.D. (lethal dose = 2 g); nortriptyline best tolerated, especially by elderly
Nortriptyline (Pamelor)	50–200		
Imipramine (Tofranil)	150–300		
Desipramine (Norpramin)	150–300		
Doxepin (Sinequan)	150–300		
Clomipramine (Anafranil)	150–300		
Mixed norepinephrine/serotonin reuptake inhibitors			
Venlafaxine (Effexor)	75–375	Nausea; dizziness; dry mouth; headaches; increased blood pressure; anxiety and insomnia	Bid-tid dosing (extended release available); lower potential for drug interactions than SSRIs; contraindicated with MAOI
Duloxetine (Cymbalta)	40–60	Nausea, dizziness, headache, insomnia, constipation	May have utility in treatment of neuropathic pain and stress incontinence
Mirtazapine (Remeron)	15–45	Somnolence; weight gain; neutropenia rare	Once daily dosing
Mixed-action drugs			
Bupropion (Wellbutrin)	250–450	Jitteriness; flushing; seizures in at-risk patients; anorexia; tachycardia; psychosis	Tid dosing, but sustained release also available; fewer sexual side effects than SSRIs or TCAs; may be useful for adult ADD

Drug	Dose (mg)	Side Effects	Comments
Trazodone (Desyrel)	200–600	Sedation; dry mouth; ventricular irritability; postural hypotension; priapism rare	Useful in low doses for sleep because of sedating effects with no anticholinergic side effects
Nefazodone (Serzone)	300–600	Sedation; headache; dry mouth; nausea; constipation	Discontinued sale in United States and several other countries due to risk of liver failure
Amoxapine (Asendin)	200–600	Sexual dysfunction	Lethality in overdose; EPS possible
MAOIs			
Phenelzine (Nardil)	45–90	Insomnia; hypotension; anorgasmia; weight gain; hypertensive crisis; toxic reactions with SSRIs	May be more effective in patients with atypical features or treatment-refractory depression
Tranylcypromine (Parnate)	20–50		
Isocarboxazid (Marplan)	20–60		
Transdermal selegiline (Emsam)	6–12	Local skin reaction; hypertension	No dietary restrictions with 6-mg dose

Note: ADD, attention deficit disorder; MAOI, monoamine oxidase inhibitor; SSRI, selective serotonin reuptake inhibitor; TCA, tricyclic antidepressant; EPS, extrapyramidal symptoms.

The TCAs, or tricyclic antidepressants, affect noradrenergic and, to a lesser extent, serotonergic neurotransmission but also have anticholinergic and antihistaminic effects. Venlafaxine, duloxetine, and mirtazapine have mixed noradrenergic and serotonergic effects. Bupropion is a novel antidepressant that enhances noradrenergic function. Trazodone and nefazodone have mixed effects on serotonin receptors and on other neurotransmitter systems. The MAOIs inhibit monoamine oxidase, the primary enzyme responsible for the degradation of monoamines in the synaptic cleft.

ADs are effective against major depression, particularly when neurovegetative symptoms and signs are present. Despite the widespread use of SSRIs, there is no convincing evidence that they are more efficacious than TCAs, although their safety profile in overdose is more favorable than that of the TCAs. ADs are also useful in treatment of panic disorder, posttraumatic stress disorder, chronic pain syndromes, and generalized anxiety disorder. The TCA clomipramine and the SSRIs successfully treat obsessive-compulsive disorder.

All ADs require at least 2 weeks at a therapeutic dose before clinical improvement is observed. All ADs also have the potential to trigger a manic episode or rapid cycling when given to a pt with bipolar disorder. The MAOIs must not be prescribed concurrently with other ADs or with narcotics, as potentially fatal reactions may occur. "Withdrawal syndromes" usually consisting of malaise can occur when ADs are stopped abruptly.

ANXIOLYTICS

Benzodiazepines bind to sites on the γ-aminobutyric acid receptor and are crosstolerant with alcohol and with barbiturates. Four clinical properties: (1) sedative, (2) anxiolytic, (3) skeletal muscle relaxant, and (4) antiepileptic. Individual drugs differ in terms of potency, onset of action, duration of action (related to half-life and presence of active metabolites), and metabolism (Table 207-2). Benzodiazepines have additive effects with alcohol; like alcohol, they can produce tolerance and physiologic dependence, with serious withdrawal syndromes (tremors, seizures, delirium, and autonomic hyperactivity) if discontinued too quickly, especially for those with short half-lives.

Buspirone is a nonbenzodiazepine anxiolytic that is nonsedating, is not cross-tolerant with alcohol, and does not induce tolerance or dependence. It requires at least 2 weeks at therapeutic doses to achieve full effects.

ANTIPSYCHOTIC MEDICATIONS

These include the typical neuroleptics, which act by blocking dopamine D_2 receptors, and the atypical neuroleptics, which act on dopamine, serotonin, and other neurotransmitter systems. Some antipsychotic effect may occur within hours or days of initiating treatment, but full effects usually require 6 weeks to several months of daily, therapeutic dosing.

Conventional Antipsychotics Useful to group into high-, mid-, and low-potency neuroleptics (Table 207-3). High-potency neuroleptics are least sedating, have almost no anticholinergic side effects, and have a strong tendency to induce extrapyramidal side effects (EPSEs). The EPSEs occur within several hours to several weeks of beginning treatment and include acute dystonias, akathisia, and pseudoparkinsonism. Extrapyramidal symptoms respond well to trihexyphenidyl, 2 mg twice daily, or benztropine mesylate, 1 to 2 mg twice daily. Akathisia may respond to beta blockers. Low-potency neuroleptics are very sedating, may cause orthostatic hypotension, are anticholinergic, and tend not to induce EPSEs frequently.

TABLE 207-2 ANXIOLYTICS

Name	Equivalent PO dose, mg	Onset of Action	Half-life, h	Comments
Benzodiazepines				
Diazepam (Valium)	5	Fast	20–70	Active metabolites; quite sedating
Flurazepam (Dalmane)	15	Fast	30–100	Flurazepam is a pro-drug; metabolites are active; quite sedating
Triazolam (Halcion)	0.25	Intermediate	1.5–5	No active metabolites; can induce confusion and delirium, especially in elderly
Lorazepam (Ativan)	1	Intermediate	10–20	No active metabolites; direct hepatic glucuronide conjugation; quite sedating
Alprazolam (Xanax)	0.5	Intermediate	12–15	Active metabolites; not too sedating; may have specific antidepressant and antipanic activity; tolerance and dependence develop easily
Chlordiazepoxide (Librium)	10	Intermediate	5–30	Active metabolites; moderately sedating
Oxazepam (Serax)	15	Slow	5–15	No active metabolites; direct glucuronide conjugation; not too sedating
Temazepam (Restoril)	15	Slow	9–12	No active metabolites; moderately sedating
Clonazepam (Klonopin)	0.5	Slow	18–50	No active metabolites; moderately sedating
Non-benzodiazepines				
Buspirone (BuSpar)	7.5	2 weeks	2–3	Active metabolites; tid dosing—usual daily dose 10–20 mg tid; nonsedating; no additive effects with alcohol; useful for agitation in demented or brain-injured patients

TABLE 207-3 ANTIPSYCHOTIC AGENTS

Name	Usual PO Daily Dose, mg	Side Effects	Sedation	Comments
First-Generation Antipsychotics				
Low-potency				
Chlorpromazine (Thorazine)	100–1000	Anticholinergic effects; orthostasis; photosensitivity; cholestasis; QT prolongation	+++	EPSEs usually not prominent; can cause anticholinergic delirium in elderly patients
Thioridazine (Mellaril)	100–600			
Clozapine (Clozaril)	150–600	Agranulocytosis (1%); weight gain; seizures; drooling; hyperthermia	++	Requires weekly WBC for first 6 months, then biweekly if stable
Mid-potency				
Trifluoperazine (Stelazine)	2–50	Fewer anticholinergic effects; fewer EPSEs than with higher potency agents.	++	Well tolerated by most patients
Perphenazine (Trilafon)	4–64	Frequent EPSEs	++	
Loxapine (Loxitane)	30–100	Frequent EPSEs	++	
Molindone (Moban)	30–100		0	Little weight gain
High-potency				
Haloperidol (Haldol)	.5–20	No anticholinergic side effects; EPSEs often prominent	0/+	Often prescribed in doses that are too high; long-acting injectable forms of haloperidol and fluphenazine available
Fluphenazine (Prolixin)	1–20	Frequent EPSEs	0/+	
Thiothixene (Navane)	2–50	Frequent EPSEs	0/+	

Second-Generation Antipsychotics

Risperidone (Risperdal)	2–8	Orthostasis	Requires slow titration; EPSEs observed with doses >6 mg qd +
Olanzapine (Zyprexa)	10–30	Weight gain	Mild prolactin elevation + +
Quetiapine (Seroquel)	350–800	Sedation; weight gain; anxiety	Bid dosing + + +
Ziprasidone (Geodon)	120–200	Orthostatic hypotension	Minimal weight gain; increases QT interval +/++
Aripiprazole (Abilify)	10–30	Nausea, anxiety, insomnia	Mixed agonist/antagonist 0/+

Note: EPSEs, extrapyramidal side effects; WBC, white blood count.

Up to 20% of pts treated with conventional antipsychotic agents for >1 year develop tardive dyskinesia (probably due to dopamine receptor supersensitivity), an abnormal involuntary movement disorder most often observed in the face and distal extremities. Treatment includes gradual withdrawal of the neuroleptic, with possible switch to a novel neuroleptic; anticholinergic agents can worsen the disorder.

Rarely, pts exposed to neuroleptics develop neuroleptic malignant syndrome (NMS), a life-threatening complication with a mortality rate as high as 25%; hyperpyrexia, autonomic hyperactivity, muscle rigidity, obtundation, and agitation are characteristic, associated with increased WBC, increased CPK, and myoglobinuria. Treatment involves immediate discontinuation of neuroleptics, supportive care, and use of dantrolene and bromocriptine.

Novel Antipsychotics A new class of agents that has become the first line of treatment (Table 207-3); efficacious in treatment-resistant pts, tend not to induce EPSEs or tardive dyskinesia, and appear to have uniquely beneficial properties on negative symptoms and cognitive dysfunction. Main problem is side effect of weight gain (most prominent in clozapine and in olanzapine; can induce diabetes). The CATIE study, a large-scale investigation of antipsychotic agents in the "real world," revealed a high rate of discontinuation of all medications over 18 months; olanzapine was modestly more effective than other agents but with a higher discontinuation rate due to side effects.

TABLE 207-4	CLINICAL PHARMACOLOGY OF MOOD STABILIZERS
Agent and Dosing	**Side Effects and Other Effects**

Lithium
    Starting dose: 300 mg bid or tid
    Therapeutic blood level:
        0.8–1.2 meq/L
	Common side effects: Nausea/anorexia/diarrhea, fine tremor, thirst, polyuria, fatigue, weight gain, acne, folliculitis, neutrophilia, hypothyroidism
	Blood level is increased by thiazides, tetracyclines, and NSAIDs
	Blood level is decreased by bronchodilators, verapamil, and carbonic anhydrase inhibitors
	Rare side effects: Neurotoxicity, renal toxicity, hypercalcemia, ECG changes

Valproic acid
    Starting dose: 250 mg tid
    Therapeutic blood level:
        50–125 µg/mL
	Common side effects: Nausea/anorexia, weight gain, sedation, tremor, rash, alopecia
	Inhibits hepatic metabolism of other medications
	Rare side effects: Pancreatitis, hepatotoxicity, Stevens-Johnson syndrome

Carbamazepine/oxcarbazepine Starting dose: 200 mg bid for carbamazepine, 150 bid for oxcarbazepine Therapeutic blood level: 4–12 µg/mL for carbamazepine	*Common side effects:* Nausea/anorexia, sedation, rash, dizziness/ataxia Carbamazepine, but not oxcarbazepine, induces hepatic metabolism of other medications *Rare side effects:* Hyponatremia, agranulocytosis, Stevens-Johnson syndrome
Lamotrigine Starting dose: 25 mg/d	*Common side effects:* Rash, dizziness, headache, tremor, sedation, nausea *Rare side effect:* Stevens-Johnson syndrome

Note: NSAID, nonsteroidal anti-inflammatory drug; ECG, electrocardiogram.

MOOD-STABILIZING AGENTS

Four mood stabilizers in common use: lithium, carbamazepine, valproic acid, and lamotrigine (Table 207-4). Lithium is the "gold standard" and the best studied, and along with carbamazepine and valproic acid, is used for treatment of acute manic episodes; 1–2 weeks to reach full effect. As prophylaxis, the mood stabilizers reduce frequency and severity of both manic and depressed episodes in cyclical mood disorders. In refractory bipolar disorder, combinations of mood stabilizers may be beneficial.

For a more detailed discussion, see Reus VI: Mental Disorders, Chap. 386, p. 2710, in HPIM-17.

208 Eating Disorders

DEFINITIONS

Anorexia nervosa is characterized by refusal to maintain normal body weight, resulting in a body weight < 85% of the expected weight for age and height. *Bulimia nervosa* is characterized by recurrent episodes of binge eating followed by abnormal compensatory behaviors, such as self-induced vomiting, laxative abuse, or excessive exercise. Weight is in the normal range or above.

Both anorexia nervosa and bulimia nervosa occur primarily among previously healthy young women who become overly concerned with body shape and weight. Binge eating and purging behavior may be present in both conditions, with the critical distinction between the two resting on the weight of the individual. The diagnostic features of each of these disorders are shown in Tables 208-1 and 208-2.

CLINICAL FEATURES

Anorexia Nervosa
- General: feeling cold
- Skin, hair, nails: alopecia, lanugo, acrocyanosis, edema

TABLE 208-1   DIAGNOSTIC FEATURES OF ANOREXIA NERVOSA

Refusal to maintain body weight at or above a minimally normal weight for age and height. (This includes a failure to achieve weight gain expected during a period of growth leading to an abnormally low body weight.)
Intense fear of weight gain or becoming fat.
Distortion of body image (e.g., feeling fat despite an objectively low weight or minimizing the seriousness of low weight).
Amenorrhea. (This criterion is met if menstrual periods occur only following hormone—e.g., estrogen—administration.)

TABLE 208-2	**DIAGNOSTIC FEATURES OF BULIMIA NERVOSA**

Recurrent episodes of binge eating, which is characterized by the consumption of a large amount of food in a short period of time and a feeling that the eating is out of control.

Recurrent inappropriate behavior to compensate for the binge eating, such as self-induced vomiting.

The occurrence of both the binge eating and the inappropriate compensatory behavior at least twice weekly, on average, for 3 months.

Overconcern with body shape and weight.

Note: If the diagnostic criteria for anorexia nervosa are simultaneously met, only the diagnosis of anorexia nervosa is given.

- Cardiovascular: bradycardia, hypotension
- Gastrointestinal: salivary gland enlargement, slow gastric emptying, constipation, elevated liver enzymes
- Hematopoietic: normochromic, normocytic anemia; leukopenia
- Fluid/electrolyte: increased blood urea nitrogen, increased creatinine, hyponatremia, hypokalemia
- Endocrine: low luteinizing hormone and follicle-stimulating hormone with secondary amenorrhea, hypoglycemia, normal thyroid-stimulating hormone with low normal thyroxine, increased plasma cortisol, osteopenia

Bulimia Nervosa

- Gastrointestinal: salivary gland enlargement, dental erosion
- Fluid/electrolyte: hypokalemia, hypochloremia, alkalosis (from vomiting) or acidosis (from laxative abuse)
- Other: loss callus on dorsum of hand

℞ Eating Disorders

Anorexia Nervosa

Weight restoration to 90% of predicted weight is the primary goal in the treatment of anorexia nervosa. The intensity of the initial treatment, including the need for hospitalization, is determined by the pt's current weight, the rapidity of recent weight loss, and the severity of medical and psychological complications (Fig. 208-1). Severe electrolyte imbalances should be identified and corrected. Nutritional restoration can almost always be successfully accomplished by oral feeding. For severely underweight pts, sufficient calories should be provided initially in divided meals as food or liquid supplements to maintain weight and to permit stabilization of fluid and electrolyte balance (1200–1800 kcal/d intake). Calories can be gradually increased to achieve a weight gain of 1–2 kg per week (3000–4000 kcal/d intake). Meals must be supervised. Intake of vitamin D (400 IU/d) and calcium (1500 mg/d) should be sufficient to minimize bone loss. The assistance of psychiatrists or psychologists experienced in the treatment of anorexia nervosa is usually necessary. No psychotropic medications are of established value in the treatment of anorexia nervosa. Medical complications occasionally occur during refeeding; most patients transiently retain excess fluid, occasionally resulting in peripheral edema. Congestive heart failure and acute gastric dilatation have been described when refeeding is rapid. Transient modest elevations in serum levels of liver enzymes occasionally occur. Low levels of magnesium and phosphate should be replaced. Mortality is 5% per decade, from either chronic starvation or suicide.

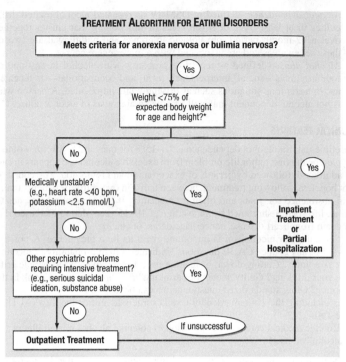

FIGURE 208-1 An algorithm for basic treatment decisions regarding patients with anorexia nervosa or bulimia nervosa. *(Based on Fig. 76-1 from HPIM 17e.)*

Bulimia Nervosa

Bulimia nervosa can usually be treated on an outpatient basis (**Fig. 208-1**). Cognitive behavioral therapy and fluoxetine (Prozac) are first-line therapies. The recommended treatment dose for fluoxetine (60 mg/d) is higher than that typically used to treat depression.

For a more detailed discussion, see Walsh TB: Eating Disorders, Chap. 76, p. 473, in HPIM-17.

209 Alcoholism

Alcoholism is a multifactorial disorder in which genetic, biologic, and sociocultural factors interact.

- *Alcohol dependence*: defined in DSM-IV as repeated alcohol-related difficulties in at least three of seven areas of functioning that cluster together over a 12-month period; physiologic tolerance and withdrawal are two of these seven areas and are associated with a more severe course.
- *Alcohol abuse*: defined as repetitive problems with alcohol in any one of four life areas—social, interpersonal, legal, and occupational—or repeated use in hazardous situations such as driving while intoxicated. A person who is not alcohol dependent may still be given a diagnosis of alcohol abuse.

CLINICAL FEATURES

Lifetime risk for alcohol dependence is 10–15% for men and 5–8% for women. Typically, the first major life problem from excessive alcohol use appears in early adulthood, followed by periods of exacerbation and remission. The course is not hopeless; following treatment, between half and two-thirds of patients maintain abstinence for years and often permanently. If the alcoholic continues to drink, life span is shortened by an average of 10–15 years due to increased risk of death from heart disease, cancer, accidents, or suicide.

Screening for alcoholism is important given its high prevalence. A positive answer to any of the "CAGE questions" indicates a high probability of alcoholism: Are you... *C*utting down, or feel the need to? *A*nnoyed when people criticize your drinking? *G*uilty about your drinking? *E*ye-opening with a drink in the morning? Other standardized questionnaires can be helpful in busy clinical practices including the 10-item Alcohol Use Disorders Identification Test (AUDIT) (see Table 209-1)

Routine medical care requires attention to potential alcohol-related illness and to alcoholism itself:

1. Neurologic—blackouts, seizures, delirium tremens, cerebellar degeneration, neuropathy, myopathy
2. Gastrointestinal—esophagitis, gastritis, pancreatitis, hepatitis, cirrhosis, GI hemorrhage
3. Cardiovascular—hypertension, cardiomyopathy
4. Hematologic—macrocytosis, folate deficiency, thrombocytopenia, leukopenia
5. Endocrine—gynecomastia, testicular atrophy, amenorrhea, infertility
6. Skeletal—fractures, osteonecrosis
7. Cancer—breast cancer, oral and esophageal cancers, rectal cancers

Alcohol Intoxication Alcohol is a CNS depressant that acts on receptors for γ-aminobutyric acid (GABA), the major inhibitory neurotransmitter in the nervous system. Behavioral, cognitive, and psychomotor changes can occur at blood alcohol levels as low as 4–7 mmol/L (20–30 mg/dL), a level achieved after the ingestion of one or two typical drinks. Mild to moderate intoxication occurs at 17–43 mmol/L (80–200 mg/dL). Incoordination, tremor, ataxia, confusion, stupor, coma, and even death occur at progressively higher blood alcohol levels.

Alcohol Withdrawal Chronic alcohol use produces CNS dependence, and the earliest sign of alcohol withdrawal is tremulousness ("shakes" or "jitters"), occurring 5–10 h after the last drink. This may be followed by generalized seizures in the first 24–48 h; these do not require initiation of antiseizure medications. With severe withdrawal, autonomic hyperactivity ensues (sweating, hypertension, tachycardia, tachypnea, fever), accompanied by insomnia, nightmares, anxiety, and GI symptoms.

Delirium Tremens (DTs) A very severe withdrawal syndrome characterized by profound autonomic hyperactivity, extreme confusion, agitation, vivid delu-

TABLE 209-1   THE ALCOHOL USE DISORDERS IDENTIFICATION TEST (AUDIT)[a]

Item	5-Point Scale (Least to Most)
1. How often do you have a drink containing alcohol?	Never (0) to 4+ per week (4)
2. How many drinks containing alcohol do you have on a typical day?	1 or 2 (0) to 10+ (4)
3. How often do you have six or more drinks on one occasion?	Never (0) to daily or almost daily (4)
4. How often during the last year have you found that you were not able to stop drinking once you had started?	Never (0) to daily or almost daily (4)
5. How often during the last year have you failed to do what was normally expected from you because of drinking?	Never (0) to daily or almost daily (4)
6. How often during the last year have you needed a first drink in the morning to get yourself going after a heavy drinking session?	Never (0) to daily or almost daily (4)
7. How often during the last year have you had a feeling of guilt or remorse after drinking?	Never (0) to daily or almost daily (4)
8. How often during the last year have you been unable to remember what happened the night before because you had been drinking?	Never (0) to daily or almost daily (4)
9. Have you or someone else been injured as a result of your drinking?	No (0) to yes, during the last year (4)
10. Has a relative, friend, doctor or other health worker been concerned about your drinking or suggested that you should cut down?	No (0) to yes, during the last year (4)

[a]Total score ≥ 8 indicates harmful alcohol use and possible alcohol dependence.
Source: Adapted from DF Reinert, GP Allen: *Alcoholism: Clinical & Experimental Research* 26:272, 2002, and from MA Schuckit, 2006.

sions, and hallucinations (often visual and tactile) that begins 3–5 days after the last drink. Mortality is 5–15%.

Wernicke's Encephalopathy   An alcohol-related syndrome characterized by ataxia, ophthalmoplegia, and confusion, often with associated nystagmus, peripheral neuropathy, cerebellar signs, and hypotension; there is impaired short-term memory, inattention, and emotional lability. Korsakoff's syndrome follows, characterized by anterograde and retrograde amnesia and confabulation. Wernicke-Korsakoff's syndrome is caused by chronic thiamine deficiency, resulting in damage to thalamic nuclei, mamillary bodies, and brainstem and cerebellar structures.

LABORATORY FINDINGS

Include mild anemia with macrocytosis, folate deficiency, thrombocytopenia, granulocytopenia, abnormal liver function tests, hyperuricemia, and elevated triglycerides. Two blood tests with between 70% and 80% sensitivity and specificity are γ-glutamyl transferase (GGT) (>35 U) and carbohydrate-deficient transferrin (CDT) (>20 U/L); the combination of the two is likely to be more accurate than either alone when screening pts for high levels of alcohol intake. Decreases in serum K, Mg, Zn, and PO_4 levels are common. A variety of diagnostic studies may show evidence of alcohol-related organ dysfunction.

Alcoholism

ACUTE WITHDRAWAL

Acute alcohol withdrawal is treated with multiple B vitamins including thiamine (50–100 mg IV or PO daily for ≥1 week) to replenish depleted stores; use the IV route if Wernicke-Korsakoff's syndrome is suspected since intestinal absorption is unreliable in alcoholics. CNS depressant drugs are used when seizures or autonomic hyperactivity is present to halt the rapid state of withdrawal in the CNS and allow for a slower, more controlled reduction of the substance. Low-potency benzodiazepines with long half-lives are the medication of choice (e.g., diazepam, chlordiazepoxide), because they produce fairly steady blood levels of drug with a wide dose range within which to work. Risks include overmedication and oversedation, which occur less commonly with shorter-acting agents (e.g., oxazepam, lorazepam). Typical doses are diazepam 10 mg or chlordiazepoxide 25–50 mg PO every 4–6 h as needed for objective signs of alcohol withdrawal (such as pulse < 90).

In severe withdrawal or DTs, high doses of benzodiazepines are usually required. Fluid and electrolyte status and blood glucose levels should be closely followed. Cardiovascular and hemodynamic monitoring are crucial, as hemodynamic collapse and cardiac arrhythmia are not uncommon. Generalized withdrawal seizures rarely require aggressive pharmacologic intervention beyond that given to the usual pt undergoing withdrawal, i.e., adequate doses of benzodiazepines.

RECOVERY AND SOBRIETY
Counseling, Education, and Cognitive Approaches

First, attempts should be made to help the alcoholic achieve and maintain a high level of motivation toward abstinence. These include education about alcoholism and instructing family and/or friends to stop protecting the person from the problems caused by alcohol. A second goal is to help the pt to readjust to life without alcohol and to reestablish a functional lifestyle through counseling, vocational rehabilitation, and self-help groups such as Alcoholics Anonymous (AA). A third component, called *relapse prevention*, helps the person to identify situations in which a return to drinking is likely, formulate ways of managing these risks, and develop coping strategies that increase the chances of a return to abstinence if a slip occurs. There is no convincing evidence that inpatient rehabilitation is more effective than outpatient care.

Drug Therapy

Several medications may be useful in alcoholic rehabilitation; usually medications are continued for 6–12 months if a positive response is seen.

- The opioid-antagonist drug naltrexone, (50–150 mg/d) decreases the probability of a return to drinking and shortens periods of relapse; a once-a-month injectable form of this drug (380 mg) has recently been developed to help improve compliance.
- A second medication, acamprosate (2 g/d), an *N*-methyl-D-aspartate receptor inhibitor, may be used; efficacy appears to be similar to naltrexone.
- Disulfiram (250 mg/d), an aldehyde dehydrogenase inhibitor, produces an unpleasant and potentially dangerous reaction in the presence of alcohol. Few controlled trials demonstrate a clear superiority over placebo.

For a more detailed discussion, see Schuckit MA: Alcohol and Alcoholism, Chap. 387, p. 2724, in HPIM-17.

210 Narcotic Abuse

Narcotics, or opiates, bind to specific opioid receptors in the CNS and elsewhere in the body. These receptors mediate the opiate effects of analgesia, euphoria, respiratory depression, and constipation. Endogenous opiate peptides (enkephalins and endorphins) are natural ligands for the opioid receptors and play a role in analgesia, memory, learning, reward, mood regulation, and stress tolerance.

The prototypic opiates, morphine and codeine, are derived from the juice of the opium poppy, *Papaver somniferum*. The semisynthetic drugs produced from morphine include hydromorphone (Dilaudid), diacetylmorphine (heroin), and oxycodone. The purely synthetic opioids and their cousins include meperidine, propoxyphene, diphenoxylate, fentanyl, buprenorphine, tramadol, methadone, and pentazocine. All of these substances produce analgesia and euphoria as well as physical dependence when taken in high enough doses for prolonged periods of time.

CLINICAL FEATURES

Close to 1 million individuals in the United States are opioid-dependent. A 2005 survey of young adults revealed that 13.5% of high school seniors had tried opioid drugs outside of a doctor's prescription. Three groups of abusers can be identified:

- "Medical" abusers. Pts with chronic pain syndromes who misuse their prescribed analgesics
- Physicians, nurses, dentists, and pharmacists with easy access to narcotics
- "Street" abusers. Typically a higher functioning individual who began by using tobacco, alcohol, marijuana, and brain depressants or stimulants and then moved on to opiates

Acute Effects All opiates have the following CNS effects: sedation, euphoria, decreased pain perception, decreased respiratory drive, and vomiting. In larger doses, markedly decreased respirations, bradycardia, pupillary miosis, stupor, and coma ensue. Additionally, the adulterants used to "cut" street drugs (quinine, phenacetin, strychnine, antipyrine, caffeine, powdered milk) can produce permanent neurologic damage, including peripheral neuropathy, amblyopia, myelopathy, and leukoencephalopathy; adulterants can also produce an "allergic-like" reaction characterized by decreased alertness, frothy pulmonary edema, and an elevation in blood eosinophil count.

Chronic Effects Chronic use of opiates will result in tolerance (requiring higher doses to achieve psychotropic effects) and physical dependence. At least 25% of street abusers die within 10–20 years of starting active opiate abuse from suicide, homicide, accidents, or infections such hepatitis or AIDS; the latter is epidemic among injection drug users, with HIV+ rates as high as 60% in some locales.

Withdrawal Withdrawal produces nausea and diarrhea, coughing, lacrimation, mydriasis, rhinorrhea, diaphoresis, twitching muscles, piloerection, fever, tachypnea, hypertension, diffuse body pain, insomnia, and yawning. Relief of these exceedingly unpleasant symptoms by narcotic administration leads to more frequent narcotic use.

With shorter-acting opiates such as heroin, morphine, or oxycodone, withdrawal signs begin 8–16 h after the last dose, peak at 36–72 h, and subside over 5–8 days. With longer-acting opiates such as methadone, withdrawal begins several days after the last dose, peaks at 7–10 days in some cases, and lasts several weeks.

℞ Narcotic Abuse

Overdose

High doses of opiates, whether taken in a suicide attempt or accidentally when its potency is misjudged, are potentially lethal. Toxicity occurs immediately after IV administration and with a variable delay after oral ingestion. Symptoms include miosis, shallow respirations, bradycardia, hypothermia, and stupor or coma. Treatment requires cardiorespiratory support, using intubation if needed, and administration of the opiate antagonist naloxone (0.4–2 mg IV or IM repeated every 2–3 min up to 10 mg, if no or only partial response). Because the effects of naloxone diminish in 2–3 h compared with longer-lasting effects of heroin (up to 24 h) or methadone (up to 72 h), pts must be observed for at least 1–3 days for reappearance of the toxic state.

Withdrawal

One treatment approach to withdrawal is the administration of any opioid (e.g., 10–25 mg of methadone twice a day) on day 1 to decrease symptoms. After several days of a stabilized drug dose, the opioid is then decreased by 10–20% of the original day's dose each day. However, detoxification with opioids is proscribed or limited in most states. Thus, pharmacologic treatments often center on relief of symptoms of diarrhea with loperamide, of "sniffles" with decongestants, and pain with nonopioid analgesics (e.g., ibuprofen). Comfort can be enhanced with administration of the α_2-adrenergic agonist clonidine in doses up to 0.3 mg given two to four times a day to decrease sympathetic nervous system overactivity. Blood pressure must be closely monitored. Some clinicians augment this regimen with low to moderate doses of benzodiazepines for 2–5 days to decrease agitation. An ultrarapid detoxification procedure using deep sedation and withdrawal precipitated by naltrexone has many inherent dangers and few, if any, advantages.

Opioid Maintenance

Methadone maintenance is a widely used treatment strategy in the management of opiate addiction. Methadone is a long-acting opioid optimally dosed at 80–120 mg/d (gradually increased over time). This level is optimally effective in blocking heroin-induced euphoria, decreasing craving, and maintaining abstinence from illegal opioids. Over three-quarters of patients in well-supervised methadone clinics are likely to remain heroin-free for ≥6 months. Methadone is administered as an oral liquid given once a day at the program, with weekend doses taken at home. After a period of maintenance (usually 6 months to ≥1 year), the clinician can work to slowly decrease the dose by about 5% per week. An additional medication that has been used for maintenance treatment involves the μ opioid agonist and antagonist buprenorphine; it has several advantages, including low overdose danger, potentially easier detoxification than with methadone, and a probable ceiling effect in which higher doses do not increase euphoria.

Opiate Antagonists

The opiate antagonists (e.g., naltrexone) compete with heroin and other opioids at receptors, reducing the effects of the opioid agonists. Administered over long periods with the intention of blocking the opioid "high," these drugs can be useful as part of an overall treatment approach that includes counseling and support. Naltrexone doses of 50 mg/d antagonize 15 mg of heroin for 24 h, and the possibly more effective higher doses (125–150 mg) block the effects of 25 mg of IV heroin for up to 3 days. To avoid precipitating a withdrawal syndrome, patients must be free of opioids for a minimum of 5 days before beginning treatment with naltrexone and should first be challenged with 0.4 or 0.8 mg of the shorter-acting agent naloxone to be certain they can tolerate the long-acting antagonist.

Drug-Free Programs

Most opioid treatment programs focus primarily on cognitive-behavioral approaches of enhancing commitment to abstinence, helping individuals to rebuild their lives without substances, and preventing relapse. Whether carried out in inpatient or outpatient settings, patients do not receive maintenance medications.

PREVENTION

Except for the terminally ill, physicians should carefully monitor opioid drug use in their patients, keeping doses as low as is practical and administering them over as short a period as the level of pain would warrant in the average person. Physicians must be vigilant regarding their own risk for opioid abuse and dependence, never prescribing these drugs for themselves. For the nonmedical intravenous drug–dependent person, all possible efforts must be made to prevent the infectious consequences of contaminated needles both through methadone maintenance and by considering needle-exchange programs.

For a more detailed discussion, see Shuckit MA: Opioid Drug Abuse and Dependence, Chap. 388, p. 2729, in HPIM-17.

DISEASE PREVENTION AND HEALTH MAINTENANCE

211 Routine Disease Screening

A primary goal of health care is to prevent disease or to detect it early enough that interventions will be more effective. In general, screening is most effective when applied to relatively common disorders that carry a large disease burden and have a long latency period. Early detection of disease has the potential to reduce both morbidity and mortality; however, screening asymptomatic individuals carries some risk. False-positive results can lead to unnecessary lab tests and invasive procedures and can increase pt anxiety. Several measurements have been derived to better assess the potential gain from screening and prevention interventions:

- Number of subjects needed to be screened to alter the outcome in one individual
- Absolute impact of screening on disease (e.g., lives saved per thousand screened)
- Relative impact of screening on disease outcome (e.g., the % reduction in deaths)
- The cost per year of life saved
- The increase in average life expectancy for a population

Current recommendations include performance of a routine health care examination every 1–3 years before age 50 and every year thereafter. History should include medication use, allergies, dietary history, use of alcohol and tobacco, sexual practices, safety practices (seat belt and helmet use, gun possession), and a thorough family history. Routine measurements should include assessments of height, weight, body-mass index, and blood pressure. Screening should also be considered for domestic violence and depression.

Counseling by health care providers should be performed at health care visits. Tobacco and alcohol use, diet, and exercise represent the vast majority of factors that influence preventable deaths. While behavioral changes are frequently difficult to achieve, it should be emphasized that studies show even brief (<5 min) tobacco counseling by physicians results in a significant rate of long-term smoking cessation. Instruction about self-examination (e.g., skin, breast, testicular) should also be provided during preventative visits.

The top causes of age-specific mortality and corresponding preventative strategies are listed in Table 211-1. Formal recommendations from the U.S. Preventive Services Task Force are listed in Table 211-2.

Specific recommendations for disease prevention can also be found in subsequent chapters on Immunization and Advice to Travelers (Chap. 212), Cardiovascular Disease Prevention (Chap. 213), Prevention and Early Detection of Cancer (Chap. 214), Smoking Cessation (Chap. 215), and Women's Health (Chap. 216).

TABLE 211-1 AGE-SPECIFIC CAUSES OF MORTALITY AND CORRESPONDING PREVENTATIVE OPTIONS

Age Group	Leading Causes of Age-Specific Mortality	Screening Prevention Interventions to Consider for Each Specific Population
15–24	1. Accident 2. Homicide 3. Suicide 4. Malignancy 5. Heart disease	• Counseling on routine seat belt use, bicycle/motorcycle/ATV helmets (1) • Counseling on diet and exercise (5) • Discuss dangers of alcohol use while driving, swimming, boating (1) • Ask about vaccination status (tetanus, diphtheria, hepatitis B, MMR, rubella, varicella, meningitis, HPV) • Ask about gun use and/or gun possession (2,3) • Assess for substance abuse history including alcohol (2,3) • Screen for domestic violence (2,3) • Screen for depression and/or suicidal/homicidal ideation (2,3) • Pap smear for cervical cancer screening, discuss STD prevention (4) • Recommend skin, breast, and testicular self-exams (4) • Recommend UV light avoidance and regular sun screen use (4) • Measurement of blood pressure, height, weight and body mass index (5) • Discuss health risks of tobacco use, consider emphasis of cosmetic and economic issues to improve quit rates for younger smokers (4,5) • *Chlamydia* screening and contraceptive counseling for sexually active females • HIV, hepatitis B, and syphilis testing if there is high-risk sexual behavior(s) or any prior history of sexually transmitted disease
25–44	1. Accident 2. Malignancy 3. Heart disease 4. Suicide 5. Homicide 6. HIV	*As above plus consider the following:* • Readdress smoking status, encourage cessation at every visit (2,3) • Obtain detailed family history of malignancies and begin early screening/prevention program if patient is at significant increased risk (2) • Assess all cardiac risk factors (including screening for diabetes and hyperlipidemia) and consider primary prevention with aspirin for patients at >3% 5-year risk of a vascular event (3) • Assess for chronic alcohol abuse, risk factors for viral hepatitis, or other risks for development of chronic liver disease • Begin breast cancer screening with mammography at age 40 (2)

(continued)

TABLE 211-1	**AGE-SPECIFIC CAUSES OF MORTALITY AND CORRESPONDING PREVENTATIVE OPTIONS (CONTINUED)**
45–64	1. Malignancy 2. Heart disease 3. Accident 4. Diabetes mellitus 5. Cerebrovascular disease 6. Chronic lower respiratory disease 7. Chronic liver disease and cirrhosis 8. Suicide	• Consider prostate cancer screen with annual PSA and digital rectal exam at age 50 (or possibly earlier in African Americans or patients with family history) (1) • Begin colorectal cancer screening at age 50 with either fecal occult blood testing, flexible sigmoidoscopy, or colonoscopy (1) • Reassess vaccination status at age 50 and give special consideration to vaccines against *Streptococcus pneumoniae*, influenza, tetanus, and viral hepatitis • Consider screening for coronary disease in higher risk patients (2,5)
≥65	1. Heart disease 2. Malignancy 3. Cerebrovascular disease 4. Chronic lower respiratory disease 5. Alzheimer's disease 6. Influenza and pneumonia 7. Diabetes mellitus 8. Kidney disease 9. Accidents 10. Septicemia	*As above plus consider the following:* • Readdress smoking status, encourage cessation at every visit (1,2,3) • One-time ultrasound for AAA in men 65–75 who have ever smoked • Consider pulmonary function testing for all long-term smokers to assess for development of chronic obstructive pulmonary disease (3,7) • Vaccinate all smokers against influenza and *S. pneumoniae* at age 50 (6) • Screen all postmenopausal women (and all men with risk factors) for osteoporosis • Reassess vaccination status at age 65, emphasis on influenza and *S. pneumoniae* (3,7) • Screen for dementia and depression (5) • Screen for visual and hearing problems, home safety issues, and elder abuse (9)

Note: The numbers in parentheses refer to areas of risk in the mortality column affected by the specified intervention.
Abbreviations: MMR, measles-mumps-rubella; HPV, human papilloma virus; STD, sexually transmitted disease; UV, ultraviolet; PSA, prostate-specific antigen; AAA, abdominal aortic aneurysm.

TABLE 211-2 **CLINICAL PREVENTIVE SERVICES FOR NORMAL-RISK ADULTS RECOMMENDED BY THE U.S. PREVENTIVE SERVICES TASK FORCE**

Test or Disorder	Population,[a] Years	Frequency
Blood pressure, height and weight	>18	Periodically
Cholesterol	Men > 35	Every 5 years
	Women > 45	Every 5 years
Diabetes	>45 or earlier, if there are additional risk factors	Every 3 years
Pap smear[b]	Within 3 years of onset of sexual activity or 21–65	Every 1–3 years
Chlamydia	Women 18–25	Every 1–2 years
Mammography[a]	Women > 40	Every 1–2 years
Colorectal cancer[a]	>50	
fecal occult blood and/or		Every year
sigmoidoscopy or		Every 5 years
colonoscopy		Every 10 years
Osteoporosis	Women > 65; >60 at risk	Periodically
Abdominal aortic aneurysm (ultrasound)	Men 65–75 who have ever smoked	Once
Alcohol use	>18	Periodically
Vision, hearing	>65	Periodically
Adult immunization		
Tetanus-diphtheria (Td)	>18	Every 10 years
Varicella (VZV)	Susceptibles only, >18	Two doses
Measles, mumps, rubella (MMR)	Women, childbearing age	One dose
Pneumococcal	>65	One dose
Influenza	>50	Yearly
Human papillomavirus (HPV)	Up to age 26	If not done prior

[a]Screening is performed earlier and more frequently when there is a strong family history. Randomized, controlled trials have documented that fecal occult blood testing (FOBT) confers a 15 to 30% reduction in colon cancer mortality. Although randomized trials have not been performed for sigmoidoscopy or colonoscopy, well-designed case-control studies suggest similar or greater efficacy relative to FOBT.
[b]In the future, Pap smear frequency may be influenced by HPV testing and the HPV vaccine.
Note: Prostate-specific antigen (PSA) testing is capable of enhancing the detection of early-stage prostate cancer, but evidence is inconclusive that it improves health outcomes. PSA testing is recommended by several professional organizations and is widely used in clinical practice, but it is not currently recommended by the U.S. Preventive Services Task Force (Chap. 81).
Source: Adapted from the U.S. Preventive Services Task Force, 2005. *Guide to Clinical Prevention Services*, 3d ed. http://www.ahrq.gov/clinic/uspstfix.htm

For a more detailed discussion, see Martin GJ: Screening and Prevention of Disease, Chap. 4, p. 24, in HPIM-17.

212 Immunization and Advice to Travelers

IMMUNIZATION

Vaccination is one of the greatest public health achievements of the twentieth century and among the most cost-effective health interventions available.

DEFINITIONS

- Immunization: induction or provision of immunity by any means

  Active immunization: administration of a vaccine consisting of either (1) live, attenuated agents (e.g., measles virus); or (2) inactivated agents (e.g., influenza virus), their constituents (e.g., *Bordetella pertussis*), or their products (e.g., hepatitis B virus)

  Passive immunization: provision of temporary immunity in a person exposed to an infectious disease who has not been actively immunized. Products used for this purpose are standard human immune serum globulin, special immune serum globulins with a known content of antibody to specific agents (e.g., hepatitis B virus or varicella-zoster immune globulin), and specific animal-derived antisera and antitoxins.

VACCINES FOR ROUTINE USE

For the recommended immunization schedule for persons age 0–6 years, see Fig. 212-1; for persons age 7–18 years, see Fig. 212-2; and for adults, see Fig. 212-3. Clinically significant adverse events that follow immunization should be reported to the Vaccine Adverse Event Reporting System (VAERS). Guidance in obtaining and completing a VAERS form is available online at www.vaers.hhs.gov or by telephone at 800-822-7967.

ADVICE FOR TRAVELERS

Travelers should be aware of various health risks that might be associated with given destinations. Information regarding country-specific risks can be obtained from the CDC publication *Health Information for International Travel*, which is available at www.cdc.gov/travel.

IMMUNIZATIONS FOR TRAVEL

There are three categories of immunization for travel.

- *Routine* immunizations (see Figs. 212-1, 212-2, and 212-3) are needed regardless of travel. However, travelers should be certain that their routine immunizations are up to date because certain diseases (e.g., diphtheria, tetanus, polio, measles) are more likely to be acquired outside the United States than at home.
- *Required* immunizations are mandated by international regulations for entry into certain areas.
- *Recommended* immunizations are advisable because they protect against illnesses acquisition of which the traveler is at increased risk. Table 212-1 lists vaccines required or recommended for travel.

Recommended Immunization Schedule for Persons Aged 0–6 Years
UNITED STATES • 2007

Vaccine ▼ Age ▶	Birth	1 month	2 months	4 months	6 months	12 months	15 months	18 months	19–23 months	2–3 years	4–6 years
Hepatitis B [1]	HepB	HepB		see footnote 1	HepB					HepB Series	
Rotavirus [2]			Rota	Rota	Rota						
Diphtheria, Tetanus, Pertussis [3]			DTaP	DTaP	DTaP		DTaP	DTaP			DTaP
Haemophilus influenzae type b [4]			Hib	Hib	Hib [4]	Hib					
Pneumococcal [5]			PCV	PCV	PCV	PCV				PCV / PPV	
Inactivated Poliovirus			IPV	IPV		IPV					IPV
Influenza [6]					Influenza (Yearly)						
Measles, Mumps, Rubella [7]						MMR					MMR
Varicella [8]						Varicella					Varicella
Hepatitis A [9]						HepA (2 doses)				HepA Series	
Meningococcal [10]											MPSV4

Legend:
- Range of recommended ages
- Catch-up immunization
- Certain high-risk groups

FIGURE 212-1 Recommended immunization schedule for persons aged 0–6 years—United States, 2006–2007. **1. Hepatitis B vaccine (HepB).** *(Minimum age: birth)* **At birth:** Administer monovalent HepB to all newborns before hospital discharge. If mother is hepatitis surface antigen (HBsAg)-positive, administer HepB and 0.5 mL of hepatitis B immune globulin (HBIG) within 12 hours of birth. If mother's HBsAg status is unknown, administer HepB within 12 hours of birth. Determine the HBsAg status as soon as possible and if HBsAg-positive, administer HBIG (no later than age 1 week). If mother is HBsAg-negative, the birth dose can only be delayed with physician's order and mother's negative HBsAg laboratory report documented in the infant's medical record. **After the birth dose:** The HepB series should be completed with either monovalent HepB or a combination vaccine containing HepB. The second dose should be administered at age 1–2 months. The final dose should be administered at age ≥24 weeks. Infants born to HBsAg-positive mothers should be tested for HBsAg and antibody to HBsAg after completion of ≥3 doses of a licensed HepB series, at age 9–18 months (generally at the next well-child visit). **4-month dose:** It is permissible to administer 4 doses of HepB when combination vaccines are administered after the birth dose. If monovalent HepB is used for doses after the birth dose, a dose at age 4 months is not needed. **2. Rotavirus vaccine (Rota).** *(Minimum age: 6 weeks)* Administer the first dose at age 6–12 weeks. Do not start the series later than age 12 weeks. Administer the final dose in the series by age 32 weeks. Do not administer a dose later than age 32 weeks. Data on safety and efficacy outside of these age ranges are insufficient. **3. Diphtheria and tetanus toxoids and acellular pertussis vaccine (DTaP).** *(Minimum age: 6 weeks)* The fourth dose of DTaP may be administered as early as age 12 months, provided 6 months have elapsed since the third dose. Administer the final dose in the series at age 4–6 years. **4.** *Haemophilus influenzae* **type b conjugate vaccine (Hib).** *(Minimum age: 6 weeks)* If PRP-OMP (Pedvax-HIB or ComVax [Merck]) is administered at ages 2 and 4 months, a dose at age 6 months is not required. TriHiBit (DTaP/Hib) combination products should not be used for primary immunization but can be used as boosters following any Hib vaccine in children aged ≥12 months. **5. Pneumococcal vaccine.** *(Minimum age: 6 weeks for pneumococcal conjugate vaccine [PCV]; 2 years for pneumococcal polysaccharide vaccine [PPV]).* Administer PCV at ages 24–59 months in certain high-risk groups. Administer PPV to children aged ≥2 years in certain high-risk groups. See MMWR 2000;49(No. RR-9):1–35. **6. Influenza vaccine.** *(Minimum age: 6 months for trivalent inactivated influenza vaccine [TIV]; 5 years for live, attenuated influenza vaccine [LAIV]).* All children aged 6–59 months and close contacts of all children aged 0–59 months are recommended to receive influenza vaccine. Influenza vaccine is recommended annually for children aged ≥59 months with certain risk factors, health-care workers, and other persons (including household members) in close contact with persons in groups at high risk. See MMWR 2006;55(No. RR-10):1–41. For healthy persons aged 5–49 years, LAIV may be used as an alternative to TIV. Children receiving TIV should receive 0.25 mL if aged 6–35 months or 0.5 mL if aged ≥3 years. Children aged <9 years who are receiving influenza vaccine for the first time should receive 2 doses (separated by ≥4 weeks for TIV and ≥6 weeks for LAIV). **7. Measles, mumps, and rubella vaccine (MMR).** *(Minimum age: 12 months)* Administer the second dose of MMR at age 4–6 years. MMR may be administered before age 4–6 years, provided ≥4 weeks have elapsed since the first dose and both doses are administered at age ≥12 months. **8. Varicella vaccine.** *(Minimum age: 12 months)* Administer the second dose of varicella vaccine at age 4–6 years. Varicella vaccine may be administered before age 4–6 years, provided that ≥3 months have elapsed since the first dose and both doses are administered at age ≥12 months. If the second dose was administered ≥28 days following the first dose, the second dose does not need to be repeated. **9. Hepatitis A vaccine (HepA).** *(Minimum age: 12 months)* HepA is recommended for all children aged 1 year (i.e., aged 12–23 months). The 2 doses in the series should be administered at least 6 months apart. Children not fully vaccinated by age 2 years can be vaccinated at subsequent visits. HepA is recommended for certain other groups of children, including in areas where vaccination programs target older children. See MMWR 2006;55(No. RR-7):1–23. **10. Meningococcal polysaccharide vaccine (MPSV4).** *(Minimum age: 2 years)* Administer MPSV4 to children aged 2–10 years with terminal complement deficiencies or anatomic or functional asplenia and certain other high-risk groups. See MMWR 2005;54(No. RR-7):1–21.

Recommended Immunization Schedule for Persons Aged 7–18 Years
UNITED STATES • 2007

Vaccine ▼ Age ▶	7–10 years	11–12 YEARS	13–14 years	15 years	16–18 years
Tetanus, Diphtheria, Pertussis [1]	see footnote 1	Tdap		Tdap	
Human Papillomavirus [2]	see footnote 2	HPV (3 doses)	HPV Series		
Meningococcal [3]	MPSV4	MCV4		MCV4 [3] MCV4	
Pneumococcal [4]		PPV			
Influenza [5]		Influenza (Yearly)			
Hepatitis A [6]		HepA Series			
Hepatitis B [7]		HepB Series			
Inactivated Poliovirus [8]		IPV Series			
Measles, Mumps, Rubella [9]		MMR Series			
Varicella [10]		Varicella Series			

Range of recommended ages

Catch-up immunization

Certain high-risk groups

1110

FIGURE 212-2 Recommended immunization schedule for persons aged 7–18 years—United States, 2006–2007. **1. Tetanus and diphtheria toxoids and acellular pertussis vaccine (Tdap).** *(Minimum age: 10 years for BOOSTRIX and 11 years for ADACEL)* Administer at age 11–12 years for those who have completed the recommended childhood DTP/DTaP vaccination series and have not received a tetanus and diphtheria toxoids vaccine (Td) booster dose. Adolescents aged 13–18 years who missed the 11–12 year Td/Tdap booster dose should also receive a single dose of Tdap if they have completed the recommended childhood DTP/DTaP vaccination series. **2. Human papillomavirus vaccine (HPV).** *(Minimum age: 9 years)* Administer the first dose of the HPV vaccine series to females at age 11–12 years. Administer the second dose 2 months after the first dose and the third dose 6 months after the first dose. Administer the HPV vaccine series to females at age 13–18 years if not previously vaccinated. **3. Meningococcal vaccine.** *(Minimum age: 11 years for meningococcal conjugate vaccine [MCV4]; 2 years for meningococcal polysaccharide vaccine [MPSV4]).* Administer MCV4 at age 11–12 years and to previously unvaccinated adolescents at high school entry (at approximately age 15 years). Administer MCV4 to previously unvaccinated college freshmen living in dormitories; MPSV4 is an acceptable alternative. Vaccination against invasive meningococcal disease is recommended for children and adolescents aged ≥2 years with terminal complement deficiencies or anatomic or functional asplenia and certain other high-risk groups. See MMWR 2005;54(No. RR-7):1–21. Use MPSV4 for children aged 2–10 years and MCV4 or MPSV4 for older children. **4. Pneumococcal polysaccharide vaccine (PPV).** *(Minimum age: 2 years)* Administer for certain high-risk groups. See MMWR 1997;46(No. RR-8):1–24, and MMWR 2000;49(No. RR-9):1–35. **5. Influenza vaccine.** *(Minimum age: 6 months for trivalent inactivated influenza vaccine [TIV]; 5 years for live, attenuated influenza vaccine [LAIV]).* Influenza vaccine is recommended annually for persons with certain risk factors, health-care workers, and other persons (including household members) in close contact with persons in groups at high risk. See MMWR 2006;55 (No. RR-10):1–41. For healthy persons aged 5–49 years, LAIV may be used as an alternative to TIV. Children aged <9 years who are receiving influenza vaccine for the first time should receive 2 doses (separated by ≥4 weeks for TIV and ≥6 weeks for LAIV). **6. Hepatitis A vaccine (HepA).** *(Minimum age: 12 months)* The 2 doses in the series should be administered at least 6 months apart. HepA is recommended for certain other groups of children, including in areas where vaccination programs target older children. See MMWR 2006;55 (No. RR-7):1–23. **7. Hepatitis B vaccine (HepB).** *(Minimum age: birth)* Administer the 3-dose series to those who were not previously vaccinated. A 2-dose series of Recombivax HB is licensed for children aged 11–15 years. **8. Inactivated poliovirus vaccine (IPV).** *(Minimum age: 6 weeks)* For children who received an all-IPV or all-oral poliovirus (OPV) series, a fourth dose is not necessary if the third dose was administered at age ≥4 years. If both OPV and IPV were administered as part of a series, a total of 4 doses should be administered, regardless of the child's current age. **9. Measles, mumps, and rubella vaccine (MMR).** *(Minimum age: 12 months)* If not previously vaccinated, administer 2 doses of MMR during any visit, with ≥4 weeks between the doses. **10. Varicella vaccine.** *(Minimum age: 12 months)* Administer 2 doses of varicella vaccine to persons without evidence of immunity. Administer 2 doses of varicella vaccine to persons aged <13 years at least 3 months apart. Do not repeat the second dose, if administered ≥28 days after the first dose. Administer 2 doses of varicella vaccine to persons aged ≥13 years at least 4 weeks apart.

Recommended Adult Immunization Schedule
United States, October 2006–September 2007

Recommended adult immunization schedule, by vaccine and age group

Vaccine ▼ Age group (yrs) ▶	19–49 years	50–64 years	≥65 years
Tetanus, diphtheria, pertussis (Td/Tdap)[1]*	1-dose Td booster every 10 yrs / Substitute 1 dose of Tdap for Td		
Human papillomavirus (HPV)[2]*	3 doses (females)		
Measles, mumps, rubella (MMR)[3]*	1 or 2 doses		1 dose
Varicella[4]*	2 doses (0, 4–8 wks)	2 doses (0, 4–8 wks)	
Influenza[5]*	1 dose annually	1 dose annually	
Pneumococcal (polysaccharide)[6,7]	1–2 doses		1 dose
Hepatitis A[8]*	2 doses (0, 6–12 mos, or 0, 6–18 mos)		
Hepatitis B[9]*	3 doses (0, 1–2, 4–6 mos)		
Meningococcal[10]	1 or more doses		

For all persons in this category who meet the age requirements and who lack evidence of immunity (e.g., lack documentation of vaccination or have no evidence of prior infection)

Recommended if some other risk factor is present (e.g., on the basis of medical, occupational, lifestyle, or other indications)

FIGURE 212-3 Recommended adult imunization schedule, by vaccine and age group—United States, 2006–2007. This schedule indicates the recommended age groups for routine administration of currently licensed vaccines for persons aged ≥19 years, as of October 1, 2006. Licensed combination vaccines may be used whenever any components of the combination are indicated and when the vaccine's other components are not contraindicated. For detailed recommendations on all vaccines, including those used primarily for travelers or that are issued during the year, consult the manufacturers' package inserts and the complete statements from the Advisory Committee on Immunization Practices (*http://www.cdc.gov/nip/publications/acip-list.htm*). Asterisk indicates vaccines covered by the Vaccine Injury Compensation Program. Report all clinically significant postvaccination reactions to the Vaccine Adverse Event Reporting System (VAERS). Reporting forms and instructions on filing a VAERs report are available at *http://vaers.hhs.gov* or by telephone, 800-822-7967. Information on how to file a Vaccine Injury Compensation Program claim is available at *http://www.hrsa.gov/vaccinecompensation* or by telephone, 800-338-2382. To file a claim for vaccine injury, contact the U.S. Court of Federal Claims, 717 Madison Place, N.W., Washington, DC, 20005; telephone, 202-357-6400. Additional information about the vaccines in this schedule and contraindications for vaccination is also available at *http://www.cdc.gov/nip* or from the CDC-INFO Contact Center at 800-CDC-INFO (800-232-4636) in English and Spanish, 24 hours a day, 7 days a week. **1. Tetanus, diphtheria, and acellular pertussis (Td/Tdap) vaccination.** Adults with uncertain histories of a complete primary vaccination series with diphtheria and tetanus toxoid–containing vaccines should begin or complete a primary vaccination series. A primary series for adults is 3 doses; administer the first 2 doses at least 4 weeks apart and the third dose 6–12 months after the second. Administer a booster dose to adults who have completed a primary series and if the last vaccination was received ≥10 years previously. Tdap or tetanus and diphtheria (Td) vaccine may be used; Tdap should replace a single dose of Td for adults aged <65 years who have not previously received a dose of Tdap (either in the primary series, as a booster, or for wound management). Only one of two Tdap products (Adacel [sanofi pasteur]) is licensed for use in adults. If the person is pregnant and received the last Td vaccination ≥10 years previously, administer Td during the second or third trimester; if the person received the last Td vaccination in <10 years, administer Tdap during the immediate postpartum period. A one-time administration of 1 dose of Tdap with an interval as short as 2 years from a previous Td vaccination is recommended for postpartum women, close contacts of infants aged <12 months, and all healthcare workers with direct patient contact. In certain situations, Td can be deferred during pregnancy and Tdap substituted in the immediate postpartum period, or Tdap can be given instead of Td to a pregnant woman after an informed discussion with the woman (see *www.cdc.gov/nip/publications/acip-list.htm*). Consult the ACIP statement for recommendations for administering Td as prophylaxis in wound management (*www.cdc.gov/mmwr/preview/mmwrhtml/00041645.htm*). **2. Human papillomavirus (HPV) vaccination.** HPV vaccination is recommended for all women aged ≤ 26 years who have not completed the vaccine series. Ideally, vaccine should be administered before potential exposure to HPV through sexual activity; however, women who are sexually active should still be vaccinated. Sexually active women who have not been infected with any of the HPV vaccine types receive the full benefit of the vaccination. Vaccination is less beneficial for women who have already been infected with one or more of the four HPV vaccine types. A complete series consists of 3 doses. The second dose should be administered 2 months after the first dose; the third dose should be administered 6 months after the first dose. Vaccination is not recommended during pregnancy. If a woman is found to be pregnant after initiating the vaccination series, the remainder of the 3-dose regimen should be delayed until after completion of the pregnancy. **3. Measles, mumps, rubella (MMR) vaccination.** *Measles component:* adults born before 1957 can be considered immune to measles. Adults born during or after 1957 should receive ≥1 dose of MMR unless they have a medical contraindication, documentation of ≥1 dose, history of measles based on healthcare provider diagnosis, or laboratory evidence of immunity. A second dose of MMR is recommended for adults who (1) have been recently exposed to measles or in an outbreak setting; (2) have been previously vaccinated with killed measles vaccine; (3) have been vaccinated with an unknown type of measles vaccine during 1963–1967; (4) are students in postsecondary educational institutions; (5) work in a healthcare facility; or (6) plan to travel internationally. Withhold MMR or other measles-containing vaccines from HIV-infected persons with severe immunosuppression. *(Continued)*

FIGURE 212-3 *(CONTINUED)* *(Mumps component:* adults born before 1957 can generally be considered immune to mumps. Adults born during or after 1957 should receive 1 dose of MMR unless they have a medical contraindication, history of mumps based on healthcare provider diagnosis, or laboratory evidence of immunity. A second dose of MMR is recommended for adults who (1) are in an age group that is affected during a mumps outbreak; (2) are students in postsecondary educational institutions; (3) work in a healthcare facility; or (4) plan to travel internationally. For unvaccinated healthcare workers born before 1957 who do not have other evidence of mumps immunity, consider giving 1 dose on a routine basis and strongly consider giving a second dose during an outbreak. *Rubella component:* administer 1 dose of MMR vaccine to women whose rubella vaccination history is unreliable or who lack laboratory evidence of immunity. For women of childbearing age, regardless of birth year, routinely determine rubella immunity and counsel women regarding congenital rubella syndrome. Do not vaccinate women who are pregnant or who might become pregnant within 4 weeks of receiving vaccine. Women who do not have evidence of immunity should receive MMR vaccine upon completion or termination of pregnancy and before discharge from the healthcare facility. **4. Varicella vaccination.** All adults without evidence of immunity to varicella should receive 2 doses of varicella vaccine. Special consideration should be given to those who (1) have close contact with persons at high risk for severe disease (e.g., healthcare workers and family contacts of immunocompromised persons) or (2) are at high risk for exposure or transmission (e.g., teachers of young children; child care employees; residents and staff members of institutional settings, including correctional institutions; college students; military personnel; adolescents and adults living in households with children; nonpregnant women of childbearing age; and international travelers). Evidence of immunity to varicella in adults includes any of the following: (1) documentation of 2 doses of varicella vaccine at least 4 weeks apart; (2) U.S.-born before 1980 (although for healthcare workers and pregnant women, birth before 1980 should not be considered evidence of immunity); (3) history of varicella based on diagnosis or verification of varicella by a healthcare provider (for a patient reporting a history of or presenting with an atypical case, a mild case, or both, healthcare providers should seek either an epidemiologic link with a typical varicella case or evidence of laboratory confirmation, if it was performed at the time of acute disease); (4) history of herpes zoster based on healthcare provider diagnosis; or (5) laboratory evidence of immunity or laboratory confirmation of disease. Do not vaccinate women who are pregnant or might become pregnant within 4 weeks of receiving the vaccine. Assess pregnant women for evidence of varicella immunity. Women who do not have evidence of immunity should receive dose 1 of varicella vaccine upon completion or termination of pregnancy and before discharge from the healthcare facility. Dose 2 should be administered 4–8 weeks after dose 1. **5. Influenza vaccination.** *Medical indications:* chronic disorders of the cardiovascular or pulmonary systems, including asthma; chronic metabolic diseases, including diabetes mellitus, renal dysfunction, hemoglobinopathies, or immunosuppression (including immunosuppression caused by medications or HIV); any condition that compromises respiratory function or the handling of respiratory secretions or that can increase the risk of aspiration (e.g., cognitive dysfunction, spinal cord injury, or seizure disorder or other neuromuscular disorder); and pregnancy during the influenza season. No data exist on the risk for severe or complicated influenza disease among persons with asplenia; however, influenza is a risk factor for secondary bacterial infections that can cause severe disease among persons with asplenia. *Occupational indications:* healthcare workers and employees of long-term–care and assisted living facilities. *Other indications:* residents of nursing homes and other long-term–care and assisted living facilities; persons likely to transmit influenza to persons at high risk (e.g., in-home household contacts and caregivers of children aged 0–59 months, or persons of all ages with high-risk conditions); and anyone who would like to be vaccinated. Healthy, nonpregnant persons aged 5–49 years without high-risk medical conditions who are not contacts of severely immunocompromised persons in special care units can receive either intranasally administered influenza vaccine (Flu-Mist) or inactivated vaccine. Other persons should receive the inactivated vaccine. *(Continued)*

FIGURE 212-3 *(CONTINUED)* **6. Pneumococcal polysaccharide vaccination.** *Medical indications:* chronic disorders of the pulmonary system (excluding asthma); cardiovascular diseases; diabetes mellitus; chronic liver diseases, including liver disease as a result of alcohol abuse (e.g., cirrhosis); chronic renal failure or nephrotic syndrome; functional or anatomic asplenia (e.g., sickle cell disease or splenectomy [if elective splenectomy is planned, vaccinate at least 2 weeks before surgery]); immunosuppressive conditions (e.g., congenital immunodeficiency, HIV infection [vaccinate as close to diagnosis as possible when CD4 cell counts are highest], leukemia, lymphoma, multiple myeloma, Hodgkin disease, generalized malignancy, or organ or bone marrow transplantation); chemotherapy with alkylating agents, antimetabolites, or high-dose, long-term corticosteroids; and cochlear implants. *Other indications:* Alaska Natives and certain American Indian populations and residents of nursing homes or other long-term–care facilities. **7. Revaccination with pneumococcal polysaccharide vaccine.** One-time revaccination after 5 years for persons with chronic renal failure or nephrotic syndrome; functional or anatomic asplenia (e.g., sickle cell disease or splenectomy); immunosuppressive conditions (e.g., congenital immunodeficiency, HIV infection, leukemia, lymphoma, multiple myeloma, Hodgkin disease, generalized malignancy, or organ or bone marrow transplantation); or chemotherapy with alkylating agents, antimetabolites, or high-dose, long-term corticosteroids. For persons aged ≥65 years, one-time revaccination if they were vaccinated ≥5 years previously and were aged <65 years at the time of primary vaccination. **8. Hepatitis A vaccination.** *Medical indications:* persons with chronic liver disease and persons who receive clotting factor concentrates. *Behavioral indications:* men who have sex with men and persons who use illegal drugs. *Occupational indications:* persons working with hepatitis A virus (HAV)–infected primates or with HAV in a research laboratory setting. *Other indications:* persons traveling to or working in countries that have high or intermediate endemicity of hepatitis A (a list of countries is available at *www.cdc.gov/travel/diseases.htm*) and any person who would wish to obtain immunity. Current vaccines should be administered in a 2-dose schedule at either 0 and 6–12 months, or 0 and 6–18 months. If the combined hepatitis A and hepatitis B vaccine is used, administer 3 doses at 0, 1, and 6 months. **9. Hepatitis B vaccination.** *Medical indications:* persons with end-stage renal disease, including patients receiving hemodialysis; persons seeking evaluation or treatment for a sexually transmitted disease (STD); persons with HIV infection; persons with chronic liver disease; and persons who receive clotting factor concentrates. *Occupational indications:* healthcare workers and public-safety workers who are exposed to blood or other potentially infectious body fluids. *Behavioral indications:* sexually active persons who are not in a long-term, mutually monogamous relationship (i.e., persons with >1 sex partner during the previous 6 months); current or recent injection-drug users; and men who have sex with men. *Other indications:* household contacts and sex partners of persons with chronic hepatitis B virus (HBV) infection; clients and staff members of institutions for persons with developmental disabilities; all clients of STD clinics; international travelers to countries with high or intermediate prevalence of chronic HBV infection (a list of countries is available at *www.cdc.gov/travel/diseases.htm*); and any adult seeking protection from HBV infection. Settings where hepatitis B vaccination is recommended for all adults: STD treatment facilities; HIV testing and treatment facilities; facilities providing drug-abuse treatment and prevention services; healthcare settings providing services for injection-drug users or men who have sex with men; correctional facilities; end-stage renal disease programs and facilities for chronic hemodialysis patients; and institutions and nonresidential daycare facilities for persons with developmental disabilities. *Special formulation indications:* for adult patients receiving hemodialysis and other immunocompromised adults, 1 dose of 40 μg/mL (Recombivax HB) or 2 doses of 20 μg/mL (Engerix-B). **10. Meningococcal vaccination.** *Medical indications:* adults with anatomic or functional asplenia, or terminal complement component deficiencies. *Other indications:* first-year college students living in dormitories; microbiologists who are routinely exposed to isolates of *Neisseria meningitidis*; military recruits; and persons who travel to or live in countries in which meningococcal disease is hyperendemic or epidemic (e.g., the "meningitis belt" of sub-Saharan Africa during the dry season [December–June]), particularly if their contact with local populations will be prolonged. Vaccination is required by the government of Saudi Arabia for all travelers to Mecca during the annual Hajj. Meningococcal conjugate vaccine is preferred for adults with any of the preceding indications who are aged ≤ 55 years, although meningococcal polysaccharide vaccine (MPSV4) is an acceptable alternative. Revaccination after 5 years might be indicated for adults previously vaccinated with MPSV4 who remain at high risk for infection (e.g., persons residing in areas in which disease is epidemic).

TABLE 212-1 **VACCINES COMMONLY USED FOR TRAVEL**

Vaccine	Primary Series	Booster Interval
Cholera, live oral (CVD 103-HgR)	1 dose	6 months
Hepatitis A (Havrix), 1440 enzyme immunoassay U/mL	2 doses, 6–12 months apart, IM	None required
Hepatitis A (VAQTA, AVAXIM, EPAXAL)	2 doses, 6–12 months apart, IM	None required
Hepatitis A/B combined (Twinrix)	3 doses at 0, 1, and 6–12 months or 0, 7, and 21 days plus booster at 1 year, IM	None required except 12 months (once only, for accelerated schedule)
Hepatitis B (Engerix B): accelerated schedule	3 doses at 0, 1, and 2 months or 0, 7, and 21 days plus booster at 1 year, IM	12 months, once only
Hepatitis B (Engerix B or Recombivax): standard schedule	3 doses at 0, 1, and 6 months, IM	None required
Immune globulin (hepatitis A prevention)	1 dose IM	Intervals of 3–5 months, depending on initial dose
Japanese encephalitis (JEV, Biken)	3 doses, 1 week apart, SC	12–18 months (first booster), then 4 years
Meningococcus, quadrivalent [Menimmune (polysaccharide), Menactra (conjugate)]	1 dose SC	>3 years (optimal booster schedule not yet determined)
Rabies (HDCV), rabies vaccine absorbed (RVA), or purified chick embryo cell vaccine (PCEC)	3 doses at 0, 7, and 21 or 28 days, IM	None required except with exposure
Typhoid Ty21a, oral live attenuated (Vivotif)	1 capsule every other day × 4 doses	5 years
Typhoid Vi capsular polysaccharide, injectable (Typhim Vi)	1 dose IM	2 years
Yellow fever	1 dose SC	10 years

PREVENTION OF MALARIA AND OTHER INSECT-BORNE DISEASES

Chemoprophylaxis against malaria and other measures may be recommended for travel. In the United States, 90% of cases of *Plasmodium falciparum* infection occur in persons returning or immigrating from Africa and Oceania. The destination helps determine the particular medication chosen (e.g., whether chloroquine-resistant *P. falciparum* is present), as does the traveler's preference and medical history. In addition, personal protective measures against mosquito bites, especially between dusk and dawn (e.g., the use of DEET-containing insect repellents, permethrin-impregnated bed nets, and screened sleeping areas), can prevent malaria and other insect-borne diseases (e.g., dengue fever).

PREVENTION OF GASTROINTESTINAL ILLNESS

Diarrhea is the leading cause of illness in travelers. The incidence is highest in parts of Africa, Central and South America, and Southeast Asia. Travelers should eat only well-cooked hot foods, peeled or cooked fruits and vegetables, and bottled or boiled liquids. Although self-limited, diarrheal illness alters travel plans and confines 20% of pts to bed. Travelers should carry medications for self-treatment. Mild to moderate diarrhea can be treated with loperamide and fluids. Moderate to severe diarrhea should be treated with a 3-day course or a single double dose of a fluoroquinolone. High rates of quinolone-resistant *Campylobacter* in Thailand make azithromycin a better choice for that country. Rifaximin, a poorly absorbed rifampin derivative, is highly effective against noninvasive bacterial pathogens such as toxigenic and enteroaggregative *E. coli*. Prophylaxis with bismuth subsalicylate is ~60% effective; a single daily dose of a quinolone or azithromycin or a once-daily rifaximin regimen during travel of <1 month's duration is 75–90% effective; however, preventive treatment usually is not recommended.

OTHER INFECTIONS

Travelers are at high risk for (1) sexually transmitted diseases preventable by condom use; (2) schistosomiasis preventable by avoidance of swimming or bathing in freshwater lakes, streams, or rivers in endemic areas; and (3) hookworm and *Strongyloides* infections preventable by the avoidance of walking barefoot outside.

TRAVEL DURING PREGNANCY

The safest part of pregnancy in which to travel is between 18 and 24 weeks. Relative contraindications to international travel during pregnancy include a history of miscarriage, premature labor, incompetent cervix, or toxemia or the presence of other general medical problems (e.g., diabetes). Areas of excessive risk (e.g., where live virus vaccines are required for travel or where multidrug-resistant malaria is endemic) should be avoided throughout pregnancy.

THE HIV-INFECTED TRAVELER

HIV-seropositive persons with depressed CD4+ T cell counts should seek counseling from a travel medicine practitioner before departure, particularly when traveling to the developing world. This consultation should include a discussion of the appropriate use of vaccines (e.g., live yellow fever vaccine is not recommended for HIV-infected persons) and prophylactic medications, potential drug interactions (e.g., between some antimalarial agents and antiretroviral treatments), and risks for certain infections. Several countries routinely deny entry to HIV-positive persons.

PROBLEMS AFTER RETURN FROM TRAVEL

- Diarrhea: After traveler's diarrhea, symptoms may persist because of the continued presence of pathogens (e.g., *Giardia lamblia*) or, more often, because of postinfectious sequelae such as lactose intolerance or irritable bowel syndrome. A trial of metronidazole for giardiasis, a lactose-free diet, or a trial of high-dose hydrophilic mucilloid (plus lactulose for constipation) may relieve symptoms.
- Fever: Malaria is the first diagnosis that should be considered when a traveler returns from an endemic area with fever. Malaria is acquired most often in Africa, dengue in Southeast Asia and the Caribbean, typhoid fever in southern Asia, and rickettsial infections in southern Africa.

- Skin conditions: Pyodermas, sunburn, insect bites, skin ulcers, and cutaneous larva migrans are the most common skin conditions in returning travelers.

For a more detailed discussion, see Keusch GT et al: Immunization Principles and Vaccine Use, Chap. 116, p. 767; and Keystone JS, Kozarsky PE: Health Advice for International Travel, Chap. 117, p. 782, in HPIM-17.

213 Cardiovascular Disease Prevention

Cardiovascular disease is the leading cause of death in developed nations; prevention is targeted at modifiable atherosclerosis risk factors (Table 213-1). Identification and control of these attributes reduce subsequent cardiovascular event rates.

ESTABLISHED RISK FACTORS

Cigarette Smoking   Cigarette smoking increases the incidence of, and mortality associated with, coronary heart disease (CHD). Observational studies show that smoking cessation reduces excess risk of coronary events within months; after 3–5 years, the risk falls to that of individuals who never smoked. Patients should be asked regularly about tobacco use, followed by counseling and, as needed, antismoking pharmacologic therapy to assist cessation.

Lipid Disorders   (See Chap. 187)   Both elevated LDL and low HDL cholesterol are associated with cardiovascular events. Each 1-mg/dL increase in serum LDL correlates with a 2–3 % rise in CHD risk; each 1-mg/dL decrease in HDL heightens risk by 3–4%. ATP III guidelines advise a fasting lipid profile [total cholesterol, triglycerides, HDL, LDL (calculated or directly measured)] in all adults, repeated every 5 years. Recommended dietary and/or pharmacologic approach depends on presence or risk of coronary artery disease (CAD) and the LDL level (Table 213-2); treatment should be most aggressive in patients with established

---

TABLE 213-1   ESTABLISHED RISK FACTORS FOR ATHEROSCLEROSIS

Modifiable Risk Factors
Cigarette smoking
Dyslipidemias (↑LDL or ↓HDL)
Hypertension
Diabetes mellitus
Obesity
Sedentary lifestyle
Unmodifiable Risk Factors
Family history of premature coronary heart disease
Age (men ≥ 45 years; women ≥ 55 years)
Male gender

TABLE 213-2	LDL CHOLESTEROL GOALS AND CUTPOINTS FOR THERAPEUTIC LIFESTYLE CHANGES (TLC) AND DRUG THERAPY IN DIFFERENT RISK CATEGORIES

	LDL Level, mmol/L (mg/dL)		
Risk Category	Goal	Initiate TLC	Consider Drug Therapy
Very high ACS, or CHD w/ DM, or mult CRF	<1.8 (<70)	≥1.8 (≥70)	≥1.8 (≥70)
High CHD or CHD risk equivalents (10-year risk > 20%) If LDL < 2.6 (<100)	<2.6 (<100) [optional goal: <1.8 (<70)] ic<1.8 (<70)	≥2.6 (≥100)	≥2.6 (≥100) [<2.6 (<100): consider drug Rx]
Moderately high 2+ risk factors (10-year risk, 10–20%)	<2.6 (<100)	≥3.4 (≥130)	≥3.4 (≥130) [2.6–3.3 (100–129): consider drug Rx]
Moderate 2+ risk factors (risk < 10%)	<3.4 (<130)	≥3.4 (≥130)	≥4.1 (≥160)
Lower 0–1 risk factor	<4.1 (<160)	≥4.1 (≥160)	≥4.9 (≥190)

Note: LDL, low-density lipoprotein; ACS, acute coronary syndrome; CHD, coronary heart disease; DM, diabetes mellitus; CRF, coronary risk factors.
Source: Adapted from S Grundy et al: Circulation 110:227, 2004.

CAD and in those with "equivalent risk" (e.g., presence of peripheral arterial disease or diabetes mellitus). Drug therapy is indicated when LDL level exceeds goal in Table 213-2 by 30 mg/dL (0.8 mmol/L). If elevated triglyceride level [>200 mg/dL (> 2.6 mmol/L)] persists after control of LDL, secondary goal is to achieve non-HDL level (calculated as total cholesterol minus HDL) ≤30 mg/dL (0.8 mmol/L) above the target values listed in Table 213-2. In patients with isolated low HDL, encourage beneficial lifestyle measures: smoking cessation, weight loss, and increased physical activity. Consider addition of fibric acid derivative or niacin to raise HDL in patients with established CAD (see Chap. 187).

Hypertension (See Chap. 124) Systolic or diastolic bp > "optimal" level of 115/75 mmHg is associated with increased risk of cardiovascular disease; each augmentation of 20 mmHg systolic, or 10 mmHg diastolic, above this value doubles the risk. Treatment of elevated blood pressure reduces the rate of stroke, congestive heart failure, and CHD events, with general goal of bp < 140/90 mmHg or <130/80 in patients with diabetes or chronic kidney disease. Cardiovascular event rates in elderly patients with isolated systolic hypertension (systolic > 160 but diastolic < 90) are also reduced by antihypertensive therapy.

See Chap. 124 for antihypertensive treatment recommendations. Patients with "prehypertension" (systolic bp 120–139 mmHg or diastolic bp 80–89 mmHg) should receive counseling about beneficial lifestyle modifications such as those listed below (e.g., low-fat diet replete with vegetables and fruit, weight loss if overweight, increased physical activity, reduction of excessive alcohol consumption).

Diabetes Mellitus/Insulin Resistance/Metabolic Syndrome (See Chaps. 125 and 182) Patients with diabetes most often succumb to cardiovascular disease. LDL levels are typically near average in diabetic pts, but LDL particles are smaller, denser, and more atherogenic; low HDL and elevated triglyceride levels are common. Tight control of serum glucose reduces microvascular diabetic complications (retinopathy, renal disease), but a decrease in macrovascular events (CAD, stroke) has not been definitively shown. Conversely, successful management of associated risk factors in diabetics (e.g., dyslipidemia and hypertension) *does* reduce cardiovascular events and should be vigorously pursued. As needed, antilipidemic (especially statin) therapy should be used to lower LDL to <100 mg/dL in diabetics, even if patient has no symptoms of CAD.

Individuals without overt diabetes but who have "metabolic syndrome" (constellation of insulin resistance, central obesity, hypertension, hypertriglyceridemia, low HDL—see Chap. 125) are also at high risk of cardiovascular events. Dietary counseling, weight loss, and increased physical activity are important in reducing the prevalence of this syndrome.

Male Gender/Postmenopausal State Coronary risk is greater in men compared to that of premenopausal women of same age, but female risk accelerates after menopause. Estrogen-replacement therapy lowers LDL and raises HDL in postmenopausal women and in observational studies has been associated with reduced coronary events. However, prospective clinical trials do not support such a benefit and hormone-replacement therapy should not be prescribed for the purpose of cardiovascular risk reduction, especially in older women.

EMERGING RISK FACTORS

May be assessed selectively in patients without above traditional risk factors who have premature vascular disease or strong family history of premature vascular disease.

Homocysteine There is a graded correlation between serum homocysteine levels and risk of cardiovascular events and stroke. Supplemental folic acid and other B vitamins lower serum levels, but prospective clinical trials have not shown that such therapy reduces cardiac events.

Inflammation Inflammatory serum markers, such as high-sensitivity C-reactive protein (CRP), correlate with the risk of coronary events. CRP prospectively predicts risk of MI and outcomes after acute coronary syndromes; its usefulness and role in prevention as an independent risk factor is currently being defined. Potential benefits of assessing other emerging risk factors [e.g., lipoprotein(a), fibrinogen, infections by *Chlamydia* or CMV] remain unproven and controversial.

PREVENTION

Antithrombotic Therapy in Primary Prevention Thrombosis at the site of disrupted atherosclerotic plaque is the most common cause of acute coronary events. In primary prevention trials, chronic low-dose aspirin therapy has reduced the risk of a first MI in men and the risk of stroke in women. The American Heart Association recommends aspirin (75–160 mg daily) for men and women who are at high cardiovascular risk (i.e., by Framingham Study criteria, for men with ≥10% 10-year risk, or women with ≥ 20% 10-year risk).

Lifestyle Modifications   Encourage beneficial exercise habits (> 30 min moderate intensity physical activity daily) and sensible diet (low in saturated and trans fat; 2–3 servings of fish/week to ensure adequate intake of omega-3 fatty acids; balance caloric consumption with energy expenditure). Advise moderation in ethanol intake (no more than 1–2 drinks/day).

For a more detailed discussion, see Libby P: The Pathogenesis, Prevention, and Treatment of Atherosclerosis, Chap. 235, p. 1501-1509; Gaziano TA and Gaziano JM: Epidemiology of Cardiovascular Disease, Chap. 218, p. 1375-1379; and Martin GJ: Screening and Prevention of Disease, Chap. 4, p. 24; in HPIM-17.

214 Prevention and Early Detection of Cancer

One of the most important functions of medical care is to prevent disease or discover it early enough that treatment might be more effective. All risk factors for cancer have not yet been defined. However, a substantial number of factors that elevate risk are within a person's control. Some of these factors are listed in Table 214-1. Every physician visit is an opportunity to teach and reinforce the elements of a healthy lifestyle.

Cancer screening in the asymptomatic population at average risk is a complicated issue. To be of value, screening must detect disease at a stage that is more readily curable than disease that is treated after symptoms appear. For cervix cancer and colon cancer, screening has been shown to save lives. For other tumors, benefit is less clear. Screening can cause harm; complications may ensue from the screening test or the tests done to validate a positive screening test or from treatments for the underlying disease. Furthermore, quality of life can be adversely affected by false-positive tests. Evaluation of screening tools can be biased and needs to rely on prospective randomized studies. *Lead-time bias* occurs when the natural history of disease is unaffected by the diagnosis, but the pt is diagnosed earlier in the course of disease than normal; thus, the pt spends more of his/her life span knowing the diagnosis. *Length bias* occurs when slow-growing cancers that might never have come to medical attention are detected during screening. *Overdiagnosis* is a form of length bias in which a

TABLE 214-1 LIFESTYLE FACTORS THAT REDUCE CANCER RISK
Do not use any tobacco products
Maintain a healthy weight; eat a well-balanced diet[a]; maintain caloric balance
Exercise at least 3 times a week
Prevent sun exposure
Avoid excessive alcohol intake
Practice safe sex; use condoms

[a]Not precisely defined, but current recommendations include 5 servings of fruits and vegetables per day, 25 g fiber, and <30% of calories coming from fat.

cancer is detected when it is not growing and is not an influence on length of survival. *Selection bias* is the term for the fact that people who volunteer for screening trials may be different from the general population. Volunteers might have family history concerns that actually elevate their risk or they may be generally more health-conscious, which can affect outcome.

The various groups that evaluate and recommend screening practice guidelines have used varying criteria to make their recommendations (Table 214-2). The absence of data on survival for a number of diseases has led to a lack of consensus. In particular, four areas are worth noting.

1. *Prostate cancer*: Prostate-specific antigen (PSA) levels are elevated in prostate cancer, but a substantial number of the cancers detected appear to be non-life-threatening. PSA screening has not been shown to improve survival. Efforts are underway to develop better tests (predominantly using bound vs. free and rate of increase of PSA) to distinguish lethal and nonlethal cancers.
2. *Breast cancer*: The data on annual mammography support its use in women over age 50 years. However, the benefit for women age 40–49 years is quite small. One study shows some advantage for women who are screened starting at age 40 that appears 15 years later; however, it is unclear if this benefit would not have also been derived by starting screening at age 50 years. Women age 40–49 years have a much lower incidence of breast cancer and a higher false-positive rate on mammography. Nearly half of women screened during their forties will have a false-positive test. Refined methods of screening are in development.
3. *Colon cancer*: Annual fecal occult blood testing after age 50 years is felt to be useful. However, colonoscopy is the gold standard in colorectal cancer detection, but it is expensive and has not been shown to be cost-effective in asymptomatic people.
4. *Lung cancer*: Chest radiographs and sputum cytology in smokers appear to identify more early-stage tumors, but paradoxically, the screened pts do not have improved survival. Spiral CT scanning is being evaluated, but it is known to have more false-positive tests.

CANCER PREVENTION IN HIGH-RISK GROUPS

BREAST CANCER

Risk factors include age, early menarche, nulliparity or late first pregnancy, high body-mass index, radiation exposure before age 30 years, hormone-replacement therapy (HRT), alcohol consumption, family history, presence of mutations in *BRCA1* or *BRCA2*, and prior history of breast neoplasia. Risk assessment models have been developed to predict an individual's likelihood of developing breast cancer (see *www.nci.nih.gov/cancertopics/pdq/genetics/breast-and-ovarian/healthprofessional#Section_66*).

Diagnosis MRI scanning is a more effective screening tool than mammography in women with a familial breast cancer risk.

Interventions Women whose risk exceeds 1.66% in the next 5 years have been shown to have a 50% reduction in breast cancer from taking tamoxifen. Raloxifene also appears to reduce the risk and may have less toxicity. Aromatase inhibitors have generally been superior to tamoxifen in the adjuvant treatment of hormone-sensitive breast cancer but are still being evaluated as preventive agents. Women with strong family histories should undergo testing for mutations in *BRCA1* and *BRCA2*. Mutations in these genes carry a lifetime probabil-

TABLE 214-2 SCREENING RECOMMENDATIONS FOR ASYMPTOMATIC NORMAL-RISK SUBJECTS[a]

Test or Procedure	USPSTF	ACS	CTFPHC
Sigmoidoscopy	Fair evidence to recommend	≥50, every 5 years	Fair evidence to consider
Fecal occult blood testing	≥50, good evidence for every 1–2 years	≥50, every year	Good evidence, age ≥50
Colonoscopy	No direct evidence	≥50, every 10 years	No direct evidence
Digital rectal examination	No recommendation	No recommendation	No recommendation
Prostate-specific antigen	Insufficient evidence to recommend	M: ≥50, every year	Recommendation against
Pap test	F: 18–65, every 1–3 years	F: with uterine cervix, beginning 3 years after first intercourse or by age 21. Yearly for standard Pap; every 2 years with liquid test.	Fair evidence to include in examination of sexually active women
Pelvic examination	No recommendation, advise adnexal palpation during exam for other reasons	F: 18–40, every 1–3 years with Pap test; >40, every year	Not considered
Breast self-examination	No recommendation	≥20, monthly	Fair evidence to exclude
Breast clinical examination	Insufficient evidence as a stand-alone without mammography	F: 20–40, every 3 years; >40, yearly	F: 50–69, every 1–2 years
Mammography	F: 40–75, every 1–2 years (fair evidence)	F: ≥40, every year	F: 50–69, every 1–2 years
Complete skin examination	Insufficient evidence for or against	Periodic exam	Poor evidence to include or exclude

[a]Summary of the screening procedures recommended for the general population by U.S. Preventive Services Task Force (USPSTF), the American Cancer Society (ACS), and the Canadian Task Force on Prevention Health Care (CTFPHC). These recommendations refer to asymptomatic persons who have no risk factors, other than age or gender, for the targeted condition. *Note:* F, female; M, male.

ity of >80% for developing breast cancer. Bilateral prophylactic mastectomy prevents at least 90% of these cancers but is a more radical prevention than the usual treatment for the disease. In addition, bilateral salpingo-oophorectomy reduces ovarian and fallopian tube cancer risk by about 96% in women with *BRCA1* or *BRCA2* mutations.

COLORECTAL CANCER

Risk factors include diets high in saturated fats and low in fruits and vegetables, smoking, and alcohol consumption. Stronger but less prevalent risk factors are the presence of inflammatory bowel disease or genetic disorders such as familial polyposis (autosomal dominant germ-line mutation in *APC*) and hereditary non-polyposis colorectal cancer (mutations in DNA mismatch repair genes *hMSH2* and *hMLH1*).

Interventions Pts with ulcerative colitis and familial polyposis generally undergo total colectomy. In familial polyposis, nonsteroidal anti-inflammatory drugs (NSAIDs) reduce the number and size of polyps. Celecoxib, sulindac, and even aspirin appear to be effective, and celecoxib is approved by the U.S. Food and Drug Administration for this indication. Calcium supplementation can lead to a decrease in the recurrence of adenomas, but it is not yet clear that the risk of colorectal cancer is decreased and survival increased. The Women's Health Study noted a significant reduction in the risk of colorectal cancer in women taking HRT, but the increase in thrombotic events and breast cancers counterbalanced this benefit. Studies are underway to assess NSAIDs with and without inhibitors of the epidermal growth factor (EGF) receptor in other risk groups.

LUNG CANCER

Risk factors include smoking, exposure to radiation, asbestos, radon.

Interventions Smoking cessation is the only effective prevention. NSAIDs and EGF receptor inhibitors are being evaluated. Carotenoids, selenium, retinoids, and α-tocopherol do not work.

PROSTATE CANCER

Risk factors include age, family history, and possibly dietary fat intake. African Americans are at increased risk. The disease is highly prevalent, with autopsy studies finding prostate cancer in 70–80% of men over age 70.

Interventions In a group of men age ≥55 years with normal rectal examinations and PSA levels <3 ng/mL, daily finasteride reduced the incidence of prostate cancer by 25%. Finasteride also prevents the progression of benign prostate hyperplasia. However, some men experience decreased libido as a side effect. The Gleason grade of tumors seen in men taking finasteride prevention was somewhat higher than the controls; however, androgen deprivation alters the morphology of the cells and it is not yet clear that the Gleason grade is a reliable indicator of tumor aggressiveness in the setting of androgen deprivation. Some data suggest that selenium and α-tocopherol may lower risk of prostate cancer. In a lung cancer prevention trial, men taking vitamin E had a 34% lower incidence of prostate cancer during the 6-year study period.

CERVICAL CANCER

Risk factors include early age at first intercourse, multiple sexual partners, smoking, and infection with human papillomavirus (HPV) types 16, 18, 45, and 56.

Interventions Regular Pap testing can detect nearly all cases of the premalignant lesion called *cervical intraepithelial neoplasia*. Untreated, the lesion can progress to carcinoma in situ and invasive cervical cancer. Surgical removal, cryotherapy, or laser therapy is used to treat the disease and is effective in 80%. Risk of recurrence is highest in women over age 30, those with prior HPV infection, and those who have had prior treatment for the same condition. A vaccine (Gardasil) containing antigens of strains 6, 11, 16, and 18 has been shown to be 100% effective in preventing HPV infections from those strains. The vaccine is recommended for all females age 9–16 years and could prevent up to 70% of all cervical cancer.

HEAD AND NECK CANCER

Risk factors include smoking, alcohol consumption, and possibly HPV infection.

Interventions Oral leukoplakia, white lesions of the oral mucosa, occur in 1–2 persons in 1000, and 2–3% of these pts go on to develop head and neck cancer. Spontaneous regression of oral leukoplakia is seen in 30–40% of pts. Retinoid treatment (13-*cis* retinoid acid) can increase the regression rate. Vitamin A induces complete remission in ~50% of pts. The use of retinoids in pts who have been diagnosed with head and neck cancer and received definitive local therapy has not produced consistent results. Initial studies claimed that retinoids prevented the development of second primary tumors, a common feature of head and neck cancer. However, large randomized studies did not confirm this benefit. Other studies are underway combining retinoids and NSAIDs with and without EGF receptor inhibitors.

PATIENT EDUCATION IN EARLY DETECTION

Pts can be taught to look for early warning signals. The American Cancer Society has identified seven major warning signs of cancer:

- A change in bowel or bladder habits
- A sore that does not heal
- Unusual bleeding or discharge
- A lump in the breast or other parts of the body
- Chronic indigestion or difficulty in swallowing
- Obvious changes in a wart or mole
- Persistent coughing or hoarseness

For a more detailed discussion, see Brawley OW, Kramer BS: Prevention and Early Detection of Cancer, Chap. 78, p. 486, in HPIM-17.

215 Smoking Cessation

Over 400,000 individuals die each year in the United States from cigarette use: one out of every five deaths nationwide. Approximately 40% of smokers will die prematurely unless they are able to quit; major diseases caused by cigarette smoking are listed in Table 215-1.

APPROACH TO THE PATIENT WITH NICOTINE ADDICTION

All pts should be asked whether they smoke, their past experience with quitting, and whether they are currently interested in quitting; those who are not interested should be encouraged and motivated to quit. Provide a clear, strong, and personalized physician message that smoking is an important health concern. A quit date should be negotiated within a few weeks of the visit, and a follow-up contact by office staff around the time of the quit date should be provided. Incorporation of cessation assistance into a practice requires a change of the care delivery infrastructure. Simple changes include:

- Adding questions about smoking and interest in cessation on patient-intake questionnaires

TABLE 215-1 **RELATIVE RISKS FOR CURRENT SMOKERS OF CIGARETTES**

Disease or Condition	Current Smokers	
	Males	Females
Coronary heart disease		
Age 35–64	2.8	3.1
Age ≥65	1.5	1.6
Cerebrovascular disease		
Age 35–64	3.3	4
Age ≥65	1.6	1.5
Aortic aneurysm	6.2	7.1
Chronic airway obstruction	10.6	13.1
Cancer		
Lung	23.3	12.7
Larynx	14.6	13
Lip, oral cavity, pharynx	10.9	5.1
Esophagus	6.8	7.8
Bladder, other urinary organs	3.3	2.2
Kidney	2.7	1.3
Pancreas	2.3	2.3
Stomach	2	1.4
Cervix		1.6
Acute myeloid leukemia	1.4	1.4
Sudden infant death syndrome		2.3
Infant respiratory distress syndrome		1.3
Low birth weight at delivery		1.8

- Asking pts whether they smoke as part of the initial vital sign measurements made by office staff
- Listing smoking as a problem in the medical record
- Automating follow-up contact with the pt on the quit date

℞ Nicotine Addiction

Clinical practice guidelines suggest a variety of pharmacologic and non-pharmacologic interventions to aid in smoking cessation (Table 215-2). There are a variety of nicotine-replacement products, including over-the-counter nicotine patches, gum, and lozenges, as well as nicotine nasal and oral inhalers available by prescription; these products can be used for 3–6 months with a gradual stepdown in dosage with increasing duration of abstinence. Prescription medications that have been shown to be effective include antidepressants such as bupropion (300 mg/d in divided doses for up to 6 months) and varenicline, a partial agonist for the nicotinic acetylcholine receptor (initial dose 0.5 mg daily increasing to 1 mg twice daily at day 8; treatment duration up to 6 months). Clonidine or nortriptyline may be useful for pts who have failed first-line therapies. Antidepressants are more effective in pts with a history of depressive symptoms. Current recommendations are to offer pharmacologic treatment, usually with nicotine replacement therapy and bupropion, to all who will accept it and to provide counseling and other support as a part of the cessation attempt.

TABLE 215-2 CLINICAL PRACTICE GUIDELINES

Physician actions
  Ask: Systematically identify all tobacco users at every visit
  Advise: Strongly urge all smokers to quit
  Identify smokers willing to quit
  Assist the patient in quitting
  Arrange follow-up contact
Effective pharmacologic interventions[a]
  First-line therapies
    Nicotine gum (1.5)
    Nicotine patch (1.9)
    Nicotine nasal inhaler (2.7)
    Nicotine oral inhaler (2.5)
    Nicotine lozenge (2.0)
    Bupropion (2.1)
    Varenicline (2.7)
  Second-line therapies
    Clonidine (2.1)
    Nortriptyline (3.2)
Other Effective Interventions[a]
  Physician or other medical personnel counseling (10 min) (1.3)
  Intensive smoking cessation programs (at least 4–7 sessions of 20–30 min duration lasting at least 2 and preferably 8 weeks) (2.3)
  Clinic-based smoking status identification system (3.1)
  Counseling by nonclinicians and social support by family and friends
  Telephone counseling (1.2)

---

[a]Numerical value following the intervention is the multiple for cessation success compared to no intervention.

PREVENTION

Approximately 90% of individuals who will become cigarette smokers initiate the behavior during adolescence; prevention must begin early, preferably in the elementary school years. Physicians who treat adolescents should be sensitive to the prevalence of this problem and screen for tobacco use, reinforcing the fact that most adolescents and adults do not smoke, and explaining that all forms of tobacco are both addictive and harmful.

 For a more detailed discussion, see Burns DM: Nicotine Addiction, Chap. 390, p. 2736, in HPIM-17.

216 Women's Health

The most common causes of death in both men and women are heart disease and cancer, with lung cancer the top cause of cancer death, despite common misperceptions that breast cancer is the most common cause of death in women. These misconceptions perpetuate inadequate attention to modifiable risk factors in women, such as dyslipidemia, hypertension, and cigarette smoking. Furthermore, since women in the Unites States live on average 5.2 years longer than men, the majority of the disease burden for many age-related disorders rests in women. For a discussion of the menopause transition and postmenopausal hormone therapy, see Chap. 184.

SEX DIFFERENCES IN HEALTH AND DISEASE

ALZHEIMER'S DISEASE   (See also Chap. 192)

Alzheimer's disease (AD) affects approximately twice as many women as men, due to larger numbers of women surviving to older ages and to sex differences in brain size, structure, and functional organization. Postmenopausal hormone therapy may worsen cognitive function and the development of AD.

CORONARY HEART DISEASE   (See also Chap. 126)

Coronary heart disease (CHD) presents differently in women, who are usually 10–15 years older than men with CHD and are more likely to have comorbidities, such as hypertension, congestive heart failure, and diabetes. Women more often have atypical symptoms, such as nausea, vomiting, indigestion, and upper back pain. Physicians are less likely to suspect heart disease in women with chest pain and are less likely to perform diagnostic and therapeutic cardiac procedures in women. The conventional risk factors for CHD are the same in both men and women, though women receive fewer interventions for modifiable risk factors than do men.

DIABETES MELLITUS   (See also Chap. 182)

The prevalence of type 2 diabetes mellitus (DM) is similar between men and women. Polycystic ovary syndrome and gestational diabetes mellitus are both common conditions in premenopausal women that carry an increased risk for type 2 DM. Premenopausal women with DM have identical rates of CHD to those of males.

HYPERTENSION   (See also Chap. 124)

Hypertension, as an age-related disorder, is more common in women than in men after age 60. Antihypertensive drugs appear to be equally effective in women and men; however, women may experience more side effects.

AUTOIMMUNE DISORDERS   (See also Chap. 167)

Most autoimmune disorders occur more commonly in women than in men; these include autoimmune thyroid and liver diseases, lupus, rheumatoid arthritis, scleroderma, multiple sclerosis, and idiopathic thrombocytopenic purpura. The mechanism for these sex differences remains obscure.

HIV INFECTION   (See also Chap. 112)

Heterosexual contact with an at-risk partner is the fastest-growing transmission category of HIV. Women with HIV have more rapid decreases in their CD4 cell counts than men do. Other sexually transmitted diseases, such as chlamydial infection and gonorrhea, are important causes of infertility in women, and papilloma virus infection predisposes to cervical cancer.

OBESITY   (See also Chap. 181)

The prevalence of obesity is higher in women than in men, in part due to the unique risk factors of pregnancy and menopause. In addition, the distribution of body fat differs by sex, with a gluteal and femoral pattern in women and a central pattern in men. Obesity increases a woman's risk for postmenopausal breast and endometrial cancer, in part because of adipose tissue aromatization of androgens to estrone.

OSTEOPOROSIS   (See also Chap. 186)

Osteoporosis is much more prevalent in postmenopausal women than in age-matched men, since men accumulate more bone mass and lose bone more slowly than do women. In addition, differences in calcium intake, vitamin D, and estrogen levels contribute to sex differences in bone formation and bone loss.

PHARMACOLOGY

On average, women have lower body weights, smaller organs, higher percent body fat, and lower total-body water than men do. Gonadal steroids, menstrual cycle phase, and pregnancy can all affect drug action. Women also take more medications than men do, including over-the-counter formulations and supplements. The greater use of medications, combined with biologic differences, may account for the reported higher frequency of adverse drug reactions in women.

PSYCHOLOGICAL DISORDERS   (See also Chaps. 206 & 208)

Depression, anxiety, and eating disorders (bulimia and anorexia nervosa) are more common in women than in men. Depression occurs in 10% of women during pregnancy and 10–15% of women during the postpartum period.

SLEEP DISORDERS (See also Chap. 45)

During sleep, women have an increased amount of slow-wave activity, differences in timing of delta activity, and an increase in the number of sleep spindles. They have a decreased prevalence of sleep apnea.

SUBSTANCE ABUSE AND TOBACCO (See also Chap. 209)

Substance abuse is more common in men than women. However, women alcoholics are less likely to be diagnosed than men and are less likely to seek help. When they do seek help, it is more likely to be from a physician than from a treatment facility. Alcoholic women drink less than alcoholic men but exhibit the same degree of impairment. More men than women smoke tobacco, but the prevalence of smoking is declining faster in men than women.

VIOLENCE AGAINST WOMEN

Domestic violence is the most common cause of physical injury in women. Women may present with symptoms of chronic abdominal pain, headaches, substance abuse, and eating disorders, in addition to obvious manifestations such as trauma. Sexual assault is one of the most common crimes against women and is more likely by a spouse, ex-spouse, or acquaintance than by a stranger.

For a more detailed discussion, see Dunaif A: Women's Health, Chap. 6, p. 39, HPIM-17.

217   Adverse Drug Reactions

Adverse drug reactions are among the most frequent problems encountered clinically and represent a common cause for hospitalization. They occur most frequently in pts receiving multiple drugs and are caused by:

- Errors in self-administration of prescribed drugs (quite common in the elderly).
- Exaggeration of intended pharmacologic effect (e.g., hypotension in a pt given antihypertensive drugs).
- Concomitant administration of drugs with synergistic effects (e.g., aspirin and warfarin).
- Cytotoxic reactions (e.g., hepatic necrosis due to acetaminophen).
- Immunologic mechanisms (e.g., quinidine-induced thrombocytopenia, hydralazine-induced SLE).
- Genetically determined enzymatic defects (e.g., primaquine-induced hemolytic anemia in G6PD deficiency).
- Idiosyncratic reactions (e.g., chloramphenicol-induced aplastic anemia).

Recognition   History is of prime importance. Consider the following:

- Nonprescription drugs and topical agents as potential offenders
- Previous reaction to identical drugs
- Temporal association between drug administration and development of clinical manifestations
- Subsidence of manifestations when the agent is discontinued or reduced in dose
- Recurrence of manifestations with cautious readministration (for less hazardous reactions)
- *Rare*: (1) biochemical abnormalities, e.g., red cell G6PD deficiency as cause of drug-induced hemolytic anemia; (2) abnormal serum antibody in pts with agranulocytosis, thrombocytopenia, hemolytic anemia.

Table 217-1 lists a number of clinical manifestations of adverse effects of drugs. It is not designed to be complete or exhaustive.

TABLE 217-1   CLINICAL MANIFESTATIONS OF ADVERSE REACTIONS TO DRUGS

Multisystem Manifestations

Anaphylaxis	**Angioedema**
Cephalosporins	ACE inhibitors
Dextran	**Drug-induced lupus erythematosus**
Insulin	Cephalosporins
Iodinated drugs or contrast media	Hydralazine
Lidocaine	Iodides
Penicillins	Isoniazid
Procaine	Methyldopa

(continued)

TABLE 217-1 **CLINICAL MANIFESTATIONS OF ADVERSE REACTIONS TO DRUGS (CONTINUED)**

Multisystem Manifestations (*Continued*)

Phenytoin	**Hyperpyrexia**
Procainamide	Antipsychotics
Quinidine	**Serum sickness**
Sulfonamides	Aspirin
Thiouracil	Penicillins
Fever	Propylthiouracil
Aminosalicylic acid	Sulfonamides
Amphotericin B	
Antihistamines	
Penicillins	

Endocrine Manifestations

Addisonian-like syndrome	Guanethidine
Busulfan	Lithium
Ketoconazole	Major tranquilizers
Galactorrhea (may also cause amenorrhea)	Methyldopa
Methyldopa	Oral contraceptives
Phenothiazines	Sedatives
Tricyclic antidepressants	**Thyroid function tests, disorders of**
Gynecomastia	Acetazolamide
Calcium channel antagonists	Amiodarone
Digitalis	Chlorpropamide
Estrogens	Clofibrate
Griseofulvin	Colestipol and nicotinic acid
Isoniazid	Gold salts
Methyldopa	Iodides
Phenytoin	Lithium
Spironolactone	Oral contraceptives
Testosterone	Phenothiazines
Sexual dysfunction	Phenylbutazone
Beta blockers	Phenytoin
Clonidine	Sulfonamides
Diuretics	Tolbutamide

Metabolic Manifestations

Hyperbilirubinemia	Oral contraceptives
Rifampin	Thiazides
Hypercalcemia	**Hypoglycemia**
Antacids with absorbable alkali	Insulin
Thiazides	Oral hypoglycemics
Vitamin D	Quinine
Hyperglycemia	**Hyperkalemia**
Chlorthalidone	ACE inhibitors
Diazoxide	Amiloride
Encainide	Cytotoxics
Ethacrynic acid	Digitalis overdose
Furosemide	Heparin
Glucocorticoids	Lithium
Growth hormone	

(continued)

Metabolic Manifestations (Continued)

Potassium preparations including salt substitute
Potassium salts of drugs
Spironolactone
Succinylcholine
Triamterene

Hypokalemia
Alkali-induced alkalosis
Amphotericin B
Diuretics
Gentamicin
Insulin
Laxative abuse
Mineralocorticoids, some glucocorticoids
Osmotic diuretics
Sympathomimetics
Tetracycline
Theophylline
Vitamin B_{12}

Hyperuricemia
Aspirin
Cytotoxics

Ethacrynic acid
Furosemide
Hyperalimentation
Thiazides

Hyponatremia
1. Dilutional
   Carbamazepine
   Chlorpropamide
   Cyclophosphamide
   Diuretics
   Vincristine
2. Salt wasting
   Diuretics
   Enemas
   Mannitol

Metabolic acidosis
Acetazolamide
Paraldehyde
Salicylates
Spironolactone

Dermatologic Manifestations

Acne
Anabolic and androgenic steroids
Bromides
Glucocorticoids
Iodides
Isoniazid
Oral contraceptives

Alopecia
Cytotoxics
Ethionamide
Heparin
Oral contraceptives (withdrawal)

Eczema
Captopril
Cream and lotion preservatives
Lanolin
Topical antihistamines
Topical antimicrobials
Topical local anesthetics

Erythema multiforme or Stevens-Johnson syndrome
Barbiturates
Chlorpropamide
Codeine
Penicillins
Phenylbutazone
Phenytoin

Salicylates
Sulfonamides
Sulfones
Tetracyclines
Thiazides

Erythema nodosum
Oral contraceptives
Penicillins
Sulfonamides

Exfoliative dermatitis
Barbiturates
Gold salts
Penicillins
Phenylbutazone
Phenytoin
Quinidine
Sulfonamides

Fixed drug eruptions
Barbiturates
Captopril
Phenylbutazone
Quinine
Salicylates
Sulfonamides

Hyperpigmentation
Bleomycin
Busulfan

(continued)

TABLE 217-1 **CLINICAL MANIFESTATIONS OF ADVERSE REACTIONS TO DRUGS (CONTINUED)**

Dermatologic Manifestations *(Continued)*

Chloroquine and other antimalarials
Corticotropin
Cyclophosphamide
Gold salts
Hypervitaminosis A
Oral contraceptives
Phenothiazines
Lichenoid eruptions
Aminosalicylic acid
Antimalarials
Chlorpropamide
Gold salts
Methyldopa
Phenothiazines
Photodermatitis
Captopril
Chlordiazepoxide
Furosemide
Griseofulvin
Nalidixic acid
Oral contraceptives
Phenothiazines
Sulfonamides
Sulfonylureas
Tetracyclines, particularly demeclocycline
Thiazides
Purpura (see also **Thrombocytopenia**)
Allopurinol
Ampicillin

Aspirin
Glucocorticoids
Rashes (nonspecific)
Allopurinol
Ampicillin
Barbiturates
Indapamide
Methyldopa
Phenytoin
Skin necrosis
Warfarin
Toxic epidermal necrolysis (bullous)
Allopurinol
Barbiturates
Bromides
Iodides
Nalidixic acid
Penicillins
Phenylbutazone
Phenytoin
Sulfonamides
Urticaria
Aspirin
Barbiturates
Captopril
Enalapril
Penicillins
Sulfonamides

Hematologic Manifestations

Agranulocytosis (see also **Pancytopenia**)
Captopril
Carbimazole
Chloramphenicol
Cytotoxics
Gold salts
Indomethacin
Methimazole
Oxyphenbutazone
Phenothiazines
Phenylbutazone
Propylthiouracil
Sulfonamides
Tolbutamide
Tricyclic antidepressants

Clotting abnormalities/ hypothrombinemia
Cefamandole
Cefoperazone
Moxalactam
Eosinophilia
Aminosalicylic acid
Chlorpropamide
Erythromycin estolate
Imipramine
L-Tryptophan
Methotrexate
Nitrofurantoin
Procarbazine
Sulfonamides

(continued)

Hematologic Manifestations (*Continued*)

Hemolytic anemia
Aminosalicylic acid
Cephalosporins
Chlorpromazine
Dapsone
Insulin
Isoniazid
Levodopa
Mefenamic acid
Melphalan
Methyldopa
Penicillins
Phenacetin
Procainamide
Quinidine
Rifampin
Sulfonamides

Hemolytic anemias in G6PD deficiency
See Table 66-3

Leukocytosis
Glucocorticoids
Lithium

Lymphadenopathy
Phenytoin
Primidone

Megaloblastic anemia
Folate antagonists
Nitrous oxide
Oral contraceptives
Phenobarbital
Phenytoin
Primidone
Triamterene
Trimethroprim

Pancytopenia (aplastic anemia)
Carbamazepine
Chloramphenicol

Cytotoxics
Gold salts
Mephenytoin
Phenylbutazone
Phenytoin
Quinacrine
Sulfonamides
Trimethadione
Zidovudine (AZT)

Pure red cell aplasia
Azathioprine
Chlorpropamide
Isoniazid
Phenytoin

Thrombocytopenia (see also
Pancytopenia)
Acetazolamine
Aspirin
Carbamazepine
Carbenicillin
Chlorpropamide
Chlorthalidone
Furosemide
Gold salts
Heparin
Indomethacin
Isoniazid
Methyldopa
Moxalactam
Phenylbutazone
Phenytoin and other hydantoins
Quinidine
Quinine
Thiazides
Ticarcillin

Cardiovascular Manifestations

Angina exacerbation
Alpha blockers
Beta blocker withdrawal
Ergotamine
Excessive thyroxine
Hydralazine
Methysergide
Minoxidil
Nifedipine
Oxytocin
Vasopressin

Arrhythmias
Adriamycin
Antiarrhythmic drugs
Atropine
Anticholinesterases
Beta blockers
Digitalis
Emetine
Lithium
Phenothiazines
Sympathomimetics

(continued)

| TABLE 217-1 | CLINICAL MANIFESTATIONS OF ADVERSE REACTIONS TO DRUGS (CONTINUED) |

Cardiovascular Manifestations (*Continued*)

Thyroid hormone
Tricyclic antidepressants
Verapamil
AV block
  Clonidine
  Methyldopa
  Verapamil
Cardiomyopathy
  Adriamycin
  Daunorubicin
  Emetine
  Lithium
  Phenothiazines
  Sulfonamides
  Sympathomimetics
Fluid retention or congestive heart failure
  Beta blockers
  Calcium antagonists
  Estrogens
  Indomethacin
  Mannitol
  Minoxidil
  Phenylbutazone
  Steroids
Hypotension
  Calcium antagonists
  Citrated blood

Diuretics
Levodopa
Morphine
Nitroglycerin
Phenothiazines
Protamine
Quinidine
Hypertension
  Clonidine withdrawal
  Corticotropin
  Cyclosporine
  Glucocorticoids
  Monoamine oxidase inhibitors with sympathomimetics
  NSAIDs
  Oral contraceptives
  Sympathomimetics
  Tricyclic antidepressants with sympathomimetics
Pericarditis
  Emetine
  Hydralazine
  Methysergide
  Procainamide
Thromboembolism
  Oral contraceptives

Respiratory Manifestations

Airway obstruction
  Beta blockers
  Cephalosporins
  Cholinergic drugs
  NSAIDs
  Penicillins
  Pentazocine
  Streptomycin
  Tartrazine (drugs with yellow dye)
Cough
  ACE inhibitors
Pulmonary edema
  Contrast media
  Heroin
  Methadone
  Propoxyphene

Pulmonary infiltrates
  Acyclovir
  Amiodarone
  Azathioprine
  Bleomycin
  Busulfan
  Carmustine (BCNU)
  Chlorambucil
  Cyclophosphamide
  Melphalan
  Methotrexate
  Methysergide
  Mitomycin C
  Nitrofurantoin
  Procarbazine
  Sulfonamides

(continued)

Gastrointestinal Manifestations

Cholestatic jaundice
  Anabolic steroids
  Androgens
  Chlorpropamide
  Erythromycin estolate
  Gold salts
  Methimazole
  Nitrofurantoin
  Oral contraceptives
  Phenothiazines
Constipation or ileus
  Aluminum hydroxide
  Barium sulfate
  Calcium carbonate
  Ferrous sulfate
  Ion exchange resins
  Opiates
  Phenothiazines
  Tricyclic antidepressants
  Verapamil
Diarrhea or colitis
  Antibiotics (broad-spectrum)
  Colchicine
  Digitalis
  Magnesium in antacids
  Methyldopa
Diffuse hepatocellular damage
  Acetaminophen (paracetamol)
  Allopurinol
  Aminosalicylic acid
  Dapsone
  Erythromycin estolate
  Ethionamide
  Glyburide
  Halothane
  Isoniazid
  Ketoconazole
  Methimazole
  Methotrexate
  Methoxyflurane
  Methyldopa
  Monoamine oxidase inhibitors
  Niacin
  Nifedipine
  Nitrofurantoin
  Phenytoin
  Propoxyphene
  Propylthiouracil
  Pyridium
  Rifampin
  Salicylates

  Sodium valproate
  Sulfonamides
  Tetracyclines
  Verapamil
  Zidovudine (AZT)
Intestinal ulceration
  Solid KCl preparations
Malabsorption
  Aminosalicylic acid
  Antibiotics (broad-spectrum)
  Cholestyramine
  Colchicine
  Colestipol
  Cytotoxics
  Neomycin
  Phenobarbital
  Phenytoin
Nausea or vomiting
  Digitalis
  Estrogens
  Ferrous sulfate
  Levodopa
  Opiates
  Potassium chloride
  Tetracyclines
  Theophylline
Oral conditions
  1. Gingival hyperplasia
       Calcium antagonists
       Cyclosporine
       Phenytoin
  2. Salivary gland swelling
       Bretylium
       Clonidine
       Guanethidine
       Iodides
       Phenylbutazone
  3. Taste disturbances
       Biguanides
       Captopril
       Griseofulvin
       Lithium
       Metronidazole
       Penicillamine
       Rifampin
  4. Ulceration
       Aspirin
       Cytotoxics
       Gentian violet
       Isoproterenol (sublingual)
       Pancreatin

(continued)

TABLE 217-1 **CLINICAL MANIFESTATIONS OF ADVERSE REACTIONS TO DRUGS (CONTINUED)**

Gastrointestinal Manifestations *(Continued)*

Pancreatitis
  Azathioprine
  Ethacrynic acid
  Furosemide
  Glucocorticoids
  Opiates
  Oral contraceptives

Sulfonamides
Thiazides
Peptic ulceration or hemorrhage
  Aspirin
  Ethacrynic acid
  Glucocorticoids
  NSAIDs

Renal/Urinary Manifestations

Bladder dysfunction
  Anticholinergics
  Disopyramide
  Monoamine oxidase inhibitors
  Tricyclic antidepressants
Calculi
  Acetazolamide
  Vitamin D
Concentrating defect with polyuria
  (or nephrogenic diabetes insipidus)
  Demeclocycline
  Lithium
  Methoxyflurane
  Vitamin D
Hemorrhagic cystitis
  Cyclophosphamide
Interstitial nephritis
  Allopurinol
  Furosemide
  Penicillins, esp. methicillin
  Phenindione
  Sulfonamides
  Thiazides
Nephropathies
  Due to analgesics (e.g., phenacetin)

Nephrotic syndrome
  Captopril
  Gold salts
  Penicillamine
  Phenindione
  Probenecid
Obstructive uropathy
  Extrarenal: methysergide
  Intrarenal: cytotoxics
Renal dysfunction
  Cyclosporine
  NSAIDS
  Triamterene
Renal tubular acidosis
  Acetazolamide
  Amphotericin B
  Degraded tetracycline
Tubular necrosis
  Aminoglycosides
  Amphotericin B
  Colistin
  Cyclosporine
  Methoxyflurane
  Polymyxins
  Radioiodinated contrast medium
  Sulfonamides
  Tetracyclines

Neurologic Manifestations

Exacerbation of myasthenia
  Aminoglycosides
  Polymyxins
Extrapyramidal effects
  Butyrophenones, e.g., haloperidol
  Levodopa
  Methyldopa
  Metoclopramide
  Oral contraceptives
  Phenothiazines
  Tricyclic antidepressants

Headache
  Ergotamine (withdrawal)
  Glyceryl trinitrate
  Hydralazine
  Indomethacin
Peripheral neuropathy
  Amiodarone
  Chloramphenicol
  Chloroquine
  Chlorpropamide
  Clofibrate
  Demeclocycline

(continued)

Neurologic Manifestations (Continued)

Disopyramide
Ethambutol
Ethionamide
Glutethimide
Hydralazine
Isoniazid
Methysergide
Metronidazole
Nalidixic acid
Nitrofurantoin
Phenytoin
Polymyxin, colistin
Procarbazine
Streptomycin
Tolbutamide
Tricyclic antidepressants
Vincristine

Pseudotumor cerebri (or intracranial hypertension)
Amiodarone
Glucocorticoids, mineralocorticoids

Hypervitaminosis A
Oral contraceptives
Tetracyclines

Seizures
Amphetamines
Analeptics
Isoniazid
Lidocaine
Lithium
Nalidixic acid
Penicillins
Phenothiazines
Physostigmine
Theophylline
Tricyclic antidepressants
Vincristine

Stroke
Oral contraceptives

Ocular Manifestations

Cataracts
Busulfan
Chlorambucil
Glucocorticoids
Phenothiazines

Color vision alteration
Barbiturates
Digitalis
Methaqualone
Streptomycin
Thiazides

Corneal edema
Oral contraceptives

Corneal opacities
Chloroquine
Indomethacin
Vitamin D

Glaucoma
Mydriatics
Sympathomimetics

Optic neuritis
Aminosalicylic acid
Chloramphenicol
Ethambutol
Isoniazid
Penicillamine
Phenothiazines
Phenylbutazone
Quinine
Streptomycin

Retinopathy
Chloroquine
Phenothiazines

Ear Manifestations

Deafness
Aminoglycosides
Aspirin
Bleomycin
Chloroquine
Erythromycin
Ethacrynic acid

Furosemide
Nortriptyline
Quinine

Vestibular disorders
Aminoglycosides
Quinine

(continued)

TABLE 217-1 **CLINICAL MANIFESTATIONS OF ADVERSE REACTIONS TO DRUGS (CONTINUED)**

Musculoskeletal Manifestations

Bone disorders	Chloroquine
1. Osteoporosis	Clofibrate
Glucocorticoids	Glucocorticoids
Heparin	Oral contraceptives
2. Osteomalacia	**Myositis**
Aluminum hydroxide	Gemfibrozil
Anticonvulsants	Lovastatin
Glutethimide	
Myopathy or myalgia	
Amphotericin B	

Psychiatric Manifestations

Delirious or confusional states	**Hallucinatory states**
Amantadine	Amantadine
Aminophylline	Beta blockers
Anticholinergics	Levodopa
Antidepressants	Meperidine
Cimetidine	Narcotics
Digitalis	Pentazocine
Glucocorticoids	Tricyclic antidepressants
Isoniazid	**Hypomania, mania, or excited**
Levodopa	**reactions**
Methyldopa	Glucocorticoids
Penicillins	Levodopa
Phenothiazines	Monoamine oxidase inhibitors
Sedatives and hypnotics	Sympathomimetics
Depression	Tricyclic antidepressants
Amphetamine withdrawal	**Schizophrenic-like or paranoid**
Beta blockers	**reactions**
Centrally acting antihypertensives	Amphetamines
(reserpine, methyldopa,	Bromides
clonidine)	Glucocorticoids
Glucocorticoids	Levodopa
Levodopa	Lysergic acid
Drowsiness	Monoamine oxidase inhibitors
Antihistamines	Tricyclic antidepressants
Anxiolytic drugs	**Sleep disturbances**
Clonidine	Anorexiants
Major tranquilizers	Levodopa
Methyldopa	Monoamine oxidase inhibitors
Tricyclic antidepressants	Sympathomimetics

Source: Adapted from AJJ Wood: HPIM-15, pp. 432–436.

For a more detailed discussion, see Roden DM: Principles of Clinical Pharmacology, Chap. 5, p. 27, in HPIM-17; Wood AJJ: Adverse Reactions to Drugs, Chap. 71, p. 430, in HPIM-15.

218 Laboratory Values of Clinical Importance

INTRODUCTORY COMMENTS

In preparing for the Appendix, the authors have taken into account the fact that the system of international units (SI, système international d'unités) is used in most countries and in some medical journals. However, clinical laboratories may continue to report values in "conventional" units. Therefore, both systems are provided in the Appendix.

REFERENCE VALUES FOR LABORATORY TESTS

(Tables 218-1 through 218-5)

TABLE 218-1 HEMATOLOGY AND COAGULATION

Analyte	Specimen[a]	SI Units	Conventional Units
D-Dimer	P	0.22–0.74 µg/mL	0.22–0.74 µg/mL
Differential blood count	WB		
Neutrophils		0.40–0.70	40–70%
Bands		0.0–0.05	0–5%
Lymphocytes		0.20–0.50	20–50%
Monocytes		0.04–0.08	4–8%
Eosinophils		0.0–0.6	0–6%
Basophils		0.0–0.02	0–2%
Eosinophil count	WB	150–300/µL	150–300/mm^3
Erythrocyte count	WB		
Adult males		$4.30–5.60 \times 10^{12}$/L	$4.30–5.60 \times 10^6$/mm^3
Adult females		$4.00–5.20 \times 10^{12}$/L	$4.00–5.20 \times 10^6$/mm^3
Erythrocyte life span	WB		
Normal survival		120 days	120 days
Chromium labeled, half life ($t_{1/2}$)		25–35 days	25–35 days
Erythrocyte sedimentation rate	WB		
Females		0–20 mm/h	0–20 mm/h
Males		0–15 mm/h	0–15 mm/h
Fibrin(ogen) degradation products	P	0–1 mg/L	0–1 µg/mL
Fibrinogen	P	2.33–4.96 g/L	233–496 mg/dL
Glucose-6-phosphate dehydrogenase (erythrocyte)	WB	< 2400 s	<40 min
Hematocrit	WB		
Adult males		0.388–0.464	38.8–46.4
Adult females		0.354–0.444	35.4–44.4

1142

Hemoglobin			
Plasma	P	6–50 mg/L	0.6–5.0 mg/dL
Whole blood	WB		
Adult males		133–162 g/L	13.3–16.2 g/dL
Adult females		120–158 g/L	12.0–15.8 g/dL
Hemoglobin electrophoresis	WB		
Hemoglobin A		0.95–0.98	95–98%
Hemoglobin A_2		0.015–0.031	1.5–3.1%
Hemoglobin F		0–0.02	0–2.0%
Hemoglobins other than A, A_2, or F		Absent	Absent
Leukocytes			
Alkaline phosphatase (LAP)	WB	0.2–1.6 μkat/L	13–100 μ/L
Count (WBC)	WB	$3.54–9.06 \times 10^9$/L	$3.54–9.06 \times 10^3$/mm^3
Mean corpuscular hemoglobin (MCH)	WB	26.7–31.9 pg/cell	26.7–31.9 pg/cell
Mean corpuscular hemoglobin concentration (MCHC)	WB	323–359 g/L	32.3–35.9 g/dL
Mean corpuscular hemoglobin of reticulocytes (CH)	WB	24–36 pg	24–36 pg
Mean corpuscular volume (MCV)	WB	79–93.3 fL	79–93.3 μm^3
Mean platelet volume (MPV)	WB	9.00–12.95 fL	9.00–12.95 μm^3
Osmotic fragility of erythrocytes	WB		
Direct		0.0035–0.0045	0.35–0.45%
Index		0.0030–0.0065	0.30–0.65%
Partial thromboplastin time, activated	P	26.3–39.4 s	26.3–39.4 s
Plasminogen	P		
Antigen		84–140 mg/L	8.4–14.0 mg/dL
Functional		0.70–1.30	70–130%
Plasminogen activator inhibitor 1	P	4–43 μg/L	4–43 ng/mL

(continued)

TABLE 218-1 HEMATOLOGY AND COAGULATION (CONTINUED)

Analyte	Specimen[a]	SI Units	Conventional Units
Platelet aggregation	PRP	Not applicable	> 65% aggregation in response to adenosine diphosphate, epinephrine, collagen, ristocetin, and arachidonic acid
Platelet count	WB	165–415 × 10⁹/L	165–415 × 10³/mm³
Platelet, mean volume	WB	6.4–11 fL	6.4–11.0 µm³
Protein C	P		
Total antigen		0.70–1.40	70–140%
Functional		0.70–1.30	70–130%
Protein S	P		
Total antigen		0.70–1.40	70–140%
Functional		0.65–1.40	65–140%
Free antigen		0.70–1.40	70–140%
Prothrombin time	P	12.7–15.4 s	12.7–15.4 s
Reticulocyte count	WB		
Adult males		0.008–0.023 red cells	0.8–2.3% red cells
Adult females		0.008–0.020 red cells	0.8–2.0% red cells
Sickle cell test	WB	Negative	Negative
Thrombin time	P	15.3–18.5 s	15.3–18.5 s
Total eosinophils	WB	150–300 × 10⁶/L	150–300/mm³
Viscosity			
Plasma	P	1.7–2.1	1.7–2.1
Serum	S	1.4–1.8	1.4–1.8

[a]P, plasma; JF, joint fluid; PRP, platelet-rich plasma; S, serum; WB, whole blood.

1144

TABLE 218-2 CLINICAL CHEMISTRY AND IMMUNOLOGY

Analyte	Specimen[a]	SI Units	Conventional Units
Acetoacetate	P	20–99 μmol/L	0.2–1.0 mg/dL
Adrenocorticotropin (ACTH)	P	1.3–16.7 pmol/L	6.0–76.0 pg/mL
Alanine aminotransferase (AST, SGPT)	S	0.12–0.70 μkat/L	7–41 U/L
Albumin	S		
Female		41–53 g/L	4.1–5.3 g/dL
Male		40–50 g/L	4.0–5.0 g/L
Aldolase	S	26–138 nkat/L	1.5–8.1 U/L
Aldosterone (adult)			
Supine, normal sodium diet	S, P	55–250 pmol/L	2–9 ng/dL
Upright, normal sodium diet	S, P		2–5-fold increase over supine value
Supine, low-sodium diet	S, P		2–5-fold increase over normal sodium diet level
	U	6.38–58.25 nmol/d	2.3–21.0 μg/24 h
Alpha fetoprotein (adult)	S	0–8.5 μg/L	0–8.5 ng/mL
Alpha$_1$ antitrypsin	S	1.0–2.0 g/L	100–200 mg/dL
Ammonia, as NH_3	P	11–35 μmol/L	19–60 μg/dL
Amylase (method dependent)	S	0.34–1.6 μkat/L	20–96 U/L
Androstenedione (adult)	S	1.75–8.73 nmol/L	50–250 ng/dL
Angiotensin-converting enzyme (ACE)	S	0.15–1.1 μkat/L	9–67 U/L
Anion gap	S	7–16 mmol/L	7–16 mmol/L
Arterial blood gases			
[HCO_3^-]		22–30 mmol/L	22–30 meq/L
P_{CO_2}		4.3–6.0 kPa	32–45 mmHg
pH		7.35–7.45	7.35–7.45
P_{O_2}		9.6–13.8 kPa	72–104 mmHg

(continued)

1145

TABLE 218-2 CLINICAL CHEMISTRY AND IMMUNOLOGY (CONTINUED)

Analyte	Specimen[a]	SI Units	Conventional Units
Aspartate aminotransferase (AST, SGOT)	S	0.20–0.65 μkat/L	12–38 U/L
B type natriuretic peptide (BNP)	P	Age and gender specific: < 167 ng/L	Age and gender specific: < 167 pg/mL
Bence Jones Protein, urine, quantitative	U		
Kappa		<25 mg/L	<2.5 mg/dL
Lambda		<50 mg/L	<5.0 mg/dL
β_2-Microglobulin			
	S	<2.7 mg/L	<0.27 mg/dL
	U	<120 μg/d	<120 μg/day
Bilirubin	S		
Total		5.1–22 μmol/L	0.3–1.3 mg/dL
Direct		1.7–6.8 μmol/L	0.1–0.4 mg/dL
Indirect		3.4–15.2 μmol/L	0.2–0.9 mg/dL
C peptide (adult)	S, P	0.17–0.66 nmol/L	0.5–2.0 ng/mL
C1-esterase-inhibitor protein	S		
Antigenic		124–250 mg/L	12.4–24.5 mg/dL
Functional		Present	Present
CA 125	S	0–35 kU/L	0–35 U/mL
CA 19-9	S	0–37 kU/L	0–37 U/mL
CA-15-3	S	0–34 kU/L	0–34 U/mL
CA27-29	S	0–40 kU/L	0–40 U/mL
Calcitonin	S		
Male		3–26 ng/L	3–26 pg/mL
Female		2–17 ng/L	2–17 pg/mL
Calcium	S	2.2–2.6 mmol/L	8.7–10.2 mg/dL
Calcium, ionized	WB	1.12–1.32 mmol/L	4.5–5.3 mg/dL

Carbon dioxide content (TCO_2)	P (sea level)	22–30 mmol/L	22–30 meq/L
Carboxyhemoglobin (carbon monoxide content)	WB		
Nonsmokers		0–0.04	0–4%
Smokers		0.04–0.09	4–9%
Onset of symptoms		0.15–0.20	15–20%
Loss of consciousness and death		>0.50	>50%
Carcinoembryonic antigen (CEA)	S		
Nonsmokers	S	0.0–3.0 µg/L	0.0–3.0 ng/mL
Smokers	S	0.0–5.0 µg/L	0.0–5.0 ng/mL
Ceruloplasmin	S	250–630 mg/L	25–63 mg/dL
Chloride	S	102–109 mmol/L	102–109 meq/L
Cholesterol: see Table 218-5			
Cholinesterase	S	5–12 kU/L	5–12 U/mL
Complement			
C3	S	0.83–1.77 g/L	83–177 mg/dL
C4	S	0.16–0.47 g/L	16–47 mg/dL
Total hemolytic complement (CH50)	S	50–150%	50–150%
Factor B	S	0.17–0.42 g/L	17–42 mg/dL
Coproporphyrins (types I and III)	U	150–470 µmol/d	100–300 µg/d
Cortisol	S		
Fasting, 8 A.M.–12 noon		138–690 nmol/L	5–25 µg/dL
12 noon–8 P.M.		138–414 nmol/L	5–15 µg/dL
8 P.M.–8 A.M.		0–276 nmol/L	0–10 µg/dL
Cortisol, free	U	55–193 nmol/24 h	20–70 µg/24 h
C-reactive protein	S	0.2–3.0 mg/L	0.2–3.0 mg/dL
Creatine kinase (total)	S		
Females		0.66–4.0 µkat/L	39–238 U/L
Males		0.87–5.0 µkat/L	51–294 U/L

(continued)

TABLE 218-2	**CLINICAL CHEMISTRY AND IMMUNOLOGY (CONTINUED)**		
Analyte	Specimen[a]	SI Units	Conventional Units
Creatine kinase-MB	S		
Mass		0.0–5.5 µg/L	0.0–5.5 ng/mL
Fraction of total activity (by electrophoresis)		0–0.04	0–4.0%
Creatinine	S		
Female		44–80 µmol/L	0.5–0.9 ng/mL
Male		53–106 µmol/L	0.6–1.2 ng/mL
Dehydroepiandrosterone (DHEA) (adult)	S		
Male		6.2–43.4 nmol/L	180–1250 ng/dL
Female		4.5–34.0 nmol/L	130–980 ng/dL
Dehydroepiandrosterone (DHEA) sulfate	S		
Male (adult)		100–6190 µg/L	10–619 µg/dL
Female (adult, premenopausal)		120–5350 µg/L	12–535 µg/dL
Female (adult, postmenopausal)		300–2600 µg/L	30–260 µg/dL
Deoxycorticosterone (DOC) (adult)	S	61–576 nmol/L	2–19 ng/dL
11-Deoxycortisol (adult) (compound S) (8:00 A.M.)	S	0.34–4.56 nmol/L	12–158 ng/dL
Dihydrotestosterone	S, P		
Male		1.03–2.92 nmol/L	30–85 ng/dL
Female		0.14–0.76 nmol/L	4–22 ng/dL
Dopamine	P	< 475 pmol/L	< 87 pg/mL
Dopamine	U	425–2610 nmol/d	65–400 µg/d
Epinephrine	P		
Supine (30 min)		< 273 pmol/L	< 50 pg/mL
Sitting		< 328 pmol/L	< 60 pg/mL
Standing (30 min)		< 491 pmol/L	< 90 pg/mL
Epinephrine	U	0–109 nmol/d	0–20 µg/d

Erythropoietin	S	4–27 U/L	4–27 U/L
Estradiol	S, P		
Female			
Menstruating:			
Follicular phase		74–532 pmol/L	<20–145 pg/mL
Mid-cycle peak		411–1626 pmol/L	112–443 pg/mL
Luteal phase		74–885 pmol/L	<20–241 pg/mL
Postmenopausal		217 pmol/L	<59 pg/mL
Male		74 pmol/L	< 20 pg/mL
Estrone	S, P		
Female			
Menstruating:			
Follicular phase		55–555 pmol/L	15–150 pg/mL
Luteal phase		55–740 pmol/L	15–200 pg/mL
Postmenopausal		55–204 pmol/L	15–55 pg/mL
Male		55–240 pmol/L	15–65 pg/mL
Fatty acids, free (nonesterified)	P	<0.28–0.89 mmol/L	<8–25 mg/dL
Ferritin	S		
Female		10–150 µg/L	10–150 ng/mL
Male		29–248 µg/L	29–248 ng/mL
Follicle stimulating hormone (FSH)	S, P		
Female			
Menstruating:			
Follicular phase		3.0–20.0 IU/L	3.0–20.0 mIU/mL
Ovulatory phase		9.0–26.0 IU/L	9.0–26.0 mIU/mL
Luteal phase		1.0–12.0 IU/L	1.0–12.0 mIU/mL
Postmenopausal		18.0–153.0 IU/L	18.0–153.0 mIU/mL
Male		1.0–12.0 IU/L	1.0–12.0 mIU/mL

(continued)

TABLE 218-2 CLINICAL CHEMISTRY AND IMMUNOLOGY (CONTINUED)

Analyte	Specimen[a]	SI Units	Conventional Units
Free testosterone, adult			
Female	S	2.1–23.6 pmol/L	0.6–6.8 pg/mL
Male		163–847 pmol/L	47–244 pg/mL
Fructosamine	S	<285 μmol/L	<285 μmol/L
Gamma glutamyltransferase	S	0.15–0.99 μkat/L	9–58 U/L
Gastrin	S	<100 ng/L	<100 pg/mL
Glucagon	P	20–100 ng/L	20–100 pg/mL
Glucose (fasting)	P		
Normal		4.2–6.1 mmol/L	75–110 mg/dL
Impaired glucose tolerance		6.2–6.9 mmol/L	111–125 mg/dL
Diabetes mellitus		>7.0 mmol/L	>125 mg/dL
Glucose, 2 h postprandial	P	3.9–6.7 mmol/L	70–120 mg/dL
Growth hormone (resting)	S	0.5–17.0 μg/L	0.5–17.0 ng/mL
Hemoglobin A$_{1c}$	WB	0.04–0.06 Hb fraction	4.0–6.0%
High-density lipoprotein (HDL) (see Table 218-5)			
Homocysteine	P	4.4–10.8 μmol/L	4.4–10.8 μmol/L
Human chorionic gonadotropin (hCG)	S		
Non-pregnant female		< 5 IU/L	< 5 mIU/mL
1–2 weeks postconception		9–130 IU/L	9–130 mIU/mL
2–3 weeks postconception		75–2600 IU/L	75–2600 mIU/mL
3–4 weeks postconception		850–20,800 IU/L	850–20,800 mIU/mL
4–5 weeks postconception		4000–100,200 IU/L	4000–100,200 mIU/mL
5–10 weeks postconception		11,500–289,000 IU/L	11,500–289,000 mIU/mL
10–14 weeks postconception		18,300–137,000 IU/L	18,300–137,000 mIU/mL
Second trimester		1400–53,000 IU/L	1400–53,000 mIU/mL
Third trimester		940–60,000 IU/L	940–60,000 mIU/mL

β-Hydroxybutyrate	P	0–290 μmol/L	0–3 mg/dL
5-Hydroxyindoleacetic acid [5-HIAA]	U	10.5–36.6 μmol/d	2–7 mg/d
17-Hydroxyprogesterone (adult)	S		
Male		0.15–7.5 nmol/L	5–250 ng/dL
Female			
Follicular phase		0.6–3.0 nmol/L	20–100 ng/dL
Midcycle peak		3–7.5 nmol/L	100–250 ng/dL
Luteal phase		3–15 nmol/L	100–500 ng/dL
Postmenopausal		≤2.1 nmol/L	≤70 ng/dL
Hydroxyproline	U, 24 hour	38–500 μmol/d	38–500 μmol/d
Immunofixation	S	Not applicable	No bands detected
Immunoglobulin, quantitation (adult)			
IgA	S	0.70–3.50 g/L	70–350 mg/dL
IgD	S	0–140 mg/L	0–14 mg/dL
IgE	S	24–430 μg/L	10–179 IU/mL
IgG	S	7.0–17.0 g/L	700–1700 mg/dL
IgG_1	S	2.7–17.4 g/L	270–1740 mg/dL
IgG_2	S	0.3–6.3 g/L	30–630 mg/dL
IgG_3	S	0.13–3.2 g/L	13–320 mg/dL
IgG_4	S	0.11–6.2 g/L	11–620 mg/dL
IgM	S	0.50–3.0 g/L	50–300 mg/dL
Insulin	S, P	14.35–143.5 pmol/L	2–20 μU/mL
Iron	S	7–25 μmol/L	41–141 μg/dL
Iron-binding capacity	S	45–73 μmol/L	251–406 μg/dL
Iron-binding capacity saturation	S	0.16–0.35	16–35%
Ketone (acetone)	S, U	Negative	Negative
17 Ketosteroids	U	0.003–0.012 g/d	3–12 mg/d

(continued)

TABLE 218-2 CLINICAL CHEMISTRY AND IMMUNOLOGY (CONTINUED)

Analyte	Specimen[a]	SI Units	Conventional Units
Lactate	P, arterial	0.5–1.6 mmol/L	4.5–14.4 mg/dL
	P, venous	0.5–2.2 mmol/L	4.5–19.8 mg/dL
Lactate dehydrogenase	S	2.0–3.8 μkat/L	115–221 U/L
Lactate dehydrogenase isoenzymes	S		
Fraction 1 (of total)		0.14–0.26	14–26%
Fraction 2		0.29–0.39	29–39%
Fraction 3		0.20–0.25	20–26%
Fraction 4		0.08–0.16	8–16%
Fraction 5		0.06–0.16	6–16%
Lipase (method dependent)	S	0.51–0.73 μkat/L	3–43 U/L
Lipids: see Table 218-5			
Lipoprotein (a)	S	0–300 mg/L	0–30 mg/dL
Low-density lipoprotein (LDL) (see Table 218-5)			
Luteinizing hormone (LH)	S, P		
Female			
Menstruating			
Follicular phase		2.0–15.0 U/L	2.0–15.0 U/L
Ovulatory phase		22.0–105.0 U/L	22.0–105.0 U/L
Luteal phase		0.6–19.0 U/L	0.6–19.0 U/L
Postmenopausal		16.0–64.0 U/L	16.0–64.0 U/L
Male		2.0–12.0 U/L	2.0–12.0 U/L
Magnesium	S	0.62–0.95 mmol/L	1.5–2.3 mg/dL
Metanephrine	P	<0.5 nmol/L	<100 pg/mL
Metanephrine	U	30–211 mmol/mol creatinine	53–367 μg/g creatinine
Methemoglobin	WB	0.0–0.01	0–1%

Microalbumin urine			
24-h urine	U	0.0–0.03 g/d	0–30 mg/24 h
Spot urine	S	0.0–0.03 g/g creatinine	0–30 µg/mg creatinine
Myoglobin			
Male		19–92 µg/L	19–92 µg/L
Female		12–76 µg/L	12–76 µg/L
Norepinephrine	U	89–473 nmol/d	15–80 µg/d
Norepinephrine	P		
Supine (30 min)		650–2423 pmol/L	110–410 pg/mL
Sitting		709–4019 pmol/L	120–680 pg/mL
Standing (30 min)		739–4137 pmol/L	125–700 pg/mL
N-telopeptide (cross linked), NTx	S		
Female, premenopausal		6.2–19.0 nmol BCE	6.2–19.0 nmol BCE
Male		5.4–24.2 nmol BCE	5.4–24.2 nmol BCE
Bone collagen equivalent (BCE)			
N-telopeptide (cross linked), NTx	U		
Female, premenopausal		17–94 nmol BCE/mmol creatinine	17–94 nmol BCE/mmol creatinine
Female, postmenopausal		26–124 nmol BCE/mmol creatinine	26–124 nmol BCE/mmol creatinine
Male		21–83 nmol BCE/mmol creatinine	21–83 nmol BCE/mmol creatinine
Bone collagen equivalent (BCE)			
5' Nucleotidase	S	0.02–0.19 µkat/L	0–11 U/L
Osmolality	P	275–295 mOsmol/kg serum water	275–295 mOsmol/kg serum water
	U	500–800 mOsmol/kg water	500–800 mOsmol/kg water
Osteocalcin	S	11–50 µg/L	11–50 ng/mL
Oxygen content	WB		
Arterial (sea level)		17–21	17–21 vol%
Venous (sea level)		10–16	10–16 vol%

(continued)

TABLE 218-2 CLINICAL CHEMISTRY AND IMMUNOLOGY (CONTINUED)

Analyte	Specimen[a]	SI Units	Conventional Units
Oxygen percent saturation (sea level)	WB		
Arterial		0.97	94–100%
Venous, arm		0.60–0.85	60–85%
Parathyroid hormone (intact)	S	8–51 ng/L	8–51 pg/mL
Phosphatase, alkaline	S	0.56–1.63 μkat/L	33–96 U/L
Phosphorus, inorganic	S	0.81–1.4 mmol/L	2.5–4.3 mg/dL
Porphobilinogen	U	None	None
Potassium	S	3.5–5.0 mmol/L	3.5–5.0 meq/L
Prealbumin	S	170–340 mg/L	17–34 mg/dL
Progesterone	S, P		
Female			
Follicular		<3.18 nmol/L	<1.0 ng/mL
Midluteal		9.54–63.6 nmol/L	3–20 ng/mL
Male		<3.18 nmol/L	< 1.0 ng/mL
Prolactin	S	0–20 μg/L	0–20 ng/mL
Prostate-specific antigen (PSA)	S		
Male			
<40 years		0.0–2.0 μg/L	0.0–2.0 ng/mL
>40 years		0.0–4.0 μg/L	0.0–4.0 ng/mL
PSA, free; in males 45–75 years, with PSA values between 4 and 20 μg/mL	S	>0.25 associated with benign prostatic hyperplasia	>25% associated with benign prostatic hyperplasia
Protein fractions	S		
Albumin		35–55 g/L	3.5–5.5 g/dL (50–60%)
Globulin		20–35 g/L	2.0–3.5 g/dL (40–50%)
Alpha₁		2–4 g/L	0.2–0.4 g/dL (4.2–7.2%)

Alpha$_2$		5–9 g/L	0.5–0.9 g/dL (6.8–12%)
Beta		6–11 g/L	0.6–1.1 g/dL (9.3–15%)
Gamma		7–17 g/L	0.7–1.7 g/dL (13–23%)
Protein, total	S	67–86 g/L	6.7–8.6 g/dL
Pyruvate	P, arterial	40–130 µmol/L	0.35–1.14 mg/dL
	P, venous	40–130 µmol/L	0.35–1.14 mg/dL
Rheumatoid factor	S, JF	<30 kIU/L	<30 IU/mL
Serotonin	WB	0.28–1.14 µmol/L	50–200 ng/mL
Sex hormone binding globulin (adult)			
Male		13–71 nmol/L	13–71 nmol/L
Female		18–114 nmol/L	18–114 nmol/L
Sodium	S	136–146 mmol/L	136–146 meq/L
Somatomedin-C (IGF-1) (adult)	S		
16–24 years		182–780 µg/L	182–780 ng/mL
25–39 years		114–492 µg/L	114–492 ng/mL
40–54 years		90–360 µg/L	90–360 ng/mL
>54 years		71–290 µg/L	71–290 ng/mL
Somatostatin	P	<25 ng/L	<25 pg/mL
Testosterone, total, morning sample	S		
Female		0.21–2.98 nmol/L	6–86 ng/dL
Male		9.36–37.10 nmol/L	270–1070 ng/dL
Thyroglobulin	S	0.5–53 µg/L	0.5–53 ng/mL
Thyroid-binding globulin	S	13–30 mg/L	1.3–3.0 mg/dL
Thyroid-stimulating hormone	S	0.34–4.25 mIU/L	0.34–4.25 µIU/mL
Thyroxine, free (fT$_4$)	S	10.3–21.9 pmol/L	0.8–1.7 ng/dL
Thyroxine, total (T$_4$)	S	70–151 nmol/L	5.4–11.7 µg/dL
(Free) thyroxine index	S	6.7–10.9	6.7–10.9
Transferrin	S	2.0–4.0 g/L	200–400 mg/dL

(continued)

TABLE 218-2 CLINICAL CHEMISTRY AND IMMUNOLOGY (CONTINUED)

Analyte	Specimen[a]	SI Units	Conventional Units
Triglycerides (see Table 218-5)	S	0.34–2.26 mmol/L	30–200 mg/dL
Triiodothyronine, free (FT$_3$)	S	3.7–6.5 pmol/L	2.4–4.2 pg/mL
Triiodothyronine, total (T$_3$)	S	1.2–2.1 nmol/L	77–135 ng/dL
Troponin I	S		
Normal population, 99 %tile		0–0.08 µg/L	0–0.08 ng/mL
Cut-off for MI		>0.4 µg/L	>0.4 ng/mL
Troponin T	S		
Normal population, 99 %tile		0–0.1 µg/L	0–0.01 ng/mL
Cut-off for MI		0–0.1 µg/L	0–0.1 ng/mL
Urea nitrogen	S	2.5–7.1 mmol/L	7–20 mg/dL
Uric acid	S		
Females		0.15–0.33 µmol/L	2.5–5.6 mg/dL
Males		0.18–0.41 µmol/L	3.1–7.0 mg/dL
Urobilinogen	U	0.09–4.2 µmol/d	0.05–25 mg/24 h
Vanillylmandelic acid (VMA)	U, 24h	<30 µmol/d	<6 mg/d
Vasoactive intestinal polypeptide	P	0–60 ng/L	0–60 pg/mL

[a]P, plasma; S, serum; U, urine; WB, whole blood; IF, joint fluid.

TABLE 218-3 TOXICOLOGY AND THERAPEUTIC DRUG MONITORING

	Therapeutic Range		Toxic Level	
Drug	SI Units	Conventional Units	SI Units	Conventional Units
Acetaminophen	66–199 μmol/L	10–30 μg/mL	>1320 μmol/L	>200 μg/mL
Amikacin				
Peak	34–51 μmol/L	20–30 μg/mL	>60 μmol/L	>35 μg/mL
Trough	0–17 μmol/L	0–10 μg/mL	>17 μmol/L	>10 μg/mL
Carbamazepine	17–42 μmol/L	4–10 μg/mL	85 μmol/L	>20 μg/mL
Cyclosporine				
Renal transplant				
0–6 months	208–312 nmol/L	250–375 ng/mL	>312 nmol/L	>375 ng/mL
6–12 months after transplant	166–250 nmol/L	200–300 ng/mL	>250 nmol/L	>300 ng/mL
>12 months	83–125 nmol/L	100–150 ng/mL	>125 nmol/L	>150 ng/mL
Cardiac transplant				
0–6 months	208–291 nmol/L	250–350 ng/mL	>291 nmol/L	>350 ng/mL
6–12 months after transplant	125–208 nmol/L	150–250 ng/mL	>208 nmol/L	>250 ng/mL
>12 months	83–125 nmol/L	100–150 ng/mL	>125 nmol/L	>150 ng/mL
Lung transplant				
0–6 months	250–374 nmol/L	300–450 ng/mL	>374 nmol/L	>450 ng/mL
Liver transplant				
0–7 days	249–333 nmol/L	300–400 ng/mL	>333 nmol/L	>400 ng/mL
2–4 weeks	208–291 nmol/L	250–350 ng/mL	>291 nmol/L	>350 ng/mL
5–8 weeks	166–249 nmol/L	200–300 ng/mL	>249 nmol/L	>300 ng/mL
9–52 weeks	125–208 nmol/L	150–250 ng/mL	>208 nmol/L	>250 ng/mL
>1 year	83–166 nmol/L	100–200 ng/mL	>166 nmol/L	>200 ng/mL
Digoxin	0.64–2.6 nmol/L	0.5–2.0 ng/mL	>3.1 nmol/L	>2.4 ng/mL

(continued)

TABLE 218-3 TOXICOLOGY AND THERAPEUTIC DRUG MONITORING (CONTINUED)

Drug	Therapeutic Range		Toxic Level	
	SI Units	Conventional Units	SI Units	Conventional Units
Ethanol				
Behavioral changes			>4.3 mmol/L	>20 mg/dL
Legal limit			≥17 mmol/L	≥80 mg/dL
Critical with acute exposure			>54 mmol/L	>250 mg/dL
Ethylene glycol				
Toxic			>2 mmol/L	>12 mg/dL
Lethal			>20 mmol/L	>120 mg/dL
Gentamicin				
Peak	10–21 µmol/mL	5–10 µg/mL	>25 µmol/mL	>12 µg/mL
Trough	0–4.2 µmol/mL	0–2 µg/mL	>4.2 µmol/mL	>2 µg/mL
Lithium	0.5–1.3 mmol/L	0.5–1.3 meq/L	>2 mmol/L	>2 meq/L
Methadone	1.3–3.2 µmol/L	0.4–1.0 µg/mL	>6.5 µmol/L	>2 µg/mL
Methamphetamine	1.3–4.0 µmol/L	2–6 µg/dL	4.0–33.5 µmol/L	60–500-1.0 µg/dL, toxic
			67.0–268.0 µmol/L	1000–4000 µg/dL, lethal
Methanol			>6 mmol/L	>20 mg/dL, toxic
			>16 mmol/L	>50 mg/dL, severe toxicity
			>28 mmol/L	>89 mg/dL, lethal
Phenobarbital	65–172 µmol/L	15–40 µg/mL	>215 µmol/L	>50 µg/mL
Phenytoin	40–79 µmol/L	10–20 µg/mL	>118 µmol/L	>30 µg/mL
Phenytoin, free	4.0–7.9 µmol/L	1–2 µg/mL	>13.9 µmol/L	>3.5 µg/mL
% Free	0.08–0.14	8–14%		
Quinidine	6.2–15.4 µmol/L	2.0–5.0 µg/mL	>31 µmol/L	>10 µg/mL
Salicylates	145–2100 µmol/L	2–29 mg/dL	>2172 µmol/L	>30 mg/dL

	Therapeutic range (SI)	Therapeutic range (conventional)	Toxic (SI)	Toxic (conventional)
Sirolimus (trough level)				
Kidney transplant	4.4–13.1 nmol/L	4–12 ng/mL	>16 nmol/L	>15 ng/mL
Tacrolimus (FK506) (trough)				
Kidney and liver				
0–2 months posttransplant	12–19 nmol/L	10–15 ng/mL	>25 nmol/L	>20 ng/mL
> 2 months posttransplant	6–12 nmol/L	5–10 ng/mL		
Heart				
0–2 months posttransplant	19–25 nmol/L	15–20 ng/mL	>25 nmol/L	>20 ng/mL
3–6 months posttransplant	12–19 nmol/L	10–15 ng/mL		
>6 months posttransplant	10–12 nmol/L	8–10 ng/mL		
Theophylline	56–111 µmol/L	10–20 µg/mL	>140 µmol/L	>25 µg/mL
Tobramycin				
Peak	11–22 µmol/L	5–10 µg/mL	>26 µmol/L	>12 µg/mL
Trough	0–4.3 µmol/L	0–2 µg/mL	>4.3 µmol/L	>2 µg/mL
Valproic acid	350–700 µmol/L	50–100 µg/mL	>1000 µmol/L	>150 µg/mL
Vancomycin				
Peak	14–28 µmol/L	20–40 µg/mL	>55 µmol/L	>80 µg/mL
Trough	3.5–10.4 µmol/L	5–15 µg/mL	>14 µmol/L	>20 µg/mL

TABLE 218-4 **VITAMINS AND SELECTED TRACE MINERALS**

Specimen	Analyte[a]	Reference Range	
		SI Units	Conventional Units
Aluminum	S	<0.2 μmol/L	<5.41 μg/L
	U, random	0.19–1.11 μmol/L	5–30 μg/L
Arsenic	WB	0.03–0.31 μmol/L	2–23 μg/L
	U, 24 h	0.07–0.67 μmol/d	5–50 μg/d
Cadmium	WB	<44.5 nmol/L	<5.0 μg/L
Coenzyme Q10 (ubiquinone)	P	433–1532 μg/L	433–1532 μg/L
β carotene	S	0.07–1.43 μmol/L	4–77 μg/dL
Copper			
	S	11–22 μmol/L	70–140 μg/dL
	U, 24 h	<0.95 μmol/d	<60 μg/d
Folic acid	RC	340–1020 nmol/L cells	150–450 ng/mL cells
Folic acid	S	12.2–40.8 nmol/L	5.4–18.0 ng/mL
Lead (adult)	S	<0.5 μmol/L	<10 μg/dL
Mercury	WB	3.0–294 nmol/L	0.6–59 μg/L
	U, 24 h	<99.8 nmol/L	<20 μg/L
Selenium	S	0.8–2.0 μmol/L	63–160 μg/L
Vitamin A	S	0.7–3.5 μmol/L	20–100 μg/dL
Vitamin B_1 (thiamine)	S	0–75 nmol/L	0–2 μg/dL
Vitamin B_2 (riboflavin)	S	106–638 nmol/L	4–24 μg/dL
Vitamin B_6	P	20–121 nmol/L	5–30 ng/mL
Vitamin B_{12}	S	206–735 pmol/L	279–996 pg/mL
Vitamin C (ascorbic acid)	S	23–57 μmol/L	0.4–1.0 mg/dL
Vitamin D_3, 1,25-dihydroxy	S	60–108 pmol/L	25–45 pg/mL
Vitamin D_3, 25-hydroxy	P		
Summer		37.4–200 nmol/L	15–80 ng/mL
Winter		34.9–105 nmol/L	14–42 ng/mL
Vitamin E	S	12–42 μmol/L	5–18 μg/mL
Vitamin K	S	0.29–2.64 nmol/L	0.13–1.19 ng/mL
Zinc	S	11.5–18.4 μmol/L	75–120 μg/dL

[a]P, plasma; RC, red cells; S, serum; WB, whole blood; U, urine.

TABLE 218-5 **CLASSIFICATION OF LDL, TOTAL, AND HDL CHOLESTEROL**

LDL cholesterol, mg/dL (mmol/L)

<70 (<1.81)	Therapeutic option for very high risk patients
<100 (<2.59)	Optimal
100–129 (2.59–3.34)	Near optimal/above optimal
130–159 (3.36–4.11)	Borderline high
160–189 (4.14–4.89)	High
≥190 (≥4.91)	Very high

Total cholesterol, mg/dL (mmol/L)

<200 (<5.17)	Desirable
200–239 (5.17–6.18)	Borderline high
≥240 (≥6.21)	High

HDL cholesterol, mg/dL (mmol/L)

<40 (<1.03)	Low
≥60 (≥1.55)	High

Note: LDL, low-density lipoprotein; HDL, high-density lipoprotein.
Source: Executive summary of the third report of the National Cholesterol Education Program (NCEP) expert panel on detection, evaluation, and treatment of high blood cholesterol in adults (adult treatment panel III). JAMA 285:2486, 2001; and Implications of recent clinical trials for the National Cholesterol Education Program Adult Treatment Panel III Guidelines: SM Grundy et al for the Coordinating Committee of the National Cholesterol Education Program. Circulation 110:227, 2004.

REFERENCE VALUES FOR SPECIFIC ANALYTES

(Tables 218-6 through 218-9)

TABLE 218-6 CEREBROSPINAL FLUID (CSF)[a]

	Reference Range	
Constituent	SI Units	Conventional Units
Osmolarity	292–297 mmol/kg water	292–297 mosmol/L
P_{CO_2}	6–7 kPa	45–49 mmHg
pH	7.31–7.34	
Glucose	2.22–3.89 mmol/L	40–70 mg/dL
Lactate	1–2 mmol/L	10–20 mg/dL
Total protein		
Lumbar	0.15–0.5 g/L	15–50 mg/dL
IgG	0.009–0.057 g/L	0.9–5.7 mg/dL
IgG index[b]	0.29–0.59	
Oligoclonal bands	<2 bands not present in matched serum sample	
CSF pressure		50–180 mmH$_2$O
Red blood cells	0	0
Leukocytes		
Total	0–5 mononuclear cells per µL	0–5 mononuclear cells per mm^3
Differential		
Lymphocytes	60–70%	
Monocytes	30–50%	
Neutrophils	None	

[a]Since cerebrospinal fluid concentrations are equilibrium values, measurements of the same parameters in blood plasma obtained at the same time are recommended. However, there is a time lag in attainment of equilibrium, and cerebrospinal levels of plasma constituents that can fluctuate rapidly (such as plasma glucose) may not achieve stable values until after a significant lag phase.
[b]IgG index = CSF IgG(mg/dL) × serum albumin(g/dL)/Serum IgG(g/dL) × CSF albumin(mg/dL).

TABLE 218-7 URINE ANALYSIS

	Reference Range	
	SI Units	Conventional Units
Acidity, titratable	20–40 mmol/d	20–40 meq/d
Ammonia	30–50 mmol/d	30–50 meq/d
Amylase		4–400 U/L
Amylase/creatinine clearance ratio $[(Cl_{am}/Cl_{cr}) \times 100]$	1–5	1–5
Calcium (10 meq/d or 200 mg/d dietary calcium)	<7.5 mmol/d	<300 mg/d
Creatine, as creatinine		
Female	<760 µmol/d	<100 mg/d
Male	<380 µmol/d	<50 mg/d
Creatinine	8.8–14 mmol/d	1.0–1.6 g/d
Eosinophils	<100,000 eosino-phils/L	<100 eosinophils/mL
Glucose (glucose oxidase method)	0.3–1.7 mmol/d	50–300 mg/d
5-Hydroxyindoleacetic acid (5-HIAA)	10–47 µmol/d	2–9 mg/d
Iodine, spot urine		
WHO classification of iodine deficiency		
Not iodine deficient	>100 µg/L	>100 µg/L
Mild iodine deficiency	50–100 µg/L	50–100 µg/L
Moderate iodine deficiency	20–49 µg/L	20–49 µg/L
Severe iodine deficiency	<20 µg/L	<20 µg/L
Microalbumin		
Normal	0.0–0.03 g/d	0–30 mg/d
Microalbuminuria	0.03–0.30 g/d	30–300 mg/d
Clinical albuminuria	>0.3 g/d	>300 mg/d
Microalbumin/creatinine ratio		
Normal	0–3.4 g/mol creatinine	0–30 µg/mg creatinine
Microalbuminuria	3.4–34 g/mol creatinine	30–300 µg/mg creatinine
Clinical albuminuria	>34 g/mol creatinine	>300 µg/mg creatinine
Oxalate		
Male	80–500 µmol/d	7–44 mg/d
Female	45–350 µmol/d	4–31 mg/d
pH	5.0–9.0	5.0–9.0
Phosphate (phosphorus) (varies with intake)	12.9–42.0 mmol/d	400–1300 mg/d
Potassium (varies with intake)	25–100 mmol/d	25–100 meq/d
Protein	<0.15 g/d	<150 mg/d
Sediment		
Red blood cells	0–2/high power field	
White blood cells	0–2/high power field	
Sodium (varies with intake)	100–260 mmol/d	100–260 meq/d
Specific gravity	1.001–1.035	1.001–1.035
Urea nitrogen	214–607 mmol/d	6–17 g/d
Uric acid (normal diet)	1.49–4.76 mmol/d	250–800 mg/d

Note: WHO, World Health Organization.

TABLE 218-8 **DIFFERENTIAL NUCLEATED CELL COUNTS OF BONE MARROW ASPIRATES[a]**

	Observed Range, %	95% Confidence Intervals, %	Mean, %
Blast cells	0–3.2	0–3.0	1.4
Promyelocytes	3.6–13.2	3.2–12.4	7.8
Neutrophil myelocytes	4–21.4	3.7–10.0	7.6
Eosinophil myelocytes	0–5.0	0–2.8	1.3
Metamyelocytes	1–7.0	2.3–5.9	4.1
Neutrophils			
Males	21.0–45.6	21.9–42.3	32.1
Females	29.6–46.6	28.8–45.9	37.4
Eosinophils	0.4–4.2	0.3–4.2	2.2
Eosinophils plus eosinophil myelocytes	0.9–7.4	0.7–6.3	3.5
Basophils	0–0.8	0–0.4	0.1
Erythroblasts			
Male	18.0–39.4	16.2–40.1	28.1
Females	14.0–31.8	13.0–32.0	22.5
Lymphocytes	4.6–22.6	6.0–20.0	13.1
Plasma cells	0–1.4	0–1.2	0.6
Monocytes	0–3.2	0–2.6	1.3
Macrophages	0–1.8	0–1.3	0.4
M:E ratio			
Males	1.1–4.0	1.1–4.1	2.1
Females	1.6–5.4	1.6–5.2	2.8

[a]Based on bone marrow aspirate from 50 healthy volunteers (30 men, 20 women).
Source: From BJ Bain: The bone marrow aspirate of healthy subjects. Br J Haematol 94(1):206, 1996.

TABLE 218-9 **STOOL ANALYSIS**

	Reference Range	
	SI Units	Conventional Units
Amount	0.1–0.2 kg/d	100–200 g/24 h
Coproporphyrin	611–1832 nmol/d	400–1200 µg/24 h
Fat		
Adult		<7 g/d
Adult on fat-free diet		<4 g/d
Fatty acids	0–21 mmol/d	0–6 g/24 h
Leukocytes	None	None
Nitrogen	<178 mmol/d	<2.5 g/24 h
pH	7.0–7.5	
Occult blood	Negative	Negative
Trypsin		20–95 U/g
Urobilinogen	85–510 µmol/d	50–300 mg/24 h
Uroporphyrins	12–48 nmol/d	10–40 µg/24 h
Water	<0.75	<75%

Source: Modified from FT Fishbach, MB Dunning III: *A Manual of Laboratory and Diagnostic Tests*, 7th ed., Lippincott Williams & Wilkins, Philadelphia, 2004.

SPECIAL FUNCTION TESTS (Tables 218-10 through 218-14)

TABLE 218-10 | RENAL FUNCTION TESTS

	Reference Range	
	SI Units	**Conventional Units**
Clearances (corrected to 1.72 m^2 body surface area)		
Measures of glomerular filtration rate		
Inulin clearance (Cl)		
Males (mean ± 1 SD)	2.1 ± 0.4 mL/s	124 ± 25.8 mL/min
Females (mean ± 1 SD)	2.0 ± 0.2 mL/s	119 ± 12.8 mL/min
Endogenous creatinine clearance	1.5–2.2 mL/s	91–130 mL/min
Measures of effective renal plasma flow and tubular function		
p-Aminohippuric acid clearance (Cl$_{PAH}$)		
Males (mean ± 1 SD)	10.9 ± 2.7 mL/s	654 ± 163 mL/min
Females (mean ± 1 SD)	9.9 ± 1.7 mL/s	594 ± 102 mL/min
Concentration and dilution test		
Specific gravity of urine		
After 12-h fluid restriction	>1.025	>1.025
After 12-h deliberate water intake	≤1.003	≤1.003
Protein excretion, urine	<0.15 g/d	<150 mg/d
Specific gravity, maximal range	1.002–1.028	1.002–1.028
Tubular reabsorption, phosphorus	0.79–0.94 of filtered load	79–94% of filtered load

TABLE 218-11 CIRCULATORY FUNCTION TESTS

	Results: Reference Range	
Test	SI Units (Range)	Conventional Units (Range)
Arteriovenous oxygen difference	30–50 mL/L	30–50 mL/L
Cardiac output (Fick)	2.5–3.6 L/m² of body surface area per min	2.5–3.6 L/m² of body surface area per min
Contractility indexes		
Max. left ventricular $dp/dt(dp/dt)/DP$ when DP = 5.3 kPa (40 mmHg) (DP, diastolic pressure)	220 kPa/s (176–250 kPa/s) (37.6 ± 12.2)/s	1650 mmHg/s (1320–1880 mmHg/s) (37.6 ± 12.2)/s
Mean normalized systolic ejection rate (angiography)	3.32 ± 0.84 end-diastolic volumes per second	3.32 ± 0.84 end-diastolic volumes per second
Mean velocity of circumferential fiber shortening (angiography)	1.83 ± 0.56 circumferences per second	1.83 ± 0.56 circumferences per second
Ejection fraction: stroke volume/end-diastolic volume (SV/EDV)	0.67 ± 0.08 (0.55–0.78)	0.67 ± 0.08 (0.55–0.78)
End-diastolic volume	70 ± 20.0 mL/m² (60–88 mL/m²)	70 ± 20.0 mL/m² (60–88 mL/m²)
End-systolic volume	25 ± 5.0 mL/m² (20–33 mL/m²)	25 ± 5.0 mL/m² (20–33 mL/m²)
Left ventricular work		
Stroke work index	50 ± 20.0 (g•m)/m² (30–110)	50 ± 20.0 (g•m)/m² (30–110)
Left ventricular minute work index	1.8–6.6 [(kg•m)/m²]/min	1.8–6.6 [(kg•m)/m²]/min
Oxygen consumption index	110–150 mL	110–150 mL
Maximum oxygen uptake	35 mL/min (20–60 mL/min)	35 mL/min (20–60 mL/min)
Pulmonary vascular resistance	2–12 (kPa•s)/L	20–130 (dyn•s)/cm⁵
Systemic vascular resistance	77–150 (kPa•s)/L	770–1600 (dyn•s)/cm⁵

Source: E Braunwald et al: *Heart Disease*, 6th ed, Philadelphia, Saunders, 2001.

1166

TABLE 218-12 **GASTROINTESTINAL TESTS**

Test	Results SI Units	Conventional Units
Absorption tests		
D-Xylose: after overnight fast, 25 g xylose given in oral aqueous solution		
Urine, collected for following 5 h	25% of ingested dose	25% of ingested dose
Serum, 2 h after dose	2.0–3.5 mmol/L	30–52 mg/dL
Vitamin A: a fasting blood specimen is obtained and 200,000 units of vitamin A in oil is given orally	Serum level should rise to twice fasting level in 3–5 h	Serum level should rise to twice fasting level in 3–5 h
Bentiromide test (pancreatic function): 500 mg bentiromide (chymex) orally; *p*-aminobenzoic acid (PABA) measured		
Plasma		>3.6 (±1.1) µg/mL at 90 min
Urine	>50% recovered in 6 h	>50% recovered in 6 h
Gastric juice		
Volume		
24 h	2–3 L	2–3 L
Nocturnal	600–700 mL	600–700 mL
Basal, fasting	30–70 mL/h	30–70 mL/h
Reaction		
pH	1.6–1.8	1.6–1.8
Titratable acidity of fasting juice	4–9 µmol/s	15–35 meq/h
Acid output		
Basal		
Females (mean ± 1 SD)	0.6 ± 0.5 µmol/s	2.0 ± 1.8 meq/h
Males (mean ± 1 SD)	0.8 ± 0.6 µmol/s	3.0 ± 2.0 meq/h
Maximal (after SC histamine acid phosphate, 0.004 mg/kg body weight, and preceded by 50 mg promethazine, or after betazole, 1.7 mg/kg body weight, or pentagastrin, 6 µg/kg body weight)		
Females (mean ± 1 SD)	4.4 ± 1.4 µmol/s	16 ± 5 meq/h
Males (mean ± 1 SD)	6.4 ± 1.4 µmol/s	23 ± 5 meq/h
Basal acid output/maximal acid output ratio	≤0.6	≤0.6
Gastrin, serum	0–200 µg/L	0–200 pg/mL
Secretin test (pancreatic exocrine function): 1 unit/kg body weight, IV		
Volume (pancreatic juice) in 80 min	>2.0 mL/kg	>2.0 mL/kg
Bicarbonate concentration	>80 mmol/L	>80 meq/L
Bicarbonate output in 30 min	>10 mmol	>10 meq

TABLE 218-13 NORMAL VALUES OF DOPPLER ECHOCARDIOGRAPHIC MEASUREMENTS IN ADULTS

	Range	Mean
RVD (cm), measured at the base in apical 4-chamber view	2.6–4.3	3.5 ± 0.4
LVID (cm), measured in the parasternal long axis view	3.6–5.4	4.7 ± 0.4
Posterior LV wall thickness (cm)	0.6–1.1	0.9 ± 0.4
IVS wall thickness (cm)	0.6–1.1	0.9 ± 0.4
Left atrial dimension (cm), antero-posterior dimension	2.3–3.8	3.0 ± 0.3
Aortic root dimension (cm)	2.0–3.5	2.4 ± 0.4
Aortic cusps separation (cm)	1.5–2.6	1.9 ± 0.4
Percentage of fractional shortening	34–44%	36%
Mitral flow (m/s)	0.6–1.3	0.9
Tricuspid flow (m/s)	0.3–0.7	0.5
Pulmonary artery (m/s)	0.6–0.9	0.75
Aorta (m/s)	1.0–1.7	1.35

Note: RVD, right ventricular dimension; LVID, left ventricular internal dimension; LV, left ventricle; IVS, interventricular septum.
Source: From A Weyman: *Principles and Practice of Echocardiography*, 2d ed., Philadelphia, Lea & Febiger, 1994.

TABLE 218-14 SUMMARY OF VALUES USEFUL IN PULMONARY PHYSIOLOGY

	Symbol	Typical Values	
		Man, Age 40, 75 kg, 175 cm Tall	Woman, Age 40, 60 kg, 160 cm Tall
Pulmonary Mechanics			
Spirometry—volume-time curves			
Forced vital capacity	FVC	4.8 L	3.3 L
Forced expiratory volume in 1 s	FEV_1	3.8 L	2.8 L
FEV_1/FVC	FEV_1%	76%	77%
Maximal midexpiratory flow	MMF (FEF 25–27)	4.8 L/s	3.6 L/s
Maximal expiratory flow rate	MEFR (FEF 200–1200)	9.4 L/s	6.1 L/s
Spirometry—flow-volume curves			
Maximal expiratory flow at 50% of expired vital capacity	V_{max} 50 (FEF 50%)	6.1 L/s	4.6 L/s
Maximal expiratory flow at 75% of expired vital capacity	V_{max} 75 (FEF 75%)	3.1 L/s	2.5 L/s
Resistance to airflow			
Pulmonary resistance	RL (R_L)	<3.0 (cmH_2O/s)/L	
Airway resistance	Raw	<2.5 (cmH_2O/s)/L	
Specific conductance	SGaw	>0.13 cmH_2O/s	
Pulmonary compliance			
Static recoil pressure at total lung capacity	Pst TLC	25 ± 5 cmH_2O	
Compliance of lungs (static)	CL	0.2 L cmH_2O	
Compliance of lungs and thorax	C(L + T)	0.1 L cmH_2O	
Dynamic compliance of 20 breaths per minute	C dyn 20	0.25 ± 0.05 L/cmH_2O	
Maximal static respiratory pressures			
Maximal inspiratory pressure	MIP	>90 cmH_2O	>50 cmH_2O
Maximal expiratory pressure	MEP	>150 cmH_2O	>120 cmH_2O

(continued)

TABLE 218-14	SUMMARY OF VALUES USEFUL IN PULMONARY PHYSIOLOGY (CONTINUED)

Lung Volumes

Total lung capacity	TLC	6.4 L	4.9 L
Functional residual capacity	FRC	2.2 L	2.6 L
Residual volume	RV	1.5 L	1.2 L
Inspiratory capacity	IC	4.8 L	3.7 L
Expiratory reserve volume	ERV	3.2 L	2.3 L
Vital capacity	VC	1.7 L	1.4 L

Gas Exchange (Sea Level)

Arterial O_2 tension	Pa_{O_2}	12.7 ± 0.7 kPa (95 ± 5 mmHg)
Arterial CO_2 tension	Pa_{CO_2}	5.3 ± 0.3 kPa (40 ± 2 mmHg)
Arterial O_2 saturation	Sa_{O_2}	0.97 ± 0.02 ($97 \pm 2\%$)
Arterial blood pH	pH	7.40 ± 0.02
Arterial bicarbonate	HCO_3^-	$24 + 2$ meq/L
Base excess	BE	0 ± 2 meq/L
Diffusing capacity for carbon monoxide (single breath)	DL_{CO}	0.42 mL CO/s/mmHg (25 mL CO/min/mmHg)
Dead space volume	V_D	2 mL/kg body wt
Physiologic dead space; dead space-tidal volume ratio	V_D/V_T	
Rest		$\leq 35\% V_T$
Exercise		$\leq 20\% V_T$
Alveolar-arterial difference for O_2	$P(A - a)_{O_2}$	≤ 2.7 kPa ≤ 20 kPa (≤ 20 mmHg)

MISCELLANEOUS (Table 218-15)

TABLE 218-15	BODY FLUIDS AND OTHER MASS DATA

	Reference Range	
	SI Units	**Conventional Units**
Ascitic fluid: See Table 44-1		
Body fluid,		
Total volume (lean) of body weight	50% (in obese) to 70%	
Intracellular	0.3–0.4 of body weight	
Extracellular	0.2–0.3 of body weight	
Blood		
Total volume		
Males	69 mL per kg body weight	
Females	65 mL per kg body weight	
Plasma volume		
Males	39 mL per kg body weight	
Females	40 mL per kg body weight	
Red blood cell volume		
Males	30 mL per kg body weight	$1.15–1.21 \text{ L/m}^2$ of body surface area
Females	25 mL per kg body weight	$0.95–1.00 \text{ L/m}^2$ of body surface area
Body mass index	$18.5–24.9 \text{ kg/m}^2$	$18.5–24.9 \text{ kg/m}^2$

Bold number indicates the start of the main discussion of the topic; numbers with "f" and "t" refer to figure and table pages.

A

Abacavir, for HIV/AIDS, 609t
Abatacept, for rheumatoid arthritis, 888
Abciximab, for thrombotic disorders, 338
Abdominal angina, 843
Abdominal pain, **179**
  acute, catastrophic, **181**
  causes of, 179t
  features of, 180–181
Abdominal radiography, **22**
  in pancreatitis, 850, 852
Abdominal wall disorders, pain in, 179t
Abiotrophia infection, **501**
Abortion, 957
Abscess. *See specific sites*
ABVD regimen, for Hodgkin's disease, 363–364
Acamprosate, for alcoholic rehabilitation, 1098
Acanthocytes, 280, 321
Acarbose, for diabetes mellitus, 945t
Accelerated idioventricular rhythm
  clinical and ECG features of, 724t
  in myocardial infarction, 704
Accessory nerve, 983
  disorders of, 1024
Accident prevention, 1104t–1105t
Acebutolol poisoning, 140t
ACE inhibitors
  for aortic regurgitation, 683
  for coronary artery disease, 716
  for diabetic nephropathy, 805
  for dilated cardiomyopathy, 685
  for glomerulonephritis, 804–805, 808
  for heart failure, 731, 732t, 733t, 735
  for hypertension, 695t, 696, 697t, 698, 796, 822, 824
  for mitral regurgitation, 679
  for myocardial infarction, 704, 706, 711–712
    preventive treatment, 709
  for systemic sclerosis, 889
  for unstable angina, 711
Acetaminophen
  for back pain, 196
  for fever, 201
  for migraine, 186t
  for osteoarthritis, 902
  for pain, 36t–37t, 38
  for tension headache, 186
  toxicity of, 130, 858
Acetazolamide
  for glaucoma, 294
  for periodic paralysis, 1074
N-Acetylcysteine, for acetaminophen overdose, 858
Acetylsalicylic acid, for pain, 36t–37t
Achalasia, **251**
Acid-base balance, **3**
Acid-base disorders, **14**
  metabolic acidosis, **16**
  metabolic alkalosis, **19**
  mixed disorders, **21**
  nomogram for, 16f

respiratory acidosis, **21**
  respiratory alkalosis, **21**
Acid-fast bacilli, 538
Acid maltase deficiency, 1073
Acidosis, **14**
Acinetobacter infection, 516
Acitretin, for psoriasis, 314
Acne, **317**
  drug-induced, 1133t
Acne rosacea, 318
Acne vulgaris, 310f, 317–318
Acoustic neuroma, 213, 1022
Acrodermatitis chronica atrophicans, 550
Acromegaly, **920**
  paraneoplastic, 405t, 406
Acrophobia, 1083
ACTH, 917, 918f
  deficiency of, 919t, 922, 922t, 936
  ectopic ACTH syndrome, 405, 405t, **406**
  hypersecretion of, 919t, 934–935
  therapy for inflammatory bowel disease, 838
Actinic keratosis, 311f
Actinobacillus actinomycetemcomitans infection. *See* HACEK group infection
Actinomycetoma, 535, 536t
Actinomycosis, **537**
  abdominal, 537
  oral-cervicofacial, 537–538
  pelvic, 537
  thoracic, 537
Action tremor, 1002
Activated charcoal
  for erythropoietic porphyria, 978
  for heavy metal poisoning, 155t
  for methylxanthine poisoning, 137t
  for paralytic shellfish poisoning, 124
  for poisoning, 135
  for toxic and drug-induced hepatitis, 858
Activated protein C therapy
  for Ebola and Marburg virus infections, 600
  for meningococcal infections, 505
  for sepsis/septic shock, 66
Acute coronary syndrome, 709, 710f
Acute disseminated encephalomyelitis (ADEM), **1041**
Acute motor axonal neuropathy, 1061
Acute respiratory distress syndrome (ARDS), **69**
  clinical course and pathophysiology of, 69–70
  definition and etiology of, 69
  outcomes of, 71
  treatment of, 70–71, 70f
Acute stress disorder, 1083
Acyclovir
  for Bell's palsy, 1022
  for HSV infections, 475, 479t, 566, 567t–568t, 569
  for viral encephalitis, 1049–1050
  for viral esophagitis, 252
  for viral meningitis, 1048

Adalimumab
    for ankylosing spondylitis, 897
    for inflammatory bowel disease, 840, 907
    for psoriatic arthritis, 898
    for rheumatoid arthritis, 887
Addison's disease, **936**
    drug-induced, 1132t
Adefovir, for chronic hepatitis B, 860t–861t,
        864
Adenoma
    adrenal, 934–935
    colonic, 383
    gastric, 381
    hepatocellular, 388
    pituitary. *See* Pituitary adenoma
    small-bowel, 382
    thyroid, **932**
Adenosine
    for arrhythmias, 728t
    for tachyarrhythmias, 722t
    for Wolff-Parkinson-White syndrome, 729
Adenosine deaminase deficiency, 882
Adenovirus infection
    pharyngoconjunctival fever, 583
    respiratory disease, **583**
Admission orders, **1**
ADMIT VITALS AND PHYSICAL EXAM
        (admissions mnemonic), 1–2
Adnexal mass, 395
Adrenal adenoma, 934–935
Adrenal carcinoma, 934–935
Adrenal gland disease, **933**
    hyperfunction, **934**
    hypofunction, **936**
Adrenal insufficiency
    paraneoplastic, **115**
    primary, 936
    secondary, 936
Adrenal mass, incidental, 937f, **938**
Adrenomyeloneuropathy, 1030–1031
Adult T cell leukemia/lymphoma, **360**
Advance directives, 47
Advanced sleep phase syndrome, 230
Adverse drug reactions, **1131**, 1131t–1140t.
        See also Drug-induced illness
Aeromonas infection, 478, **516**
Affective disorder, major, **1077**
African tick-bite fever, 555
Agammaglobulinemia
    autosomal, 884
    X-linked, 883
Agglutination, 636
Agitation, in terminally ill patient, 53t
AGMA inducers, poisoning, 147t
Agoraphobia, 1081, 1083
Agranulocytosis, drug-induced, 1134t
AIDS. *See also* HIV/AIDS
    definition of, 600
Airborne precautions, 429
Airway obstruction
    drug-induced, 1136t
    dyspnea in, 231
Alanine aminotransferase (ALT), 268, 268t
Albendazole
    for ascariasis, 650
    for echinococcosis, 657
    for enterobiasis, 651
    for hookworm infection, 650

for larva migrans, 649
    for lymphatic filariasis, 652
    for strongyloidiasis, 651
    for taeniasis solium and cysticercosis, 656
    for trichinellosis, 649
Albumin
    intravenous, for hepatorenal syndrome,
        274
    serum, in liver disease, 269, 269t
    serum-ascites gradient, 273t
    urine, 278
Albuterol
    for COPD, 761–763
    for hyperkalemia, 15t
    poisoning, 136t
Alcohol abuse, 1096
Alcohol dependence, 1096
Alcoholic ketoacidosis, 17t, 18
Alcoholic liver disease, **869**
Alcoholic polyneuropathy, 1016
Alcohol intoxication, 1096
Alcoholism, **1095**, 1104t
    chronic, 852
    dementia in, 996t
    metabolic consequences of, 870
    treatment of
        acute withdrawal, 1098
        drug therapy, 1098
        recovery and sobriety, 1098
        relapse prevention, 1098
Alcohol Use Disorder Screening Test
        (AUDIT), 1096, 1097t
Alcohol withdrawal, 1096, 1098
Aldosteronism, **935**
    primary, 935
    secondary, 935
Alefacept
    for psoriasis, 314
    for psoriatic arthritis, 898
Alemtuzumab, for CLL, 356
Alendronate, for osteoporosis, 967
Alkaline diuresis, for poisoning, 149t, 160
Alkaline phosphatase, 268, 269t, 850
Alkali therapy, for nephrolithiasis, 828t
Alkalosis, **14**
Alkylating agents, toxicities of, 341t
Allergic angiitis and granulomatosis, **891**
Allergic bronchopulmonary aspergillosis,
        622, 624t
Allergic disease, immediate type hypersensi-
        tivity, **877**
Allergy
    anaphylaxis, **116**
    to insect sting, 127
    leukocytosis in, 330
Allodynia, 34, 1018
Alloimmunization, 44
Allopurinol
    for CML, 349
    for gout, 905
    for nephrolithiasis, 828t
Allylamines, for dermatophyte infections, 317
Almotriptan, for migraine, 185t, 187t
Alopecia, drug-induced, 341t, 1133t
Alosetron, for irritable bowel syndrome, 841,
        842t
Alpha-adrenergic antagonists, for vasospastic
        disorders, 740

Alpha radiation, 171
Alpha-tocopherol, for prostate cancer prevention, 1124
Alprazolam
  dosage and action of, 1089t
  poisoning, 143t
Alprostadil injection, for erectile dysfunction, 951
Alteplase, for thrombotic disorders, 338
Aluminum phosphate binders, for hyperphosphatemia, 964
Alveolar-arterial oxygen gradient, 749–750
Alveolar hemorrhage syndrome, 774, **776**
Alveolar hypoventilation, **781**, 782t
Alveolar ventilation, 749
Alzheimer's disease, 995, 996t, **998**
  differentiation of major dementias, 997t
  familial, 998
  in women, 1128
Amantadine
  for influenza, 579t, 580
  for Parkinson's disease, 1004, 1007
  poisoning, 138t, 153t
Amaurosis fugax, 80, 215
Amebiasis, 420t, **460**
Ameboma, 460–461
Amenorrhea, **952**, 952f
  primary, 952
  secondary, 952
Amikacin
  for gram-negative enteric bacterial infections, 516
  indications for, 426t
  for Klebsiella infections, 515
  for nocardiosis, 536t
  for nontuberculous mycobacterial infections, 548
  for P. aeruginosa infections, 519t
  for pneumonia, 766t, 767t
  resistance to, 426t
Amiloride
  for diabetes insipidus, 8
  for edema, 243t
  for hypertension, 695t
  for Liddle's syndrome, 20
Aminoglycosides, adverse reactions to, 424
Aminophylline, for anaphylaxis, 117
Aminosalicylates, for inflammatory bowel disease, 838
Aminotransferases, 268, 268t
Amiodarone
  for arrhythmias, 728t
  for dilated cardiomyopathy, 685
  for tachyarrhythmias, 723t–724t
  for ventricular tachycardia, 704
Amiodarone-induced thyrotoxicosis, **931**
Amitriptyline
  for ciguatera poisoning, 124
  dosage and adverse effects of, 138t, 141t, 1086t
  for irritable bowel syndrome, 841
  for migraine prevention, 188t
  for multiple sclerosis, 1041
  for pain, 36t–37t
Ammonia, blood, in liver disease, 269–270
Amodiaquine, for malaria, 638t
Amoxapine, 1087t

Amoxicillin
  for anthrax, 164t
  during COPD exacerbations, 763
  for H. pylori eradication, 833t
  indications for, 425t
  for leptospirosis, 553
  for Lyme borreliosis, 550
  for otitis media, 303t, 305
  for pharyngitis, 304t
  for pneumococcal infections, 488
  for pneumonia, 766t
  for pyelonephritis, 818t
  resistance to, 425t
  for sinusitis, 303t
Amoxicillin-clavulanate
  for animal bite infections, 119t, 479t
  for H. influenzae infections, 509
  for otitis media, 303t
  for pneumonia, 766t
  for sinusitis, 303t
Amphetamine poisoning, 136t, 152t
Amphotericin B, **619**
  for blastomycosis, 631
  for candidiasis, 252, 621
  for coccidioidomycosis, 630
  for cryptococcosis, 626
  for febrile neutropenia in cancer patient, 115
  for fusariosis, 632
  for histoplasmosis, 629t
  for leishmaniasis, 643–644
  for mucormycosis, 627
  for penicilliosis, 632
  for sporotrichosis, 631
Ampicillin
  for actinomycosis, 538
  for bacterial meningitis, 1046t, 1047t
  for diverticulitis, 842
  for enterococcal infections, 501
  for HACEK group infections, 512t
  indications for, 425t
  for infective endocarditis, 444t, 446
  for leptospirosis, 553
  for listerial infections, 507
  for necrotizing fasciitis, 480t
  for osteomyelitis, 485t
  for pneumonia, 766t
  for Proteus infections, 515
  resistance to, 425t
  for urinary tract infections, 819t
Ampicillin-clavulanate, for diverticulitis, 842
Ampicillin-sulbactam
  for animal bite infections, 119t
  for cellulitis, 479t
  for cholecystitis, 847
  for epiglottitis, 306
  for HACEK group infections, 512t
  for human bite infections, 119t
  for infective endocarditis, 445t
  for myositis/myonecrosis, 481
  for osteomyelitis, 485t
  for pneumonia, 767t
  for snakebite, 120t
Amprenavir, for HIV/AIDS, 613t
Amrinone
  for beta blocker poisoning, 140t
  for calcium channel blocker poisoning, 140t
Amylase, serum, 849

Amylase-creatinine clearance ratio, urinary, 849
Amyl nitrite, for cytochrome oxidase inhibitor poisoning, 145t
Amyloid angiopathy, 82t
Amyloidosis, **913**
  AA (secondary), 913–915, 914f
  Aβ2M, 913–915, 914f
  AL (primary), 812t, 813, 913–915, 914f
  autonomic involvement in, 1016
  clinical features of, 913–914
  diagnosis of, 914, 914f
  familial, 913–915, 914f
  glomerular disease in, 807t
Amyotrophic lateral sclerosis (ALS), **1010**
  familial, 1010
  treatment of, 1013
Anaerobic bacteria, 528
Anaerobic infection, **528**
  bacteremia, 534
  bone and joint, 533
  botulism, **529**
  brain abscess, 533
  mixed, **532**
    treatment of, 534, 534t
  of mouth, head, and neck, 532
  osteomyelitis, 485t
  pelvic, 533
  skin/soft tissue, 533
  specimen collection and transport, 418t
  tetanus, **528**
Anakinra, for rheumatoid arthritis, 888
Anal cancer, **387**
Anal fissure, **844**
Analgesia, 34
Analgesic(s), 36t–37t, 38
Analgesic nephropathy, 811–812
Anaphylaxis, **116**
  drug-induced, 1131t
  prevention of, 117
  related to hymenoptera sting, 127
Anaplasmosis, 125
  human granulocytotropic (HGA), **558**
Anastrozole
  for breast cancer, 378–379
  toxicity of, 342t
Ancylostoma braziliense infection, **649**
Ancylostoma duodenale infection. *See* Hookworm infection
Androgen(s), adrenal, **933**
Androgen abuse, 950
Androgen deficiency, **947**
Androgen deprivation, for prostate cancer, 401
Androgen excess, in female, 955
Anemia, **280**. *See also specific types*
  blood loss, **326**
  drug-induced, 325, 327, 327t, 344, 1135t
  in hypometabolic states, 325t
  hypoproliferative, 282, **323**, 325t
  in inflammation, 325t
  microcytic, 324f, 325, 325t
  parvovirus infection, 588
  physiologic classification of, 281, 281f
  refractory, 325
  in renal failure, 325t
  treatment of, 328–329
Anemia of chronic disease, 324, 328

Aneurysm. *See specific types*
Angina pectoris, 175, **712**
  chronic stable, **712**
  drug-induced, 1135t
  Prinzmetal's variant, **716**
  recurrent, 708, 714
  treatment of
    drug therapy, 714–716, 715t
    long-term suppression, 715–716
    mechanical revascularization, 716, 717t
  unstable, **709**
Angiodysplasia, 261, 263
  colonic, **843**
Angioedema, 241, **878**
  classification of, 878, 878t
  drug-induced, 1131t
Angiography, hepatobiliary, 270–271
Angiotensin receptor blockers
  for diabetic nephropathy, 805–806
  for dilated cardiomyopathy, 685
  for glomerulonephritis, 805, 808
  for heart failure, 732t, 733t
  for hypertension, 695t, 696, 697t, 698, 796, 822
  for myocardial infarction, 704
  preventive treatment, 709
Anidulafungin, **620**
Anilines, 146t
Animal bite
  rabies, 592
  treatment of, 479t
Animal-borne viral infection, **592**
Anion gap, 16, 17t, 21
  calculation of, 19
Anion-gap metabolic alkalosis (AGMA) inducers, 131t
Anisocytosis, 321
Anistreplase, for thrombotic disorders, 338
Ankle-brachial index, 661, 739
Ankylosing spondylitis, **895**, 896f, 897
Ann Arbor staging system, for Hodgkin's disease, 363, 363t
Annular skin lesion, 309
Anomia, 225t
Anorectal disease, **844**
Anorexia, in terminally ill patient, 52t
Anorexia nervosa, 247, **1093**, 1093t, 1095f
Anosmia, 1002
Anosognosia, 80
Antacids
  for erosive gastropathies, 834
  for indigestion, 247
  for peptic ulcer disease, 833
  for systemic sclerosis, 889
Anterior ischemic optic neuropathy (AION), 216f, 217
Anthrax, **162**, 201
  as bioweapon, 162, 164t
  cutaneous, 162
  gastrointestinal, 162
  inhalation, 111, 162
  prevention of, 163
  treatment of, 163, 164t
Antiarrhythmics, 720, 727t–728t
  for pain, 36t–37t, 38
  poisoning, 153t
  selection of, 729f

Antibacterial resistance, **422**
  emerging problems, 432
Antibacterial therapy, **422**
  adverse reactions to, **424**
  choice of antibacterial agents, 424,
    425t–427t
  mechanisms of drug action, 422
  pharmacokinetics of antibiotics, 423
  principles of, 423
  susceptibility testing, 413
  toxicity of, 342t
Antibody detection, tissue parasites, 421
Anticholinergics
  for asthma, 754–755
  for COPD, 761–763
  for diverticular disease, 842
  for irritable bowel syndrome, 841
  for Parkinson's disease, 1004
  poisoning, 131t
Anticholinesterase drugs
  for myasthenia gravis, 1066
  poisoning, 142t
Anticoagulants
  for deep venous thrombosis, 770–771
  for myocardial infarction, 702
  for pulmonary embolism, 770–771
  for SLE, 886
  for stroke, 84
    preventive treatment, 85
  for thrombotic disorders, 336–337, 337t
Anticonvulsants
  for pain, 36t–37t, 38
  poisoning, 143t
  for polyneuropathy, 1061
  for subarachnoid hemorrhage, 89
Antidepressants, **1085**
  for Alzheimer's disease, 1000
  for chronic fatigue syndrome, 291
  for depression, 1079
  for fibromyalgia, 909
  for insomnia, 228
  for irritable bowel syndrome, 842t
  for pain, 36t–37t, 38
  for panic disorder, 1081
  poisoning, 138t
  for smoking cessation, 1127
  withdrawal syndromes, 1088
Antidotes, 133
Antiepileptic drugs, 992t–994t
Antifungal agents, **619**
  topical, 620
Antigen detection
  bacterial and viral infections, **411**
  tissue parasites, 421
Antigenic drift, 577
Antigenic shift, 577
Anti-glomerular basement membrane disease,
  802, **803**
Antihistamines
  for allergic rhinitis, 880
  for antivenom reaction, 122
  for chronic fatigue syndrome, 291
  for erythema multiforme, 318
  for hymenoptera sting, 126
  for nausea and vomiting, 245
  for pityriasis rosea, 314
  poisoning, 138t, 149t, 153t
  for scombroid poisoning, 124

  for systemic mastocytosis, 881
  for urticaria/angioedema, 879
Anti-LKM antibodies, 867
Antimalarials, 638t, 639t
  poisoning, 146t, 153t
  for SLE, 886
Antimetabolites, toxicities of, 341t
Antimonial compounds, for leishmaniasis,
  643–644
Antineuronal antibodies, paraneoplastic, 407,
  409t
Antineutrophil cytoplasmic autoantibodies
  (ANCA), 892
  glomerulonephritis, **803**
Antinuclear antibodies, 743, 774, 865, 867
Antiplatelet agents
  for stroke, 84
    preventive treatment, 85
  for thrombotic disorders, 338
Antipsychotics, **1088**, 1090t–1091t
  for Alzheimer's disease, 1000
  conventional, 1081, 1088–1092, 1090t
  for ergot alkaloid poisoning, 137t
  novel, 1081, 1091t, 1092
  poisoning, 138t, 149t, 153t
  for schizophrenia, 1081
Antipyretics, 201
Antiretroviral therapy, 606–617, 607t–615t,
  617t
Antisocial personality disorder, 1084
Antithrombotic drugs
  for myocardial infarction, 710–711
  for unstable angina, 710–711
Antithymocyte globulin, for aplastic anemia,
  329
α_1-Antitrypsin deficiency, 761
Antitussive agents, 235
Antivenom
  for snakebite, 121–122
  sources of, 123
Antrectomy, 833t
Anuria, 276
Anxiety attack, **210**
Anxiety disorder, **1081**
Anxiolytics, **1088**, 1089t
Aorta
  abdominal, occlusive disease of, 738
  coarctation of, **676**, 693
  diseases of, **736**
    echocardiography in, 671, 672t
Aortic aneurysm, **736**
Aortic dissection, **736**, 738t
  chest pain in, 176, 177f
  classification of, 736–737, 737f
Aortic regurgitation, 662t, **681**
  echocardiography in, 671f
Aortic stenosis, 662t, **681**, 682f
  echocardiography in, 671f
Aortography, 736
Aphasia, **224**, 225t
Aplastic anemia, 323, 329, 331
Aplastic crisis, parvovirus infections,
  587–588
Apnea, in terminally ill patient, 53t
Apo B-100, familial defective, 969t, **970**
Apo CII deficiency, 969t, **973**
Aprepitant, for nausea and vomiting, 48, 246,
  344

Arachnoiditis, lumbar, pain in, 193
Arbovirus infection, **595**, 596t–597t
Arcanobacterium haemolyticum infection, 503
Argatroban
 for heparin-induced thrombocytopenia, 334
 for thrombotic disorders, 337
Argentine hemorrhagic fever, 598
Aripiprazole
 dosage and adverse effects of, 1091t
 for schizophrenia, 1081
Aromatase inhibitors, for breast cancer, 376, 378–379
Arrhythmia
 bradyarrhythmia, **717**
 drug-induced, 1135t
 in myocardial infarction, 704
 serum magnesium and, 704
 syncope in, 208, 209t
 tachyarrhythmias, **720**
Arsenic poisoning, 154t–155t
Arsenic trioxide, for AML, 346
Artemether, for malaria, 639t
Artemether-lumefantrine, for malaria, 638t
Artemis gene, 882
Artemisinin derivatives, for malaria, 637, 638t
Arterial blood gases (ABG), 749
 in acid-base disorders, 16, 20
Arterial embolism, **739**
Arteriosclerosis, of peripheral arteries, **739**
Arteriovenous fistula, dural, 82t
Arteriovenous malformation, 1030
 intracranial hemorrhage in, 82t
 subarachnoid hemorrhage in, 88
Arteritis, 891–892
Artesunate, for malaria, 637, 638t–639t
Arthritis. *See also specific types*
 gonococcal, 469, 481–482
 infectious, **481**
  HACEK group, 511
  S. aureus, 491, 496
  streptococcal, 499–500
  treatment of, 482
 mycoplasmal, 471
 nongonococcal bacterial, 481
 noninfectious inflammatory, 482
 rash and, arboviral disease, 595–596
 synovial fluid analysis in, 482
Arthritis mutilans, 898t
Arthropod bite/sting, 124
Arthropod-borne disease
 protozoan infections, **636**
 viral infections, **593**
Arthropod ectoparasites, **657**
Arthroscopic therapy, for osteoarthritis, 902
Asbestosis, 757
Asbestos-related disease, **757**
Ascariasis, **649**
Ascites, 241, **271**
 chylous, 272, 273t
 cirrhotic, **272**, 273t
 complications of, 272–274
 fluid characteristics, 273t
 pancreatic, 852
 paracentesis, 28–29

primary bacterial peritonitis and, **448**
 refractory, 272
 serum-ascites albumin gradient, 273t
L-Asparaginase, for acute lymphoblastic leukemia and lymphoblastic lymphoma, 359
Aspartate aminotransferase (AST), 268, 268t, 850
Aspergilloma, 622–623, 624t
Aspergillosis, 432, **621**
 allergic bronchopulmonary, 622, 624t
 cerebral, 622
 disseminated, 622
 pulmonary
  chronic, 622–623, 625t
  invasive, 622, 624t
 sinusitis, 622–623
 treatment of, 623, 624t–625t
Asphyxiants, poisoning, 131t, 145t
Aspirin
 for angina pectoris, 716
 for atrial fibrillation, 726
 for cardiovascular disease prevention, 1120
 for colon cancer prevention, 1124
 for fever, 201
 low-dose, 1120
 for migraine, 185t
 for myocardial infarction, 701–702, 710, 712
  preventive treatment, 709
 for pain, 36t–37t, 38
 for pericarditis, 688
 for rheumatoid arthritis, 887
 for stroke, 84
  preventive treatment, 86, 87t
 for superficial thrombophlebitis, 740
 for tension headache, 186
 for thrombotic disorders, 338
 for unstable angina, 710
Assist-control ventilation, 72, 73t
Assisted reproductive technology, 958
Asterixis, 224
Asthma, **753**
 chronic, 754–755
 dyspnea in, 233
 intrinsic, 753
 occupational, 753, 758
 pulmonary function tests in, 753–754
 sleep disorders in, 227, 229t
Asthma exacerbations, **755**
Astrocytoma, **1032**, 1032f
Asystole, 57, 58f
Ataxia, **1007**
 acute, 1008t
 approach to, 1007–1009, 1008t, 1009f
 chronic, 1008t
 inherited, 1009
 subacute, 1008t
Ataxia-telangiectasia, 883
Atazanavir, for HIV/AIDS, 613t
Atenolol
 for hypertension, 695t
 poisoning, 140t
 for thyrotoxicosis, 929
 for vasovagal syncope, 210
Atheroembolism, **740**
 renal, **821**

Atherosclerosis
  C. pneumoniae infection and, 563
  prevention of complications of, 974
  risk factors for, **1118,** 1118t
Athetosis, 223
Atorvastatin
  for hyperlipidemia, 972t
  for myocardial infarction, 711
    preventive treatment, 709
  for unstable angina, 711
Atovaquone
  for babesiosis, 107t, 642
  for *Pneumocystis* infections, 634t, 635
    preventive treatment, 635t
Atovaquone-proguanil, for malaria, 638t
  preventive treatment, 640t
Atrial fibrillation, 721f, 723t
  antithrombotic prophylaxis in, 85–86, 87t
  chronic, **726**
Atrial flutter, 721f, 723t
Atrial premature beats, 722t
Atrial septal defect, **674**
  ostium primum, 674
  ostium secundum, 674
Atrial tachycardia, 722t
  with block, 721f
  multifocal, 723t
Atrioventricular (AV) block, **718**
  causes of, 718t
  drug-induced, 718t, 1136t
  first degree, 719, 719f
  in myocardial infarction, 704
  second degree
    Mobitz I, 719, 719f
    Mobitz II, 719, 719f
  third degree (complete), 719, 719f
Atrophy (skin lesion), 313t
Atropine
  for beta blocker poisoning, 140t
  for bradycardia, 702
  for calcium channel blocker poisoning, 140t
  for cardiac glycoside poisoning, 141t
  for cholinergic poisoning, 142t
  for inflammatory bowel disease, 838
  for nerve agent exposure, 169–171, 170t
  poisoning, 138t
  for sympatholytic poisoning, 139t
  for tachyarrhythmias, 724t
Audiologic assessment, 298
Auer rods, 322
Auscultation, **663**
Autoantibody disorders, 46
Autoimmune disease
  leukopenia in, 331
  thrombocytopenia in, 332
  in women, 1129
Autoimmune hemolysis, 329
Autologous transfusion, **45**
Automated external defibrillator, 55–56
Autonomic nervous system (ANS)
  activation of, 1015t
  anatomy of, 1014f
  function tests, 1016
Autonomic nervous system (ANS) disease, **1013**
  approach to, 1015
  autoimmune, 1016–1018

  with brain involvement, 1017t
  classification of, 1017t–1018t
  drug-induced, 1015
  with multisystem degeneration, 1017t
  with spinal cord involvement, 1017t
  treatment of, 1019
Avascular necrosis, **909**
Avoidant personality disorder, 1085
Axillary lymph node, carcinoma in, 402
5-Azacytidine, for myelodysplastic syndromes, 350
Azathioprine
  for autoimmune hepatitis, 867
  for inflammatory bowel disease, 838
  for inflammatory myopathy, 1072
  for multiple sclerosis, 1039
  for myasthenia gravis, 1066
  for myocarditis, 687
  for polyneuropathy, 1061
  for reactive arthritis, 900
  for rheumatoid arthritis, 888
  for SLE, 803, 886
  toxicity of, 341t
  for vasculitis, 894
Azelastine, for allergic rhinitis, 880
Azithromycin
  for babesiosis, 107t, 642
  for *Bartonella* infections, 526t
  for chancroid, 476
  for cholera, 453
  for *C. pneumoniae* infections, 563
  for *C. trachomatis* infections, 562
  for diarrhea, 1117
  for donovanosis, 476
  for *H. influenzae* infections, 509
  indications for, 426t
  for *Legionella* infections, 522
  for meningococcal disease prevention, 506t
  for *M. pneumoniae* infections, 560
  for nontuberculous mycobacterial infections, 548
  for otitis media, 303t
  for pertussis, 510
  for pneumonia, 766t
  resistance to, 426t
  for shigellosis, 459
  for traveler's diarrhea, 451
  for urethritis in men, 463
Azotemia, **274,** 275f
  intrinsic renal, 792t
  prerenal, 276, 791, 792t
Aztreonam
  indications for, 426t
  for pyelonephritis, 818t
  resistance to, 426t
  for sepsis/septic shock, 65t
  for urinary tract infections, 819t

B
Babesiosis, 106, 107t, 125, 420t, **642**
Babinski sign, 219t, 984
Bacillary angiomatosis, 479t, 526t, **527**
Bacillary peliosis, 526t, **527**
Bacille Calmette-Guérin, intravesical instillation of, 392
Bacillus anthracis infection. *See* Anthrax
Bacillus cereus infection, 453

Back pain, **189.** *See also* Low back pain
  approach to, 114f
  cancer patient with, 114f
Baclofen
  for dystonia, 223
  poisoning, 144t
  for trigeminal neuralgia, 1020
Bacteremia
  Aeromonas, 516
  anaerobic, 534
  clostridial, 531
  E. coli, 514
  Klebsiella, 515
  listerial, 507
  P. aeruginosa, 517, 519t
  S. aureus, 491
  streptococcal, 498–499
Bacterial infection
  anaerobic. *See* Anaerobic infection
  diagnosis of, **411**
Bacterial vaginosis, 464, 471, 533
Bacteriuria, asymptomatic, 815, 817
Bacteroides fragilis infection, **532**
Balanitis, circinate, 899
Balkan endemic nephropathy, 812
Balloon dilatation, for esophageal disorders,
  251
Balloon tamponade, for esophageal varices,
  874
Barbiturate(s)
  for isoniazid poisoning, 150t
  poisoning, 143t
  for sedative-hypnotic poisoning, 143t
Barbiturate coma, 92t
Bariatric surgery, 940–941, 941f
Barium contrast x-ray study, 256
Barium enema, air-contrast, 387
Barium radiography, for GI bleeding, 260
Barium swallow, 250–251, 380–381
Barotrauma, 74
Barrett's esophagus, 246, 379
Barrier contraception, 957
Bartonella infection, **526,** 526t
Bartter's syndrome, 788
Basal cell carcinoma, **366**
  keratotic, 366
  morpheaform, 366
  noduloulcerative, 366
  pigmented, 366
  superficial, 366
Basal energy expenditure, 39, 39f
Basic life support, 55–57, 56f–58f
Basophilia, **330**
Basophilic stippling, 321
Bechterew's disease. *See* Ankylosing
      spondylitis
Beclomethasone
  for allergic rhinitis, 880
  for asthma, 755
Bed nets, 1116
Beer potomania, 3
Bee sting, 126
Belladonna alkaloid poisoning, 138t
Bell's palsy, 565, **1021**
Belsey procedure, 247
Benign paroxysmal positional vertigo, 213,
      213t, 214t
Bentiromide test, 852

Benzathine penicillin
  for diphtheria prevention, 503
  for endemic treponematosis, 551
  for pharyngitis, 304t
  for rheumatic fever prevention, 678
  for streptococcal infections, 498t
  for syphilis, 474t
Benzene derivative poisoning, 858
Benznidazole, for Chagas' disease, 645
Benzodiazepines, 1088
  for alcohol withdrawal, 1098
  dosage and action of, 1089t
  for dystonia, 223
  for generalized anxiety disorder, 1082
  for narcotic withdrawal, 1100
  for panic disorder, 1082
  poisoning, 143t
  for sedative-hypnotic poisoning, 143t
  for sympathomimetic poisoning, 136t
Benzoyl peroxide, for acne, 318
Benztropine
  for extrapyramidal reactions, 149t
  for Parkinson's disease, 1004
Berylliosis, **758**
Beta agonists
  for asthma, 754
  for COPD, 761–762
Beta blockers
  for angina pectoris, 715
  for aortic dissection, 738, 738t
  for cardiomyopathy, 685–686
  for glaucoma, 295
  for heart failure, 731–732, 732t, 733t,
      735
  for hypertension, 695, 695t, 697t
  for mitral regurgitation, 679
  for mitral stenosis, 678
  for mitral valve prolapse, 681
  for myocardial infarction, 702, 711–712
      preventive treatment, 709
  poisoning, 140t, 153t
  for sinus tachycardia, 704
  for tachyarrhythmias, 722t–724t
  for thyrotoxicosis, 929–930
  for unstable angina, 711
  for Wolff-Parkinson-White syndrome,
      729
Beta-carotene, for erythropoietic porphyria,
      978
Betamethasone, 938–939, 938t
Beta radiation, 171
Bethanecol
  for multiple sclerosis, 1041
  poisoning, 142t
Bevacizumab
  for colorectal cancer, 387
  for kidney cancer, 393
  toxicity of, 342t
Bicarbonate, renal retention of, 19
Bicarbonate therapy
  for metabolic acidosis, 19, 62
  for renal tubular acidosis, 814–815
  for tumor lysis syndrome, 116
Bichloroacetic acid, for HPV infection, 476
Bicuspid aortic valve, congenital, **676**
Bile ducts, diagnostic evaluation of, 846t
Bile salt deficiency, 259t
Biliary colic, 844–845

Biliary disease
  gram-negative enteric bacteria, 516
  infections in cancer patients, 433t
Bilirubin, serum, **263**, 850
  conjugated fraction (direct), 264, 264t, 267
  unconjugated fraction (indirect), 264, 264t, 267
Binge eating, 1093
Biopsy. *See also specific organs*
  collection and transport of, 417t
Bioterrorism
  chemical, **168**
  microbial, **160**
  radiation, **171**
Bipolar disorder, **1079**
Bisacodyl, for constipation, 48t
Bismuth subsalicylate
  for diarrhea, 1117
  for *H. pylori* eradication, 833t
Bisoprolol, for heart failure, 733t
Bisphosphonates
  for breast cancer, 379
  for hypercalcemia, 406
  for osteoporosis, 967
Bite
  arthropod, **124**
  mammalian, **117**
    treatment of, 121
  management of wound infections, 119t–120t
  snakebite, **121**
Bladder cancer, **391**
Blastomycosis, **630**
  South American, **631**
Bleeding disorders, **332**
  blood vessel wall defects, **334**
  coagulation disorders, **334**
  gastrointestinal, **259**
  platelet disorders, **332**
  treatment of, 334–335
Bleomycin
  for germ cell tumor, 402
  for testicular cancer, 394
  toxicity of, 342t
Blepharoconjunctivitis, 294
Blepharospasm, 1022–1023
Blocking agents, for radionuclide contamination, 174
Blood
  reference values for laboratory tests, **1141**
  specimen collection and transport, 414t
  toxicologic analysis of, 133, 1157t–1159t
Blood loss
  anemia in, **280, 326**
  symptoms of, 260
Blood smear, **321**
  erythrocyte abnormalities, 321–322
  leukocyte abnormalities, 322
  platelet abnormalities, 322
Blood urea nitrogen, 274
Blood vessel wall defects, **334**
Blood volume, disorders of, 209t
Blue toe syndrome, 740
Body fluids
  reference ranges for volumes of, 1171t
  specimen collection and transport, 416t
Body louse, 658–659
Body mass index (BMI), 39, **939,** 1171t

Body temperature, 199
Body weight. *See* Weight *entries*
Bolivian hemorrhagic fever, 598
Bone density, 967
Bone disease
  anaerobic infections, 533
  drug-induced, 1140t
  neck pain in, 198
  osteomalacia, **967**
  osteoporosis, **967**
  P. aeruginosa infections, 517, 519t
Bone marrow
  cellularity of, 323
  damage causing anemia, 323–324
  erythroid:granulocytic ratio, 323
  examination of, 282, **322**
Bone marrow aspirate, 322
  reference values for specific analytes, 1164t
Bone marrow failure, 331
Bone marrow transplant, 883
  for acute lymphoblastic leukemia and lymphoblastic lymphoma, 359
  for AML, 346–347
  for CML, 347
  for myelodysplastic syndromes, 350
Bone metastasis, osteoblastic, in men, **404**
Borderline personality disorder, 1084
Bordetella pertussis infection. *See* Pertussis
Bornholm disease, 590
Borrelia burgdorferi infection. *See* Lyme borreliosis
Borrelia recurrentis infection, 553
Bortezomib
  for multiple myeloma, 361
  toxicity of, 342t
Bosentan, for systemic sclerosis, 889
Botulinum toxin
  for achalasia, 251
  for anal fissures, 844
  as bioweapon, 165t, 167
  for dystonia, 223
  for hemifacial spasm or blepharospasm, 1023
Botulism, **529,** 1018
  as bioweapon, 530
  food-borne, 530
  intestinal, 530
  treatment of, 165t, 530
  wound, 530
Botulism antitoxin, 530
Botulism immune globulin, 530
Bounding pulse, 661, 661f
Bowen's disease, 366
BPM regimen, for Burkitt's lymphoma/leukemia, 360
Brachial neuritis, acute, 198
Brachial plexus, injury to, 198
Brachytherapy, interstitial, 1032
Bradyarrhythmia, 209t, **717**
  approach to, 57, 58f
  in myocardial infarction, 704
Bradycardia, **717**
Bradykinesia, 218, 222
Brain abscess, 109t, 111, 1042, **1050**
  anaerobic, 533
  nocardiosis, 535–536
  streptococcal, 501

Brain death, 79
Brain herniation, 90, 91f
Brain metastasis, 1033, 1034t
Brain natriuretic peptide, 685, 730
Brainstem auditory evoked responses (BAER), 298
Brainstem lesion, 219t, 220t
Brain tumor, 998
    approach to, 1031
    headache in, 183t
    intracranial, **1032**
    metastatic, 82t
    treatment of, 1031–1032
Brazilian hemorrhagic fever, 598
BRCA genes, 374–375, 379, 395, 1122
Breast cancer, **374**
    carcinoma in axillary lymph node, **402**
    diagnosis of, 375–376
    estrogen receptor status of, 376, 378–379
    genetic factors in, 374–375
    infections in cancer patients, 433t
    locally advanced, 376
    metastatic, 376, 378
    oncologic emergencies, 112–113
    operable, 376
    paraneoplastic syndromes in, 409t
    prevention of, 379, 1122–1123
    prognosis by stage, 376, 378t
    risk factors for, 1122
    screening for, 1104t, 1122, 1123t
    staging of, 376, 377t–378t
    treatment of, 376–379
Breast mass, approach to, 375, 375f
Breast self-examination, 1123t
Brenner tumor, 395
Bretylium, for cardiac glycoside poisoning, 141t
Brill-Zinsser disease, 557
Broca's aphasia, 225, 225t
Bromocriptine
    for hyperprolactinemia, 920
    for Parkinson's disease, 1006t
    poisoning, 137t
Bronchial aspirate, 415t
Bronchiolitis
    human RSV, 582
    respiratory, 775
Bronchiolitis obliterans with organizing pneumonia, 774
Bronchitis
    dyspnea in, 231
    hemoptysis in, 236
Bronchoalveolar lavage, 752
Bronchodilators
    for asthma, 754–756
    for COPD, 761–763
    for cor pulmonale, 735
    poisoning, 136t
Bronchoscopy, 237, 751–752, 774
Brown-Séquard syndrome, 220t, 1026
Brucellosis, **522**
    tuberculosis vs., 523, 523t
Brugada syndrome, 720
Brugia infection. See Filariasis
Bruton's tyrosine kinase gene, 883
Budd-Chiari syndrome, 272
Budesonide, for asthma, 755
Bulimia nervosa, **1093**, 1094t, 1095f

Bullae (skin lesion), 313t, 477
Bumetanide
    for edema, 243t
    for heart failure, 733t
    for hypertension, 698
    for pulmonary edema, 68
Bundle branch block
    left, 667f, 668t, 720, 726t
    right, 667f, 720, 726t
"Bundled interventions," 430t
Buprenorphine
    narcotic abuse, **1099**
    for opioid maintenance, 1100
Bupropion
    dosage and adverse effects of, 1086t
    for smoking cessation, 1127
    for vasovagal syncope, 210
Burkholderia cepacia infection, **518,** 520t
Burkholderia mallei infection, 518–521, 520t
Burkholderia pseudomallei infection, 518, 520t
Burkitt's lymphoma, **359,** 575–576, 576t
Burn patient
    hypothermia in, 128t
    neutrophilia in, 329
Bursitis, **909**
Buruli ulcer, 549
Buspirone, 1088
    dosage and action of, 1089t
    for generalized anxiety disorder, 1082
Busulfan, 341t
Butabarbital poisoning, 143t
Butorphanol
    for migraine, 186t
    for pain, 36t–37t
Butterfly rash, 885

C

Cabergoline
    for hyperprolactinemia, 920
    for Parkinson's disease, 1006t
Cadmium poisoning, 154t–155t
CaEDTA, for lead poisoning, 157t
Caffeine poisoning, 137t
CAGE questions, 1096
Calamine lotion, for insect stings, 126
Calcipotriol, for psoriasis, 314
Calcitonin, for hypercalcemia, 962t
Calcitriol
    for hypoparathyroidism, 964
    for osteomalacia, 968
Calcium apatite deposition disease, **906**
    conditions associated with, 906t
Calcium carbonate, for hyperphosphatemia, 796
Calcium channel blockers
    for angina pectoris, 715
    for hypertension, 695t, 696–698, 697t, 822
    for mitral stenosis, 678
    poisoning, 140t
    for pulmonary hypertension, 745
    for systemic sclerosis, 889
    for vasospastic disorders, 740
Calcium docusate, for constipation, 48t
Calcium gluconate
    for GI bleeding, 263
    for hypocalcemia, 963
    for muscle spasms, 123

Calcium oxalate deposition disease, **907**
Calcium oxalate stones, 827, 828t
Calcium phosphate stones, 827, 828t
Calcium polycarbophil, for irritable bowel syndrome, 842t
Calcium therapy
    for beta blocker poisoning, 140t
    for calcium channel blocker poisoning, 140t
    for colon cancer prevention, 1124
    for hyperkalemia, 15t
    for hypermagnesemia, 965
    for hypocalcemia, 963–964
    for hypoparathyroidism, 964
    for osteoporosis, 967
    for primary sclerosing cholangitis, 848
Calicivirus infection, diarrhea, **454**
Calorics, 211
Calvert formula, 397
Campylobacteriosis, **458**
    proctocolitis, 468
Cancer. *See also specific types and sites*
    depression in, 1078
    detection of, **1121**
    fatigue in, 289t
    infections in cancer patients, **432,** 433t
    leukocytosis in, 330
    lifestyle factors that reduce risk of, 1121t
    oncologic emergencies, **112**
    paraneoplastic syndromes
        endocrine, **405**
        neurologic, 407, 408t
    prevention of, 1104t–1105t, **1121**
        in high-risk groups, **1122**
    screening for, 1104t–1105t, **1121**
        lead-time bias, 1121
        length bias, 1121
        overdiagnosis, 1121–1122
        selection bias, 1122
    spinal cord compression in, **94**
    tumor growth, 339
    vaccination of cancer patients, 438t
    warning signs of, 1125
Cancer chemotherapy, **339**
    categories of agents, 339
    complications of, 340–343
    curability of cancers with, 340t
    development of drug resistance, 339
    leukopenia in, 331
    nausea and vomiting in, 245t, 246
    toxicities of agents, 339, 341t–342t
        management of, 343–344
Cancer of unknown primary site, **401**
    cytogenetics in, 403t
    cytokeratin markers, 402, 404f
    histology of, 402, 403t
    pathologic evaluation of biopsy specimens from, 403t–404t
    prognosis for, 402
Cancrum oris, 532
Candesartan
    for heart failure, 733t
    for hypertension, 695t
    for myocardial infarction, 704
Candidemia, 621
Candidiasis, **317, 620**
    cutaneous, 311, 620–621

    deeply invasive, 621
    disseminated, 201
    esophageal, 252, 620–621
    mucocutaneous, 620, 884
    thrush, 620–621
    urinary tract, 620
    vulvovaginal, 317, 464, 620–621
Capecitabine
    for breast cancer, 379
    for pancreatic cancer, 389
    toxicity of, 341t
Capillary telangiectasia, 82t
Capnocytophaga canimorsus infection, 110, 118, 119t
Capsaicin cream
    for osteoarthritis, 902
    for polyneuropathy, 1061
Capsulitis, adhesive, 910
Captopril
    for ergot alkaloid poisoning, 137t
    for heart failure, 731, 733t
    for hypertension, 695t, 696
    for myocardial infarction, 704
        preventive treatment, 709
Carbamazepine
    for bipolar disorder, 1080
    dosage and adverse effects of, 143t, 153t, 1092t
    for glossopharyngeal neuralgia, 1024
    for multiple sclerosis, 1041
    for pain, 36t–37t
    for seizures, 992t–993t, 994t
    for trigeminal neuralgia, 1020
Carbidopa/levodopa, for Parkinson's disease, 1004, 1005t
Carbimazole, for thyrotoxicosis, 929
Carbon monoxide poisoning, 98, 130, 145t, 758
Carbon tetrachloride poisoning, 858
Carboplatin
    for bladder cancer, 392
    for head and neck cancer, 368
    for ovarian cancer, 397
    toxicity of, 341t
Carbuncle, 491
Carcinoid syndrome, 389, 390t
Carcinoid tumor, **389**
    paraneoplastic syndromes in, 405t
Carcinomatosis, peritoneal, in women, **402**
Cardiac arrest, **55**
    follow-up of, 57–58
    management of, 55–57, 56f–58f
Cardiac biomarkers, in myocardial infarction, 700–701, 709
Cardiac catheterization
    in cardiac tamponade, 689
    in cardiomyopathy, 684t, 686
    in constrictive pericarditis, 691
    in pulmonary hypertension, 743–744
Cardiac disease. *See* Heart disease
Cardiac glycoside poisoning, 141t
Cardiac tamponade, 60t, **689**
Cardiac toxicity, 733
Cardiobacterium hominis infection. *See* HACEK group infection
Cardiogenic shock, 30, 31f, 59t, 60t, 62, 706t, **707**

Cardiomyopathy, **684**
　dilated, **684**
　　laboratory evaluation of, 684t, 685
　　drug-induced, 1136t
　hypertrophic, 662t, **686**
　　ECG in, 666, 668t
　　laboratory evaluation of, 684t, 686
　restrictive, **685,** 692t
　　laboratory evaluation of, 684t, 686
Cardiopulmonary resuscitation, 55–57, 56f
　for hypothermia, 128
Cardiovascular collapse, **55,** 55t
Cardiovascular disease. *See also* Heart dis-
　　ease
　drug-induced, 1135t–1136t
　prevention of, **1118**
　　antithrombotic therapy, 1120
　　lifestyle modifications, 1121
　risk factors for, 1118–1120
　syncope in, 208, 209t
　syphilis, 473
Carisoprodol poisoning, 144t
Carnitine palmitoyltransferase deficiency,
　　1073
Carotene, serum, 264
Carotene supplementation, for macular de-
　　generation, 296
Carotid artery pulse, **661,** 661f
Carotid endarterectomy, 86
Carotid sinus hypersensitivity, 209t
Carotid stenosis
　asymptomatic, 87
　symptomatic, 86
Carpal tunnel syndrome, 1055, 1062t
Carvedilol
　for heart failure, 732, 733t
　for hypertension, 695t
　poisoning, 140t
Caspofungin, **620**
　for candidiasis, 621
Castleman's disease, multicentric, 572
Cast nephropathy, 812t, 813
Cataplexy, 228, 229t, 230, 230t
Cataract, **295**
　drug-induced, 1139t
Cat bite, **118,** 119t, 478, 527
Catfish envenomation, 123
Catheter-related infection, 434
Cat-scratch disease, 118, 478, 526t, **527**
Cauda equina syndrome, 190, 1028
Causalgia, 34
Cavernous angioma, 82t
Cavernous sinus, anatomy of, 1025f
Cavernous sinus syndrome, 1025
Cefazolin
　for cellulitis, 479t
　indications for, 425t
　for infective endocarditis, 445t
　for osteomyelitis, 485t
　for peritonitis, 449
　resistance to, 425t
　for staphylococcal infections, 494t
Cefdinir, for otitis media, 303t
Cefepime
　for bacterial meningitis, 1046t, 1047t
　indications for, 425t
　for *P. aeruginosa* infections, 519t
　for pneumococcal infections, 488

　for pneumonia, 766t, 767t
　resistance to, 425t
　for sepsis/septic shock, 65t, 107t
Cefixime
　for gonococcal infections, 470t
　for urethritis in men, 463
Cefotaxime
　for bacterial meningitis, 1046t, 1047t
　for brain abscess, 1051
　for gonococcal infections, 470t
　for meningococcal infections, 506t
　for nocardiosis, 536t
　for pneumococcal infections, 488
　for pneumonia, 766t
　for sepsis/septic shock, 65t
　for spontaneous bacterial peritonitis, 274
Cefotetan
　for gonococcal infections, 470t
　indications for, 425t
　for pelvic inflammatory disease, 466
　resistance to, 425t
Cefoxitin
　for animal bite infections, 479t
　for gas gangrene, 480t
　for gonococcal infections, 470t
　for human bite infections, 119t
　for nontuberculous mycobacterial infec-
　　tions, 548
　for pelvic inflammatory disease, 466
Cefpodoxime
　for pneumococcal infections, 488
　for pneumonia, 766t
　for pyelonephritis, 818t
　for urethritis in men, 463
Ceftazidime
　for bacterial meningitis, 1046t, 1047t
　for brain abscess, 1051
　for febrile neutropenia in cancer patient,
　　115
　indications for, 425t
　for neutropenia, 346
　for osteomyelitis, 485t
　for otitis externa, 305
　for *P. aeruginosa* infections, 519t
　for peritonitis, 449
　for pneumonia, 767t
　resistance to, 425t
Ceftizoxime
　for gonococcal infections, 470t
　for nocardiosis, 536t
Ceftriaxone
　for arthritis, infectious, 482
　for bacterial meningitis, 108t, 1046t, 1047t
　for *Bartonella* infections, 526t
　for brain abscess, 109t, 1051
　for chancroid, 476
　for epididymitis, 463
　for epidural abscess, 109t
　for gonococcal infections, 470t
　for HACEK group infections, 512t
　for *H. influenzae* infections, 509
　indications for, 425t
　for infective endocarditis, 109t, 444t–445t,
　　446
　for leptospirosis, 553
　for Lyme borreliosis, 550–551
　for meningococcal infections, 506t
　　preventive treatment, 506t, 1045

for meningococcemia, 107t
for nocardiosis, 536t
for osteomyelitis, 485t
for otitis media, 303t
for pelvic inflammatory disease, 466
for peritonitis, 448
for pneumococcal infections, 488
for pneumonia, 766t, 767t
for post-splenectomy sepsis, 107t
for purpura fulminans, 108t
for pyelonephritis, 818t
resistance to, 425t
for sepsis/septic shock, 65t
for shigellosis, 459
for typhoid fever, 457
for urethritis in men, 463
for urinary tract infections, 819t
Cefuroxime
for otitis media, 303t
for pneumonia, 766t
Celecoxib
for colon cancer prevention, 1124
for pain, 36t–37t, 38
Celiac arteriography, 873
Cellophane tape methods, 421
Cellulitis, **478,** 479t
anaerobic, 531
auricular, 304
clostridial, 531
E. coli, 513–514
Klebsiella, 515
nocardiosis, 535, 536t
streptococcal, 478, 498–500, 498t
Central catheter, clotted, 112
Central European encephalitis, 596t–597t
Central nervous system (CNS) disease
cryptococcal, **623**
histoplasmosis, 629t
infections in immunocompromised patients, 434, 436t
listerial, 507
measles virus, 584–585
P. aeruginosa infections, 517, 519t
paraneoplastic, 407–408, 408t
syphilis, 473
toxoplasmosis, 646
Central pontine myelinolysis, 6
Central venous catheter infection, 430t
Cephalexin, for streptococcal infections, 498
Cerebellar degeneration, paraneoplastic, 407, 408t, 409t
Cerebral angiography, 88
Cerebral edema, 859
Cerebral herniation, 90, 91f
Cerebral palsy, 223
Cerebral perfusion pressure (CPP), 90
Cerebral salt wasting, 89
Cerebritis, 1042, 1050
Cerebrospinal fluid analysis
in bacterial meningitis, 1044–1045, 1045t
in chronic meningitis, 1052–1053
lumbar puncture, 27–28, 28f
reference values for specific analytes, 1162t
specimen collection and transport, 416t
in viral meningitis, 1046–1047
Cernunnos gene, 882

Ceruloplasmin, serum, 978
Cerumen impaction, 297–300
Cervical angina syndrome, 198
Cervical cancer, **397**
prevention of, 398, 477, 1124–1125
risk factors for, 1124
screening for, 398, 1123t
staging and prognosis in, 396t, 398
Cervical intraepithelial neoplasia, 1125
Cervical lymph node metastasis, **404**
Cervical spine disease, pain in, 176f, 178, 196
Cervicitis
chlamydial, 471
gonococcal, 465, 468
mucopurulent, **465**
Cestode infection, **655**
Cetirizine
for allergic rhinitis, 880
for urticaria/angioedema, 879
Cetuximab
for colorectal cancer, 387
for head and neck cancer, 368
toxicity of, 342t
Cevimeline, for Sjögren's syndrome, 891
Chagas' disease, **644**
acute, 644–645
chronic, 644–645
Chagoma, 644
Chancre, syphilitic, 472
Chancroid, **475,** 478
features of genital ulcers, 467t
Channelopathy, 1074
Charcoal, activated. *See* Activated charcoal
Charcot's joint, 473, 908
Charcot's triad, 848
Chelation therapy
for heavy metal poisoning, 157t, 159t
for hemochromatosis, 975
for radionuclide contamination, 174
Chemical bioterrorism, **168**
Chemotherapy, cancer. *See* Cancer chemotherapy
Chest pain, **175**
approach to, 177f, 178
causes of, 175–178, 175t
differential diagnosis of, 176f
in myocardial infarction, 700
noncardiac, **250**
Chest tube, 778, 780
Chest wall disease, 231, 748t, 782
Chest wall pain, 175t, 176f, 178
Chest x-ray
in cardiomyopathy, **684,** 684t
in congenital heart disease, **674**
in cor pulmonale, 735
in hemoptysis, 237
indications for, **22**
in interstitial lung disease, 774
in myocarditis, 687
normal radiograph, 23f
in pericardial disease, **688**
in pneumonia, 765
in pulmonary embolism, 770
in respiratory disease, 751
in superior vena cava syndrome, 112
utility of, **22**
in valvular heart disease, **678**
Cheyne-Stokes respiration, 53t

Chickenpox, **569**. *See also* Varicella-zoster virus infection
Chikungunya virus infection, 596
Child-Pugh classification, of cirrhosis, 869t
Chinese herbal nephropathy, 812
Chlamydial infection, **469, 561**
  cervicitis, 465, 471
  epididymitis, 463, 471
  pelvic inflammatory disease, 465, 471
  proctitis, 468, 471
  salpingitis, 471
  urethritis, 463–464, 471
Chlamydia pneumoniae infection, **563**
  atherosclerosis and, 563
Chlamydia psittaci infection, **562**
Chlamydia trachomatis infection, **469, 561**
Chloral hydrate poisoning, 144t
Chlorambucil, 341t
Chloramphenicol
  for *Bartonella* infections, 526t
  for meningococcal infections, 506t
  for plague, 164t, 526
  for relapsing fever, 553
  for Rocky Mountain spotted fever, 555
  for scrub typhus, 557
  for tick-borne spotted fevers, 555
  for tularemia, 165t, 524
Chlordiazepoxide
  dosage and action of, 1089t
  poisoning, 143t
Chloroquine
  for inflammatory bowel disease, 840
  for malaria, 638t
    preventive treatment, 640t
  poisoning, 153t
  for porphyria cutanea tarda, 977
Chlorpheniramine
  for allergic rhinitis, 880
  for urticaria/angioedema, 879
Chlorpromazine
  for delirium, 50t
  dosage and adverse effects of, 138t, 139t, 1091t
  for migraine, 186t
  for serotonin syndrome, 152t
Chlorthalidone
  for edema, 243t
  for hypertension, 695t
Cholangiography, 270
Cholangiopancreatography, 846t, 848
Cholangitis, **847**
  E. coli, 513
  primary sclerosing, **848**
Cholecystectomy, 845, 847–848
Cholecystitis
  acute, **845**
  chronic, **847**
Choledocholithiasis, **847**
Cholelithiasis, **844**, 846t
Cholera, **453**
Cholera vaccine, 1116t
Cholestasis, liver function tests in, 268t
Cholesteatoma, 298
Cholesterol
  blood
    cardiovascular disease and, 1118–1119, 1119t

    goals and cutpoints for therapeutic intervention, 1119t
    reference values for laboratory tests, 1161t
  HDL, 968–970, 969t
  LDL, 968–970, 969t
  total, 968–970, 969t
Cholesterol emboli, 821
Cholesterol gallstones, 844
Cholestyramine
  for erythropoietic porphyria, 978
  for hyperlipidemia, 972t
  for irritable bowel syndrome, 841, 842t
  for nephrolithiasis, 828t
  for primary biliary cirrhosis, 871
  for primary sclerosing cholangitis, 848
  for toxic and drug-induced hepatitis, 858
  for viral hepatitis, 858
Cholinergic crisis, 169
Cholinergic poisoning, 131t, 142t
Cholinesterase inhibitors, for Alzheimer's disease, 1000
CHOP regimen, for follicular lymphoma, 357
Choreoathetosis, 223
Choriocarcinoma, 393
Chronic fatigue syndrome, **290**, 1078
  CDC criteria for diagnosis of, 290t
Chronic kidney disease, **794**
Chronic obstructive pulmonary disease (COPD), **759**
  dyspnea in, 231, 233
  pulmonary function tests in, 759, 760t, 761
  sleep disorders in, 228
  treatment of
    exacerbations of, 762–763
    outpatient therapy, 761–762
    surgery, 762
Chronic progressive external ophthalmoplegia (CPEO), 1074
Churg-Strauss syndrome, **891**
Chvostek's sign, 963
Chylothorax, **780**
Ciclopirox olamine, 620
  for dermatophyte infections, 317
Cidofovir
  for adenovirus infections, 583
  for cytomegalovirus infections, 574
Ciguatera poisoning, **123**
Cilostazol, for arteriosclerosis, 739
Cimetidine
  for antivenom reaction, 122
  for erosive gastropathies, 834
Ciprofloxacin
  for *Aeromonas* infections, 516
  for animal bite infections, 119t, 479t
  for anthrax, 164t
  for arthritis, infectious, 482
  for *Bartonella* infections, 526t
  for campylobacteriosis, 458
  for chancroid, 476
  for cholecystitis, 847
  for cholera, 453
  for diverticulitis, 842
  indications for, 427t
  for inflammatory bowel disease, 840
  for intestinal pseudoobstruction, 843

for meningococcal disease prevention, 506t, 1045
for necrotizing fasciitis, 480t
for osteomyelitis, 485t
for *P. aeruginosa* infections, 519t–520t
for perichondritis, 304
for peritonitis prevention, 449
for plague, 526
for pneumonia, 766t, 767t
for Q fever, 559
resistance to, 427t
for sepsis/septic shock, 65t
for shigellosis, 459
for staphylococcal infections, 494t, 496
for tick-borne spotted fevers, 555
for tuberculosis, 542
for tularemia, 165t
for typhoid fever, 457
Circadian rhythm disorder, 226, **230**
Circulatory function tests, reference values for, 1166t
Circulatory overload, 44
Cirrhosis, **868**
ascites in, **272**, 273t
causes of, 868t
Child-Pugh classification of, 869t
complications of, 868, 869t
edema in, 241, 243
liver function tests in, 268t
primary bacterial peritonitis in, **448**
primary biliary, **870**
Cisplatin
for bladder cancer, 392
for cervical cancer, 398
for endometrial cancer, 397
for extragonadal germ cell tumor, 402
for gastric cancer, 381
for head and neck cancer, 368
for lung cancer, 371
for ovarian cancer, 397
for testicular cancer, 394
toxicity of, 341t
Citalopram
for depression, 50
dosage and adverse effects of, 1086t
Citrate therapy
for nephrolithiasis, 828t
for renal tubular acidosis, 815
Citrobacter infection, 516
Cladribine
for follicular lymphoma, 357
toxicity of, 341t
Clarithromycin
for *H. influenzae* infections, 509
for *H. pylori* eradication, 833t
indications for, 426t
for *Legionella* infections, 522
for *M. pneumoniae* infections, 560
for nontuberculous mycobacterial infections, 548–549
for pertussis, 510
for pneumonia, 766t
resistance to, 426t
Claustrophobia, 1083
Clenched-fist injury, 118, 119t
Clindamycin
for actinomycosis, 538
adverse reactions to, 424

for anaerobic infections, 534
for animal bite infections, 119t, 479t
for anthrax, 164t
for babesiosis, 107t, 642
for bacterial vaginosis, 464
for cellulitis, 479t
for clostridial infections, 108t, 532
for diphtheria, 502
for erythroderma, 108t
for gas gangrene, 480t
indications for, 426t
for malaria, 638t
for necrotizing fasciitis, 108t, 479t–480t
for osteomyelitis, 485t
for otitis media, 303t
for pelvic inflammatory disease, 466
for pneumococcal infections, 488
for *Pneumocystis* infections, 634t, 635
resistance to, 426t
for sepsis/septic shock, 65t
for staphylococcal infections, 496
for streptococcal infections, 498t
for toxic shock syndrome, 108t
for toxoplasmosis, 647
Clinical chemistry, reference values for laboratory tests, 1145t–1156t
Clofazimine, for leprosy, 547
Clomiphene citrate, for female infertility, 958
Clomipramine
for daytime sleepiness, 230
dosage and adverse effects of, 1086t
for OCD, 1082
Clonazepam
dosage and action of, 1089t
for dyspnea, 49t
for myoclonus, 224
for pain, 37t
poisoning, 143t
for posthypoxic myoclonus, 98
for seizures, 994t
for vertigo, 214t
Clonidine
for menopausal symptoms, 957
for narcotic withdrawal, 1100
poisoning, 139t
for smoking cessation, 1127
for tics, 224
Clonorchiasis, 654
Clopidogrel
for angina pectoris, 716
for myocardial infarction, 710, 712
preventive treatment, 709
for stroke prevention, 85
for thrombotic disorders, 338
for unstable angina, 710
Clostridial infection, **530**
bacteremia and sepsis, 531
food poisoning, 453
myonecrosis. *See* Gas gangrene
skin/soft tissue, 531
Clostridium botulinum infection. *See* Botulism
Clostridium difficile-associated disease (CDAD), 431, **461**
Clostridium tetani infection. *See* Tetanus
Clotrimazole, 620
for candidiasis, 252, 464

Clozapine
dosage and adverse effects of, 139t, 1091t
for schizophrenia, 1081
Clubbing, 239, 369
Cluster headache, 183–184, 183t
CMV regimen, for bladder cancer, 392
Coagulase-negative staphylococci, **493**
Coagulation disorders, **334**
dilutional, 334
drug-induced, 1134t
intracranial hemorrhage in, 82t
in liver disease, 269
reference values for laboratory tests, 1142t–1144t
Coal tar shampoo, 315
Coal worker's pneumoconiosis, **758**
Coarctation of the aorta, **676**
hypertension in, 693
Cocaine, 136t, 152t, 153t
Coccidioidomycosis, **628**
cavitary pulmonary, 630
disseminated, 630
meningitis, 630
primary pulmonary, 629–630
Cochlear implant, 300
Cockcroft-Gault formula, 276
Codeine
for cough, 235
for dyspnea, 49t
for hemoptysis, 238
narcotic abuse, **1099**
for pain, 36t–37t
CODOX-M regimen, for Burkitt's lymphoma, 360
Cognitive-behavioral psychotherapy, 1082
Cogwheeling, 1002
Colchicine
for amyloidosis, 915
for gout, 904
for pericarditis, 688
for pseudogout, 906
Colectomy, 383, 840, 1124
Colesevelam, for hyperlipidemia, 972t
Colestipol, for hyperlipidemia, 972t
Colitis
amebic, 460–461
drug-induced, 1137t–1138t
ischemic, 843
ulcerative. *See* Ulcerative colitis
Colon cut-off sign, 850
Colonic angiodysplasia, **843**
Colonic disease, **840**
Colonic polyps, **383**
hereditary syndromes, **383,** 384t
Colonoscopy, 387, 1122, 1123t
for colonic polyps, 383
in diarrhea, 256
for GI bleeding, 261
virtual, 387
Color vision, drug-induced abnormalities, 1139t
Colorectal cancer, **385**
advanced tumor, 387
local disease, 387
pathology of, 385, 386f
prevention of, 387, 1124
risk factors for, 1124

screening for, 387, 1105t, 1122, 1123t
staging and prognosis for, 386f
Coma, **74**
approach to, 77–79
differential diagnosis of, 76t
eye movements in, 78–79
in head trauma, 93
hyperosmolar, **100**
myxedema, 927–928
pupillary signs in, 78
respiratory patterns in, 79
responsiveness in, 78
Common cold, 301
coronavirus, 581
human RSV, 582
rhinovirus, 581
Common variable immunodeficiency, 884
Complete transposition of the great arteries, **677**
Complex regional pain syndrome, **1018**
Compulsive personality disorder, 1084
Computed tomography (CT)
in coma, 79
in heart disease, 672t, 673
hepatobiliary, 270, 846t
in increased intracranial pressure, 91
indications for, **24**
neuroimaging, 986, 987t
in osteomyelitis, 484t
in poisoning, 133
in respiratory disease, 751
in stroke, 80, 85
in subarachnoid hemorrhage, 88
utility of, **24**
Concussion, 91, 93
Conduction aphasia, 225–226
Condyloma acuminatum, 310f
Condylomata lata, 472
Confusion, **74**
Congenital heart disease, **674**
acyanotic lesions with left-to-right shunt, **674**
acyanotic lesions without shunt, **676**
complex heart lesions, **677**
echocardiography in, 671
endocarditis prophylaxis in, **677**
pulmonary hypertension in, 675
Congenital rubella syndrome, 585–586
Conjunctivitis
acute hemorrhagic, enterovirus, 590
adult inclusion, **561**
Connective tissue disease, **885**
interstitial lung disease in, 775–776
mixed, **890**
rheumatoid arthritis, **886**
Sjögren's syndrome, **890**
SLE, 885
systemic sclerosis, **888**
Consciousness, disorders of, **74,** 91
Constipation, **257**
causes of, 257–258
drug-induced, 257, 1137t–1138t
irritable bowel syndrome, **840,** 842t
in terminally ill patient, 48
treatment of, 48, 48t, 258–259
Contact precautions, 429
Continuous renal replacement therapy, 793
Contraception, **957**

Controller therapy, for asthma, 755
Conversion disorder, 1083
Coordination, testing of, **986**
Copper metabolism, 978
Coprolalia, 223
Corneal abrasion, 294
Coronary arteriography, 711, 714
Coronary artery bypass surgery, 711, 716, 717t
Coronary artery disease (CAD), 709, 710f, 712
    laboratory features of, 713–714, 713f, 714t
    stress testing in, 713–714, 713f, 714t
    treatment of
        drug therapy, 714–716, 715t
        mechanical revascularization, 716, 717t
Coronary artery spasm, 714
Coronary vasospasm, **716**
Coronavirus infection, **581**
Cor pulmonale, **735**
Corrosive ingestion, 135
Corticosteroid therapy
    for asthma, 754–756
    for COPD, 762
Cortisol, excess of, **934**
Cortisone
    for hypopituitarism, 922t
    steroid preparations, 938–939, 938t
Corynebacterium diphtheriae infection. See Diphtheria
Corynebacterium infection, nondiphtherial species, **503**
Costochondral pain, 178
Cough, **233**
    approach to, 234–235, 234f
    drug-induced, 1136t
    treatment of, 235, 236f
Cough headache, 189
Cover test, 217
COX-2 inhibitors, for osteoarthritis, 902
Coxiella burnetii infection. See Q fever
Coxsackievirus infection, **588**. See also Enteroviral infection
C-PAP, nasal, 784
CPPD deposition disease. See Pseudogout
Cranial nerves
    CN I. See Olfactory nerve
    CN II, 979–980
    CN III, 981–982
    CN IV, 981–982
    CN V. See Trigeminal nerve
    CN VI, 981–982
    CN VII. See Facial nerve
    CN VIII, 982–984
    CN IX, 984
    CN X. See Vagus nerve
    CN XI. See Accessory nerve
    CN XII. See Hypoglossal nerve
    disorders of, **1020**
        multiple cranial nerve palsies, **1024**
    examination of, **979**
C-reactive protein, 1120
Creatinine, serum, 795
Creatinine clearance, 274, 276
Crescent sign, 909
CREST syndrome, 889
Creutzfeldt-Jakob disease, 997t, 998, **1002**
Crimean Congo hemorrhagic fever, 598

Critical care medicine, **30**
Critically ill patient, **30**
    initial evaluation of, 30
    limitation or withdrawal of care, 33
    mechanical ventilation, **30**
    monitoring in ICU, **32**
    multiorgan system failure, **32**
    neurologic dysfunction, 33
    prevention of complications, **33**
    shock, **30**
Crocodile tears, 1021
Crohn's disease, **837**
    epidemiology of, 836, 836t
    extraintestinal manifestations of, 838
    treatment of, 838, 839f, 840
Cromolyn sodium
    for allergic rhinitis, 880
    for asthma, 755
    for systemic mastocytosis, 881
Crossed SLR sign, 190
Croup, **306**, 583–584
Crust (skin lesion), 313t, 477
Cryoglobulinemia, 807t
    essential mixed, **892**
Cryoprecipitate, 45, 335
Cryotherapy
    for HPV infection, 476
    for warts, 317
Cryptococcoma, 623
Cryptococcosis, 201, **623**
    pulmonary, 623, 626
Cryptosporidiosis, 420t, 421, **455**
Crystalloids, for antivenom reaction, 122
Cullen's sign, 849
Culture
    diagnosis of infectious disease, 411–413
    specimen collection and transport for, 414t–419t
CURB-65, 765
Cushing's syndrome, 694, **934**
    paraneoplastic, 405, 935
Cyanide poisoning, 145t
Cyanosis, **239**
    causes of, 240t
    central, 239, 240t
    peripheral, 239, 240t
Cyclic adenosine monophosphate eyedrops, 891
Cyclic vomiting syndrome, 245t
Cyclobenzaprine
    for back pain, 196
    for multiple sclerosis, 1041
    poisoning, 138t, 144t
Cyclopentolate, for corneal abrasion, 294
Cyclophosphamide
    for acute renal failure, 793
    for breast cancer, 376, 378
    for Burkitt's lymphoma/leukemia, 359
    for CLL, 356
    for gastric cancer, 381
    for idiopathic thrombocytopenic purpura, 335
    for inflammatory myopathy, 1072
    for multiple sclerosis, 1039
    for myasthenia gravis, 1066
    for polyneuropathy, 1061
    for rheumatoid arthritis, 888
    for SLE, 803, 886

Cyclophosphamide (*Cont.*):
  for systemic sclerosis, 889
  toxicity of, 341t
  for vasculitis, 894
Cyclosarin, 169–171
Cyclosporiasis, **456**
Cyclosporine
  for aplastic anemia, 329
  immunosuppression for renal transplant, 799–800
  for inflammatory bowel disease, 840
  for inflammatory myopathy, 1072
  for membranous glomerulonephritis, 804
  for myasthenia gravis, 1066
  for polyneuropathy, 1061
  for primary sclerosing cholangitis, 849
  for psoriasis, 314
  for rheumatoid arthritis, 888
Cyclosporine eyedrops, 890–891
Cyproheptadine
  for ergot alkaloid poisoning, 137t
  for serotonin syndrome, 152t
  for urticaria/angioedema, 879
Cystectomy, 392
Cysticercosis, **655**, 656t
Cystine stones, 827, 828t
Cystitis, **815**, 818t
  hemorrhagic, drug-induced, 341t, 1138t
Cytarabine
  for acute lymphoblastic leukemia and lym-
      phoblastic lymphoma, 359
  for AML, 346
  toxicity of, 341t
Cytoadherence, 636
Cytokeratin, in cancer of unknown primary,
      402, 404f
Cytomegalic inclusion disease, 573
Cytomegalovirus immune globulin, 574
Cytomegalovirus infection, **572**
  congenital, 573
  in HIV/AIDS, 573–574
  in immunocompromised host, 573, 800
  mononucleosis, 573
  neurologic disease, 573
  perinatal, 573
  pneumonia, 573–574
  retinitis, 573

D

Dacarbazine
  for melanoma, 365
  toxicity of, 341t
Dactinomycin, 342t
Dalbavancin, for staphylococcal infections,
      494t
Dalteparin, for thrombotic disorders, 336
Danazol, for autoimmune hemolysis, 329
Dantrolene
  for malignant hyperthermia, 203
  for multiple sclerosis, 1041
Dapsone
  for leprosy, 547
  for *Pneumocystis* infections, 634t, 635
    preventive treatment, 635t
  poisoning, 146t
  for recluse spider bite, 125
Daptomycin
  adverse reactions to, 424

  for enterococcal infections, 501
  indications for, 426t
  resistance to, 426t
  for staphylococcal infections, 493, 494t
Darunavir, for HIV/AIDS, 614t
Dasatinib
  for CML, 349
  toxicity of, 342t
Daunorubicin
  for acute lymphoblastic leukemia and lym-
      phoblastic lymphoma, 350
  for AML, 346
  toxicity of, 341t
Daytime sleepiness, excessive, 226, **228,**
      229t, 784
DDAVP
  for hypernatremia, 7
  for hyponatremia, 7
  for von Willebrand disease, 335
Death and dying, **46**
  brain death, 79
  leading causes of death by age, 1103,
      1104t–1105t
Death rattle, 52t
Debranching enzyme deficiency, 1073
Decerebration, 78
Decitabine, for myelodysplastic syndromes,
      350
Decongestants
  for chronic fatigue syndrome, 291
  poisoning, 136t, 139t
  for sinusitis, 302
Decontamination, after nerve agent exposure,
      169
Decortication, 78
Deep-brain stimulation, 223, 1007
Deep venous thrombosis, **741, 769**
  causes of, 741, 741t
  prevention of, 731, 741
  thrombotic disorders, **336**
  treatment of, 336–338, 337t, 741, 770–772
Defecation, 253
Deferasirox, for thalassemia, 328
Deferoxamine
  for hemochromatosis, 975
  for iron poisoning, 147t
  for thalassemia, 328
Dehydration, in terminally ill patient, 52t
Delavirdine, for HIV/AIDS, 606, 609t
Delayed sleep phase syndrome, 226, 230
Delirium, **74,** 75t
  drug-induced, 75t, 1140t
  step-wise evaluation of, 75–76, 77t
  in terminally ill patient, 50, 53t
  treatment of, 50, 50t, 76
Delirium tremens, 1096–1098
Demeclocycline
  for hyponatremia, 406
  for SIADH, 114, 406, 925
Dementia, **995.** See also *specific types*
  diagnosis of, 995, 996t, 997t, 999t
  differentiation of major types, 997t
  sleep disorders in, 227
Dementia with Lewy bodies, 995–998, 997t,
      1001
Dengue fever, **595,** 1116
Dengue hemorrhagic fever/dengue toxic
      shock syndrome, 110, **599**

Denileukin diftitox, 342t
Dental procedures, endocarditis prophylaxis before, 447t, 448
Dependent personality disorder, 1084
Depression
  drug-induced, 1078, 1140t
  major, **1077**
  with medical illness, 1078
  in terminally ill patient, 49–50
  treatment of, 50, 1078–1079, 1079f, 1088
  weight loss in, 247
Dermatitis, **315**
  allergic contact, 315
  atopic, 310f, 311f, 315
  drug-induced, 1133t
  irritant contact, 315
  seborrheic, 315
  stasis, 311f
Dermatofibroma, 311f
Dermatomes, 982f–983f
Dermatomyositis, 1072, 1073t
Dermatophyte infections, 311, **317**
Desipramine
  dosage and adverse effects of, 1086t
  for pain, 36t–37t
Desloradine, for allergic rhinitis, 880
Desmopressin
  for diabetes insipidus, 924–925
  for hypopituitarism, 922t
Device-related infections, **429**
Devic's syndrome, 1041
Dexamethasone
  for bacterial meningitis, 1045
  for brain tumor, 1031
  for *H. influenzae* infections, 509
  for hirsutism, 955
  for increased intracranial pressure, 92t
  for multiple myeloma, 361
  for nausea and vomiting, 343–344
  for spinal cord compression, 95, 113
  steroid preparations, 938–939, 938t
  for typhoid fever, 457
Dexamethasone test, 934
Dextroamphetamine, for daytime sleepiness, 230
Dextromethorphan
  for cough, 235
  poisoning, 152t
Diabetes insipidus, **923**
  central, 7, 276t, 277, 923
  drug-induced, 8, 1138t
  gestational, 923
  nephrogenic, 7, 276t, 277–278, 788, 923
  treatment of, 7–8, 924–925
Diabetes mellitus, **942**
  cardiovascular disease and, 1120
  clinical features of, 942–943
  depression in, 1078
  diagnosis of, 942, 943t
  nephropathy, **805,** 945
  neuropathy in, 1016, 1061
  retinopathy in, **296,** 297f
  risk factors for, 943t
  treatment of, 943–947, 944t–946t, 1120
    hospitalized patient, 946–947, 946t
  type 1, 942
  type 2, 942
  in women, 1129

Diabetic ketoacidosis, 21, **100,** 943, 947
  laboratory values in, 100f, 101
  treatment of, 19, 101, 102t
Dialysis, **796**
  for acute renal failure, 793
  hemodialysis, **797**
  for hypercalcemia, 962t
  peritoneal, **797**
Diarrhea, **254**
  from altered intestinal motility, 254
  C. difficile-associated disease, **461**
  chronic, physical examination in, 255t
  from decreased absorptive state, 254, 259t
  drug-induced, 1137t–1138t
  exudative, 254
  hemorrhagic, adenovirus, 583
  infectious, 254–255, 255t, **451**
    inflammatory, 452t, **456**
    noninflammatory, **451,** 452t
    pathogens causing, 452t
    penetrating, 452t
  irritable bowel syndrome, **840,** 842t
  metabolic acidosis in, 17t, 18
  nosocomial, 431
  osmotic, 254, 256
  in returned traveler, 1117
  secretory, 254
  stool examination, 256
  treatment of, 256, 257f, 258f
Diascopy, 312
Diastolic failure, 730
Diazepam
  for alcohol withdrawal, 1098
  dosage and action of, 1089t
  for isoniazid poisoning, 150t
  for multiple sclerosis, 1041
  for muscle spasms, 123
  for myocardial infarction, 702
  for nerve agent exposure, 170t, 171
  poisoning, 143t
  for tetanus, 529
  for vertigo, 214t
Dichloralphenazone, for migraine, 186t
Dicloxacillin
  for auricular cellulitis, 304
  for streptococcal infections, 498
Dicyclomine
  for diverticular disease, 842
  for irritable bowel syndrome, 841
  poisoning, 138t
Didanosine, for HIV/AIDS, 607t
Dietary reference intake (DRI), 39
Diethylcarbamazine, for filariasis, 652
Diethylstilbestrol, 342t
Diffuse large B cell lymphoma, 358, 380–381
Diffuse white matter disease, 996t, 1000–1001, 1001f
DiGeorge's syndrome, 883
Digitalis
  for heart failure, 732t
  for mitral stenosis, 678
Digitalis toxicity, 722t, 733–734
Digital rectal exam, 387, 399–400, 400f, 1123t, 1124
Digoxin
  for arrhythmias, 728t, 736
  for atrial fibrillation, 726
  for heart failure, 732–733

Digoxin (*Cont.*):
for mitral regurgitation, 679
poisoning, 141t
for supraventricular arrhythmias, 704
for tachyarrhythmias, 722t–723t
Digoxin-specific antibody fragments, 141t
Dihydroergotamine, for migraine, 185t–186t, 187t
Diltiazem
for aortic dissection, 738
for arrhythmias, 728t
for atrial fibrillation, 726
for hypertension, 695t
for hypertrophic cardiomyopathy, 686
for mitral stenosis, 678
for myocardial infarction, 711
poisoning, 140t
for supraventricular arrhythmias, 704
for tachyarrhythmias, 722t–723t
for unstable angina, 711
for Wolff-Parkinson-White syndrome, 729
Diluting agent, for radionuclide contamination, 174
Dimenhydrinate
for nausea and vomiting, 245
for vertigo, 214t
Dimercaprol
for arsenic poisoning, 155t
for heavy metal poisoning, 157t, 159t
Dioctyl sodium sulfosuccinate, for hemorrhoids, 844
Diphenhydramine
for allergic rhinitis, 880
for anaphylaxis, 117
for antivenom reaction, 122
for extrapyramidal reactions, 149t
poisoning, 138t, 153t
for urticaria/angioedema, 879
Diphenoxylate
for diarrhea, 256
for inflammatory bowel disease, 838
for irritable bowel syndrome, 841
narcotic abuse, **1099**
Diphtheria, **501**
Diphtheria antitoxin, 502
Diphtheria-tetanus vaccine, 438t
Diphtheria toxin, 501
Diphtheria vaccine, 503
Diphyllobothriasis, **657**
Dipyrimadole
for stroke prevention, 85
for thrombotic disorders, 338
Disease prevention, **1103**
immunization, **1107**
U.S. Preventive Services Task Force recommendations, 1106t
Disequilibrium syndrome, dialysis, 797
Disopyramide
for angina pectoris, 715
for arrhythmias, 727t
for hypertrophic cardiomyopathy, 686
Disseminated intravascular coagulation (DIC), 332–335
Distributive shock, 59t, 60t
Disulfiram, for alcoholic rehabilitation, 1098
Diuresis, osmotic, 276t
Diuretics
for ascites, 272

for chronic glomerulonephritis, 808
complications of, 10, 244t
for cor pulmonale, 735
for diabetic nephropathy, 806
for edema, 243, 243t
for heart failure, 731, 732t, 733t, 735
for hypertension, 695–696, 695t, 697t, 796
for mitral regurgitation, 679
for myocardial infarction, 705, 706t
for nephrolithiasis, 828t
for pulmonary hypertension, 745
for restrictive cardiomyopathy, 686
for tricuspid regurgitation, 683
Divalproex, for generalized anxiety disorder, 1082
Diverticular disease, **841**
asymptomatic, 841
hemorrhage in, 842
Diverticulitis, 841–842
Diverticulosis, 261, 263
Dizziness, **211**
DLCO (diffusing capacity of lung), 749–750
DNA-dependent tyrosine kinase gene, 882
Dobutamine
for beta blocker poisoning, 140t
for heart failure, 734, 734t
for myocardial infarction, 705, 705t, 706t
for pulmonary edema, 68
for shock, 62, 62t, 66
Docetaxel, 341t
Docusate salts
for constipation, 48t, 259
for myocardial infarction, 702
Dofetilide, for arrhythmias, 728t
Dog bite, **117**, 119t, 478
Döhle bodies, 322
Domestic violence, 1130
Donepezil, for Alzheimer's disease, 1000
Donovanosis, **476**
features of genital ulcers, 467t
Dopamine
for anaphylaxis, 117
for beta blocker poisoning, 140t
for calcium channel blocker poisoning, 140t
for cardiac glycoside poisoning, 141t
for heart failure, 734, 734t
for increased intracranial pressure, 92t
for myocardial infarction, 705, 705t, 706t
for shock, 62, 62t, 707
for sympatholytic poisoning, 139t
Dopamine agonists
for hyperprolactinemia, 920
for Parkinson's disease, 1003–1004, 1005t–1006t
Dorsal root ganglionopathy, paraneoplastic, 407–408, 408t
Dothiepin, for migraine prevention, 188t
Double vision, **217**, 218t, 293
monocular, 217
Doxepin
dosage and adverse effects of, 138t, 141t, 1086t
for pain, 36t–37t
Doxorubicin
for bladder cancer, 392
for breast cancer, 376, 378
for Burkitt's lymphoma/leukemia, 360

for carcinoid tumor, 389
for endometrial cancer, 397
for gastric cancer, 381
for islet-cell tumors, 391
for multiple myeloma, 361
toxicity of, 341t
for Zollinger-Ellison syndrome, 836
Doxycycline
for animal bite infections, 479t
for anthrax, 164t
for bacillary angiomatosis, 479t
for *Bartonella* infections, 526t
for *B. cepacia*, 518
for brucellosis, 523
for cholera, 453
during COPD exacerbations, 763
for *C. psittaci* infections, 563
for *C. trachomatis* infections, 562
for donovanosis, 476
for endemic treponematosis, 551
for epididymitis, 463
for human granulocytotropic anaplasmosis, 558
indications for, 426t
for *Legionella* infections, 522
for leptospirosis, 553
for Lyme borreliosis, 550
for lymphatic filariasis, 652
for lymphogranuloma venereum, 471
for malaria, 638t
preventive treatment, 640t
for *M. pneumoniae* infections, 560
for murine typhus, 556
for onchocerciasis, 653
for pelvic inflammatory disease, 466
for plague, 164t, 526
for pneumococcal infections, 488
for pneumonia, 766t
for Q fever, 559
for relapsing fever, 553
resistance to, 426t
for rickettsialpox, 556
for Rocky Mountain spotted fever, 108t, 555
for rodent bite infections, 120t
for staphylococcal infections, 494t, 496
for syphilis, 474t
for tick-borne spotted fevers, 555
for tularemia, 165t
for typhus, 557
for urethritis in men, 463
Doxylamine poisoning, 138t
Dronabinol, for weight loss, 248
Droplet precautions, 429
Drowsiness, drug-induced, 1140t
Drug-induced illness
acne, 1133t
Addison's disease, 1132t
agranulocytosis, 1134t
airway obstruction, 1136t
alopecia, 341t, 1133t
anaphylaxis, 1131t
anemia, 325, 327, 327t, 344, 1135t
angina, 1135t
angioedema, 1131t
arrhythmia, 1135t
autonomic nervous system disease, 1015
AV block, 718t, 1136t

bladder dysfunction, 1138t
bone disease, 1140t
cardiomyopathy, 1136t
cataract, 1139t
coagulation disorders, 1134t
colitis, 1137t
color vision disturbance, 1139t
constipation/ileus, 257, 1137t
cough, 1136t
delirium, 75t
depression, 1078, 1140t
dermatitis, 1133t–1134t
diabetes insipidus, 8
diarrhea, 1137t
drowsiness, 1140t
eczema, 1133t
edema, 241t, 342t
eosinophilia, 1134t
erythema multiforme, 1133t
erythema nodosum, 1133t
extrapyramidal effects, 1138t
fatigue, 289, 289t
fever, 1132t
fluid retention, 1136t
galactorrhea, 1132t
glaucoma, 1139t
gynecomastia, 342t, 1132t
hallucinations, 1140t
headache, 1138t
hearing loss, 300, 1139t
heart disease, 342t
heat stroke, 203
hemorrhagic cystitis, 341t, 1138t
hepatitis, 858
hirsutism, 955
hyperbilirubinemia, 1132t
hypercalcemia, 1132t
hyperglycemia, 1132t
hyperkalemia, 10, 12t, 13f, 1132t
hyperpigmentation, 1133t
hyperprolactinemia, 919
hyperpyrexia, 1132t
hypertension, 1136t
hyperuricemia, 1133t
hypocalcemia, 342t
hypoglycemia, 103, 1132t
hypokalemia, 10, 1133t
hypomania, 1140t
hyponatremia, 1133t
hypotension, 1136t
hypothermia, 128t
hypothrombinemia, 1134t
insomnia, 227
interstitial lung disease, 774
intracranial hemorrhage in, 82t
jaundice, 266t, 1137t
leukemia, 341t
leukocytosis, 1135t
leukopenia, 331
lichenoid eruptions, 1134t
liver disease, 1137t
lupus, 885, 1131t
lymphadenopathy, 1135t
malabsorption, 1137t
mania, 1140t
metabolic acidosis, 17t, 1133t
myalgia, 1140t
myelosuppression, 341t–342t

Drug-induced illness (*Cont.*):
  myopathy, **1074**, 1075t, 1140t
  myositis, 1140t
  nausea and vomiting, 245t, 341t–342t,
      343–344, 1137t
  nephritis, 810–812, 811t, 1138t
  nephropathy, 1138t
  nephrotic syndrome, 1138t
  neutropenia, 329, 344
  obesity, 940
  optic neuritis, 1139t
  oral conditions, 1137t
  pancreatitis, 1138t
  pancytopenia, 1135t
  peptic ulcer disease, 1138t
  pericarditis, 1136t
  peripheral neuropathy, 341t, 1138t
  pill-related esophagitis, 252
  pseudotumor cerebri, 1139t
  pulmonary edema, 1136t
  pulmonary fibrosis, 341t–342t
  pulmonary infiltrate, 1136t
  pure red cell aplasia, 1135t
  purpura, 1134t
  renal tubular acidosis, 1138t
  retinopathy, 1139t
  schizophrenic-like reactions, 1140t
  seizure, 990t, 1139t
  serum sickness, 1132t
  sexual dysfunction, 1132t
  SIADH, 341t
  skin disorders, 319, 1134t
  sleep disorders, 1140t
  stroke, 1139t
  thrombocytopenia, 332, 344, 1135t
  thromboembolism, 1136t
  thyroid disease, 1132t
  toxic epidermal necrolysis, 1134t
  treatment of, 343–344
  urinary calculi, 1138t
  urinary tract obstruction, 1138t
  urticaria, 1134t
  vestibular disorders, 1139t
  weight loss, 248t
Drug monitoring, therapeutic, reference val-
      ues for laboratory tests,
      1157t–1159t
Drug overdose, **130**. *See also* Poisoning
  reference values for laboratory tests,
      1157t–1159t
  treatment of, 133–160, 134t, 136t–159t
Drusen, 296, 296f
DTaP vaccine, 503, 1108t–1109t
Dual-energy x-ray absorptiometry, 967, 967t
Duchenne dystrophy, **1068**
Ductal carcinoma in situ, 376
Duke criteria, for infective endocarditis, 442,
      443t
Duloxetine
  dosage and adverse effects of, 1086t
  for pain, 36t–37t
  for polyneuropathy, 1061
Duodenal ulcer, 831–834 833t
Durable attorney for health care, 47
Durie-Salmon staging, for multiple my-
      eloma, 362t
Dysautonomia, 1013, 1018
Dysbetalipoproteinemia, 969t, **974**

Dysentery, 452t, 453
  amebic, 460–461
Dysfunctional uterine bleeding, 952
Dyskinesia, 1004
Dyslipidemia, **968**
  in diabetes mellitus, 945–946
  metabolic syndrome, **699**, 700t
Dysmenorrhea
  primary, 954
  secondary, 954
Dyspepsia, 246
  functional, 246
  peptic ulcer disease, 246
Dysphagia, **249, 1024**
  esophageal, 250
  oropharyngeal, 250
  in terminally ill patient, 52t
Dysphonia, **1024**
Dyspnea, **231**
  approach to, 68f, 232f, 233
  ARDS, **69**
  cardiac vs. pulmonary, 232t
  paroxysmal nocturnal, 228, 233
  pulmonary edema, acute, **66**
  in terminally ill patient, 49, 53t
  treatment of, 49, 49t
Dystonia, 223
  focal, 223
  generalized, 223
  idiopathic torsional, 223

E
Ear disease
  anaerobic infections, 533
  drug-induced, 1139t
  external ear infections, **304**
  hearing loss, **297**
  middle ear infections, **305**
Eastern equine encephalitis, **595**, 596t–597t
Eating disorder, **1093**
  clinical features of, 1093–1094
  treatment of, 1094–1095, 1095f
  in women, 1129
Ebola virus infection, 110, **599**
Ebstein anomaly, **677**
Echinocandins, **620**
Echinococcosis, **656**
Echinocytes, 321
Echocardiography, **669**
  in aortic disease, 671, 672t, 736, 738
  in cardiac mass, 670, 672t
  in cardiomyopathy, **684**, 684t
  chamber size and ventricular performance,
      669
  clinical uses of, 669t, 670, 671f
  in congenital heart disease, 671, **674**
  in coronary artery disease, 713–714, 714t
  in cor pulmonale, 735
  2-D echo, 669t, 670f
  Doppler, 669t
      normal values in adults, 1168t
  in endocarditis, 442
  in heart failure, **730**
  in myocardial infarction, 701
  in myocarditis, 687
  in pericardial disease, 670, 672t, **688**, 691,
      691f
  in pericardial effusion/tamponade, 112

in pulmonary embolism, 770
in pulmonary hypertension, 742–743
stress, 669t, 671
in stroke, 85
transesophageal, 669t
in valvular heart disease, 670, 671f, 672t, **678**
Echolalia, 223
Echovirus infection, **588.** *See also* Enteroviral infection
Ecstasy (MDMA), 6
Ecthyma gangrenosum, 110, 478, 516–517
Ectoparasites, **657**
Ectopic atrial contractions, 721f
Ectopic ventricular contractions, 721f
Eczema, **315**
asteatotic, 311f
drug-induced, 1133t
dyshidrotic, 310f
hand, 310f
Eczema herpeticum, 565
Edema, **240,** 242f
drug-induced, 241t, 342t
generalized, 241–242
in heart failure, 730
idiopathic, 242
localized, 241
lymphedema, **742**
treatment of, 242–243, 243t, 244t
Efalizumab, for psoriasis, 314
Efavirenz, for HIV/AIDS, 606, 610t
Effective circulating volume, 3, 3t
Eflornithine, for sleeping sickness, 646
Ehrlichiosis, 125
ehrlichiosis ewingii, **558**
human monocytotropic, **557**
Eikenella corrodens infection. *See* HACEK group infection
Eisenmenger syndrome, 675
Elderly, joint pain in, 207
Electrocardiography (ECG), **665**
approach to, 665–669
in bradyarrhythmias, **717**
in cardiac hypertrophy, 666, 668t
in cardiomyopathy, **684,** 684t
in congenital heart disease, **674**
in coronary artery disease, 713
in cor pulmonale, 735
heart rate, 665
in hyperkalemia, 12–13, 13f, 14f
in hypothermia, 127
lead system, 666f
mean axis in, 665
in myocardial infarction, 178, 666–667, 667f, 668t, 668t, 689t, 700, **709**
in myocarditis, 687
in pericardial disease, **688**
in pericarditis, 688, 689t, 690f, 691
in poisoning, 133
PR interval, 666
in pulmonary hypertension, 742
QRS interval, 666
QT interval, 666
rhythm, 665
ST-T waves, 667–669
in subarachnoid hemorrhage, 89
in tachyarrhythmias, **720,** 721f, 722t–725t

in valvular heart disease, **678**
in variant angina, 716
Electrocochleography, 298
Electroconvulsive therapy, 1079
Electrodiagnosis
of mononeuropathy, 1062t–1064t
of muscle disease, 1068
of peripheral neuropathy, 1059–1060
Electroencephalography (EEG)
in brain death, 79
in coma, 79
in seizure, 990–991
in status epilepticus, 98
Electrolyte balance, 3
Electronystagmography, 211
Elephantiasis, 652
Eletriptan, for migraine, 185t, 187t
Elliptocytes, 321
Embolectomy, 772
Embryonal carcinoma, 393
Emergencies, medical, **55**
anaphylaxis, **116**
ARDS, **69**
bioterrorism, **160**
bites, venoms, and stings, **117**
cardiovascular collapse, **55**
diabetic ketoacidosis, **100**
drug overdose, **130**
frostbite, **128**
head trauma, **90**
hyperosmolar coma, **100**
hypoglycemia, **103**
hypothermia, **127**
increased intracranial pressure, **90**
infectious disease, **105**
oncologic, **112**
poisoning, 117, **130**
pulmonary edema, acute, **66**
respiratory failure, **71**
septic shock, **63**
shock, **58**
spinal cord compression, 94
status epilepticus, **98**
stroke, **79**
stupor and coma, **74**
subarachnoid hemorrhage, **88**
Emergency contraceptive pills, 957
Emerging disease, **431**
Emphysema
dyspnea in, 231, 233
mediastinal, chest pain in, 176
Empyema, 498, 498t, 533, 777–778
Emtricitabine, for HIV/AIDS, 609t
Enalapril/enalaprilat
for heart failure, 733t
for hypertensive emergencies, 698t
Encephalitis. *See also specific types*
acute, **1042**
approach to, 1042, 1043f–1044f
arbovirus, 595, 596t–597t
cytomegalovirus, 573
enterovirus, 590
HSV, 565
insect-borne disease, **595**
measles, 584
paraneoplastic, 407, 408t, 409t
viral, 1047t, **1048**
diagnosis of, 1049, 1049f

Encephalitis. *See also specific types (Cont.)*:
    pathogens, 1048
    treatment of, 1049–1050
Encephalopathy
    hepatic, **874**
    hypoxic-ischemic, **96**, 97f
Endocarditis
    culture-negative, *Bartonella*, 526t, **527**
    infective, **440**
        acute, 109t, 111, 440
        causes of, 440
        definite, 442
        diagnosis of, 442, 443t
        enterococcal, 444t, 446, 500–501
        gonococcal, 470t
        HACEK group, 445t, 511
        noncardiac manifestations of,
            441–442
        nosocomial, 442, 492
        P. aeruginosa, 517, 519t
        paravalvular, 442
        pathogenesis of, 440–441, 441f
        pneumococcal, 487–488
        possible, 442
        prevention of, 447–448, 447t
        prophylaxis before dental procedures,
            447t, 448
        prophylaxis in congenital heart disease,
            677
        staphylococcal, 445t, 446, 491–492,
            496
        streptococcal, 443, 444t, 499–500
        subacute, 440
        treatment of, 442–447, 444t–446t, 470t
        tricuspid valve, 442
Endocrine disease
    adrenal, **933**
    diabetes mellitus, **942**
    drug-induced, 1132t
    hypothermia in, 128t
    leukocytosis in, 330
    muscle disorders in, **1074**
    nausea and vomiting in, 245t
    paraneoplastic, **405**
    pituitary, **917, 923**
    reproductive system disorders
        female, **952**
        male, **947**
    shock in, 59t
    thyroid, **925**
    tumors of GI tract and pancreas, **389**
    weight loss in, 248t
Endodermal sinus tumor, 393
End-of-life care, **46**. *See also* Terminally ill
    patient
Endometrial cancer, 396t, **397**
Endometritis, 465
Endophthalmitis
    Candida, 621
    Klebsiella, 515
Endoscopic retrograde cholangiopancreatog-
    raphy, 846t, 848, 852
Endoscopic variceal ligation, 873
Endoscopy
    in gastropathies, 834
    in GI bleeding, 260, 262
    in peptic ulcer disease, 832
Enfuvirtide, for HIV/AIDS, 606, 614t

Enoxaparin
    for deep venous thrombosis prevention,
        741
    for myocardial infarction, 701–702
    for thrombotic disorders, 336
    for venous disease, 741
    for venous thromboembolism, 770
    for venous thrombosis prevention, 731
Entacapone, for Parkinson's disease, 1004
Entamoeba histolytica infection. *See* Amebiasis
Entecavir, for chronic hepatitis B, 860t–861t,
    864
Enteral nutrition, **41**
    decision tree for initiating, 42f
    formulas for, 42–43
Enteric bacilli, **513**
Enteric fever, 452t
    salmonellosis, **456**
Enteritis, **466**
Enterobacter infection, 516
    osteomyelitis, 485t
Enterobiasis, 421, **651**
Enteroclysis, 383
Enterococcal infection, **500**
    endocarditis, 444t, 446, 500–501
    urinary tract, 500
Enterocolitis, **466**
    infectious, 837
Enteropathic arthritis, 896f, **907**
Enteroviral infection, **588**
    encephalitis, 590
    exanthems, 590
    generalized disease of the newborn, 590
    hand-foot-and-mouth disease, 590
    hemorrhagic conjunctivitis, 590
    herpangina, 590
    meningitis, 590
    myocarditis/pericarditis, 590
    pleurodynia, 590
    prevention of, 591
    treatment of, 591
Envenomations, **122**
Enzyme immunoassay (EIA), 411
Eosinopenia, **331**
Eosinophilia, **330**
    drug-induced, 1134t
    pulmonary infiltrates with, 776
Ependymoma, **1033**
Ephedrine
    poisoning, 136t
    for vertigo, 214t
Epidemic disease, **431**
Epidermal inclusion cyst, 310f
Epididymitis, **463**
    chlamydial, 471
    treatment of, 463–464, 470t
Epidural abscess
    neck pain in, 198
    S. aureus, 491
    spinal, **95**, 109t, 483, 1029
Epidural hematoma, 93
    spinal, **95**, 1029
Epiglottitis, **306**
    H. influenzae, 509
Epilepsy, **988**
    sleep disorders in, 227
    status epilepticus, **98**
    treatment of, 992t–994t, 994–995

Epinephrine
  for anaphylaxis, 117
  for antivenom reaction, 122
  for beta blocker poisoning, 140t
  for calcium channel blocker poisoning,
    140t
  for cardiac glycoside poisoning, 141t
  for heart failure, 734t
  for hymenoptera sting, 127
  for MAO inhibitor poisoning, 138t
Epiphysitis, brucellosis vs. tuberculosis, 523,
  523t
Epirubicin
  for gastric cancer, 381
  toxicity of, 341t
Episcleritis, 294
Eplerenone
  for aldosteronism, 935
  for heart failure, 733t
  for hyperaldosteronism, 21
  for hypertension, 695t
  for myocardial infarction, 707
Epley procedure, 213
Epoprostenol
  for pulmonary hypertension, 745
  for systemic sclerosis, 889
Eprodisate, for amyloidosis, 915
Epstein-Barr virus infection, **574**
  cancer associated with, 353, 575–576,
    576t
  mononucleosis, 574–577, 576t
  posttransplantation lymphoproliferative
    disease, 575, 577
  in transplant recipients, 800
Eptifibatide
  for myocardial infarction, 711
  for thrombotic disorders, 338
  for unstable angina, 711
Erectile dysfunction, **950**, 951f
Ergot alkaloid poisoning, 137t
Ergotamine
  for cluster headache prevention, 187
  for migraine, 185t, 187t
  poisoning, 137t
Erlotinib
  for lung cancer, 374
  for pancreatic cancer, 389
  toxicity of, 342t
Erosion (skin lesion), 313t
Ertapenem, for pneumonia, 766t, 767t
Eruptive xanthoma, 973
Erysipelas, **316**, 478, 498, 498t
Erysipelothrix rhusiopathiae infection, 478
Erythema infectiosum, 587
Erythema migrans, 549
Erythema multiforme, **318**, 565, 568t
  drug-induced, 1133t
Erythema nodosum, 201, **318**
  drug-induced, 1133t
Erythema nodosum leprosum, 544, 547
Erythrocytosis. See Polycythemia
Erythroderma, 108t, 110
Erythroid:granulocytic ratio, bone marrow,
  323
Erythroleukemia, 345t
Erythromycin
  for acne, 318
  for bacillary angiomatosis, 479t

  for *Bartonella* infections, 526t
  for campylobacteriosis, 458
  for cellulitis, 479t
  for chancroid, 476
  for *C. pneumoniae* infections, 563
  for *C. psittaci* infections, 563
  for diphtheria, 502
    preventive treatment, 503
  for *H. pylori* eradication, 247
  for human bite infections, 119t
  indications for, 426t
  for leptospirosis, 553
  for Lyme borreliosis, 550
  for lymphogranuloma venereum, 471
  for nausea and vomiting, 246
  for pertussis, 510
  for pharyngitis, 304t
  for relapsing fever, 553
  resistance to, 426t
Erythroplakia, 367
Erythropoiesis, 281
Erythropoietin, decreased level of, 324
Erythropoietin therapy
  for anemia, 328, 344
  for chronic kidney disease, 795–796
Eschar, 201, 478
Escherichia coli infection
  E. coli O157:H7, 459, 514
  enteroaggregative and diffusely adherent
    (EAEC), 514
  enteropathogenic (EPEC), 514
  enterotoxigenic (ETEC), 514
  extraintestinal (ExPEC), **513**
  intestinal, **514**
  osteomyelitis, 485t
  Shiga toxin-producing/enterohemorrhagic
    (STEC/EHEC), **458**, 514
Escitalopram, 1086t
Esmolol
  for aortic dissection, 738t
  for arrhythmias, 727t
  for hypertensive emergencies, 698t
  for MAO inhibitor poisoning, 138t
  poisoning, 140t
  for sympathomimetic poisoning, 136t
Esophageal cancer, **379**
  adenocarcinoma, 379–380
  squamous cell carcinoma, 379–380
Esophageal inflammation, **252**
Esophageal manometry, 250
Esophageal motility disorders, **250**
Esophageal pain, 175t, 176f, 178
Esophageal spasm, **251**
Esophageal ulcer, 253
Esophageal varices, **873**
  prevention of initial bleed, 874
  treatment of
    acute bleeding, 873–874
    prevention of recurrent bleeds, 874
Esophagitis, **252**
  Candida, 252
  eosinophilic, 252–253
  HSV infections, 566, 568t
  pill-related, 252
  viral, 252
Esophagogastroscopy, 250, 380, 873
Esophagus, rupture of, 177f
Estazolam poisoning, 143t

Estramustine
for prostate cancer, 401
toxicity of, 341t
Estrogen therapy
for amenorrhea, 953
for hypopituitarism, 922t
for menopausal symptoms, 957
oral contraceptives, 957
for osteoporosis, 967
Etanercept
for ankylosing spondylitis, 897
for psoriasis, 314
for psoriatic arthritis, 898
for rheumatoid arthritis, 887
Ethacrynic acid, for edema, 243t
Ethambutol
for nontuberculous mycobacterial infections, 548–549
for tuberculosis, 541, 543t
Ethanol, for AGMA inducer poisoning,
147t
Ethchlorvynol poisoning, 144t
Ethosuximide
poisoning, 143t
for seizures, 992t–993t
Ethylene glycol poisoning, 17t, 18–19, 147t
Ethylestradiol/norethisterone, for GI telang-
iectasis, 263
Etomidate poisoning, 144t
Etoposide
for AML, 346
for extragonadal germ cell tumor, 402
for lung cancer, 371
for testicular cancer, 394
toxicity of, 341t
Etravirine, for HIV/AIDS, 606, 610t
Eustachian tube dysfunction, 298–300, **305**
Exanthem, enterovirus, 590
Exanthem subitum, **571**
Exchange transfusion, 44, 160
Excoriation, 313t
Exemestane
for breast cancer, 378
toxicity of, 342t
Exenatide, for diabetes mellitus, 944
Exercise habits, 1121
Exercise testing, in coronary artery disease,
713–714, 713f, 714t
Exertional headache, 183t, 189
External contamination, radiation, 172
Extrapyramidal side effects, 149t, 1088,
1138t
Eye disease, **293**
drug-induced, 1139t
HSV infections, 565, 568t
infections, 294
inflammation, 294
larva migrans, 649
in malnutrition, 41
nocardiosis, 535, 536t
P. aeruginosa infections, 517, 519t
paraneoplastic, 408t
red or painful eye, **293**, 293t
toxoplasmosis, 647
tumors, **296**
Eye movements, in coma, 78–79
Eye trauma, 293–294
Ezetimibe, for hyperlipidemia, 972t

F
FAB classification, of AML, 345t
Facial diplegia, 1025
Facial masking, 1002
Facial myokymia, 1021
Facial nerve, disorders of, **1021**, 1022f
Facial numbness, **1020**
Facial pain, **189**, **1020**
Facial weakness, **1021**
bilateral, 1022
Facioscapulohumeral dystrophy, **1071**
Factitious illness, 1084
Facultative bacteria, 528
Faintness, 207, **211**
Famciclovir, for HSV infections, 475, 479t,
567t–568t, 569
Familial polyposis coli, 383
Familial spastic paraplegia, 1030
Famotidine, for erosive gastropathies, 834
Fanconi syndrome, 788, 812t, 813
Farmer's lung, **758**
Fasciculations, 219t, 220t, 984
Fascioliasis, 654
Fatigability, 218
Fatigue
chronic fatigue syndrome, **290**
drug-induced, 289, 289t
generalized, **288**, 289t
in muscle disease, 1068
in terminally ill patient, 52t
Fatty liver, 869
Fecal antigen test, *H. pylori,* 832, 832t
Fecal incontinence, 53t, 254–256
Fecal occult blood test, 260, 385–387, 1122,
1123t
Felbamate
poisoning, 143t
for seizures, 994t
Femoral neuropathy, 1063t
Fenofibrate, for hyperlipidemia, 972t
Fenoprofen, for pain, 36t–37t
Fentanyl
narcotic abuse, **1099**
for pain, 36t–37t, 38
Fever, **199**
approach to, 200–201, 435–436, 435f
in cancer patient, 115
causes of, 200
drug-induced, 1132t
with myalgia, viral disease, 594–595
with rash, 200
recurrent, 201
in returned traveler, 1117
treatment of, 201
Fever of unknown origin
approach to, 201, 202f
classic, 199
HIV-associated, 199–200
neutropenic, 199–200
nosocomial, 199–200
treatment of, 201
Fexofenadine
for allergic rhinitis, 880
for urticaria/angioedema, 879
Fiber, dietary, 258, 842
Fibrinogen deficiency, 334
Fibrinolytic therapy
for myocardial infarction, 701, 702f, 703f

for thrombotic disorders, 338
for venous thromboembolism, 772
Fibromyalgia, **908**, 1078
Fifth disease, 587
Filariasis, 421, **651**
lymphatic, **652**
nocturnally periodic, 652
subperiodic, 652
Finasteride
for prostate cancer prevention, 1124
for prostate hyperplasia, 399
Fire coral, 122
Fisher syndrome, 1061
Fish oil supplementation
for hyperlipidemia, 972t
for IgA nephropathy, 808
for inflammatory bowel disease, 840
Fitz-Hugh-Curtis syndrome, 465
Fixed drug eruption, 1133t
Flatworm infection, **653**
Flecainide, for arrhythmias, 727t
Floxuridine, for colorectal cancer, 387
Fluconazole, **619**
for blastomycosis, 631
for candidiasis, 252, 317, 464, 621
preventive treatment, 621
for coccidioidomycosis, 630
for cryptococcosis, 626
Flucortisone, for adrenal insufficiency,
115
Flucytosine, **620**
for cryptococcosis, 626
Fludarabine
for CLL, 356
for follicular lymphoma, 357
for idiopathic thrombocytopenic purpura,
335
toxicity of, 341t
Fludrocortisone
for Addison's disease, 936
for hypoaldosteronism, 937
for orthostatic hypotension, 1019
for SIADH, 925
Fluid absorption, in GI tract, 253
Fluid restriction
for hyponatremia, 406
for SIADH, 114, 925
Fluid retention, drug-induced, 1136t
Fluke infection
blood flukes, 420t
liver (biliary) flukes, **654**
lung flukes, **654**
Flumazenil, for sedative-hypnotic poisoning,
143t
Flunarizine, for migraine prevention, 188t
Flunisolide, for asthma, 755
Flunitrazepam poisoning, 143t
5-Fluorouracil (5-FU)
for anal cancer, 388
for breast cancer, 378
for carcinoid tumor, 389
for cervical cancer, 398
for colorectal cancer, 387
for gastric cancer, 381
for head and neck cancer, 368
for pancreatic cancer, 389
toxicity of, 341t
for Zollinger-Ellison syndrome, 836

Fluoxetine
for depression, 50
for daytime sleepiness, 230
dosage and adverse effects of, 1086t
for menopausal symptoms, 957
for OCD, 1082
for systemic sclerosis, 889
Fluphenazine, 1091t
Flurazepam
dosage and action of, 1089t
poisoning, 143t
Flutamide
for prostate cancer, 401
toxicity of, 342t
Fluticasone
for allergic rhinitis, 880
for asthma, 755
for esophagitis, 253
Fluvastatin, for hyperlipidemia, 972t
Fluvoxamine
dosage and adverse effects of, 1086t
for OCD, 1082
Folate
deficiency, anemia in, 325, 328
for methanol poisoning, 148t
FOLFIRI regimen, for colorectal cancer, 387
FOLFOX regimen, for colorectal cancer, 387
Folinic acid, for methanol poisoning, 148t
Follicle-stimulating hormone, 917, 917f
Follicular lymphoma, 354f, 355, **357**
Folliculitis, 310f, 478, 490
hot-tub, 478
Fomepizole, for AGMA inducer poisoning,
147t
Fondaparinux
for thrombotic disorders, 337
for venous thromboembolism, 770
Food poisoning
bacterial, **453**
clostridial, 541
S. aureus, 492
Foot, muscles and innervation of, 980t–981t
Foramen magnum, lesions near, 1027
Forearm, muscles and innervation of,
980t–981t
Formoterol, for asthma, 754
Fosamprenavir, for HIV/AIDS, 613t
Foscarnet
for cytomegalovirus infections, 574
for viral esophagitis, 252
Fosphenytoin, for status epilepticus, 99f
Fournier's gangrene, 533
Foxglove, 141t
Fracture, osteoporotic, 965–966, 966t
Francisella tularensis infection. *See* Tulare-
mia
Fresh-frozen plasma (FFP), 44–45
for bleeding disorders, 335
for warfarin reversal, 336
Friedreich's ataxia, 1009–1010
Frontotemporal dementia, 995, 997t, 998,
1001
Frostbite, **128**, 129t
Frovatriptan, for migraine, 185t, 187t
Frozen shoulder, 910
Fungal infection, **618**
diagnosis of, **411**
specimen collection and transport, 417t

Fungus ball, 302
Furosemide
    for ascites, 272
    for edema, 243t
    for heart failure, 731, 733t
    for hypercalcemia, 406, 962t
    for hyperkalemia, 15t
    for hypertension, 695t, 698
    for myocardial infarction, 705, 706t
    for pulmonary edema, 68
    for SIADH, 114
Furuncle, 490
Furunculosis, 316
Fusariosis, 632
Fusobacterium infection, 532

G
Gabapentin
    for generalized anxiety disorder, 1082
    for menopausal symptoms, 957
    for migraine prevention, 188t
    for multiple sclerosis, 1041
    for pain, 37t, 38
    poisoning, 143t
    for polyneuropathy, 1061
    for seizures, 994t
Gait analysis, 986
Galactorrhea, drug-induced, 1132t
Galantamine, for Alzheimer's disease, 1000
Gallstones, 175t
Gametocyte, 636
Gamma-glutamyltranspeptidase (GGT), 269
Gamma knife radiosurgery, 1020–1021,
    1032
Gamma radiation, 171
Ganciclovir
    for cytomegalovirus infections, 574
    for viral esophagitis, 252
Gardasil, 398
Gardner's syndrome, 381, 384, 384t
Gas exchange, disturbances of, 749
Gas gangrene, 108t, 111, 477, 480t, 531–532
Gastrectomy, 381, 833
Gastric aspiration, 148t
Gastric atrophy, 834
Gastric cancer, 380
    adenocarcinoma, 380–381
    diffuse infiltrative, 380
    intestinal type, 380
    staging of, 382t
    superficial spreading, 380
Gastric lavage, 135, 858
Gastric tumor, benign, 381
Gastric ulcer, 831–833
Gastrinoma, 389, 390t, 391, 835
Gastritis, 834
    atrophic, 834
    chronic, 834
    superficial, 834
    treatment of, 263
    types A and B, 834–835
Gastroenteritis
    Aeromonas, 516
    campylobacteriosis, 458
Gastroesophageal reflux disease (GERD),
    246
    sleep disorders in, 228
Gastroesophageal varices, 260, 263

Gastrointestinal bleeding, 259
    anemia in, 326
    drug-induced, 1138t
    lower GI tract, 261–263, 262f
    upper GI tract, 260–263, 261f
Gastrointestinal cancer, 379
Gastrointestinal decontamination, 135
Gastrointestinal disease
    cholecystitis
        acute, 845
        chronic, 847
    choledocholithiasis/cholangitis, 847
    cholelithiasis, 844
    cirrhosis, 868
    colonic angiodysplasia, 843
    colonic polyps, 383
    diarrhea, infectious, 451
    diverticular disease, 841
    drug-induced, 1137t–1138t
    endocrine tumors, 389
    esophageal varices, 873
    gastric tumors, 381
    gastropathies, 834
    hepatic failure, 858
    hepatitis
        acute, 854
        chronic, 859
    infections in immunocompromised pa-
        tients, 434, 436t
    inflammatory bowel disease, 836
    intestinal parasites, 421
    intestinal pseudoobstruction, 842
    irritable bowel syndrome, 840
    listerial, 507
    liver tumors, 388
    measles virus, 585
    nausea and vomiting in, 245t
    pain in, 175t, 176f, 179t
    pancreatitis, 849
    peptic ulcer disease, 831
    portal hypertension, 872
    primary sclerosing cholangitis, 848
    small-bowel tumors, 382
    in travelers, 1117
    tuberculosis, 540
    vascular, 843
    weight loss in, 247, 248t
    Zollinger-Ellison syndrome, 835
Gastrointestinal function, normal, 253, 1167t
Gastrointestinal stromal cell tumor (GIST),
    380
Gastrointestinal telangiectasis, 263
Gastropathies, 834
    erosive, 834
Gastroscopy, 381
Gefitinib
    for lung cancer, 374
    toxicity of, 342t
Gemcitabine
    for bladder cancer, 392
    for breast cancer, 379
    for pancreatic cancer, 389
Gemfibrozil, for hyperlipidemia, 972t
Gemifloxacin, for pneumonia, 766t
Gemtuzumab ozogamicin, 342t
Generalized anxiety disorder, 1082, 1088
Generalized disease of the newborn, enterovi-
    rus, 590

Genital herpes, 464, **475, 565**
   features of genital ulcers, 467t
   treatment of, 475, 479t, 567t–568t
Genital lesion, ulcerative, **466,** 467t
Genital warts, 844
Genitourinary tract cancer, **391**
Gentamicin
   for *Abiotrophia* infections, 501
   for bacterial meningitis, 1046t, 1047t
   for *Bartonella* infections, 526t
   for brucellosis, 523
   for enterococcal infections, 501
   for gram-negative enteric bacteria infec-
      tions, 516
   indications for, 426t
   for infective endocarditis, 444t–445t, 446
   for listerial infections, 508
   for necrotizing fasciitis, 108t
   for pelvic inflammatory disease, 466
   for plague, 164t, 526
   for pneumonia, 767t
   for pyelonephritis, 818t
   resistance to, 426t
   for sepsis/septic shock, 65t, 107t
   for staphylococcal infections, 496
   for streptococcal infections, 499
   for tularemia, 165t, 524
   for urinary tract infections, 819t
German measles. *See* Rubella
Germ cell tumor, 395
   extragonadal, unrecognized, **402**
   paraneoplastic syndromes in, 409t
GHB, 132t, 144t
   for daytime sleepiness, 230
Giant cell arteritis, 217, **892**
Giardiasis, 420t, 421, **454**
   enteritis, 468
Gilbert's syndrome, 265, 268t
Gingivitis, 532
   necrotizing ulcerative, 532
Gingivostomatitis, HSV infections, 564
Gitelman's syndrome, 788
Glanders, 518–521, 520t
Glatiramer acetate, for multiple sclerosis,
   1039
Glaucoma, 216f, **295,** 295f
   acute angle-closure, **294**
   drug-induced, 1139t
   open-angle, 295
Glimepiride, for diabetes mellitus, 945t
Glioma, 1032
Glipizide, for diabetes mellitus, 945t
Global aphasia, 225, 225t
Globin, in liver disease, 269
Globus pharyngeus, 249
Glomerular disease, **801**
   serologic findings in multisystem diseases
      causing, 807t
Glomerular filtration rate (GFR), 274, 275t,
   794, 797
   eGFR, 795
   estimation of, 276
Glomerulonephritis
   acute, 785, **801,** 801t
   ANCA-associated, **803**
   chronic, **808**
   membranoproliferative, **805**
   membranous, **804**

postinfectious, **801**
poststreptococcal, 280, **801**
rapidly progressive, 785, **802**
   with ant-GBM antibodies, 802–803
   causes of, 802t
   immune complex-associated, 802
   pauci-immune, 802–803
   in SLE, 803
Glossopharyngeal neuralgia, **1023**
Glucagon
   for beta blocker poisoning, 140t
   for calcium channel blocker poisoning,
      140t
   for hypoglycemia, 105
Glucagonoma, 389, 390t, 391
Glucocorticoids, adrenal, **933**
Glucocorticoid therapy
   for acute disseminated encephalomyelitis,
      1041
   for acute renal failure, 793
   for adult T cell leukemia/lymphoma, 260
   for amiodarone-induced thyrotoxicosis,
      931
   for amyloidosis, 915
   for anaphylaxis, 117
   for ankylosing spondylitis, 897
   for ataxia, 1010
   for autoimmune hemolysis, 329
   for autoimmune hepatitis, 867
   for brain tumor, 1031
   clinical uses of, **938,** 938t
   for CLL, 356
   for dermatitis, 315
   for eczema, 315
   epidural, for back pain, 196
   for Epstein-Barr virus infections, 577
   for erythema nodosum, 318
   for fever, 201
   for gout, 904
   for histoplasmosis, 629t
   for hymenoptera sting, 127
   for hypercalcemia, 113, 962t
   for increased intracranial pressure, 92t
   for inflammatory bowel disease, 838
   for inflammatory myopathy, 1072
   for interstitial lung disease, 775
   for larva migrans, 649
   for leishmaniasis, 644
   for lichen planus, 314
   for meningococcal infections, 505
   for minimal change disease, 804
   for muscular dystrophy, 1071
   for myasthenia gravis, 1066
   nasal, for allergic rhinitis, 880
   for optic neuritis, 217
   for osteoarthritis, 902
   for parainfluenza virus infections, 583
   for pityriasis rosea, 314
   for polyneuropathy, 1061
   for primary sclerosing cholangitis, 849
   for pseudogout, 906
   for psoriasis, 314
   for psoriatic arthritis, 898
   for reactive arthritis, 900
   for rosacea, 318
   for sarcoidosis, 912
   for schistosomiasis, 654
   for Sjögren's syndrome, 891

Glucocorticoid therapy (*Cont.*):
for SLE, 803, 886
for spinal cord compression, 95
steroid preparations, 938–939, 938t
for systemic mastocytosis, 881
for systemic sclerosis, 889
for taeniasis solium and cysticercosis, 656
topical, for inflamed eye, 294
for trichinellosis, 649
for vasculitis, 893
for vertigo, 214t
Gluconate, for hyperkalemia, 15t
Glucosamine and chondroitin, for osteoarthritis, 902
Glucose-lowering agents, oral, 944–945, 945t
Glucose-6-phosphate dehydrogenase deficiency, 326, 327t, 328–329
Glucose therapy
for hypoglycemia, 105
for salicylate poisoning, 149t
Gluten-free diet, 1010
Glutethimide poisoning, 144t
Glyburide, for diabetes mellitus, 945t
Glycocholic breath test, 256
Glycolytic defects, 1073
Glycylcyclines, 424
Goiter, 926, 931
nontoxic, **931**
toxic multinodular, 928–930, **931**
Gold compounds, for rheumatoid arthritis, 887
Golytely, 135
Gonadotropin(s)
deficiency of, 919t, 922, 922t
hypersecretion of, 919t, **921**
Gonadotropin-releasing hormone deficiency, 947
Gonococcemia, 201
Gonorrhea, **468**
anorectal, 469
arthritis, 469, 481–482
cervicitis, 465, 468
disseminated infection, 469, 470t
epididymitis, 463, 470t
ocular, 469
pelvic inflammatory disease, 465, 469, 470t
pharyngeal, 469
in pregnancy, 469
proctitis, 468
treatment of, 463, 470t
urethritis, 463–464, 468
Goodpasture's syndrome, 807t
Goserelin, for prostate cancer, 401
Gout, **903**
Gouty arthritis, acute, 903–904
GP IIb/IIIa antagonists
for myocardial infarction, 711
for unstable angina, 711
Graft-versus-host disease, 44
Grain(s), 537
Grain dust, **758**
Gram-negative bacilli
enteric, **513**
miscellaneous, **522**
Gram's stain, 411, 412f, 482
Granisetron, for nausea and vomiting, 246

Granulocyte colony-stimulating factor, 343t, 368
Granulocyte-macrophage colony-stimulating factor, 343t
Granuloma inguinale, **476**
Granulomatous disease, leukocytosis in, 330
Granuloma venereum, **476**
Graphesthesia, 985
Graves' disease, 928–930
Graves' ophthalmopathy, 1074
Gray (radiation unit), 171
Griseofulvin, **620**
for dermatophyte infections, 317
Growth hormone, 917, 918f
deficiency of, 919t, 922, 922t
hypersecretion of, 919t, 920–921
therapy for weight loss, 248
Guanabenz poisoning, 139t
Guanfacine, for tics, 224
Guillain-Barré syndrome, 1016, 1061
Gumma, 473
Gynecologic cancer, **395**
Gynecomastia
drug-induced, 342t, 1132t
evaluation of, 949f
paraneoplastic, 405t

H
HAART therapy, **606**
HACEK group infection, **511,** 512t
endocarditis, 445t
Haemophilus ducreyi infection. *See* Chancroid
Haemophilus influenzae infection, **508**
epiglottitis, 509
Hib, **508**
meningitis, 508–509
nontypable strains, 508–509
pneumonia, 509
Haemophilus influenzae type b vaccine, 438t, 509, 1108t–1109t
Haemophilus species infection. *See* HACEK group infection
Hallucinations
drug-induced, 1140t
hypnagogic, 229t, 230, 230t
Hallucinogens, 131t
Haloperidol
for delirium, 50t
dosage and adverse effects of, 139t, 1091t
for nausea and vomiting, 49, 245
Haloprogin, for dermatophyte infections, 317
Hand, muscles and innervation of, 980t–981t
Hand-foot-and-mouth disease, 590
Hand hygiene, 429, 493, 591
Hantavirus hemorrhagic fever with renal syndrome, 110
Hantavirus pulmonary syndrome, 111, **598**
Harris and Benedict formula, 39, 39f
Headache, **183.** *See also specific types*
causes of, 183t
drug-induced, 1138t
symptoms suggesting serious underlying disorder, 184t
Head and neck cancer, **367**
infections in cancer patients, 433t
local disease, 368
locally advanced disease, 368

oncologic emergencies, 112–113
paraneoplastic syndromes in, 405t, 406
prevention of, 368, 1125
recurrent or metastatic, 368
Head and neck infection, anaerobic, 532
Head louse, 658–659
Head trauma, **91**, 996t, 998
approach to, 93
hearing loss in, 297
increased intracranial pressure in, 90
intracranial hemorrhage in, 82t
post-concussion headache, 183t, 187–189
subarachnoid hemorrhage in, **88**
Health care-associated infections, **428**
Health care worker, HIV/AIDS in, 617–618
Hearing aid, 297–298, 300
Hearing loss, 212–213, **297**
approach to, 297–298, 299f
causes of, 298–300
conductive, 297, **298**, 301
drug-induced, 300, 1139t
noise-induced, 301
prevention of, 301
sensorineural, 297–298, **300**
treatment of, 300–301
Heart
chamber size and ventricular performance, 669
noninvasive examination of, **669**
physical examination of, **661**
Heartburn, **246**
Heart disease. *See also* Cardiovascular disease
cardiac mass, 670, 672t
computed tomography in, 672t, 673
congenital. *See* Congenital heart disease
cyanosis in, **239**, 240t
depression in, 1078
drug-induced, 342t, 1135t–1136t
dyspnea in, 231–233, 232t
echocardiography in, **669**
edema in, 241
endocarditis prophylaxis, 447t, 448
fatigue in, 289t
Lyme borreliosis, 550–551
MRI in, 672t, 673
nausea and vomiting in, 245t
nuclear cardiology, **671**
prevention of, 1104t–1105t, **1118**
risk factors for, 709, 1118–1120
screening for, 1105t
valvular. *See* Valvular heart disease
weight loss in, 248t
in women, 1128
Heart failure, **730**
ascites in, **271**, 273t
conditions that mimic, 730
drug-induced, 1136t
edema in, 241, 243, 730
myocardial infarction and, 705, 705t, 706t
precipitating factors, 730
treatment of, 705, 705t, 706t, 730–735, 731f, 732t–734t
Heart murmur, 662t, **665**
diastolic, 662t, 664f, 665
effects of physiologic and pharmacologic interventions, 663t

systolic, 662t, 664f, 665
Heart rate, 665
Heart sounds, 662f, **663**
effects of physiologic and pharmacologic interventions, 663t
ejection click, 664
midsystolic click, 665
opening snap, 664
S_1 through S_4, 663–664
Heart transplant, infections in recipients, 437–439
Heat stroke, **201**
drug-induced, 203
exertional, 201
nonexertional, 203
Heavy chain deposition disease, 812t
Heavy metal poisoning, 154t–160t
Height, ideal weight for height, 40t
Heinz bodies, 322
Helicobacter pylori infection
detection of, 832, 832t
eradication of, 247, 832, 833t
indigestion, **246**
lymphoid malignancies and, 355
peptic ulcer disease, **831**
Helminth ectoparasites, **657**
Helminth infection, **648**
intestinal, 421
Hemapheresis, **46**
Hematemesis, 259
Hematin, for porphyria, 977
Hematochezia, 260
Hematocrit, 280
Hematologic disease
bleeding disorders, **332**
blood smear, **321**
bone marrow examination, **322**
drug-induced, 1134t
fatigue in, 289t
leukocytosis and leukopenia, **329**
red cell disorders, **323**
reference values for laboratory tests, 1142t–1144t
thrombotic disorders, **336**
Hematomyelia, **96**
Hematopoietic cell transplant
for amyloidosis, 915
for CLL, 356
for follicular lymphoma, 357
infections in recipients, 436–437, 436t
vaccination of recipients, 438t, 439
Hematuria, **280**, 392–393, 787, 806–807
approach to, 279f
causes of, 278t
gross, 280
microscopic, 280
Heme preparations
for acute intermittent porphyria, 977
for erythropoietic porphyria, 978
Hemianopia
bitemporal, 215, 216f
homonymous, 215, 216f, 220t
Hemiballismus, 223
Hemiblock, 667f
Hemicrania, paroxysmal, 189
Hemicrania continua, 189
Hemifacial spasm, 1022–1023
Hemiparesis, 80, 93, 220t, 221f

Hemochromatosis, 44, **975**
  HFE-associated, 975, 976f
  screening for, 975f
Hemodialysis
  complications of, 797, 797t
  for hyperkalemia, 15t
  intermittent, 793
  for poisoning, 137t, 143t, 147t, 148t, 149t,
    151t, 160
  for tumor lysis syndrome, 116
Hemoglobin
  abnormal, 239, 326, 326t
  blood concentration, 280
  unstable variants, 326
Hemolysis, 280
  leukemoid reaction in, 330
  leukoerythroblastic reaction in, 330
Hemolytic anemia, **280, 326**
  classification of, 326t
  drug-induced, 1135t
  microangiopathic, 825
Hemolytic pattern
  α-hemolysis, 497
  β-hemolysis, 497
  γ-hemolysis, 497
Hemolytic uremic syndrome (HUS), 326t,
  459, 824–826
Hemoperfusion
  for methylxanthine poisoning, 137t
  for sedative-hypnotic poisoning, 143t
Hemophilia A, 334–335
Hemophilia B, 334–335
Hemoptysis, **235**, 238f
Hemorrhage. *See also specific types and sites*
  with extensive transfusion, 333
  leukoerythroblastic reaction in, 330
Hemorrhagic fever, viral, 110, **596**
Hemorrhagic fever with renal syndrome,
  598
Hemorrhoids, 310f, **844**
Hemostatic disorders, 335
Hemothorax, **780**
Henbane, 138t
Henoch-Schönlein purpura, **803**, 807t, **892**
Heparin
  for arterial embolism, 739
  for deep venous thrombosis prevention,
    741
  for DIC, 335
  for myocardial infarction, 701–702, 711
  for thrombotic disorders, 336–337, 337t
  for unstable angina, 711
  for venous disease, 741
  for venous thromboembolism, 770–771
    preventive treatment, 731
Heparin-induced thrombocytopenia, 332,
  334, 770
Hepatic artery embolization, 389
Hepatic disease. *See* Liver disease
Hepatic encephalopathy, **874**
Hepatitis
  acute, **854**
  alcoholic, 268t, 869
  autoimmune, 269, **865**
    treatment of, 867
    type I, 865
    type II, 865–867
    type III, 867

  chronic, **859**
    depression in, 1078
    grading of, 859
    staging of, 859
  toxic/drug-induced, **858**
  viral, **854**, 855t, 858
Hepatitis A
  acute, **854,** 855t, 856f
  prevention of, 854
Hepatitis A vaccine, 438t, 854, 865,
  1108t–1112t, 1115t, 1116t
Hepatitis B, 388
  acute, **854,** 855t, 856f
  chronic, 860t–863t, **861**
  prevention of, 856
Hepatitis B immune globulin, 856
Hepatitis B vaccine, 438t, 856, 1108t–1112t,
  1115t, 1116t
Hepatitis C, 388
  acute, 855t, **857,** 857f
  chronic, **864,** 865t–867t
  prevention of, 857
Hepatitis D, 855t, **857**
Hepatitis E, 855t, **857**
Hepatobiliary disorders
  imaging in, **270,** 846t
  liver function tests in, 268t
Hepatocellular carcinoma, **388**
Hepatocellular disorders, liver function tests
  in, 268t
Hepatorenal syndrome, **274**
Hepatotoxins, 858
Hereditary elliptocytosis, 326
Hereditary spherocytosis, 326, 328
Heroin abuse, **1099**
Herpangina, 590
Herpanginia, 590
Herpes gladiatorum, **565**
Herpes simplex virus (HSV) infection, 310f,
  311, **475, 564**
  acyclovir-resistant, 568–569, 568t
  Bell's palsy, 1021–1022
  eye infection, 565, 568t
  genital. *See* Genital herpes
  in immunocompromised host, 564–565,
    567t
  neonatal, 566, 568t
  neurologic disease, 565–566, 568t
  oral-facial, 564, 567t–568t
  proctitis, 468
  reactivation of, 564
  skin disease, 316
  treatment of, 316, 475, 479t, 566–569,
    567t–568t
  visceral infections, 566, 568t
  whitlow, 565, 568t
Herpesvirus infection, **564**
Herpes zoster, 310f, 311, **316, 570**
  neck pain in, 198
  treatment of, 316, 479t, 571
Herpes zoster vaccine, 571
Herpetiform lesion, 309
Heterophile test, 576
Hirsutism, **955,** 956f
  drug-induced, 955
Histoplasmosis, **627**
  acute pulmonary, 627, 629t
  African, 628
  chronic cavitary, 628, 629t

CNS disease, 629t
mediastinitis, 628
progressive disseminated, 627–628, 629t
treatment of, 628, 629t
Histotoxic hypoxia, 96
Histrionic personality disorder, 1084
HIV/AIDS, **600**
acute retroviral syndrome, 604 605
advanced HIV disease, 602
asymptomatic infection, 605
chronic and persistent infection, 601–602
clinical features of, 604–605, 604t
cytomegalovirus infections in, 573–574
depression in, 1078
diagnosis of, 603, 603f
epidemiology of, 601
etiology of, 600–601
fever of unknown origin in, 199–200
health care workers and, 617–618
immune response to HIV, 602
infected travelers, 1117
laboratory monitoring of, 603–604
neoplasms in, 605
pathophysiology and immunopathogenesis of, 601–602
Pneumocystis infections in, **633**
postexposure prophylaxis, 617–618
prevention of, 618, 1104t
primary infection, 601–602
secondary infectious diseases in, 605, 617
symptomatic disease, 605
treatment of, **605**
antiretroviral therapy, 606–617, 607t–615t, 617t
prevention of secondary infections, 617
principles of, 616t
tuberculosis and, 538–540, 542, 545t–546t
vacuolar myelopathy, 1029
in women, 1129
HIV entry inhibitors, 606, 614t–615t
HIV vaccine, 618
Hodgkin's disease, 353t, **361,** 575
infections in, 433t
paraneoplastic syndromes in, 409t
staging of, 363, 363t
vaccination in, 438t
Homocysteine, 1120
Hookworm infection, 649, **650,** 1117
Hormones, ectopic production of, **405**
Hornet sting, 126
Hospitalized patient. *See also* Nosocomial infections
care of
acid-base balance, **3**
admission orders, **1**
critical care medicine, **30**
electrolyte balance, **3**
end-of-life care, **46**
enteral nutrition, **41**
imaging, **22**
pain and its management, **34**
palliative care, **46**
parenteral nutrition, **41**
procedures performed by internists, **25**
transfusion and pheresis therapy, **44**
Howell-Jolly bodies, 321

H$_2$ receptor antagonists
for erosive gastropathies, 834
for peptic ulcer disease, 833
Human bite, **118,** 119t, 478, 511
Human herpesvirus 6 infection, **571**
Human herpesvirus 7 infection, **571**
Human herpesvirus 8 infection, 353, **571**
Human papillomavirus (HPV) infection, **476**
cervical cancer and, 398
warts, 317
Human papillomavirus (HPV) vaccine, 398, 477, 1110t–1113t, 1125
Human respiratory syncytial virus (RSV) infection, **582**
Human T-lymphotropic virus infection, 353
Hunt-Hess Scale, for subarachnoid hemorrhage, 88t
Huntington's disease, **223,** 998, **1002**
Hydralazine
for heart failure, 731, 733t
for hypertension, 698, 698t
for myocardial infarction, 706–707
Hydralazine-nitrate, for dilated cardiomyopathy, 685
Hydrocephalus
normal-pressure, 998, **1001**
in subarachnoid hemorrhage, 89–90
Hydrochlorothiazide
for diabetes insipidus, 8
for edema, 243t
for heart failure, 733t
for hypertension, 695, 695t
Hydrocodone
for dyspnea, 49t
for hemoptysis, 238
Hydrocortisone
for Addison's disease, 936
for adrenal insufficiency, 115
for hypopituitarism, 922t
for inflammatory bowel disease, 838
for meningococcal infections, 505
for myxedema coma, 928
for sepsis/septic shock, 66
steroid preparations, 938–939, 938t
Hydrofludrocortisone, for syncope, 210
Hydrogen sulfide, 145t
Hydromorphone
for dyspnea, 49t
narcotic abuse, **1099**
for pain, 36t–37t
Hydrops fetalis, 588
Hydrothorax, 241
Hydroxychloroquine
for malaria prevention, 640t
poisoning, 153t
for porphyria cutanea tarda, 977
for Q fever, 559
for rheumatoid arthritis, 887
for Sjögren's syndrome, 891
for SLE, 886
5-Hydroxyindoleacetic acid, urinary, 389
Hydroxyprogesterone, for endometrial cancer, 397
Hydroxyurea
for cervical cancer, 398
for sickle cell anemia, 328
for systemic mastocytosis, 881
toxicity of, 341t

Hydroxyzine
  for ciguatera poisoning, 124
  for urticaria/angioedema, 879
Hymenoptera sting, **126**
Hyoscyamine
  for irritable bowel syndrome, 841
  poisoning, 138t
Hypalgesia, 34
Hyperaldosteronism
  hypertension in, 693–694
  treatment of, 20–21
Hyperalgesia, 34
Hyperbaric oxygen
  for cytochrome oxidase inhibitor poison-
    ing, 145t
  for gas gangrene, 532
Hyperbilirubinemia, **263**, 264t
  conjugated (direct), 264, 264t, 267
  drug-induced, 1132t
  unconjugated (indirect), 264, 264t, 267
Hypercalcemia, 812t, **959**, 960f
  diagnosis of, 960, 961t
  drug-induced, 1132t
  familial hypocalciuric, 959–960, 961t, 963
  paraneoplastic, **113**, 405, 405t, **406**, 959,
    963
  treatment of, 113–114, 961–963, 962t
Hypercalciuria, 827, 960
Hypercapnia, 21, 750
Hypercarbia, 71–72
Hypercholesterolemia, **968**
  approach to, 971f
  cardiovascular disease and, 1118–1119,
    1119t
  familial, 969t, **970**
  with hypertriglyceridemia, 969t, 973–974
  isolated, 969t, **970**
  polygenic, 969t, **970**
  treatment of, 970, 971f, 972t
Hypereosinophilic syndromes, 330
Hyperesthesia, 34
Hyperglobulinemia, 269
Hyperglycemia, drug-induced, 1132t
Hyperglycemic hyperosmolar state, **100**,
    100f, 943
Hyperhidrosis, 1013, 1018
Hyper-IgE syndrome, 884
Hyperkalemia, **10**
  approach to, 13f
  causes of, 12t
  drug-induced, 10, 12t, 13f, 1132t
  ECG in, 12–13, 13f, 14f
  treatment of, 12–14, 15t, 796
Hyperlipidemia, **968**, 969t
  familial combined, 969t, **973**
Hyperlipoproteinemia, **968**
Hypermagnesemia, **965**
Hypernatremia, **7**, 8t
Hyperoxaluria, 827
Hyperparathyroidism
  primary, 959–960, 961t, 963
  secondary, 959, 961t, 963
Hyperpathia, 1018
Hyperphosphatemia, **964**
  treatment of, 796
Hyperpigmentation, drug-induced, 1133t
Hyperprolactinemia, **919**
  drug-induced, 919

Hyperpyrexia, 199
  drug-induced, 1132t
Hypersensitivity disorder, immediate type,
    877
  allergic rhinitis, **879**
  angioedema, **878**
  pathophysiology of, 877–878, 877f
  systemic mastocytosis, **880**
  urticaria, **878**
Hypersomnia, **228**, 229t
Hypersplenism, 287, 328, 331
Hypertension, **693**
  approach to, 693–694
  cardiovascular disease and, 1119–1120
  in coarctation of the aorta, 693
  drug-induced, 1136t
  essential, 693
  in hyperaldosteronism, 693–694, 935
  malignant, 83, 215, 698–699, 698t, 822
  metabolic syndrome, **699**, 700t
  in pheochromocytoma, 693–694
  portal. *See* Portal hypertension
  in pregnancy, 698
  pulmonary. *See* Pulmonary hypertension
  in renal disease, 693, 698, 786t, 788,
    795–796
  renovascular, 693–694, 821–824
  secondary, **693**
  supine nocturnal, 1019
  treatment of, 694–698, 695t, 696f, 697t,
    698t, 1119–1120
    blood pressure goals, 694, 1119
  in women, 1129
Hypertensive emergency, 698–699, 698t
Hyperthermia, **201**
  malignant, 203
Hyperthyroidism
  depression in, 1078
  muscle disorders in, 1074
  primary, 928–930
  secondary, 928–930
  sleep disorders in, 228
  subclinical, 931
  weight loss in, 247
Hypertransfusion therapy, 44
Hypertriglyceridemia, **968**
  approach to, 971f
  familial, 969t, **973**
  with hypercholesterolemia, 969t,
    973–974
  isolated, 969t, **970**
  treatment of, 971f, 972t, 973
Hypertrophic osteoarthropathy, **908**
Hyperuricemia, 903
  asymptomatic, 904
  drug-induced, 1133t
Hyperventilation, **783**
  treatment for increased intracranial pres-
    sure, 91, 92t
Hyperviscosity syndrome, 46, 283, 812t
Hypervolemia, 3
Hypnozoite, 636
Hypoalbuminemia, 242, 269, 272, 963
Hypoaldosteronism, **936**
Hypocalcemia, **963**
  drug-induced, 342t
Hypochondriasis, 1083–1084
Hypocuric myelopathy, 1030

Hypoglossal nerve, 984
  disorders of, 1024
Hypoglycemia, **103,** 104f, 210
  diagnosis of, 103–104, 105t
  drug-induced, 103, 1132t
  paraneoplastic, 405, 405t
  reactive, 103f
Hypoglycemic unawareness, 103–104
Hypogonadism, 953
  hypogonadotropic, 947
  primary, 947, 949
  secondary, 947, 949
  treatment of, 948
Hypohidrosis, 1013
Hypokalemia, **9**
  approach to, 11f
  causes of, 9t, 10
  drug-induced, 10, 1133t
Hypomagnesemia, 963, **964**
Hypomania, 1080
  drug-induced, 1140t
Hyponatremia, **3**
  acute symptomatic, 6–7
  approach to, 4f
  chronic, 5–7
  drug-induced, 1133t
  euvolemic, 3, 4f, 6
  hypervolemic, 3, 4f, 5–7
  hypovolemic, 3, 4f, 5
  paraneoplastic, **406**
  in subarachnoid hemorrhage, 89
  treatment of, 6–7
Hypoparathyroidism, 963–964
Hypophosphatemia, **946**
Hypopituitarism, **921,** 922t
Hypopnea, 783
Hypotension
  drug-induced, 1136t
  in myocardial infarction, 706, 707f,
    708
  orthostatic. *See* Orthostatic hypotension
Hypothalamic hormones, 918f
Hypothermia, **127**
  drug-induced, 128t
  risk factors for, 127, 128t
  therapeutic
    for hypoxic-ischemic encephalopathy,
      98
    for increased intracranial pressure,
      92t
    for stroke, 84
  treatment of, 128
Hypothrombinemia, drug-induced, 1134t
Hypothyroidism, 925, **926,** 827f
  clinical or overt, 926
  depression in, 1078
  edema in, 242
  muscle disorders in, 1074
  primary, 926, 926t
  secondary, 926, 926t
  subclinical or mild, 926
  transient, 926, 926t
Hypoventilation syndromes, 782t, **783**
  alveolar, **781**
  neuromuscular, 783
  obesity-hypoventilation, **783**
Hypovolemia, 3, 5
  in myocardial infarction, 706t

Hypoxemia, 71–72, 743t, 749, 782
  approach to, 750f
  mechanisms of, 750
Hypoxia, 96
  histotoxic, 96
  hypoxic-ischemic encephalopathy, **96**
Hysterectomy, 398
Hysterical fainting, 210

I
Ibandronate, for osteoporosis, 967
Ibritumomab tiuxetan
  for follicular lymphoma, 357
  toxicity of, 342t
Ibuprofen
  for frostbite, 129, 129t
  for migraine, 185t
  for narcotic withdrawal, 1100
  for pain, 36t–37t
  for pericarditis, 688
  for SLE, 886
Ibutilide
  for arrhythmias, 728t
  for Wolff-Parkinson-White syndrome, 729
Icterus. *See* Jaundice
ICU patient. *See* Critically ill patient
Idarubicin
  for AML, 346
  toxicity of, 341t
Idebenone, for ataxia, 1010
Idoxuridine, for HSV infections, 568t
Ifosfamide
  for cervical cancer, 398
  toxicity of, 341t
IgA deficiency, isolated, 884
IgA nephropathy, **808**
IgG subclass deficiency, 884
Ileal pouch-anal anastomosis, 840
Ileoproctostomy, 383
Ileus, drug-induced, 1137t–1138t
Imaging, diagnostic, **22,** 484t
Imatinib
  for CML, 349
  for gastric cancer, 381
  toxicity of, 342t
Imidazoles, **619**
  for dermatophyte infections, 317
Imipenem
  for anaerobic infections, 534t
  for cholecystitis, 847
  for enterococcal infections, 501
  for gram-negative enteric bacteria infec-
    tions, 516
  for human bite infections, 119t
  indications for, 425t
  for nocardiosis, 536t
  for nontuberculous mycobacterial infec-
    tions, 548
  for *P. aeruginosa* infections, 519t
  for pneumonia, 766t, 767t
  resistance to, 425t
Imipenem-cilastatin
  for pancreatitis, 851
  for sepsis/septic shock, 65t
  for urinary tract infections, 819t
Imipramine
  dosage and adverse effects of, 138t, 141t,
    1086t

Imipramine (*Cont.*):
for noncardiac chest pain, 250
for pain, 36t–37t
Imiquimod
for HPV infections, 476
for warts, 317
Immune-complex disorders, 46
Immune globulin, intramuscular, for hepatitis A, 854
Immune-mediated myelopathy, 1029
Immunization, **1107**
of immunosuppressed patients, 438t, **439**
recommendations for, 1104t–1105t
schedule
for adults, 1112t–1115t
for children, 1108t–1111t
for travelers, **1107**, 1116t
Immunocompromised host
cytomegalovirus infections in, 573
HSV infections in, 564–565, 567t
infections in, **432**
varicella-zoster virus infections in, 570
Immunodeficiency disease
definition of, 881
diagnosis of, 882t
immunoglobulin deficiency syndromes, **883**
leukopenia in, 331
primary, **881**
secondary, 881
severe combined immunodeficiency, **881**
T cell immunodeficiency, **883**
Immunodeficiency with hyper IgM, X-linked, 884
Immunofluorescent stain, 411
Immunoglobulin deficiency syndromes, **883**
Immunohemolytic anemia, 327–328
cold antibody, 327
warm antibody, 327
Immunology, reference values for laboratory tests, 1145t–1156t
Immunoproliferative small-intestinal disease (IPSID), 382
Immunosuppressive agents
for inflammatory bowel disease, 838
for liver transplant, 872
for renal transplant, 799–800
Impetigo, **316**, 477
bullous, 316, 477
streptococcal, 498, 498t
Impetigo contagiosa, 477
Incidentaloma, 937f, **938**
Inclusion body myositis, 1072, 1073t
India ink, 411
Indigestion, **246**
Indinavir, for HIV/AIDS, 612t
Indomethacin
for ankylosing spondylitis, 897
for pain, 36t–37t
for pericarditis, 688
for reactive arthritis, 900
Indomethacin-responsive headache, 189
Infant botulism, 529–530
Infections
leukemoid reaction in, 330
lymphocytosis in, 330
monocytosis in, 330
neutrophilia in, 329

skin disease, **316**
weight loss in, 248t
Infectious disease. *See also* Sepsis; *specific diseases and pathogens*
diagnosis of, **411**
antigen detection, 411
culture, 411–413
microscopy, 411
fatigue in, 289t
focal infections with fulminant course, 109t, 111
in immunocompromised host, **432**, 800
medical emergencies, **105**
treatment of, 106, 107t–109t
Infectious mononucleosis
cytomegalovirus, 573
Epstein-Barr virus, 574–577, 576t
Infectious myelopathy, 1029
Inferior vena cava filter, 772
Infertility
female, **958**
male, **949**
Inflammatory bowel disease, **836**
Crohn's disease, **837**
diagnosis of, 837–838, 896f
enteropathic arthritis, **907**
epidemiology of, 836, 836t
extraintestinal manifestations of, 838
treatment of, 838, 839f, 840
ulcerative colitis, **837**
Infliximab
for ankylosing spondylitis, 897
for inflammatory bowel disease, 840, 907
for psoriatic arthritis, 898
for rheumatoid arthritis, 887
Influenza, **577**
avian, 111, 577–578
complications of, 578
epidemic and emerging problems, 431
pneumonia, 578
prevention of, 580–581
treatment of, 579–580, 579t
Influenza vaccine, 438t, 580–581, 1108t–1112t, 1114t
recommendations, 580t
Influenza virus
antigenic variation, 577
as bioweapon, 167
Insect-borne disease
protozoan infections, **636**
viral infections, **593**
Insecticide poisoning, 142t
Insomnia, **226**, 229t
adjustment (acute), 227
drug-induced, 227
long-term (chronic), 227
psychophysiologic, 227
rebound, 227
short-term, 227
sleep-offset, 227
sleep-onset, 226
transient, 227
Insulin
combinations, 944t
long-acting preparations, 944t
short-acting preparations, 944t
Insulinoma, 103, 104f, 105t, 389, 390t

Insulin resistance syndrome. *See* Metabolic syndrome
Insulin therapy
    for beta blocker poisoning, 140t
    for calcium channel blocker poisoning, 140t
    for diabetes mellitus, 943–947, 944t, 946f
    for diabetic ketoacidosis, 102t
    for hyperglycemic hyperosmolar state, 101–102
    for hyperkalemia, 15t
Integrase inhibitors, for HIV/AIDS, 606, 615t
Interferon-alpha therapy
    for carcinoid tumor, 389
    for chronic hepatitis B, 864
    for essential thrombocytosis, 351–352
    for follicular lymphoma, 357
    for islet-cell tumors, 391
    for kidney cancer, 393
    for melanoma, 365
    for membranoproliferative glomerulonephritis, 805
    for Zollinger-Ellison syndrome, 836
Interferon-beta therapy, for multiple sclerosis, 1039
Interferon therapy
    for adult T cell leukemia/lymphoma, 260
    for HSV infections, 568t
    for squamous cell carcinoma, 366
    toxicity of, 342t
Interleukin-2 therapy
    for kidney cancer, 393
    for melanoma, 365
    toxicity of, 342t
Internal contamination, radiation, 172
International travel. *See* Travelers
Internist, procedures commonly performed by, **25**
Intestinal decompression, 843
Intestinal motility, 253
    altered, 254
Intestinal pseudoobstruction, **842**
    primary, 843
    secondary, 843
Intraabdominal abscess, **449,** 513
Intraabdominal infection, **448**
    clostridial, 531
    Klebsiella, 515
Intracerebral hemorrhage, 88
    in head trauma, 93
    intracranial pressure in, 90
    treatment of, 84–85
Intracranial aneurysm, 82t, 88
Intracranial hemorrhage, 80, 82t
Intracranial infection, 109t
Intracranial pressure (ICP)
    increased, **90**
        clinical features of, 90
        treatment of, 90–91, 92t
    monitoring of, 91, 92f, 92t
Intracranial tumor, **1032**
Intracytoplasmic sperm injection, 950, 958
Intraocular pressure, 295
Intraperitoneal abscess, **449**
Intrauterine contraceptive device, 537, 957
Intrauterine insemination, 958
Intravascular device infection, 431, 516

Intravenous immunoglobulin
    for *C. difficile*-associated disease, 462
    for CLL, 356
    for idiopathic thrombocytopenic purpura, 335
    for immunoglobulin deficiency, 884
    for inflammatory myopathy, 1072
    for multiple sclerosis, 1041
    for myasthenia gravis, 1066
    for parvovirus infections, 588
    for polyneuropathy, 1061
    for RSV infections, 583
    for streptococcal infections, 498t
In vitro fertilization (IVF), 958
Involucrum, 483
Iodine, radioactive, bioterrorism, 174
Iodine deficiency, 926t, 931
Iodine excess, 928
Iodoquinol, for amebiasis, 460
Ipecac, syrup of, 135, 155t
Ipratropium
    for COPD, 761–763
    for cough, 235
Irbesartan, for heart failure, 733t
Iridocyclitis, 294
Irinotecan
    for breast cancer, 379
    for cervical cancer, 398
    for colorectal cancer, 387
    toxicity of, 341t
Iris lesion, 309
Iritis, 294
Iron
    hemochromatosis, **975**
    poisoning, 147t
Iron-deficiency anemia, 324f, 325, 325t, 328
Iron overload, 44
Irritable bowel syndrome, **840,** 841t, 842t
Ischemia, hypoxic-ischemic encephalopathy, **96**
Islet-cell tumor
    pancreatic, **389,** 390t
    paraneoplastic syndromes in, 405t
Isocarboxazid, 1087t
Isolation techniques, 429
Isomethepteue, for migraine, 186t
Isoniazid
    for nontuberculous mycobacterial infections, 548
    poisoning, 150t
    for tuberculosis, 541, 543t, 545t
Isoproterenol
    for antipsychotic poisoning, 139t
    for beta blocker poisoning, 140t
    for calcium channel blocker poisoning, 140t
    for membrane-active agent poisoning, 153t
    for tachyarrhythmias, 725t
Isosorbide dinitrate
    for achalasia, 251
    for angina pectoris, 715t
    for esophageal spasm, 251
Isosorbide mononitrate, for angina pectoris, 715t
Isosporiasis, 420t, **456**
Isotretinoin, for acne, 318
Itch mite, **658**

Itraconazole, **619**
  for aspergillosis, 623, 624t–625t
  for blastomycosis, 631
  for candidiasis, 252, 621
  for coccidioidomycosis, 630
  for histoplasmosis, 629t
  for penicilliosis, 632
  for sporotrichosis, 631
Ivermectin
  for larva migrans, 649
  for onchocerciasis, 653
  for pediculiasis, 658
  for scabies, 658
  for strongyloidiasis, 651

J
Japanese encephalitis, **595,** 596t–597t
Japanese encephalitis vaccine, 1116t
Jarisch-Herxheimer reaction, 474
Jaundice, **263**
  approach to, 265f
  causes of, 264, 264t
  cholestatic conditions that produce, 267t
  drug-induced, 266t, 1137t–1138t
  hepatocellular conditions that produce, 266t
  obstructive, 268t
JC virus, 1051
Jellyfish sting, 122
Jet-lag disorder, 226–227, 230
Jimson weed, 138t
Joint(s), muscles and innervation of, 980t
Joint disease
  anaerobic infections, 533
  neuropathic, **908**
  P. aeruginosa infections, 517
Joint pain, **203**
  assessment of, 204–205, 204f
  diagnostic imaging in, 206–207, 207t
  in elderly, 207
  laboratory features in, 205–206
  physical examination in, 205
Joint replacement surgery, 902
Jugular foramen syndrome, 1024
Jugular venous pulsation, **661,** 662f
Juvenile polyposis, 384, 384t

K
Kaolin-pectin, for diarrhea, 256
Kaposi's sarcoma, 572, 605
Katayama fever, 654
Kayexalate, for hyperkalemia, 15t
Kenya tick typhus, 555
Keratitis, 294
Keratoconjunctivitis, 583
Keratoconjunctivitis sicca, 890
Keratoderma blenorrhagica, 899
Keratosis pilaris, 311f
Ketoacidosis. *See specific types*
Ketoconazole
  for *Candida* esophagitis, 252
  for ectopic ACTH syndrome, 407
Ketorolac
  for frostbite, 129t
  for pain, 36t–37t
Kidney cancer, **392**
  infections in cancer patients, 433t
  oncologic emergencies, 113
  paraneoplastic syndromes in, 393, 405t

Kidney disease. *See* Renal disease
Kidney stones, 450
Kingella kingae infection. *See* HACEK group
  infection
Klebsiella granulomatosis infection, **476**
Klebsiella infection, **514**
Klinefelter's syndrome, 947
Koplik's spots, 584
Korsakoff's syndrome, 1097
Kussmaul's sign, 662
Kwashiorkor, 40
Kyphoscoliosis, 231

L
Labetalol
  for aortic dissection, 738t
  for hypertension, 695t, 698, 698t, 822
  poisoning, 140t
  for sympathomimetic poisoning, 136t
Laboratory tests, reference values for, **1141**
Labyrinthine dysfunction
  acute bilateral, 212–213
  acute unilateral, 212
  recurrent, 213
Labyrinthitis, 212, 245t
La Crosse encephalitis, 596t–597t
Lactic acidosis, 17t, 18–19
D-Lactic acidosis, 17t, 18–19
Lactose hydrogen breath test, 256
Lactulose
  for constipation, 48t, 259
  for hepatic encephalopathy, 874
  for irritable bowel syndrome, 842t
Lacunar syndromes, 80, 85
Lambert-Eaton myasthenic syndrome, 408t,
  409, 409t
Laminectomy, decompressive, 95
Lamivudine
  for chronic hepatitis B, 858, 860t–861t,
    864
  for HIV/AIDS, 608t
Lamotrigine
  for bipolar disorder, 1080
  dosage and adverse effects of, 143t, 1092t
  for seizures, 992t–993t, 994t
Lansoprazole, for *H. pylori* eradication, 833t
Larva migrans
  cutaneous, **649**
  ocular, **649**
  visceral, **649**
Laryngeal cancer, **367**
Laryngeal palsy, 1024
Laryngitis, **306**
Laser therapy
  for diabetic retinopathy, 296
  for glaucoma, 295
Lassa fever, 110, 597–598
Latex agglutination assay, 411
Laxatives
  for constipation, 259
  for hemorrhoids, 844
Lead poisoning, 156t–157t
Leech infestation, **659**
Leflunomide
  for psoriatic arthritis, 898
  for rheumatoid arthritis, 888
Left ventricular function, assessment by nu-
  clear cardiology, 671, 672t

Legionella infection, **521**
  specimen collection and transport, 418t
Legionnaires' disease, 521
Leiomyoma
  gastric, 381
  small-bowel, 382
Leiomyosarcoma, gastric, 380–381
Leishmaniasis, **642**
  cutaneous, 643–644
  mucosal, 643–644
  visceral, 643–644
Lemierre syndrome, 533
Lenalidomide, for myelodysplastic syndromes, 350
Lepirudin
  for heparin-induced thrombocytopenia, 334
  for thrombotic disorders, 337
Leprosy, **542**
  complications of, 544–545
  lepromatous, 544
  treatment of, 546–547
  tuberculoid, 544
Leptomeningeal metastasis, **1034**, 1034t
Leptospirosis, **551**
  anicteric, 552
  icteric, 552
Leriche syndrome, 738
Letrozole
  for breast cancer, 378–379
  toxicity of, 342t
Leucovorin
  for *Pneumocystis* infections, 634t
    preventive treatment, 635t
  for toxoplasmosis, 647
Leukapheresis, **46**
Leukemia. *See also specific types*
  definition of, 352
  drug-induced, 341t
  infections in cancer patients, 433t
  monocytopenia in, 331
Leukemoid reaction, **330**
Leukocytes
  inclusion and nuclear abnormalities, 322
  normal values in blood, 329t
Leukocytosis, **329**
  drug-induced, 1135t
Leukoerythroblastic reaction, **330**
Leukopenia, **330**
  drug-induced, 331
Leukoplakia, 367
  oral, 1125
Leuprolide
  for prostate cancer, 401
  toxicity of, 342t
Levetiracetam
  poisoning, 143t
  for seizures, 994t
Levodopa, for Parkinson's disease, 1004, 1005t–1006t
Levofloxacin
  for *C. pneumoniae* infections, 563
  indications for, 427t
  for *Legionella* infections, 522
  for *M. pneumoniae* infections, 560
  for *P. aeruginosa* infections, 519t–520t
  for pelvic inflammatory disease, 466
  for pneumococcal infections, 488

  for pneumonia, 766t, 767t
  resistance to, 427t
  for sepsis/septic shock, 65t
  for sinusitis, 303t
  for *S. maltophilia,* 518
  for staphylococcal infections, 494t
  for tuberculosis, 542
Levorphanol, for pain, 36t–37t, 38
Levosimendan, for heart failure, 734t
Levothyroxine, for hypothyroidism, 927–930
Lewisite, 168
Lhermitte's symptom, 1036
Lice, human, **658**
Lichenification, 313t
Lichenoid eruption, drug-induced, 1134t
Lichen planus, 310f, **314**
Lichen simplex chronicus, 311f
Liddle's syndrome, 20
Lidocaine
  for antidepressant poisoning, 141t
  for antipsychotic poisoning, 139t
  for arrhythmias, 727t
  for cardiac glycoside poisoning, 141t
  for membrane-active agent poisoning, 153t
  for polyneuropathy, 1061
  for tachyarrhythmias, 724t–725t
Ligase IV gene, 882
Light chain deposition disease, 812t, 813
Limb dystonia, 223
Limb-girdle dystrophy, **1071**
Limbic encephalitis, paraneoplastic, 407, 408t
Linear skin lesion, 309
Linezolid
  adverse reactions to, 428
  for enterococcal infections, 501
  indications for, 427t
  for MRSA infections, 479t
  for nocardiosis, 536t
  for osteomyelitis, 485t
  for pneumonia, 766t, 767t
  resistance to, 427t
  for staphylococcal infections, 494t, 496
Lioresal, for multiple sclerosis, 1041
Lipase, serum, 849
Lipemia retinalis, 973
Lipodystrophy syndrome, 606
Lipoma, small-bowel, 382
Lipoprotein analysis, 968–970, 969t
Lipoprotein lipase deficiency, 969t, **973**
Liquid nitrogen, for warts, 317
Lisinopril
  for heart failure, 733t
  for hypertension, 695t
Listerial infection, **507**
  in pregnancy, 507
Lithium, 1093
  for bipolar disorder, 1080
  for cluster headache prevention, 187
  dosage and adverse effects of, 8, 151t, 1092t
Liver abscess, **450**
  amebic, 460–461
  streptococcal, 501
Liver biopsy, percutaneous, 271
Liver disease
  alcoholic, **869**
  benign tumors, **388**

Liver disease (*Cont.*):
  coagulation disorders in, 334–335
  drug-induced, 1137t–1138t
  hepatobiliary imaging in, **270**
  jaundice in, **263**
Liver failure
  acute, **858**
  adverse prognostic indicators, 859
  fulminant, 90
  sleep disorders in, 228
Liver flap, 224
Liver function tests, 266f, **267**, 268t
Liver transplant, 858–859, 862t, 870, **871,**
    915, 978
  for ascites, 272
  contraindications to, 872t
  immunosuppressive agents for, 872
  indications for, 871t
  infections in recipients, 439
  medical complications after, 872
Lobeline, 142t
Local anesthetics, 146t, 153t
Lockjaw, 528
Löffler's syndrome, 650
Löfgren's syndrome, 911
Loperamide
  for diarrhea, 256, 1117
  for inflammatory bowel disease, 838
  for irritable bowel syndrome, 841, 842t
  for narcotic withdrawal, 1100
  for traveler's diarrhea, 453
Lopinavir/ritonavir, for HIV/AIDS, 613t
Loratadine, for allergic rhinitis, 880
Lorazepam
  for alcohol withdrawal, 1098
  for delirium, 50t
  dosage and action of, 1089t
  for dyspnea, 49t
  for myocardial infarction, 702
  for nausea, 49
  poisoning, 143t
  for status epilepticus, 99f
Losartan
  for heart failure, 733t
  for hypertension, 695t
  for systemic sclerosis, 889
Lovastatin, for hyperlipidemia, 972t
Low back pain, **189**
  acute, 193–196, 194f–195f
  causes of, 190–191
    visceral, 193, 193t
  chronic, 196
  examination in, 190, 191t
  risk factors for structural cause, 192t
  types of, 190
Low back strain/sprain, 192
Lower esophageal sphincter, disorders of, 251
Low-molecular-weight heparin
  for thrombotic disorders, 336, 337t
  for venous disease, 741
  for venous thromboembolism, 770–771
Loxapine, 1091t
Lubiprostone, for irritable bowel syndrome,
    842t
Ludwig's angina, 532
Lumbar disk disease, back pain in, 190
Lumbar puncture, **27**, 28f, 416t
Lumbar puncture headache, 189

Lumpectomy, 376
Lung abscess, 533, 767
Lung biopsy, 774
Lung cancer, **368**
  adenocarcinoma, 369, 372t–373t
  bronchoalveolar, 374
  causes of, 369, 756–757
  diagnosis of, 751
  epidermoid (squamous), 369
  large cell, 369
  non-small cell, 372t
  oncologic emergencies, 112–113
  paraneoplastic syndromes in, 369, 405t,
    406–407, 409t
  prevention of, 1124
  screening for, 1122
  small cell (oat cell), 369, 371–374, 372t
  staging of, 369–371, 370t–371t
  treatment of, 371–374, 372t–373t
Lung disease. *See also* Respiratory disease
  anaerobic infections, 533
  cor pulmonale, **735**
  cyanosis in, **239,** 240t
  diffuse parenchymal, 231
  dyspnea, 231–233, 232t
  environmental, **756**
    inorganic dusts, 757
    occupational exposures, **757**
    organic dusts, **758**
    toxic chemicals, **758**
  fatigue in, 289t
  interstitial, **772**
    with alveolitis, inflammation, and fi-
      brosis, 772, 773t
    in connective tissue disorders, 775–776
    drug-induced, 774
    with granulomatous reaction, 772, 773t
  nocardiosis, 535, 536t
  nontuberculous mycobacterial infections,
    547
  pulmonary hypertension in, 743t
Lung transplant
  for COPD, 762
  infections in recipients, 439
Lung volume(s), 747f
Lung volume reduction surgery, 762
Lupus, drug-induced, 885, 1131t
Luteinizing hormone, 917, 918f
Lyme borreliosis, 125, **549,** 558
  arthritis, 550–551
  disseminated infection, 550–551
  localized infection, 549
  persistent infection, 550–551
Lymphadenitis, in tuberculosis, 539
Lymphadenopathy, **283**
  diseases associated with, 284t
  drug-induced, 1135t
  due to hyperplasia, 284–285
  due to infiltration, 285
  in HIV/AIDS, 605
Lymphangiectasia, intestinal, 331
Lymphedema, **742**
Lymphocutaneous syndrome, nocardiosis,
    535, 536t
Lymphocytic choriomeningitis, **594**
Lymphocytic leukemia, chronic (CLL), **355**
  staging of, 355, 356t
Lymphocytosis, **330**

Lymphoepithelioma, 367
Lymphogranuloma venereum, 468, 471
    features of genital ulcers, 467t
Lymphoid leukemia/lymphoma
    acute (ALL), 353t, 354f, **359**
        adult T cell leukemia/lymphoma, **360**
        acute lymphoblastic leukemia and lym-
            phoblastic lymphoma, **359**
    chronic, 353t, 354f, **355**
Lymphoid malignancy, **352**
    classification of, 352, 353t
    diagnosis and staging of, 355
    incidence and etiology of, 352–355, 354f
Lymphoma, **352**, 572. *See also specific types*
    aggressive, 353t, 355, **357**
    definition of, 352
    indolent, 353t, 355, **357**
    infections in patients, 433t
    oncologic emergencies, 112–113
    primary CNS, **1033**
Lymphopenia, **331**
Lymphoproliferative disease
    posttransplantation, 575, 577
    X-linked, 884
Lynch syndrome, 384, 384t

M
Macular degeneration, 215, 216f, **296**, 296f
    dry, 296
    wet, 296
Macule, 313t
Maculopapular rash, 106, 200
Magnesium, serum, arrhythmias and, 704
Magnesium citrate
    for constipation, 48t
    for poisoning, 135
Magnesium hydroxide (Milk of Magnesia)
    for constipation, 48t
    for irritable bowel syndrome, 842t
Magnesium therapy
    for antipsychotic poisoning, 139t
    for cardiac glycoside poisoning, 141t
    for hypomagnesemia, 965
    for membrane-active agent poisoning,
        153t
    for torsades de pointes, 725t
Magnetic resonance angiography, in stroke,
        80, 85
Magnetic resonance imaging (MRI)
    in coma, 79
    in heart disease, 672t, 673
    hepatobiliary, 270, 846t
    indications for, **24**
    in myocardial infarction, 701
    neuroimaging, 986, 987t
    in osteomyelitis, 484t
    in poisoning, 133
    in respiratory disease, 751
    in spinal cord disorders, 94–95
    utility of, **24**
Malabsorption syndromes, **256**
    causes of, 259t
    drug-induced, 1137t–1138t
Malaria, 421, 636
    cerebral, 109t, 636
    in children, 637
    diagnosis of, 420t
    in pregnancy, 637

prevention of, 639, 640t–641t, 1116
    transfusion, 637
    treatment of, 637–639, 638t–639t
Malassezia infection, **631**
Malathion, for pediculiasis, 658
Maldigestion, 259t
Male gender, cardiovascular disease and,
        1120
Malingering, 1084
Malnutrition, **39**
    ascites in, 272
    eye disease in, 294
MALT lymphoma, 355, 380–382, 835
Mammography, 375
    screening, 375–376, 1122, 1123t
Mandibular positioning device, 784
Mania, 1080
    drug-induced, 1140t
Manic depressive illness. *See* Bipolar disorder
Mannitol therapy
    for increased intracranial pressure, 90–91,
        92t
    for poisoning, 135
    for stroke, 83
MAO inhibitor poisoning, 138t, 152t
Marasmus, 40
Maraviroc, for HIV/AIDS, 606, 615t
Marburg virus infection, 110, **599**
March hemoglobinuria, 328
Marie-Strumpell disease. *See* Ankylosing
        spondylitis
Marine envenomations, **122**
    invertebrate, 122–123
    vertebrate, 123
Marine poisoning, **123**
Mastectomy
    bilateral prophylactic, 1124
    for breast cancer, 376
Mastitis, staphylococcal, 491
Mastocytosis, systemic, **880**, 880t
Mastoiditis, **305**
M component, 360–361
Measles vaccine, 585
Measles virus infection, **584**
    atypical measles, 585
    CNS disease, 584–585
    gastrointestinal disease, 585
    postexposure prophylaxis, 585
    respiratory disease, 584
    subacute sclerosing panencephalitis, 585
Mebendazole
    for ascariasis, 650
    for enterobiasis, 651
    for hookworm, 650
    for trichinellosis, 649
Mechanical ventilation. *See* Ventilatory sup-
        port
Mechlorethamine, 341t
Meclizine
    for nausea and vomiting, 48, 245
    for vertigo, 214t
Mediastinal mass, **781**
Mediastinitis, **781**
Mediastinoscopy, 752
Medical emergencies. *See* Emergencies, med-
        ical
Medicinal leech, 659
Mediterranean spotted fever, 110, 555

Medrol, for anaphylaxis, 117
Medroxyprogesterone
    for amenorrhea, 953
    for menopausal symptoms, 957
    toxicity of, 342t
Mefloquine, for malaria, 638t
    preventive treatment, 639, 641t
Megestrol
    for endometrial cancer, 397
    for weight loss, 248
Meglumine antimonate, for leishmaniasis,
        643
Melanoma, **364**
    acral lentiginous, 364–365
    of eye, 296
    lentigo maligna, 364
    metastatic, 365
    nodular, 365
    paraneoplastic syndromes in, 409t
    risk factors for, 364, 365t
    superficial spreading, 364
Melarsoprol, for sleeping sickness, 646
Melena, 259
Meleney's gangrene, 533
Melioidosis, 518, 520t
Melphalan
    for amyloidosis, 915
    for multiple myeloma, 361
    toxicity of, 341t
Memantine, for Alzheimer's disease, 1000
Mendelson's syndrome, 533
Ménière's disease, 213, 214t, 300
Meningioma, 216f, **1033**, 1034f
Meningitis
    acute, **1042**
        approach to, 1042, 1043f–1044f
    acute bacterial, **1042**
        clinical features of, 1044
        laboratory features of, 1044–1045,
            1045t
        pathogens, 1042, 1047t
        treatment of, 1045, 1046t, 1047t
    aseptic
        enterovirus, 590
        HSV, 565–566, 567t–568t
        poliovirus, 589
    bacterial, 108t, 111
    chronic, **1052**
        approach to, 1052–1055
        causes of, 1053, 1054t, 1055t
        clinical features of, 1052, 1053t
    coccidioidomycosis, 630
    E. coli, 513
    enterococcal, 501
    gonococcal, 470t
    H. influenzae, 508
    listerial, 507
    lumbar puncture, 27–28, 28f
    meningococcal, 504–506
    Mollaret's, 566
    pneumococcal, 487–488
    streptococcal, 500
    viral, **1046**
        pathogens, 1047t
        treatment of, 1048
Meningococcal infection, **504,** 506t
    meningitis, 504–506
    respiratory disease, 504

Meningococcal vaccine, 438t, 505–506, 506t,
        1108t–1112t, 1115t, 1116t
Meningococcemia, 106, 107t, 201, 504–506
Meningoencephalitis
    cryptococcal, 623, 626
    listerial, 507
Menopause, **956**
    sleep disorders in, 228
Mental status exam, **979,** 979t
Meperidine
    for cholecystitis, 847
    narcotic abuse, **1099**
    for pain, 36t–37t
    for pancreatitis, 851
    poisoning, 152t, 153t
Meprobamate poisoning, 144t
Meralgia paresthetica, 1063t
6-Mercaptopurine
    for Burkitt's lymphoma, 359–360
    for inflammatory bowel disease, 838
Mercury poisoning, 158t–159t
Meropenem
    for anaerobic infections, 534t
    for bacterial meningitis, 1046t, 1047t
    for *B. cepacia* infections, 518, 520t
    for brain abscess, 1051
    for cholecystitis, 847
    indications for, 425t
    for meningococcal infections, 506t
    for *P. aeruginosa* infections, 519t
    for pneumonia, 767t
    resistance to, 425t
Merozoite, 636
Mesalamine enema, for inflammatory bowel
        disease, 838
Mesenteric arteriography, 260, 873
Mesenteric insufficiency, chronic, 843
Mesenteric ischemia, acute, 843
Mesothelioma, 757
Metabolic acidosis, **16**
    anion-gap, 17t, 18–19, 21
    causes of, 16–18, 17t
    drug-induced, 17t, 1133t
    hyperchloremic, 19
    non-anion-gap, 17t, 18, 21
Metabolic alkalosis, **19,** 20f
    chloride-resistant, 19–20, 20f
    chloride-responsive, 19–20, 20f
Metabolic disease
    abdominal pain in, 179t
    drug-induced, 1132t
    weight loss in, 248t
Metabolic syndrome, **699**
    NCEP:ATPIII 2001 and IDF criteria for,
        700t
Metabolism disruptors, 132t
Metapneumovirus infection, **583**
Metformin
    for diabetes mellitus, 944–945, 945t
    for obesity, 940
Methadone, 1099
    for narcotic withdrawal, 1100
    for opioid maintenance, 1100
    for pain, 36t–37t, 38
Methanol poisoning, 17t, 18–19, 148t
Methemoglobinemia, 239
Methemoglobin inducers, 146t
Methenamine, for nephrolithiasis, 828t

Methimazole, for thyrotoxicosis, 928–929
Methotrexate
    for ankylosing spondylitis, 897
    for bladder cancer, 392
    for head and neck cancer, 368
    for inflammatory bowel disease, 840
    for inflammatory myopathy, 1072
    for multiple sclerosis, 1039
    for polyneuropathy, 1061
    for primary sclerosing cholangitis, 849
    for psoriasis, 314
    for psoriatic arthritis, 898
    for reactive arthritis, 900
    for rheumatoid arthritis, 887
    toxicity of, 341t
    for vasculitis, 894
Methyl cellulose, for irritable bowel syn-
        drome, 842t
Methyldopa, for hypertension, 698
Methylene blue, for methemoglobin, 146t
Methylphenidate, for daytime sleepiness,
        229t, 230
Methylprednisolone
    for asthma, 756
    for multiple sclerosis, 1039, 1041
    for optic neuritis, 217
    for renal transplant rejection, 799
    steroid preparations, 938–939, 938t
Methylsergide
    for migraine prevention, 188t
    poisoning, 137t
Methylxanthine poisoning, 137t
Metoclopramide
    for H. pylori eradication, 247
    for migraine, 186t
    for nausea and vomiting, 246
    for systemic sclerosis, 889
Metolazone
    for edema, 243t
    for heart failure, 731, 733t
    for hypertension, 698
Metoprolol
    for arrhythmias, 727t
    for heart failure, 733t
    for hypertension, 695, 695t
    for myocardial infarction, 702, 711
        preventive treatment, 709
    poisoning, 140t
    for sympathomimetic poisoning, 136t
    for unstable angina, 711
    for vasovagal syncope, 210
Metronidazole
    for acne, 318
    adverse reactions to, 428
    for amebiasis, 461
    for anaerobic infections, 534, 534t
    for bacterial meningitis, 1046t, 1047t
    for brain abscess, 109t, 1051
    for C. difficile-associated disease,
        461–462
    for diverticulitis, 842
    for giardiasis, 455
    for hepatic encephalopathy, 874
    for H. pylori eradication, 833t
    indications for, 427t
    for inflammatory bowel disease, 838–839
    for intestinal pseudoobstruction, 843
    for necrotizing fasciitis, 480t

    for osteomyelitis, 485t
    for pelvic inflammatory disease, 466
    resistance to, 427t
    for tetanus, 529
    for trichomoniasis, 464
    for urethritis in men, 463
Metyrapone, for ectopic ACTH syndrome,
        407
Mexiletine
    for arrhythmias, 727t
    for myotonic dystrophy, 1071
MHC class II deficiency, 883
Micafungin, 620
    for candidiasis, 621
Miconazole, 620
    for candidiasis, 464
Microaerophilic bacteria, 528
Microbial bioterrorism, 160, 432
    CDC category A agents, 161t, 162–167
    CDC category B agents, 161t, 167
    CDC category C agents, 161t, 167
    features of bioweapons, 161t
    prevention and preparedness, 167
Micrographia, 1002
Micronutrient deficiency, 43t, 44
Microscopic polyangiitis, 892
Microscopy, diagnostic, 411
Midazolam
    for delirium, 50t
    for dyspnea, 49t
    for increased intracranial pressure, 92t
    poisoning, 143t
    for scorpion sting, 126
    for status epilepticus, 99f
Midodrine
    for hepatorenal syndrome, 274
    for orthostatic hypotension, 1019
Mifepristone, for emergency contraception,
        957
Miglitol, for diabetes mellitus, 945t
Migraine, 183, 183t
    diagnosis of, 184t
    prevention of, 188t
    sleep disorders and, 227
    treatment of, 184, 185t–187t
    vertigo in, 213, 214t
    visual loss in, 215
Migrating motor complex, 253
Milk alkali syndrome, 19
Milrinone
    for heart failure, 734t, 735
    for myocardial infarction, 705, 705t
Miltefosine, for leishmaniasis, 643–644
Milwaukee shoulder, 906
Mineral(s)
    therapy for mineral deficiencies, 43t
    trace, reference values for laboratory tests,
        1160t
Mineralocorticoids, 933
Mineral oil, for constipation, 259
Minimal change disease, 804
Mini-mental status examination, 979t, 995
Mini-transplant, 356
Minocycline
    for actinomycosis, 538
    indications for, 426t
    for leprosy, 547
    for nocardiosis, 536t

Minocycline (*Cont.*):
  resistance to, 426t
  for staphylococcal infections, 493, 494t
Mirtazapine, 1086t
Misoprostol, for erosive gastropathies, 834
Mithramycin, 342t
Mitochondrial myopathies, **1074**
Mitomycin
  for anal cancer, 388
  toxicity of, 342t
Mitotane, for adrenal carcinoma, 934
Mitoxantrone
  for multiple sclerosis, 1039
  for prostate cancer, 401
  toxicity of, 341t
Mitral regurgitation, 662t, **678**, 680f
  echocardiography in, 671f
  in myocardial infarction, 708
Mitral stenosis, 662t
  echocardiography in, 671f
  treatment of, 678, 679f
Mitral valve prolapse, 662t, **680**
Mittelschmerz, 954
Mixed anaerobic infection, **532**
Mixed connective tissue disease, **890**
MMR vaccine, 438t, 585–586, 1108t–1113t
MMRV vaccine, 585
Mobilizing agent, for radionuclide contamination, 174
Modafinil
  for circadian rhythm disorders, 230
  for daytime sleepiness, 229t, 230
  for depression, 50
Moh's micrographic surgery, 366
Molindone, 1091t
Molluscum contagiosum, 477
Monkey bite, 118, 119t
Monoamine oxidase inhibitors (MAOI), 1087t, 1088
Monoclonal gammopathy of uncertain significance (MGUS), 361
Monocytopenia, **331**
Monocytosis, **330**
Mononeuritis multiplex, 1061
Mononeuropathy, 1055, 1062t–1064t, **1065**
Mononeuropathy multiplex, 1061
Montelukast
  for allergic rhinitis, 880
  for asthma, 755
  for urticaria/angioedema, 879
Mood disorder, **1077**
Mood stabilizers, 1092t, **1093**
MOPP-ABV regimen, for Hodgkin's disease, 364
MOPP regimen, for Hodgkin's disease, 364
Moraxella catarrhalis infection, **510**
Morbilliform lesion, 309
Morganella infection, 516
Morphine
  for dyspnea, 49t
  for increased intracranial pressure, 92t
  for myocardial infarction, 702, 711
  narcotic abuse, **1099**
  for pain, 36t–37t, 38
  for pulmonary edema, 68
  for unstable angina, 711
Mortality, age-specific, 1103, 1104t–1105t
Mosquito-borne viral infection, **593**

Motion sickness, 214t, 245, 245t
Motor exam, **984**
Motor fluctuations, 1004
Motor neuron disease, **1010**
  etiology and investigation of, 1012t
  lower motor neurons, 219t, 220t, 1011t
  secondary, 1011t
  sporadic, 1011t
  upper motor neurons, 219t, 220, 220t, 1011t
Motor unit disorders, 220, 220t
Movement disorders, **222**
  insomnia and, 227
Moxifloxacin
  indications for, 427t
  for *Legionella* infections, 522
  for pneumonia, 766t, 767t
  resistance to, 427t
  for tuberculosis, 542
Mucormycosis, **626**
  pulmonary, 627
  rhinocerebral, 111, 626–627
Mucositis, acute necrotizing ulcerative, 532
Mucous membranes
  dry, in terminally ill patient, 53t
  in malnutrition, 41
Mucous patch, 472
Multifocal motor neuropathy with conduction block, 1011, 1011t
Multi-infarct dementia, 1000–1001
Multiorgan system failure, **32**
Multiple cranial nerve palsies, **1024**
Multiple endocrine neoplasia type 1, 389, 835–836, 959
Multiple myeloma, 355, **360**
  glomerular disease in, 807t
  infections in patients, 433t
  oncologic emergencies, 113
  paraneoplastic syndromes in, 405t
  staging of, 361, 362t
Multiple sclerosis (MS), **1035**
  acute (Marburg's variant), 1041
  clinical features of, 1035–1036
  clinical variants of, **1041**
  definite, 1036t
  diagnostic criteria for, 1036–1037, 1036t
  disorders that mimic, 1037t
  facial nerve involvement in, 1022
  laboratory features of, 1037–1038, 1038f
  primary progressive, 1037, 1040f
  probable, 1036t
  progressive-relapsing, 1037
  relapsing-remitting, 1037, 1040f
  at risk for, 1036t
  secondary progressive, 1037, 1039, 1040f
  spinal cord involvement in, 1030
  treatment of, 1039–1041, 1040f
    acute relapses, 1039
    disease-modifying therapies, 1039
    progressive symptoms, 1039–1040
    symptomatic therapy, 1041
Multiple sleep latency test, 228, 229t
Multiple system atrophy, 1016
Mumps virus infection, **586**
  orchitis, 587
  parotitis, 586–587
Munchausen's syndrome, 1084

Mupirocin, 427t
Murmur. *See* Heart murmur
Murphy's sign, 845
Muscle contracture, 1068
Muscle cramp, 1068
Muscle disease, **1068**
    approach to, 1068, 1069f–1070f
    disorders of energy metabolism, **1072**
    drug-induced, **1074**, 1075t, 1140t
    endocrine and metabolic myopathies, **1074**
    inflammatory myopathies, **1072**, 1073t
    mitochondrial myopathies, **1074**
    muscular dystrophies, **1068**
    paraneoplastic, 408–409, 408t
    periodic paralysis, **1074**
Muscle relaxant poisoning, 138t, 139t, 144t
Muscle spasm, back pain in, 190
Muscular dystrophy
    Duchenne, **1068**
    facioscapulohumeral, **1071**
    limb-girdle, **1071**
    myotonic dystrophy, **1071**
    oculopharyngeal, **1072**
Musculoskeletal complaints, **203**
Musculoskeletal infection
    E. coli, 513
    S. aureus, 491
Mushrooms, poisonous, 138t, 142t, 858
M-VAC regimen, for bladder cancer, 392
Myalgia, 1068
    drug-induced, 1140t
Myasthenia gravis (MG), **1065**
    differential diagnosis of, 1066
    diplopia in, 217
    paraneoplastic, 408t, 409t
    treatment of, 1066–1067, 1067f
Myasthenic crisis, 1066–1067
Mycetoma, 302
Mycobacterium abscessus infection, **548**
Mycobacterium chelonae infection, **548**
Mycobacterium fortuitum infection, **548**
Mycobacterium infection, 417t
Mycobacterium kansasii infection, **548**
Mycobacterium leprae infection. *See* Leprosy
Mycobacterium marinum infection, **549**
Mycobacterium tuberculosis infection. *See*
        Tuberculosis
Mycobacterium ulcerans infection, **549**
Mycophenolate mofetil
    immunosuppression for renal transplant,
        800
    for inflammatory myopathy, 1072
    for myasthenia gravis, 1066
    for SLE, 803, 886
Mycoplasma genitalium infection, **471**
    cervicitis, 465
    urethritis in men, 463
Mycoplasmal infection, **471**
    arthritis, 471
    bacterial vaginosis, 471
    pelvic inflammatory disease, 465, 471–472
    urethritis, 471
Mycoplasma pneumoniae infection, **560**
Mycotic aneurysm, 88
Myelitis, paraneoplastic, 408t
Myelodysplastic syndrome, 325, 345t, **350**
    classification of, 348t–349t
    with isolated del(5q), 348t–349t

prognostic scoring system for, 350, 350t
    unclassified, 348t–349t
Myelofibrosis, 330
    idiopathic, **351**
Myelography, 986
Myeloid leukemia
    acute (AML), **344**
        classification of, 345t
    chronic (CML), **347**
        response criteria for, 348t
Myelopathy. *See also specific types*
    retrovirus-associated, 1029
Myelophthisis, 330
Myeloproliferative syndrome, **351**
    leukocytosis in, 329–330
Myelosuppression, drug-induced, 341t–342t
Myiasis, **659**
Myocardial infarction
    anterior, 704
    arrhythmias in, 704
    cardiogenic shock in, 706t, 707
    chest pain in, 175, 177f
    complications of, 704–705
        acute mechanical complications, 708
        hemodynamic, 706t
    ECG in, 666–667, 667f, 668f, 668t, 689t
    heart failure and, 705, 705t, 706t
    hypotension in, 706, 707f, 708
    hypovolemia in, 706t
    laboratory features of, 700–701, 709
    non-ST-elevation (non-Q-wave), 666–667,
        667f, 668t, 689t, 700, **709**
        treatment of, 709–712, 710f
    pericarditis in, 708
    secondary prevention of, 708–709
    ST-segment elevation (Q-wave), 666–667,
        667f, 668t, 689t, **700**
        treatment of, 701–704, 702f, 703f
    syncope in, 208
    TIMI Risk Score for, 709–710, 711f
    treatment of, 337t, 338
    ventricular aneurysm and, 708
Myocardial ischemia
    chest pain in, 175, 175t, 176f
    sleep disruption in, 228
Myocarditis, **687**
    enterovirus, 590
Myoclonus, 224
    posthypoxic, 98
Myonecrosis, **481**
    clostridial. *See* Gas gangrene
Myopathy, 1068. *See also specific types*
    drug-induced, 1074, 1075t, 1140t
    inflammatory, **1072**, 1073t
    weakness in, 219t, 220t
Myophosphorylase deficiency, 1073
Myositis, **481**. *See also specific types*
    drug-induced, 1140t
Myotonia, 1068
Myotonic dystrophy, **1071**
Myringitis, bullous, 560
Myxedema coma, 927–928

N
Nadolol
    poisoning, 140t
    for variceal bleeding, 263
    for vasovagal syncope, 210

Nafcillin
  for bacterial meningitis, 1046t, 1047t
  for cellulitis, 479t
  indications for, 425t
  for infective endocarditis, 445t
  for osteomyelitis, 485t
  for perichondritis, 304
  resistance to, 425t
  for sepsis/septic shock, 65t
  for staphylococcal infections, 494t
Nailbed, in cyanosis, 239
Nail lesions, 311
Naloxone
  for membrane-active agent poisoning, 153t
  for opiate overdose, 1100
  for sympatholytic poisoning, 139t
Naltrexone
  for alcoholic rehabilitation, 1098
  for primary biliary cirrhosis, 871
Naproxen
  for migraine, 185t
  for pain, 36t–37t
Naratriptan, for migraine, 185t, 187t
Narcissistic personality disorder, 1084
Narcolepsy, 226, 228, 229t, 230t
Narcotic(s), 36t–37t, 38
  for abdominal pain, 182
  for frostbite, 129, 129t
  for migraine, 186t
Narcotic abuse, **1099**
  clinical features of, 1099–1100
  prevention of, 1101
  treatment of, 1100–1101
    drug-free programs, 1101
    opiate antagonists, 1100–1101
    opioid maintenance, 1100
    overdose, 1100
    withdrawal, 1099–1100
Nasal swab, 414t
Nasopharyngeal cancer, **367,** 575–576, 576t
Nasopharynx, *S. pneumoniae* carriage, 486
Nataglinide, for diabetes mellitus, 945t
Natalizumab, for multiple sclerosis, 1039
Nausea and vomiting, **244**
  causes of, 244–245, 245t
  drug-induced, 245t, 341t–342t, 343–344, 1137t–1138t
  in terminally ill patient, 48
  treatment of, 48–49, 245–246, 343–344
Necator americanus infection. *See* Hook-
    worm infection
Neck infections, 307
Neck pain, **196**
Neck weakness, 1024
Necrotizing fasciitis, 108t, 110, 477, **478**
  mixed anaerobic-aerobic infection, 533
  streptococcal, 497–498, 498t
  treatment of, 479t–480t, 480
Necrotizing myelopathy, acute, 408
Nedocromil sodium, for asthma, 755
Nefazodone, 1087t
Negri bodies, 592
Neisseria gonorrhoeae infection. *See* Gonor-
    rhea
Neisseria meningitidis infection. *See* Menin-
    gococcal infection
Nelfinavir, for HIV/AIDS, 612t

Nematocysts, 122
Nematode infection, **648**
  filarial worms, **651**
  intestinal, **649**
  tissue nematodes, **648**
Neomycin, for hepatic encephalopathy, 874
Neonatal disease
  cytomegalovirus infections, 573
  generalized disease of the newborn, 590
  HSV infections, 566, 568t
  streptococcal infections, 500
Neostigmine poisoning, 142t
Nephrectomy, 393
Nephritic syndrome, 280, **801**
Nephritis
  acute interstitial, **810,** 811t
  chronic interstitial, **811**
  drug-induced, 810–811, 811t, 1138t
Nephrolithiasis, 786t, 788, **826,** 828t, 904
  stone composition, 826–827
Nephropathy. *See also specific types*
  drug-induced, 1138t
  ischemic, **821,** 823f
Nephrosclerosis, arteriolar, **824**
Nephrostomy tube, 830
Nephrotic syndrome, 279, **803**
  ascites in, 273t
  causes of, 804, 804t
  drug-induced, 1138t
  evaluation of, 806t
Nerve agents, **169,** 170t
  clinical features of exposure, 169
  treatment of, 169–171, 170t
Nerve gas, 142t
Nervous system tumor, **1031**
  metastasis to nervous system, 1033–1034, 1034t
Nesiritide, for heart failure, 734, 734t
Neuralgia, 34. *See also specific types*
Neuritis. *See specific types*
Neuroborreliosis, 550
Neurocysticercosis, 655–656
Neurogenic shock, 59t
Neuroimaging, **986,** 987t, 994
Neuroleptic malignant syndrome, 203, 1092
Neurologic disease
  abdominal pain in, 179t
  ataxia, **1007**
  autonomic nervous system disorders, **1013**
  brain abscess, **1050**
  cranial nerve disorders, **1020**
  in critically ill patient, 33
  cytomegalovirus infections, 573
  dementia, **995**
  depression in, 1078
  diphtheria, 502
  drug-induced, 341t, 1138t–1139t
  encephalitis, acute, **1042**
  epilepsy, **988**
  Epstein-Barr virus infections, 575
  fatigue in, 289t
  HSV infections, 565–566, 568t
  in HIV/AIDS, 605
  hypothermia in, 128t
  infections, 108t–109t, 111
  in leprosy, 546
  Lyme borreliosis, 550
  in malnutrition, 41

meningitis
  acute, **1042**
  chronic, **1052**
motor neuron disease, **1010**
multiple sclerosis, **1035**
myasthenia gravis, **1065**
paraneoplastic, **407,** 408t
Parkinson's disease, **1002**
peripheral neuropathy, **1055**
progressive multifocal leukoencephalopathy, **1051**
seizure, **988**
sleep disorders in, 227
spinal cord disease, **1026**
tuberculosis, 540
tumors of nervous system, **1031**
varicella-zoster virus infections, 570
weakness and paralysis in, **218**
weight loss in, 248t
Neurologic examination, **979**
  anatomic localization of problem, 985t, 986
  coordination and gait, **986**
  cranial nerve exam, **979**
  in head trauma, 93
  in low back pain, 190, 191t
  mental status exam, **979,** 979t
  motor exam, **984**
  reflexes, **984**
  sensory exam, **985**
Neuromuscular blockers, 31
Neuromuscular junction disorders, 219t, 220t
Neuromyelitis optica, 217, 1041
Neuropathy. *See specific types*
  paraneoplastic, 408t, 409t
Neuroprotection, for stroke, 84
Neurosyphilis, 473, 474t, 475
Neutron particles, 171
Neutropenia, **331**
  in cancer patient, 115
  drug-induced, 329, 344
  febrile, 331
    approach to, 435–436, 435f
    P. aeruginosa infections, 518
  treatment of, 115, 331
Neutrophilia, **329**
Nevirapine, for HIV/AIDS, 606, 609t
Niacin deficiency, 43t
Nicardipine, for hypertensive emergencies, 698t
Nicotine, 142t
  for inflammatory bowel disease, 840
Nicotine addiction, **1126.** *See also* Smoking cessation
  in women, 1130
Nicotine-replacement products, 1127, 1127t
Nicotinic acid, for hyperlipidemia, 972t
Nifedipine
  for achalasia, 251
  for aortic regurgitation, 683
  for ergot alkaloid poisoning, 137t
  for esophageal spasm, 251
  for hypertension, 695t, 698
  poisoning, 140t
  for systemic sclerosis, 889
  for vasospastic disorders, 740
Nightshade, 138t

Nilotinib
  for CML, 349
  toxicity of, 342t
Nimodipine, for subarachnoid hemorrhage with vasospasm, 89
Nissen fundoplication, 247
Nit(s), 658–659
Nitazoxanide
  for cryptosporidiosis, 455
  for giardiasis, 455
Nitrates
  for angina pectoris, 714–715, 715t
  for heart failure, 731, 733t
  for myocardial infarction, 705–706
  poisoning, 146t
Nitrite poisoning, 146t
Nitrofurantoin
  for cystitis, 818t
  for urinary tract infection prevention, 817
Nitrogen mustard, 168
Nitrogen oxides, poisoning, 146t
Nitroglycerin
  for anal fissures, 844
  for angina pectoris, 714–715, 715t
  for ergot alkaloid poisoning, 137t
  for hypertensive emergencies, 698t
  for myocardial infarction, 702, 705, 705t, 706t, 711
  for systemic sclerosis, 889
  for unstable angina, 711
Nitroprusside
  for aortic dissection, 738, 738t
  for ergot alkaloid poisoning, 137t
  for heart failure, 734, 734t
  for hypertension, 698t, 822
  for MAO inhibitor poisoning, 138t
  for mitral regurgitation, 680
  for myocardial infarction, 705, 705t, 706t, 708
Nitrosourea, 341t
Nocardiosis, **535,** 536t
  eye infections, 535, 536t
  pulmonary disease, 535
  skin/soft tissue infections, 535, 536t
Nodule (skin lesion), 201, 313t, 478
Noma, 532
Non-Hodgkin's lymphoma, 354f, 355
  international prognostic index for, 358, 358t
Nonpolyposis syndrome, 384, 384t
Nonsteroidal anti-inflammatory drugs (NSAID)
  for ankylosing spondylitis, 897
  for calcium apatite deposition disease, 907
  for cholecystitis, 847
  for chronic fatigue syndrome, 291
  for colon cancer prevention, 1124
  for colonic polyps, 383
  for diabetes insipidus, 8
  for enteropathic arthritis, 907
  for erythema multiforme, 318
  for erythema nodosum, 318
  for fever, 201
  for fibromyalgia, 909
  for gout, 904
  for low back pain, 196
  for migraine, 184, 185t
  for osteoarthritis, 902

Nonsteroidal anti-inflammatory drugs
    (NSAID) (*Cont.*):
  for osteonecrosis, 909
  for pain, 36t–37t, 38, 955
  for pseudogout, 906
  for psoriatic arthritis, 898
  for reactive arthritis, 900
  for rheumatoid arthritis, 887
  for SLE, 886
  for systemic mastocytosis, 881
  for tension headache, 186
Nontuberculous mycobacterial infection, **547**
  disseminated disease, 548
  lung disease, 547
Norepinephrine
  for beta blocker poisoning, 140t
  for calcium channel blocker poisoning,
      140t
  for increased intracranial pressure, 92t
  for MAO inhibitor poisoning, 138t
  for shock, 62, 62t
  for subarachnoid hemorrhage with vaso-
      spasm, 89
  for sympatholytic poisoning, 139t
Norovirus infection, 431
  diarrhea, **454**
Nortriptyline
  dosage and adverse effects of, 1086t
  for migraine prevention, 188t
  for pain, 36t–37t, 38
  for smoking cessation, 1127
Nosocomial infections, **428**
  endocarditis, 442
  prevention of, 428–429, 430t
Nuclear cardiology, **671,** 672t, 684t
Nuclear medicine imaging, in respiratory dis-
    ease, 751
Nuclear myocardial perfusion assessment,
    673, 701, 714t
Nucleoside analogues, for HIV/AIDS, 606
5'-Nucleotidase, 268
Nude syndrome, 883
Nummular lesion, 309
Nutcracker esophagus, 251
Nutrients, absorption in GI tract, 253
Nutritional status, assessment of, **39**
Nutritional support, **41**
  decision tree for initiating, 42f
  enteral nutrition, 42–43
  parenteral nutrition, 43
Nystagmus, 211–213
Nystatin, 620
  for candidiasis, 252, 317, 621

O
Obesity, **939,** 939t
  central, 939
  drug-induced, 940
  extreme, 939t
  metabolic syndrome, **699,** 700t
  sleep disorders in, 229t
  treatment of, 940–941
      bariatric surgery, 940–941, 941f
      in women, 1129
Obesity-hypoventilation syndrome, **783**
Obsessive-compulsive disorder (OCD), **1082,**
    1088
Obstructive shock, extracardiac, 59t

Obturator neuropathy, 1063t
Occipital neuralgia, 189
Occlusional injury, 118, 119t
Octreotide
  for acromegaly, 406, 921
  for carcinoid tumor, 389
  for esophageal varices, 874
  for hepatorenal syndrome, 274
  for islet-cell tumors, 391
  for variceal bleeding, 263
Octreotide scintigraphy, 389
Ocular motor nerve palsy, 217–218
Oculopharyngeal dystrophy, **1072**
Odynophagia, 249
Ofloxacin
  for leprosy, 547
  for meningococcal disease prevention, 506t
  for pelvic inflammatory disease, 466
Olanzapine
  for delirium, 50t
  dosage and adverse effects of, 138t, 1091t
  for schizophrenia, 1081
Olfactory nerve, 979
  disorders of, **1023,** 1023t
Oligemic shock, 59t, 60t
Oligoamenorrhea, 952
Oligoanuria, 276
Oligoblastic leukemia, 350
Oligodendroglioma, **1033**
Oliguria, **276**
Omalizumab, for asthma, 755
Omeprazole
  for *H. pylori* eradication, 833t
  for indigestion, 247
  for systemic sclerosis, 889
Onchocerciasis, **652**
Onchocercomata, 652
Oncologic emergencies, **112**
  paraneoplastic syndromes, **113**
  structural/obstructive, **112**
  treatment complications, **115**
Ondansetron, for nausea and vomiting, 246,
    343
Ophthalmia neonatorum, 469, 470t
Ophthalmoplegia, 1025
  chronic progressive external, 1074
  progressive external, **1072**
Ophthalmoscopic examination, 215
Opiates
  narcotic abuse, **1099**
  poisoning, 131t
Opisthorchiasis, 654
Opisthotonus, 528
Opsoclonus-myoclonus syndrome, 408, 408t
Optic neuritis, 216f, 217
  drug-induced, 1139t
Optic neuropathy, 216f
Oral contraceptives, 955, 957
Oral disease
  drug-induced, 1137t–1138t
  infections, 306
      anaerobic, 532
  in malnutrition, 41
  oral cavity cancer, **367**
Oral dissolution therapy, for gallstones, 845
Oral hairy leukoplakia, 575
Oral rehydration solution (ORS), 453
Orchiectomy, 394

Orchitis, mumps, 587
Orientia tsutsugamushi infection. *See* Typhus, scrub
Oritavancin, for staphylococcal infections, 494t
Orlistat, for obesity, 940
Oroya fever, 526t, **527**
Orphenadrine poisoning, 138t, 144t, 153t
Orthostatic hypotension, 209t, 210, 1015
  evaluation of, 1016
  neurogenic, 1015
  in pheochromocytoma, 693
  treatment of, 1019, 1019t
Osborn (J) waves, 127
Oseltamivir, for influenza, 579, 579t
  preventive treatment, 580–581
Osmolar gap, 18
Osmoregulation, 3t
Osmotic demyelination syndrome, 6–7
Osteoarthritis, **900**
  low back pain in, 192
Osteomalacia, **967**
  drug-induced, 1140t
Osteomyelitis, **483**
  acute hematogenous, 483–484
  chronic, 483, 486
  contiguous-focus, 483, 486
  diagnosis of, 483–484, 484t
  E. coli, 514
  HACEK group, 511
  Klebsiella, 515
  neck pain in, 198
  S. aureus, 491, 496
  treatment of, 484–486, 485t
  vertebral, 483–484
    low back pain in, 193
Osteonecrosis, **909**
Osteoporosis, 957, **965**
  diseases associated with, 966t
  drug-induced, 1140t
  fracture risk in, 965–966, 966t
  low back pain in, 192–193
  screening for, 967, 1105t
  in women, 1129
Otitis externa
  acute diffuse, 304
  acute localized, 304
  chronic, 305
  malignant or necrotizing, 305, 518, 519t
Otitis media, 298
  acute, 298, 302t, 305
  chronic, 298, 305
  M. catarrhalis, 510
  measles, 584
  pneumococcal, 487
  serous, 298, 305
Otoacoustic emissions, 298
Otosclerosis, 298
Otoscopy, 300
Ovarian cancer, **395**
  paraneoplastic syndromes in, 409t
  staging and prognosis in, 395, 396t
Ovarian cyst, 395
Ovarian tumor, 395
Overdosage, 130
Oxacillin
  for arthritis, infectious, 482
  indications for, 425t

for infective endocarditis, 445t
  for osteomyelitis, 485t
  resistance to, 425t
  for sepsis/septic shock, 65t
  for staphylococcal infections, 494t
Oxaliplatin
  for colorectal cancer, 387
  toxicity of, 341t
Oxazepam
  dosage and action of, 1089t
  for myocardial infarction, 702
  poisoning, 143t
Oxcarbazepine
  dosage and adverse effects of, 143t, 1092t
  for generalized anxiety disorder, 1082
  for seizures, 992t–993t, 994t
Oxcarbazine, for pain, 36t–37t
5-Oxoprolinuria, 17t, 18–19
Oxybutinin, for multiple sclerosis, 1041
Oxycodone
  for dyspnea, 49t
  for pain, 36t–37t
Oxygen therapy
  for anaphylaxis, 117
  for asthma, 756
  for COPD, 762–763
  for cor pulmonale, 735
  for cytochrome oxidase inhibitor poisoning, 145t
  for interstitial lung disease, 775
  for methemoglobin inducer poisoning, 146t
  for myocardial infarction, 702, 705
  for pulmonary edema, 68
  for pulmonary hypertension, 745
  for shock, 62, 707
Oxytocin, 923

P
Packed red blood cell transfusion, 44
Paclitaxel
  for bladder cancer, 392
  for breast cancer, 376
  for head and neck cancer, 368
  for ovarian cancer, 397
  toxicity of, 341t
Pain. *See also specific types and sites*
  approach to, 34–35
  chronic, 35
    chronic pelvic pain syndrome, **820**
    treatment of, 38, 1088
  drugs for relief of, 36t–37t, 38
  management of, **34,** 36t–37t, 38
    terminally ill patient, 47
  neuropathic, 34, 34t, 38
  organization of pain pathways, **35,** 35f
  somatic, 34, 34t, 38, 180
  spontaneous, 1018
  visceral, 34, 34t, 180
Palivizumab, for human RSV infections, 583
Palliative care, **46**
Palmar xanthoma, 974
Palpation, precordial, 662f, **663**
Pamidronate, for hypercalcemia, 113, 406, 962t
Pancreatectomy, 853
Pancreatic abscess, 852
Pancreatic cancer, **388**

Pancreatic endocrine tumors, **389**
Pancreatic enzyme replacement, 853
Pancreatic exocrine insufficiency, 852–853, 853t
Pancreatic necrosis, 852
Pancreatic pseudocyst, 852
Pancreatitis, **849**
  acute, **849**
    causes of, 850t
    complications of, 851–852
    risk factors that adversely affect survival, 851t
  ascites in, 273t
  chronic, **852**
    complications of, 853
    TIGAR-O classification of, 853t
  diagnosis of, 587
  drug-induced, 1138t
  interstitial, 849
  necrotizing, 849
Pancytopenia, drug-induced, 1135t
Panic disorder, **1081**, 1088
Panitumumab, for colorectal cancer, 387
Pantoprazole
  for erosive gastropathies, 834
  for *H. pylori* eradication, 833t
Papillary necrosis, **817**
Papilledema, 216
Pappenheimer bodies, 321
Pap smear, 397–398, 1123t, 1125
Papule (skin lesion), 313t, 478
Papulosquamous disorder, **314**
Paracentesis, **28**, 272
Paracoccidioidomycosis, **631**
Paragonimus infection. *See* Fluke infection, lung flukes
Parainfluenza virus infection, **583**
Paralysis, **218**
  periodic, **1074**
  site of responsible lesion, 219, 219t
Paralytic shellfish poisoning, **124**
Paraneoplastic syndromes
  emergent, **113**
  endocrine, **405**
  neurologic, **407**, 408t
Paranoid personality disorder, 1084
Paraparesis, 220t, 221f
Parasitic infection
  blood, 322, **421**
  diagnosis of, **413**, 420t
  eosinophilia in, 330
  intestinal, **421**
  tissue, **421**
Parasympathetic system, 1014f, 1015t
Parathyroidectomy, 963
Paravertebral abscess, brucellosis vs. tuberculosis, 523, 523t
Parcopa, for Parkinson's disease, 1005t
Parenteral nutrition, **41**
  decision tree for initiating, 42f
Paresis, 218
Parkinsonism, 222, 1002
Parkinson's disease, **1002**, 1003t, 1016
  dementia in, 996t, 998
  treatment of, 1003–1007, 1005t–1006t
  tremor in, 222
Paromomycin, for amebiasis, 460
Parotitis, mumps, 586–587

Paroxetine
  for depression, 50
  dosage and adverse effects of, 1086t
  for irritable bowel syndrome, 841
  for menopausal symptoms, 957
  for vasovagal syncope, 210
Paroxysmal nocturnal hemoglobinuria, 323, 326, 326t
Parvovirus B19 infection, **587**
Patch (skin lesion), 313t
Patch tests, 312
Patent ductus arteriosus, 662t, **675**
Peau d'orange appearance, 316
Pediculiasis, **658**
Pegvisomant, for acromegaly, 921
Pegylated interferon
  for chronic hepatitis B, 860t–861t, 864
  for chronic hepatitis C, 864, 865t–866t
Pelger-Hüet anomaly, 322
Pelvic infection, anaerobic, 533
Pelvic inflammatory disease (PID), **465,** 469
  chlamydial, 465, 471
  mycoplasmal, 465, 471–472
  pain in, 954
  treatment of, 466, 470t
Pelvic pain, **953**
  acute, 954
  causes of, 953–954, 954t
  chronic, 954
  cyclic, 954, 954t
  noncyclic, 954, 954t
Pemetrexed
  for lung cancer, 371
  toxicity of, 341t
Pemoline, for depression, 50
Penciclovir, for HSV infections, 568t
Penetrating radiation, 171
Penicillamine
  for lead poisoning, 159t
  for nephrolithiasis, 828t
  for rheumatoid arthritis, 887
  for systemic sclerosis, 889
Penicillin/penicillin G/penicillin V
  for actinomycosis, 538
  for anaerobic infections, 534
  for bacterial meningitis, 1046t, 1047t
  for clostridial infections, 108t, 480t, 532
  for diphtheria, 502
  for enterococcal infections, 501
  for HACEK group infections, 512t
  indications for, 425t
  for infective endocarditis, 444t
  for leptospirosis, 553
  for meningococcal infections, 107t, 506t
  for necrotizing fasciitis, 108t, 479t
  for osteomyelitis, 485t
  for perichondritis, 304
  for pharyngitis, 304t
  for pneumococcal infections, 488
  resistance to, 425t
  for rheumatic fever prevention, 678
  for rodent bite infections, 120t
  for staphylococcal infections, 493, 494t
  for streptococcal infections, 498t, 499–500
  for syphilis, 474t
  for tetanus, 529
Penicilliosis, **632**

Pentamidine
for *Pneumocystis* infections, 634t, 635
preventive treatment, 635t
for sleeping sickness, 646
Pentazocine abuse, **1099**
Pentobarb coma, 92t
Pentobarbital
poisoning, 143t
for status epilepticus, 99f
Pentostatin, 341t
Pentoxifylline
for alcoholic liver disease, 870
for arteriosclerosis, 739
Peptic ulcer disease (PUD), 389, **831**
bleeding in, 260
causes and risk factors for, 831
diagnosis of, 835t
drug-induced, 1138t
duodenal, 831–833
gastric, 831–833
treatment of, 832–834, 833t
Peptostreptococcus infection, **532**
Percutaneous coronary intervention (PCI),
701, 702f, 711, 712t, 716, 717t
Percutaneous needle aspiration, of lung, 752
Pergolide
for Parkinson's disease, 1006t
poisoning, 137t
Periappendicitis, 465
Periarticular disorder, **909**
Pericardial disease, **688**
echocardiography in, 670, 672t
Pericardial effusion
approach to, 692
oncologic emergency, **112**
treatment of, 113
Pericardial stripping/window, 113
Pericardial tamponade, oncologic emergency, **112**
Pericarditis
acute, **688**
causes of, 688t
chest pain in, 175t, 177f, 178
laboratory features of, 688, 689t, 690f
constrictive, 112, **689**, 692t
laboratory features of, 691, 691f
drug-induced, 1136t
enterovirus, 590
in myocardial infarction, 708
in tuberculosis, 540
Perichondritis, 304
Perihepatitis, 465
Perimenopause, 956
Perimeter, 215
Perinephric abscess, **450**
Periodic leg movements of sleep, 226–227
Periodic paralysis, **1074**
hyperkalemic, 1074
hypokalemic, 1074
Periodontal disease, 511, 532
Periorbital edema, 241
Peripheral edema, 730
Peripheral nerves, cutaneous areas supplied
by, 982f–983f
Peripheral neuropathy, **1055**
approach to, 1055–1058, 1056f
autonomic involvement in, 1016, 1018t
causes of, 1057, 1060t

classification of
by fiber type, 1057, 1058t
by histopathology, 1057, 1059t
by time course, 1057, 1059t
clinical features of, 1057t
diagnosis of, 1057t, 1058–1060
drug-induced, 341t, 1138t
mononeuropathy, 1062t–1064t, **1065**
motor-predominant, 1011t
paraneoplastic, 408t, 409, 409t
polyneuropathy, 1055, **1058**
weakness in, 219t, 220t
Peripheral vascular disease, **739**
arteriosclerosis of arteries, **739**
Peristalsis, 253
Peritoneal carcinomatosis, in women, **402**
Peritoneal dialysis, 160, 793, **797**
complications of, 798, 798t
Peritoneal disease
ascites in, 271
pain in, 179t
Peritoneal fluid, paracentesis, 28–29
Peritonitis, **448**
E. coli, 513
primary bacterial, **272, 448**
pyogenic, 273t
secondary, 448, **449**
tuberculous, 273t
Peritonsillar abscess, 532
Permethrin cream
for pediculiasis, 658
for scabies, 658
Peroneal nerve entrapment, 1064t
Perphenazine, 1091t
Personality disorder, **1084**
cluster A, **1084**
cluster B, **1084**
cluster C, **1084**
Pertussis, **509**
catarrhal phase of, 510
convalescent phase of, 510
paroxysmal phase of, 510
Petechiae, 106
Peutz-Jeghers syndrome, 381, 384t, 385
Pharmacologic stress testing, 713–714, 714t
Pharyngitis
acute, **306**
Epstein-Barr virus, 575
HSV, 564
streptococcal, 497, 498t
treatment of, 304t, 497, 498t
Pharyngoconjunctival fever, 583
Phenazopyridine, 146t
Phenelzine, 138t, 1087t
Phenobarbital
poisoning, 143t
for seizures, 994t
for status epilepticus, 99f
Phentolamine
for hypertensive emergencies, 698t
for sympathomimetic poisoning, 136t
Phenylephrine
for heart failure, 734t
for increased intracranial pressure, 92t
poisoning, 136t
for shock, 62, 62t
for subarachnoid hemorrhage with vasospasm, 89

Phenylpropanolamine, 136t
Phenytoin
    for antidepressant poisoning, 141t
    for cardiac glycoside poisoning, 141t
    for multiple sclerosis, 1041
    for myotonic dystrophy, 1071
    for pain, 36t–37t
    poisoning, 143t
    for seizures, 992t–993t, 994t
    for status epilepticus, 99f
    for trigeminal neuralgia, 1020
Pheochromocytoma, 693–694
Pheresis therapy, **44**
Phlebotomy, 283, 351, 975, 977
Phobic disorder, **1083**
Phosphofructokinase deficiency, 1073
Photodermatitis, drug-induced, 1134t
Physostigmine
    for anticholinergic poisoning, 138t
    for membrane-active agent poisoning,
        153t
    poisoning, 142t
Pigment gallstones, 844
Pill rolling, 1002
Pilocarpine
    for glaucoma, 294
    poisoning, 142t
    for Sjögren's syndrome, 891
Pindolol, 140t
Pink eye, 294
Pinta, 551
Pinworm. See Enterobiasis
Pioglitazone, for diabetes mellitus, 945t
Piperacillin
    for osteomyelitis, 485t
    for otitis externa, 305
Piperacillin-tazobactam
    for anaerobic infections, 534t
    indications for, 425t
    for osteomyelitis, 485t
    for P. aeruginosa infections, 519t
    for peritonitis, 448
    for pneumonia, 766t, 767t
    resistance to, 425t
    for septic shock, 107t
Piracetam, for myoclonus, 224
Pitting, 287
Pituitary adenoma, **917**
    ACTH-secreting, 917, 919t, 934–935
    gonadotropin-secreting, 919t, 921
    growth hormone-secreting, 917, 919t,
        920–921
    hormonal evaluation of, 919t
    macroadenoma, 917
    microadenoma, 917
    prolactin-secreting, 917, 919–920, 919t
    thyroid-stimulating hormone-secreting,
        919t, **921,** 928
Pituitary apoplexy, 917, 919
Pituitary disease
    anterior pituitary, **917**
    hormone hypersecretion syndromes, **919,**
        919t
    posterior, **923**
Pituitary hormones, 917, 918f
Pituitary tumor, 216f, 296–297, **917**
Pityriasis rosea, 310f, **314,** 572
Pivmecillinam, for shigellosis, 459

Pizotifen, for migraine prevention, 188t
Plague, 106, 478, **525**
    as bioweapon, 163, 164t, 526
    bubonic, 525–526
    pneumonic, 163, 164t, 525–526
    septicemic, 525–526
    treatment of, 164t, 526
Plantar reflex, 984
Plaque (lesion of MS), 1035
Plaque (skin lesion), 313t
Plasma cell disorders, 353t, 354f, **360**
Plasmacytoma, 361
Plasma exchange
    for acute renal failure, 793
    for multiple sclerosis, 1039
Plasmapheresis, **46**
    for acute renal failure, 793
    for autoimmune hemolysis, 329
    for myasthenia gravis, 1066
    for polyneuropathy, 1061
    for primary biliary cirrhosis, 871
    for thrombotic microangiopathy, 826
    for thrombotic thrombocytopenic purpura,
        335
    for vasculitis, 894
Plasmodium infection. See Malaria
Platelet clumping, 322
Platelet disorders, **332**
    platelet function disorders, 334–335
Plateletpheresis, **46**
Platelet transfusion, **45**
    for thrombocytopenia, 344
Platinum compounds, 341t
    for breast cancer, 379
Pleural biopsy, 752
Pleural effusion, 767, **777**
    approach to, 779f
    causes of, 778t
    chylothorax, 780
    exudative, 777, 778t
    malignant, 778–780
    in pancreatitis, 852
    parapneumonic, 777–778
    related to pulmonary embolism, 780
    thoracentesis, 26–27, 26f
    transudative, 777, 778t
Pleuritis, tuberculous, 780
Pleurodesis, 780
Pleurodynia, enterovirus, 590
Pleuropulmonary infection, anaerobic, 533
Plummer's nails, 928
Pneumatic compression stockings, 89
Pneumococcal infection, **486**
    endocarditis, 488
    meningitis, 487–488
    otitis media, 487
    pneumonia, 487–488
Pneumococcal vaccine, 438t, 488–489,
        1108t–1112t, 1115t
Pneumocystis infection, **633**
    prevention of, 635, 635t
    treatment of, 634–635, 634t
Pneumonia, **764**
    acute interstitial, 774
    adenovirus, 583
    aspiration, 533
    causes of, 764
    community-acquired, 491, **764**

antibiotic therapy, 765, 766t
complications of, 766–767
site of care, 765, 766t
C. pneumoniae, 563
cryptogenic organizing, 774, **776**
cytomegalovirus, 573–574
E. coli, 513
eosinophilic, 774, 776
gram-negative enteric bacteria, 516
health care-associated, 764, **767**
hemoptysis in, 236
H. influenzae, 509
hospital-acquired, **769**
human RSV, 582
influenza virus, 578
Klebsiella, 515
laboratory features of, 765
M. catarrhalis, 510
measles virus, 584
M. pneumoniae, **560**
nocardiosis, 535, 536t
nosocomial, 429–430, 430t, 491
P. aeruginosa, 517, 519t
pathophysiology of, 764
pneumococcal, 487–488
Pneumocystis, **633**
S. aureus, 491
secondary bacterial, 578
streptococcal, 498, 498t, 500
toxoplasmosis, 646
varicella-zoster virus, 570–571
ventilator-associated, 74, 430t, 517, **767**
pathogenic mechanisms, 768t
prevention of, 768t
treatment of, 767t, 768
Pneumonia Severity Index, 765
Pneumonitis
HSV infections, 566, 568t
hypersensitivity, 774–775, **776**
necrotizing, 533
Pneumothorax, 177f, 774, **780**
Podagra, 903
Podofilox, for HPV infections, 476
Podophyllin
for HPV infections, 476
for warts, 317
Poikilocytosis, 321
Poison control center, 123, 160
Poisoning
diagnosis of, 130–133, 131t–132t
heavy metals, 154t–160t
marine, **123**
reference values for laboratory tests, 1157t–1159t
treatment of, 133–160, 134t, 136t–159t
enhancement of elimination, 134t, 160
prevention of poison absorption, 134t, 135
Poliovirus infection, **588**
meningitis, 589
paralytic disease, 589
postpolio syndrome, 589
Poliovirus vaccine, 438t, 589, 591, 1108t–1111t
Polyangiitis, microscopic, **892**
Polyarteritis, glomerular disease in, 807t
Polyarteritis nodosa, **891**
Polyarthropathy, parvovirus, 587

Polychondritis, relapsing, **908**
Polycystic kidney disease, **813**
autosomal dominant, 813–814
Polycystic ovarian syndrome, 953, 955
Polycythemia, **282,** 282f, 351
Polycythemia vera, 283, **351**
Polydipsia, primary, 923
Polyethylene glycol-containing solution
for constipation, 259
for irritable bowel syndrome, 842t
Polymyalgia rheumatica, **909**
Polymyositis, 1072, 1073t
Polymyxin-bacitracin-neomycin, for eye infections, 294
Polymyxin E (colistin)
indications for, 427t
for *P. aeruginosa* infections, 520t
resistance to, 427t
Polyneuropathy, 1055, **1058**
acute inflammatory demyelinating, 1061
chronic inflammatory demyelinating, 1061
Polyp(s)
colonic. *See* Colonic polyps
gastric, 381
Polyposis syndromes, 381
hereditary, **383,** 384t
Polysomnography, 229t
Polystyrene sulfonate
for diabetic nephropathy, 806
for hyperkalemia, 796
Polyuria, 276t, **277,** 277f
Pontiac fever, 521
Porphyria, **976**
acute intermittent, **976,** 1016
erythropoietic, 976, **977**
hepatic, 976
Porphyria cutanea tarda, **977**
Porphyromonas infection, **532**
Portal hypertension, 287, **872**
complications of, 873
hepatic, 873t
posthepatic, 873t
prehepatic, 873t
Portuguese man-of-war injury, 122
Posaconazole, **619**
for aspergillosis, 623
for mucormycosis, 627
Positive end-expiratory pressure (PEEP), 71, 74
Post-concussion headache, 183t, 187–189
Postherpetic neuralgia, 316, 570–571
Postmenopausal hormone therapy, 956
Postmenopausal state, 1120
Postpolio syndrome, 589
Postradiation fibrosis, 198
Posttraumatic stress disorder (PTSD), **1083,** 1088
Postural orthostatic tachycardia syndrome, 1018
Potassium, disorders of, **8**
Potassium chloride
for hypokalemia, 10
for periodic paralysis, 1074
Potassium hydroxide preparation, 311, 411
Potassium iodide, for radioactive iodine exposure, 174
Potassium perchlorate, for amiodarone-induced thyrotoxicosis, 931

Pott's disease, 540
Pott's puffy tumor, 302
Powassan encephalitis, 596t–597t
2-Pralidoxime chloride
  for cholinergic poisoning, 142t
  for nerve agent exposure, 170t, 171
Pramipexole
  for Parkinson's disease, 1006t
  for restless legs syndrome, 227, 229t
Pravastatin, for hyperlipidemia, 972t
Praziquantel
  for echinococcosis, 657
  for fluke infection, 654–655
  for schistosomiasis, 654
  for taeniasis solium and cysticercosis, 656
  for tapeworm infection, 655
Prazosin
  for ergot alkaloid poisoning, 137t
  for vasospastic disorders, 740
Precordial palpation, 662f, **663**
Prednisolone
  for alcoholic liver disease, 870
  for autoimmune hepatitis, 867
Prednisone
  for acute lymphoblastic leukemia and lym-
      phoblastic lymphoma, 350
  for alcoholic liver disease, 870
  for autoimmune hepatitis, 867
  for Bell's palsy, 1022
  for Burkitt's lymphoma/leukemia, 360
  for cluster headache prevention, 187
  for gastric cancer, 381
  for hirsutism, 955
  for hypercalcemia, 962t
  for hypopituitarism, 922t
  for idiopathic thrombocytopenic purpura,
      335
  immunosuppression for renal transplant,
      800
  for inflammatory bowel disease, 838
  for inflammatory myopathy, 1072
  for interstitial lung disease, 775
  for multiple myeloma, 361
  for multiple sclerosis, 1039
  for muscular dystrophy, 1071
  for myasthenia gravis, 1066
  for optic neuritis, 217
  for pericarditis, 688
  for *Pneumocystis* infections, 634t
  for polymyalgia rheumatica, 909
  for relapsing polychondritis, 908
  for sarcoidosis, 912
  steroid preparations, 938–939, 938t
  for thyrotoxicosis, 930
  for vasculitis, 894
Preexcitation syndrome. *See* Wolff-Parkin-
    son-White syndrome
Pregabalin, 37t
  for generalized anxiety disorder, 1082
  for multiple sclerosis, 1041
Pregnancy
  ectopic, 954–955
  gonorrhea in, 469
  hypertension in, 698
  listerial infections in, 507
  malaria in, 637
  streptococcal infections in, 500
  syphilis in, 474t

  toxemia of, **826**
  toxoplasmosis in, 646
  travel during, 1117
Prehypertension, 1119
Preleukemia, 350
Premenstrual syndrome (PMS), 954–955
Presbycusis, 300
Pressure-control ventilation (PCV), 72, 73t
Pressure-support ventilation (PSV), 72, 73t,
    74
Preventive medicine, **1103**
Preventive Services Task Force, U.S., recom-
    mendations of, 1106t
Prevotella infection, **532**
Primaquine
  for malaria, 638t
    preventive treatment, 641t
  for *Pneumocystis* infections, 634t, 635
Primary (spontaneous) bacterial peritonitis,
    448
Primary biliary cirrhosis, **870**
Primary lateral sclerosis, 1011t
Primary sclerosing cholangitis, **848**
Primidone
  for myoclonus, 224
  poisoning, 143t
  for seizures, 994t
  for tremor, 222
Primitive neuro-ectodermal tumor, **1033**
Prinzmetal's variant angina, **716**
Proamatine, for vasovagal syncope, 210
Probenecid
  for gonococcal infections, 470t
  for gout, 905
  for syphilis, 474t
Procainamide
  for arrhythmias, 727t
  for malignant hyperthermia, 203
  for tachyarrhythmias, 724t
  for Wolff-Parkinson-White syndrome, 729
Procaine penicillin
  for diphtheria prevention, 502
  for streptococcal infections, 498t
Prochlorperazine
  for migraine, 186t
  for nausea and vomiting, 246, 343
  for vertigo, 214t
Proctitis, **466,** 471
  HSV, 568t
Proctocolitis, **466**
Progressive multifocal leukoencephalopathy
    (PML), **1051**
Progressive systemic sclerosis, 775
Prolactin, 917, 917f
  deficiency of, 919t
  hypersecretion of, **919,** 919t
Prolactinoma, 297, 919–920
Promethazine, for vertigo, 214t
Prometrium, for amenorrhea, 953
Promyelocytic leukemia, acute, 344, 345t
Propafenone, for arrhythmias, 727t
Propionibacterium acnes infection, **532**
Propofol
  for delirium, 50t
  for increased intracranial pressure, 92t
  poisoning, 144t
  for status epilepticus, 99f
  for sympathomimetic poisoning, 136t

Propoxyphene
  narcotic abuse, **1099**
  poisoning, 153t
Propranolol
  for aortic dissection, 738t
  for hypertension, 695t
  for methylxanthine poisoning, 137t
  for migraine prevention, 188t
  poisoning, 140t
  for sympathomimetic poisoning, 136t
  for thyrotoxicosis, 929
  for tremor, 222
  for variceal bleeding, 263
Propylene glycol poisoning, 17t, 18
Propylthiouracil, for thyrotoxicosis, 930
Prostascint scanning, 401
Prostate biopsy, transrectal ultrasound, 400,
    400f
Prostate cancer, **399**
  oncologic emergencies, 113
  osteoblastic bone metastasis, **404**
  prevention of, 1124
  risk factors for, 1124
  screening for, 1105t, 1122, 1123t
Prostatectomy, radical retropubic, 400–401
Prostate hyperplasia, **399**
Prostate-specific antigen (PSA), 399, 400f,
    1122, 1123t, 1124
  bound, 400
  free, 400
Prostatitis, **820**
  acute bacterial, **820**
  chronic bacterial, **820**
Prosthetic device-related infection, 481–482,
    492–493
Prosthetic-valve endocarditis, 492, 496
Protamine, to reverse anticoagulation, 336,
    771
Protease inhibitors, for HIV/AIDS, 606,
    611t–614t
Protein-losing enteropathy, 272
Protein malnutrition, 40–41
Protein restriction, in renal failure, 796
Proteinuria, **278,** 787
  nephrotic range, 279
Proteus infection, **515**
Prothrombin time, 269, 269t
Proto-oncogenes, 339
Protozoal infection, **636**
  blood, 420t
  intestinal, 420t, 421
  tissue, 420t
Protriptyline, for daytime sleepiness, 229t,
    230
Providencia infection, 516
Prune juice, 48t
Pruritus ani, **844**
Pseudallescheriasis, **632**
Pseudocyst, pancreatic, 273t, 852
Pseudodementia, 998
Pseudoephedrine, for allergic rhinitis, 880
Pseudogout, **905**
  conditions associated with, 905t
Pseudohyponatremia, 5
Pseudomelena, 259
Pseudomonas aeruginosa infection, **517**
  osteomyelitis, 485t
  treatment of, 518, 519t–520t

Pseudothrombocytopenia, **333**
Pseudotumor cerebri, 216–217
  drug-induced, 1139t
Psittacosis, **562**
Psoas abscess, **451**
  brucellosis vs. tuberculosis, 523, 523t
Psoriasis, 310f, 311f, **314**
Psoriatic arthritis, 896t, **897**
  patterns of joint involvement in, 898t
Psychiatric disorder, **117**
  anxiety disorders, **1081**
  diagnosis of, 999t
  drug-induced, 1140t
  DSM-IV Axis I, **1077**
  DSM-IV Axis II, 1077, **1084**
  eating disorders, **1093**
  fatigue in, 289t
  mood disorders, **1077**
  nausea and vomiting in, 245t
  personality disorders, **1084**
  psychotic disorders, **1080**
  schizophrenia, **1080**
  sleep disorders and, 227
  treatment of, **1085**
  weight loss in, 248t
  in women, 1129
Psychiatric medication, **1085**
  antidepressants, **1085**
  antipsychotics, **1088**
  anxiolytics, **1088**
  mood stabilizers, 1092t, **1093**
  principles of use of, 1085
Psychotic disorder, **1080**
Psyllium
  for diverticular disease, 842
  for hemorrhoids, 844
  for irritable bowel syndrome, 841,
    842t
PTH(1–34), for osteoporosis, 967
Pubic louse, 658–659
Puddle sign, 271
Puerperal sepsis, 499
Pulmonary alveolar proteinosis, **776**
Pulmonary angiography, 751
Pulmonary artery pressure, 748
Pulmonary circulation
  cor pulmonale, **734**
  disturbances of, 748
Pulmonary disease. *See* Lung disease
Pulmonary edema, 241, 243
  acute, **66**
  approach to, 68f
  cardiogenic, 67–68
  causes of, 67t
  drug-induced, 1136t
  noncardiogenic, 67t, 68
  precipitants of, 67t
  treatment of, 67–69
Pulmonary embolism, **769**
  chest pain in, 175t, 176, 177f
  dyspnea in, 231
  hemodynamic profiles in, 60t
  hemoptysis in, 236
  pleural effusion related to, 780
  pulmonary hypertension in, 743t
  thrombotic disorders, **336**
  treatment of, 336–338, 337t, 770–772,
    772f

Pulmonary fibrosis
  drug-induced, 341t–342t
  idiopathic, 774, **775**
  progressive massive, 758
Pulmonary function tests, 747, 751
  in asthma, 753–754
  in COPD, 759, 760t, 761
  in pulmonary hypertension, 743
  reference values for, 1169t–1170t
Pulmonary hypertension, **742,** 749
  approach to, 744f
  arterial, 743t
  causes of, 743t
  in congenital heart disease, 675
  differential diagnosis of, 743–744
  laboratory features of, 742–743
  primary, **743**
  venous, 743t
Pulmonary infiltrate
  drug-induced, 1136t
  with eosinophilia, **776**
Pulmonary Langerhans cell histiocytosis, 774–775, **776**
Pulmonary nodule, solitary, 371, 373f
Pulmonary rehabilitation, 761, 775
Pulmonary vascular resistance, 748
Pulmonic stenosis, 662t, **676**
Pulmonic valve regurgitation, 662t
Pulseless disease, **738**
Pulseless electrical activity, 57, 58f
Pulse oximetry, 749
Pulsus alternans, 661, 661f
Pulsus biferiens, 661, 661f
Pulsus paradoxus, 661, 661f
Pulsus parvus, 661, 661f
Pulsus tardus, 661, 661f
Pupillary signs, in coma, 78
Pure alexia, 225t
Pure red cell aplasia
  drug-induced, 1135t
  parvovirus infections, 588
Pure tone audiometry, 298
Pure word deafness, 225t
Purging behavior, 1093
Purine nucleoside phosphorylase deficiency, 883
Purpura, 201. *See also specific types*
  drug-induced, 1134t
  palpable, 319
Purpura fulminans, 108t, 110
Pustule, 313t
PUVA, for psoriasis, 314
Pyelonephritis, 450, **815,** 818t
  emphysematous, **817**
Pyloroplasty, 833t
Pyomyositis, 481
Pyrantel pamoate
  for ascariasis, 650
  for enterobiasis, 651
  for hookworm infection, 650
Pyrazinamide, for tuberculosis, 541, 543t, 546t
Pyridostigmine
  for myasthenia gravis, 1066
  for orthostatic hypotension, 1019
Pyridoxine, for isoniazid poisoning, 150t
Pyridoxine deficiency, 43t
Pyrilamine, 138t

Pyrimethamine
  for isosporiasis, 456
  for pneumocystosis prevention, 635t
  for toxoplasmosis, 647
Pyroglutamic aciduria, 17t, 18–19
Pyruvate kinase deficiency, 326
Pyuria, **280,** 787
  sterile, 787

Q
Q fever, **558**
  acute, 559
  chronic, 559
Quadrantanopia, 220t
Quadrantopia, 216f
Quadriparesis, 220t, 221f
Quantitative sudomotor axon reflex test (QSART), 1016
Quetiapine
  dosage and adverse effects of, 138t, 1091t
  for schizophrenia, 1081
Quinidine
  for arrhythmias, 727t
  for malaria, 637, 639t
Quinine
  for babesiosis, 107t, 642
  for malaria, 109t, 638t–639t
Quinolones
  for cystitis, 818t
  for tuberculosis, 543t
  for urinary tract infections, 818t–819t
Quinsy, 532
Quinupristin-dalfopristin
  for enterococcal infections, 501
  indications for, 427t
  resistance to, 427t
  for staphylococcal infections, 493, 494t

R
Rabies, 118, **592**
  encephalitic form, 592
  paralytic form, 593
  postexposure prophylaxis, 121, 593, 594f
  preexposure prophylaxis, 593
  prodrome, 592
Rabies immune globulin, 121, 593, 594f
Rabies vaccine, 121, 593, 1116t
Rad, 171
Radial neuropathy at spiral groove, 1063t
Radiation bioterrorism, **171**
  acute radiation sickness, **172**
  treatment of casualties, 173f
  types of exposure, 172
  types of radiation, 171
Radiation sickness, acute, **172,** 173f
Radiation therapy
  for anal cancer, 388
  for bladder cancer, 392
  for brain tumor, 1032–1033
  for breast cancer, 379
  for cervical cancer, 398
  for colorectal cancer, 387
  complications of, 342t, 1035
  for endometrial cancer, 397
  for follicular lymphoma, 357
  for gastric cancer, 381
  for head and neck cancer, 368
  for Hodgkin's disease, 363–364

leukopenia in, 331
for lung cancer, 371
for prostate cancer, 400–401
for spinal cord compression, 95, 113
for testicular cancer, 394, 394t
Radiculopathy
cervical, 197t
nonprogressive, 198–199
lumbosacral, 191t
subacute, 196
Radiography
in joint pain, 206–207, 207t
in osteomyelitis, 484t
in spinal cord compression, 113
Radioiodine
for nontoxic goiter, 931
for thyroid neoplasms, 932–933
for thyrotoxicosis, 928–930
for toxic adenoma, 932
for toxic multinodular goiter, 932
Radionuclide contamination, 174
Radionuclide scan
hepatobiliary imaging, 270
for osteomyelitis, 484t
Ragged red fibers, 1074
Raloxifene
for breast cancer prevention, 1122
for osteoporosis, 967
toxicity of, 342t
Raltegravir, for HIV/AIDS, 606, 615t
Ramipril
for heart failure, 733t
for hypertension, 695t
Ramsay Hunt syndrome, 1022
Ranitidine
for H. pylori eradication, 833t
for indigestion, 247
for urticaria/angioedema, 879
Ranolazine, for angina pectoris, 715–716
Rapid eye movement (REM) behavioral disorder, 226
Rapid shallow breathing index, 32
Rapid urease test, 832, 832t
Rasagiline, for Parkinson's disease, 1004
Rasburicase, for tumor lysis syndrome, 116
Rat-bite fever, 118
Raynaud's disease, 740t
Raynaud's phenomenon, 740, 740t
Reactive arthritis, 896f, 899
Recluse spider bite, 125
Recombinase activating gene deficiency, 882
Recommended dietary allowance (RDA), 39
Rectal cancer, 387
Red blood cell(s)
inclusions, 321–322
increased RBC mass, 351
morphology of, 321
RBC indices, 281–282
Red blood cell disorders, 323
anemia, 280, 323, 326
intracellular abnormalities, 326
maturation disorders, 325
membrane abnormalities, 326
polycythemia, 282
Red blood cell transfusion, 44
Red eye, 293, 293t
Reentrant AV nodal tachycardia, 721f, 722t

Referred pain, 34
abdominal pain, 179t
low back pain, 190
shoulder pain, 198
Reflexes, testing of, 984
Reflex sympathetic dystrophy, 1018
Refractory anemia, 348t–349t
with excess blasts, 348t–349t
with ringed sideroblasts, 348t–349t
Refractory cytopenia with multilineage dysplasia, 348t–349t
with ringed sideroblasts, 348t–349t
Regurgitation, 244, 246
Rehydration, in diarrhea, 256
Reiter's arthritis, 482
Reiter's syndrome, 471
Relapsing fever, 553
chill phase of, 553
flush phase of, 553
louse-borne, 553
tick-borne, 553
Relapsing polychondritis, 908
Renal abscess, 450
Renal artery occlusion, 820
Renal artery stenosis, 821
approach to, 823f
clinical features of, 822, 822t
hypertension in, 693–694, 821–824
Renal artery thrombosis, 821
Renal atheroembolism, 821
Renal cancer. See Kidney cancer
Renal disease
approach to, 785
azotemia, 274
chronic
classification of, 275t
treatment of, 795–796
clinical and laboratory database for, 786t
dialysis in, 796
drug-induced, 341t, 1138t
end-stage, 794
renal transplant in, 798
fatigue in, 289t
glomerular, 785, 801
hypertension in, 693, 698, 786t, 788, 795–796
infections in immunocompromised patients, 434, 436t
metabolic acidosis in, 17t, 18
monoclonal immunoglobulins and, 812, 812t
nephrolithiasis, 786t, 788, 826
nephrotic syndrome, 786t, 787
reference values for renal function tests, 1165t
renal tubular disease, 786t, 787–788, 808
renovascular disease, 820
urinary abnormalities in, 276
urinary tract infection. See Urinary tract infection
urinary tract obstruction, 786t, 788, 829
Renal failure
acute, 785, 786t, 789
approach to, 791–792, 792t
causes of, 790t
dialysis for, 793
intrinsic, 789–791, 790t, 792t

Renal failure (*Cont.*):
    postrenal, 789, 790t, 791
    prerenal, 789, 790t, 791, 792t
  chronic, 786t, 787, **794**
    causes of, 794–795, 794t
    sleep disorders in, 228
    slowing progression of, 796
  edema in, 242
Renal transplant, 796, **798**
  complications of, 800
  contraindications to, 799t
  factors influencing graft survival, 799t
  immunosuppressive therapy for, 799–800
  infections in recipients, 437
  rejection of, 799
Renal tubular acidosis, 17t, 788, **814**
  distal (type I), 814
  drug-induced, 1138t
  proximal (type II), 814
  type IV, 814–815
Renal tubular disease, 786t, 787–788, **808**
  causes of, 809t–810t
  transport dysfunction in, 810t
Renovascular disease, **820**
  arteriolar nephrosclerosis, **824**
  renal artery occlusion, **820**
  renal artery stenosis, **821**
  renal vein thrombosis, **821**
  in scleroderma, 824
  sickle cell nephropathy, **826**
  thrombotic microangiopathy, **824**
  toxemia of pregnancy, **826**
Repaglinide, for diabetes mellitus, 945t
Repositioning exercises, for vertigo, 213, 214t
Reproductive system disease
  female, **952**
  male, **947**
Reproductive tract infection, **462**
Respiratory acidosis, **21**
Respiratory alkalosis, **21**
Respiratory disease. *See also* Lung disease
  bronchoalveolar lavage in, 752
  bronchoscopy in, 751–752
  chest x-ray in, 751
  computed tomography in, 751
  diagnosis of, 751
  drug-induced, 1136t
  emergencies, 111
  extraparenchymal, 748, 748t
  infections in immunocompromised patients, 434, 436t
  meningococcal, 504
  M. pneumoniae, **560**
  MRI in, 751
  nuclear medicine imaging in, 751
  obstructive, 747–748, 748t
  P. aeruginosa, 517
  parenchymal, 748, 748t
  pulmonary function tests in, 751
  restrictive, 747–748, 748t
  sputum exam in, 751
  upper respiratory infections, **301**
  viral, **577**
  weight loss in, 248t
Respiratory failure, **71,** 73t
  hypercarbic, 71–72
  hypoxemic, 71–72

Respiratory function, **747**
  in coma, 79
  disturbances of, **751**
Respiratory muscle dysfunction, 231
Respiratory rate, 749
Respiratory syncytial virus (RSV), human.
    See Human respiratory syncytial
    virus infection
Respiratory syncytial virus (RSV) immune
    globulin, 583
Respiratory tract, 414t–415t
Resting energy expenditure, 39
Restless legs syndrome, 227, 229t
Retching, 244
Reteplase, for thrombotic disorders, 338
Reticulocyte(s), 321
Reticulocyte index, 281
Retinal artery occlusion, 216f
Retinal detachment, 216
Retinal vein occlusion, 215, 216f
Retinitis, cytomegalovirus, 573
Retinoic acid
  for acne, 318
  for head and neck cancer prevention, 1125
  for squamous cell carcinoma, 366
Retinopathy
  diabetic, **296,** 297f
  drug-induced, 1139t
  paraneoplastic, 408, 408t
Reverse SLR sign, 190
Reverse transcriptase inhibitors, for HIV/
    AIDS, 606, 607t–610t
Rewarming
  active, 128
  external, 128
  internal, 128
  passive, 128
Reye's syndrome, 578
Rhabdomyolysis, 280
Rheumatic (Sydenham's) chorea, 223
Rheumatic fever, prophylaxis for, 678
Rheumatic heart disease, 678
Rheumatoid arthritis, 775, 780, **886**
  neck pain in, 198
  treatment of, 887–888, 888t
Rheumatoid factor, 774, 887
Rhinitis, allergic, **879**
Rhinovirus infection, **581**
Rhizomucor infection. *See* Mucormycosis
Rhizopus infection. *See* Mucormycosis
Rhodococcus infection, 503
Ribavirin
  for adenovirus infections, 583
  for chronic hepatitis C, 864, 865t–866t
  for human RSV infections, 582–583
  for measles, 585
  for membranoproliferative glomerulone-
    phritis, 805
  for viral hemorrhagic fevers, 165t
Richter's syndrome, 355
Rickettsia africae infection, 555
Rickettsia akari infection, **555**
Rickettsia conorii infection, 555
Rickettsial disease, 106, 108t, 110, 201, **554**
  flea- and louse-borne typhus, **556**
Rickettsialpox, **555**
Rickettsia prowazekii infection. *See* Typhus,
    epidemic

Rickettsia rickettsii infection. *See* Rocky Mountain spotted fever
Rickettsia typhi infection. *See* Typhus, endemic murine
Rifabutin, for tuberculosis, 541–542
Rifampin
  adverse reactions to, 428
  for anthrax, 164t
  for arthritis, infectious, 482
  for *Bartonella* infections, 526t
  for brucellosis, 523
  for diphtheria, 502
  for human granulocytotropic anaplasmosis, 558
  indications for, 427t
  for infective endocarditis, 445t
  for *Legionella* infections, 522
  for leprosy, 546–547
  for meningococcal disease prevention, 506t, 1045
  for nontuberculous mycobacterial infections, 548
  for osteomyelitis, 485t
  for primary biliary cirrhosis, 871
  for Q fever, 559
  resistance to, 427t
  for staphylococcal infections, 496
  for tuberculosis, 541, 543t, 545t–546t
Rifapentine, for tuberculosis, 542
Rifaximin
  for *C. difficile*-associated disease, 462
  for diarrhea, 1117
  for hepatic encephalopathy, 875
Rift Valley fever, 598
Right ventricular systolic pressure, 669
Riluzole, for ALS, 1013
Rimantadine, for influenza, 579t, 580
Ringer's lactate, for cholera, 453
Ringworm, 317
Rinne test, 298
Risedronate, for osteoporosis, 967
Risperidone
  for delirium, 50t
  dosage and adverse effects of, 139t, 1091t
  for schizophrenia, 1081
Risus sardonicus, 528
Ritonavir, for HIV/AIDS, 611t
Rituximab
  for autoimmune hemolysis, 329
  for CLL, 356
  for gastric cancer, 381
  for idiopathic thrombocytopenic purpura, 335
  for inflammatory myopathy, 1072
  for lymphoma, 357–358
  for membranous glomerulonephritis, 804
  for rheumatoid arthritis, 888
  toxicity of, 342t
Rivastigmine, for Alzheimer's disease, 1000
River blindness, **652**
Rizatriptan, for migraine, 185t, 187t
Rocky Mountain spotted fever, 108t, 110, 200, **554**
Rodent bite, 118, 120t
Rodent-borne viral infection, **593**
Romaña's sign, 644
Romberg sign, 986

Ropinirole
  for Parkinson's disease, 1006t
  for restless legs syndrome, 227, 229t
Rosacea. *See* Acne rosacea
Roseola infantum, **571**
Rose spots, 457
Rosetting, 636
Rosiglitazone, for diabetes mellitus, 945t
Ross River virus infection, 596
Rosuvastatin, for hyperlipidemia, 972t
Rotavirus infection, diarrhea, **454**
Rotavirus vaccine, 454, 1108t–1109t
Rotigotine, for Parkinson's disease, 1006t
Rouleaux formation, 321
Roundworm infection. *See also* Nematode infection
  intestinal, 420t
Rubella, **585**
  congenital rubella syndrome, 585–586
Rubella vaccine, 585
Rumination, 244
Russian spring-summer encephalitis, 596t–597t

S
Saccharomyces boulardii therapy, 462
Sacroiliitis, 898t
St. Louis encephalitis, 596t–597t
Salicylates
  for osteoarthritis, 902
  poisoning, 149t
Salicylic acid
  for seborrheic dermatitis, 315
  for warts, 317
Saline therapy
  for hypercalcemia, 113, 406, 962t
  for hyperglycemic hyperosmolar state, 101
  for hypernatremia, 7
  for hyponatremia, 6–7
  for increased intracranial pressure, 92t
  for membrane-active agent poisoning, 153t
  for metabolic alkalosis, 20
  for SIADH, 114
  for tumor lysis syndrome, 116
Salmeterol, for asthma, 754
Salmonellosis, **456**
  nontyphoidal, 457
  typhoid fever, 456–457
Salpingitis, 465, 469, 471
Samarium-153 EDTMP, 342t
Saquinavir, for HIV/AIDS, 611t
Sarcoidosis, 774, **910,** 912f
  acute, 912f
  chronic, 912f
Sarcoma, paraneoplastic syndromes in, 405t
Sarcoptes scabiei infestation. *See* Scabies
Sarin, 142t, 169–171
SARS coronavirus, as bioweapon, 167
Scabies, **658**
Scale (skin lesion), 313t
Scar, 313t
Scar carcinoma, 366
Scarlet fever, **497**
Scedosporiosis, **632**
Schilling test, 256
Schistocytes, 321

Schistosomiasis, 391, 420t, 421, **653**, 1117
  acute, 654
  chronic, 654
Schizoaffective disorder, 1081
Schizoid personality disorder, 1084
Schizophrenia, **1080**
  drug-induced schizophrenic reactions,
    1140t
Schizophreniform disorder, 1081
Schizotypal personality disorder, 1084
Schwannoma, **1033**
  vestibular, 300
Sciatica, 196
Sciatic neuropathy, 1064t
Scleritis, 294
Sclerodactyly, 889
Scleroderma. *See* Systemic sclerosis
Scombroid poisoning, **124**
Scopolamine
  for nausea and vomiting, 48, 245
  poisoning, 138t
  for vertigo, 214t
Scorpionfish envenomation, 123
Scorpion sting, **126**
Scotoma, 215, 216f, 295
Screening recommendations, **1103**
Sea anemone injury, 122
Seborrheic keratosis, 311f
Secobarbital, 143t
Sedative-hypnotics, poisoning, 131t, 143t
Seizure, **988**. *See also* Epilepsy
  absence (petit mal), 988, 988t, 992t–994t
  approach to, 988, 991f
  causes of, 989, 989t, 990t
  complex-partial, 988, 988t
  differential diagnosis of, 990t
  drug-induced, 990t, 1139t
  EEG in, 990–991
  febrile, 201
  generalized, 988, 988t
  neuroimaging in, 994
  partial, 988, 988t
  in poisoning, 135
  simple-partial, 988, 988t
  syncope vs., 210
  tonic-clonic (grand mal), 988, 988t,
    992t–994t
  treatment of, 992t–994t, 994–995
Selective serotonin reuptake inhibitors, 1085,
    1086t
Selegiline
  for Alzheimer's disease, 1000
  dosage and adverse effects of, 138t, 1087t
  for Parkinson's disease, 1004
Selenium, for prostate cancer prevention,
    1124
Selenium sulfide, for seborrheic dermatitis,
    315
Semen analysis, 950
Seminoma, 393–394, 394t
Senna, for constipation, 48t
Sensitization, 34
Sensory exam, **985**
Sensory level, 113
Sensory loss, 220t
  proprioceptive, 218
Sentinel loop, 850
Sentinel node biopsy, in breast cancer, 376

Sepsis, **63**
  Aeromonas, 516
  without clear focus of primary infection,
    106, 107t
  clostridial, 531
  infectious disease emergencies, **105**
  post-splenectomy, 106, 107t
  puerperal, 499
  S. aureus, 491
  severe, 63
  with skin manifestations, 106, 107t–108t, 110
  with soft tissue/muscle findings, 108t,
    110–111
  treatment of, 64–66, 65t
Septic shock, 30, 31f, 59t, 60, **63**, 106, 107t
  infectious disease emergencies, **105**
  pathogenesis and pathology of, 63–64
  treatment of, 64–66, 65t
Sequestra, 483
Serotonin syndrome, 152t
Serratia infection, 516
Sertraline
  dosage and adverse effects of, 1086t
  for vasovagal syncope, 210
Serum sickness, 201
  drug-induced, 1132t
Sevelamer, for hyperphosphatemia, 964
Severe acute respiratory infection (SARS),
    581
Severe combined immunodeficiency, **881**
  X-linked, 882–883
Sexual assault, 1130
Sexual dysfunction, drug-induced, 1132t
Sexually transmitted disease, **462**
  in travelers, 1117
Shift work, 226, 230
Shigellosis, **458**
  proctocolitis, 468
Shingles, 316, **570**
Shock, **30, 58**. *See also specific types*
  approach to, 31f, 59–60
  forms of, 59t
  in GI bleeding, 260
  hemodynamic profiles in, 60t, 61f
  high cardiac output/low systemic vascular
    resistance, 30, 31f
  hypovolemic, 30, 31f
  treatment of, 60–62, 62t
Shoulder
  adhesive capsulitis, 910
  muscles and innervation of, 980t–981t
Shoulder pain, **196**
  causes of, 196–198
  mechanical, 198
  treatment of, 198–199
Shunting, hypoxemia in, 750
Sibutramine, for obesity, 940
Sick euthyroid syndrome, **930**
Sickle cell anemia, 326, 328
  pathophysiology of sickle cell crisis, 327f
Sickle cell nephropathy, **826**
Sickled cells, 321
Sick sinus syndrome, 717–718
Sideroblastic anemia, 325, 325t
Sigmoidoscopy, 387, 1123t
  in diarrhea, 256
  in GI bleeding, 261
"Sign of the groove," 471

Sildenafil
  for achalasia, 251
  for erectile dysfunction, 951
  for systemic sclerosis, 889
Silent ischemia, 714
Silicosis, **757**
Simple phobia, 1083
Simvastatin, for hyperlipidemia, 972t
Sindbis virus infection, 596
Sinoatrial node dysfunction, **717**
  extrinsic, 717
  intrinsic, 717
Sinusitis, **301**
  acute, 302
  anaerobic, 533
  aspergillosis, 622–623
  bacterial, 302
  chronic, 302
  fungal, 302
  Klebsiella, 515
  M. catarrhalis, 510
  nosocomial, 302
  treatment of, 302, 303t
Sinus rhythm, 665
Sinus tachycardia, 704, 721f, 722t
Sirolimus, immunosuppression for renal
    transplant, 800
Sister Mary Joseph's nodule, 271
Sitagliptin, for diabetes mellitus, 945t
Sjögren's syndrome, **890**
Skin, examination of, **309**
Skin biopsy, 311
Skin cancer, **364**
  basal cell carcinoma, **366**
  melanoma. *See* Melanoma
  prevention of, 364, 367, 1104t
  screening for, 1123t
  squamous cell carcinoma, **366**
Skin disease
  acne, **317**
  arrangement and shape of lesions, 309,
    310f–312f
  in cancer patients, 432
  diagnosis of, 311–313
  distribution of lesions, 309
  drug-induced, 319, 342t, 1133t–1134t
  eczematous, 315
  history in, 310
  lesion characteristics, 309, 310f–312f
  in malnutrition, 41
  papulosquamous, **314**
  primary lesions, 309, 313t
  in returned traveler, 1118
  secondary lesions, 309, 313t
  sepsis-associated, 106
  vascular disorders, **318**
Skin infection, **316, 477**
  anaerobic, 533
  clostridial, 531
  P. aeruginosa, 518
  S. aureus, 490–491, 496
  in transplant recipients, 436t
  treatment of, 479t–480t
Skin tag, 311f
Skull fracture, 91
Sleep, nonrestorative, 227
Sleep apnea, 226, 228, **228, 783,** 784t
  central, 228, 783

mixed, 228
  obstructive, 228, 229t, 783, 784t
Sleep disorder, **226,** 289t
  drug-induced, 1140t
  in women, 1130
Sleep hygiene, 227
  inadequate, 227
Sleeping sickness, **645**
  East African, 645–646
  West African, 645–646
Sleep paralysis, 229t, 230, 230t
Sleepwalking, 226
Slit-lamp examination, 215, 294
Slow low-efficiency dialysis, 793
Slow-reacting substance of anaphylaxis, 877,
    877f
Small-bowel cancer, **382**
Small-bowel tumor, **382**
Smallpox
  as bioweapon, 163–166, 164t
  hemorrhagic, 166
  malignant, 166
  microbiology and clinical features of,
    163–166
  treatment of, 164t, 166
  vaccination and prevention, 166
Smell, disorders of sense of, **1023,** 1023t
Smoke inhalation, 758
Smoking, 369, 391–392
  cough and, 234–235
  prevention of, 1128
  relative risks for current smokers, 1126t
Smoking cessation, 368, 374, 759, 761, 775,
    1103, 1104t–1105t, 1118, 1124,
    1126
  approach to, 1126–1127
  clinical practice guidelines, 1127, 1127t
  methods of, 1126, 1127t
  quit date, 1126–1127
Snakebite, 120t, **121**
  field management of, 121
  hospital management of, 121–122
Snoring, 229t
Social phobia, 1083
Sodium, disorders of, **3**
Sodium bicarbonate
  for AGMA inducer poisoning, 147t
  for antidepressant poisoning, 141t
  for antipsychotic poisoning, 139t
  for iron poisoning, 147t
  for membrane-active agent poisoning,
    153t
  for metabolic acidosis, 19
  for methanol poisoning, 148t
  for poisoning, 160
  for salicylate poisoning, 149t
Sodium citrate, for metabolic acidosis, 19
Sodium deficit, 7
Sodium nitrite, for cytochrome oxidase inhib-
    itor poisoning, 145t
Sodium phosphate enema, for constipation,
    48t
Sodium restriction
  for aldosteronism, 935
  for ascites, 272
  for cor pulmonale, 735
  for edema, 243
  for heart failure, 731, 735

Sodium restriction (*Cont.*):
  for hypertension, 694
  for restrictive cardiomyopathy, 686
  for vertigo, 213, 214t
Sodium stibogluconate, for leishmaniasis, 643
Sodium thiosulfate, for cytochrome oxidase
    inhibitor poisoning, 145t
Soft tissue infection, **477**
  anaerobic, 533
  clostridial, 531
  HACEK group, 511
  Klebsiella, 515
  P. aeruginosa, 518
  S. aureus, 490–491, 496
Solid organ transplant
  infections in recipients, 437–438
  vaccination of recipients, 439
Soman, 142t
Somatization disorder, 1083
Somatoform disorder, **1083**
Somatostatinoma, 389, 390t, 391
Somatostatin therapy, for esophageal varices,
    874
Somatotropin, for hypopituitarism, 922t
Sorafenib
  for kidney cancer, 393
  toxicity of, 342t
Sorbitol
  for irritable bowel syndrome, 842t
  for paralytic shellfish poisoning, 124
  for poisoning, 135
Sotalol
  for arrhythmias, 728t
  poisoning, 140t
South American hemorrhagic fevers, **598**
Soy-based products, 957
Spastic colon, **840**
Specimen collection, 414t–419t
Specimen transport, 414t–419t
Spectinomycin, for gonococcal infections,
    470t
Speech audiometry, 298
Spermatogenesis, 949–950
Spherocytes, 321
Spider bite, **125**
Spinal cord, anatomy of, 1027f
Spinal cord compression, **94**
  brucellosis vs. tuberculosis, 523, 523t
  epidural abscess, **95**
  epidural hematoma, **95**
  hematomyelia, **96**
  from metastases, 1034–1035, 1034t
  neoplastic, **94**, 1028, 1028f
  oncologic emergency, **113**
  treatment of, 95, 113, 114f
Spinal cord disease, **1026**
  acute, **1028**
  autonomic dysfunction in, 1016, 1027
  cauda equina, 1028
  cervical cord, 1027
  chronic, **1029**
  complications of, 1031
  extramedullary, 1028
  intramedullary, 1028
  lumbar cord, 1028
  sacral cord, 1028
  subacute, **1028**
  thoracic cord, 1028
    trauma, 94
    treatable, 1026t
    weakness in, 219t
Spinal cord infarction, 1029
Spinal stenosis, 906
  back pain in, 190–191
Spinocerebellar ataxia, 1009
Spirillum minor infection, 118
Spirochetal infection, nonsyphilitic, **549**
Spirometry, 747, 759
Spironolactone
  for aldosteronism, 21, 935
  for ascites, 272
  for dilated cardiomyopathy, 685
  for edema, 243, 243t
  for heart failure, 732, 732t, 733t
  for hirsutism, 955
  for hypertension, 695t
  for myocardial infarction, 707
Splenectomy, 288, 356, 450, 577
  post-splenectomy infections, 106, 107t
Splenic abscess, **450**
Splenomegaly, **285**
  diseases associated with, 286t–287t
  mechanism of, 286t–287t, 287
  tropical, 637
Spondylitic myelopathy, 199, 1029
Spondylitis, 898t
Spondyloarthritides, 896f
Spondylosis, cervical, 198–199
Spontaneous breathing trial, 32
Sporotrichosis, **631**
  disseminated, 631
  lymphocutaneous, 631
  osteoarticular, 631
  plaque disease, 631
  pulmonary, 631
Sporozoite, 636
Spotted fever
  mite-borne, **554**
  tick-borne, **554**
Spur cell anemia, 326
Sputum analysis
  in pneumonia, 765
  in respiratory disease, 751
  specimen collection and transport, 415t
Sputum clearance, 235
Squamous cell carcinoma, **366**
  infections in cancer patients, 433t
Stabbing headache, primary, 183t, 189
Stain, 411
Staphylococcal infection, **489**
  cellulitis, 478
  coagulase-negative staphylococci, **493**
  endocarditis, 445t, 446
  food poisoning, 453
  treatment of, 493–496, 494t–495t
Staphylococcal scalded-skin syndrome, 477,
    492
Staphylococcus aureus infection, **489**
  bacteremia and sepsis, 491
  endocarditis, 491–492, 496
  impetigo, 316
  invasive disease, 490
  methicillin-resistant (MRSA), 65t, 477,
    485t, 489–493, 494t–495t, 496
  musculoskeletal, 491, 496
  osteomyelitis, 483, 485t

prosthetic device-related, 492–493
respiratory tract, 491
risk of, 490
skin/soft tissue, 477, 490–491, 496
spinal epidural abscess, 95
toxin-mediated disease, 490, 492
treatment of, 493–496, 494t–495t
urinary tract, 492
Starvation, 40
Stasis ulcer, 311f
Stat DRIP (medication pneumonic), 2
Statins
for aortic stenosis, 681
for hyperlipidemia, 972t
for myocardial infarction, 711–712
for unstable angina, 711
Status epilepticus, **98,** 99f
GCSE, 98–100
after hypoxic-ischemic insult, 98
nonconvulsive, 98–99
Stauffer's syndrome, 393
Stavudine, for HIV/AIDS, 608t
Steatorrhea, 256
Stellate ganglion blockade, 1019
Stenotrophomonas maltophilia infection, **518,**
520t
Stenting, vascular
for angina pectoris, 716, 717t
for superior vena cava syndrome, 112
Stereognosis, 985
Sterilization, 957
Stevens-Johnson syndrome, 318, 1133t
Stiff-person syndrome, 408t
Stingray envenomation, 123
Stomatitis, HACEK group, 511
Stonefish envenomation, 123
Stool analysis, 256
parasites, 421
reference values for specific analytes,
1164t
specimen collection and transport, 415t
Stool softeners, 48t, 844
Straight leg raising sign, 190
Streptobacillus moniliformis infection, 118
Streptococcal infection, **496**
arthritis, 499–500
bacteremia, 498–499
brain abscess, 501
cellulitis, 498–500, 498t
empyema, 498, 498t
endocarditis, 443, 444t, 499–500
erysipelas, 316, 498, 498t
group A, 316, **497,** 498t
group B, **499**
groups C and G, **499**
hemolytic patterns, 497
impetigo, 498, 498t
liver abscess, 501
meningitis, 500
necrotizing fasciitis, 497–498, 498t
neonatal, 500
nutritionally variant streptococci, **501**
osteomyelitis, 485t
pharyngitis, 497, 498t
pneumonia, 498, 498t, 500
poststreptococcal glomerulonephritis, 801
in pregnancy, 500
puerperal sepsis, 499

scarlet fever, **497**
toxic shock syndrome, 497, 498t, 499
urinary tract, 500
viridans streptococci, **501**
Streptococcus pneumoniae infection. *See*
Pneumococcal infection
Streptococcus pyogenes infection
erysipelas, 478
necrotizing fasciitis, **478**
Streptokinase
for myocardial infarction, 701
for thrombotic disorders, 338
Streptomycin
for *Bartonella* infections, 526t
for brucellosis, 523
for enterococcal infections, 501
for nontuberculous mycobacterial infections, 548
for plague, 164t, 526
for tuberculosis, 541
for tularemia, 165t, 524
Streptozotocin
for carcinoid tumor, 389
for islet-cell tumors, 391
for Zollinger-Ellison syndrome, 836
Stress testing, in coronary artery disease,
713–714, 713f, 714t
Stroke, **79**
anatomic localization in, 81t
causes of, determination of, 85
drug-induced, 1139t
embolic, prevention of, 85–86, 87t
hemorrhagic, 80
ischemic, 80
causes of, 86t
treatment of, 81–84, 84t
prevention of, 85–87, 87t
risk factors for, 85, 87t
small-vessel, 80
treatment of, 80–85, 83f
Strongyloidiasis, 420t, 421, **650,** 1117
Strontium-89 therapy, 342t
Struvite stones, 827, 828t
Stupor, **74**
Subacute sclerosing panencephalitis, 585
Subarachnoid hemorrhage (SAH), **88**
grading scales for, 88, 88t
headache in, 183t
with hydrocephalus, 89–90
lumbar puncture, 27–28, 28f
vasospasm in, 89
Subdural hematoma, 93
Substance abuse, 1104t
alcoholism, **1095**
narcotic abuse, **1099**
in women, 1130
Succimer, for heavy metal poisoning, 157t,
159t
Sucralfate
for erosive gastropathies, 834
for peptic ulcer disease, 833
Sudden death, **55**
differential diagnosis of, 55t
Suicide, 1078, 1080
prevention of, 1104t–1105t
Suicide attempt, 130
Sulfacetamide, for eye infections, 294
Sulfadiazine, for toxoplasmosis, 647

Sulfadoxine-pyrimethamine, for malaria, 638t
Sulfasalazine
 for ankylosing spondylitis, 897
 for enteropathic arthritis, 907
 for inflammatory bowel disease, 838
 for psoriatic arthritis, 898
 for reactive arthritis, 900
 for rheumatoid arthritis, 887
Sulfhemoglobinemia, 239
Sulfinpyrazone, for gout, 905
Sulfonamides
 adverse reactions to, 428
 indications for, 426t
 poisoning, 146t
 resistance to, 426t
Sulfonylurea, for diabetes mellitus, 944, 945t
Sulfur granules, 537
Sulfur mustard, 168–169
Sulindac
 for colon cancer prevention, 1124
 for colonic polyps, 383
Sumatriptan
 for cluster headache, 187
 for migraine, 185t–186t, 187t
Summer grippe, 589–590
Sunitinib
 for kidney cancer, 393
 toxicity of, 342t
Superior vena cava syndrome, **112**
Supraventricular arrhythmia, 736
 in myocardial infarction, 704
Supraventricular tachycardia, 720, 725t
 in poisoning, 134
Suramin, for sleeping sickness, 645–646
Swallowing studies, 250
Sweet's syndrome, 201, 432
Swimmer's ear, 304, 518
Swimmer's itch, 478, 653
Swinging flashlight test, 215
Sympathetic poisoning, 131t
Sympathetic system, 1014f, 1015t
Sympatholytic poisoning, 131t–132t
Sympathomimetic poisoning, 131t, 136t
Synchronized intermittent mandatory ventila-
 tion (SIMV), 72, 73t
Syncope, **207**
 approach to, 207–208, 208f
 causes of, 208–210, 209t
 neurocardiogenic, 208, 209t
 situational, 209t
 treatment of, 210–211
 vasodepressor, 208
 vasovagal, 208, 210
Syndrome of inappropriate ADH (SIADH),
 925
 causes of, 924t
 drug-induced, 341t
 hyponatremia in, 6
 paraneoplastic, **114**, 405t, 406
 treatment of, 114–115, 406, 925
Syndrome X. *See* Metabolic syndrome
Synkinesis, 1021
Synovial fluid analysis, 205–206, 206f, 482,
 904, 906
Synovitis, symmetric proliferative, 906
Syphilis, 468, **472**, 474t, 478
 congenital, 473
 endemic, 551

 features of genital ulcers, 467t
 late, 473–475, 474t
 latent, 472, 474–475, 474t
 in pregnancy, 474t
 primary, 472, 474, 474t
 secondary, 200, 472, 474, 474t
 tertiary, 1030
Syringomyelia, 1029
Systemic inflammatory response syndrome
 (SIRS), 63
Systemic lupus erythematosus (SLE), 776,
 885
 glomerular disease in, 803, 807t
 treatment of, 886
Systemic sclerosis, **888**
 diffuse cutaneous, 889
 esophageal disorders in, 251–252
 limited cutaneous, 889
 renovascular disease in, 824
Systemic vascular resistance, 705

T

Tabes dorsalis, 473, 1030
Tabun, 142t, 169–171
Tache noire, 555
Tachyarrhythmia, 209t, **720**
 clinical and ECG features of, 721f,
 722t–725t, 726t
 narrow QRS complex, 722t–723t
 wide QRS complex, 724t–725t
Tachycardia, 717
Tacrine
 for Alzheimer's disease, 1000
 poisoning, 142t
Tacrolimus
 immunosuppression for renal transplant,
 799–800
 for inflammatory myopathy, 1072
Tadalafil, for erectile dysfunction, 951
Taeniasis saginata, 421, **655**
Taeniasis solium, **655**
Takayasu's arteritis, **738, 892**
Tamoxifen
 for breast cancer, 376, 378–379
 preventive treatment, 379, 1122
 for endometrial cancer, 397
 for melanoma, 365
 toxicity of, 342t
Tapeworm infection, **655**
Tardive dyskinesia, 223, 1092
Target cells, 321
Target lesion, 309
Tarsal tunnel syndrome, 1064t
Taxanes, for prostate cancer, 401
Tazarotene, for psoriasis, 314
T cell immunodeficiency, **883**
T cell receptor complex deficiency, 883
Tdap vaccine, 529, 1110t–1113t
Td vaccine, 503
Teardrop cells, 321
Telangiectasia, 313t
Telavancin, for staphylococcal infections,
 494t
Temazepam, 1089t
 poisoning, 143t
Temozolomide, for melanoma, 365
Temperature, 199
Temporal arteritis. *See* Giant cell arteritis

Temsirolimus
  for kidney cancer, 393
  toxicity of, 342t
Tendinitis, **910**
  calcific, 910
Tendon reflexes, 219t
Tendon xanthoma, 970
Tenecteplase, for thrombotic disorders, 338
Tenofovir, for HIV/AIDS, 609t
Tension headache, 183t, 186
Teratogenesis, of cancer chemotherapy,
    340–342
Teratoma, 393
Terazosin, for prostate hyperplasia, 399
Terbinafine, **620**
Terbutaline poisoning, 136t
Terminally ill patient, **46**
  anorexia in, 52t
  apnea in, 53t
  care during last hours, 50–51, 52t–53t
  clinical courses in last days, 51f
  constipation in, 48
  death rattle in, 52t
  dehydration in, 52t
  delirium in, 50, 53t
  depression in, 49–50
  dysphagia in, 52t
  dyspnea in, 49, 53t
  fatigue in, 52t
  incontinence in, 53t
  mucosal membranes in, 53t
  nausea and vomiting in, 48
  pain management in, 47
  physical symptoms of, 47, 47t
  psychological symptoms of, 47, 47t
  withdrawal of care, 33
Testicular cancer, **393**, 394t
  paraneoplastic syndromes in, 405t
Testosterone deficiency, 947–949
Testosterone therapy
  for androgen deficiency, 948
  for hypopituitarism, 922t
Tetanus, 118, **528**
  generalized, 528–529
  local, 529
  neonatal, 528–529
Tetanus and diphtheria toxoid (Td), 529
Tetanus booster, 121
Tetanus immune globulin, 529
Tetracycline
  for acne, 318
  adverse reactions to, 424
  for C. pneumoniae infections, 563
  for C. psittaci infections, 563
  for H. pylori eradication, 833t
  for intestinal pseudoobstruction, 843
  for malaria, 109t, 638t
  for syphilis, 474t
  for tularemia, 524
Tetralogy of Fallot, **677**
Tetrathiomolybdate, for Wilson's disease,
    978
Thalassemia, 325–326, 325t, 328
Thalidomide
  for leprosy, 547
  for multiple myeloma, 361
Theophylline
  for asthma, 754–755

for COPD, 761–762
  poisoning, 137t
Thermoregulatory sweat test, 1016
Thiamine deficiency, 43t
Thiamine therapy, for alcohol withdrawal,
    1098
Thiazolidinedione, for diabetes mellitus, 945,
    945t
Thigh, muscles and innervation of, 980t–981t
Thin basement membrane nephropathy,
    808
Thiocyanate toxicity, 734
Thioguanine, 341t
Thioridazine
  for delirium, 50t
  dosage and adverse effects of, 138t, 139t,
    1091t
Thiothixene, 1091t
Thoracentesis, **26**, 26f, 752
Thoracic outlet syndrome, 1063t
  arterial, 198
  disputed, 198
  true neurogenic, 198
Thoracic spine disease, chest pain in, 176f,
    178
Thoracic surgery, video-assisted (VATS),
    752, 775
Throat specimen, collection and transport of,
    414t
Thrombocytopenia, **332**, 333f
  drug-induced, 332, 344, 1135t
Thrombocytopenic purpura
  idiopathic (ITP), 332, 335
  thrombotic (TTP), 333, 335, 459,
    824–826
  treatment of, 335
Thrombocytosis, **333**
  essential, **351**
Thrombolytic therapy
  for arterial embolism, 739
  for stroke, 83
Thrombophlebitis, superficial, **740**
Thrombotic disorders, **336**
  treatment of, 336–338, 337t
Thrombotic microangiopathy, **824**, 825t
Thrush, 620–621
Thumb, muscles and innervation of,
    980t–981t
Thymectomy, 1066
Thymoma, 409t
Thymus, myasthenia gravis, **1065**
Thyroid adenoma, **932**
Thyroid carcinoma, **932**
Thyroid disease, **925**
  drug-induced, 1132t
  hypothyroidism, **926**
  neoplasms, **932**
  nontoxic goiter, **931**
  sick euthyroid syndrome, **930**
  thyrotoxicosis, **928**
  toxic adenoma, **932**
  toxic multinodular goiter, **931**
Thyroidectomy, 932
Thyroid function tests, 929
Thyroiditis
  silent, 928–930
  subacute, 928–930, 930f
Thyroid nodule, 933f

Thyroid-stimulating hormone, 917, 918f
  deficiency of, 919t, 922, 922t
  hypersecretion of, 919t, **921**
Thyroid storm, 928, 930
Thyrotoxic crisis, 928, 930
Thyrotoxicosis, 925, **928**, 929f
  amiodarone-induced, **931**
Thyroxine, **925**
  for hypopituitarism, 922t
Tiagabine
  for generalized anxiety disorder, 1082
  poisoning, 143t
  for seizures, 994t
Tic(s), **223**
Ticarcillin-clavulanate
  for anaerobic infections, 534t
  for sepsis/septic shock, 65t
  for *S. maltophilia* infections, 518, 520t
  for urinary tract infections, 819t
Tic douloureux. *See* Trigeminal neuralgia
Tick, removal of, 125
Tick bite, **124**
Tick paralysis, **124**
Ticlopidine, for thrombotic disorders, 338
TIGAR-O classification, of pancreatic dis-
     ease, 853t
Tigecycline
  for enterococcal infections, 501
  for *Klebsiella* infections, 515
  for staphylococcal infections, 493, 494t
Tilt-table test, 1016
TIMI Risk Score, 709–710, 711f
Timolol
  for myocardial infarction prevention, 709
  poisoning, 140t
Tinea capitis, 317
Tinea cruris, 311f, 317
Tinea pedis, 310f, 311f
Tinea unguium, 317
Tinea (pityriasis) versicolor, 311, 631
Tinidazole
  for amebiasis, 461
  for *H. pylori* eradication, 833t
  for trichomoniasis, 464
  for urethritis in men, 463
Tinnitus, 212–213, 297, **300**
Tinzaparin, for venous thromboembolism,
    770
Tipranavir, for HIV/AIDS, 614t
Tirofiban
  for myocardial infarction, 711
  for thrombotic disorders, 338
  for unstable angina, 711
Tissue necrosis, 329
Tissue plasminogen activator
  for frostbite, 129
  for stroke, 83, 84t
  for thrombotic disorders, 338
Tizanidine
  for multiple sclerosis, 1041
  poisoning, 139t, 144t
TNM staging
  for breast cancer, 376, 377t–378t
  for lung cancer, 369, 370t–371t
Toad skin secretions, 141t
Tobramycin
  indications for, 426t
  for osteomyelitis, 485t

  for *P. aeruginosa* infections, 519t
  for pneumonia, 767t
  resistance to, 426t
  for sepsis/septic shock, 65t
Toes, muscles and innervation of, 980t–981t
Tolcapone, for Parkinson's disease, 1004
Tolfenamic acid, for migraine, 185t
Tolnaftate, for dermatophyte infections, 317
Tolosa-Hunt syndrome, 1025
Tongue paralysis, 1024
Topiramate
  for migraine prevention, 188t
  poisoning, 143t
  for seizures, 992t–993t, 994t
Topoisomerase inhibitors, 341t
Topotecan, 341t
Torsades de pointes, 725t
Torsemide, for heart failure, 733t
Torticollis, 223
Tositumomab
  for follicular lymphoma, 357
  toxicity of, 342t
Tourette syndrome, 223
Toxemia of pregnancy, **826**
Toxic adenoma, **932**
Toxic epidermal necrolysis, 477
  drug-induced, 1134t
Toxic granulations, 322
Toxicology, reference values for laboratory
    tests, 1157t–1159t
Toxic shock syndrome, 108t, 110, 200
  dengue, 599
  staphylococcal, 490, 492, 496
  streptococcal, 497, 498t, 499
Toxocara canis infection. *See* Larva migrans
Toxoplasmosis, **646**
  CNS disease, 646
  congenital, 646–647
  diagnosis of, 420t
  ocular, 647
  pneumonia, 646
  in pregnancy, 646
  prevention of, 647
Tracheobronchitis
  human RSV, 582
  M. catarrhalis, 510
Trachoma, 294, **561**
Tramadol
  narcotic abuse, **1099**
  for osteoarthritis, 902
  for pain, 36t–37t
  poisoning, 152t
Trandolapril, for heart failure, 733t
Transaminases, 268, 268t
Transfusion therapy, **44**
  for AML, 346
  autologous transfusion, **45**
  complications of, 44, 45t
  plasma components, **45**
  platelet transfusion, **45**
  red blood cell transfusion, **44**
  whole blood, **44**
Transient hypogammaglobulinemia of in-
    fancy, 884
Transient ischemic attack (TIA), **79**, 83f
Transient monocular blindness, 215
Transjugular intrahepatic portosystemic shunt
    (TIPS), 263, 272, 874

Transplant recipient
  cytomegalovirus infection in, 573
  infections in, **436,** 800
Transsphenoidal surgery, 919, 934
trans-Tretinoic acid, for AML, 346
Transtubular potassium gradient, 10, 11f, 13f
Transurethral microwave thermotherapy
      (TUMT), 399
Transurethral resection of prostate (TURP),
      399
Tranylcypromine, 138t, 1087t
Trastuzumab
  for breast cancer, 379
  toxicity of, 342t
Travelers
  gastrointestinal illness, 1117
  HIV-infected, 1117
  immunizations for, **1107,** 1116t
  insect-borne disease prevention, 1116
  malaria prevention, 1116
  pregnant, 1117
  problems after return, 1117–1118
  sexually transmitted diseases in, 1117
Traveler's diarrhea, **451,** 454
  prevention of, 1117
Trazodone
  dosage and adverse effects of, 1087t
  for PTSD, 1083
Trematode infection, **653**
Tremor, **222**
  essential, 222, 222t
  intention, 222
  Parkinsonian, 222, 222t
  postural, 222
  at rest, 222
Trench fever, 526t, **527**
Trench mouth, 532
Treponema pallidum infection. *See* Syphilis
Treponematosis, endemic, **551**
Treprostinil, for pulmonary hypertension, 745
Tretinoin, 342t
Triamcinolone
  for asthma, 755
  for cough, 235
  steroid preparations, 938–939, 938t
Triamterene
  for edema, 243t
  for hypertension, 695t
Triazolam
  dosage and action of, 1089t
  for insomnia, 228
  poisoning, 143t
Triazoles, **619**
  for dermatophyte infections, 317
Trichinellosis, **648**
Trichloroacetic acid, for HPV infection, 476
Trichomoniasis, 464
Triclabendazole, for liver flukes, 654
Tricuspid regurgitation, 662t, **683**
Tricuspid stenosis, 662t, **683**
Tricuspid valve endocarditis, 442
Tricuspid valve prolapse, 662t
Tricyclic antidepressants, 1086t, 1088
  for irritable bowel syndrome, 842t
  for migraine prevention, 184
  poisoning, 141t, 149t, 152t, 153t
  for polyneuropathy, 1061
Trientine, for Wilson's disease, 978

Trifluoperazine, 1091t
Trifluorothymidine, for HSV infections, 568t
Trigeminal nerve, 982
  sensory divisions of, 1020f
Trigeminal neuralgia, 189, **1020**
Trigeminal neuropathy, 1021, 1021t
Trigger points, 1020
Triglycerides, **968**
Trihexyphenidyl
  for dystonia, 223
  for Parkinson's disease, 1004
Triiodothyronine, **925**
Trimethoprim, for urinary tract infection pre-
      vention, 817
Trimethoprim-polymyxin, for eye infections,
      294
Trimethoprim-sulfamethoxazole
  for *Aeromonas* infections, 516
  for animal bite infections, 119t
  for *B. cepacia* infections, 518, 520t
  for brucellosis, 523
  during COPD exacerbations, 763
  for cyclosporiasis, 456
  for cystitis, 818t
  for diverticulitis, 842
  for *E. coli* infections, 514
  indications for, 426t
  for isosporiasis, 456
  for *Legionella* infections, 522
  for listerial infections, 508
  for nephrolithiasis, 828t
  for nocardiosis, 536, 536t
  for peritonitis prevention, 449
  for pertussis, 510
  for plague, 526
  for *Pneumocystis* infections, 634, 634t
    preventive treatment, 635, 635t
  for Q fever, 559
  resistance to, 426t
  for sinusitis, 303t
  for *S. maltophilia,* 518, 520t
  for snakebite, 120t
  for staphylococcal infections, 493, 494t,
      496
  for streptococcal infections, 501
  for toxoplasmosis prevention, 647
  for typhoid fever, 457
  for urinary tract infections, 819t
    preventive treatment, 817
Trimetrexate, for *Pneumocystis* infections,
      634t, 635
Triolein breath test, 256
Triple-H therapy, for subarachnoid hemor-
      rhage with vasospasm, 89
Triptans
  for migraine, 185t
  poisoning, 152t
Tritium contamination, 174
Trophozoite, 636
Troponins, cardiac-specific, 700–701
Trousseau's sign, 963
Trypanosomiasis, 421, **644**
Tryptophan poisoning, 152t
Tuberculin skin test, 539
Tuberculosis, **538**
  ascites in, **271,** 273t
  brucellosis vs., 523, 523t
  extrapulmonary, 539–540

Tuberculosis (*Cont.*):
  gastrointestinal disease in, 540
  genitourinary, 540
  HIV/AIDS and, 538–540, 542, 545t–546t
  meningitis in, 540
  miliary disease, 540
  multidrug-resistant, **538**
  nosocomial, 432
  pericarditis in, 540
  pleural involvement in, 539, 780
  postprimary, 539
  prevention of, 542
  primary, 539
  pulmonary, 539
  skeletal disease in, 540
  treatment of, 541–542, 543t
    latent infection, 542, 544t–546t
Tuberoeruptive xanthoma, 974
Tuberous sclerosis/lymphangioleiomyomatosis, 774
Tuberous xanthoma, 970
Tube thoracostomy, 778
Tubulin poisons, 341t
Tubulointerstitial disease, **808**
Tubulointerstitial nephritis and uveitis syndrome, 811
Tularemia, 106, 118, 201, 478, **524**
  as bioweapon, 165t, 166
  oculoglandular, 524
  oculopharyngeal and gastrointestinal, 524
  pulmonary, 524
  treatment of, 165t, 524–525
  typhoidal, 524
  ulceroglandular/glandular, 524
Tumor (skin lesion), 313t
Tumor lysis syndrome, **116**, 359
Tumor-suppressor genes, 339
Turcot's syndrome, 384, 384t
Turner's sign, 849
Twitching, 984
Two-point discrimination, 985
Tympanic membrane perforation, 298–300
Tympanometry, 298
Typhoid fever. *See* Enteric fever
Typhoid vaccine, 1116t
Typhus
  endemic murine (flea-borne), **556**
  epidemic (louse-borne), 110, **556**
  scrub, 110, 201, **557**
Tzanck preparation, 311–313

U
Ulcer, 313t
  cutaneous, 201, 478
  genital, **466**, 467t
Ulcer (skin lesion), 313t
Ulcerative colitis, **837**
  epidemiology of, 836, 836t
  extraintestinal manifestations of, 838
  treatment of, 838, 839f, 840
Ulnar nerve entrapment, 1062t
Ultrasonography
  diagnostic, **24**
  endoscopic, 380, 846t, 847
  hepatobiliary, 270, 846t, 847–848
  neuroimaging, 987t
  in osteomyelitis, 484t
  in pancreatitis, 851–852

renal, 794
  in stroke, 85
  venous, 770
Undecylenic acid, for dermatophyte infections, 317
Underweight, 939t
Undulating fever, 522–523
Unfractionated heparin
  for thrombotic disorders, 336
  for venous thromboembolism, 770–771
Unstable angina, **709**
  TIMI Risk Score for, 709–710, 711f
  treatment of, 709–712, 710f
Upper respiratory infection (URI), **301,** 303t–304t
Urate nephropathy, 903
Urea breath test, 832, 832t
Ureaplasma infection, **471**
Ureidopenicillin, for cholecystitis, 847
Uremia, 276, 794, **795**
Uremic syndrome, **795**
Ureteral obstruction, 830
Urethral syndrome, **464**
Urethritis, **815**
  chlamydial, 471
  gonococcal, 464, 468
  in men, **463**
  nongonococcal, 463, 471, 482
  treatment of, 463, 816–817
  in women, **464**
Uric-acid lowering agents, 905
Uric acid stones, 827, 828t, 904
Uricosuric drugs, for gout, 905
Urinalysis, 816
  reference values for specific analytes, 1163t
Urinary incontinence, in terminally ill patient, 53t
Urinary retention, 399
Urinary stones, drug-induced, 1138t
Urinary tract infection, 786t, 787, **815**
  acute, **815**
  in cancer patients, 434
  candidiasis, 620
  catheter-associated, 816
  causes of, 815, 818t–819t
  complicated, 819t
  E. coli, 513
  enterococcal, 500
  gram-negative enteric bacteria, 516
  Klebsiella, 515
  nosocomial, 429, 430t
  P. aeruginosa, 518, 520t
  prevention of, 817
  Proteus, 515
  S. aureus, 492
  streptococcal, 500
  treatment of, 816–817, 818t–819t
Urinary tract obstruction, 786t, 788, **829,** 830f
  drug-induced, 1138t
Urine
  abnormalities
    asymptomatic, 786t, 787, **806,** 806t
    of composition, **278**
    of volume, **276**
  specimen collection and transport, 416t
  toxicologic analysis of, 133
Urogenital tract, 416t

Urokinase, for thrombotic disorders, 338
Ursodeoxycholic acid
　for primary biliary cirrhosis, 871
　for primary sclerosing cholangitis, 849
Urticaria, 201, **319, 878**
　classification of, 878, 878t
　drug-induced, 1134t
UV-B phototherapy, for pityriasis rosea, 314
Uveitis, 294
Uvulopalatopharyngoplasty, 784

V
Vaccination. *See* Immunization
Vaccine Adverse Event Reporting System
　　(VAERS), 1107
Vaginal discharge, 464
Vagotomy, for peptic ulcer disease, 833t
Vagus nerve, 984
　disorders of, 1024
Vagus nerve stimulation, 1079
Valacyclovir
　for Bell's palsy, 1022
　for HSV infections, 475, 479t, 567t–568t,
　　569
Valdecoxib, for pain, 36t–37t
Valganciclovir
　for cytomegalovirus infections, 574
　for viral esophagitis, 252
Valproate/valproic acid
　for bipolar disorder, 1080
　dosage and adverse effects of, 1092t
　for migraine prevention, 188t
　for myoclonus, 224
　poisoning, 143t
　for posthypoxic myoclonus, 98
　for seizures, 992t–993t, 994t
　for status epilepticus, 99f
Valsalva maneuver, 663t, 1016
Valsalva ratio, 1016
Valsartan
　for heart failure, 733t
　for hypertension, 695t
　for myocardial infarction, 704
Valvular heart disease, **678**
　echocardiography in, 670, 671f, 672t
　murmurs in, 662t
Vancomycin
　for acute bacterial endocarditis, 109t
　adverse reactions to, 424
　for arthritis, infectious, 482
　for bacterial meningitis, 108t, 1046t, 1047t
　for brain abscess, 109t, 1051
　for C. difficile-associated disease,
　　461–462
　for enterococcal infections, 501
　for epidural abscess, 109t
　for erythroderma, 108t
　indications for, 426t
　for infective endocarditis, 443, 444t–445t,
　　446
　for MRSA infections, 479t
　for necrotizing fasciitis, 480t
　for osteomyelitis, 485t
　for peritonitis, 449
　for pneumococcal infections, 488
　for pneumonia, 766t, 767t
　for post-splenectomy sepsis, 107t
　for purpura fulminans, 108t
　for pyomyositis, 481
　resistance to, 426t
　for sepsis/septic shock, 65t, 107t
　for staphylococcal infections, 493,
　　494t–495t, 496
　for toxic shock syndrome, 108t
Vardenafil, for erectile dysfunction, 951
Varenicline, for smoking cessation, 1127
Varicella vaccine, 571, 1108t–1112t, 1114t
Varicella-zoster immune globulin, 571
Varicella-zoster vaccine, 438t
Varicella-zoster virus infection, **569**
　chickenpox, **569**
　epidemic and emerging problems,
　　431–432
　in immunocompromised host, 570
　shingles, **570**
Varicocele, 950
Variola major, 163–166
Variola minor, 163–166
Vascular dementia, 996t, 997t, 998, **1000**
Vascular disease
　abdominal pain in, 179t
　gastrointestinal, **843**
　headache in, 183t
　malabsorption in, 259t
　peripheral, **738**
　skin diseases, **318**
Vascular malformation, myelopathy in, 1029,
　　1030f
Vascular shunting, anatomic, 239
Vascular tone, disorders of, 208, 209t
Vasculitis, 319, **891**
　approach to, 892, 893f
　conditions that mimic, 894t
　cutaneous, 319, 892
　neuropathy in, 1061
　primary vasculitis syndrome, 891–892
　renal complications of, 826
　secondary vasculitis syndromes, 892
　treatment of, 319, 893–894
　urticarial, 319
Vasoconstrictors, for heart failure, 734t
Vasodilators
　for aortic regurgitation, 683
　for heart failure, 734, 734t
　for myocardial infarction, 705, 705t, 708
　for pulmonary hypertension, 745
Vasopressin, 923
　deficiency of, 922t
　for heart failure, 734t
　interarterial, for diverticulosis, 263
　for shock, 62, 62t
Vasopressin antagonists, for hyponatremia, 7
Vasospasm, in subarachnoid hemorrhage, 89
Vasospastic disorders, 740
Venezuelan equine encephalitis, 596t–597t,
　　598
Venlafaxine
　dosage and adverse effects of, 1086t
　for menopausal symptoms, 957
　for pain, 36t–37t
Venous disease, **740**
Venous insufficiency, chronic, **741**
Venous thromboembolism, **769**
　drug-induced, 1136t
Ventilation, disorders of, **781**
Ventilation/perfusion lung scan, 743, 770

Ventilation/perfusion mismatch, 750
Ventilatory function, disturbances in, 747–748
  extraparenchymal, 748, 748t
  obstructive, 747–748, 748t
  parenchymal, 748, 748t
  restrictive, 747–748, 748t
Ventilatory support
  in ALS, 1013
  in ARDS, 70–71, 70f
  care of ventilated patient, 31–32
  complications of, 74
  during COPD exacerbations, 763
  for critically ill patient, **30**
  management of mechanically ventilated patients, 72–74
  mechanical ventilation, **30**
  modes of mechanical ventilation, 72–74, 73t
  monitoring of respiratory mechanics, 32
  after nerve agent exposure, 169
  in respiratory failure, 72–74, 73t
  weaning from mechanical ventilation, 32
Ventricular aneurysm
  in myocardial infarction, 708
  pseudoaneurysm, 708
  true, 708
Ventricular arrhythmia, in myocardial infarction, 704
Ventricular fibrillation, 721f, 724t
  management of, 57f
  in myocardial infarction, 704
Ventricular premature beats, 724t
Ventricular septal defect, 662t, **674**
Ventricular septal rupture, 708
Ventricular tachycardia, 720, 721f, 724t, 726t
  hypotensive, 57, 57f
  in myocardial infarction, 704
  in poisoning, 134–135
Ventriculoencephalitis, cytomegalovirus, 573
Verapamil
  for angina pectoris, 715
  for aortic dissection, 738
  for arrhythmias, 728t, 736
  for atrial fibrillation, 726
  for cluster headache prevention, 187
  for hypertension, 695t, 696–698
  for hypertrophic cardiomyopathy, 686
  for migraine prevention, 184, 188t
  for mitral stenosis, 678
  for myocardial infarction, 711
  poisoning, 140t
  for supraventricular arrhythmias, 704
  for tachyarrhythmias, 722t–724t
  for unstable angina, 711
  for Wolff-Parkinson-White syndrome, 729
Verruca plana, 310f
Verruca vulgaris, 311f
Verrucous carcinoma, 366
Verruga (skin lesion), 528
Verruga peruana, 526t, **527**
Vertebral disk herniation
  acute, 1029
  cervical disk, 196, 198
  lumbar disk, 190
Vertebral fracture, 192
Vertebral metastasis, 192
Vertebrobasilar insufficiency, 215

Vertigo, **211,** 214t, 297
  central, 213, 213t
  pathologic, 212
  peripheral, 212–213, 212t
  physiologic, 212
  provocative tests to reproduce, 211
  psychogenic, 213
Vesicants, **168**
Vesicle (skin lesion), 313t, 477
Vesiculobullous eruptions, 200
Vestibular disorder
  drug-induced, 1139t
  vertigo, **211**
Vestibular function tests, 211
Vestibular neuritis, 212
Vibrio cholerae infection. *See also* Cholera
  non-01, **453**
Vibrio parahaemolyticus infection, **453**
Vibrio vulnificus infection, 110, 477
Vidarabine, for HSV infections, 568t
Vinblastine
  for bladder cancer, 392
  for lung cancer, 371
  toxicity of, 341t
Vincent's angina, 532
Vincristine
  for acute lymphoblastic leukemia and lymphoblastic lymphoma, 359
  for Burkitt's lymphoma/leukemia, 359
  for gastric cancer, 381
  for idiopathic thrombocytopenic purpura, 335
  for multiple myeloma, 361
  toxicity of, 341t
Vindesine, for lung cancer, 371
Vinorelbine
  for breast cancer, 379
  for lung cancer, 371
  toxicity of, 341t
VIPoma, 389, 390t, 391
Viral disease
  diagnosis of, **411**
  specimen collection and transport, 418t
Viral hemorrhagic fevers
  as bioweapon, 165t, 166–167
  treatment of, 165t
Virilization, 955
Visceral abscess, **450**
Visceral disease, back pain in, 193, 193t
Visceral spasm, 179t
Visual acuity, 215
Visual field mapping, 215, 216f
Visual loss, 293
  acute, approach to, 215
  chronic, progressive, **295,** 295t
  transient or sudden, **215**
Vitamin(s)
  reference values for laboratory tests, 1160t
  therapy for vitamin deficiencies, 43t
Vitamin A deficiency, 43t
Vitamin A supplementation
  for head and neck cancer prevention, 1125
  for measles, 585
Vitamin B_{12} deficiency, 657, 998, 1030, 1061
  anemia in, 325, 328
Vitamin C deficiency, 43t

Vitamin C supplementation
  for macular degeneration, 296
  for nephrolithiasis, 828t
Vitamin D deficiency, 963, 968
Vitamin D supplementation
  for osteomalacia, 968
  for osteoporosis, 967
  for primary sclerosing cholangitis, 848
  for psoriasis, 314
Vitamin E deficiency, 43t, 1009
Vitamin E supplementation
  for macular degeneration, 296
  for menopausal symptoms, 957
Vitamin K deficiency, 43t, 334–335
Vitamin K supplementation
  for vitamin K deficiency, 335
  for warfarin reversal, 336
Vitiligo, 310f
Vitreous detachment, 215–216
Vitreous hemorrhage, 216
Volume regulation, 3t
Volume status, assessment of, 4f
Vomiting. *See* Nausea and vomiting
von Hippel-Lindau disease, 392
von Willebrand disease, 334–335
Voriconazole, **619**
  for aspergillosis, 623, 624t
  for fusariosis, 632
Vulvovaginal infection, **464**
VX gas, 142t, 169–171

W
Waldenström's macroglobulinemia, 807t
Warfarin
  for atrial fibrillation, 726, 929
  for deep venous thrombosis prevention,
    741
  for dilated cardiomyopathy, 685
  for mitral stenosis, 678
  for pulmonary hypertension, 736, 745
  for renal vein thrombosis, 821
  for stroke prevention, 85, 87t
  for thrombotic disorders, 336–337
  for venous disease, 741
  for venous thromboembolism, 770–771
Warts, **317**
Wasp sting, 126
Weakness, **218,** 288
  approach to, 218–219, 221f
  causes of, 219t
  diagnostic evaluation of, 1069f–1070f
  site of responsible lesion, 219, 219t
Weaning, from mechanical ventilation, 32
Weaponization, 161
Weber test, 298
Wegener's granulomatosis, 807t, **891**
Weight, ideal weight for height, 40t
Weight loss, **247,** 248t
  drug-induced, 248
  for hypertension, 694
  in malnutrition, 39
  for metabolic syndrome, 699
  for obesity, 940–941
  for sleep apnea, 784
Weil's syndrome, 552
Wernicke's aphasia, **224,** 225t
Wernicke's encephalopathy, 1097
Western equine encephalitis, 596t–597t

West Nile virus encephalitis, **595,** 596t–597t,
    1048–1049
Wet mount, 411
WFNS Scale, for subarachnoid hemorrhage,
    88t
Wheal, 313t
Whiplash injury, 196
Whipple's disease, **907**
Whipple's triad, 103, 104f, 389
Whitlow, herpetic, **565,** 568t
WHO classification
  of AML, 345t
  of CML, 348t–349t
Whole blood transfusion, **44**
Whole-body radiation exposure, 172
Whole-bowel irrigation, 135, 147t, 151t
Widow spider bite, **125**
Wilson's disease, **978**
Winking owl sign, 113
Winterbottom's sign, 645
Winter's formula, 16
Withdrawal of care, 33
Withdrawal syndrome, 131t–132t
Wolbachia endosymbiont, 652–653
Wolff-Parkinson-White syndrome, 668t, 720,
    721f, **729**
Women's health, **1128**
  Alzheimer's disease, 1128
  autoimmune disease, 1129
  coronary heart disease, 1128
  diabetes mellitus, 1129
  HIV infection, 1129
  hypertension, 1129
  nicotine addiction, 1130
  obesity, 1129
  osteoporosis, 1129
  pharmacology, 1129
  psychiatric disease, 1129
  sleep disorders, 1130
  substance abuse, 1130
  violence, 1130
Wood's light examination, 312
Work hardening, 196
Wound infection
  specimen collection and transport, 417t
  surgical, 430–431, 430t
Wrist, muscles and innervation of, 980t–981t
Wuchereria bancrofti infection. *See* Filariasis

X
Xanthelasma, 970
Xanthoma, 970, 973–974
Xerostomia, 890–891
D-Xylose absorption test, 256
D-Xylose urinary excretion test, 852

Y
Yaws, 551
Yellow fever, 110, **599**
Yellow fever vaccine, 1116t
Yellow jacket sting, 126
Yersinia pestis infection. *See* Plague
Yersiniosis, **459**

Z
Zafirlukast
  for asthma, 755
  for urticaria/angioedema, 879

Zalcitabine, for HIV/AIDS, 608t
Zaleplon
for insomnia, 228
poisoning, 143t
Zanamivir, for influenza, 579, 579t
preventive treatment, 580–581
Zap70 kinase deficiency, 883
Zidovudine
for adult T cell leukemia/lymphoma, 260
for HIV/AIDS, 607t
Zieve's syndrome, 868
Zinc deficiency, 43t
Zinc supplementation
for hepatic encephalopathy, 875
for macular degeneration, 296
for Wilson's disease, 978

Ziprasidone
dosage and adverse effects of, 1091t
for schizophrenia, 1081
Zoledronate
for hypercalcemia, 113, 406, 962t
for osteoporosis, 967
Zollinger-Ellison syndrome, 389, 390t, **835,**
835t
Zolmitriptan, for migraine, 185t, 187t
Zolpidem
for insomnia, 228
poisoning, 143t
Zonisamide
poisoning, 143t
for seizures, 994t
Zoster ophthalmicus, 570–571